DIAGNOSES IN ASSYRIAN AND BABYLONIAN MEDICINE

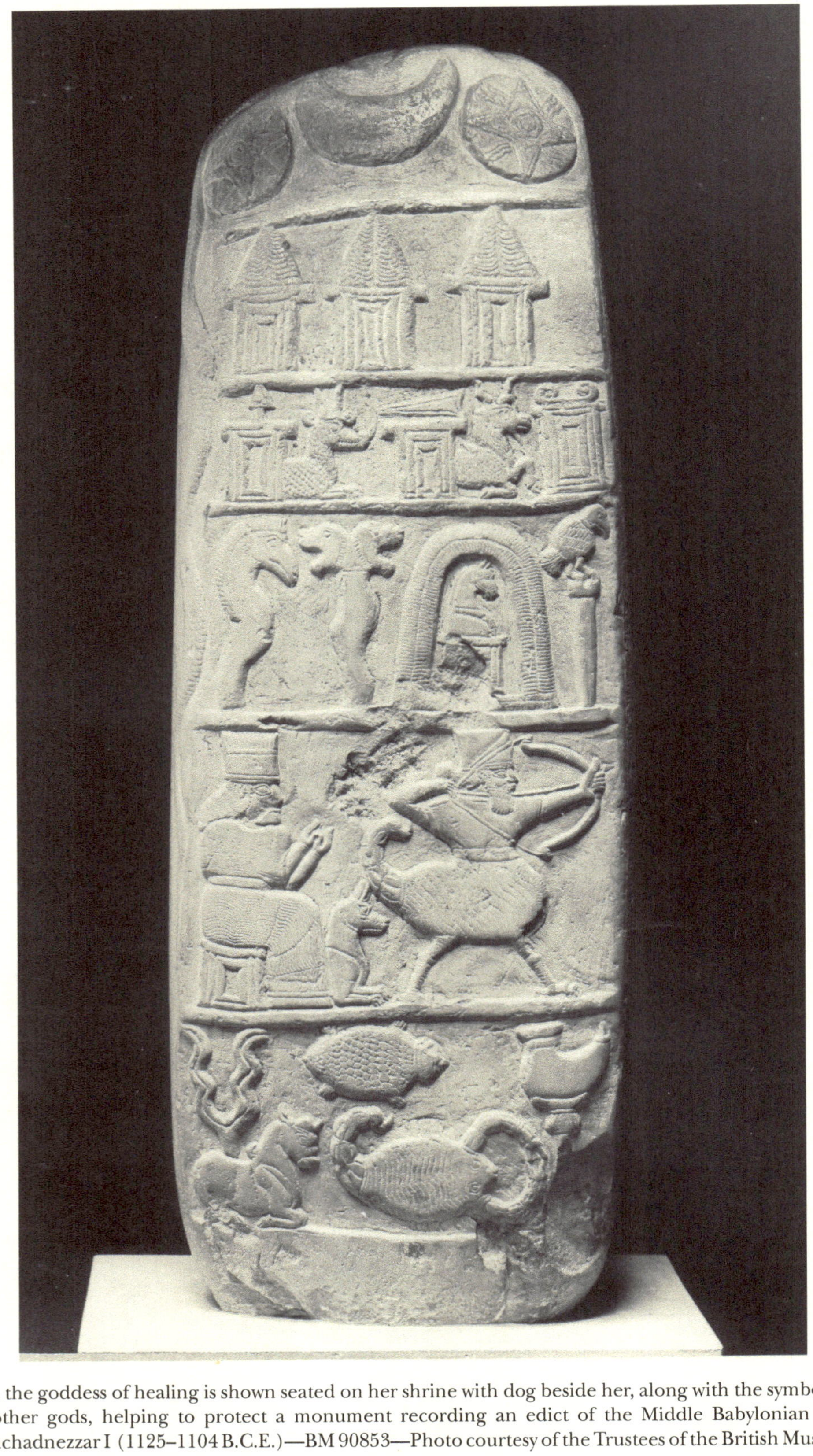

Gula, the goddess of healing is shown seated on her shrine with dog beside her, along with the symbols of the other gods, helping to protect a monument recording an edict of the Middle Babylonian king Nebuchadnezzar I (1125–1104 B.C.E.)—BM 90853—Photo courtesy of the Trustees of the British Museum

Diagnoses in Assyrian and Babylonian Medicine

Ancient Sources, Translations, and Modern Medical Analyses

TRANSLATED AND WITH COMMENTARY BY

JoAnn Scurlock, PhD

Burton R. Andersen, MD

UNIVERSITY OF ILLINOIS PRESS

URBANA AND CHICAGO

♾ This book is printed on acid-free paper.

Library of Congress Cataloging-in-Publication Data

Scurlock, Jo Ann, 1953–
Diagnoses in Assyrian and Babylonian medicine: ancient sources,
translations, and modern medical analyses / translated, and with
commentary by Jo Ann Scurlock and Burton R. Andersen
p. cm.
ISBN 0-252-02956-9 (cl. : alk. paper)
1. Medicine, Assyro-Babylonian. I. Andersen, Burton R., 1932– II. Title.
R135.3S286 2004
610'.p35—dc22 2004058037

The authors and the University of Illinois Press
gratefully acknowledge that publication of this volume
has been assisted by the generous support of
the following philanthropic Assyrians:

Norman Solhkhah, Ph.D. & Vallo Benjamin, M.D.

In addition, Dr. Solhkhah would like to acknowledge
the support of the following contributors:

Edison Ishaya, DDS
Assyrian National Council
John Budin, Esq.
Renee & Juliette George
Mark Mkrdichian, DDS
Ashurbanipal & Sharrukin DeKelaita
Marina & Sam Shapira
Jonathan S. Davidson, MD
Samir D. Johna, MD
Odisho B. Khoshaba, MD
Sabah & Nada Shamoon
Baito Malek Chikko

The donors have contributed to this project
to honor Assyrians throughout the world.

Contents

Acknowledgments

We wish to thank the National Endowment for the Humanities for their generous support without which this book would have been impossible.

We would also like to thank the following people who read drafts of some or all of the chapters and who made many valuable suggestions. They are not, of course, responsible for any mistakes that may remain.

Our spouses deserve special thanks for their encouragement and tolerance. Susan Andersen, BFA, MBA, reviewed the manuscript and made many helpful suggestions. Richard H. Beal, PhD, aided in collating the original cuneiform tablets, reviewed and made many suggestions for various drafts of the manuscript, labored in the construction of the chart and indexes, and helped with the reference checking and copy editing.

We also thank Annie Attia MD, Paris; Val Beasley DVM PhD, University of Illinois at Champaign-Urbana; Ellen C. Benya MD, Northwestern University; Gilles Buisson MD, Paris; Arlene Chapman MD, Emory University; Julia A. DeBroux MS, University of Washington; John T. Dunn MD, University of Washington; Arthur L. Frank MD, University of Illinois at Chicago; Thomas H. Jobe MD, University of Illinois at Chicago; Eileen M. Martin PhD, University of Illinois at Chicago; Tammy Novak MD, Evanston Northwestern Health Care, Evanston, IL; Andrew Poznanski MD, Childrens Memorial Hospital, Chicago; Mary Louise Tamyanovich MD, University of Illinois at Chicago.

We wish to thank the Trustees of the British Museum for permission to use and publish the texts stored in that museum. We also wish to thank Christopher Walker (British Museum, London), Joachim Marzahn (Vorderasiatisches Museum, Berlin), Béatrice André-Salvini and Alain Duclos (Louvre, Paris), Jean-Marie Durand (École Pratique des Hautes Études and Collège de France, Paris), Walter Farber and Jonathan Tinney (Oriental Institute, Chicago), Benjamin Foster and Ulla Kasten (Yale, New Haven), Eric Gubel (Musée du Cinquentenaire, Brussels) and Gretchen Worden (Mutter Museum of the College of Physicians of Philadelphia). A special thanks goes to Sarah Collins of the British Museum, Catherine Giraudon of the Louvre, and Thomas Urban of the Oriental Institute.

We would also like to thank Dr. Willis Regier, director of the University of Illinois Press, for being tolerant of our foibles (and manuscript size), for helping us in every way possible, and for having confidence in our project. Kristine Ding has labored to ensure a remarkably smooth glide through the production process. BookComp, Inc., did a masterful job getting our computer files converted for publication. Finally we would like to thank Maria denBoer, our editor at BookComp, for restraining the authors' tendency to be innovative in matters of English spelling, grammar, and punctuation.

Concordance of Sigla

The sigla used for DPS (Diagnostic and Prognostic Series) are based on the numbers and letters assigned by Nils Heeßel, *Babylonisch-assyrische Diagnostik,* Alter Orient und Altes Testament 43: 140–146. The first number after the equals sign is the museum number; the volume in which the hand copy (if one exists) is published is given in parentheses. All unpublished texts were read from the original tablets by J. A. Scurlock. Most of the published texts were checked against the originals by J. A. Scurlock.

III A = BM 33424
III B = BM 46139
III C = MLC 2639 (Goetze, *JCS* 2 [1948]: 305–308)
III D = VAT 14554 (*LKU* 90)
III E_1 = VAT 14553 (*LKU* 91) +
III E_2 = W 17360k (*TDP* LXVII)
III F = W 17360ac (*AUWE* 23.323)
III G = VAT 14552 (*LKU* 89)

IV A = K 2723 + K 3872 obv. + K 4051 (*TDP* IV–V) +
IV A_2 = K 3872 rev. (*AMT* 107/1) +
IV A_3 = K 10602+
IV A_4 = K 13842+
IV A_5 = K 10592(+)
IV A_6 = K 19432
IV B = AO 6682 (*TDP* VI–VIII)
IV C = ND 4405/35 (*CTN* 4.77)
IV D = VAT 14550 (*LKU* 79)
IV E = W 22761 (*SpTU* 3.88) line nos. follow translit.
IV F = *LKU* 77
IV G = VAT 14567 (*LKU* 94)
IV H = W 17360c (*TDP* LXVI)

V A = K 6629 (*AMT* 75/2)
V B = K 6737 (*CT* 37.50)
V C = K 13985 (*TDP* IX)
V D = K 10570 (*TDP* IX)
V E = W 17360g (*TDP* LXVI)
V F = K 3957 + K 6347 + K 9350 (*AMT* 105/2)
V G = K 7099 (*CT* 37.50)

VI A = K 2243 + Rm 248 + Rm 481 (*TDP* X–XI)
VI B_1 = K 10343 (*TDP* XI)+
VI B_2 = K 12539 + K 12897 (both *KMI* 35) (+)
VI B_3 = K 12899 (+)
VI B_4 = K 13959 (*CT* 28:18 & *TBP* = *AfO Beih.* 3.31) +
VI B_5 = K 18289
VI C = BM 34071 obv.
VI D = VAT 14557 (*LKU* 95)
VI E = K 4977 (*TDP* X) + K 11858 (*TDP* XI)
VI F = W 17360p (*TDP* LXVII)

VII A = K 2949 + K 12856 (*CT* 37:37 & *KMI* 41)
VII B = K 2952 + K 3678 (*CT* 37:40)
VII C = K 34071 rev.

VIII = K 4080 + Sm 552 + K 9254 + K 11774 (*TDP* XII)
+ K 14851 (*AMT* 69/6)

IX A = AO 6681 (*TDP* XIII–XIV)
IX B = K 261 (*TDP* XV–XVII)
IX C = VAT 14561 (*LKU* 99)

X A = AO 6679 (*TDP* XIX–XX)
X B = K 3687 + K 6389 + Sm 951 (*TDP* XXI–XXIII = *AMT* 106/2, 107/2)
X C = (*LKU* 86)
X D = VAT 14544 (*LKU* 75)

XI A = BM 65698 (*TDP* XXIV–XXVIII)
XI B = W 22307/1 (*SpTU* 1.34)
XI C = Sm 1210 (*TBP* = *AfO Beih.* 3.29)

XII A = Sm 232 (*TDP* XXIX)
XII B = K 6704
XII C = W 22307/56 (*SpTU* 1.35)

XII D = A 3442 (iii & iv only in *TDP* XXXI)
XII E = BE 35828 (*TDP* XXX)
XII F = K 7286 + Sm 856
XII G_1 = VAT 14537 (*LKU* 85) +
XII G_2 = VAT 14598 (*LKU* 83)

XIII A = K 18019
XIII B = A 3506 (*TDP* XXXII–XXXIV)
XIII C = K 5670
XIII D = K 3743 (*CT* 37:41)
XIII E = K 19906
XIII F = K 9250
XIII G_1 = K 1756 (+)
XIII G_2 = K 3693 + K 6290 + Rm 102 (*CT* 37.38–39)
XIII H = W 17360n (*TDP* LXVII)
XIII I = VAT 14551 (*LKU* 88)
XIII J = VAT 14564 (*LKU* 102)

XIV A = K 2006 + K 3795 + K 4014 + K 4083 + K 4094a
+ K 11294 + K 14000 (+) K 3826 (*TDP* XXXV–XXXVI) (+)
XIV A_2 = K 3826 (*CT* 37.44 + *TDP* XXXVI)
XIV B = VAT 14542 (*LKU* 73)
XIV C = VAT 303 + VAT 404 + VAT 579 + VAT 589
(*SBH* 148 no. 10 only part copied)[1]

XIV D = VAT 14543 (*LKU* 74)
XIV E = VAT 14545 (*LKU* 76)
XIV F = BM 38655
XIV G = VAT 14540 (*LKU* 70)
XIV H = VAT 14541 (*LKU* 71)
XIV I = VAT 14547 (*LKU* 82)
XIV J = VAT 14548 (*LKU* 84)
XIV K = W17360o (*TDP* LXVII)
XIV L = *LKU* 65

For DPS XV through XXXV, the transliterations follow the edition of Heeßel pp. 150–373, unless otherwise indicated.

XXXVI A = BM 92694 (*TDP* LII–LVI)
XXXVI B = BM 65450 + BM 76497
XXXVI C = W 17360f (*TDP* LXVI)
XXXVI D = K 7071

XXXVII A = A 3438 (*TDP* LVII)
XXXVII B = W 17360q (*TDP* LXVIII)

XL A = BM 92690 (*TDP* LVIII–LXII)
XL B = BM 46228 (*TDP* LXIII, variants only)
XL C = VAT 14563 (*LKU* 101)
XL D = VAT 14549 (*LKU* 87)

Translator's Notes

Abbreviations

The abbreviations used in this work correspond to those generally used in Assyriology and medicine. Full citations of all works cited are given in the bibliography. Lists of standard Assyriological abbreviations can be found in the "Register Assyriologie"; in the journal *Archiv für Orientforschung* 40/41 (1993–1994), and augmented annually thereafter; in the "Keilschriftbibliographie" published annually in the journal *Orientalia*; in R. Borger's *Handbuch der Keilschriftliteratur* vols. 1–2; at the end of W. von Soden's *Assyrisches Handwörterbuch*; and in *The Assyrian Dictionary of the Oriental Institute of the University of Chicago.*

Format of Quotations from Ancient Texts

In accordance with the conventions of Assyriology, Akkadian words or phonetic complements appear in italics separated by hyphens (e.g., *še-pa-ša ka-ṣa-a*: "her feet are cold") whereas Sumerian word-signs[1] appearing in the text are rendered in capital letters separated by periods (e.g., ZÉ.GIG: "sick gall bladder"). Since a number of different Sumerian words sounded the same to the Akkadian ear, there may be many homophonous signs. When modern scholars transcribe these signs into the Roman alphabet, they differentiate them by giving the most common value no diacritic mark, the next most common an acute accent, the third a grave accent, and all subsequent homophones a number subscript, for example, SIG "weak," SÍG "wool, hair," SÌG "strike, beat," SIG_4 "brick," SIG_5 "good," SIG_7 "yellow/green." To avoid confusion, certain Sumerian words (GIŠ = "wood," Ú = "plant," ŠEM = "aromatic," and NA_4 = "stone") were used as determinatives to mark certain classes of nouns. These are rendered in transcription as superscripted capital letters set just before or just after the word that they classify.

Readings of Sumerian signs are in accordance with R. Borger, *Assyrisch-babylonische Zeichenliste* with one notable exception: SI+A is read DIRI when it means "full" or "to be full" and SA_5 when it means "red" or "to redden." Restoration of text lost in lacunae is indicated by square brackets; partially effaced signs and partially preserved words are marked with half brackets; additions to the translation necessary to make the meaning of the original clearer to the modern reader appear in parentheses. An ellipsis in square brackets indicates a missing section of text whose restoration is uncertain. Simple ellipses indicate passages preserved in the text but omitted from transliteration and/or translation. A sign accidentally omitted by the ancient scribe is restored within pointed brackets, whereas an extraneous sign is indicated by double pointed brackets. An exclamation point indicates an emendation (correction by the modern scholar of the ancient text)—in rare cases ancient scribes apparently miswrote or miscopied signs.[2] In many cases, more than one copy of a given text has come down to us. Although scored transliterations were either prepared by J. Scurlock or taken from N. Heeßel, *Babylonisch-assyrische Diagnostik* (AOAT 43), we have chosen to save space and to avoid unduly confusing the non-Assyriologist reader by presenting citations as combined editions with a single line of text representing what is maximally preserved. In the transliteration, the presence of a slash (/) between two words without an intervening space (e.g., DU-*ka*/DU.MEŠ) indicates a significant variant in one of the texts used to make the combined edition; with a space, the slash indicates a line break. The slash thus serves the same function as a mark used by ancient copyists and known to Assyriologists as a "glossenkeil." Where the ancient copyist used a glossenkeil to indicate a significant variant in the texts that he was copying, this is rendered in the transliteration with a colon.

The Enclitic Particle -*ma*

A problem that plagues all current translations of ancient medical texts and that comes up so frequently in references as to merit foregrounding is the issue of the use in medical texts of the enclitic particle -*ma*. Most commonly this appears in the expression GÍD-*ma* GAM, which is often misinterpreted as "he will linger and then die" or "after a long time he will die."[3] The correct translation of this phrase is: "(if) it is prolonged, he will die." For this use of the enclitic -*ma* to indicate a subordinate "if" clause, see two standard grammars of Akkadian, Von Soden, *GAG* § 160 and Huehnergard, *A Grammar of Akkadian* § 7.4c.

Introduction

Prospectus

It is our objective to provide a comprehensive review and analysis of all available ancient Mesopotamian texts dealing with medical diagnosis or prognosis. Unfortunately, some of the references are so fragmented, damaged, or limited in information that nothing useful can be said about them. In these cases, we have chosen to exclude these texts from further consideration.

Some texts are available in hand copies of the original cuneiform tablets, while others are as yet unpublished and had to be studied by J. A. Scurlock in the student's room of the British Museum. This material represents only a fraction of the original corpus of texts, since some tablets were scattered or destroyed in antiquity, some have yet to be catalogued and are thus unavailable for study, and even more have yet to be uncovered. We look forward to additions, improvements, and corrections as new texts are discovered and as new eyes review this material. This is an inquiring and exploratory study with a view to interesting others in joining us in rescuing lost medical texts; this is not, nor does it intend to be, a definitive and final book on Mesopotamian medicine.

Methodology

Processing ancient Mesopotamian medical texts requires its own special methodology. Among the founding fathers of Assyriology,[1] it was agreed that the proper way to translate Akkadian words was to gather together all references in ancient texts where the word to be studied appeared and to use a combination of etymology (i.e., the meaning of the root in related languages) and the context provided by the assembled material to puzzle out the meaning. It was further agreed that of the two possible sources for determining meaning, etymology and context, the latter was the most reliable. After a century and a half of work, the general meanings of most Akkadian words have now been established.

Our own methodology builds upon this basic foundation. Certain terms in Akkadian were used to describe medical signs and symptoms. This provides a further medical context for translation, which should be the most reliable source for determining meaning if it can be correctly recovered. Great care must obviously be exercised in this enterprise to avoid circular arguments. The way in which we approached this problem was to begin by making a rough translation of all of the medical texts, using the basic meaning suggested by non-medical context as given in the two dictionaries, W. von Soden's *Akkadisches Handwörterbuch* (*AHw*) and *The Chicago Assyrian Dictionary* (*CAD*) and as refined by subsequent scholarship. Part of this information comes from therapeutic texts, and part from an ancient reference work that explained the basic principles of diagnosis and prognosis by specific example.

We carved these texts up in accordance with the individual entries contained in them (taking care to note series of sequenced references that were clearly meant to refer to a single condition; see below), sorted these entries by subject matter, and tried to figure out what condition or conditions each entry was describing.[2] In doing this, our goal was to determine which diseases still recognized by modern science were in fact suffered by ancient Mesopotamians. We did not begin with a list of modern diseases and proceed deductively to fit ancient descriptions to modern context. Instead, we proceeded inductively, finding modern equivalent descriptions to match as many ancient texts as possible, taking into consideration the possibility that the course of diseases might have altered and that what are now rare diseases might once have been much more common (and common diseases rare or even nonexistent) in antiquity. In spite of numerous uncertainties, the fullness of documentation and the care exercised by ancient observers makes it possible to make reasonable inferences from these ancient texts.

Armed with these identifications, we went back to see if our provisional translations could be refined. For example, there are a number of words that have long been known to refer to some form of involuntary movement. Ancient Mesopotamian medical texts are anything but literary; they are written in a cramped style packed with technical vocabulary, and contain nary a word beyond what was thought necessary to make an accurate diagnosis or prognosis. The different terms used to describe involuntary movement, then, are not mere synonyms but represent some observed difference in the type of movement being made by the patient. But what sort of difference?

One of these words appears in an entry which, to judge from the other signs and symptoms mentioned in it, is a reference to what we call Parkinson's disease. This allows us to understand that the specific word used to render "trembling" in this context is the ancient physician's way of describing what we call a Parkinsonian tremor (see Chapter 13). The suggested new translation was then rigorously tested against all other references in which the term appeared to make sure that it was appropriate.

The last question to be asked (see Chapter 19) was the most fascinating of all. Now that we had some idea of what the ancient physician was talking about, just how good was he? When he assigned a single diagnosis to thirty-odd entries in the diagnostic/prognostic handbook was he, in fact, describing a single modern disease? Without the benefit of modern lab tests, rarely if ever. But was there still "modern" sense to be made of these diagnoses; in other words, if some terrible catastrophe were to occur and we suddenly had to rely on our five unaided senses alone, might we not also assign some of the same sets of entries to a single diagnostic category? What was the principle of diagnosis and how much of it relied on the presumed proclivities of the gods, ghosts, or demons who are so often blamed? Here the expertise of one of the authors in ancient Mesopotamian magical and religious texts was particularly helpful.

None of this often tedious but very necessary work (the skeletal foundation, as it were) is actually visible in the finished product. Wisely or unwisely, the authors have chosen the historian's convention of presenting only their conclusions, with corroborative notes, and not taking the reader through every step of the interpretive process. In this, we echo the method of presentation of ancient Mesopotamian scholarship. Esagil-kīn-apli, redactor of the diagnostic/prognostic handbook (see below), has similarly left us only his conclusions; ours is the unenviable task of reconstructing the logic that must have animated them.

Only when this process was completed did we begin to look at the extensive secondary literature of the last fifty years on ancient Mesopotamian medicine. Looking too soon at the work of other scholars prejudices the results, since what tends to happen is that previous theories are unconsciously read into the evidence. However, the authors have endeavored to make a thorough survey of previous scholarship, to note agreements and disagreements, and to change our opinions where we found ourselves convinced. Where we agree, we have endeavored to give others full credit for having anticipated our conclusions. Where we disagree, we have endeavored always to explain our reasoning. The authors apologize if anyone's ideas have been inadvertently overlooked or not given the attention they deserve.

Signs and Symptoms

Modern physicians use the terms *signs* and *symptoms* to distinguish between the doctor's findings and the patient's complaints, respectively. Ancient Mesopotamian physicians were certainly aware that there could be a discrepancy between their observations and what they were told by their patients. For example, they recognized that a patient's sensation of heat (symptom) does not always correspond to an actual elevation of temperature (sign), as in the following reference.

> **0.1** DIŠ NA KÚ[M o]-⸢*šú*⸣ K[ÚM.M]EŠ ŠED$_7$.MEŠ NINDA KÚ KAŠ NAG-*ma* [*i*]-*ár-rù i-t*[*a-na-š*]*a-áš e-*⸢*li*⸣*-u-na* UZU.MEŠ-*šú* ŠED$_7$ [*ša*]*p-la-nu e-ṣ*[*e-e*]*n-ta-šú ṣar-pa* NA BI [UD.D]A TAB.BA-*ma l*[*i*]-ʾ*-ba* TUKU *ana* TI-*šú* . . . (*BAM* 146:43′–46′)
>
> **If fever [. . .] a person (and) he continually gets ⸢hot⸣ and gets cold, when he eats bread and drinks beer, [he] vomits (and his stomach) ⸢is continually upset⸣, the flesh above is cold (but) his ⸢bones below⸣ feel burning hot, that person is burned by ⸢*ṣētu*⸣ (enteric fever; see Chapter 3) and has *li*ʾ*bu*, to cure him . . .

In some cases, a distinction was made in terminology between signs and symptoms. For example, the *āšipu* (physician; see Chapter 1) used two different words, both meaning "to go round" and sharing the same Sumerogram (NIGIN) to distinguish the sign that the patient's eyes were spinning (*lamû*) "like a spindle whorl" (i.e., ocular bobbing) from the symptom that the patient was experiencing a spinning sensation (*ṣâdu*; i.e., dizziness, vertigo). Unfortunately, these distinctions are not always made, making interpretation of some references difficult. This also adds an element of uncertainty to the diagnoses that have been made, a fact of which readers should be aware.

Retrospective Diagnosis

In reading through the secondary literature on ancient medicine one sometimes encounters the argument that those who attempt to identify illnesses described in ancient texts are engaged in retrospective diagnosis, a reckless and false process.[3] In fact, modern physicians have much to gain by attempting to understand the nature of a patient's past illnesses. If there is an adequate amount of good information, the possibility of achieving a correct diagnosis is excellent. Some ancient Mesopotamian texts contain a great deal of useful information permitting us to be close to certain about the nature of the illnesses described. About others we cannot be as confident; we have tried in all cases to indicate our level of conviction in the suggested diagnosis.

Reliability of Sources for Ancient Mesopotamian Medicine

THE DIAGNOSTIC/PROGNOSTIC HANDBOOK

The most reliable sources for ancient medicine are the descriptions of illnesses found as individual entries in therapeutic texts and in the diagnostic/prognostic handbook. The latter is often denigrated or ignored on the grounds that it is a "sorcerer's manual" containing nothing more than omens "predicting the future of the patient."[4] However, the *āšipu* was not a sorcerer,[5] and his diagnostic/prognostic handbook is not a collection of omens.[6] Instead, the entries represent the distillation of millennia of firsthand observations. With these texts, it is not a question of retrospective diagnosis, since the illnesses described have already been diagnosed, but of attempting to correlate ancient and modern systems of classification. The main difficulty here is in determining when different entries with the same ancient diagnosis should be taken as referring to the same illness as opposed to different illnesses falling into a single diagnostic category. With the exception of Chapter 19, where the issue of ancient diagnostic categories had to be addressed directly, we have generally assumed individual entries to be self-contained except with what we refer to as "sequenced references." There are places in the diagnostic/prognostic handbook where a series of entries with only one or two signs or symptoms and the same diagnosis are listed one after the other. What appears to have happened in some of these cases is that the ancient physician chose to represent a single illness with somewhat variable signs and symptoms as a series of short, sequenced entries rather than one exceedingly long "monster" entry.

0.2 DIŠ DIB-*su ina* AN.USAN DIB.DIB-*su* DIB GIDIM$_7$ / DIŠ DIB-*su ina* AN.USAN DIB.DIB-*su* SAG.ŠÀ-*šú* MÚ.MEŠ-*aḫ u* GÌR^{II}-*šú* ÍL-*a* DIB GIDIM$_7$ / DIŠ DIB-*su ina* AN.USAN DIB.DIB-*su* ŠÀ.MEŠ-*šú* MÚ.MEŠ-*ḫu* EN EN.NUN.MURUB$_4$.BA *id-lip* DIB GIDIM$_7$ / DIŠ DIB-*su ina* AN.USAN DIB.DIB-*su* IGI^{II}-*šú ur-ru-pa* GEŠTU^{II}-*šú* GÙ.DÉ.MEŠ DIB GIDIM$_7$ / DIŠ DIB-*su ina* AN.USAN DIB.DIB-*su* GEŠTU^{II}-*šú* GÙ.DÉ.MEŠ DIB GIDIM$_7$ / DIŠ DIB-*su ina* AN.USAN DIB.DIB-*su u* GEŠTU^{II}-*šú i-šam-ma-ma-šú* DIB GIDIM$_7$ / DIŠ DIB-*su ina* AN.USAN DIB.DIB-*su u* SAG.KI-*šú* KÚ-*šú* DIB GID[IM$_7$] / DIŠ KI.MIN U$_4$ DIB-*šú* KÚM TA EN.NUN.AN.USAN EN

EN.NUN.MURUB$_4$.BA *id-da-lip-šú* DIB GID[IM$_7$] (DPS XXVI:31′–38′ [AOAT 43.281])

**If his affliction always afflicts him in the evening, affliction by a ghost. If his affliction always afflicts him in the evening (and) his upper abdomen (epigastrium) is continually bloated and his feet are raised up, affliction by a ghost. If his affliction always afflicts him in the evening (and) his insides are continually bloated (and) it keeps (him) awake until the middle watch, affliction by a ghost. If his affliction always afflicts him in the evening (and) his eyes are clouded (and) his ears roar, affliction by a ghost. If his affliction always afflicts him in the evening (and) his ears roar, affliction by a ghost. If his affliction always afflicts him in the evening and his ears go numb, affliction by a ghost. If his affliction always afflicts him in the evening and his temples continually hurt him, affliction by a ghost. If (his affliction always afflicts him in the evening and) when it afflicts him, fever keeps him awake from the evening watch until the middle watch of the night, affliction by a ⌜ghost⌝.

As to why this format was chosen, the obvious suggestion is that the presence of multiple signs or symptoms in a single entry would have implied that a person should not be diagnosed with whatever it was unless *all* of the signs or symptoms listed were present, whereas with the signs or symptoms listed in sequence it was obvious that any individual patient might not be exhibiting all of the listed signs or symptoms at any one time. For example, the following sequence of references describing infant "hand" of Gula would seem to indicate that any given patient might be choking, or choking and refusing to eat, and might or might not also be jaundiced at the same time.

0.3 DIŠ LÚ.TUR *ur-us-su ḫa-niq* ŠU ^{d}*Gu-la* / DIŠ LÚ.TUR *ú-nap-paq u* UZU.MEŠ-*šú* SIG$_7$ ŠU ^{d}*Gu-la* / DIŠ LÚ.TUR *ú-nap-paq* UBUR NU NAG *u* SU-*šú* SIG$_7$ ŠU ^{d}*Gu-la* / DIŠ LÚ.TUR *ú-nap-paq* UBUR NU NAG ŠU ^{d}*Gu-la* (DPS XL A 91–94 = *TDP* 228:91–94)

**If an infant's larynx is constricted, "hand" of Gula. If an infant chokes and his flesh is yellow, "hand" of Gula. If an infant chokes (and) will not drink from the breast and his body is yellow, "hand" of Gula. If an infant chokes (and) will not drink from the breast, "hand" of Gula.

Also helpful to keep in mind when dealing with the diagnostic/prognostic handbook is that it was not merely a listing of medical syndromes logically organized into a sort of ancient medical dictionary but also, like modern medical textbooks, a didactic tool for instructing novices in ancient medicine. Therefore, in addition to the head-to-toe order and sequenced references, there is a consistent pattern, particularly noticeable in the sections of the diagnostic/prognostic handbook rearranged by Esagil-kīn-apli,[7] of placing different diseases together for the purpose of comparing and contrasting important findings that would be useful in separating these different conditions. Thus, in Tablet III of the diagnostic series, lines 22–23 and 24–26 explain the difference between nonfatal and fatal headaches characterized by severe pain and lines 40 and 41–42 the difference between physical and psychosomatic pain. Lines 65 and 66–67 explain the difference between fevers with gastrointestinal symptoms and peritonitis and lines 78 and 79–80 the difference between remittent and biphasic fevers. Lines 105–106 and 107–108 explain the difference between cataplexy and a mild coma.

Usually, the contrasted references are simply listed side by side, but there is also a common pattern of sandwiching references to one disease or medical condition between references to the disease or medical condition to which it is being contrasted. For example, again in Tablet III, lines 51 and 54 on the one hand and lines 52–53 on the other explain by contrast the difference between shaking chills and Parkinson's tremor. Tablet IV, lines 27 and 29–30 on the one hand and 28 on the other explain by contrast the difference between different types of optic neuropathy.[8]

LETTERS AND RECITATIONS

The quality of medical information contained in ancient letters is of considerably less value than either the therapeutic texts or the diagnostic/prognostic handbook. The reason for this is that, in letters, individual cases are typically described by medically untrained patients or interested relatives. Somewhat more helpful are letters from doctors attempting to explain illnesses to their patients. Particularly problematic is the medical correspondence of Assyrian king Esarhaddon. Since it is impossible to determine whether these letters are describing a single illness or multiple illnesses, we have chosen not to deal with the issue of Esarhaddon's illness, otherwise much discussed in the literature.[9]

Even less reliable are the recitations that accompanied medical treatments in ancient Mesopotamia. Some of these recitations were specific to a particular illness, but recitations were often used for more than one medical condition recognized by the ancient physician. Of these multiuse recitations, some enumerated a specific range of illnesses for which they were deemed appropriate[10] and a few were actually created by a process of cut-and-paste in which two or more originally separate recitations were combined into one.[11] It is for this reason that signs and symptoms mentioned in recitations have been quoted only when we are reasonably sure that only one medical condition is being described. It is astonishing to note how many modern scholars deny the possibility that findings appearing as part of a single entry in the diagnostic/prognostic handbook or even the therapeutic texts could represent a syndrome.[12] And yet many of these same scholars place complete confidence in identifications of complex diseases on the basis of recitations or even literary texts that clearly refer to a number of different illnesses.[13]

RIGHT HAND, LEFT HAND

In modern medical writing, it is necessary to identify on which side of the body a particular sign or symptom is located. This was also the case in the ancient Mesopotamia. However, their convention was not the same as ours. Modern physicians identify the location by the right or left hand of the patient. The ancient Mesopotamian physician used his own hand orientation to localize the findings.

0.4 SA[G.K]I-*šú šá* 15 ⌜KÚ-*šú*⌝ ŠU ^{d}UTU DIN [SAG.KI-*šú šá* 1]50 KÚ-*šú* ŠU ⌜^{d}⌝15 DIN : IGI 15 : ^{d}15 : IGI 150 : ^{d}UTU (*SpTU* 1.30 obv. 11–12)

**(If) his "right" ⌜temple⌝ hurts him, "hand" of Šamaš. [(If) his] ⌜"left"⌝ [temple] hurts him, "hand" of Ištar. (This is because) the right side (of the face) is "hand" of Ištar (and) the left side (of the face) is "hand" of Šamaš.

In order to minimize confusion for a modern audience, the English translation has been altered to reflect the modern convention in all of the references quoted in this book. The transliteration, by contrast, retains the "right," "left" assignments as given in the original texts.

Another issue is the prejudice that is universally linked to handedness. There are many ancient Mesopotamian medical texts that list signs or symptoms that occur on either the right or left side of the body. The overwhelming majority of these references assign a less favorable prognosis when the abnormality occurs on the left side (from the perspective of the observer, that is, the patient's right) than when it occurs on the right side (from the perspective of the observer, that is, the patient's left).

0.5 DIŠ *gir-ri* 15-*šú* SA_5 DIN / DIŠ *gir-ri* 150-*šú* SA_5 DUGUD-*ma* DIN / DIŠ ⌜*gir*⌝-*ra-šú* SA_5.ME DIN / DIŠ *gir-ri* 15-*šú* SIG_7 GIG-*su* GÍD / DIŠ *gir-ri* 150-*šú* SIG_7 GAM / DIŠ *gir-ra-šú* SIG_7.MEŠ GÍD.DA-*ma* GAM / DIŠ *gir-ri* 15-*šú* GI_6 GIG-*su* MAN-*ni* / DIŠ *gir-ri* 150-*šú* GI_6 GIG-*su* GÍD / DIŠ *gir-ra-šú* GI_6.MEŠ GAM / DIŠ *gir-ri* 15-*šú tar-kát* GIG-*su ú-šá-an-na-aḫ* / [DIŠ *g*]*ir-ri* 150-*šú tar-kát* GAM / DIŠ *gir-ra-šú tar-ka* GAM / DIŠ *gir-ri* 15-*šú nap-ḫat* DIN / DIŠ *gir-ri* 150-*šú nap-ḫat* GAM (DPS X A obv. 41–46 = *TDP* 86:41–46)

**If the left side of his throat is red, he will get well. If the right side of his throat is red, (even if) it becomes difficult for him, he will get well . . . If the left side of his throat is yellow, his illness will be prolonged. If the right side of his throat is yellow, he will die . . . If the left side of his throat is black, his illness will alter (for the worse). If the right side of his throat is black, his illness will be prolonged . . . If the left side of his throat is dark, his illness will weaken (him). [If] the right side of his ⌜throat⌝ is dark, he will die . . . If the left side of his throat is swollen, he will get well. If the right side of his throat is swollen, he will die.

With very few exceptions, there is no basis in medical science that can justify predictions of outcome based on the side of the body on which the abnormality occurred. It seems clear that these predictions are founded on the hand preference that can be seen in many cultures, including our own.

Male, Female

As a general rule, ancient Mesopotamian medical texts refer specifically to female patients only in connection with conditions that do not affect male patients (as, e.g., pregnancy). Otherwise, the masculine LÚ and NA (but not the specifically male NITA/NÍTA) are used to refer to both sexes.

DIAGNOSES IN ASSYRIAN AND BABYLONIAN MEDICINE

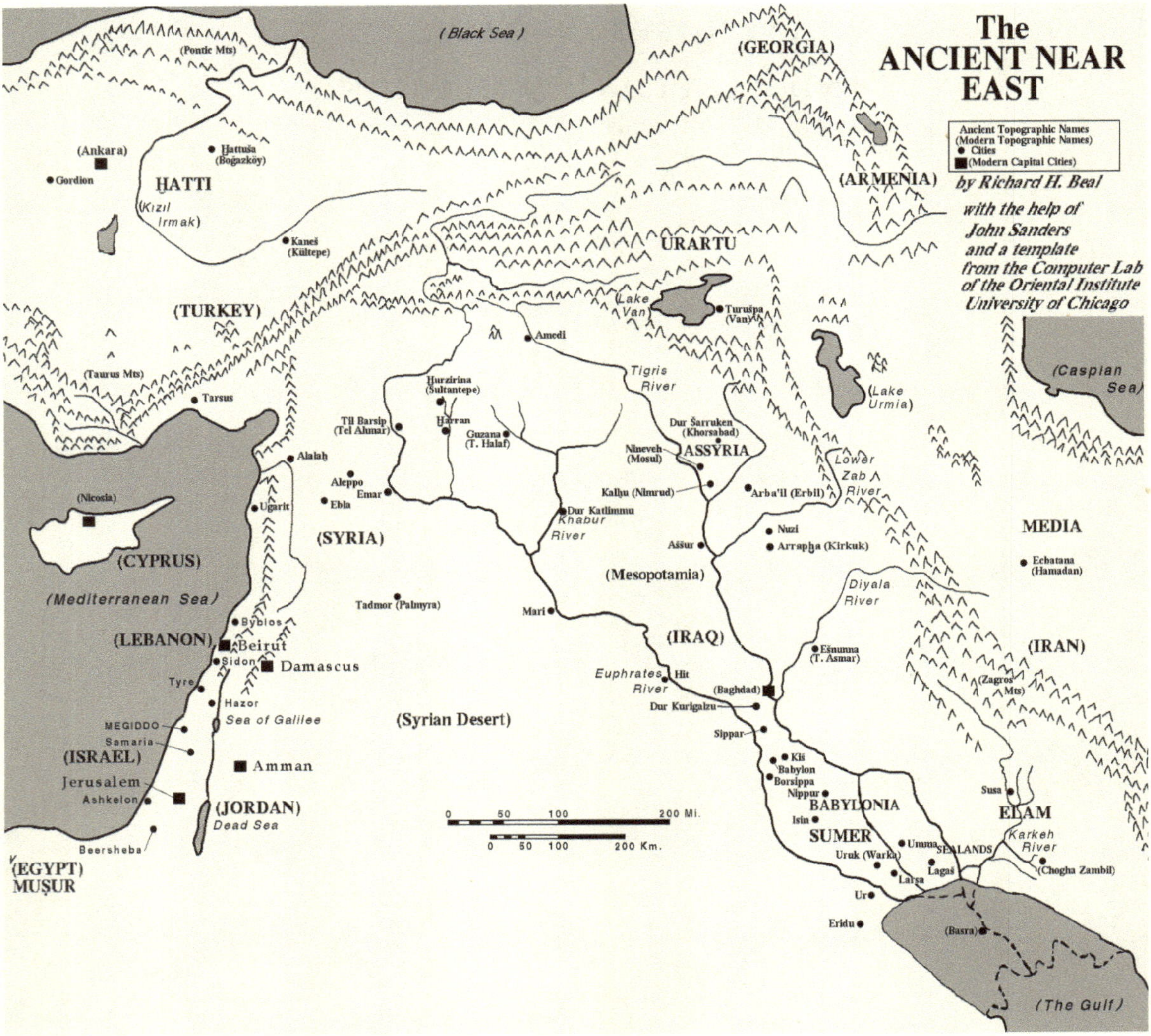
The ANCIENT NEAR EAST
Ancient Topographic Names
(Modern Topographic Names)
Cities
(Modern Capital Cities)
by Richard H. Beal
with the help of
John Sanders
and a template
from the Computer Lab
of the Oriental Institute
University of Chicago
(Black Sea)
(Pontic Mts)
(GEORGIA)
(Ankara)
Gordion
Hattuša
(Boğazköy)
HATTI
(Kızıl
Irmak)
Kaneš
(Kültepe)
(ARMENIA)
URARTU
(Lake
Van)
Turušpa
(Van)
(TURKEY)
(Taurus Mts)
Tarsus
Amedi
Tigris
River
(Lake
Urmia)
(Caspian
Sea)
Hurzirina
(Sultantepe)
Harran
Til Barsip
(Tel Ahmar)
Guzana
(T. Halaf)
Dur Šarruken
(Khorsabad)
Nineveh
(Mosul)
ASSYRIA
Lower
Zab
River
Alalah
Aleppo
Emar
Ebla
Ugarit
(Nicosia)
Kalhu (Nimrud)
Arba'il (Erbil)
Dur Katlimmu
Khabur
River
(SYRIA)
Nuzi
Aššur
Arrapha (Kirkuk)
MEDIA
(CYPRUS)
Ecbatana
(Hamadan)
(Mesopotamia)
(Mediterranean Sea)
Diyala
River
Tadmor (Palmyra)
Mari
Byblos
(LEBANON)
Beirut
Sidon
Damascus
(IRAQ)
Ešnunna
(T. Asmar)
(IRAN)
Tyre
Hazor
Sea of Galilee
Euphrates
River
Hit
(Baghdad)
(Zagros
Mts)
Dur Kurigalzu
MEGIDDO
Samaria
(Syrian Desert)
Sippar
(ISRAEL)
Amman
Kiš
Babylon
Borsippa
Jerusalem
Nippur
Ashkelon
(JORDAN)
Dead Sea
BABYLONIA
Susa
ELAM
0 50 100 200 Mi.
0 50 100 200 Km.
Isin
SUMER
Umma
SEALANDS
Karkeh
River
Beersheba
Uruk (Warka)
Lagaš
(Chogha Zambil)
(EGYPT)
MUṢUR
Larsa
Ur
Eridu
(Basra)
(The Gulf)

CHAPTER 1

The Ancient Mesopotamian Context

A sore without an *asû* (pharmacist)
is like hunger without food.
—W. G. Lambert, *BWL* 242–243 ii 35–37[1]

Ancient Mesopotamia, the "cradle of civilization," is one of the sources of our own Western medical tradition.[2] It vies with ancient Egypt for the honor of having produced the world's earliest recorded medical texts. And yet, even the most basic questions remain unanswered. From what diseases did ancient Mesopotamians suffer? Without the benefit of modern technology, how well were they able to distinguish one illness from another? What herbs or other medicinal substances did they use to treat their patients? In view of the antiquity of this medical tradition, a surprisingly large amount of information is available to answer these questions. In addition to a little over half of the three thousand or so entries originally contained in the forty tablets of the diagnostic/prognostic handbook, there are over nine hundred tablets or tablet fragments containing instructions for the preparation of treatments.

This book aims to bring our knowledge of ancient Mesopotamian medicine to the same level as that enjoyed by other medical traditions of the ancient world. Previously, of pre-Greek medical traditions in the ancient Near East, only that of ancient Egypt was well known outside its own field.[3] This is in part due to the presence of special types of evidence in Egypt (such as mummies) which allow the existence of various modern diseases in ancient times to be independently established.

Such archaeologically recoverable sources of information do not currently exist for ancient Mesopotamia, although the science of bone analysis, still in its infancy and suffering badly from a lack of relevant skeletal material, may yet provide precisely this missing link. Nonetheless, the presence in ancient Mesopotamia of a corpus of texts that were designed for the training and use of ancient physicians allows for a type of study that is possible nowhere else in the ancient world, including Greece. Parchment is highly perishable, and we have every reason to believe that what we have of Hippocratic medicine is only a fraction of what originally existed. In addition, there is the vexing question of which manuscripts actually belong to Hippocrates of Kos and his followers and which to competing traditions such as that of Knidos.

Moreover, we have a decisive advantage in approaching ancient Mesopotamian medical texts not available to the eighteenth- and nineteenth-century founding fathers of Assyriology and quite apart from the subsequent accumulation of material and great advances made in the basic interpretation of texts. Our own modern system of medicine was founded on the premise that the rationalist and deductive approach pioneered by ancient Greek physicians was henceforth to be scrapped in favor of an inductive approach and an empiricist philosophy of "whatever works." This new development came at a cost to the history of medicine, since, as time progresses, the way in which modern physicians approach their patients, diagnose illnesses, and recommend treatments will inevitably diverge further and further from the Hippocratic norm, making the treatises attributed to the "father of medicine" and the elaborations of Galen ever more foreign and incomprehensible to modern practitioners of medicine.

The ancient Greeks' loss is, however, ancient Mesopotamia's gain. As has long been recognized, an inductive, empiricist approach is precisely that taken by ancient Mesopotamian physicians to their patients. What this means is that, once the absence of lab tests has been accounted for, the types of clinical information collected by ancient Mesopotamian physicians are comprehensible to modern doctors in ways that ancient Greek descriptions of diseases will now never be.

The Sumerian Legacy

The oldest known ancient Mesopotamian medical text is a therapeutic manual, written in Sumerian, which dates from the Ur III period (2112–2004 B.C.E.). This text is, in turn, part of a long tradition of scholarship whose beginnings may be traced back in Mesopotamia to the production of the earliest written records in the mid-fourth millennium B.C.E. or earlier.

The Sumerians, a people speaking an agglutinative language with no known relatives, and their northerly neighbors the Akkadians, a people speaking a Semitic language distantly related to Hebrew, Aramaic, and Arabic, created their civilizations from the most unpromising of materials: mud, clay, and water. Rising in the Armenian Taurus ranges near Mount Ararat, the Euphrates River meanders for 2,780 km across the modern states of Turkey, Syria, and Iraq to the Persian Gulf. The comparatively shorter Tigris (only 1,950 km long) flows immediately southward from its sources just south of Lake Van in eastern Turkey. Both rivers slow as the gradient lessens, and form a number of shifting channels in what is now southern Iraq before losing themselves in a maze of swampy wetlands at the head of the Persian Gulf.[4] These marshes were home to wild boar and waterfowl, various types of reeds and grasses, and innumerable mosquitoes.

Aside from these marshes and a strip of green along the rivers, the land up to the latitude of ancient Aššur (modern Qalat Šerqat) was a desert, whose parched earth received less than the 200 mm of annual rainfall necessary to sustain agriculture. The climate was dry and subtropical, as is still the case today, with temperatures reaching 49°C (120°F) in summer. In contrast to the situation in ancient Egypt, the natural river floods came at the wrong time to benefit the crops. Irrigating the heartlands of Sumer and Akkad therefore required a network of man-made canals, ditches, reservoirs, and sluice-gates to store and distribute the precious water. Without this system, ancient Mesopotamia would not have been able to produce sufficient food to support the population levels necessary for urban civilization. With it, there was not only enough wheat and barley to maintain the population, but a surplus that provided an important item for trade to obtain materials that were lacking in Mesopotamia. Stone and wood (apart from palm logs) were not immediately available for building, nor were there local sources of iron, copper, or tin for making tools.

The Development of Writing

Mesopotamia's only natural resources, apart from water, were clay and mud, and of these the Sumerians took full advantage. In addition to more mundane uses as building material for houses and to make pots, clay was pressed into service to provide a writing surface for record keeping. A lump of clay was shaped into a tablet, which was inscribed with a stylus made of reed from the southern marshes. The resulting document was allowed to dry or, more rarely, was baked.

For short passages, a small tablet of a size to be conveniently held in one hand was all that was needed. For longer texts, it was necessary to form larger, multicolumn tablets or to write smaller or both. Some of the texts were inscribed with such tiny signs that it is difficult to read them without a magnifying glass. There is, however, a natural limit to the size of tablet beyond which they become too heavy and too unwieldy for convenient use. Longer compositions were, therefore, copied onto a number of separate tablets (as with our volumes). Mistakes were easy to correct by simply rubbing out an error while the clay was still wet. The materials were cheap and readily available, which encouraged evolution from the use of writing for purely practical inventories of goods to more esoteric uses such as recording political events and preserving literary and scientific materials for posterity.

Before the invention of writing, the education of the young consisted of learning the basics of civilized life from their parents and grandparents, often through stories and proverbs. Boys would master a craft or profession, usually by some form of on-the-job training as assistants or apprentices. The initial invention of writing did not change this pattern greatly; most people (including kings) had no use for reading and writing beyond what a notary public or a secretary could conveniently provide. What did emerge was a new profession, that of scribe. Scribes, like members of other professions, began their training in childhood. There is a fascinating set of school texts in Sumerian describing the process.[5] Those scribes who were not fortunate enough to have fathers and grandfathers who were attached to some institution sat in the public square and wrote contracts and letters or read them to illiterate customers for a set fee.

By the Neo-Assyrian period (934–609 B.C.E.), records were being kept not only on clay tablets (in Akkadian) and papyrus scrolls (in Aramaic) but also on writing boards of wood or ivory, coated with a thin layer of beeswax to provide a smooth and erasable surface. What was written on scrolls or writing boards is probably lost to us forever. On the other hand, clay tablets are virtually indestructible. Where archaeologists have managed to find these tablets, whatever was recorded by ancient scribes (with allowances for breakage and abraded surfaces) is available for us to study.

As writing developed, objects, ideas, and numbers were initially represented by pictures (as of a donkey) or abstract symbols (such as circles or triangles) laboriously drawn onto the clay with a sharpened stylus. Eventually, it dawned on some frustrated scribe that the process could be considerably sped up if the tip of the stylus were cut off and jabbed into the clay in a rough approximation of the drawing. The resulting "wedge-shaped" (cuneiform) signs gradually changed and developed over time. These changes allow for a rough dating of tablets by sign-form, just as medieval English may be distinguished from modern English on purely calligraphic grounds.

Akkadian speakers adapted this writing system for their own language by using the pictograms as word-signs and by creating a syllabary by the simple expedient of exploiting the syllabic value of the Sumerian or Akkadian word or words represented by the pictograms. For example, the Sumerian word for "hand" is ŠU, written with a sign that originally looked like a hand. Akkadian speakers used this sign to represent the concept "hand" (Akkadian *qātu*) but also for the syllables "šu" and "qat."

The Development and Spread of Ancient Mesopotamian Culture

The culture created by Sumerians and Akkadians spread along the trade routes that were developed to supply the "land between the rivers" with the supplies of wood, metal, and stone that it lacked. As early as the Uruk period (fourth millennium B.C.E.), close cultural contacts had been established over much of the area that was eventually to form the Assyrian empire (see below), and lapis lazuli (a blue semi-precious stone) was being traded all the way from Afghanistan to Egypt by way of Sumer and Akkad. In the early second millennium B.C.E., Old Assyrian merchant colonies centered in Kaneš near modern Kayseri supplied Anatolia with Afghani tin and Babylonian or Assyrian textiles manufactured to order at a considerable profit. By the Old Babylonian period (1894–1595 B.C.E.), seaborne traffic had reached up the Persian Gulf past the island of Dilmun (Bahrain and its coastal hinterland) to Oman and India. A flourishing Mediterranean trade reaching Greece was firmly established by the mid-second millennium B.C.E. Successive empires continued this far-flung trade; the ruler of Izki in Oman and kings of "Ionia" "paid tribute" (i.e., sent gifts) to Neo-Assyrian monarchs. With the domestication of the camel in the mid-first millennium B.C.E., incense and other goods from the Arabian peninsula flowed into southern Mesopotamia. So important was this particular trade route that the last Neo-Babylonian king, Nabonidus (555–539 B.C.E.), secured it by moving his place of residence to a palace that he built for himself in Teima in the Hijaz.

Included in this developing Sumero-Akkadian cultural sphere were the Assyrians. The Assyrians are so-called because they spoke a separate dialect of Akkadian, "Assyrian," as opposed to the "Babylonian" dialect of the south. They lived to the north of Babylonia on the eastern end of what the Arabs call al-Jazirah ("the island"), a fertile plain some 400 km wide. This area is blessed with adequate rainfall, numerous wells supplied by mountain snowmelt, and two additional rivers between the Euphrates and Tigris, the Balikh and the Khabur. Beyond the Tigris to the east and north of Assyria, the land rises in a series of rolling foothills beside the Upper and Lower Zab, the Adheim and the Diyala rivers. It was in these "hilly flanks" and the neighboring Levant that agriculture was first developed and sheep and goats domesticated. Beyond them to the east lie the rugged, snow-covered peaks of the Zagros range (2,500 to 3,600 m) and, to the north, the Taurus mountains (1,800–4,100 m). The climate of Assyria is hot in summer but cool enough in winter to require the use of movable braziers to heat large rooms.

Between 1363 and 609 B.C.E., the Assyrians gradually united the modern countries of Iraq, Syria, Lebanon, Israel, Palestine, and parts of Iran and Turkey into a single political entity. Always respectful of the culture and traditions of their southern neighbors while creating their own distinctive civilization, Assyrian monarchs went to great pains to collect the combined wisdom of Assyrian and Babylonian scholars into palace archives of which the "library" of Aššurbanipal (668–627 B.C.E.) is the best known. This collective knowledge was, by a supreme irony of history, partially preserved for us when Aššurbanipal's palace was sacked by the Medes[6] and the tablets, though scattered, baked to the hardness of stone in the flames.

Assyrian monarchs also made collections of unusual plants and animals that they encountered on their campaigns. One of them, Sennacherib (704–681 B.C.E.), took a particular interest in scientific matters, importing cotton plants (presumably from India), and growing them in the palace gardens with a view to making them into garments.

The Neo-Babylonian dynasty that overthrew the Assyrians with the help of the Medes in 612 B.C.E. practiced a brutal policy of ethnic cleansing in areas that refused to submit to their rule. The people of Jerusalem were lucky to be carried off into Babylonian captivity; Assyrians were simply slaughtered and buried in mass graves. Not only did the Assyrians disappear from history as a result, but every major settlement in the section of northern Mesopotamia that was slated to go to the Medes was so thoroughly destroyed that most did not recover until the Persian (538–331 B.C.E.) or Hellenistic (330–141 B.C.E.) period. The Babylonians, however, continued to rule the southern part of Mesopotamia as a unit and preserved at least a portion of the common tradition to pass along to Persian kings.

When Alexander the Great died in 307 B.C.E., the empire that he had conquered from the Persians was fought over and eventually divided among his generals, one of whom was Seleucus (305–281 B.C.E.). Along with other spoils of war, Seleucus and his successors fell heir to a rich collection of medical and scientific texts that continued to be preserved and copied in the temples of Babylon, Borsippa, Sippar, Uruk, and Nippur through the subsequent Parthian period until at least the first[7] and possibly as late as the third century C.E.[8]

The Recording of a Medical Tradition

Sumerian died out as a spoken language sometime in the third millennium B.C.E. but so embedded was it in the writing system that it survived as a scholarly language, learned and even spoken by the educated Akkadian scribe with the help of the world's oldest dictionaries and grammars, much as Latin was learned and to some extent spoken in medieval universities. Sumerian words came to be used as a sort of scientific shorthand in a purely Akkadian context, as Latin and Greek are used in our own tradition. We must, therefore, not be too hasty to assume that, because a particular set of symptoms is given a Sumerian name, that the Sumerians were the first to recognize or describe it, although this will more often have been the case than with our Greek and Latin terminology. That Akkadian speakers made refinements in diagnostic categories over time is readily demonstrable from the appearance of purely Akkadian terms in the texts. One such term is *bennu*, one of the first neurological terms to be encountered by beginning students in Assyriology for the simple reason that it is found in the Old Babylonian Laws of Ḫammurapi.[9]

Ancient Mesopotamian healers were among the first to appreciate the advantages of a recorded medical tradition, where what could not be committed to memory could be "written so as not to be forgotten,"[10] to be copied out as needed when performing an unfamiliar procedure or treating an unfamiliar disease. As a result, the experiments of one generation of scholars were not doomed to be endlessly repeated by their successors. Through the medium of written tablets, knowledge could also readily be shared between one center of learning in, say, Hittite Ḫattuša, and another in Elamite Susa.

As we have mentioned, the oldest known ancient Mesopotamian medical text is a therapeutic manual, written in Sumerian, which dates from the Ur III period (2112–2004 B.C.E.). It contained instructions for the treatment of patients but no written diagnoses (at least not in the preserved sections of the text). Such manuals were presumably intended for the use of an expert known as the AZU who was the ancestor of the later *asû* (for whom, see below).

An inventory text from third-millennium Ebla indicates that the AZU had in his tool kit, in addition to straight and curved bronze blades each weighing 2 to 3 shekels (16 to 24 g) and bronze needles and tweezers (forceps)[11] of similar dimensions, small bronze hammers (DUB.NAGAR),[12] which to judge from later texts were intended for testing reflexes (see Chapter 13). Also available to ancient physicians were magnifying glasses made of polished rock crystal that could have been used for closer examination of skin and other tissues.[13]

By the Old Babylonian period (1894–1595 B.C.E.), Mesopotamian therapeutic texts had begun to include descriptions of signs and symptoms and/or diagnoses with instructions for the preparation and administration of medications. It is often asserted that all medical knowledge that would ever be present in Mesopotamia had been discovered by this period. Allegedly, this body of knowledge was recorded directly from oral tradition in the Middle Babylonian period and was subsequently copied in "fossilized" form until the end of Mesopotamian civilization. There is no basis in fact for these beliefs. As is readily demonstrable from the Old Babylonian medical texts that we possess, there was a complete change in format and wording of medical texts between the Old Babylonian and the Middle Babylonian periods. There is also internal evidence for later improvements and additions.[14]

By the Middle Assyrian and Middle Babylonian periods (ca. 1430–1050 B.C.E.), there seems to have been sufficient elaboration of medical knowledge to justify the preparation of a separate diagnostic and prognostic handbook. Apparently simultaneous with these developments was an emerging division of labor between two separate healing experts. One of these was known as the *āšipu*, for whose training and eventual use the diagnostic and prognostic handbook was intended. The other, called an *asû*, seems to have played the role of pharmacist (and bone setter and performer of minor surgery) to the *āšipu's* physician.[15]

Under the patronage of Adad-apla-iddina (1068–1047 B.C.E.), the Borsippan scholar Esagil-kīn-apli redacted the *āšipu's* diagnostic and prognostic handbook, apportioning the available material among forty tablets of varying length by subject matter to allow for future additions and corrections. The first subseries (Tablets I–II) contained all of the ominous occurrences that might take place as the *āšipu* was on his way to the patient's house. Tablets III–XIV constituted the second subseries, which began with headaches and progressed down the body in head-to-toe order. Tablets XV–XVI contained entries organized in accordance with the number of days the patient had been sick. Tablet XVII was concerned with phases of illness and times of day. Tablet XVIII was a discussion of fevers and of attendant signs and symptoms. For example, lines 1–14 described fevers with potential mental status changes followed by a discussion of mental status changes in a nonfebrile context and in lines 39′–42′, a description of *ṣētu* (enteric fever), which as we know from other references (see Chapter 3) could cause urinary tract problems or petechiae and diarrhea, was followed by a discussion of urinary tract problems, petechiae, and diarrhea that were not caused by *ṣētu*. Tablets XIX/XX and XXI divided off illnesses with fever (XIX/XX) from illnesses where the pulse rate was normal (XXI). Tablets XXII and XXIII rounded out the third subseries which was devoted for the most part to infectious diseases. Tablets XXVI–XXX constituted the fourth subseries, which collected together entries relating to neurology, an apparent subspecialty of the *āšipu's* craft. The fifth subseries consisted of two surviving tablets: XXXI, which was devoted to enteric fever (*ṣētu*; see Chapter 3), and XXXIII, which gave detailed descriptions of skin lesions. Tablets XXXVI, XXXVII, and LX (and the missing XXXVIII and XXXIX) formed the sixth subseries, which contained entries dealing with women and infants.

Of the entries originally contained in this series, we have a little less than half and that due largely to the scholarly interests of the Assyrian king Aššurbanipal (668–627 B.C.E.) who also preserved at his capital Nineveh a large collection of therapeutic texts. Included in the collection was an herbal handbook for the *asû*, complete with descriptions of plants, possible substitutions, and brief instructions for preparation and use. Another substantial archive, also Neo-Assyrian in date, was found in a private house excavated at the original capital of Assyria, the city of Aššur. Some of these tablets, which have colophons[16] preserved, show them to stem from the activities of Kiṣir-Aššur son of Nabû-bēssunu and his nephew Kiṣir-Nabû son of Šamaš-ibni, both *āšipus* attached to the temple of Aššur, chief god of Assyria. Smaller caches come from Kalḫu and provincial Ḫuzirīna.

To judge from developments in other fields of science, the Neo-Assyrian court should have provided fertile ground for new discoveries in medicine. In astronomy, for example, the late eighth to seventh centuries B.C.E. brought about what has been described as a "revolution of wisdom" or "paradigm shift involving evolution from a celestial divination that did not incorporate the accurate prediction of celestial phenomena to a celestial divination / astrology / astronomy that did."[17]

Like this new science of astronomy,[18] Assyrian medical knowledge survived the fall of Assyria and the conquest of Babylon by Cyrus. The last dated exemplar of the diagnostic handbook is from the eleventh year of the Persian king Artaxerxes I (453 B.C.E.), but some copies can be attributed to the Seleucid era on the basis of sign-forms and prosopography[19] and one exemplar may have been produced after 153 B.C.E.[20] The venerable city of Uruk in particular seems to have flourished under Seleucid rule, and excavations there have revealed a number of copies of tablets of the diagnostic series, as well as commentaries and therapeutic texts.

The Earliest Physicians

Āšipus were generally associated with temples and, in addition to their medical duties, performed purification rites in connection with calendric celebrations or the consecration of cult statues. They were not, however, responsible for any of the various chores associated with the daily cult (feeding, bathing, and clothing the god/goddess). Alongside other cultic personnel, they formed part of an extensive staff that included the priests, administrators, and record keepers and numerous butchers, bakers, craftsmen, musicians, and singers.

Those with access to the temple were required to maintain a high degree of cleanliness, including shaving off head and body hair, to avoid offending the god/goddess into whose house they were entering.[21] The gods/goddesses residing in a temple were fed twice daily, with extra helpings on feast days. The gods/goddesses, of course, took only the essence of the sacrifice, leaving the remainder to be divided up among the temple personnel as a sort of salary. Bread, meat, and fruit from such offerings were so plentiful that enterprising citizens of Old Babylonian Ur[22] and Late Babylonian Uruk[23] sold entitlements to shares of the benefits of minor temple offices such as butcher and courtyard sweeper on the open market.

What this tells us is not only that the *āšipu* was very unlikely to have approached a patient with dirty hands, but that the basic service that he provided was probably free. This does not of course count the cost of medicines, equipment, and animals sacrificed in the more elaborate rituals, part of which was eaten by the participants and part of which was the god's/goddess's share and hence taken by the *āšipu*.

In addition to a number of what we would characterize as purely "magical" duties (such as the exorcism of haunted houses), it was the task of the *āšipu* to treat diseases, as these were understood by Mesopotamians. This means that he was responsible for dealing with the spirit or malfunctioning body part whose irritation or malevolent activities were producing the observed symptoms (see below). He was, his "magical" duties excluded, a close equivalent to a modern "physician."

The physicians of ancient Mesopotamia were careful observers of clinical symptoms, frequently visiting patients in their houses and questioning them and those who had attended them in their illnesses. The detailed medical information that they obtained included past venereal contact, travel to areas where illness was common, activities or behaviors to be associated with illness, and family histories of illness. They also laid hands on patients, testing the temperature (of which they recognized five grades) and noting the color of feces and urine, if unusual. There is recorded evidence that physicians used all of their five senses except taste in observing their patients. They looked carefully at the patient's color, general appearance, and movement; listened to breathing and bowel sounds; felt temperature and body configuration; and described the odor of the patient's breath and of infected wounds.

It is unclear whether the *āšipu* added to his medical knowledge by performing autopsies, since the dissection of human corpses is not mentioned in any of the extant medical texts. However, the *āšipu* had a colleague, the diviner (*barû*), who shared the same patron deity (Gula) and whose job was the regular sacrifice and dissection of animals for purposes of divination (extispicy).[24] A great deal was undoubtedly learned about anatomy and animal pathology by this practice. From the idea of dissecting animals for extispicy, it seems logical to suppose that the idea of dissecting patients who died of mysterious illnesses to discern, as it were, the messages that the gods/goddesses had written in diseased human internal organs would have suggested itself quite naturally.

Anatomical knowledge would also have been gained by observing trauma victims and wounds produced by wars, which in some periods as, for example, the reign of Sargon II of Assyria (721–705 B.C.E.) were an almost yearly occurrence. Some of the medical texts discussed in subsequent chapters demonstrate a knowledge of organ pathology that could only have been gained from direct examination, that is, during a surgical procedure or in the course of an autopsy. Ancient Egyptians had no qualms about cutting open bodies and removing internal organs before burial; it may be that taboos on dissection are neither as universal nor as ancient as we imagine.

Ancient Mesopotamian *āšipus* generated a special vocabulary to describe medically significant signs (e.g., different types of pain, paralysis, spontaneous movement, and skin lesions). The depth of this vocabulary shows that the healing specialists' observations were performed with great attention to detail, and that precision in such matters was considered to be of the utmost importance. They also devised a number of diagnostic maneuvers such as the test that modern physicians call the Moro test that is used to evaluate the neurologic system of infants (see 13.281).

It is quite clear from a number of references in ancient Mesopotamian medicine that physicians must at some point have taken case histories. For example, there is a therapeutic text that attributes the appearance of arthritis in a person before the expected age to the fact that he had had another disease in his childhood (see 6.187). There is also a tablet of the diagnostic/prognostic handbook (XXXI) which judges the number of days a patient has been sick with some form of enteric fever (see Chapter 3) by the symptoms that have to that date appeared (e.g., chills on the third day and epistaxis on the seventh). Neither of these pieces of information would have been possible without the gathering of some form of case history.[25] We do not have these case histories for the simple reason that medicine had advanced beyond that stage by the time diagnoses and prognoses began to be systematically recorded.

Like modern doctors, ancient Mesopotamian physicians made prognoses as well as diagnoses, and also administered[26] or recommended treatments. In this book, we describe symptoms, physical findings, diagnosis, and prognosis only. We hope to publish a subsequent book containing an analysis of the treatment sections of these texts. Regarding prognosis, the following possible outcomes are listed: "he will die" or "he will not get well" (a hopeless case); "he will not straighten up" (incurable paralytic conditions); "he will not do well" (not an immediate death sentence but not really curable either); "his illness will take a change (for the worse)," "his illness will be difficult," or "it is worrisome" (bad but not hopeless); "it is of no consequence" (there is nothing actually wrong); "he will get up" (the problem is psychological not physical); he will get well (a treatable ailment); and "he will get well but afterward he will get sick again" (epilepsy—treatable but not curable).

No treatment intended for cure (as opposed to medicines to relieve symptoms such as pain) was offered in cases that the ancient Mesopotamian healer knew to be incurable.[27] Ailments that were incurable were nonetheless studied and described with as much care as curable ones. Diagnoses, prognoses, and therapeutic treatments[28] were organized into written handbooks (see above) that were arranged in a logical fashion and subdivided into tablets by subject matter so that one might actually have had some hope[29] of looking up what one needed in them.[30]

The *āšipu* was not likely to have had time to acquire more than a basic working knowledge of the medicines that he used. He was a very busy man with a host of duties to perform and, unlike modern physicians, he did make house calls.[31] In his labors he was, therefore, aided by a second healing specialist known as the *asû*.

The *asû* operated out of his shop. Herbs were kept in jars that lined the shelves. Each jar had a label on the side indicating its contents.[32] The *asû* also kept shelf lists. The Laws of Ḫammurapi attempted to regulate the fees that he could charge. As in Indian and Chinese medicine to this day, these fees were graded in accordance with the patient's ability to pay.[33] Like the modern pharmacist, the *asû* compounded drugs that were observed to have practical value in relieving the complaints of patients. He also knew how to set bones, bandage wounds, lance boils, and stop nosebleeds, none of which require a particularly sophisticated knowledge of medicine. It would also have been his responsibility to recognize medicinal plants, to know where they grew, when best to gather them, and how to store and prepare them.

What the *asû* did not do was to diagnose complex illnesses. If the *asû* was ever called upon to treat a patient with an illness requiring a diagnosis, he could only have done so with the cooperation, perhaps even the consent,[34] of his colleague, the *āšipu*. It is not hard, then, to understand why, except for minor problems with which the *asû* could deal by himself, these specialists typically combined their efforts in the treatment of illness in ancient Mesopotamia. This mirrors modern physicians and pharmacists, who still cooperate in the treatment of illness.

Definitions of Disease

Signs and symptoms may appear by themselves in the texts, but they were also grouped into syndromes to which descriptive names might be given. Some treatments were designed to deal with a sign or symptom wherever it might appear, others with a sign or symptom that was a subset of a particular syndrome. Other treatments were meant to deal with syndromes as a whole. A few of these syndromes correspond to modern diseases. More commonly, the texts describe syndromes (jaundice and wasting or fever with a rash), which make rational sense as a clinical category but which modern physicians know to be caused by more than one disease.

The ancient Mesopotamian concept of disease differs strikingly from the familiar Hippocratic notion,[35] that illness results from an imbalance of internal "humors." The ancient Mesopotamian physician was always open to the possibility that the symptoms that he was observing were due to an invisible external force. In his terms, the cause might be a god/goddess, a demon/demoness or some angry ghost attacking the patient.

Disease entities attributed to what we would call an external cause were imagined as being brought about by physical contact between an afflicting spirit and his victim. As would have been the case with a human enemy, such a spirit might inflict injury through "touch" or "seizing" or even "striking" the patient, with the obvious difference that, unlike his human counterpart, the spirit did his or her dirty work invisibly. It is presumably for this reason that disease entities tend to be literally attributed to the "hand" of the disease-causing spirit as, for example, "hand" of Ištar for sexually transmitted diseases (see Chapter 4).

This is not to say that ancient Mesopotamians did not realize that it was possible for a person's body to malfunction on its own; a number of ancient syndromes are given the diagnosis "sick" liver, gall bladder, or other organs (see Chapter 6). Organs with a sufficient independence of mind to malfunction, however, readily came to be viewed not as inanimate matter but as a lower order of spirit. Like their more obviously demonic fellow trouble-causers, malfunctioning body parts might be sparked by other spirits but they could also, theoretically at least, misbehave on their own. For example, a person could have his head "seize" him or a ghost could cause his head to "seize" him or an angry god could cause the ghost to cause his head to "seize" him, or a sorcerer could get the god angry so that he caused the ghost to cause his head to "seize" him, and so on.

Symptoms are nonetheless listed in diagnostic handbooks in a way which shows that it was the symptoms that were generating the diagnosis, however "supernatural" that diagnosis may look to us. Indeed, it was because of rather than in spite of this tendency to proffer "supernatural" explanations that the approach of the *āšipu* to both diagnosis and treatment was fully grounded in analysis of prior observations. There is no inherent conflict between the ancient Mesopotamian belief that malevolent spirits are causers of disease and the observed beneficial effects of herbs, tree resins, and minerals. One need only suppose that the malfunctioning body part, or the god/goddesses, ghost, or demon/demoness who was believed to be causing a particular set of symptoms, was fond of the particular set of medicines that were observed to relieve those symptoms.

Spirits could be assumed to have their preferences in terms of offerings (or to put it in ancient Mesopotamian terms, to have things that were "special" [*ikkibu*] to them), but also to welcome some variety in their diet. An excellent way in which a particular god, ghost, or demon could communicate exactly what it was that he wanted at any particular moment was to induce a particular set of symptoms that he knew to be treated with the desired medicines. It, therefore, followed that the way to determine the cure for a particular ailment was to try out various medicines or combinations of medicines until something worked, and to keep trying until all possible treatments had been discovered.

With many illnesses, buying off the spirit or placating the malfunctioning body part with offerings in the form of medicines seems to have been sufficient, with perhaps a generic Sumerian or "Subarean"[36] incantation and the odd "special" ingredient added to increase the chance of success. More elaborate (and expensive) rituals involving the manipulation of figurines, the preparation of libations, or other "magical" procedures were available on demand. All this may sound very strange to modern ears, but the fact is that attributing diseases to spirits is considerably closer to the modern theory of infection by organisms invisible to the naked eye attacking the body from without than is the Hippocratic notion of imbalance of humors.[37]

This appreciation of the potential for external causes for disease also led to the development of such sanitary practices as handwashing before a meal and taking baths. For more details on this and other subjects relating to public health, see Chapter 2.

Modern Understanding of the Assyro-Babylonian Medical Tradition

As mentioned above, this medical tradition with its roots in Sumer and Akkad and developed by Assyrians and Babylonians survived until at least the first and possibly as late as the third century C.E. From that point in time, however, knowledge even of the existence of this ancient Mesopotamian medical tradition dropped from awareness, only to resurface a century ago. Since that time, there has been a growing interest in Assyriology as knowledge of the language has grown.

Unfortunately, interest in the medical literature has developed more slowly. Physicians and medical specialists with an interest in exploring ancient Mesopotamian medicine soon discover that most of this fascinating material is available only in hand copies[38] of the original cuneiform texts, which are impenetrable without years of hard study. What is available in English translation by R. Campbell Thompson is outdated by the current standards of cuneiform studies, since this is a relatively new and rapidly developing field. Numerous misinterpretations and occasional misreadings make this an unreliable source of information for those who cannot read the texts in the original. There are editions of a few of the most important texts,[39] as well as scattered articles on the meanings of specific technical terms or the identification of specific plants or diseases; however, no systematic study of all of the available material by a cuneiformist working hand in hand with trained medical doctors has yet appeared. This book hopes to remedy this problem, and to make the descriptions of symptoms contained in ancient Mesopotamian medical texts available to doctors of both Assyriology and medicine as well as educated laypersons.

The readers of this monograph may be astonished at the level of sophistication of the clinical observations found in these ancient texts.[40] Since they did not become available to modern scholars until the last century, we are only now beginning to realize their significance. It is no exaggeration to say that the skill of ancient Mesopotamians in diagnosis and therapy was only surpassed in the late nineteenth century C.E., a startling tribute to the potential of the human mind to reason, if armed with an observation-based approach and an attitude of "use whatever works." As other texts are rescued from the soil, and the uncatalogued tablets languishing in the basements of museums are gradually published, we expect even greater treasures to be revealed.

CHAPTER 2

General Health and Public Health Practices

Nobody is to drink from the cup from which she drinks;
nobody is to sit on the seat on which she sits and
nobody is to lie on the bed on which she lies and
many women are ⌜not⌝ to mingle with her.
That ⌜illness⌝ is contagious.

—*ARM*[*T*] 10.129:11–20

The general level of health in a society is less influenced by the quality of its medical care than it is by the quality of its nutrition, public and personal hygiene, and the techniques used to prevent and control contagious diseases. Using these measures, ancient Mesopotamians deserve high marks.

Nutrition

Although information about the quality of the diet of ancient Mesopotamians is incomplete, it was certainly better than that of the average nineteenth-century European peasant. Plants native to and first cultivated in the Near East included not only barley (from which a rich and nutritious beer was made) and bread wheat, but also chick peas, lentils, peas, fava beans, apricots, dates, figs, grapes, olives, almonds, pistachio nuts, and walnuts. Archaeological deposits from ancient sites in Iraq have also yielded remains of various vetches (pea family),[1] acorns, dried crab apples, capers, hackberry and pomegranate seeds, hazelnuts, and the pods of *Prosopis stephaniana*, another member of the pea or bean family.[2] There were also several varieties of onions and garlic, cucumbers and melons, various types of greens, root vegetables, and spices, including cumin, coriander, and fenugreek. The average ancient Mesopotamian probably did not eat a great deal of beef or mutton, but less expensive meat sources were available, including poultry, ducks and geese, pigs and wild boar, deer and gazelles, birds, and bandicoot rats, the latter apparently particularly flavorful.[3] Locusts were skewer-roasted to provide crisp finger food.[4] Fish and shellfish of all varieties were eaten, or made into what the Romans later called garum (a sort of salty fish paste) and used as a condiment.[5] To round out the diet, there were vegetable oils (sesame and olive), goose and hen eggs, honey, and various sorts of milk products (cheese, yogurt, and clarified butter).[6] Certainly these foods, if taken in proper proportions, would have provided an excellent diet.[7]

Ancient recipes from the Old Babylonian period[8] give some idea of the richness of ancient stews and pies. Texts from Emar mention one such pie, which was manufactured from flour and oil, and which contained no less than forty birds, plus correspondingly large quantities of raisins, figs, and pistachio nuts, a combination reminiscent of Moroccan bisteeya, and perhaps its ultimate ancestor.[9]

Starvation and protein malnutrition, however, were known and described (Chapter 7). During sieges an entire city might be reduced to eating leather straps and even human flesh to survive. Some years, due to inadequate rainfall in the highlands north of Mesopotamia, the flood waters were inadequate. In other years, they were too plentiful and sometimes produced catastrophic floods. Also, marginal agricultural land on the periphery of the "fertile crescent" lacked irrigation and was always susceptible to drought and therefore starvation. Areas within reach of irrigation eventually experienced a buildup of salt in the soil and had to be allowed to go unirrigated to permit the polluted soil to dry up and be blown off by the wind. Some of these problems were remedied by stockpiling grain, dates, and the like[10] to ensure that there was an ample supply of food throughout the year and in years of drought.

Climate

The climate throughout much of ancient Mesopotamia would have been hot and dry during the summer, but cooler and wetter in the winter. Humidity would have been higher near the Persian Gulf. In Babylon, which is located near the center of the Mesopotamian floodplain, the mean daily maximum temperature is still 57.2° F, or 14.0° C, in January and 107° F or 43.7° C in August, while the mean relative humidity varies from 22 to 67 percent.[11] Sandstorms are relatively common in summer, whereas rainstorms with thunder and lightning occur more commonly in winter. The prevailing dryness would have been a benefit in dessicating contaminated excrement and animal residue, helping to prevent the spread of microorganisms. Other effects of heat, dryness, sun, wind, and sandstorms on health are discussed in the infectious disease and skin chapters (Chapters 3, 10).

Public Health Practices

GARBAGE DISPOSAL

Mesopotamian housewives prided themselves on keeping their houses swept clean.[12] That this practice was understood as preventive is clear from the use of sweeping in apotropaic[13] rites.

2.1 É.BI *ina* ^{GIŠ}AN.NA.GIŠIMMAR *šá* IM.SI.SÁ *tu-še-šir šu-šu-rat* É *ana* ÍD ŠUB-*di* (*SpTU* 5.246 iii 21′–22′)[14]

**You sweep that house with a palm frond from the north side (of the tree); you throw the sweepings of the house into the river. (This is a rite designed to keep evils including epidemics from entering the house.)

Unfortunately, this often merely resulted in the transfer of the refuse from the house to the street.[15] As in modern India, pigs and feral dogs, and an occasional cow and goat, seem to have served as impromptu garbage disposals. Dogs ran in packs, howled in the streets,[16] and were a danger to unattended children and unguarded graves. Adoption contracts describing abandoned babies "brought in from the street"[17] sometimes refer to them as "snatched from the mouths of the dogs."[18]

The animals kept the streets clear of food scraps, and the dung was doubtless eventually collected for use as fertilizer, but in the meantime, street animals made city living a somewhat malodorous experience.

2.2 ŠAḪ *la qa-šid* [. . . *mu-bal-l*]*il ar-ki mu-ba-ḫi-iš su-qa-ni* x [*mu*]-*ṭa-an-ni-pu* É.MEŠ (Lambert, *BWL* 215 iii 13-14)

**The pig is unholy [. . . it] ⌜defiles⌝ everything behind it, makes the streets stink [. . .] besmirches the houses.

2.3 DIŠ UR.GI$_7$ GI$_6$ *ana* UGU LÚ GÌR *iš-ši-ma* KÀŠ-*šú iš-tin* . . . (*CT* 39.1:67)

**If a black dog lifts its leg and urinates on a person . . .

2.4 DIŠ U$_8$ *ina* ^{GIŠ}NÁ NÁ *lu* A.GAR.GAR *lu* ⌜KÀŠ⌝ *it-bu-*[*ka*] . . . (*CT* 28.38 (K 4079a) obv. 12)

**If a ewe discharges (its) dung or urine in a person's bed . . .

Burial of the dead was the normal practice, but bodies were occasionally left unburied or dumped into the river as a form of punishment. In times of war it was often difficult to give prompt burial to casualties. At the end of a long siege, the first task of a victorious army was to clean out the dead bodies choking the streets and polluting the water supply.

SEWAGE DISPOSAL

Bathrooms are a distinctive and readily recognizable feature of ancient Mesopotamian houses. In addition to a basin for washing (whence they were referred to as "lavatories"),[19] these contained emplacements for urination and/or defecation. Bathrooms were connected by means of an elaborate drainage system to underground sewers, which also carried off excess rainwater.[20] Archaeological evidence also reveals the existence of sump pits[21] which, taken together with sewers and drains, would have given ancient Mesopotamians a supply of drinking water cleaner than that available to many Londoners in the 1850s. Since, however, at least part of the organic waste would inevitably have found its way sooner or later into the river, river water[22] was supplemented wherever possible by digging wells. Contamination of wells by sump pits may sometimes have been a problem, although the dry climate and the absence of flush toilets would have helped in this regard. Meals were washed down with sweet Mesopotamian beer or imported wine, the alcoholic content of which would have helped reduce bacterial contaminants (see Chapter 3).

WASHING AND THE USE OF SOAP

Ancient Mesopotamians understood the importance of cleanliness and recognized the fact that attention to personal hygiene could help to prevent some illnesses. In the second reference below, the condition caused by the dirty hands was probably conjunctivitis due either to a chemical irritant or a microorganism present on the hands.

2.5 *a-na* É *mu-sa-a-tú* NU KU$_4$-*ub* : ^{d}*Šu-lak* SÌG-*su* / ^{d}*Šu-lak šá* E-*ú* : ŠU : *qa-tu*$_4$: LA : *la-a* : KÙ : *el-lu* / DIŠ É *mu-sa-a-tú* KU$_4$-*ub* ŠU^{II}-*šú* NU KÙ *ana* UGU *qa-bi* (*SpTU* 1.47 obv. 3–5)

**He should not enter a lavatory (or) Šulak (the lavatory demon) will strike him. When they say "Šulak" (what they mean is) ŠU = "hand", LA = "not" (and) KÙ = "clean." If he enters a lavatory, his hands will not be clean. That is why this is said.

2.6 DIŠ ŠU^{II}-*šú* NU LUḪ.MEŠ IGI^{II}.MEŠ-*šú ik-*[*pur*] EN ⸢U$_4$⸣-*um* TI.LA IGI^{II}-*šú mar-*[*ṣa*] . . . DIŠ ŠU^{II}-*šú* LUḪ.MEŠ-*ma* IGI^{II}.MEŠ-*šú ik-pur* ^{d}LAMMA TUKU-*ši* (*STT* 324:10–11, 13)[23]

**If he ⸢rubs⸣ his eyes with his unwashed hands, as long as he lives, his eyes will be ⸢sore⸣. . . . If he washes his hands and then rubs his eyes, he will have a protective spirit.[24]

Ancient texts contain frequent references to washing hands, feet, hair, and clothing with water and plant-based alkali soap.[25] Facilities were available for soaking baths for the whole body or merely the lower extremities.[26] Otherwise, baths were taken by the simple expedient of dipping in the river or pouring the water over the part to be washed. It was customary to wash one's hands before a meal,[27] and Assyrian palace rooms where banquets were held were provided with a waterproof emplacement for the requisite water jar.[28] Washing before religious rituals was also an expected practice.

STERILIZATION

It is interesting to note the frequency with which medicines were baked or boiled before use, suggesting at least some empirical knowledge of the virtues of sterilization. Frequent dressing changes for wounds (3.188) also suggests a recognition of the importance of cleanliness. We are unaware of special cleaning or sterilization for surgical instruments, although it is interesting that it was customary to cut the umbilical cord of a newborn child with a sliver of reed, essentially a one-use disposable knife blade.[29] In the text below, we believe that moving the patient from room to room served to keep the patient in a clean environment and thus encouraged recovery.

2.7 DIŠ SA SAG.KI^{II}-*šú* ŠU^{II}-*šú* RI.MEŠ GAR.MEŠ -*ma* PA IGI^{II}-*šú* DIB.DIB-*tu* ŠU.LUḪ[30] *ina* KI DIB-*tu* TA É *ana* É KÚR-*šú-ma* DIN (DPS IV A r. 2–3+A$_4$ r. 1–2//B r. 15 = *TDP* 42 r. 35–36)[31]

**If the blood vessels of his temples and hands are present in tandem and his eyelids are "seized," you wash (him). He is at an acute stage of the illness;[32] (if) you move him from one room to another, he will get well.

An extension of the *āšipu*'s awareness of cleanliness is his appreciation of the value of fresh air in aiding recovery. Assyrian palaces were provided with air shafts to ensure the ventilation of larger rooms,[33] and "wind doors" were a standard feature of traditional Iraqi houses until the arrival of modern air conditioners. In the quote below, we cannot determine the nature of the illness, but the outcome was considered to be worse in cold weather when the patient could not go outside. (In summer, it would have been possible to sleep on the roof at night.) Complicating secondary infection would be more likely if the patient occupied a confined space, possibly with poor ventilation and other occupants.

2.8 DIŠ SAL.KALAG.GA IGI-*ma ib-luṭ* EGIR *ib-lu-ṭu* GÌR^{II}-*šú it-te-né-eb-ṭa-ni* GIG.BI *šum-ma*[34] É.MEŠ EN LÍL-*šú i-qat-*⸢*tu*⸣*-ú* EN.TE.NA RI-*šum-ma* NU DIN (DPS XXII:69–70 [AOAT 43.257])

**If he experiences a mighty illness and then gets well (and) after he gets well, his feet are continually cramped, if the summer finishes before his illness does, the cold season will fall upon him so that he will not get well.

CONTAGION

Mesopotamian physicians attributed illnesses to gods/goddesses, demons/demonesses, and ghosts, rather than an imbalance of internal humors as Hippocratic physicians believed. Thus, they were open to the possibility of practical associations between illnesses and surrounding events and circumstances. They noted, for example, a greater likelihood for a person to become ill when in contact with someone with certain diseases; lexical texts equate "infected" with "place that has been touched."[35] In the first reference, a letter, the writer advises against person-to-person contact as well as the reuse of the patient's household articles,[36] while the second reference recommends both hygienic measures and quarantine.

2.9 [*a-na*] ⸢^{f}⸣*Ši-ib-tu* [*qí-b*]*í-ma* [*um-m*]*a be-el-ki-i-ma eš-me-e-ma* ^{f}*Na-an-na-me sí-im-ma-am mar-ṣa-at ù it-ti* É.GAL-*lim ma-ga-al wa-aš-ba-at-ma* MUNUS.MEŠ *ma-da-tim it-ti-ša-ma i-sa-ab-bi-ik i-na-an-na dan-na-tim šu-uk-ni-ma i-na ka-ás i-ša-at-tu-ú ma-am-ma-an la i-ša-at-ti i-na* ^{GIŠ}GU.ZA *ša úš-ša-bu ma-am-ma-an la úš-ša-ab ù i-na* ^{GIŠ}NÁ *ša it-ti-il-lu ma-am-ma-an la it-te-e-el-ma* MUNUS.MEŠ *ma-da-tim it-ti-*⸢*ša*⸣*-ma* [*l*]*a i-sa-ab-bi-ik* [*si-im-m*]*u-*⸢*um*⸣ *šu-ú mu-uš-ta-aḫ-ḫi-iz* (*ARM*[*T*] 10.129:1–20)

**[To] Šibtu, ⸢speak⸣, ⸢thus⸣ speaks your lord. I have heard that Nanname is ill with an illness, yet she is about the palace a lot and many of the women mingle with her. Now give stern orders that nobody is to drink from the cup from which she drinks; nobody is to sit on the seat on which she sits and nobody is to lie on the bed on which she lies and many women are ⸢not⸣ to mingle with her. That ⸢illness⸣ is contagious.[37]

2.10 Á.KÁ[R] *tu-na-kar-šu* ^{SÍG}*a-za-mi-il-la tu-ka-par-šu ša qú-ut-tu-ri tu-qat-tar-šu ṣi-tam na-pi-ir-tam la i-im-mar ma-am-man it-ti-šu la i-dub-bu-ub a-šar na-du-ú ma-am-man la ir-ru-ub* (BM 64526:26-31)[38]

**You remove his gear. You wipe him off with a rough cloth. You fumigate him with fumigants. He is not to see either daylight or torchlight. Nobody is to speak with him. Nobody is to enter the place where he has been put.

Ancient Mesopotamian physicians recognized that the death of a child by infection could be followed by the death of another child or of the mother or father. It is likely that both parents and children died of the same contagious infectious disease.

2.11 DIŠ ZI.ḪA.ZA SAG.ÚS DIB.DIB-*su u i-ṭa-mu* ÚŠ-*ma* EGIR-*šú* AMA-*šú* [GAM] / DIŠ ZI.ḪA.ZA SAG.ÚS DIB.DIB-*su u* GÙ.⌜DÉ⌝.ME ÚŠ-*ma* EGIR-*šú* ŠEŠ-*šú* [GAM] (DPS X A obv. 39–40 = *TDP* 84:39–40)[39]

**If persistent "grabbing of the throat"[40] continually afflicts him and he twists, if he dies afterward his mother [will die]. If persistent "grabbing of the throat" continually afflicts him and he continually roars, if he dies afterward his brother [will die].

2.12 DIŠ *ina šèr-ti* KÚM-*em ina le-lá-a-ti* ŠED$_7$ *ina* ⌜GI$_6$⌝ *ma-šil ù*ʾ DUG$_4$.GA ŠEŠ-*šú ma-a-a-ta-nu* KI-*šú* KEŠDA (DPS XVII:91–92 [AOAT 43.204])

**If in the morning he is hot, in the evening he is cold, (and) in middle of the night he says, "Ua," his dying brother is bound with him.

In the following reference, a man chooses to live separately from his diseased wife. Whatever the cause of her problem, living separately appears to be intended to prevent the disease from spreading.

2.13 *šum-ma a-wi-lum aš-ša-tam i-ḫu-uz-ma la-aḫ-bu-um iṣ-ṣa-ba-as-sí a-na ša-ni-tim a-ḫa-zi-im pa-ni-šu iš-ta-ka-an i-iḫ-ḫa-az aš-ša-sú ša la-aḫ-bu-um iṣ-ba-tu ú-ul i-iz-zi-ib-ši i-na* É *i-pu-šu uš-ša-am-ma a-di ba-al-ṭa-at it-ta-na-aš-ši-ši* (Laws of Ḫammurapi § 148)

**If a man marries a wife and *li*ʾ*bu* (see 10.136) afflicts her (and) he sets his mind on marrying another wife, he may marry her (but) he may not divorce his wife whom *li*ʾ*bu* afflicts; she shall live in a house that he builds (for her) and as long as she lives he shall support her.

Compare also the following extracts from a letter, an omen text, and a medical prognosis.

2.14 *ša* MUNUS *ša-a-ti* MUNUS.MEŠ *ma-da-[tum] sí-im-ma-am ša-a-tu i-ma-ar-ra-ṣ[a!] i+na* 1 É-*tim pa-ar-si-im* MUNUS *ši-i* ⌜*li*⌝-[*ši-ib*] *ma-am-ma-an la i-ir-ru-ub-ši-im* (*ARM*[*T*] 10.130:2′–5′)

**From that woman many women will become ill with that sickness. Let that woman stay in an isolated room. Nobody is to go in to where she is.

2.15 *mu-ta-nu da-an-nu-tum ib-ba-aš-šu-ú-ma a-ḫu-um a-na bi-it a-ḫi-im ú-ul i-*⌜*ru*⌝*-ub* (YOS 10.56 iii 3–5)

**There will be a serious epidemic (lit. "dying") and, consequently, one person will not enter another person's house.

2.16 DIŠ ZI-*bi-ma* ŠU *ti-iṣ-bat* LÚ.TU.RA.BI ÚŠ-*ma* EGIR-*šú* GIG GÁL-*ši* (DPS XXII:65 [AOAT 43.256])

**If he gets up and (his) hand is grasped (by others), if that patient dies, there will be another patient after him.

The references cited above show that ancient physicians realized that some illnesses were subject to person-to-person transmission. The substance transmitted may have been considered to be a spirit or ghost, but they knew that transmission required close physical contact. There was also some recognition of the fact that the act of defecation can be associated with disease, as seen in the text below.

2.17 *a-na* É *ši-ti-im ú-ul i-ru-ub li-bu it-ta-na-an-pa-ḫu* (H 77:17 [Cavigneaux and al-Rawi, *Iraq* 55.100–104])[41]

**He should not enter a room for defecation (or) there will be an outbreak[42] of *liʾbu*-fever (see Chapter 3).

Sexual activity, as may be seen below, was also known to transmit illness (see Chapter 4).

2.18 DIŠ NA GÌŠ-*šú u* SAG ŠÀ-*šú* KÚM *ṣar-ḫa ú-kal* TÙN ŠÀ-*šú* KÚ-*šú u* ŠÀ-*šú ma-ḫu* Á^{II}-*šú* GÌR^{II}-*šú u* ŠÀ-*šú* KÚM-*em* NA BI GIG *na-a-ki* GIG ŠU ^{d}15 (DPS XXII:14–15 [AOAT 43.251]; cf. DPS XIV A ii 34–36//C ii 10–11 = *TDP* 134 ii 34–36)[43]

**If a person's penis and his upper abdomen (epigastrium)[44] hold burning fever, his liver[45] hurts him, and his stomach goes crazy (and) his arms, his feet, and his stomach are hot, that person is sick with a disease of sexual intercourse, "hand" of Ištar.[46]

Another text cites the association of foot infection with the use of dirty bath water (mycetoma; see Chapter 3).

2.19 [DIŠ NA G]IG *ka-[bar-ti]m ša* A.TU$_5$ *ik-bu-us* . . . (*AMT* 100/3 i 8)[47]

**[If a person has] ⸢*muruṣ kabbarti*⸣ from stepping in (dirty) bath water . . .

Contaminated food was recognized to cause disease.

2.20 [DIŠ NA NINDA] ⸢KÚ!-*ma*⸣ KAŠ NAG-*ma ina* ŠÀ-*šú la ina-aḫ* [. . .] *is-sal-la-a* A.MEŠ *ir-ta-na-muk* [. . .] *ik-ka-šú ik-ta-na-ru* [. . .]-*ka-ak* NA BI *lu-a-te* KI NINDA KÚ *u* KAŠ [NAG *lu*]-*a-te* KI A.MEŠ NAG . . . (*BAM* 90:3′–5′//*AMT* 48/2:11–14)[48]

**[If a person eats bread and] drinks beer and then in his stomach he is not at ease [. . .], he becomes ill, he continually bathes in water [. . .], he is continually short of breath [. . .] that person has eaten or drunk dirty substances[49] with the bread he ate and the beer [he drank or] ⸢dirty⸣ substances with the water he drank . . .

The text below directs the burning of bandages from a patient with *saḫaršubbû* (see Chapter 10 with 10.131–10.136). From this it seems safe to conclude that the bandages were viewed as contaminated with something dangerous that might transmit the infection.

2.21 *ki-i-me-e* TI-*uṭ u mi-nu-me-e na-aṣ-ma-da-tu*$_4$ *ša ir-ta-na-ka-sú ina* IZI *ú-qa-al-la-šu-nu-ti* (Tsukimoto, *Priests and Officials* 199–200:85–86)

**When he gets well, then they burn with fire whatever bandages were used to bandage him.

EPIDEMICS

In addition to examples of small-scale person-to-person spread of infections, there are references that document larger epidemics of diseases that were probably infectious in nature. Shown below is an example of an outbreak of an unknown illness that caused many deaths in the vicinity of Old Babylonian Mari.

2.22 *aš-šum ú-ku-ul-ti* DINGIR-*lim* [*š*]*a be-lí iš-pu-ra-am i-*[*n*]*a Tu-ut-tu-ul*^{KI} *mu-*[*u*]*r-ṣa-nu-ma mu-tum wa-qa-ar i-na Du-un-nim*^{KI} *ša ša-ap-la-an La-as-qí-im ku-ru-ul-lum* ⌜*i*⌝*-na bi-ri-it* U_4.2.KAM [*ṣ*]*a-bu-um ki-i* 20 LÚ.MEŠ *i-mu-ut ù* [*du-u*]*n-*[*na-iu*]$^{⌜\text{KI}⌝}$ *a-lam i-*[*zi-bu-ma*] *a-na* ^{KUR}*La-as-*[*qí-im*] *it-ta-al-k*[*u*] (*ARM* 26/1.259:5–18)

**As for the plague (lit. "eating of the god") ⌜about which⌝ my lord wrote (me)— in Tuttul, there were cases of illness but death(s) were few. In Dunnu, which is below Lasqu, catastrophe—within two days, some twenty soldiers died and the people of Dunnu ⌜abandoned⌝ the city and went to Mount Lasqu.

Environmental Hazards

BODY PARASITES

These parasites were of concern to the *āšipu* not only because of local skin irritation, but because they were associated with more serious infectious diseases. Parasites such as fleas, lice, and crabs can transmit infections including typhus and plague. They also disrupt the skin, making it easier for bacteria and fungi to penetrate. It is interesting that ancient Mesopotamian physicians used the term *crabs* for the louse that infects the groin, *Phthirus pubis*. Modern physicians use this same informal name for the simple reason that they look like tiny crabs. The texts below document the presence of lice and crabs.

BODY LICE

2.23 Ú UḪ.MEŠ *ina* SU NA NU GÁL . . . (*BAM* 1 iii 33//*CT* 14.43 [S. 60+]:9′)[50]

**Plant for there to be no lice on a person's body . . .

HEAD LICE

2.24 DIŠ NA SAG.DU-*su kal-ma-tú ma-tu-uq-ta ma-li* . . . (*BAM* 494 i 30′; Labat, *RA* 53.10–11 obv. 35; *SpTU* 1.51:1)[51]

**If a person's head is full of "sweet" louse (bites) . . .

PHTHIRIS PUBIS (CRABS)

2.25 [DIŠ MUNUS *a*]*l-lu-tú* GIG . . . (*BAM* 237 iv 15)

**[If a woman] is sick with ⌜crabs⌝ . . .

SIKKATU

The following references cite a disease called *sikkatu,* which caused skin lesions that spread through a flock of sheep and involved human handlers as well. This may be the disease which today is called orf or some other pox virus such as cowpox. Pox viruses infect sheep, goats, and cattle, but can also infect humans through skin abrasions.[52]

2.26 *sí-ik-ka-⸢tum⸣ im-ta-qú-ut e-li ka-li bu-li-im úḫ-ta-am-mi-⸢iṭ⸣ la-a-le-e ka-lu-mi ù ṣe-eḫ-ḫe-ru-tim i-na bu-⸢ú⸣-ud ta-ri-i-tim* ... KA.INIM.MA UDU.GAG.ŠUB.BA ... (YOS 11.7:3–7, 17)[53]

**The *sikkatu* fell on all the herds; it made the kids, lambs, and babies in the arms of the nurse burn (with fever) ... recitation for *sikkatu* falling on sheep ...

2.27 KAK.MEŠ *ina* SU NA *id-[d]a-a-ki-a it-ta-ši-na* [. . .] BABBAR.MEŠ GAL.MEŠ *e-la-a ana* ZI.MEŠ*-ši-na* ... (*BAM* 268 iii 6′–7′ // *BAM* 582 i 3′–4′)

**(If) *sikkatu* are transferred to the body of a person (and) their characteristic feature (is that they are) [. . .] white, large, (and) they come up; to remove them ...

BITES AND STINGS

Ancient Mesopotamians had to deal with the stings of scorpions and the bites of several varieties of venomous snake (see Chapter 15 with 15.34–15.39).[54] There was also the danger of being bitten by a wild dog or gored by a stray ox in the narrow streets of ancient cities.

2.28 6,40[55] *a-wi-lum ka-al-ba-am na-ši-ik* ... (*BAM* 393 r. 5)

**If a person is bitten by a dog ...

2.29 Ú ZÚ UR.GI$_7$ ... (*CT* 14.23 [K 9283]:1–3 // *STT* 92 i 1–3; *BAM* 423 i 27′; *KADP* 1 v 1, 4, 9; BM 68046:1–3)[56]

**Plant for dog bite...

2.30 *šum-ma* GUD *sú-qá-am i-na a-la-ki-šu a-wi-lam ik-ki-ip-ma uš-ta-mi-it di-nu-um šu-ú ru-gu-um-ma-am ú-ul i-šu* (Laws of Ḫammurapi § 250)

**If an ox while going in the street gores a person and so causes his death, that case has no claim.

The *āšipu* was aware that victims of dog bite also risked contracting rabies.[57] Since the clinical illness of rabies may take weeks or even months to develop after the bite of a rabid dog or wolf, careful histories must have been obtained in order to make this association. One reference to rabies comes from Ešnunna in a collection of laws. It seeks to punish the owner of a rabid dog that caused illness in others. The second is in a poetic passage from an Old Babylonian recitation describing a rabid dog.

2.31 *šum-ma* UR.GI$_7$ *še-gi-ma* ... LÚ *iš-šu-uk-ma uš-ta-mi-it* (Laws of Ešnunna §§ 56/57 A iv 20, 22)

**If a dog rages ... and bites a person and so causes his death (the owner of the dog shall pay two-thirds mina of silver).

2.32 *ur-ru-uk bi-ir-ki-šu a-ru-uḫ la-sa-ma-am i-iṣ bu-bu-tam et-nu-uš a-ka-lam i-na ši-in-ni-šu e-ʾi-il ni-il-šu a-šar iš-šu-ku ma-ra-šu i-zi-ib* (Whiting, *ZA* 75.182:1–9)

**He is long of leg, quick at running. He is short of sustenance, poor in food. His semen is suspended from his teeth; wherever he bites, he leaves behind his child.[58]

It was also known that rabies could be spread to oxen, sheep, and equids.

2.33 UR.GI$_7$.MEŠ BAD.MEŠ-*ma* [NAM.LÚ.U$_{18}$.LU] GUD UDU.NÍTA ANŠE *ú-na-šá-ku šá ú-na-šá-ku ul* [TI] (*ACh Supp.* Ištar 37 iii 32–33; cf. Borger, *BiOr* 28.8 ii 10–11)

**Dogs will become enraged and bite [people], oxen, sheep, (or) equids; those whom they bite will not [recover].

The clinical presentation of rabies is quite dramatic and the outcome is usually death. Early clinical findings include pain, numbness, and tingling near the site of the bite. Vomiting, fever, abdominal pain, muscle pain, headache, and weakness also are early occurrences. As the disease progresses, hyperactivity, restlessness, and agitation develop. Hydrophobia is not always present, and it is not true fear of water. It is, instead, reflex gagging produced by attempts to swallow or by an attendant's touch that makes it impossible to take fluids orally. Mental status continues to deteriorate, and an ascending paralysis may develop. The patient usually lapses into a coma, and then dies. The following reference lists many of the characteristics of clinical rabies.[59]

2.34 DIŠ NA SAG.DU-*su* ⸢DIB⸣.[DIB-*su*] IGI.MEŠ-*šú* NIGIN-*du mi-na-tu-šú it-ta-n*[*a-á*]*š-pa-ka a-šu-uš-tum* TUKU-*ši* DUG$_4$-*šú* LÙ.LÙ-*aḫ* ŠÀ-⸢*šú*⸣ *šá-pil ik-ka-šú ku-ri* KÚM *mu-un-ga li-ʾ-*⸢*ba*⸣ *ta-dir-tú* TUKU-*ši* GABA-*su u šá-*[*šal-l*]*a-šú* KÚ.MEŠ-*šú* SA x x su ŠU^{II}-*šú u* [GÌ]R^{II}-*šú* KÚ.MEŠ-*šú šá-pu-la-šú* BAL.B[AL]-*šú ana* ZI-*e* GUB-*zi u* DUG$_4$.DUG$_4$ *mu-uq* SA GÚ-[*šú*] KÚ.MEŠ-*šú* ŠED$_7$.MEŠ *ina* KI.NÁ-*šú il-la-tu-šú* D[U].MEŠ-*šú* BAL.BAL-*at uš-ta-na-aḫ* [*i*!-*t*]*a-na-áš-a-áš* DUG$_4$-*šú* KÚR.K[Ú]R-*te qí-bit* KA-*šú im-ta-na-ši* [M]ÁŠ.GI$_6$.MEŠ-*šú ma-ʾ-da* MÁŠ.G[I$_6$].MEŠ IGI *la ú-kal* [^{LÚ}ÚŠ].MEŠ IGI.IGI KI ŠÀ-*šú* DUG$_4$.DUG$_4$-*ub* ŠÀ-*šú iʾ-áš-ma* [*l*]*a i-ár-ru mi-na-at* UZU.MEŠ-*šú* SÌG.MEŠ *ú-zaq-qa-ta-š*[*u* . . .] ⸢*i*⸣-*raš-ši-*[*šu*]*m-ma* dug [. . .] ⸢*ni*⸣-*ip-qu-šú qer-b*[*u ʾu-a*] ⸢*i*⸣-*qab-bi a-a i-še*[*s-si*] NINDA *u* KAŠ LA[L NA.B]I *ka-šip* A.MEŠ ZI.KU$_5$.RU.[D]A-*šú ḫi-pu-ú* [. . .]-*su a-na* ^{d}GIŠ.GÍN.M[AŠ . . .] ⸢*ina*⸣ KU$_4$-*ib* ITI.NE NU.MEŠ-*šú ip*[. . .] *ana* ITI.3.KAM U$_4$.10+x.KAM *ú-za-b*[*a-al-ma* . . .] (*BAM* 231 i 1–18)

**If his head continually ⸢afflicts⸣ [him], his face seems to be spinning, his limbs are continually tense,[60] he has depression, his words are troubled, his heart is down, his breath is short, he has fever, *mungu*-stiffness, *liʾbu*-fever, and apprehensiveness, his breast and his ⸢back⸣ continually hurt him, the muscles of his [. . .], hands and ⸢feet⸣ continually hurt him, his inguinal regions continually shift under him, he is slow to get up, to stand, and to speak, [his] neck muscles continually hurt him, he is continually cold, his saliva continually flows in his bed, he continually has mood swings, is dejected, (and) disturbed, his words are unintelligible, he continually forgets what he has said, his ⸢dreams⸣ are numerous (but) he cannot remember the ⸢dreams⸣ that he sees, he continually sees [dead person]s, he continually talks to himself, his stomach heaves but then he does ⸢not⸣ vomit, his flesh gives him a jabbing pain and stings him [. . .] reddens [. . .] he has closely spaced fits of choking, he says "oh" (and) cries: "ah," (and) his appetite for bread and beer is diminished, that person is hexed, his ⸢*zikurudû*⸣ waters have been drawn[61] [. . .] to Gilgamesh at the beginning of Abu his figurines [. . .] (If) for three months and 10+x days he ⌜carries⌝ it [. . .][62]

The last phrase in the text above mentions a three-month period. Most patients with rabies die within ten days, so this reference cannot be to rabies if the three months is understood to be the duration of clinical symptoms. *Zubbulu* means literally "to carry," and usually refers to illnesses of long duration (as opposed to those that end in speedy death or quick recovery).[63] If the patient could be said to "carry" the disease without actually displaying symptoms, the three months might be referring to the incubation period, a duration that is quite consistent with rabies.

UNDRAINED MARSHES AND SWAMPS

River lowlands and swamps were known to be associated with "infectious diseases" (*liʾbu*).

2.35 *ana ú-šal-li* ÍD *la* DU-*ak la-ʾ-bu i-la-ʾ-ib-šú* (*KAR* 177 r. ii 34//Hulin, *Iraq* 21.52:47)

**He must not go into the lowlands by the river or an infectious disease will infect him.

2.36 ⌜Ú⌝ *ḫa-am-me* . . . (*BAM* 1 i 44)

**Plant for swamp (fever?) . . .

RIVER TOXINS

There is an interesting group of twelve references that identify illnesses associated with exposure to river water. Six texts mention patients being in the water for bathing or some other purpose. The remaining six texts indicate that the patient had drunk water from a hoisting device used to move river water onto irrigated garden plots. Most of the references describe neurologic abnormalities, including seizures, vertigo (spinning), paralysis (immobilization), twisting (athetoid movement), and altered mentation, and are probably due to the ingestion of neurotoxins (see Chapter 15 with 15.26–15.33).

SPRINGLESS CHARIOTS

Riding in ancient Mesopotamian chariots must have been a punishing experience. The original Sumerian model with fixed solid wooden wheels had been modernized over time and, by the Neo-Assyrian period, had a relatively spacious four-man cab set on a pair of eight-spoked turning composite wheels with metal treads for better traction. No device that we know of, however, absorbed the shock of the ride. As the following references indicate, "jostling in a chariot" could cause the worsening of a number of underlying conditions, including liver and abdominal pain, and arthritis.

2.37 [DIŠ NA] *di-kiš* ^{GIŠ}GIGIR GIG-*ma* ŠÀ-*šú u* TÙN-*šú* KÚ.MEŠ-*šú* . . . (*AMT* 96/1:17, cf. 20)

**[If a person] is sick with needling pain after (riding in) a chariot and his abdomen and liver[64] continually hurt him . . .

2.38 DIŠ NA IGI^{II}-*šú* [. . .] x [. . .] ŠÀ-*šú* x x [. . .] *it-te-*[. . .] *bur-ka-šú tab*?!-*ka* a ga? zi x [. . .] ⌜*u*⌝ *it-ta-*⌜*na*⌝-*an-*⌜*ga*⌝-*ag* GABA.MEŠ-*šú* TAG.GA[-*šú*] *u* SAG.MEŠ-*šú e-te-nen-nu u* IM *ina* ŠÀ-*šú i-le-eb-bu ni-ḫi-is* ^{GIŠ}GIGIR NU ÍL NA.BI ^{d}NAM.ÉRIM DIB-⌜*su*⌝ *ana* TI-*šú* . . . (*BAM* 49:1′–6′//*BAM* 50 obv. 1–7)

**If a person's eyes [. . .], his stomach [. . .], his knees are tense(?) [. . .] and is continually stiff, his breasts hurt [him] intensely, he keeps changing the (side of his) head (he sleeps on), "wind" groans in his stomach, (and) he is unable to bear being jostled in a chariot,[65] "hand" of curse afflicts that person, to cure him . . .

2.39 [DIŠ N]A MURUB$_4$ *u* ÚR GIG *mun-ga* TUKU *ni-ḫi-is* ^{GIŠ}GIGIR *a-ni-iḫ ana* TI-[*šú*] . . . (*AMT* 69/3:6′–7′+*AMT* 26/5:2′–3′)

**[If a person's] hip and thigh have *mungu* (stiffness; see Chapter 11) (and) he is tired (after) jostling in a chariot, to cure [him] . . .

Longevity

Precise information about the life spans of ancient Mesopotamians is currently unavailable,[66] but we can get some idea of longevity from the observations of ancient scholars. Conventional wisdom in ancient Mesopotamia had it that 40 years was a human's prime, 60 was the age of full maturity; dying at 50 meant a short life and at 70 a long one.[67] Eighty years was old age; 90 extreme old age; and the longest life span possible for humans had been set by the gods after the flood at 120 years.[68]

Lest we be too skeptical of the figures, we know that the mother of the Neo-Babylonian king Nabonidus, Adad-Guppi, was born in the tenth year of Aššurbanipal (649 B.C.E.) and died in the ninth year of the reign of her son Nabonidus (547 B.C.E.), at the ripe old age of 102,[69] which also means that her son must have been in his sixties when he came to the throne. The studies of M. A. Dandamayev suggest that one scribe, Apla, son of Bel-iddina, descendant of Egibi, had an active career spanning no less than 68 years and that, in the late first millennium B.C.E., life spans of 50-60 years were not uncommon, even among slaves.[70]

The medical texts also suggest that many persons lived to a respectable age. For example, there is a text discussing women who are past the childbearing age (see 12.9). There are also texts that appears to describe Parkinson's disease, and the average age of onset of this disease entity at the present time is sixty years (see 13.262–13.263).

A section of the diagnostic/prognostic series describes in some detail mental attitudes and conditions that the ancient physician associated with old age.

2.40 DIŠ U$_4$.MEŠ-*šú* GÍD.DA.MEŠ-*ma ana* É-*šú u* DUMU.MEŠ-*šú* ÍR GAM (DPS XVI:88′ [AOAT 43.180])[71]

**If he is in his seventies[72] and he wails for his household and his children, he will die.

2.41 DIŠ KI.MIN IGI^{II}.MEŠ-*šú* GIN$_7$ *si-ka-a-ti ana* GA.RAŠ^{SAR} SIG$_7$.ME GAM (DPS XVI:91′ [AOAT 43.180])[73]

**If (he is in his seventies and) his eyes are as yellow as the "peg"[74] on a leek, he will die.

2.42 DIŠ KI.MIN ŠU^{II}-*šú u* GÌR^{II}-*šú* ŠED$_7$?! GIG-*su* KÚR-*šum-ma* UGU-*šú i-sap-pi-du-ma* DIN (DPS XVI:93′ [AOAT 43.180])

**If (he is in his seventies and) his hands and feet are cold,[75] (even if) his illness changes on him so that they beat their breasts over him (in mourning), he will get well.

2.43 DIŠ KI.MIN ŠU^{II}-*šú u* GÌR^{II}-*šú ik-ra-a* GIG-*su* KÚR-*šum-ma* UGU-*šú* KI.MIN DIN (DPS XVI:95′ [AOAT 43.180])[76]

**If (he is in his seventies) and his hands and feet become shrunken,[77] (even if) his illness changes on him so that they (beat their breasts) over him (in mourning), he will get well.

2.44 DIŠ KI.MIN MÚD *ina* KIR$_4$ DU-*ku* DIN / DIŠ KI.MIN KÚ *u* NAG NU ZU ŠUK KI.MAḪ-*šú* (*ḫi-pi*) (DPS XVI:96′–97′ [AOAT 43.180])[78]

**If (he is in his seventies and) blood flows from his nose, he will get well. If (he is in his seventies and) he is unable to eat or drink, [he has eaten] provisions for his grave; [he will die].

2.45 [DIŠ NA] *lu-u ina* ⌜ŠU⌝.GI.MEŠ *lu-ú ina* ^{GIŠ}GIDRU *lu-u ina ḫi-miṭ* UD.DA [*lu*]-*ú ina ni-ḫi-is* ^{GIŠ}GIGIR *a-na* MUNUS *a-la-ka mu-uṭ-ṭú a-na* ŠÀ.ZI.GA *šur-ši-šu-ma ana* MUNUS DU-*šu* . . . (*AMT* 88/3:1–3 [see Biggs, *ŠÀ.ZI.GA* 52])

**[If a person], either as a result of being in his eighties,[79] or burning pain or burning of *ṣētu* (enteric fever)[80] ⌜or⌝ jostling in a chariot has diminished desire for a woman, to cause him to have an erection and to let him go to a woman . . .

Summary

The success of ancient Mesopotamians in developing a highly productive agricultural system by using ingenious irrigating methods made it possible to build the first large urban centers. The conquest of drought with this complex but highly successful irrigation system may have provided this society with the insight and inventiveness to approach other environmental problems involving public and personal hygiene with ingenuity and the application of technical approaches.[81] In periods of peace, social tranquility, and favorable weather, ancient Mesopotamian nutrition appears to have been excellent. In many areas, public and personal hygiene was ahead of its time. Awareness of the contagiousness of certain diseases and how to control them was impressive. These successes were reflected in significant numbers of adults having life spans that are comparable to those of persons in modern industrialized societies.

CHAPTER 3

Infectious Diseases

If he has been sick for six days and, on the seventh, chills continually fall upon him (and) after the chills, there is sweat from his head to his shins, his illness will let up and he will get well.

—DPS XVI:65′–66′ [AOAT 43.178]

Tools of modern medicine allow us to differentiate many infectious diseases that have similar signs and symptoms. Some of these tools are the light and electron microscopes, techniques of growing infectious agents in culture media, and DNA and RNA analysis. Based purely on careful clinical observations, the physicians of ancient Mesopotamia built a body of knowledge about infectious diseases that appears to contain relatively accurate descriptions of many types of infections.

There are, however, limitations to our interpretation of infectious diseases as described in our sources. Both microorganisms and humans are subject to evolution and selective forces of nature. It is possible that modern diseases are caused by different organisms than infections in the past, and that humans respond differently because of changes in their immune defense mechanisms. Organisms may mutate, or genetically recombine with other organisms; older ones may disappear, and new ones appear. Some seem to be more stable, and appear to have been capable of infecting humans for many thousands of years, such as tuberculosis. Others are new arrivals, such as the HIV virus, which jumped from simian sources to humans as recently as thirty to fifty years ago. In spite of the uncertainty that the passage of time engenders, there are descriptions of signs and symptoms that closely parallel modern infectious diseases.[1] Ancient physicians clearly took great pains to differentiate and classify infections in order to apply what they considered to be appropriate and effective treatments.

Fever (KÚM/*ummu*)[2]

The frequency of infections made fever an important physical finding. The ancient Mesopotamian physician had a keen appreciation of its importance as a sign of illness even though his only means of measuring it was his hand touching the patient. The temperature courses in some cases lasted many days or even weeks, strongly suggesting that not only were a physician's patients closely followed during their illnesses but that the physician was generally not afraid to touch his patients.

Although the modern physician has the means to measure core or central body temperature, the Mesopotamian physician focused on what could be evaluated on the skin surface. He tracked not only general changes in temperature but also regional temperature differences. These regional differences we now know to be due to many factors, including localized soft tissue infections, circulatory diseases, and shock.

3.1 DIŠ SAG.DU-*su* KÚM-*im* SAG KIR$_4$-*šú* ŠU^{II}-*šú* *u* GÌR^{II}-*šú* ŠED$_7$ DIḪ KUR DIB-*su* KI.MIN *kiš-pi* DIB.MEŠ[-*šú*. . .] (DPS III C obv. 51 = *TDP* 24:51)

**If his head is hot (and) the bulb of his nose, his hands, and his feet are cold, *liʾbu* (*ṣibit*) *šadî* (see Chapter 19) afflicts him. Alternatively, *kišpu* (see Chapter 15) continually afflicts him [. . .].

3.2 [*i-na*] *ši-mi-ti um-m*[*u iṣ*]-*ṣa-ba-as-si-m*[*a i-n*]*a na-*⸢*ma*⸣*-ri šam-ma á*[*š-qí-ši u*]*m-ma-ša mi-*⸢*it*⸣*-ḫa-a*[*r*] ⸢*še-pa*⸣*-ša ka-ṣa-*⸢*a*⸣ *ša pa-na i-*⸢*ge-en*⸣*-ni-*[*ḫu*] ⸢*i-na-an-na*⸣ [*ul i-ge-en-ni-iḫ*] (*BE* 17/1.32:8–14, apud Parpola, *LAS* 2 p. 493)[3]

**[In] the evening, a ⸢fever afflicted⸣ her ⸢and⸣ [at] dawn I gave [her] a plant [to drink]. Her ⸢temperature⸣ is ⸢normal⸣ (but) her feet are cold. Whereas before she ⸢coughed⸣, [she does not cough] now.

LEVELS OF FEVER

Temperature was subdivided into five levels: normal (*mitḫaru*), warm but not very hot (lukewarm; *la ḫaḫḫaš*), hot (*ummu*), high or very hot (*dannu* or *ḫaḫḫaš*), and burning (*ṣarḫu*).[4] These categories are clearly subjective, but any modern physician with significant clinical experience will appreciate the relative validity of these observations.

NORMAL

3.3 DIŠ SAG.KI^{II}-*šú šá* 15 *u* 150 KÚ.MEŠ-*šú-ma* KÚM-*šú mit-ḫar* ŠU DINGIR-*šú* DIN (DPS IV B obv. 32//E i 12 = *TDP* 36:33//*SpTU* 3.88 i 12)[5]

**If his left and right temples hurt him and his temperature is normal, "hand" of his god; he will get well.

LUKEWARM

3.4 DIŠ SAG ŠÀ-*šú i-kàṣ-ṣa-su* ŠÀ-*šú* KÚM *ú-kal* KÚM *la ḫa-ḫaš* ÚḪ GI$_6$ ŠUB.ŠUB-*a u i-ta-nar-ru* NA BI NAM.ÉRIM DIB-*su* (DPS XXII:31–32 [AOAT 43.254])[6]

**If his upper abdomen (epigastrium) gnaws at him, fever grips his stomach, his temperature is lukewarm, he continually produces black phlegm, and he continually vomits, a curse afflicts that person.

HOT

3.5 DIŠ SAG.KI^{II}-*šú* GEŠTU^{II}-*šú* KÚ.MEŠ-*šú u* AD$_6$-*šú* KÚM *šá-né-e* ^{d}30 (DPS IV A obv. 60//E ii 5 = *TDP* 38:60//*SpTU* 3.88 ii 5)

**If his temples (and) his ears continually hurt him and his body is hot, deputy of Sîn.

HIGH OR VERY HOT

3.6 DIŠ NA KÚM *dan-nu* DIB-*su* . . . *li-ʾ-bu šá iṣ-ba-tu-šú* ZI-*aḫ* (*BAM* 147 obv. 1, 5//*BAM* 148 obv. 1, 5)[7]

**If a high fever afflicts a person . . . the *liʾbu* (see below) that afflicts him will be removed.

3.7 DIŠ SAG.DU-*su* KÚM *ḫa-ḫaš* SA.ME SAG.KI^{II}-*šú* ZI.MEŠ KÚM-*im u* ŠED$_7$ ŠU DINGIR-*š*[*u*][8] (DPS III C obv. 50 = *TDP* 24:50)[9]

**If his head (has) a very hot temperature, the blood vessels of his temples seem to pulsate, (and) he gets hot and then cold, "hand" of ⌜his⌝ god.

BURNING

3.8 DIŠ U$_4$.1.KÁM U$_4$.2.KÁM U$_4$.3.KÁM GIG-*ma* KÚM ÚḪ *ina* SU-*šú* DU$_8$-*ma* EGIR DU$_8$ KÚM ÚḪ *ina* SAG.DU-*šú* NU DU$_8$ *ana* U$_4$.3.KÁM *ana* U$_4$.6.KÁM GAM (DPS XVI:19–20 [AOAT 43.173–174])[10]

**If he is sick for one, two, (and then) three days and subsequently the burning fever lets up from his body but after it has left, the burning fever[11] does not let up from his head[12] (and he continues this way) for three days (or) for six days (altogether), he will die.

FEVER PATTERNS

Many fever patterns were identified and followed by these early physicians, even though their measurement technique was not very sensitive. For example, the insensitivity of this measurement technique was unlikely to have permitted the Mesopotamian physician to know that normal humans have a diurnal temperature course, with the lowest temperatures in the early morning hours and the highest in the late afternoon and evening. This diurnal course, however, is exaggerated in many infections so that the highest temperatures occur in the afternoon/evening with little or no fever during the rest of the day. This fever pattern was noted and described.

3.9 DIŠ KI.MIN U$_4$ DIB-*šú* KÚM TA EN.NUN.AN.USAN EN EN.NUN. MURUB$_4$.BA *id-da-lip-šú* DIB GID [IM$_7$] (DPS XXVI:38′ [AOAT 43.281])

**If (his affliction always afflicts him in the evening and) when it afflicts him, fever keeps him awake from the evening watch until the middle watch of the night, affliction by a ⌜ghost⌝.

A fever course that is classically seen in malaria and typhoid, but may occur with many infections begins with the sensation of being cold or chilled. It is followed by violent muscle contractions that generate heat to produce the high fever. The patient then sweats profusely until the temperature falls to normal, leaving the patient relieved, exhausted, and often sleeping. These ancient physicians gave excellent descriptions of this evolving fever spike.

3.10 DIŠ U$_4$.2.KÁM ŠUB-*šú-ma ina* U$_4$.3.KÁM DIB-*su* U$_4$-*ma* DIB-*šú im-ta-na-ag-ga-gu* EGIR *im-ta-na-gag-ga ra-ʾ-i-ba* TUKU-*ši* UB.MEŠ-*šú* KÚ.MEŠ-*šú* ŠU^{II}-*šú u* GÌR^{II}-*šú* ŠED$_7$-*a* EGIR-*nu* KÚM 1-*niš i-rak-kab-šú* : *i-re-eḫ-ḫi-šú u* IR ŠUB-*su-ma ina-aḫ* DIB KUR-*i* DIB-*su* (DPS XVI:25–27 [AOAT 43.174–175])

**If it falls upon him for two days and then afflicts him on the third day and when it afflicts him, he continually becomes rigid and after he continually becomes rigid, he has a trembling, his limbs continually hurt him, his hands and his feet are cold, (and) afterward fever rides (var. flows) over him everywhere at once and sweat falls upon him and then he finds relief, *ṣibit šadî* (see Chapter 19 with 19.216–19.221) afflicts him.

3.11 [DIŠ NA *li-ʾ*]-*bu ṣi-bit* KUR-*i* DIB-*su-ma* [*ú-maš-šir*]-*šu-ma ina* U$_4$.3.KÁM DIB-*su ir-te-dá-aš-šu um-ma ṣa-ar-ḫa li-ʾ-ba dá-an-na ù zu-ʾ-ta-am ma-ʾ-tam* TUKU.MEŠ-*ši si-li-ʾ-ta-šu ú-ta-ar-ri-ik-ma it-ta-dim-šu* . . . (Meier, *ZA* 45.208 v 15–20)[13]

**[If] ⌜*liʾbu*⌝ *ṣibit šadî* afflicts [a person] and then [it releases] him and then, on the third day, it afflicts him (and) pursues him, he continually has burning fever, severe *liʾbu* (see below), and lots of sweat, his illness has been prolonged and has knocked him down . . .

In the sequenced references below, another fever paroxysm is described. It interesting to note that before the fever rises, the temporal blood vessels are "calm,"[14] which means that the pulse rate is normal (see Chapter 8). The elevation in pulse rate that accompanies a fever is known to modern physicians and this set of references indicates that it was also known to the *āšipu*.

3.12 DIŠ UGU-*šú* KÚM-*im u* ⌜SAG⌝.KI^{II}-*šú ne-eḫ-a* . . . DIŠ UGU-*šú* KÚM-*im u* SAG.KI^{II}-*šú* KÚM *la-aḫ-ḫa-ḫa-šá* . . . DIŠ [U]GU-*šú* KÚM-*im u* SAG.KI^{II}-*šú* KÚM-*ma* . . . DIŠ [UG]U-*šú* KÚM-*im u* SAG.KI^{II}-*šú* KÚM *u* IR *ú-kal-la* . . . (DPS III A obv. 5–8//B 5–8)[15]

**If his skull is hot (but the blood vessels of) his temples are calm . . . If his skull is hot and his temples are lukewarm . . . "If his ⌜skull⌝ is hot and his temples are also hot . . . If his ⌜skull⌝ is hot and his temples are hot and hold sweat . . .

LIʾBU

Liʾbu (Sumerian: DIḪ) is from the verb *laʾābu* ("to infect").[16] Etymologically related to Hebrew *lahab*, "flame," *liʾbu* and *laʾbu* are equated in synonym lists with Akkadian words for fever: *ummu* and *ḫunṭu*, an equation confirmed by the following references.[17]

3.13 DIŠ NA KÚM *dan-nu* DIB-*su* . . . *li-ʾ-bu šá iṣ-ba-tu-šú* ZI-*aḫ* (*BAM* 147 obv. 1, 5//*BAM* 148 obv. 1, 5)

**If a high fever afflicts a person . . . the *liʾbu* that afflicts him will be removed.

3.14 DIŠ NA *li-bu-um dan-nu* DIB-*su* . . . (BM 42431+:9, cf. 1 [Finkel, *Fs. Lambert* 208–209 (with parallels)])

**If a high *liʾbu* afflicts a person . . .

3.15 DIŠ SAG.DU-*su* KÚM-*em* SAG KIR$_4$-*šú* ŠU^{II}-*šú u* GÌR^{II}-*šú* ŠED$_7$ DIḪ KUR DIB-*su* KI.MIN *kiš-pi* DIB.MEŠ[-*šú* . . .] (DPS III C obv. 51 = *TDP* 24:51)

**If his head is hot (and) the bulb of his nose, his hands, and his feet are cold, the *liʾbu* (*ṣibit*) *šadî* afflicts him. [. . .]

Liʾbu is used to describe the fevers produced by *ṣibit šadî* (see above) and Lamaštu (see below).

3.16 DIŠ LÚ.TUR *um-ma li-ʾ-ba ú-kal u ik-ta-na-aṣ-ṣa* DIB ^{d}DÌM.ME : ŠU DUMU.MUNUS ^{d}*A-nim* (DPS XL A 51 = *TDP* 224:51)

**If *liʾbu* fever (*um-ma li-ʾ-ba*) grips an infant and he is continually cold, affliction by Lamaštu (var. "hand" of the daughter of Anu).

Most references to *liʾbu* mention only fever. However, lexical equations show that some forms of *liʾbu* were associated with a skin lesion known as *ziʾpu*.[18] *Ziʾpu* is a term used to describe generalized red spots (probably flat or macular; see Chapter 10 with 10.66–10.67). This skin lesion plus the *liʾbu* type of fever is compatible with enteric fever (see below), especially typhoid and typhus, as in the following references.

3.17 DIŠ NA KÚ[M o]-⌜*šú*⌝ K[ÚM.M]EŠ ŠED$_7$.MEŠ NINDA KÚ KAŠ NAG-*ma* [*i*]-*ár-rù i-t*[*a-na-š*]*a-áš e*-⌜*li*⌝-*u-na* UZU.MEŠ-*šú* ŠED$_7$ [*ša*]*p-la-nu e-ṣ*[*e-e*]*n-ta-šú ṣar-pa* NA.BI [UD.D]A TAB.BA-*ma l*[*i*]-ʾ-*ba* TUKU *ana* TI-*šú* . . . (*BAM* 146 rev. 43′–46′)

**If fever [. . .] a person (and) he continually gets ⌜hot⌝ and gets cold, when he eats bread and drinks beer, [he] vomits (and his stomach) ⌜is continually upset⌝, the flesh above is cold (but) his ⌜bones below⌝ feel burning hot, that person is burned by ⌜*ṣētu*⌝ (enteric fever; see below) and has *liʾbu*, to cure him . . .

3.18 [DIŠ KI].⌜MIN *za*⌝-*mar* KÚM-*em za-mar* ŠED$_7$ *liʾba* TUKU-*ši u* IR NU TUKU NA.BI ITI.1.KÁM GIG *ana* GIG-*su* NU GÍD.DA . . . (DPS XXXI:12–13 [AOAT 43.342]//*BAM* 66 obv. 10–11)

**If (*ṣētu* [enteric fever] burns him and) sometimes he is hot, sometimes he is cold, he has *liʾbu* but he does not have sweat, that person has been sick for a month; in order for his illness not to be prolonged . . .

It appears, therefore, that *liʾbu* may have been used for a small group of infectious diseases characterized by a fever of a particular type.[19] Ancient Mesopotamian physicians sometimes describe this pattern as "one day it afflicts him and one day it releases him."[20]

3.19 DIŠ NA NAM.ÉRIM DIB-*su-ma* KÚM *u* IR *ma-gal* TUKU.MEŠ U$_4$.1.KAM DIB-[*su*] U$_4$.1.KAM BAR-*šú ḫa-a-a-at-ti* KÚM TUKU.MEŠ KÚM *la ḫa-aḫ-ḫaš* DIB-*su-ma ana* KÚM *u ṣir-ḫa* TAR-*si* . . . (*BAM* 174 r. 29–31)

**If curse afflicts a person so that he has fever and a lot of sweat (and) one day it afflicts [him] (and) one day it releases him (and) he has a febrile confusional state (and) a lukewarm temperature afflicts him, to keep away fever and burning heat . . .

3.20 DIŠ U$_4$.1.KÁM DIB-*su* U$_4$.1.KÁM BAR-*šú* U$_4$ LÁ-*šú* LÁ-*šú* UB.MEŠ-*šú* KÚ.MEŠ-*šú* KÚM-*ma i-ra-ʾu-ub* IR ŠUB-*su-ma ina-aḫ u* A *ana* NAG *ma-gal* APIN.MEŠ ŠU ^{d}DÌM.ME DIN (DPS XVI:14–15 [AOAT 43.173])[21]

**If one day it afflicts him and one day it releases him (and) when his confusional state comes over him, his limbs continually hurt him, he is feverish and trembles, sweat falls upon him, and then he finds relief and continually asks for a great deal of water to drink, "hand" of Lamaštu; he will get well.

From the above references, it appears that "(the fever) flows over him" means that the patient had fever without shaking chills, while "(the fever) afflicts" him indicates the presence of shaking chills. In spite of the absence of shaking chills when the fever "flows over him," the patient may have stupor or mental confusion (which are also said to "flow over"; see Chapter 13), and he may still be quite ill. This is demonstrated by the first reference below in which the patient has two days of shaking chills and on the third day, the fever "flows over him" and he dies. Had the patient been bright and alert and obviously recovering, the prognosis would have been good, as in the second reference.

3.21 DIŠ U$_4$.2.KÁM DIB-*su-*⸢*ma*⸣ *ina* U$_4$.3.KÁM *i-re-eḫ-ḫi-šú* DIB-*it* KUR-*i* : GAM (DPS XVI:28 [AOAT 43.175])

**If it afflicts him for two days and flows over him on the third day, *ṣibit šadî* (var. he will die).

3.22 DIŠ GIG-*ma ina* GIG-*šú* GIN$_7$ *šá* DIN-*šú* KI DAM-*šú* DUMU-*šú* DUMU.MUNUS-*šú* SIG$_5$-*iš i-ta-mu* NINDA NU KÚ *di-ḫu* D[IN] (DPS XVII:41–42 [AOAT 43.199]; Labat, *Syria* 33.121–126 obv. 15)

**If he is sick and, during his sickness, he speaks in a friendly way with his wife, son, (and) daughter just as if he were feeling well (but) he does not eat bread, *diʾu*; he will get ⸢well⸣.

The *āšipu* also commented separately on shaking chills and sweats.

3.23 DIŠ *ina šèr-ti* KÚM-*ma* ŠU^{II}-*šú u* GÌR^{II}-*šú i-ra-ʾ-ú-ba* ŠU ^{d}30 (DPS XVII:94 [AOAT 43.204])[22]

**If in the morning he is hot and his hands and his feet tremble, "hand" of Sîn.

3.24 U$_4$ GIG *um-ma-šu ṣa-ru-uḫ zu-ʾ-ta ki me-e ra-mi-ik* ŠU ^{d}UTU ŠU *ik-ri-bi-šu* (Labat, *MDP* 57.11 iii 4)[23]

**If the patient burns with fever (and) is bathed in sweat like water, "hand" of Šamaš, "hand" of his vow.

Most varieties of *li*ʾ*bu* fever were not accompanied by jaundice. An exception is a febrile illness named after its causal agent, the demoness Lamaštu (see 19.223–19.232), which we believe could be typhoid or typhus. The fever tended to be continuously present throughout the day,[24] producing mental status changes and sometimes jaundice.

3.25 DIŠ SAG.DU-*su* DIB.DIB-*su* *u* KÚM TÉŠ.BI UNU-*su*[25] GIG-*su* TAK$_4$-*šum-ma* NÍG.NIGIN TUKU *šu*[*m-ma* KI] ⌜LAL⌝[26]-*šú* LAL-*šú* UŠ$_4$-*šú* KÚR-*šum-ma ina* NU ZU-*ú ú-rap-pad* GIN$_7$ DIB-*it* GIDIM$_7$ ^{d}DIM$_8$.ME ⌜DIB⌝-[*su uš*]-*te-zib*[27] (DPS III C obv. 36–37 = *TDP* 22:36–37)

**If his head continually afflicts him and fever (has) its seat[28] equally all over (and) when his illness leaves him, he has dizziness (and) ⌜if⌝, [when a confusional state] comes over him, his mentation is altered so that he wanders about without knowing (where he is) as in affliction by a ghost, Lamaštu afflicts [him]. He will come through.

3.26 DIŠ IGI.MEŠ-*šú* SIG$_7$.MEŠ ^{d}DIM$_{11}$.ME DIB-*su* (DPS IX A 11 = *TDP* 72:11)

**If his face is yellow, Lamaštu afflicts him.

BIPHASIC FEVER

There are a number of infections that manifest fever and illness for four to ten days, with marked improvement for three or four days, only to be followed by another period of fever and illness. Some of these diseases include dengue, brucellosis, and two infections caused by spirochetes, relapsing fever and leptospirosis. These relapsing or biphasic patterns of illness were also recognized by Mesopotamian physicians.

3.27 DIŠ U$_4$.6.KÁM GIG-*ma u* UZU.MEŠ-*šú šal-mu ana* GIG-*šú* GUR-*ma ni-kit-tú* TUKU-*ši* ŠÀ-*šú* DIB.DIB-*su* GAM (DPS XVI:61′ [AOAT 43.177])[29]

**If he is sick for six days and his flesh is normal (i.e., he is not jaundiced), (if) he returns into his illness and has a turn for the worse (and) his abdomen continually afflicts him, he will die.

Ancient Mesopotamian physicians sometimes describe this pattern as "over the course of a day it leaves him and then (later) it overpowers him (and) flows over him for two days."[30]

3.28 DIŠ SAG.DU-*su* KÚM *ḫa-ḫaš*[31] U$_4$.1.KÁM TAK$_4$-*šum-ma* U$_4$.2.KÁM DUGUD-*su i-re-ḫi-*[*šum-ma*] Á.ÚR.MEŠ-*šú* 1-*niš* KÚ.ME-*šú u* A *ana* NAG APIN ŠU [. . .] (DPS III C obv. 46–47 = *TDP* 22:46–47)

**If his head (has) a very hot temperature (and) over the course of a day it leaves him and then (later) it overpowers him (and) flows over [him] for two days [so that] his limbs all hurt him at once and he asks for water to drink, "hand" of [. . .]

Within this category of fever, ancient Mesopotamian physicians recognized two subcategories, one with jaundice (*aḫḫāzu*; see Chapter 6) and one without jaundice (Labaṣu).[32] We know that the biphasic fevers may in some cases have jaundice because of liver involvement. Leptospirosis is probably the best example of an infection that can present with or without jaundice. This striking physical finding must have led the *āšipu* to conclude that those individuals had a separate disease entity. It should be noted that although modern physicians do not regard it as a separate disease, even they continue to use a separate term, Weil's syndrome, for severe leptospirosis with jaundice. The distinction is more useful in the case of relapsing fevers, which are divided into two epidemiologic varieties, louse-borne (*Borrelia recurrentis*) and tick-borne (many *Borrelia* species). Jaundice, secondary to hepato-cellular injury, occurs in 10 to 80 percent of cases of relapsing fever, but is more common in louse-borne disease.

BIPHASIC FEVERS WITHOUT JAUNDICE (*LABAṢU*)

3.29 DIŠ U$_4$.6.KÁM GIG-*ma ina* U$_4$.7.KÁM *ḫur-ba-šú* ŠUB.ŠUB-*su* EGIR *ḫur-ba-šú* IR TA SAG.DU-*šú* EN *kin-ṣi-šú*[33] GÁL GIG-*su* DU$_8$-*ár-ma* DIN (DPS XVI:65'–66' [AOAT 43.178])

**If he has been sick for six days and, on the seventh, chills continually fall upon him (and) after the chills, there is sweat from his head to his shins, his illness will let up and he will get well.

BIPHASIC FEVERS WITH JAUNDICE (*AḪḪĀZU*)

3.30 DIŠ *ina* SAG.DU-*šú* KÚM ÚḪ U$_4$.1.KÁM TAK$_4$-*šum-ma* U$_4$.2.KÁM DUGUD-*su i-re-eḫ-ḫi-šum-ma* DIB-*i*[*t* GIDIM$_7$] KI.TA![34] GÌR^{II}-*šú* ŠED$_7$ *ina* BAR-*šú* ŠU^{II}-*šú u* GÌR^{II}-*šú* ⌜KÚM-*ma*⌝ GIN$_7$ DIB-*it* GIDIM$_7$ ^{d}DIM$_{10}$.ME.LAGAB *i-sa-dir*-[*ma* DIN] (DPS III C r. 10–11//E$_1$ r. 11–12+E$_2$ r. 7–8 = *TDP* 26:70–71)[35]

**If in his head he burns with fever[36] (and) over the course of a day it leaves him and then (later) it overpowers him (and) flows over him for two days (as in) affliction by [a ghost] and the plantar surfaces[37] of his feet (feel) cold, (and) when (the fever) releases him, his hands and his feet are hot as in affliction by a ghost, *aḫḫāzu*, [(if)] (the course of the fever) is regular, [he will get well].[38]

3.31 DIŠ U$_4$.4.KÁM U$_4$.5.KÁM GIG-*ma* IR ŠUB.ŠUB-*su* DU$_8$-*ár* GIG / DIŠ U$_4$.4.KÁM U$_4$.5.KÁM GIG-*aṣ* ŠU DIM.ME.LAGAB (DPS XVI:44'–45' [AOAT 43.176])

**If he is sick for four or five days and subsequently sweat continually falls upon him, letting up of the illness. If he has been sick for four or five days, "hand" of *aḫḫāzu*.

The *āšipu* observed that the patients with biphasic fevers who develop abdominal or epi-gastric pain are more likely to die, as the examples below indicate.

3.32 DIŠ U$_4$.6.KÁM GIG-*ma* UZU.MEŠ-*šú šal-mu ana* GIG-*šú* GUR-*ma ni-kit-tú* TUKU-*ši* ŠÀ-*šú* DIB.DIB-*su* GAM / DIŠ U$_4$.6.KÁM U$_4$.10.KÁM NÍG.GI[39] TUKU-*ši šum-ma* SAG ŠÀ-*šú* DIB-*su* GAM (DPS XVI:61'–62' [AOAT 43.177])

**If he is sick for six days and his flesh is normal, (if) he returns into his illness and has a turn for the worse (and) his abdomen continually afflicts him, he will die. If in six days or ten days he has a return (of the illness and) if his upper abdomen (epigastrium) afflicts him, he will die.

3.33 DIŠ U_4.6.KÁM GIG-*ma ina* U_4.7.KÁM *ḫur-ba-šú* ŠUB.ŠUB-*su* EGIR *ḫur-ba-šú* IR TA SAG.DU-*šú* EN *kin-ṣi-šú*[40] GÁL GIG-*su* DU_8-*ár-ma* DIN (DPS XVI:65′–66′ [AOAT 43.178])

**If he has been sick for six days and, on the seventh, chills continually fall upon him (and) after the chills, there is sweat from his head to his shins, his illness will let up and he will get well.

3.34 [DIŠ U_4.6.KÁM] GI[G]-*ma ina* U_4.7.KÁM DIN-*uṭ* ⸢GIG⸣ TI U_4-*ma* TI GIG[41] SAG ŠÀ-*šú* DIB-*su* GAM (DPS XVI:69′ [AOAT 43.178])[42]

**[If] he has been ⸢sick⸣ [for six days] and, on the seventh, he gets well (and) he recovers from the illness (but) when he has recovered, he gets sick (again and) his upper abdomen (epigastrium) afflicts him, he will die.

Modern physicians describe abdominal pain in patients with biphasic illnesses such as relapsing fever and leptospirosis. Since fatal cases may have liver or spleen enlargement or heart involvement (myocarditis), it seems likely that the more severe forms of these diseases would cause greater organ enlargement with associated pain, or pain caused by heart infection. Another possibility is that a marked drop in blood pressure that commonly occurs with an overwhelming infection would cause angina because of inadequate blood flow to the heart (see Chapter 8).

In one of the references to biphasic fevers, where the term *labaṣu* is used, the *āšipu* mentions "bloody toes." We think it a good possibility that he is describing rat-bite fever, another infection that may be recurrent or biphasic. It is caused by the spirochete, *Spirillum minus*, which is inoculated at the time of a rat bite. The "bloody toes" might refer to blood from the bite, or to the redness around the bite site that develops after a few days' incubation.

3.35 DIŠ U.MEŠ GÌR^{II}-*šú* MÚD DIRI.MEŠ-*ma* ⸢KÚ⸣.MEŠ-*šú ana la-ba-aṣ* GUR-*šum-ma* GAM (DPS XIV A iv 10–11//C_2 iv 12//K 5 = *TDP* 144 iv 45′–46′)

**If his toes are continually full of blood and continually hurt him, (if) it turns to *labaṣu* on him, he will die.

There also was a recognition of some of the complications of fever including hair loss.

3.36 DIŠ NA SAG.DU-*su* KÚM-*ma* S[ÍG] SAG.DU-*šú i-šaḫ-ḫu-uḫ ana* KÚM SAG.DU [ZI-*ḫi*] *u* SÍG DU-*tú* GUB-*zi* . . . (*BAM* 480 iii 22–23)[43]

**If a person's head is hot and, as a result, the ⸢hair⸣ of his head falls out, to [remove] the fever of his head and to make the hair that is going[44] stand firm . . .

DECREASED TEMPERATURES

In addition to elevated temperature, the ancient physician was aware of decreased temperature, which was also graded. The levels described are cold mixed with warm, cold ($ŠED_7$/*kaṣû*), chilled (*ḫurbašu*), and cold as frost (*šurpû*/*šuruppû*).[45] In some cases, the physician is describing the patient's sensation of cold, which commonly occurs just prior to an increase in body temperature. In other cases, he is noting the skin surface temperature, which can be decreased because of a reduced blood supply or vasoconstriction when the body is attempting to conserve heat.

COLD MIXED WITH WARM

3.37 DIŠ SAG KIR$_4$-*šú ku-uṣ ba-lil ina* U$_4$-*mi-šú-ma* EGIR MAŠ.MAŠ LÍL-*ma* DIN (DPS VI A obv. 24//C i 8–9 = *TDP* 56:24)[46]

**If the bulb of his nose is cold mixed (with warm),[47] (if) on the same day, after treatment, he gets worse, he will get well (in the end).

COLD

3.38 DIŠ GIG-*ma* AD$_6$-*šú* UL$_4$.GAL ŠED$_7$ GIG-*su* GÍD-*ma* GAM (DPS XVII:51 [AOAT 43.200])

**If he is sick and his body is very cold, (if) his illness is prolonged, he will die.

3.39 DIŠ KI.MIN-*ma* ŠU-*su ina* LI.DUR-*šú* GAR-*at-ma* ŠU^{II}-*šú u* GÌR^{II}-*šú ka-ṣa-a ina* NU ⌜ZU-*e*⌝ [DUG$_4$.DUG$_4$-*ub*] ZI-*bi u* TÚŠ-*ab ina* LI.DUR-*šú* SÌG-*iṣ* ŠU ^{d}*Dil-bat* [GAM] (DPS XV:13–14 [AOAT 43.151]; cf. DPS XI A obv. 9//B 8 = *TDP* 90:9//*SpTU* 1.34:8)[48]

**If (it is the first day he is sick) and his hand is placed on his navel and his hands and his feet are cold, [he talks] without knowing (what he is saying and) he gets up and sits down (again), he was wounded on his navel. "Hand" of *Dilbat* (Ištar); [he will die].

CHILLED

3.40 DIŠ U$_4$.6.KÁM GIG-*ma ina* U$_4$.7.KÁM *ḫur-ba-šú* ŠUB.ŠUB-*su* EGIR *ḫur-ba-šú* IR TA SAG.DU-*šú* EN *kin-ṣi-šú*[49] GÁL GIG-*su* DU$_8$-*ár-ma* DIN (DPS XVI:65′–66′ [AOAT 43.178])[50]

**If he has been sick for six days and, on the seventh, chills continually fall upon him (and) after the chills, there is sweat from his head to his shins, his illness will let up and he will get well.

COLD AS FROST

3.41 DIŠ *ina* GIG-*šú i-leb-bu* GIG A.ZA.AD GIG DIN (DPS XVII:14 [AOAT 43.196])

**If during his illness he groans (and) he is sick with an illness of cold as frost, he will get well.

3.42 *di-i šu-ru-up-pu-ú šá ina zu-mur-šú li-né-síḫ* . . . (*SpTU* 3.65 r. 12; cf. *SpTU* 2.2:58, 165)[51]

**Let the *di*ʾ*u*-fever (see below) (with) cold as frost which is in his body be removed . . .

The attention that ancient Mesopotamian physicians paid to body temperature and its various manifestations attests to their skills as observers, and makes it easier to identify certain infections and syndromes.

MALARIA

Since malaria is spread by mosquito bites, it is a disease that is associated with areas of standing water where these insects breed. The following text associates this type of region with contracting an infectious illness. Although there are other febrile diseases associated with water, malaria is likely to be the disease described.

3.43 *ana ú-šal-lì* ÍD *la* DU-*ak la-ʾi-bu i-la-ʾ-ib-šú* (*KAR* 177 r. ii 33–34//Hulin, *Iraq* 21.52:47)

**He must not go into the lowlands by the river or an infectious disease will infect him.

Another clue to the presence of malaria in ancient Mesopotamia is the clear description of a tertian fever pattern in the reference below. Every other day fever spikes are seen in *Plasmodium vivax* and *Plasmodium ovale*; in the case of *Plasmodium malariae*, the spikes are separated by two intervening afebrile days. The following is very suggestive of *Plasmodium vivax* or *P. ovale* infection.[52]

3.44 DIŠ U_4.6.KÁM GIG-*ma ina* U_4.7.KÁM DIN-*uṭ ina* U_4.8.KÁM GIG-*ma ina* U_4.9.KÁM DIN-*uṭ ina* U_4.10.KÁM GIG-*ma ina* U_4.11.KÁM DIN-*uṭ* GIG-*su ni-kit-tú* TUKU-*ši* MAŠ.MAŠ *ana* TI-*šú* ME.A NU GAR-*an* (DPS XVI:73′–74′ [AOAT 43.178])

**If he is sick for six days and on the seventh he gets well, on the eighth day he is sick and on the ninth he gets well, on the tenth day he is sick and on the eleventh he gets well (and) his illness has a turn for the worse, the *āšipu* shall not make a prognosis as to his recovery.

One species of malaria parasite, *Plasmodium falciparum*, is much more prone than the other species to cause a high morbidity and mortality rate. Brain involvement is a very serious form of the infection, with a high rate of death and permanent neurologic damage, especially in children. A recent review of this problem by Newton and Warrell[53] lists many of the neurologic signs in patients with cerebral malaria. These include lethargy, seizures, disorders of conjugate gaze, transient ocular bobbing, horizontal and vertical nystagmus (jerking eye movements), eye muscle paralysis, forcible closure of the mouth, teeth grinding, abnormal posturing, muscle rigidity and arching of the back (opisthotonos), and coma. There are a series of ancient references with problems attributed to the "hand" of ^{d}LUGAL.GÌR.RA (and ^{d}MES.LAM.TA.È.A). We believe that these may be cases of cerebral malaria since they are attributed to a single cause, and the neurologic signs appear to be quite similar to the modern descriptions. It is also worth noting that ^{d}LUGAL.GÌR.RA and ^{d}MES.LAM.TA.È.A are twins and by-forms/associates of the god Nergal, the god of pestilence.[54]

3.45 DIŠ IGI.MEŠ-*šú* NIGIN.ME SAG.DU-*su* ŠU^{II}-*šú u* GÌR^{II}-*šú i-tar-ru-ra* ŠU ^{d}LUGAL.GÌR.RA *u* ^{d}MES.LAM.TA.È.A (DPS IX A 57–58 = *TDP* 76:57–58)

**If his face seems continually to be spinning (and) his head, his hands, and his feet tremble, "hand" of ^{d}LUGAL.GÌR.RA and ^{d}MES.LAM.TA.È.A.

3.46 DIŠ IGI.MEŠ-*šú* NIGIN.ME UB.NÍGIN.NA-*šú* *i-tar-ru-ra u i-ṭa-ma-a* ŠU ᵈLUGAL.GÌR.RA *u* ᵈMES.LAM.TA.È.A : ᵈLUGAL.BÀN.DA (DPS IX A 64–65//B r. 10 = *TDP* 76:64–65)

**If his face seems continually to be spinning (and) his limbs tremble and twist, "hand" of ᵈLUGAL.GÌR.RA and ᵈMEŠ.LAM.TA.È.A (var. ᵈLUGAL.BÀN.DA).

3.47 DIŠ U_4 UD.⌜DU-*šú*⌝ IGI-*šú šá* 15/150 GIN_7 ᴳᴵŠBAL *i-lam-[mi]* IGI-*šú šá* 150/ZAG MÚD DIRI-*at* KA-*šú* BAD.BAD-*te* EME-[*šú*] *ú-na-šak* ᵈLUGAL.GÌR.RA DIB-*su* (*STT* 89:103–105a,109–112 [Stol, *Epilepsy* 91–92])

**If when it ⌜comes⌝ over him, his left/right eye (makes bobbing movements similar to what) a spindle (does) when it spins (and) his right/left eye is full of blood, he continually opens his mouth (and) he bites [his] tongue, ᵈLUGAL.GÌR.RA afflicts him.

3.48 DIŠ TE-*su šá* 150 SIG_7-*at šá* 15 SA_5-*a*[*t*. . .] *i-šaq-qar-šú* $UŠ_4$-*šú* NU [DI]B *u* IR [. . .] ᵈLUGAL.GÌR.RA DIB-*s*[*u*] *ana* 50 [U_4-*me*] MAŠ.MAŠ-*su* DÙ-*uš-ma* [DIN?] (*STT* 89:124–127 [Stol, *Epilepsy* 93])[55]

**If his right cheek is pale (and) the left one is flushed [. . .] gives him a piercing pain, he is not [in full] possession of his faculties and [he . . .] sweat [. . .] ᵈLUGAL.GÌR.RA afflicts ⌜him⌝. If you treat him for fifty [days], [. . .].

3.49 DIŠ U_4 UD.DU-*šú* ŠU-*su šá* 150 IGI-*šú šá* [. . .] GIN_7 $UR.GI_7$ *i-šag-gúm* ZÚ.MEŠ-*šú* [. . .] IGIᴵᴵ-*šú gal!-ta* ᵈLUGAL.GÌR.RA DIB-*su ana* TI.LA-*šú qí-ba* NU GAR-*an* (*STT* 89:133–136a [Stol, *Epilepsy* 93])[56]

**If when it comes over him, his right hand (and) the [left] side of his face [. . .] he growls like a dog, [he grinds?] his teeth, (and) his eyes jerk, ᵈLUGAL.GÌR.RA afflicts him, the *āšipu* should not make a prognostication as to his recovery.

In these references we believe that the *āšipu* was describing nystagmus (jerking eye movements), eye muscle paralysis, teeth grinding, lethargy, mental status change, abnormal posturing, and seizures. We cannot say with certainty that these were cases of cerebral malaria, but we are reasonably certain that malaria was present during that period.[57] If the malaria included *P. falciparum*, then neurologic signs as described above would commonly have been seen.

Throat and Upper Airway Infections

THROAT INFECTIONS (PHARYNGITIS)

Infections of the throat can have both bacterial and viral causes. We have all experienced this common infection, which causes sore throat and difficulty swallowing. Pharyngitis is often associated with fever and chills, and it generally resolves in five to ten days. *Streptococcus pyogenes* (strep throat) is the most common bacterial cause of pharyngitis, and it may lead to other more serious complications, such as scarlet fever, rheumatic fever, and kidney disease (glomerulonephritis) in a small percentage of cases.

Ancient Mesopotamian physicians described patients with pharyngitis as seen in the quotes below, but it is not possible to know the causative organisms. We believe that their term *skinned* refers to a red, raw looking pharynx which is commonly seen with strep throat but may occasionally be seen in some patients with viral pharyngitis.

3.50 DIŠ *gir-ri* 15-*šú šu-uḫ-ḫu-ṭa-at ú-šá-an-na-aḫ-ma* DIN (DPS X A obv. 49 = *TDP* 86:49)[58]

**If the left side of his throat[59] (looks) skinned, it will exhaust him but he will get well.

3.51 DIŠ *gir-ra-šú šu-uḫ-ḫu-ṭa u* UZU.ME-*šú šal-mu* DIN : *na-kid* (DPS X A obv. 51 = *TDP* 86:51)

**If both sides of his throat (look) skinned and his flesh is healthy, he will get well (var. it is worrisome).

The following reference describes pharyngitis and skin lesions that are suggestive of scarlet fever, which means that this would have been a strep throat.

3.52 DIŠ *gir-ra-šú šu-uḫ-ḫu-ṭa u* UZU.ME-*šú* ŠUB-*tu u ṣi-rip-tu* ŠUB.ŠUB-*a* [KI.MI]N (DPS X A obv. 52//D 12 = *TDP* 86:52)

**If both sides of his throat (look) skinned and his flesh (looks) terrible[60] and is unevenly colored with red dye spots, ⌜(it is worrisome)⌝.

The next reference describes signs that are indicative of glomerulonephritis, suggesting that streptococcal pharyngitis may have been the predisposing condition.

3.53 *e-na-a-šu bur-kà-a-šu ke-er-ra-a-šu k*[*i . . . mì-i*]*t-ḫa-ri-iš ik-kà-la-a-šu ul-tu mu-ra-sú it-ta*-⌜*ab*!⌝-*šu a-na* [. . .] *ti₇-ik ša-me-e* BA.Ú[Š] (StBoT 36.23 r. 6′–8′)

**(If) his eyes, his knees, his throat, (and) [his] ⌜legs?⌝ all hurt him at once (and) after his illness? comes about [it turns] into [*agannutillû* (anasarca: generalized swelling)], ⌜he will die⌝ [on a day] when it is hailing.[61]

The text below may be describing the acute arthritis that is often seen when patients with a strep throat develop rheumatic fever.

3.54 DIŠ GEŠTU^{II}-*šú kir-ra-šu u ki-ṣir* 1.KÙŠ.M[EŠ-š]*ú* TA GIG-*su* TAK$_4$-⌜*šu*⌝ 1-*niš*! KÚ.MEŠ-*šú ki*-⌜*ma* DU$_8$?-*ra*⌝ (coll.) GIG-[*su* GUR-*m*]*a ana* É.MEŠ GUR-*šú-ma* GIG SAL.KALAG.GA IGI-*ma* DIN [o o o o] DIŠ ŠU^{II}-*šú u* GÌR^{II}-*šú ana* x-x[. . .] GIG.BI *šum$_4$-ma* É.MEŠ [. . .] (DPS VIII 18–21 = *TDP* 70:18–21)

**If after his illness has left him his ears, his throat, and his elbows all hurt him at the same time (and) after it has let up, [his] illness [returns] ⌜and⌝ comes back inside him so that he gets sick (again), he may have a difficult time of it, but he will get well. [. . .] If his hands and feet [. . .]. If his illness [comes back] inside him [a third time . . .]

EPIGLOTTITIS

Although infections of the throat and upper airway are common, only certain organisms seem likely to cause severe tissue swelling that may lead to airway obstruction and death from suffocation. In the recent past, the bacterium *Hemophilus influenzae* often caused this problem, but with the widespread use of *Hemophilus influenzae* vaccine, this is becoming very rare. Since the vaccine was not available in ancient Mesopotamia, this disease may have been seen by the *āšipu*.

Epiglottitis can occur at any age, but it is most common in children ages two to six years. It often develops very rapidly with fever, irritability, sore throat, very loud and labored breathing especially on inspiration (stridor), and loss of voice. In patients with diphtheria (see below) there may also be airway obstruction and death, but the patient's breathing does not have the loud, stridorous character of epiglottitis. The patients with epiglottitis appear anxious, their throat is red and swollen, and they prefer to sit leaning forward to facilitate breathing. They drool, unwilling to swallow saliva because of pain and respiratory distress. Death occurs if the swelling completely obstructs the airway.

3.55 DIŠ LÚ.TUR GÚ.MUR-*su ḫa-niq šá-niš* GUB-*ma ina šu-ba-as-su im-qut* . . . (BM 62376:1–2)

**If an infant's larynx is constricted and moreover he stands up and then falls down on his seat . . .

3.56 DIŠ *gir-ri* 150-*šú* MÚ.ME GIG-*su* DUGUD / DIŠ *gir-ra-šú* MÚ.ME GAM (DPS X A obv. 48 = *TDP* 86:48)[62]

**If the right side of his throat is continually swollen, his illness will be difficult. If both sides of his throat are continually swollen, he will die.

3.57 DIŠ *ina* ZI-*šú* GÚ.MUR-*su i-ḫar-ru-ur* GAM / DIŠ *ni-ip-qú-šú qit-ru-bu u* UŠ$_4$-*šú* NU DIB [GAM] (DPS X A obv. 34 = *TDP* 84:34; cf. DPS XV:8 [AOAT 43.151])

**If his larynx makes a croaking noise when he breathes, he will die. If his chokings[63] come close together and he is not in full possession of his faculties, [he will die].

3.58 DIŠ GÚ.MUR-*su i-ḫar-ru-ur* GAM (DPS X A obv. 29//B obv. 33 = *TDP* 84:29)

**If his larynx makes a croaking noise he will die.

3.59 DIŠ ZI.ḪA.ZA SAG.ÚS DIB.DIB-*su u i-ṭa-mu* ÚŠ-*ma* EGIR-*šú* AMA-*šú* [GAM] (DPS X A obv. 39 = *TDP* 84:39)[64]

**If persistent "grabbing of the throat" continually afflicts him and he twists, if he dies afterward his mother [will die].

3.60 DIŠ ZI.ḪA.ZA SAG.ÚS DIB.DIB-*su u* GÚ.⌜DÈ!⌝.ME ÚŠ-*ma* EGIR-*šú* ŠEŠ-*šú* [GAM] (DPS X A obv. 40 = *TDP* 84:40)[65]

**If persistent "grabbing of the throat" continually afflicts him and he roars, if he dies afterward his brother [will die].[66]

These references indicate that the *āšipu* knew that blockage of the airway was occurring, that the disease was causing very loud (roaring) respirations, and that mental changes and death were a consequence of the illness. It is also clear that they knew that it was contagious, since relatives were also dying.

BUʾŠĀNU

Ancient physicians distinguished three types of *buʾšānu*[67] (BI.LU in Sumerian): one that "set up its throne in the windpipe (trachea and/or bronchi)," one that "set up its throne in the hard and soft palates,"[68] and one that "set up its throne among the teeth" (see below).[69] We believe that these three types of *buʾšānu* refer to three separate diseases: diphtheria, oral infection with *Herpes simplex* virus type 1 (HSV1), and anaerobic infection of the gingiva and throat (Vincent's angina, or trench mouth), respectively.[70] Cases of the viral infection infectious mononucleosis can mimic diphtheria, and cases of scurvy (see Chapter 7 with 7.19–7.20)[71] can mimic Vincent's angina. These may therefore also be included among the *buʾšānu* references. What these three categories have in common, apart from the fact that all are infections of the mouth or throat, is that patients exhibit a noticeably foul odor (*buʾšānu* literally means "stinking") and have lesions or exudate that are grayish in contradistinction to the bright red (skinned) appearance of strep and other throat infections.

DIPHTHERIA Diphtheria is caused by the bacterium *Corynebacterium diphtheria.* This is an acute infectious disease of the tonsils, pharynx, nose, and occasionally the skin. A gray-white pseudomembrane may cover involved areas. The underlying tissue usually bleeds if the pseudomembrane is pulled away. The typical tonsillar form of diphtheria can spread upward to the uvula and soft palate, and it may spread to the larynx, producing hoarseness and a nonproductive cough. Anterior nasal diphtheria occurs when the infection spreads through the nose producing a persistent, thin, sometimes bloody nasal discharge that is irritating and gives the upper lip a raw appearance. Usually there is a low-grade fever. Patients may die from suffocation secondary to obstruction of the airway, and/or heart failure caused by a bacterial toxin. The *buʾšānu* references below are likely to be describing this infection.

3.61 *bu-ʾ-šá-nu da-an* DIB-*su* GIN$_7$ U[R.M]AḪ *nap-šá-ra iṣ-b*[*at*] GIN$_7$ UR.BAR.RA *iṣ-ṣa-bat nu-ur-za iṣ-bat nu-*[*ur-ba*] *iṣ-ṣa-bat* EME *ina* GI.GÍD ḪAR.MEŠ *it-ta-di* ^{GIŠ}GU.ZA-*šú* . . . (*SpTU* 1.44:55–57//*BAM* 543 iii 43′–45′//*BAM* 536:6′–9′//*BAM* 537 r. 1′–3′//*BAM* 533:36–40)

**Mighty is the affliction of *buʾšānu.* It ⌜seized⌝ the uvula like a ⌜lion⌝; it seized the hard palate like a wolf. It seized the ⌜soft palate⌝; it seized the tongue. It set up its throne in the windpipe (trachea and/or bronchi) . . .

3.62 DIŠ [NA KA]-*šú bu-ʾ-šá-nu* DIB-*ma na-ḫi-ra-šú* KÚ.MEŠ-*šú* GIG.MEŠ DIRI.MEŠ . . . *šum*$_4$*-ma ina na-ḫi-ri-šú in-ni-iṣ-ṣ*[*in* . . .] (*SpTU* 1.44:29, 32)[72]

**If *buʾšānu* has seized [a person]'s [nose/mouth] so that his nostrils hurt him and are full of sores . . . if (something) smells in his nostrils [. . .]

3.63 DIŠ NA *ap-pa-šú u* ⌜KA-*šú bu-ʾ-šá*⌝*-nu* DIB-*it-ma* ŠÀ.ME-*šú nap-ḫu* . . . (*SpTU* 1.44:26//*BAM* 543 ii 19)[73]

**If *buʾšānu* has seized a person's nose and his mouth and his insides are bloated . . .

HERPETIC STOMATITIS (HSV1) On the skin, HSV1 typically causes small water blisters (vesicles; *bubuʾtu* in Akkadian), with surrounding redness and pain. In the mouth, the vesicles break quickly and leave shallow, painful ulcers with a gray base and surrounding redness. Since HSV1 may occasionally involve the nose, some of the references above could be either HSV1 or diphtheria. The *buʾšānu* references below are likely to be describing HSV1 infection.

3.64 [DIŠ KA-*šú bu-bu-ʾ*]-*ta* DIRI *u il-la-tu-šu il-*⸢*la*⸣-*ka bu-ʾ-šá-nu* MU.[NI] (DPS XXXIII: 87 [AOAT 43.357])

**[If his mouth] is full of ⸢*bubuʾtu*⸣ and his saliva flows, [it] is called *buʾšānu*.

3.65 DIŠ KA-*šú* U$_4$.BU.BU.UL DIRI *u il-la-tu-šú* [DU-*ka* . . .] (DPS VII B obv. 4′ = *TDP* 64:43′)[74]

**If his mouth is full of *bubuʾtu* and his saliva [flows . . .]

3.66 DIŠ NA KA-*šú* GIG . . . [DIŠ K]A-*šú bu-bu-tú* [DIRI] . . . (BM 76515 obv. 9, 12)

**If a person's mouth is sore . . . [If] his ⸢mouth⸣ [is full] of *bubuʾtu* . . .

VINCENT'S ANGINA (TRENCH MOUTH) Vincent's angina is caused by anaerobic bacteria in the mouth, but especially in the gums (gingiva) surrounding the teeth. It is an acute illness, with painful, swollen and gray membranes, and bleeding of the gums, as well as bad breath. In some cases, the teeth become loose. Patients often experience fever and weakness. The *buʾšānu* references below are likely to be describing this infection.

3.67 *da-an šá bu-ʾ-šá-nu* DIB-*su* GIN$_7$ UR.MAḪ SAG.DU *i*[*ṣ-bat* GIN$_7$ UR.BAR.RA *iṣ*]-*bat lu-ʾ-*[*ḫa*] *iṣ-bat* KA *iṣ-bat* EME *ina* ⸢*bi*⸣-*rit* ZÚ.MEŠ *it-ta-di* ^{GI}[^{Š}GU.ZA-*šú*] (*SpTU* 1.44:65–66//*BAM* 543 iii 58′–59′)

**Mighty is the affliction of *buʾšānu*. It [seized] the head like a lion; [it] ⸢seized⸣ the ⸢throat⸣ [like a wolf]. It seized the mouth; it seized the tongue. It set up its ⸢throne⸣ among the teeth.

3.68 [DIŠ NA KA-*šú b*]*u-šá-nu* DIB-*it ina re-be-et* ZÚ.MEŠ-*šú* [. . .] (*BAM* 157 obv. 10′)

**[If] ⸢*buʾšānu*⸣ seizes [a person's mouth] and [. . .] in the "square" of his teeth [. . .]

3.69 DIŠ NA ZÚ.MEŠ-*šú mu-nu u bu-ʾ-šá-nu* (*ḫe-pi eš-šu*) <DIB>-*al ina* DAL.BA.AN.NA ZÚ.MEŠ-*šú* MÚD È.MEŠ-*ni* . . . (*SpTU* 1.44:80–81)[75]

**If *munu*-sores (see Chapter 10) and *buʾšānu* grip a person's teeth (and) blood comes out between his teeth . . .

The following picturesque recitation notes a relationship between *buʾšānu* and hurting teeth or bleeding gums (the tooth worm; see Chapter 18 with 18.11–18.16). It is intended for an infant whose mouth problems are preventing him from nursing. Vincent's angina would be unlikely to occur in what we consider infants. However, the ancient Mesopotamian term that we are translating "infant" includes children with teeth who are old enough to talk (see Chapter 17).

3.70 ^{d}*A-nu ir-ḫi-a-am ša-me-e ša-mu-ú er-ṣe-tam ul-d*[*u-n*] *im er-ṣe-tum ú-li-id bu-ša-am bu-šum ú-li-id lu-ḫu-ma-a-am lu-ḫu-mu-um ú-li-id zu-ba zu-u*[*b*]-*bu ú-li-id tu-ul-tam tu-ul-tum*

DUMU.SA[L] [d]*Gu-la lu-ul-lu-um-tam lu-ub-bu-ša-at da-mi ḫa-ab-ra-at a*⌜xx⌝*-lu? da-mi ṣe-eḫ-ri-im ú-bi-el-li-a-am i-ni-i-šu*⌜*id-di ši-ip-tam* [d]*Da-mu ù* [d]*Gu-la*⌝ *ú-ni-ra*⌜*tu?-ul?-tam?*⌝ [. . .] *iṭ-bu-uḫ-šu-nu-*⌜*ti*⌝ *a-na* ⌜*mu-uḫ-ḫi*⌝ [. . .] *ip-te pí-i-šu iṣ-ṣa-bat tu-la-a-am iš-ši-i-ma i-ni-šu i-*[. . .] *ši-ip-tum ú-ul ia-a-tum ši-pa-at* [d]*Da-mu ù* [d]*Gu-la* [d]*Da-mu* [*i*]*d-di-ma a-na-ku el-qé* (*YOS* 11.5:1–8)

**Anu inseminated the heavens; the heavens ⌜gave birth⌝ to the earth. The earth gave birth to *buʾšu*, *buʾšu* gave birth to the mud, the mud gave birth to the fly, the fly gave birth to the tooth worm. The tooth worm is the ⌜daughter⌝ of Gula (goddess of healing associated with *buʾšānu* in infants; see Chapter 19 with 19.330). She is dressed in *lulumtu* (a type of garment but also a plant for toothache).[76] She is thick[77] with blood. [. . .] the blood of the infant; she extinguished his eyes. Damu cast a spell and Gula killed the tooth worm(?). She slaughtered them (the tooth worm and [. . .]) upon [. . .] (The infant) opened his mouth (and) took the breast. He raised his eyes and [. . .] This spell is not mine; it is the spell of Damu and Gula. Damu cast it, and I took it.[78]

Lung Infections

Since the lungs are well known as being the target of many types of infections in modern times, we can be certain that the same was true in ancient Mesopotamia. This is confirmed by the numerous references to patients with "sick lungs" (ḪAR.MEŠ GIG)[79] as well as signs and symptoms compatible with lung infection.

SPUTUM

Expectorated material was described as being white, thick, colored, and bloody, all characteristics that are found in certain types of pneumonia.

3.71 DIŠ NA KI.MIN *su-a-lam* BABBAR ŠUB.MEŠ-*a ù ip-te-ne-er-ru* NA.BI x [. . .] KI A.MEŠ *šá-qi ana* TI-*šú* . . . (*AMT* 50/3:6–7)

**If a person . . . continually produces white *suʾālu*-cough phlegm[80] and he continually vomits, that person was made to drink [. . .] with the water, to cure him . . .

3.72 *sa-ḫu-nu* MU-*ša ana ki-ṣir-te* ḪAR.MEŠ DÙ.A.BI SIG$_5$ . . . (*BAM* 555 ii 14)[81]

**It is called a *saḫunu*-potion; it is good for any sort of thick sputum[82] in the lungs . . .

3.73 DIŠ NA *ši-i-qu lu-ḫu-ʾ* GIG . . . (BM 78963:55)[83]

**If a person is sick with dirty *šīqu* (colored sputum)[84] . . .

3.74 DIŠ NA GABA-*su* G[IG-*m*]*a* NINDA *u* A *ina* GABA-*šú* GUB.MEŠ-*zu ḫa-aḫ-ḫa* TUKU.MEŠ . . . (*BAM* 547 iv 13′)[85]

**If a person's breast is ⌜sore and⌝ bread and water stick in his chest (and) he continually has *ḫaḫḫu* (bloody sputum)[86] . . .

Some of the quotes, however, present a dilemma. They describe certain characteristics of the lungs and chest that would be difficult for a physician to learn without performing surgery or an autopsy. For example, in the following reference the "lungs solidified with clay" could quite possibly be describing cheesy (caseous) necrosis seen in chronic tuberculosis.

3.75 DIŠ NA ḪAR^{II}-*šú* IM *it-pu-qa*... (*BAM* 558 iv 1)[87]

**If a person's lungs are solidified with "clay"...

Eventually some of this material might be coughed up, but it seems unlikely that this would have led to the conclusion that the lung was solidified. Another quote refers to a solid mass in the lungs that involved the ribs.

3.76 DIŠ NA ḪAR.MEŠ-*šú* KI KAK.TI-*šú* *it-pu-qu ana* TI-*šú*... (*BAM* 558 iv 3; *BAM* 558 iv 7//*BAM* 174 obv. 11′; *BAM* 174 obv. 17′)

**If a person's lungs form a solid mass with his rib(s),[88] to cure him...

Some chronic lung infections such as tuberculosis, actinomycosis, and some fungi may secondarily involve the chest wall, but lung cancer can also evolve and spread in this manner. But how did physicians make these observations? We do know that some chest surgery was performed (see below). It is likely, therefore, that some descriptions came from observations of the lung and chest wall at the time of surgery. Although autopsies were never written about (except for animals), we believe that some must have been performed in fatal cases of pneumonia in order to gain more information.

BACTERIAL PNEUMONIA

Pneumonia occurs more commonly in the winter months.

3.77 [DIŠ NA] *lu ki-ṣir-te* ḪAR.MEŠ *lu su-alu* GIG [...] ... *ana* ḪAR.MEŠ DÙ.A.BI SIG$_5$ [...] 1-*tú šá* EN.TE.NA (*BAM* 44:22′, 31′, 32′//*BAM* 555 ii 25)

**[If a person] is sick either with thick sputum in the lungs or *suʾālu*-cough (barking; see Chapter 8) ... it is good for any type of lung (problems), [...] for the cold season.

3.78 [Ú ḪA]R^{II}.MEŠ *ša* EN.TE.NA... (*BAM* 430 v 41′//*BAM* 431 v 36′)[89]

**[Plants for the] ⌜lungs⌝ for the cold season...

CURSE PNEUMONIA

Pneumonia, often due to *Streptococcus pneumoniae* (pneumococcal pneumonia), *Hemophilus influenzae*, or *Staphylococcus aureus*, causes fever, cough, and sputum (phlegm) that is commonly yellow or green, and occasionally dark brown or bloody. The patient may also have abnormal breath sounds, shortness of breath, and chest pain. Occasionally, abdominal and shoulder pain and nausea can occur. The three references below appear in the diagnostic series as part of a section devoted to symptoms attributed to "curse." We believe that these represent a single entity, namely, bacterial pneumonia. It is impossible to determine the specific organism, and it is possible that some of the cases might have been due to a viral (i.e., influenza) or fungal (i.e., histoplasmosis) infection. "Curses" were believed to cause other medical conditions in addition to pneumonia (see Chapter 19 with 19.307–19.318).

3.79 DIŠ NA KÚM-*em* ŠÀ-*šú i-ta-na-aš ú-gan-na-aḫ u ki-ṣir-ta-šú* GI_6 NA BI *ma-mit* GIG (DPS XXII:25 [AOAT 43.253])

**If a person is feverish, his stomach is continually nauseous, he *guḫḫu*-coughs (brassy; see Chapter 8) and his thick sputum is dark, that person is sick with a curse.[90]

3.80 DIŠ NA KÚM *ma-dam* TUKU-*ma la i-na-aḫ ú-na-ḫaṭ u i-sa-ul u* ŠÀ-*šú a-na a-re-e i-ta-na-šá-a* NAM.ÉRIM GIG (DPS XXII:26–27 [AOAT 43.253/254])

**If a person is very feverish and cannot find rest, he breathes deeply[91] and *suʾālu*-coughs (barking; see Chapter 8) and his stomach is nauseous to the point of vomiting, he is sick with a curse.

3.81 DIŠ SAG ŠÀ-*šú i-kàṣ-ṣa-su* ŠÀ-*šú* KÚM⸢*ú*⸣-*kal* KÚM *la ḫa-ḫaš* ÚḪ GI_6 ŠUB.ŠUB-*a u i-ta-nar-ru* NA BI NAM.ÉRIM DIB-*su* (DPS XXII:31–32 [AOAT 43.254])[92]

**If his upper abdomen (epigastrium) gnaws at him, fever grips his stomach, his temperature is lukewarm, he continually produces dark phlegm, and he continually vomits, a curse afflicts that person.

KIŠPU PNEUMONIA

The following references mention chest pain, fever, phlegm, and "sick lungs." Pneumonia is the likely underlying cause. One of the texts indicates that the patient had "eaten or drunk" *kišpu* (sorcery). More precisely, as we know from *Maqlû* and similar sorcery-expelling magic, some victims of direct sorcery (as opposed to sorcery by the manipulation of figurines or the sending of ghosts) were supposed to have come into contact with the sorcerer's contaminated spittle (*ruḫû*). Since pneumonia is indeed spread by the aspiration of infected mucus, it would appear that the *āšipu* had some idea as to the source (if not the exact method of delivery) of the infection.

3.82 DIŠ NA GABA-*su* KÚ-*šú* SAG ŠÀ-*šú ú-ṣa-rap-šú* ŠÀ.MEŠ-*šú* [MÚ.MÚ] NA.BI ḪAR.MEŠ GIG $UŠ_{11}$ KÚ *u* NAG *ana* TI-*šú* . . . (*AMT* 48/4 r. 8–9)[93]

**If a person's breast hurts him, his upper abdomen (epigastrium) burns him hotly, (and) his insides [are continually bloated], (and) that person has "sick lungs," he has eaten or drunk *kišpu*; to cure him . . .

3.83 [DIŠ. . .] ḪAR.MEŠ-*šú* KÚM.MEŠ-*šú la-ʾ-ba* DIRI *u* Ú[Ḫ . . . Ḫ]AR.MEŠ GIG $UŠ_{11}$ DIB-*uš ana* TI-*šú* . . . (*AMT* 55/2:4′–5′)[94]

**[If. . .] his lungs are continually feverish, he is full of *liʾbu*-fever and ⸢phlegm⸣[95] [. . .] (and he has) "sick ⸢lungs⸣", *kišpu* afflicts him; to cure him . . .

3.84 DIŠ NA KI.MIN *su-a-lam* BABBAR ŠUB.MEŠ-*a ù ip-te-né-er-ru* NA.BI [. . .] KI A.MEŠ *šá-qi ana* TI-*šú* . . . DIŠ NA GABA-*su u* MAŠ.SÌLA.MEŠ-*šú* KÚ.MEŠ-*šú ip-te-né-ru* NA.BI $UŠ_{11}$ DIB-*šú* . . . (*AMT* 50/3:6–7,11; cf. 1–2)

**If a person . . . continually produces white *suʾālu*-phlegm and he continually vomits, that person was made to drink [. . .] with the water; to cure him . . . If a person's breast and shoulders continually hurt him (and) he continually vomits, *kišpu* afflicts that person . . .

3.85 DIŠ NA *lu* ÚḪ *lu-ba-ṭi ru-pu-uš*-⌜*tu*$_4$⌝ *lu sa-a-ḫu* ŠUB.ŠUB-*di*⌜KA⌝-*šú ù* EME-*šú ru-a-tu-šú* ŠUB.ŠUB-*di-a* ⌜NA⌝.BI NÍG.KÌD.KÌD.⌜DA⌝ *nak-mu-ti šá* ⌜*pu*⌝-*uz-ru šu-kul* . . . (BM 42328+:1–4//BM 42550:1–5//BM 43123+ obv. 1–3 [Finkel, *Fs. Lambert* 204–205])

**If a person either continually produces phlegm, bouts of sweating, and mucus (in the upper abdomen) or he continually produces *saḫḫu* (liquid from the lungs) (and) his mouth and his tongue continually produce his phlegm, that person has been made to eat substances contaminated by one ritual (of *kišpu*) after the other performed in secret . . .

What may have differentiated *kišpu*-pneumonia from "curse" pneumonia in the mind of the *āšipu* was that a victim of the former was expected to produce "white *suʾālu*-phlegm" (*AMT* 50/3:6–7) whereas what the latter coughed up was "dark" phlegm (DPS XXII:31–32 [AOAT 43.254]) or "dark thick sputum" (DPS XXII:25 [AOAT 43.253]). Dark phlegm (sputum) in general contains blood. Pneumococcal pneumonia commonly has blood containing mucoid sputum, but other types of bacterial pneumonia occasionally will have this finding.

SECONDARY PNEUMONIA

Pneumonia is frequently a secondary complication of other diseases. The cause is usually bacterial. Listed below are cases of diphtheria (*buʾšānu*; see above under throat infections) or enteric fever (*ṣētu*; see below) complicated by pneumonia.

3.86 DIŠ NA ḪAR.MEŠ-*ma* KA-*šú bu-ʾ-ša-nu* DIB-*it* . . . (*BAM* 558 i 14′//*BAM* 44:14′)

**If a person's lungs are sick and *buʾšānu* afflicts his nose/mouth . . .

3.87 [DIŠ N]A GABA-*su* SAG ⌜ŠÀ⌝ MAŠ.SÌLA.MEŠ-*šú* KÚ.MEŠ-*šú* [UD].DA SÁ.SÁ *šum*$_4$-*ma ú-ga-na-aḫ* [ḪA]R.ME GIG . . . (*CTN* 4.114 r. 7′–9′)[96]

**[If] a ⌜person's⌝ breast, upper abdomen (epigastrium), (and) shoulders continually hurt him, he was "gotten" by *ṣētu*. If he *guḫḫu* (brassy-coughs), (he has) sick ⌜lungs⌝ . . .

PNEUMONIA-ASSOCIATED PAIN

Pneumonia, when it causes inflammation of the pleural surfaces, often presents with symptoms of pain, especially when taking a deep breath (pleuritic pain). Chest pain is the most common, but when the pleural surface covering the diaphragm is inflammed, the pain may be felt in the shoulder and/or abdomen since the nerve to the diaphragm also serves these other areas. The texts below appear to be describing this pain.

3.88 [DIŠ NA] SAG ŠÀ-*šú* M[AŠ.SÌ]LA.MEŠ-*šú* KÚ.MEŠ-*šú ú-gan-na-aḫ* [NA B]I ḪAR.MEŠ G[I]G UD.DA SÁ.SÁ *ana* TI-*šú* (*BAM* 564 ii 14′–15′)[97]

**[If a person]'s upper abdomen (epigastrium) (and) his ⌜shoulders⌝ continually hurt him (and) he *guḫḫu* (brassy-coughs), ⌜that⌝ [person] has "sick lungs"; he was "gotten" by *ṣētu* (enteric fever) to cure him . . .

3.89 DIŠ NA GABA-*su* SAG ŠÀ-*šú* MAŠ.SÌLA^{II}-*šú* KÚ.MEŠ-*šú* [. . .] ḪAR.MEŠ GIG (*AMT* 49/4 obv. 1–2; cf. *AMT* 48/4 r. 13′)[98]

**If a person's breast, his upper abdomen (epigastrium), (and) his shoulders continually hurt him [. . .] "sick lungs."

3.90 DIŠ NA GABA-*su u* MAŠ.SÌLA.⌜MEŠ-*šú*⌝ K[Ú.MEŠ-*šú* . . .] *ú-ga-ḫab* [. . . *ana* T]I-*šú* . . . (*AMT* 49/1 ii 11–13//*AMT* 48/5:8–10)[99]

**If a person's breast and shoulders [continually] ⌜hurt⌝ [him . . .] he coughs [(and) . . .] [to] ⌜cure⌝ him . . .

3.91 DIŠ NA *ki-ṣir-te* ḪAR.MEŠ GIG *ana di-ik-ši* [GUR-*šú*] . . . (*BAM* 554 i 10′)

**If a person is sick with thick sputum in the lungs (and) [it turns] into a stabbing pain . . .

EMPYEMA

The bacteria that cause pneumonia may occasionally spread to the space between the lungs and chest wall (pleural space). This infection may lead to the development of pus in the pleural space, also called empyema. As indicated in the references below, the *āšipu* was aware of this problem, and knew how to treat it surgically. It is not clear how they detected this problem, but in some cases the pus drains spontaneously through the chest wall.

3.92 [DIŠ N]A ḪAR.MEŠ-*šú* [GIG!-*ma e-nu-ma*] ḪAR.MEŠ-*šú i-sa-ri-ma*? DIŠ NA ḪAR.MEŠ-*šú* MÚD *ú-k*[*al ù*] MÚD.BABBAR ŠUB.⌜MEŠ⌝-*a* [SAG-*šú i*]-*te-né-na-a* . . . ⌜*e*⌝-*nu-ma ina su-a-li-šú* MÚD *i-a*-⌜*ru*⌝ . . . *šum*$_4$-*ma* TIL DUGUD-*šú* . . . (*BAM* 557:11′–12′, 14′, 16′//*BAM* 564 ii 28′–29′, 31′–32′)[100]

**[If] a ⌜person's⌝ lungs [are sick and when (the *āšipu*)] makes an incision(?) in his lungs, if the person's lungs ⌜hold⌝ blood [and] continually produce pus (and) he continually changes (the side of) [his head] (he sleeps on) . . . when he vomits blood while coughing . . . if it is difficult for him to stop . . .

The reference below describes the surgical and medical treatment of this condition.

3.93 [DIŠ KI].MIN KÚM ⌜*ina* SU-*šú*⌝ [*la-zi-iz-ma u ma-gal i-le*]-*ḫi-ib* NA.BI *bit-qu*$_5$ [. . . *u* IR TUKU][101] [. . . *tu-sa*]-*ba*-ʾ-*šu-ma* 3 UZU.TI.MEŠ [. . . *ina* ^{NA}4]ZÚ *ina* 4 UZU.TI BAD-*te* A.MEŠ *u* MÚD [. . .] 5 *qa* A GAZI^{SAR} ŠEG$_6$-*šal ta-šá-ḫal* [. . .] *tu-sa-ba*-ʾ-*šu-ma tu-za-ak* GUR-[*ma* . . .] 1-*niš tu-šá-ḫa-an ana* ŠÀ-*šú* DUB-*ak* [. . .] NAM.SI.SÁ A.BÁR DÙ-*uš ina* TÚG.GADA *ta-ša-kak ana* ŠÀ-*šú* GAR *rib-ku ina* A GAZI^{SAR} ŠEG$_6$.⌜GÁ⌝ ŠID-*aš* LÁL-*su-ma* T[I] (*BAM* 39:2′–9′//*AMT* 49/4 r. 1–9)

**If (a mild headache afflicts a person and) fever persists in his body and also he makes a loud growling noise, that person has a "cleft"[102] [. . .] and sweat, [to cure him, you] ⌜spill⌝[103] [. . .] over him and three ribs [. . .]. You make an opening in the fourth rib[104] [with] a flint knife. Water and blood [. . .] You boil five *qû* of *kasû* juice; you filter it. [. . .] You spill it over him and you clear it away. Once again you [. . .]. You heat it together and pour it in. [. . .] You make a lead drainage instrument. You thread it on a linen cloth and put it in. You boil the decoction in *kasû* juice. You make it into a dough. (If) you bandage him with it, ⌜he should recover⌝.

Another interesting aspect of the preceding reference was the treatment of empyema (pus between the lungs and chest wall) by means of a lead drain. The Sumerians and Akkadians were excellent metallurgists who manufactured, in addition to the drain tube mentioned here, pipettes for the instillation of medicine, lead spoons for the application of eye ointments, and several varieties of straight and curved bronze surgical knives.

TUBERCULOSIS

Tuberculosis is a disease of great antiquity. Lesions that were almost certainly tuberculous in nature have been found in the vertebrae of neolithic man in Europe, and Egyptian mummies possibly as early as 3700 B.C.E. and two skeletons found in a Bronze Age cemetery (3150–3000 B.C.E.) at Bab Edh-Dha in Jordan also show signs of skeletal tuberculosis.[105] Lymph node specimens from a pre-Columbian Peruvian mummy have been shown to contain DNA sequences unique to the *Mycobacterium* complex.[106]

Caused by *Mycobacterium tuberculosis*, this chronic infection has protean manifestations. The primary infection is located in the lungs, and is initiated by inhaled droplets containing the organisms that have been coughed up by someone with active lung disease. A similar disease in cattle (*Mycobacterium bovis*) can also cause a tuberculosis-like disease in humans. From the lungs the infection may spread by intrabronchial dissemination or by direct extension or may be carried in the blood to many different organs throughout the body causing destructive lesions at the time of the dissemination or after long periods of latency. In tuberculosis, the sputum generally contains pus (purulent) and small or large amounts of blood. Other bacterial causes of lung infection are likely to produce a more acute form of pneumonia than tuberculosis, and are less likely to produce bloody sputum.

The following references are likely to be describing patients with tuberculosis. The first two imply that the process is chronic or long-term, which is certainly consistent with most cases of tuberculosis.

3.94 DIŠ NA *g*[*i-na-a*] ḪAR.MEŠ GIG-*ma ú-gan-na-aḫ ul-tú* ÚḪ-*šú* MÚD ŠUB-*a*... (*BAM* 44:16′)

**If a person ⌜constantly⌝ has sick lungs so that he *guḫḫu* (brassy-coughs) (and) produces blood with his spittle...

3.95 [DIŠ NA . . . KI ÚḪ-*š*]*u* MÚD.MEŠ ŠUB.MEŠ-*a* NA BI *ana mal-da-riš ú-sa-al* . . . (*BAM* 555 iii 55′; cf. *BAM* 575 iv 34 [AOAT 43.331])

**[If a person ...] produces blood [with his spittle] (and) that person *suʾālu* (barking-coughs) one (cough) right after the other...

3.96 DIŠ NA *em-bu-bu ḫa-še-e* GIG-*ma ú-gan-na-aḫ* KI *ru-ṭi-šú* MÚD ŠUB-*a* . . . (BM 78963:40)

**If a person (has) a sore windpipe (trachea and/or bronchi) so that he *guḫḫu* (brassy-coughs) (and) he produces blood with his spittle...

PERTUSSIS

Pertussis, or whooping cough, is caused by *Bordatella pertussis.* It causes severe bronchitis and bronchopneumonia in infants and young children, with a significant mortality. Adults can also become infected, but severe illness and death is unusual in adults. Pertussis is suggested by the following quotes, although asthma (see Chapter 8) is also a strong possibility for the second reference.

3.97 DIŠ NA *su-alu ṭup-šu-su* GIG . . . (BM 78963:45)

**If a young child (lit. a person who still has baby fat) is sick with *suʾālu* (barking-coughs) . . .

3.98 DIŠ NA *su-alu šá ši-ḫi* GIG-*ma* GI.GÍD ḪAR.MEŠ-*šú* IM DIRI *ú-sa-al ú-gan-na-aḫ* ÚḪ TUKU-*ši* . . . (Labat and Tournay, *RA* 40.116 obv. 8–9)

**If a person is sick with wheezing *suʾālu* (barking-coughs) so that his windpipe (trachea and/or bronchi) is full of wind, he coughs (and) coughs (and) has phlegm . . .[107]

ANAEROBIC LUNG ABSCESS

Anaerobic lung abscesses commonly occur following grand mal epileptic seizures, alcohol intoxication, or any neurological impairment that permits the aspiration of gastric contents into the lungs. The combination of high acidity and anaerobic organisms from the GI tract and mouth causes intense pneumonia with lung destruction and abscess formation. As with other anaerobic infections, the pus smells very bad, which explains why anaerobic lung infections are also referred to as putrid lung abscess. High fever and large volumes of sputum are also quite common. The following quote is suggestive of an anaerobic lung abscess.

3.99 DIŠ NA IM *ina* ŠÀ-*šú uš-tar-ʾ-ab ù i-le-ḫi-ib* SU-*šú* še pi bi GABA-*su u* MAŠ.SÌLA.MEŠ-*šú* KÚ.MEŠ-*šú* UZU.MEŠ-*šú ú-šam-ma-mu-šú u* GÍR.GÍR-*šú* UZU^{II}-*šú áš-ṭu u ni-ip-še* DIRI SAG.MEŠ-*šú i-ta-na-nu-ú* KÚM.MEŠ *ina kal* U$_4$-*me ú-kal-šú ana* TI-*šú* . . . (*BAM* 575 iii 30–32//*BAM* 55:1–7//*BAM* 56 r. 8′–10′//*BAM* 57:1′–5′)

**If "wind" rumbles in a person's insides, he makes a growling noise, his body . . . , his breast and shoulders continually hurt him, his flesh is numb, continually stings him and is stiff and he is full of stink, he continually changes (what side of) his head (he sleeps on) and he is gripped by fever all day, to cure him . . .

In the text below, it appears that "sick lungs" and "teeth oozing blood" were linked by the *āšipu.* Teeth that ooze blood are most commonly caused by periodontal infection (see Chapter 18) and anaerobic organisms are the major cause of periodontal infection. Periodontitis is, therefore, commonly associated with anaerobic lung abscess, a fact of which the *āšipu* seems to have been aware.

3.100 DIŠ NA DAL.BA MAŠ.SÌLA^{II}-*šú* TAG.GA-*su* ZÚ.MEŠ MÚD *i-ḫi-il-la* NA.BI ḪAR.MEŠ GIG UŠ$_{11}$.ZU *šu-kul u šá-qí ana* TI-*šú* . . . (*STT* 102:1–3)[108]

**If the area between a person's shoulders hurts him intensely (and) his teeth ooze blood, that person has "sick lungs"; he has eaten or drunk *kišpu,* to cure him . . .

Infectious Causes of Diarrhea

CHOLERA

Of all the causes of diarrhea, cholera is the most feared. It can produce profound loss of fluids and salt in a very short time, reducing the patient to a shrunken and listless shadow of his former self with death a frequent outcome. It is caused by a toxin produced by the bacterium *Vibrio comma*. Humans are the only natural host, and transmission is by ingesting food or water contaminated by infected fecal matter. Since the organism does not invade the intestinal wall and the problems are caused entirely by the toxin, patients in the current era can be cured in most cases simply by replacing the water and salt that are lost in the stool.

In severe cases, after an incubation period of one to five days, there is a rapid onset of diarrhea, which may be associated with abdominal cramping. The diarrhea, watery with flecks of white mucus, is called "ricewater stool." Fever is unusual except in children and is of brief duration. Ancient physicians seem to have attributed this illness to "hand" of ghost, possibly because the dehydration creates a shrunken body with a skeletal look.

3.101 [D]IŠ U$_4$ LÁ-*šú* UB.NÍGIN.NA-*šú i-šaḫ-ḫu-ḫa* ŠÀ-*šú* DIB.DIB-*su* ŠÀ.MEŠ-*šú* SI.SÁ.MEŠ-*šú* ŠU GIDIM$_7$ (DPS XXVI:19′ [AOAT 43.279/280])

**⌜If⌝ when (a confusional state) comes over him, his limbs waste away (and) his abdomen continually afflicts him (and) the bowels are continually loose, "hand" of ghost.[109]

3.102 DIŠ *ip-ru-ur-ma uš-ḫa-ri-ir* GIG BI GIDIM$_7$.MEŠ *ir*?-*t*[*e*?-*né-du-šú*] / DIŠ *uṣ-ṣu-ub* A.MEŠ APIN.MEŠ-*iš* KÚM *mit-ḫar* SA.MEŠ ŠU^{II}-*šú* DU-*k*[*a*] TA *taš-rit* GI$_6$ EN SA$_9$ EN.NUN *i-leb-bu* ŠU GIDIM$_7$ (DPS XXVII:26–28 [AOAT 43.299])[110]

**If he is powerless and dazed, ghosts ⌜continually pursue (?)⌝[111] that patient. If he keeps asking for more and more water[112] (but) his temperature is normal, the blood vessels of his hands "go," (and) he groans from the beginning of the night until the middle of the watch, "hand" of ghost.

DEHYDRATION

Most of the abnormalities seen in cholera are due to inadequate fluid volume or dehydration. In cholera, this problem is caused by fluid loss due to diarrhea, but inadequate fluid intake and fluid loss from sweating and urination can cause similar signs and symptoms. Other diseases that lead to dehydration will, therefore, have findings that overlap with cholera. These include shriveling of the skin, dry mouth with shriveled tongue and mouth surfaces, sunken eyes, and a gaunt face.

3.103 [DIŠ SA]G ŠÀ-*šú* DIB.DIB-*su u* EME-*šú ḫe-em-ret ana* KI GIG GAM (DPS XIII B i 8′ = *TDP* 110 i 12′)[113]

**[If] his ⌜upper abdomen (epigastrium)⌝ continually afflicts him and his tongue is shriveled, he is at an acute stage of the illness;[114] he will die.

3.104 DIŠ E[M]E-*šú it-ta-nab-bal* [. . .] / DIŠ EME-*šú u liq* KA-*šú* [. . .] (DPS VII A obv. 12–13 = *TDP* 62:12–13)

**If his ⸢tongue⸣ keeps drying out [. . .]. If his tongue and palate [keep drying out? . . .]

3.105 DIŠ *liq* KA-*šú šá-bu-ul la-ga-a* ŠUB.ŠUB ^{GIŠ}GIDRU ⸢*šá* ^{d}x⸣ [. . .] / DIŠ *liq* KA-*šú* ⸢*i*⸣-*ta-nab-bal* ŠÀ.MEŠ-*šú* MÚ.ME[Š . . .] (DPS VII B obv. 15′–16′ = *TDP* 64:54′–55′)[115]

**If his palate has dried up (and) is dotted with (what looks like) slag, scepter of [. . .]. If his palate continually dries out (and) his insides are continually bloated [. . .]

3.106 DIŠ IGI.MEŠ-*šú* SIG$_7$.MEŠ *u* IGI^{II}-*šú šap-la* GAM (DPS IX A 12 = *TDP* 72:12)

**If his face is yellowish and his eyes are sunken, he will die.[116]

As the condition worsens, circulation collapses with the pulse becoming weak and rapid. Muscles may cramp, and the patient becomes weak, confused, and listless.

3.107 DIŠ LÚ.TUR *ma-la* KÚ *i-ḫa-ḫu* KI.MIN *iṣ-ṣa-na-aḫ* ŠU^{II}-*šú u* GÌR^{II}-*šú it-te-ṣi-la-šú qí-bit* KA *ana* ^{d}30 TUKU-*ši* (DPS XL A 48 = *TDP* 222:48)[117]

**If an infant vomits as much as he eats; alternatively (if) he has diarrhea (and) his hands and his feet become sluggish, there is an (unfulfilled) promise to Sîn.[118]

3.108 [DIŠ NA Š]À(!).MEŠ-*šú it-te*-⸢*nem*⸣-*mi-ru liq* KA-*šú i-ta-nab-b*[*al*] [Á^{II}.MEŠ]-*šú šim-ma-tú* TUKU.MEŠ-*a i-ge-eš-šú az-zu-za-a bi-bil* ŠÀ TUKU.MEŠ [IGI.DU]$_8$-*ma* UGU-*šú* NU DÙG.GA MUNUS ŠÀ-*šú ḫa-šiḫ-ma* MUNUS IGI.DU$_8$-*ma* ŠÀ-*šú* NU ÍL-*šú* [ŠÀ-*šú a*]-*na da-ba-bi ša-pil* NA.BI ŠU.GIDIM.MA ÚS-*šú ana* TI-*šú* . . . (*AMT* 76/1:4–7)

**[If a person's] ⸢insides⸣ are continually colicky, his palate continually ⸢dries up⸣, his [arms] are continually numb, he belches, he has plenty of appetite (for food), but when [he sees it], it does not please him; he wants a woman, but when he sees a woman, he cannot get an erection;[119] [his heart] is (too) depressed (for him) to speak— "hand" of ghost is pursuing that person; to cure him . . .

Death will inevitably result unless fluid and salt replacement occurs.

3.109 DIŠ ŠÀ.MEŠ-*šú i-tab-lu* GAM (DPS XIII B ii 43 = *TDP* 120 ii 43)

**If his insides have dried up, he will die.

3.110 DIŠ SAG.DU-*su* AD$_6$-*šú* SAG KIR$_4$-*šú* SÌG.SÌG-*su* NUND[UN.MEŠ-*šú i-ta-na-zu*] *u* ZI.IR.MEŠ *ina ni-šu-ti-šú* GIDIM$_7$ *šá ina ṣu-um-m*[*a-mi* ÚŠ DIB-*su*] (DPS III C r. 3–4//E$_1$ r. 4–5+E$_2$ r. 1 = *TDP* 24:63–64)[120]

**If his head, his body, (and) the bulb of his nose continually give him a jabbing pain, [his] ⸢lips⸣ [continually make strange noises],[121] and (his stomach) is continually upset,[122] among his people, the ghost of (one who) [died] of ⸢thirst⸣ [afflicts him].

3.111 DIŠ U[$_4$] LÁ-*šú* UB.NÍGIN.NA-*šú i-šam-ma-ma-šú* IGI.MEŠ-*šú* NIGIN.MEŠ-*du* ŠÀ-*šú i-šaḫ-ḫu-uḫ u mim-ma šá ana* KA-*šú* GAR-*nu ina* U$_4$-*me-šú ma-ti-ma ina* DÚR-*šú* ŠUB-*šú* ŠU GIDIM$_7$ *šá ina šag-gaš-ti* GAM (DPS XXVI:20′–21′ [AOAT 43.280])

**If ⸢when⸣ (a confusional state) comes over him, his limbs go numb, his face seems continually to spin, his abdomen wastes away, and whatever he puts to his mouth is always excreted from his anus on the very same day,[123] "hand" of a ghost who died through murder.[124]

3.112 DIŠ KI.MIN-*ma* GIG-*su* DUGUD-*su-ma* ZU-*šú* NU *ú-ad-da* GAM (DPS XVI:11 [AOAT 43.172])[125]

**If (it is the first day he is sick) and his illness becomes so difficult for him that he does not recognize those known to him, he will die.

DIARRHEAL DISEASES OTHER THAN CHOLERA

There are other organisms that produce a similar toxin and disease, but they usually are milder than cholera. Other organisms cause diarrhea by invading and damaging the intestinal wall. These organisms generally cause more pain and cramping, and often cause intestinal bleeding and produce white blood cells in the stool. In many cases, the information provided by the ancient Mesoptamian physician will not permit us to decide whether the disease is due to a toxin-producing organism or an invasive one, but in some cases, we can make a pretty good guess. Ancient physicians distinguish two types of diarrhea: "loose bowels" and "flowing[126] of the bowels." The former term, *loose bowels*, is used to describe the diarrhea of cholera. Most references make no mention of any pain, and none describe blood or pus in the stools. This would seem to indicate that *loose bowels* is the term that ancient physicians used to describe enterotoxic (cholera-like) diarrhea.

ENTEROTOXIC DIARRHEA

3.113 DIŠ GIG-*ma* DIN EGIR DIN ŠÀ-*šú* SI.SÁ-*šú* U_4.3.KÁM U_4.4.KÁM *ka-ma-su u la sa-ka-pu* GAR.GAR-*šú* *ana* U_4.5.KÁM : *ana* U_4.6.KÁM [. . .] (DPS XVII:48-49 [AOAT 43.199])

**If he is sick and then well (and) after he gets well his bowels are loose for three or four days and squatting but not lying down to rest are established for him (and he is sick) for five days (var. six days) [. . .].

3.114 [*ana* ŠÀ SI.S]Á *ka-le-e* . . . ŠÀ SI.SÁ *dan-nu šá la ik-kal-ú ik-kal-la* (BM 59626:1, 11–12)

**[To] hold back ⌜bowel movements⌝ . . . the prodigious loose bowel movements that cannot be held back will be held back.

3.115 DIŠ NA ŠÀ SI.SÁ TUKU-*ma* NU TAR-*as* . . . (BM 59623:1 [Leichty, *Mem. Sachs* 263–264])[127]

**If a person's bowels are loose and will not stop . . .

3.116 [D]IŠ U_4 LÁ-*šú* UB.NÍGIN.NA-*šú* *i-šaḫ-ḫu-ḫa* ŠÀ-*šú* DIB.DIB-*su* ŠÀ.MEŠ-*šú* SI.SÁ.MEŠ-*šú* ŠU GIDIM$_7$ (DPS XXVI:19′ [AOAT 43.279/280])

**⌜If⌝ when (a confusional state) comes over him, his limbs waste away (and) his abdomen continually afflicts him (and) his bowels are continually loose, "hand" of ghost.

ENTEROINVASIVE DIARRHEA Some gastrointestinal infections invade the intestinal lining and, while they cause diarrhea, they are more likely to cause severe abdominal cramping and stools with blood and pus than the toxin-induced diarrhea of cholera. This type of diarrhea is referred to as dysentery. Causative organisms include shigella, salmonella, *Entameba histolytica,* and some strains of *Escherichia coli* (*E. coli*). The term *flowing*[128] *of the bowels* is used to describe diarrhea accompanied by cramping and blood in the stools.[129] It is, therefore, probably the term which ancient physicians used to describe enteroinvasive diarrhea (dysentery).

3.117 [DIŠ N]A NINDA KÚ KAŠ NAG-*ma* ŠÀ-*šú in-nim-me-ru in-ne-*[*e*]*n-bi-ṭú re-du-ut ir-ri* TUKU UD.DA SÁ.SÁ . . . (*AMT* 48/1:12′+ *AMT* 78/3:9′; *AMT* 44/6:1–2)[130]

**[If] a ⌜person⌝ eats bread (and) drinks beer and subsequently his stomach is colicky, he has ⌜cramps⌝ (and) he has a "flowing of the bowels," *ṣētu* (enteric fever) has "gotten" him . . .

3.118 DIŠ NA MÚD *ina* DÚR-*šú* GIN$_7$ MUNUS *ša na-aḫ-ša-te* ŠUB.ŠUB-*a ta-ḫi-iz-zu-ma* DÚR.GIG.GA.KÁM NU TUKU-*ši tir-di-it ir-ri-šú* GIG . . . (*BAM* 99:19–20//*BAM* 100:2′–4′; *BAM* 99:42–43//*AMT* 43/1 iii 3′–4′)[131]

**If blood emits from a person's anus like a woman upon whom *naḫšātu* (menorrhagia) continually falls but he does not have DÚR.GIG (see Chapter 6), he is sick with "flowing of the bowels" . . .[132]

In the second reference, the diagnosis of "flowing of the bowels" is arrived at only after the exclusion of another possibility, namely DÚR.GIG. We believe that DÚR.GIG (see Chapter 6 with 6.176–187) refers to a group of diseases which includes ulcerative colitis, a condition that can mimic dysentery.

3.119 DIŠ NA *ina-aṭ-ma lu ni-ṭa lu* MÚD.BABBAR *lu nik-ma-tu* ⌜*šá* DÚR⌝.GIG *ú-tab-ba-ka ana* TI-*šú* . . . (*BAM* 159 ii 49–50)[133]

**If a person has bloody stools and pours out bloody excrement or pus or the pent-up (wind) of DÚR.GIG, to cure him . . .

DIARRHEA IN INFANTS Infants also have infectious diarrhea, which can be viral or bacterial in etiology. In the reference below, the infant has both cramping and diarrhea and is likely to be dehydrated as is demonstrated by the "crushed" appearance.

3.120 DIŠ LÚ.TUR ITI.1.KÁM ITI.2.KÁM ITI.3.KÁM *mur-ṣu* DIB-*su-ma* U$_4$ *u* GI$_6$ *ú-šam-šá* UZU.MEŠ *im-taq-tu* ŠÀ.MEŠ-*šú eb-ṭú ir-ru-šú i-šá-ru u uḫ-ta-taš-ši-il mi-iḫ-ru* ⌜DIB⌝-*su* (coll.) (DPS XL A 8–9//C 10–11 = *TDP* 218:8–9)[134]

**If an illness afflicts an infant of one, two, (and then) three months so that it keeps him awake day and night, his flesh (looks) terrible, his insides are cramped, his bowels are loose, and he is completely crushed, *meḫru*[135] afflicts him.

Enteric Fever and Conditions That Mimic Enteric Fever

Modern physicians tend to include a number of different infections under the term *enteric fever,* since the signs and symptoms are very similar and the causative organisms invade via the gastrointestinal tract. Enteric fever is characterized by fever, headache, abdominal pain, constipation or diarrhea, and occasionally skin rash, cough, nosebleeds, and red eyes (conjunctivitis). Pneumonia with its typical signs and symptoms may also be seen in patients with enteric fever. In more severe forms of the disease, rectal bleeding and neuropsychiatric manifestations, including psychosis, confusion, and delirium, occur. Although many organisms may be included under this term, some of the most common are *Salmonella typhi*, other *Salmonella* species, *Yersinia enterocolitica*, and *Campylobacter fetus*. Epidemic, endemic, and scrub typhus are not considered enteric fever since the organisms do not invade via the gastrointestinal tract. However, they closely mimic this syndrome.

Since physicians today cannot identify which of the possible causative organisms is responsible for any particular case of enteric fever without modern laboratory diagnostic procedures, it is no surprise that ancient physicians would have considered this a single entity. It appears likely to us that the Akkadian word *ṣētu* is equivalent to "enteric fever."[136] Listed below are some *ṣētu* references that help define this syndrome.

ṢĒTU

GENERAL DESCRIPTION

3.121 [DIŠ NA U]D.DA TAB.⌜BA⌝-*ma* SÍG SAG.DU-*šú* GUB.GUB-*az* IGI.MEŠ-*šú* NIGIN.MEŠ-⌜*du*⌝-*šú*-[*ma*] *it-ta-na-aṣ-ra-ḫu* SU-*šú ta-ni-ḫu* TUKU.TUKU-*ši* KÚM *la ḫa-aḫ-ḫa-áš su-a-lam* TUKU.TUKU-*ši* ŠÀ-*šú e-ta-na-áš-šá-áš il-la-tu-šú* DU-*ku* ŠÀ-*šú ig-da-na-ru-ur re-du-ut ir-ri* GIG *u ú-šar-da e-le-nu* UZU-*šú* $ŠED_7$ *ša*[*p-l*]*a-nu* GÌR.PAD.MEŠ-*šú ṣar-ḫa ina* [*su-a*]*-li-šú i-ni-*ʾ*-i* GI.GÍD ḪAR.MEŠ-*šú it-*[*t*]*e-né-es-*⌜*kir*⌝ [*ú*]*-ga-na-aḫ/ ú-ga-áš-ši ṣi-ri-iḫ-ti* KÚM ŠÀ TUKU.MEŠ NA BI UD.DA.TAB.BA *ana* TI-*šú* . . . (*BAM* 145:1–17//*BAM* 146:29′–38′)[137]

**[If] *ṣētu* burns [a person] so that the hair of his head continually stands on end, his face seems continually to spin, [and] he continually feels burning hot, his body is continually tired (and he has) a lukewarm temperature, he continually has *su*ʾ*ālu* (barking-coughs), his stomach is continually upset, his saliva flows, his stomach turns over and over, he is sick with "flowing" of the intestines and makes (one bowel movement) follow (another), the flesh above is cold (but) his bones below (feel) burning hot, when he tries to cough,[138] (his breath) turns back (and) his windpipe (trachea and/or bronchi) continually closes up, he coughs/belches, (and) he continually has burning internal fever, that person is burned by *ṣētu*, to cure him . . .[139]

FEVER

3.122 DIŠ KI.MIN IR *ma-gal* TUKU.TUKU-*ši u* IR GIN_7 A.MEŠ x [. . .] *ut-ta-na-tak*⌜NA BI GIG⌝ *là-zi*⌜DIB⌝-[*su* . . .] (*BAM* 66 obv. 24–28//DPS XXXI:19′ [AOAT 43.343])[140]

**If (*ṣētu* "gets" a person and) he has a great deal of sweat and he drips sweat like [. . .] water, a persistent illness afflicts that person [. . .]

MENTAL STATUS CHANGE This problem occurs commonly in enteric fever (as in the first reference below), but mental status change, primarily confusion, can occur occasionally with very high fever of any cause and especially at the extremes of age (see the second reference below). Meningitis and encephalitis (see Chapter 13) are febrile illnesses where mental status change occurs in almost every case.

3.123 DIŠ U$_4$-*mi-šam ana* GIZKIM-*šú* LÁ-*šú u* BAR-*šú* U$_4$ LÁ-*šú* KÚM-*ma* SA.MEŠ-*šú* KÚ.MEŠ-*šú* IR ŠUB-*su-ma ina-aḫ* LÁ-*ti* UD.DA (DPS XVI:81′–82′ [AOAT 43.179])[141]

**If daily, at the expected time, it comes over him and leaves him (and) when it comes over him, he becomes hot and his muscles continually hurt him (and) sweat comes out on him and then he finds relief, it is a confusional state due to *ṣētu*.

3.124 DIŠ KA-*šú* KÚR.KÚR-*ir* [*u*] KÚM DIB.DIB-*su u ú-rap-pad ana* U$_4$.3.K[ÁM . . .] (DPS VII B r. 6 = *TDP* 66:62′)

**If his words are unintelligible [and] fever continually afflicts him and he wanders about (and he has been sick) for three days [. . .]

HEADACHE

3.125 DIŠ NA SAG.DU-*su* UD.DA TAB-*ma*[142] <TUKU> SÍG SAG.DU-*šú*/UGU-*šú i-šaḫ-ḫu-uḫ* ZI SAG.KI TUKU.TUKU-*ši*. . . (*BAM* 3 ii 27–28//*BAM* 480 iii 8//*BAM* 9:23–24)[143]

**If a person's head is burned by *ṣētu* so that the hair of his head/scalp falls out (and) he continually experiences pulsating of the temples . . .

CHILLY SENSATIONS/CHILLS

3.126 DIŠ NA MIN *ku-ṣú ḫur-ba-šu* ŠUB.ŠUB-*su ana* TI.BI . . . (*BAM* 66 r. 10′//*AMT* 45/1:6′//*AMT* 14/7:7)[144]

**If (*ṣētu* "gets") a person (and) cold (and) chills keep falling on him, to cure him . . .

RED OR PETECHIAL RASH In the second text, the time of onset of the lesions would have been helpful in interpreting them, but unfortunately the tablet was damaged, and the time was lost in the resulting lacuna.

3.127 DIŠ NA ŠÀ-*šú* GIG-*ma* ŠÀ GÌR.PAD.DU-*šú* SIG$_7$ ŠUB-*a* ŠÀ-*šú* [G]IG.MEŠ DIRI NA.BI UD.DA SÁ.SÁ . . . (*BAM* 575 i 21//*BAM* 52:63–64)

**If a person's stomach is sick, yellow is dotted along his bones, and his abdomen is full of ⸢spots⸣, that person was gotten by *ṣētu* . . .

3.128 DIŠ UD.DA TAB-*su-ma* SU-*šu i-raš-ši-šum-ma e-ki-*[*ik* . . .] *ana* GIG-*su* NU GÍD.DA . . . (DPS XXXI:32′–33′ [AOAT 43.343])

**If *ṣētu* burns him so that his skin is reddish and he scratches [. . . that person has been sick for x days]; in order that his illness not be prolonged . . .

MUSCLE PAIN (MYALGIA)

3.129 ⸢DIŠ⸣ TA *giš-ši-šú* EN ŠU.SI.⸢MEŠ GÌR^{II}-*šú* SA⸣.MEŠ-*šú it-te-nen-ṣi-l*[*a-šú k*]*i*-⸢*iṣ-ṣat*⸣ UD.D[A MU.NI] (DPS XXXIII:102 [AOAT 43.357]; cf. DPS XIV A i 30–31 = *TDP* 130 i 30–31; StBoT 36.48 D 2 obv. 13′)[145]

**If from his hips[146] to his toes, his muscles are continually ⌜sluggish⌝, [it is called] the ⌜gnawing⌝[147] of *ṣētu* (enteric fever).

3.130 DIŠ NA SAG ŠÀ-*šú* DIB.DIB-*su* ŠÀ-*šú* MÚ.MÚ.MEŠ-*ḫu u* IM *e-ri* SA.MEŠ *šá* ⌜MURGU⌝-*šú šad-du* $MURUB_4$.MEŠ-*šú aš-ṭa kin-ṣa-a-šú* KÚ.MEŠ-*šú i-na pa-ni ma-ka-le-e* MÚ.MÚ-*aḫ u i-šá-a*[*q-qa*?] NA.BI *ni-kim-tú* IM *u* UD.DA GIG *la-am ana* GIG *la-az-zi* GUR-*šú* (BM 29254:1–6)

**If a person's epigastrium continually afflicts him, his stomach is continually bloated and he is pregnant with "wind," the muscles of his neck and shoulders are drawn taut, his hips are stiff, his legs continually hurt him, he is bloated before eating, and (his stomach) ⌜rises up⌝ (to vomit), that person is sick with pent-up "wind" and *ṣētu* . . .

ABDOMINAL DISCOMFORT AND BLOATING

3.131 [DIŠ NA NINDA KÚ] KAŠ NAG-*ma* ŠÀ-*šú in-nen-me-er nap-ḫu* A *ma-gal* NAG UD.DA SÁ.SÁ . . . (*AMT* 48/3:8+*AMT* 23/5:7; *AMT* 48/1:7+*AMT* 78/3:4)[148]

**[If a person eats bread] (and) drinks beer and subsequently his stomach is colicky and bloated (and) he drinks a lot of water, *ṣētu* has "gotten" him . . .

INTERNAL FEVER (see Chapter 6 with 6.73–6.80)

3.132 DIŠ NA KÚM ŠÀ TUKU.TUKU-*ši* UD.DA SÁ.SÁ [. . .] (*BAM* 579 i 30)

**If a person continually has internal fever, *ṣētu* has "gotten" him [. . .]

VOMITING, DIARRHEA

3.133 DIŠ GIG ZÉ *ip-ru* UD.DA TAB.BA ŠU DINGIR AD-*šú* (DPS XXIII:1 [AOAT 43.272]//DPS XXII:79 [AOAT 43.257 (catchline)])[149]

**If the patient vomits bile (and) he burns with *ṣētu*, "hand" of his father's god.

3.134 [DIŠ N]A NINDA KÚ KAŠ NAG-*ma* ŠÀ-*šú in-nim-me-ru in-ne-*[*e*]*n-bi-tu re-du-ut ir-ri* TUKU UD.DA SÁ.SÁ . . . (*AMT* 48/1:12′+ *AMT* 78/3:9′; *AMT* 44/6:1–2)

**[If] a ⌜person⌝ eats bread (and) drinks beer and subsequently his stomach is colicky, he has ⌜cramps⌝ (and) he has a "flowing of the bowels," *ṣētu* (enteric fever) has "gotten" him . . .

PNEUMONIA

3.135 [DIŠ N]A GABA-*su* SAG ⌜ŠÀ⌝ MAŠ.SÌLA.MEŠ-*šú* KÚ.MEŠ-*šú* [UD].DA SÁ.SÁ *šum₄-ma ú-ga-na-aḫ* [ḪAR].ME GIG . . . (*CTN* 4.114 r. 7′–9′)[150]

**[If] a ⌜person's⌝ breast, upper abdomen (epigastrium), (and) shoulders continually hurt him, he was "gotten" by *ṣētu*. If he coughs, (he has) sick ⌜lungs⌝ . . .

3.136 DIŠ NA ŠÀ-*šú* NINDA *u* KAŠ *la i-ma-ḫ*[*ar*] KI ÚḪ-*šú* MÚD ŠUB.ŠUB-*a* NA.BI UD.DA SÁ.SÁ *ana* TI-*šú* . . . (*BAM* 174 obv. 28′–29′)[151]

**If a person's insides will not ⌜accept⌝ bread or beer (and) he continually produces blood with his spittle, *ṣētu* has "gotten" that person; to cure him . . .

3.137 DIŠ NA *na-piš* KA-*šú* DUGUD *ṣi-in-*[*na-aḫ*] *ti-ru ḫi-miṭ* UD.[DA . . .] (*SpTU* 1.44:1)

**If a person's breathing is difficult (and) [he has] diarrhea and burning of *ṣētu* [. . .]

NOSE BLEED (EPISTAXIS) Epistaxis is an occasional complication of high fevers, including fevers found with this syndrome.

3.138 DIŠ U$_4$.5.KÁM U$_4$.10.KÁM GIG *dan-na* GIG-*ma uš-tar-di-ma* MÚD *ka-a-an-na* U$_4$.5.KÁM *ina* KIR$_4$-*šú* DU-*ku u ik-ka-la* GIG-*su* DU$_8$-*ár* UD.DA *ḫa-miṭ ba-liṭ* PA NU TUKU (DPS XVI:50′–51′ [AOAT 43.176])[152]

**If he has been sick with a mighty sickness for five or ten days and he remains (sick and now) blood continually flows for five days from his nose but it stops, his illness will let up; he burns with *ṣētu*; he will get well; it is of no consequence.[153]

INTESTINAL HEMORRHAGE

3.139 DIŠ U$_4$-*mi ma-ʾ-du-ti* GIG-*ma* A.MEŠ SA$_5$.MEŠ *ina* DÚR-*šú* DU-*ku* GIG-*su* DU$_8$ UD.DA TAB.BA DIN U$_4$.MEŠ-*šú* GÍD.DA.MEŠ PA NU TUKU (DPS XVI:83′–84′ [AOAT 43.179])[154]

**If he has been sick for a long time and red liquid flows from his anus, his illness will let up. He burns with *ṣētu*; he will get well. His days will be long; it is of no consequence.[155]

PUFFY FACE AND BLOOD VISIBLE IN THE EYES (CONJUNCTIVITIS OR CONJUNCTIVAL HEMORRHAGE)

3.140 DIŠ NA SAG.DU-*su* UD.DA TAB-*ma u* SU-*šú* KÚ-*šú* SAG.DU-*su nu-pu-uḫ* . . . (*BAM* 481 obv. 6′//*BAM* 480 iii 17)[156]

**If *ṣētu* burns a person's head and his body hurts him (and) his head is swollen . . .

3.141 [DIŠ NA U]GU-*šú* UD.DA TAB-*ma* [IGI^{II}-*šú i-bar-r*]*u-ra ù* MÚD DIRI-*a* . . . (*BAM* 480 ii 21)[157]

**[If a person]'s ⌜skull⌝ is burned by *ṣētu* so that [his eyes] ⌜become dimmed⌝ and look full of blood . . .

The references below list not only the patient's signs and symptoms, but the day that they appeared during the course of the disease. The fact that the *āšipu* took the trouble to note the course of the illness suggests that he considered this information valuable in understanding the nature of the disease. It also indicates that the ancient Mesopotamian physician was a sophisticated and insightful observer. The first two texts below describe the early phase of the infection, characterized by a frontal headache.

3.142 DIŠ U$_4$.1.KÁM GIG-*ma* SAG.DU-*su* KÚ-*šú* UD.DA TAB.BA ŠU DINGIR AD.A.NI DIN GAM (DPS XVI:1 [AOAT 43.171/172]; cf. DPS XV:93 [AOAT 43.155]; catchline)

**If it is the first day he is sick and his head hurts him, he burns with *ṣētu* (or) "hand" of his father's god; he will get well or die.

3.143 DIŠ *ina taš-rit* GIG-*šú* ⌜SAG.KI^{II}⌝-*šú um-ma*⌜*ub*⌝-*la-nim-ma* EGIR KÚM *u* IR *it-tab-la-ni* LÍL-*ti* UD.DA U$_4$.2.KÁM U$_4$.3.KÁM LÍL-*ma* DIN (DPS XVII:8–9 [AOAT 43.195])

**If at the beginning of his illness his temples produce heat so that afterward it has brought fever and sweat, an illness of *ṣētu* of two days; (if) he is ill for three days, he will get well.[158]

The following texts describe the course of the fever and the associated bleeding. The patient's temperature was observed to rise over the course of the first two weeks (with "chills" at day 3 and "burning fever" by day 14). Nosebleeds were observed to occur during that interval.

3.144 [DIŠ NA UD.DA TAB-*s*]*u-ma ina* U$_4$-*mi-šú-ma* ŠED$_7$ NA BI U$_4$.3.KAM GIG [*ana* GIG-*su*] NU GÍD.DA . . . (DPS XXXI:1–2 [AOAT 43.342])

**[If *ṣētu* burns a person] (and) on the day (you see the patient), he has chills, that person has been sick for three days; [in order that] ⌜his⌝ [illness] not be prolonged . . .

3.145 DIŠ NA MIN SAG.KI.MEŠ [ZI.ZI]-*bi* NA.BI 6 U$_4$.MEŠ GIG *ana* GIG-*šu* NU GÍD.DA . . . (*BAM* 66 obv. 13–14)

**If (*ṣētu* "gets") a person (and) his temples [(continually feel like they)] are ⌜pulsating⌝, that person has been sick for six days; in order for his illness not to be prolonged . . .

3.146 [DIŠ KI.MIN MÚD] *ina* KIR$_4$-*šú ina* U$_4$-*mi-šú-ma uš-tar-ru-nim-ma* DU-⌜*ku*⌝ NA BI ⌜U$_4$.7.K[ÁM] GIG⌝ [*ana* GIG-*s*]*u* NU GÍD.DA . . . (DPS XXXI:3–4 [AOAT 43.342])

**[If (*ṣētu* burns a person)] (and) on the same day [blood] continually begins to flow from his nose, that person has been sick for seven days; [in order for] ⌜his⌝ [illness] not to be prolonged . . .

3.147 DIŠ KI.MIN *i-tar-rak i-sa-kip-šú u* KÚM *ṣar-ḫa* TUKU-*ši* NA BI U$_4$.14.KÁM GIG *ana* GIG-*su* NU GÍD.DA . . . (DPS XXXI:6–7 [AOAT 43.342])[159]

**If (*ṣētu* burns a person and) it throbs (and) knocks him down and he has a burning fever, that person has been sick for fourteen days; in order for his illness not to be prolonged . . .

By the third week, the fever has stabilized into a regular pattern, and the patient is flushed and groaning.

3.148 DIŠ KI.MIN U$_4$-*mi-šam-ma ana* GIZKIM-*šú i-ḫi-iṭ-*[*a-áš-šú u ú-maš-šar-šú*] *e-nu-ma i-ḫi-iṭ-ṭa-áš-šú* KÚM *ṣar-ḫa* [TUKU-*ši* SA.MEŠ-*šú* KÚ.MEŠ-*šú*][160] IR ŠUB-*su-ma ina-aḫ* NA BI U$_4$.21.K[ÁM GIG *ana* GIG.BI NU GÍD.DA] . . . (DPS XXXI:35′–37′ [AOAT 43.343])

**If (*ṣētu* burns a person and) daily, at the expected time, it comes [over him and leaves him] (and) when it comes over him, [he has] burning fever [and his muscles continually hurt him] (and) sweat comes out on him and then he finds relief, that person [has been sick] for twenty-one days; [in order for his illness not to be prolonged] . . .

3.149 [DIŠ K]I.MIN *pa-nu-šu* GIN$_7$ *šá* KAŠ NAG *ma-gal* S[A$_5$ . . .] GIG NA BI GIG U$_4$.21 GIG *ana* G[IG-*su* NU GÍD.DA] . . . (DPS XXXI:25′–26′ [AOAT 43.343])

**[If ⸢(*ṣētu* "gets" a person and)⸣ his face is very ⸢red⸣[161] like one who drinks beer [. . .] that person is sick with an illness of twenty-one days; in order for [his] ⸢illness⸣ [not to be prolonged] . . .

3.150 DIŠ KI.MIN *ka-la* U_4-*mi u* GI_6 *i*-⸢*le*⸣-*eb-bu* NA.BI U_4.21.KÁM GIG *ana* GIG-*su* NU GÍD.DA . . . (DPS XXXI:50′–51′ [AOAT 43.344])

**If (*ṣētu* burns him and) he groans all day and all night, that person has been sick for twenty-one days; in order for his illness not to be prolonged . . .

In the texts below the patients have been feverish for long periods of time (twenty-five days to a month), and there are signs that they are beginning to recover. Their temperatures have begun to return to normal and they are beginning to have a return of appetite. There are still some serious complications that can occur. In the case of typhoid fever, patients may have late-onset bleeding from the lower small intestine. This is usually manifested by rectal bleeding (see the first reference below), and can be fatal. The *āšipu*'s choice of the verb *to flow* to describe the bleeding indicates a quantity larger than a "drip" but less copious than would be indicated by "pouring out."

3.151 DIŠ U_4-*mi ma-ʾ-du-ti* GIG-*ma* A.MEŠ SA_5.MEŠ *ina* DÚR-*šú* DU-*ku* GIG-*su* DU_8 UD.DA TAB.BA DIN U_4.MEŠ-*šú* GÍD.DA.MEŠ PA NU TUKU (DPS XVI:83′–84′ [AOAT 43.179])[162]

**If he has been sick for a long time and red liquid flows from his anus, his illness will let up. He burns with *ṣētu*; he will get well. His days will be long; it is of no consequence.[163]

3.152 [DIŠ KI].⸢MIN *za*⸣-*mar* KÚM-*em za-mar* $ŠED_7$ *li-ʾ-ba* TUKU-*ši u* IR NU TUKU NA.BI ITI.1.KÁM GIG *ana* GIG-*šu* NU GÍD.DA . . . (DPS XXXI:12–13 [AOAT 43.342]; cf. *BAM* 66 obv. 10–11)

**[If (*ṣētu* burns him)] (and) sometimes he is hot, sometimes he is cold, he has *liʾbu* but he does not have sweat, that person has been sick for a month; in order for his illness not to be prolonged . . .

3.153 ⸢DIŠ KI⸣.MIN *ka-la* U_4-*mi u* GI_6 *i-le-eb-bu-ma la i-ṣal-lal* [NINDA] *u* KAŠ (coll.) *la i-maḫ-ḫar* GURUN KÚ *u* A NAG NA BI ITI.1.KÁM GIG [*ana*] GIG-*su* NU GÍD.DA . . . (DPS XXXI:52′–54′ [AOAT 43.344])

**If (*ṣētu* burns him and) groans all day and all night so that he cannot sleep, (his insides) do not accept [bread] and beer (but) he can eat fruit and drink water, that person has been sick for a month; in order for his illness not to be prolonged . . .

The texts below could be describing cases of typhoid fever relapse.

3.154 [DIŠ KI.MIN NINDA] ⸢*u*⸣ [K]AŠ *la i-maḫ-*[*ḫar ḫ*]*i-ši-iḫ-ti* (coll.) ŠÀ TUKU-*ma* NU [. . . N]A.BI U_4.44.KÁM G[IG *ana* GI]G-*su* NU GÍD.DA . . . (DPS XXXI:46′–47′ [AOAT 43.344])

**[If (*ṣētu* burns him and)] (his insides) will not ⸢accept⸣ [bread or] ⸢beer⸣, he has (food) ⸢cravings⸣ but then does not [. . . that] ⸢person⸣ has been ⸢sick⸣ for forty-four days; [in order for] his ⸢illness⸣ not to be prolonged . . .

3.155 DIŠ NA MIN U_4.1.KÁM GIG U_4.1.KÁM TI NA.BI 50 U_4.MEŠ [G]IG *ana* GIG-*šu* NU GÍD.D[A] . . . (*BAM* 66 obv. 17–20)

**If (*ṣētu* "gets") a person (and) he is sick one day and well one day, that person has been ⌜sick⌝ for fifty days; in order for his illness not to be prolonged . . .

3.156 [DIŠ KI.MIN . . .] -*ši ma-gal ra-ʾi-ba* TUKU-*ši* [. . . NA BI U_4].52.KÁM GIG *ana* GIG-*su* [N]U GÍD.D[A] . . . (DPS XXXI:43′–44′ [AOAT 43.344])

**[If (*ṣētu* burns him and) . . .] (and) he has a lot of trembling [. . . that person] has been sick for fifty-two [days]; in order for his illness ⌜not⌝ to be prolonged . . .

DIʾU

Another syndrome, *diʾu*, is closely linked to *ṣētu*,[164] and would also be classified as enteric fever by modern physicians.[165] The use of the Sumerogram SAG.GIG "sick head" for *diʾu* indicates that this typically started out with a sudden, very intense headache,[166] presumably due to an extremely rapid rise in temperature at the onset of the illness.

FEVER

3.157 *di-ʾu* NAM.[ÉRIM . . .] ÉN *ḫu-un-ṭ*[*i* . . .] IR *um-ma* me [. . .] (K 11758:5′–7′)

***diʾu* (or) ⌜curse⌝ [. . .] Recitation: "Burning [. . .] sweat, fever [. . .]

SHAKING CHILLS (RIGORS)

3.158 DIŠ *ú-ta-at-tal u im-ta-nag-ga-ag ina di-ʾi* TAG-*it* (DPS XXII:67 [AOAT 43.256])

**If he continually lays himself down[167] and he continually becomes rigid, he was "touched" by *diʾu*.

CHILLY SENSATIONS/CHILLS

3.159 *di-ʾu šu-ru-up-pu-ú ki-ma šá-a-ri ana šú-a-tú it-taš-kin* . . . (*SpTU* 2.2:58–59, cf. 165 [bilingual])

***diʾu* (and) ice cold have been placed on that one as (by) a wind . . .

3.160 *di-i šu-ru-up-pu-ú šá ina zu-mur-šú li-né-siḫ* . . . (*SpTU* 3.65 r. 12)

**Let the *diʾu* (with) ice cold that is in his body be removed . . .

ABDOMINAL DISCOMFORT AND BLOATING; MYALGIAS

3.161 DIŠ NA ŠÀ.MEŠ-*šú* MÚ.MEŠ-*ḫu ir-ru-šú i-ár-ru-ru* IGI.MEŠ-*šú* NIGIN.MEŠ-*du* [SA].MEŠ-*šú tab-ka-ma* TA! GÌR^{II}-*šu* <EN> MURUB$_4$.MEŠ-*šú* ZI-*ma kin-ṣa-a-šú* KÚ.MEŠ-*šú* [*mim-ma*] KÚ *u* NAG UGU-*šú* NU DU-*ak* NA BI GIG *di-ʾu* GIG ⌜*šum-ma*⌝ NA BI TI.LA *ḫa-ši-iḫ ana* TI-*šú* . . . (*BAM* 106 obv. 1–4//*BAM* 108 r. 2′–8′//*AMT* 39/4 r. 3′–5′//*BAM* 52:101; BM 42298:23–25 [Finkel, *Fs. Lambert* 181])

**If a person's insides are continually bloated, his intestines rumble, his face seems continually to spin, his [blood vessels] are tense and pulsate from his feet <to> his hip region and consequently his legs continually hurt him, (and) [whatever] he eats and drinks does not agree with him, that person is sick with *di'u*; if that person wants to live, to cure him . . .

LOSS OF APPETITE

3.162 DIŠ GIG-*ma ina* GIG-*šú* GIN$_7$ *šá* DIN-*šú* KI DAM-*šú* DUMU-*šú* DUMU.MUNUS-*šú* SIG$_5$-*iš i-ta-mu* NINDA NU KÚ *di-ḫu* D[IN] (DPS XVII:41–42 [AOAT 43.199]; cf. Labat, *Syria* 33.121–126 obv. 15)

**If he is sick and, during his sickness, he speaks in a friendly way with his wife, son, (and) daughter just as if he were feeling well (but) he does not eat bread, it is *di'u*; he will get ⌜well⌝.

In texts of differential diagnosis, *di'u* and *ṣētu* are often compared.

3.163 DIŠ *ina taš-rit* GIG-*šú* TA TAG-*šú* ⌜EN *ik*⌝-*lu-ú* 1-*is-su* KÚM 1-*is-su* ŠED$_7$ *a-ḫu ma-la a-ḫi* TUKU.MEŠ-*ši* EGIR KÚM *u* IR *ip-ṭú-ru* UB.NÍGIN.NA-*šú um-ma ub-la-nim-ma um-ma ma-la um-mi maḫ-ri-i ir-ši-ma ip-ta-ṭar* EGIR-*nu* ŠED$_7$ *u* IR *ir-ta-ši di-ḫu e-ri-bu wa-ṣu-u* UD.DA TAB.BA U$_4$.7.KÁM LÍL-*ma* DIN (DPS XVII.4–7 [AOAT 43.195])

**If at the beginning of his illness from the time it "touches" him until it stops, he continually has now fever, now chills in equal proportions (and) after the fever and sweat have left, his limbs produce heat so that he has a fever to the same degree as the previous fever and it leaves (and) afterward he has chills and sweat, it is *di'u* coming in and going out (or) he burns with *ṣētu*; (if) he is ill for seven days, he will get well.[168]

3.164 DIŠ TA *šèr-ti* EN *le-lá-a-ti di-ḫu ina* ZU-*šú ú-šar-r*[*i*]-*ma* LÍL-*ti* ŠÀ *ir-ta-ši ir-ra-šú i-te-šír ina* KA-*šú ig-de-šá-a ina* DÚR-*šú uš-te-ši-ra* TAG-*ti* UD.DA *šá ina mi-ni-a-ti-šú la rak-sat* GIG.BI LÍL-*ti* U$_4$.1.KÁM / DIŠ *uq-ta-ta*$_5$ *ina šèr-ti* GIG-*ma* ŠU^{II}-*šú i-nap-pa-aṣ* GÌR^{II}-*šú* KÚM-*ma* GIG-*su* KI.TA E$_{11}$-*šú* DU-*ak* (DPS XVII:100–105 [AOAT 43.205])

**If from morning until evening, *di'u* starts in his body so that he gets an illness of the stomach (and when) his bowels move, he belches from his mouth and emits (wind) from his anus, "touch" of *ṣētu* which is not (yet) bound to his limbs; his sickness is an illness of a day. If it (seems to) have finished,[169] (but) on the (next) morning, he is so sick that his hands thrash around (and) his feet are hot, his sickness is going down and up on him.

We analyzed and compared all of the references that use these terms in order to understand what factors were important to the Mesopotamian physician in establishing these two syndromes. The differences seem to relate to conditions that lead to dehydration,[170] namely, very high temperatures, sweating, diarrhea and vomiting, as well as the signs of dehydration, which include thirst, dry lips, reduced urine volume, and dark yellow (concentrated) urine. All of the above are found in patients with *ṣētu* and are generally lacking in patients with *di'u*.

THIRST OR DRY LIPS

3.165 [DIŠ NA *it-t*]*a-na-ša-aš a-šu-uš-*tu_4 ŠUB.ŠUB-*su di-ḫu* UD.DA (coll.) TAG.TAG-*su* ÚḪ-*šú ma-a-d*[*a di-ḫu*] [A *ma-gal*] NAG UD.DA SÁ.SÁ . . . (*AMT* 48/3:6–7+*AMT* 23/5:5–6)[171]

**[If a person's (stomach)] is ⌜continually⌝ upset (and) depression continually falls on him, *diʾu* or *ṣētu* continually "touches" him. (If) he has plenty of saliva, [*diʾu*; (if)] he drinks [a lot of water], *ṣētu* has "gotten" him . . .

3.166 DIŠ NA <*it*>*-ta-na-ša-aš a-šu-uš-tú* ŠU[B.ŠUB]-*su* NUNDUN.MEŠ-*šú i-ta-na-*[*ba-l*]*a* [A.MEŠ] *ma-gal* NAG UD.DA SÁ.S[Á] . . . (*BAM* 174 obv. 25′–26′)

**If a person's (stomach) is continually upset (and) depression ⌜continually falls⌝ on him, his lips continually get ⌜dry⌝ (and) he drinks a lot [of water], *ṣētu* has "gotten" him . . .

REDUCED URINE VOLUME OR CONCENTRATED URINE

3.167 DIŠ NA NINDA KÚ KAŠ NAG-*ma* ŠÀ.ME-*šú in-nem-me-ru* KÀŠ.[MEŠ]-*šú* DIB.DIB-*at* UD.DA SÁ.SÁ . . . (*AMT* 48/1:10+*AMT* 78/3:7)[172]

**If a person eats bread (and) drinks beer and subsequently his stomach is colicky (and) his urine is continually held in, *ṣētu* has "gotten" him . . .

3.168 DIŠ KÀŠ.MEŠ-*šú* SIG$_7$.MEŠ GIG-*su* GÍD KI.MIN UD.DA TAB-*iṭ* GAM (DPS XIV A ii 40 = *TDP* 136 ii 40)[173]

**If his urine is (dark) yellow, his illness will be prolonged. Alternatively, he burns with *ṣētu*; he will die.

Modern physicians do not subdivide enteric fever by the presence or absence of dehydration. Ancient Mesopotamian physicians, however, must have found this differentiation useful. Whether they clearly understood that patients with *ṣētu* lacked water can only be a matter of speculation.

The text below describes symptoms that look quite compatible with urinary tract infection to which the *āšipu* attached the diagnosis of *ṣētu*. This suggests that they either included urinary tract infection under the diagnosis of *ṣētu* or that this and similar references may represent true enteric fever complicated by urinary tract infections. A complicating urinary tract infection would be more likely in an area where *Schistosomiasis hematobium* infection with associated kidney stones was common (see Chapter 5).

3.169 [DIŠ NA *ṣi*]*-ri-iḫ-ti* ŠÀ TUKU*-ma* ⌜GÌŠ⌝ KÚM *ú-kal mi-n*[*a-tu-šú* DUB GABA-*su i-ka-sa-su*] NA BI UD.DA *ḫa-miṭ ana* DIN-*šú* . . . (BM 78963:1–2)[174]

**[If a person has] ⌜burning⌝ internal fever and his penis is gripped by fever and his ⌜limbs⌝ [are tense and his breast gnaws at him], that person burns with *ṣētu*, to cure him . . .

Wound and Soft Tissue Infections (*Samānu* and Related Conditions)

Soft tissue infections refer to muscle, skin, and surrounding tissue, exclusive of bone, which becomes infected usually because of some wound or disruption of the protective barrier of skin. When only the skin and the adjacent subcutaneous tissue is infected, it is referred to as cellulitis. If bone is near the soft tissue infection, it may become secondarily infected, in which case it is called osteomyelitis.

Injuries to a finger or toe can result in loss of a nail, as is described in the following reference. Infection can also cause nail loss, although this is less common.

3.170 DIŠ NA UMBIN-*šú lu na-da-at* . . . (*AMT* 100/3 r. 7, 11, cf. r. 4)

**If a person's nail either falls off or . . .

In addition to work-related injuries, ancient Mesopotamian societies were frequently at war, producing wounds in large numbers. Physicians' experience with infected war wounds must have been extensive, and they undoubtedly recognized similar signs and symptoms when soft tissue infections occurred in the absence of a preceding wound. The *āšipu* also described many neurologic complications of war wounds, for which see Chapter 13.[175]

Soldiers attempted to prevent the development of wound infections by treating their wounds themselves on the field of battle. In the following reference, which is a curse, a soldier who has broken his oath is imagined as finding himself in battle with none of the usual medicaments available. A modern equivalent curse might be "When you cut yourself, may there be no cleansing solution to put on the wound!"

3.171 *ki-i* LÚ.KUR-*ku-nu ú-pa-ta-ḫu-ka-nu-ni* LÀL Ì.MEŠ *zi-in-za-ru-ʾu* MÚD ^{GIŠ}ERIN *ana šá-kan pi-it-ḫi-ku-nu li-iḫ-liq* (Parpola and Watanabe, SAA 2 no. 6:643–645)

**When your enemy stabs you, may there be a dearth of honey, oil, ginger, and cedar resin to put on your stab wounds!

Samānu, as indicated in the reference below, is the Akkadian term for soft tissue infections.[176] Important signs and symptoms of wounds or soft tissue infections include fever, pain, local temperature changes, changes in the appearance of the surrounding skin and tissues, and, in some infections, a bad odor.

3.172 DIŠ GIG GAR-*šú* SA_5 *e-em* MÚ-*iḫ u* DU-*ak sa-ma-nu* [MU.NI] (DPS XXXIII:23 [AOAT 43.354])[177]

**If the nature of the sore is that it is red, hot, swollen, and flows, [it is called] *samānu.*

The local heat described above is due to vasodilitation caused by the wound infection, but generalized fever would also commonly be present, as in the following example.

3.173 DIŠ GIG GAR-*šú* SA_5 LÚ KÚM.KÚM-*im u i-ta-nar-rù sa-ma-nu* [MU.NI] (DPS XXXIII:24 [AOAT 43.354])

**If the nature of the sore is that it is red (and) the person is continually feverish and continually vomits, [it is called] *samānu.*

Abnormal appearance of the skin and tissues within the wound include redness (erythema), blanching or paleness of the tissues due to poor circulation, dark red or dusky color that often precedes necrosis with a resulting black color, and wound secretions of varying color including white, yellow, green, black, and bloody.

3.174 DIŠ NA SAG.⌜DU-*su*⌝ *sa-ma-nu* DIB-*it i-raš-ši-šum-ma i-na-saḫ i-na-aḫ* ⌜EGIR⌝-*nu* (coll.) GAL-*bi* . . . (*BAM* 494 i 35′)[178]

**If *samānu* afflicts a person's head (and) it is reddish (and) it retracts and calms down (but) afterward it increases (again) . . .

3.175 DIŠ NA *sa-ma-nu lu-ú* SA$_5$ *lu-ú* GI$_6$ *lu-ú* SIG$_7$ *lu-ú* [BABBAR] *lu-ú ṣi-tu lu-ú mi-ḫi-iṣ* ^{GIŠ}IGI.KAK *it-tab-*[*ši*] . . . *šum-ma* MÚD *u* MÚD.BABBAR ŠUB.MEŠ . . . (*BAM* 409 obv. 11′–12′, 16′)[179]

**If there is (for) a person either red *samānu* or black or yellow/green or [white] or wheals (see Chapter 10) or prick from a thorn . . . If it continually produces blood and pus . . .

3.176 DIŠ GIG GAR-*šú* GIN$_7$ *ṣe-e-tim-ma sa-ḫi-ip ina sa-ḫi-pi-šú* IGI.MEŠ-*šú* GI$_6$ ŠUB-*ú gal-lu-ú* MU.NI (DPS XXXIII:56 [AOAT 43.356]//K 3526 r. 6–7)

**If the nature of the sore is that it is like a growth and it is coated and in its coating, the entire surface is unevenly colored with black, it is called "the ghoul."

3.177 [DIŠ GIG GAR-*šú* SA$_5$ BAB]BAR MÚD.BABBAR È-*ma* x [. . .] *šàḫ-šàḫ-ḫu* MU.NI (DPS XXXIII:58 [AOAT 43.356]; cf. *BAM* 580 iii 31′)

**[If the nature of the sore is that it is red] (or) ⌜white⌝ (and) produces pus [. . .], it is called "the slanderer."

Wound secretions also vary in consistency from thick pus to thin serum. In general, the early fluid tends to be thin, and then, as the white blood cells increase in number, the fluid becomes thicker and either white or green in color.

3.178 [DIŠ GIG GAR-*šú*] *ina* ŠÀ-*šú* GIN$_7$ A *šur*!*-de-e-tu*$_4$ DU.MEŠ GI[G *l*]*a-az-za* [. . . MU.N]I (DPS XXXIII:50 [AOAT 43.355])

**[If the nature of the sore] is that what looks like canal overflow water flows from inside it (and it is) a ⌜persistent sore, it⌝ [is called . . .].

3.179 *šum*$_4$*-ma* GIG *im-šid-ma* SA.MEŠ-*šú* A.MEŠ *ú-šal-la-ku* . . . (*BAM* 32:5′//*BAM* 417 obv. 4)

**If he was stricken with a sore and his blood vessels make liquid flow (out of it) . . .[180]

The following recitations against *samānu* describe it as being dressed in garments of lapis, presumably a reference to the greenish color of the serum. Also mentioned are typical locations where *samānu* occurs and the fact that *di'u* (see above) may follow in *samānu*'s train. Staphylococcal infections of the skin commonly occur on the thighs and produce carbuncles on the back of the neck and upper part of the back which may be accompanied by fever and prostration as well as by bacteria invading the bloodstream (bacteremia).[181]

3.180 ÉN É.NU.RU *sa-ma-⌜nu⌝ ḫa-lip sa-an-ti la-biš lu-bu-ši ša* NA_4.ZA.GÌN . . . (Finkel, *Fs. Borger* 94–96:1–2)

***Samānu*, wrapped in scarlet, clad in garments of lapis . . .

3.181 KI.SIKIL.LÁ GABA ŠÚ.BA.GIN_7 GURUŠ GÚ ŠÚ.BA.GIN_7 ANŠE x ÉRIN.BA ŠÚ.BA GU_4 Á.GUR_7.BA ŠÚ.BA . . . (6 NT 145 [Finkel, *Fs. Borger* 76–78]:14–17)

**Because you have fallen on the breast of the young woman, on the neck of the young man, on the yoke of the donkey, on the thick shoulders of the ox . . .

3.182 *sa-ma-nu iš-tu šá-de-e ur-da sa-ma-nu na-a-ri e-te-bir sa-ma-nu di-ʾu a-na ni-ši ṣal-mat qaq-qa-di ki-ma me-e na-a-ri id-di-i al-pu ina qar-ni-šú iṣ-bat im-me-ru ina ṣu-up-ri-šú iṣ-bat eṭ-lu ina [š]ap-ri-šú i[ṣ-bat] ár-da-ta ina ši-ti-iq ir-ti-šá i[ṣ-bat] šer-ru e-niq ši-iz-bi ina la-[ba-ni-šú]*[182] *iṣ-bat* (Finkel, *Fs. Borger* 87–92:9–17)

***Samānu* came down from the mountains; *samānu* crossed the river. *Samānu* poured *diʾu* like water down over the black-headed people. It afflicted the ox on his horn, the donkey on his hoof, the young man on his thigh, the young woman on her breastbone, the suckling infant on the muscles of his neck.

The following reference does not describe the changes in the appearance of the patient's "flesh," but it clearly indicates that it is getting progressively worse. It is likely that it started with redness, and eventually became black (necrotic) with drainage of pus. Incidentally, the wound in this case appears to involve the severing of the Achilles tendon, a term that would not have been used by the Mesopotamian physician since the story of Achilles and his mortal heel is a Greek cultural artifact. For other possible references to tissue necrosis, see Chapter 10.

3.183 [DIŠ N]A *[t]u-ḫar eq-bi-šu ka-bíl* IGI UZU.MEŠ-*šú* KÚR.KÚR GIG [. . . G]A DUGUD . . . (*BAM* 124 i 50–51)

**[If a person]'s Achilles tendon[183] is immobilized (and) his flesh looks worse and worse, the illness [. . .] is difficult . . .

There are references to wounds that "stink," and we can be fairly certain that these wounds were infected with anaerobic organisms (ones that thrive and multiply only in the absence of oxygen). Anaerobic wound infections are common when the local blood supply is compromised and the wound is heavily contaminated with soil, a frequent situation in war wounds. Other types of wound infections may have odors, some of which are less than pleasant, but anaerobic infections truly are putrid with a stink of a feculant nature.

3.184 DIŠ NA *ni-ip-še* GIG [. . .] (*BAM* 268 iii 3′)

**If a person is sick with stink [. . .]

3.185 DIŠ NA KA.È GIG : *ni-ip-šú šá sim-me* (Uruanna IV i 4)[184]

**If a person is sick with stink, (that means) stink said of a wound.

Pus is often produced in soft tissue infections, typically collecting in abscesses that "point" (superficial whitening and outpouching) just prior to spontaneous drainage of the pus.[185] In the following reference, we believe that "bird *ḫindūru*" refers to the "pointing" abscess, comparing it to some feature of a bird's anatomy such as a cockspur.

3.186 *šum*$_4$*-ma* GIG *ḫi-dúr* MUŠEN ŠUB-*ma* IGI GIG *ṣa-bit* . . . (*BAM* 32:7′//*BAM* 417 obv. 6)[186]

**If a sore produces a "bird *ḫindūru*" and it takes up a position on top of the sore . . .

Just prior to pointing, as the abscess fills with pus the tissue becomes tense with the fluid. The physician in the reference below provides an imaginative comparison of an abscess filling with pus to a leech attached to a human or animal as it fills, expands, and becomes distended with blood.

3.187 [DIŠ N]A GIG GIN$_7$ *il-qí ú-ma-gag* . . . (*AMT* 16/5 ii 9)

**[If] a ⸢person⸣('s) sore stiffens like a leech . . .

The following quotes provide both a very clear indication of the *āšipu*'s understanding of the evolution of wound abscesses and also his knowledge of the value of heat to localize and quicken the development of the abscess and the importance of surgical drainage in curing the infection. It is also evident that the *āšipu* knew that it was important to keep the wound clean with frequent dressing changes and to use oil to keep the dressings from sticking.

3.188 DIŠ NA UGU-*šú* A ⸢*ú*⸣-[*kal*] ŠU.SI-*ka* GAL-*ti a-šar* A.MEŠ *ú-kal-lu* TAG.TAG-*at šum-ma* UZU.GIŠ-*šú bi-*ʾ*-ša*[*t* [A.MEŠ *šá gul-gu*]*l-li-šú it-tar-du* BAD-*ma gul-gul-la-šú te-ser-rim* A *ša gul-gul-li-šú t*[*u-bal* ^{TÚG}GADA A L]UḪ-*si* Ì.GIŠ SUD *ana* UGU GIG GAR-*an* KU.KU ^{GIŠ}KÍN ŠÈ BÁḪAR SÚD *ana* UGU GIG [GAR-*an* . . .] x ^{TÚG}GADA A LUḪ-*si* Ì.GIŠ SUD *ana* UGU GIG GAR-*an* ^{TÚG}*na-al-ti-ip-ti* [. . . U$_4$].2.KÁM LAL DU$_8$-*ma* ^{TÚG}GADA A LUḪ-*si* Ì.GIŠ SUD *ana* UGU GIG GAR-*an* [. . .] x GAZI^{SAR} BÍL-*ti* KI ZÌ.ŠE.SA.A ḪI.ḪI *ana* UGU GIG MAR U$_4$.1.KÁM LAL DU$_8$-*ma* [. . .^{Š}]^{EM}LI GAZ KI ZÌ.KUM ḪI.ḪI *ina* A GAZI^{SAR} ŠID-*aš* LAL IGI GIG *tu-gal-lab* EN TI.LA LÁL [. . .] x *šum*$_4$*-ma* TAG-*ma* UZU.GIŠ-*šú la bi-*ʾ*-šat ana li-mit* SAG.DU-*šú* IZI NA$_4$.MEŠ GAR-*an* (*BAM* 480 iii 57–64)

**If a man's scalp ⸢contains⸣ liquid, you continually touch the place where it contains liquid with your thumb. If his ear[187] stinks, [liquid] has come down [from his] ⸢skull⸣. You open up and make an incision in his skull. You [dry up] the liquid of his skull. You ⸢wash⸣ [a linen cloth with water]. You sprinkle (it) with oil (and) put it on the wound. You grind powdered *kiškanû* and potter's grog. [You put] (it) on the wound [. . .] You wash a linen cloth with water. You sprinkle (it) with oil (and) put (it) on the wound. You [. . .] a *naltiptu*-bandage (and) bandage (him) for two days. You take (it) off and you wash a linen cloth with water. You sprinkle (it) with oil (and) put (it) on the wound [. . .] You mix roasted *kasû* with roasted grain flour (and) daub it on the wound. You bandage (him) for one day. You take it off and [. . .] You crush *burāšu*. You mix (it) with *isqūqu*-flour. You make it into a dough with *kasû* juice (and) bandage (him with it). You shave the surface of the wound. You bandage him until he recovers [. . .] If you touch (the place where it contains liquid) and his ear does not stink, you put red-hot coals around his head (to ripen the abscess).

3.189 DIŠ NA *a-bu-ut-ta-šú* A *ú-kal*... U$_4$.7.KÁM LAL *ina* U$_4$.8.KÁM *ab-bu-ut-ta-šú* 3-*šú te-*[*ser-rim ka-a*]-*na-am* LÁL (*BAM* 480 iv 6–7)

**If a person's forelock area contains liquid . . . you bandage it for seven days. On the eighth day, you [make] three [incisions] in his forelock area. You ⌜continually⌝ bandage (the wound).

3.190 DIŠ NA SAG.DU-*su* A.MEŠ DIB-*al* <MURUB$_4$ SAG.DU-*šú* SAG.KI^{II}-*šú* TAG.MEŠ-*šú*> UGU *da-da-ni-šú ti-ik-ki-šú* DÈ GAR-*ma* A-*šú ub-bal* (*BAM* 3 ii 7–8//*BAM* 480 iv 5)[188]

**If a person's head contains liquid <(and) the middle of his head (and) his temples continually hurt him intensely> you put embers over the muscles on the back of his neck and it will dry up his liquid.[189]

Some wound infections were not rapidly fatal, but could become chronic problems requiring long-term care.

3.191 *šum$_4$-ma ina* ŠÀ KEŠDA *maḫ-re-e la iš-ta-qu-*[*ú*] KEŠDA GAR-*na-ma* LAL-*su ina* ŠÀ KEŠDA MÚD.BABBAR-*ma* GAR ŠÀ-*bi-šú*... (*AMT* 16/5 ii 4–5)

**If (the sore) has not risen during the previous bindings (or if when) the bindings are put on and bandaged on, during the binding, there is still pus inside it (after forty-five days of bandaging) . . .

Some wounds did not seem to respond to standard treatments. In the two texts below, a *midru* could be any infection of the skin and deeper soft tissues that has caused inflammation but has not produced an abscess with pus.

3.192 DIŠ GIG GAR-*šú da-an* TAB x-*ma ina* IGI-*ka la i-na-aš mid-ru*[190] KI.MIN *sa-ma-nu* [MU.NI] (DPS XXXIII:25 [AOAT 43.354])[191]

**If the nature of the sore is that it is hard, it burns [...] and does not respond to (your treatment), [it is called] a *midru* (or) alternatively *samānu* (cellulitis).

3.193 Ú GIG *mi-id-ri*... (*CT* 14.43 [S. 60]:3′–4′; *BAM* 380:6–7//*STT* 92 iii 21′–22′)

**Plant for *midru*-sore . . .

Other wounds appeared to heal, only to have later complications. In the case described below, the wound may have been contaminated with fungal spores that led to a slowly evolving fungal infection after the initial apparent wound healing. The fungal infection, chromoblastomycosis, is the likely cause of the black dots described below.[192]

3.194 GIG-*šú ib-lu-uṭ-ma* IGI GIG-*šú* GI$_6$ ŠUB-*ú*... (*BAM* 32:16′//*CTN* 4.116 obv. 16)[193]

**If his sore heals and subsequently the surface of his sore is dotted with black . . .

TETANUS (*ŠAŠŠAṬU*)[194]

In the quotes below, ancient physicians applied the term *šaššaṭu*[195] to patients with muscle jerking, spasms, and rigidity.[196] Tetanus was almost certainly a common problem given the absence of tetanus vaccine and the tendency of workers to go barefoot in fields that must have been heavily contaminated with tetanus spores. Although the references do not mention the wound infection that normally precedes tetanus, these wounds can be small and might have been overlooked. Tetanus is caused by a neurotoxin produced by the bacterium *Clostridium tetanus*. It leads to uncontrollable muscle spasms that may occur spontaneously or be triggered by sudden noises or lights. Tetanus is often fatal, but milder cases may gradually resolve with or without treatment.

3.195 *šá* LÚ *šu-a-tú meš-re-ti-šú šá-áš-šá-ṭu iṣ-ṣa-bat ki-ma ṣe-ri šá qaq-qa-su a*! *-me*! *-lu*! *i-te-eṭ-ṭi a-kal ṭa-a-bi ul ik-ka-lu* A.MEŠ *ṭa-bu-ti ul i-šat-ti šit-tú ṭa-ab-tu*$_4$ *ul i-ṣal-lal ina ú-a-a-a u*$_4$*-mi-šam uš-ta-bar-ra meš-re-ti-šú ul ú-ta-ar bi-na-ti-šú a-ḫe-e up-ta-ri-*ʾ*i ki-ma ur-ba-tu*$_4$ *ni-il-tu*$_4$ *ki-šad-su iq-ta-da-du* . . . (*SpTU* 2.2:60–72 [bilingual])

***Šaššaṭu* afflicts that one's limbs like a snake whose head a man has beaten. He does not eat good bread, he does not drink good water, he does not sleep good sleep. He spends every day in woe. He cannot turn his limbs; they (feel as if they) have been cut apart the way a lying rush bends its neck . . .

3.196 DIŠ TA SA.GÚ-*šú* EN SÌL.MUD-*šú* SA.MEŠ-*šú šag-gu šu-*ʾ*-ra-šú kaṣ-ra* ME.ZÉ-*šú hé-sa*$_5$ SA.DUGUD (DPS X A obv. 27//B obv. 30–31 = *TDP* 82:27; cf. DPS XXXIII:97 [AOAT 43.357]; Arnaud, *Emar* VI/4.694:6′)

**If a person's muscles are stiff from his neck muscles to his heel, his eyebrows are knitted, (and) his jaws (feel like they) are pressured, *šaššaṭu.*

3.197 DIŠ ⌜GÚ⌝-*su i-zur-ma* IGI-*šú gal-ta-át pi-qam* NU *pi-qam* LUḪ-*ut*/MUD-*u*[*d*] SA.DUGUD (DPS X A obv. 11//B obv. 11 = *TDP* 80:11; cf. DPS XXXIII:96 [AOAT 43.357])

**If he twists his neck and his eye jerks (and) he jerks (var. A: shudders) incessantly, *šaššaṭu.*

3.198 DIŠ SAG.DU-*su ti-*⌜*ik-ka*⌝*-šú u šá-šal-la-šú* 1-*niš* KÚ.ME-*šú* SA.[DUGUD][197] (DPS III C obv. 31 = *TDP* 20:31; cf. DPS XXXIII:94 [AOAT 43.357])

**If his head, his neck, and his back[198] all continually hurt him at the same time, ⌜*šaššaṭu*⌝.

3.199 DIŠ GÚ-*su* MU[R]UB$_4$.MEŠ-*šú* ŠU^{II}-*šú u* GÌR^{II}-*šú aš-ṭa* SA.DUGUD (DPS X A obv. 10//B obv. 10 = *TDP* 80:10; cf. DPS XXXIII:95 [AOAT 43.357])[199]

**If his neck, his ⌜hips⌝, his hands, and his feet are stiff, *šaššaṭu.*

3.200 DIŠ ⌜TA![200] SAG⌝.DU-*šú* EN *šuk-lul-ti-šú*[201] SA.MEŠ-*šú i-nu-uš-šu* NU DIN (DPS III C r. 25 = *TDP* 28:85)

**If from his head to his toes(?)[202] his muscles shake, he will not get well.

There are many causes of muscle spasms besides tetanus. Some are relatively benign, like the common "Charlie horse" and rapid breathing (respiratory alkalosis). Others, such as strychnine poisoning, are more serious illnesses. The text below indicates not only muscle spasm but also dizziness. Therefore, respiratory alkalosis seems a likely possibility. The *āšipu* clearly understood that the muscle spasms (tetany), although resembling tetanus (*šaššaṭu*), were not caused by tetanus.

3.201 U$_4$ GIG SAG-*sú* NIGIN-*šu ri-ta-šu ù* GÌR.MEŠ-*šu i-ra-ú-ba* ŠU *ra-bi-ti šà ki šà-aš-šà-ṭì-ma* (*MDP* 57.11 v 21′–24′)

**If the patient's head seems to spin (and) his hands or feet tremble, "hand" of the great one[203] who is like *šaššaṭu* (tetanus).

PERITONITIS

Abdominal wounds have some unusual characteristics. Although they may have an associated abdominal wall soft tissue infection, if the abdominal wall was penetrated as commonly occurs in war wounds, and especially if the intestines were also entered, the nature of the infection becomes much more serious. Abdominal muscles become rigid or spastic; intestinal motility ceases, resulting in constipation; abdominal fluid (ascites) develops (referred to as "puffed up" abdomen by the *āšipu*; see below); and fever is usually present. In the following reference, the upper abdomen being "puffed up" and the lower abdomen being hard seems to be the *āšipu*'s way of saying that the patient's entire abdomen was "puffed up" and hard at the same time.[204]

3.202 DIŠ SAG.DU-*su u* ŠÀ-*šú* KÚM-*em* SA SAG.KI^{II}-*šú* ŠU^{II}-*šú u* [GÌR^{II}-*šú* 1-*niš* ZI.MEŠ] SAG ŠÀ-*šú na-ši* ḪÁŠ-*su da-an* ŠE [D$_7$ . . .] (DPS III C obv. 57–58 = *TDP* 24:57–58)

**If his head and abdomen are hot (and) the blood vessel(s) of his temples, his hands and [his feet all seem to pulsate together], his upper abdomen (epigastrium) is puffed up, his lower abdomen (hypogastric region)[205] is hard, he has ⸢chills⸣ [. . .]

Abdominal cavity infection (peritonitis) without modern antibiotics and early surgery is frequently fatal. This fact was well understood by the ancient Mesopotamian physician, who expressed a dismal prognosis when such wounds occurred.

3.203 DIŠ *ir-ru-šú paṭ-ru na-kid* (DPS XIII D r. 17 = *TDP* 128 iv 26′)

**If his intestines were (cut) loose, it is worrisome.

3.204 DIŠ KI.MIN-*ma ina* ŠÀ-*šú* SÌG-*iṣ-ma e-mir u e-sil* GAM / DIŠ KI.MIN-*ma ina* ŠÀ-*šú* SÌG-*iṣ-ma u* ZI.IR.MEŠ ŠU ^{d}MAŠ.TAB.BA GAM (DPS XV:35–36 [AOAT 43.152]; cf. DPS XIII B ii 19 = *TDP* 118 ii 19)

**If (it is the first day he is sick) and he was wounded on his abdomen and consequently (it) is colicky and constipated, he will die. If (it is the first day he is sick) and he was wounded on his abdomen and consequently (it) is continually upset, "hand" of the twin gods; he will die.

3.205 DIŠ *ina re-biti-šú* SÌG-*iṣ-ma ina* KA-*šú* MÚD MUD ŠUB.ŠUB-*a* ŠU ^{d}IM GAM (DPS XIV A iii 17 = *TDP* 140 iii 51′)[206]

**If he was wounded on the side of his abdomen and consequently he continually produces black blood from his mouth, "hand" of Adad; he will die.

3.206 DIŠ KI.MIN-*ma re-biti-su šá* 150 *nap-ḫat-ma* GI$_6$-*át ina* NU ZU *ú-rap-pad* ŠU ^{d}*dil-bat ina šat ur-ri* SÌG-[*i*]*ṣ* GAM (DPS XV:53 [AOAT 43.153]; cf. DPS XIV A iii 12–13//C$_2$ iii 4//I 8–9 = *TDP* 140 iii 46′–47′)[207]

**If (it is the first day he is sick) and the right side of his abdomen is swollen and dark (and) he wanders about without knowing (where he is), "hand" of Dilbat (Ištar). <If> he was wounded in the dawn watch; he will die.

There were rare exceptions, however, where survival was possible even when the abdominal wall was opened. The reference below implies that early dressing of the wound would provide some hope of survival.

3.207 DIŠ *ir-ru-šu paṭ-ru-ma* U$_4$.2.KÁM U$_4$.3.KÁM U$_4$.4.KÁM U$_4$.5.KÁM *la i-sà-*⌜*ir*BA.ÚŠ⌝ / DIŠ *e-pi-ra ina* DÚR-*šu it-ta-na-aṣ-ṣa-am mu-ru-*⌜*uṣ*⌝ *ḫa-še-e* ⌜*šu*⌝*-ru-b*[*u* BA.ÚŠ] / DIŠ LI.DUR-*su iṣ-bat-ma ù* ZÉ GI$_6$ *ina* KA-*šu it-tab-ka* [BA.ÚŠ] / DIŠ DÚR D[U]L-*ma ù* IM *ina* DÚR-*šu it-te-es-kir* [BA.ÚŠ] (*PBS* 2/2.104:6–9)

**If his intestines were (cut) loose and he does not plaster (them) for two, three, four, or five days, he will die. If dirt continually comes out of his anus, they have been entered by a disease of the entrails;[208] [he will die]. If he grasps his navel and black bile pours from his mouth, [he will die]. If his anus is closed and wind is blocked up in his anus, [he will die].

The following texts appear to be describing abdominal rigidity, loss of intestinal motility, and ascites, characteristic signs of peritonitis.

3.208 DIŠ KI.MIN-*ma* ŠÀ.MEŠ-*šú* GI$_6$.MEŠ-*ma* SA ŠÀ-*šú šu-ud-du-du ina* KA-*šú* IM *ú-ga-áš-šá ana* U$_4$.3.KÁM GAM (DPS XV:37 [AOAT 43.152]; cf. DPS XIII B ii 38–39 = *TDP* 120 ii 38–39)[209]

**If (it is the first day he is sick) and his chest and abdomen are black,[210] the muscles of his abdomen are pulled taut,[211] (and) he belches "wind" from his mouth (after he has been sick) for three days, he will die.

3.209 DIŠ *ina re-biti-šú* SÌG-*iṣ-ma* DÚR-*šú* BAD.BAD-*ir* ŠU ^{d}*Nin-giš-zi-da* / DIŠ *ina re-biti-šú* SÌG-*iṣ-ma* MÚŠ-*šú uš-qa-ma-am-ma ina* EDIN TAG-⌜*it*⌝ KI.MIN (DPS XIV A iii 18–19 = *TDP* 140 iii 52′–53′)

**If he was wounded on the side of his abdomen and consequently his anus is continually stopped up, "hand" of Ningišzida. If he was wounded on the side of his abdomen and consequently his countenance becomes subdued and he is "touched in the steppe"[212] ("hand" of Ningišzida).

3.210 DIŠ KI.MIN-*ma* ŠU^{II}-*šú ina* SAG.DU-*šú* GAR.MEŠ-*ma la ur-ra-da-ni* ŠÀ.MEŠ-*šú* ÍL.MEŠ KÚM ÚḪ *ina* SAG ⌜ŠÀ-*šú*⌝ [SÌG-*iṣ* GAM] (DPS XV:15 [AOAT 43.151]; cf. DPS XI A obv. 25//B 24 = *TDP* 90:25//*SpTU* 1.34:24)

**If (it is the first day he is sick) and his hands are continually placed on his head and he does not bring them down, his insides are puffed up (and) he burns with fever,[213] [he was wounded] on his upper abdomen (epigastrium); [he will die].

CHRONIC PERITONITIS

The cases of peritonitis described above are predominately acute bacterial peritonitis. In patients that have a slowly progressive form of this disease, tuberculosis is the usual cause.

Without antibiotics, this also is usually a fatal disease. Abdominal findings are variable; some patients have abdominal fluid, distension, and tenderness while others have little distension but a doughy feeling on abdominal examination. The texts below were probably considered by the *āšipu* to be variations of the same disease, since they appear close together in Tablet XIII of the diagnostic/prognostic series and since they all bear the same diagnosis: "hand" of a tithe owed to the great (gods). Since the patients in these references have abdominal findings similar to cases of chronic peritonitis and since the process is identified as chronic in three of the texts, it seems appropriate to consider this diagnosis.

3.211 [DIŠ S]AG ŠÀ-*šú* DIB.DIB-*su u* ŠÀ.MEŠ-*šú* MÚ.MEŠ-*ḫu* GIG-*su* GÍD.DA *ana* UD.31.KAM ŠU ZAG 10 GAL.MEŠ (DPS XIII B i 9′–10′ = *TDP* 112 i 13′–14′)

** [If] his ⸢upper abdomen (epigastrium)⸣ continually afflicts him and his insides are bloated, his illness will be prolonged. (If he has been sick) for thirty-one days, "hand" of a tithe owed to the great (gods).

3.212 DIŠ SAG ŠÀ-*šú* ÍL-*ma* ḪÁŠ-*su da-an* U_4.27.KÁM GIG ŠU ZAG.ME GAL.MEŠ (DPS XIII B i 19′ = *TDP* 112 i 23′)

**If his upper abdomen (epigastrium) is puffed up and his lower abdomen (hypogastric region) is hard (and) he has been sick for twenty-seven days, "hand" of a tithe owed to the great (gods).

3.213 DIŠ SAG ŠÀ-*šú* ÍL-*ma* ḪÁŠ-*su* DIG-*ub* ŠU ZAG 10 GAL.MEŠ / DIŠ SAG ŠÀ-*šú* DU_8-*ma* ḪÁŠ-*su da-an* U_4.27.KÁM ŠU ZAG 10 GAL.MEŠ / DIŠ SAG ŠÀ-*šú* DU_8-*ma i-ár-ra-ár* ŠU ZAG 10 GAL.MEŠ (DPS XIII B i 22′–24′ = *TDP* 112 i 26′–28′)

**If his upper abdomen (epigastrium) is puffed up and his lower abdomen (hypogastric region) is soft, "hand" of a tithe owed to the great (gods). If his upper abdomen (epigastrium) is uncongested and his lower abdomen (hypogastric region) is hard (and he has been sick for) twenty-seven days, "hand" of a tithe owed to the great (gods). If his upper abdomen (epigastrium) is uncongested (but) rumbles, "hand" of a tithe owed to the great (gods)

Hansen's Disease (Leprosy)

Hansen's disease, a chronic bacterial infection caused by *Mycobacterium leprae*, is associated with great social stigma, primarily because of its effect on the face of the patient as well as unsightly skin changes on other parts of the body and the loss of fingers and toes. It is a very complex disease with interactions between the organism and host immunity producing varying clinical syndromes.

Hansen's disease primarily affects the skin, eyes, peripheral nervous system, and testicles. In lepromatous leprosy, when the face is involved, it may include the loss of eyebrows and the thickening of ears as well as the facial skin. Eye complications of leprosy include paralysis of eyelid muscles and chronic infection of the iris causing pinpoint pupils. Both of these may lead to blindness. Skin of the back, buttocks, arms, and legs is often affected. The nerves of the hands and feet may be thickened and very painful, but the disease ultimately results in loss of sensation and paralysis.

In later stages there may be resorption of the small distal bones of hands and feet. Ulcers commonly develop on the hands and feet secondary to loss of sensation because the patient is unaware of temperature extremes and injuries result. We believe that the following quotes are likely to be describing lepromatous leprosy.

3.214 DIŠ NU *pa-tan* UZU.MEŠ-*šu* *uš-ta-nak-ta-tu* *i-reš-ti* SUM^{SAR} : ^{Ú}[Z]AG.ḪI.LI^{SAR} UGU-*šu* GIG *ap-*[*p*]*at* U.MEŠ ŠU^{II}-*šu* *u* GÌR^{II}-*šu* *ḫu-ul-la-a* ŠU NAM.ÉRIM.MA (DPS XXII:22–23 [AOAT 43.253])

**If, without (his) having eaten, his flesh is continually thickened,[214] the smell of garlic (var. *saḫlû*) bothers him, (and) the tips of his fingers and his toes (appear to be) made to dissolve,[215] "hand" of curse.

3.215 [DIŠ U].MEŠ ŠU^{II}-*šú* *pa-áš-ṭa* [...] (DPS XI A r. 32 = *TDP* 96 r.32)

**[If the finger]s of his hands are rubbed off [...]

The first quote above almost certainly is describing Hansen's disease, and it rather accurately depicts the dissolution of fingers and toes. It is rare for other diseases to cause this phenomenon. The digits are slowly resorbed and end up markedly foreshortened. Inexperienced observers often think that the fingers and toes have fallen off. The ancient physician, however, understood that the digits gradually disappeared over time. The mention of the "smell of garlic" bothering the patient in the first reference must have been due to the common involvement of the nasal membranes by the lepra bacillus.

The following three references mention constriction of the pupils and loss of eyebrows or eyelashes. These findings are compatible with Hansen's disease, but other diseases can cause them as well.

3.216 DIŠ IGI^{II}-*šú* *iz-za-naq*!-*qá*!-*p*[*a*! ...] (DPS V F 11 = *TDP* 50 F 11)[216]

**If (the pupils of) his eyes are continually ⌜constricted⌝ [...].

3.217 DIŠ *a-na* IGI^{II}.MEŠ *ki-ṣa-a-ti* *bu*[*l*]-⌜*lu*⌝-*ṭi* *u* *kap-pi* IGI^{II}-*šú* *šu-ṣi-i* ... (*BAM* 22:32′–33′)

**If you want to cure eyes with *kiṣṣatu* and to make his eyelashes/eyebrows sprout...

3.218 PA IGI^{II}-*šú* GÁL-*ši* (*BAM* 515 ii 25)

**(After treatment) he will have eyelashes/eyebrows.

The skin lesions of lepromatous leprosy are possibly included in *saḫaršubbû* (see Chapter 10), a term that seems to have referred to generalized lesions of two specific types: hypopigmented granular lesions (*garābu*) and variously colored thickenings of the skin (*epqu*). The lesions of *saḫaršubbû* could be white or red or, less commonly, yellow or black, variations that were accounted for by attributing them to the "hands" of different divinities (see Chapter 19 with 19.93).

3.219 KI.MIN SAḪAR.ŠUB.BA SIG$_7$ SA$_5$ ŠU ^{d}30 *ana* ZI-*šú* ... (Tsukimoto, *Priests and Officials* 199–200:60)

**(If the patient has) yellow and red *saḫaršubbû*, "hand" of Sîn, to remove it...

3.220 KI.MIN SAḪAR.ŠUB.BA SA_5 BABBAR GI_6 ŠU DINGIR LÚ *ana* ZI-*šú* . . . (Tsukimoto, *Priests and Officials* 199–200:61, 70)

**(If the patient has) red, white, and black *saḫaršubbû*, "hand" of the person's god, to remove it . . .

Syphilis, tuberculosis, and Hansen's disease all produce lesions covering a broad spectrum of colors, shapes, and distributions. All three diseases (and Hansen's disease in particular) have an acute inflammatory state called erythema nodosum. This is characterized by tender nodules 2 to 5 cm in diameter or larger that appear in crops. As the lesion develops, it becomes red, then purple, and finally varying shades of green or yellow which suggest a bruise. During healing, a fine cigarette-paper scale may appear on the surface, possibly the "falling dust" that gave *saḫaršubbû* its name. Interesting in view of the fact that erythema nodosum is still treated with salicylates or other analgesics is the fact that two of the treatments for *saḫaršubbû* contain *ḫilēpu*, which is almost certainly "willow," a source of salicylates.[217]

Saḫaršubbû was thought to be infectious, and covered the body "like a garment" (see 10.134–10.135). Lexical equations also indicate that, like *buʾšānu* (see above), *garābu* was associated with an unpleasant odor.[218] An unpleasant odor might be expected in patients with Hansen's disease because of the chronic upper airway problems and frequent ulcers of the hands and feet with secondary infections.

3.221 GIG.ḪAB : *ga-ra-bu bu-⸢šá-a-nu⸣ ḫap-pu*! (2R.44 no. 2 [K 4177+]:13–15, apud *CAD* G 46a)

**"Stinking disease" means *garābu*, *buʾšānu*, (or) "stinking."

Also interesting to note is the fact that the spell chosen by the ancient physician to recite before approaching patients with *šaḫaršubbû*[219] was otherwise reserved for cases of numbness, typically a numb hand or foot on one side, as in the second reference below.

3.222 *a-di-ni a-na* UGU-*ḫi* SAḪAR.ŠUB.BA NU *qé-re-bi* ÉN ME.ŠÈ.PA.DA.RI 3-*šú a-na* UGU-*ḫi-šú* ŠID-*nu* (Tsukimoto, *Priests and Officials* 199–200:41–42)

**Before you approach (a patient with) *šaḫaršubbû*, recite over him the spell ME.ŠÈ.BA.DA.RI three times.

3.223 ÉN ME.ŠÈ.BA.DA.(ŠI).RI ŠID-*nu ina* ŠU 15-*šú* KEŠDA . . . ÉN ME.ŠÈ.BA.DA.ŠI.RI KA.INIM.MA *šá šim-ma-ti* (*BE* 31.60(+) ii 37–43//K 3274 r. 1′, 5′//*BAM* 354 iv 6//*SpTU* 4.129 i 4–5)

**You recite the spell ME.ŠÈ.BA.DA.(ŠI).RI and bind (the amulet) on his left hand. The spell ME.ŠÈ.BA.DA.ŠI.RI (etc.) is a recitation for numbness.

These references would seem to indicate that at least some of the cases of *saḫaršubbû* must have been Hansen's disease, since only leprosy (and not tuberculosis or syphilis, or indeed any of the other diseases that have been proposed for *saḫaršubbû*) has nerve involvement that would produce this type of insensitivity.

There is a milder form of Hansen's disease, tuberculoid leprosy, which has a variable number of flat white (depigmented) skin patches with reduced pain and touch sensation occurring anywhere on the body. It has been suggested by Kinnier Wilson that the following quote is a reference to this form of Hansen's disease (see Chapter 10).[220]

3.224 DIŠ LÚ *pa-ga-ar ši-ru-šu pu-ṣa-am ku-ul-lu-u*[*m*]*-ma ù nu-uq-di i-ta-ad-du* LÚ *šu-ú it-ti i-lí-šu sà-ki-ip it-ti a-wi-l*[*u-t*] *i sà-ki-ip* (Köcher and Oppenheim, *AfO* 18.66 ii 42–45 [physiognomic omens])

**If a person's body (and) his flesh contain white spots and is spotted with "points," that man is rejected by his god; he is rejected by mankind.

Plague (*Šadānu*)

In the fourteenth century C.E., plague swept across Europe killing between one-third and one-fourth of the population.[221] It has been found on all continents, and many pandemics have been recorded. Plague is caused by the bacterium *Yersinia pestis* and is transmitted by infected rat fleas.

Following the bite of the infected flea, the organisms are spread throughout the body via the lymphatics and blood. Most people develop the bubonic form of plague in which case the most prominent lesions are swollen and extremely painful lymph nodes called bubos. These nodes are hard and matted, and sometimes as large as hen's eggs. The nodes most commonly affected are in the inguinal/femoral (groin) region; frequent incapacitation of the leg occurs because of pain. Other nodes that can be affected are in the cervical (neck) and axillary (armpit) regions. The spleen is sometimes enlarged. In addition to the bubos, there can be high fever and chills, headache, vomiting, unsteady gait, and even delirium. There is a marked hemorrhagic tendency so that subcutaneous bleeding and bleeding from other sites can occur. The Akkadian term, *šadānu*, appears to include plague. The texts below may not all be cases of the plague, since other infections can cause lymph node enlargement. However, when lymph nodes[222] are particularly large, hard, and painful, plague should be strongly suspected.

3.225 DIŠ GIG GAR-*šú ana* TAG *da-an* KÚM-*em ṣa-ri-iḫ ṭu-*⌈*ù-lim*⌉[223] ÍL-*šú* NINDA *u* KAŠ LAL-*ṭi šá-da-nu* MU.NI TAG ^{d}[...] (DPS XXXIII:30 [AOAT 43.354]; cf. *BAM* 409 obv. 26′–29′)

**If the nature of the sore is that it is hard to the touch, he burns with fever, his spleen is very puffed up, (and) his appetite for bread and beer is diminished, its name is *šadānu*; "touch" of [...][224]

3.226 DIŠ GIG GAR-*šú ki-ma* NA$_4$ *da-an qer-bé-nu-um-ma* GAL *qer-bé-nu-um-ma* DU-*ak* ÍL-*šú* ⌈ZI!⌉-*a* [*u*] DU.ME[Š GUB-*za*] *la i-le-eʾ-e šá-da-nu* MU.NI TAG ^{d}AMAR.UTU *u* [^{d}NIN.IB] (DPS XXXIII:31 [AOAT 43.354/355]; cf. *BAM* 409 obv. 33′–36′)

**If the nature of his sore is that it is hard as a rock, as it grows down inside, it continually goes down inside (and) he is not able to lift (his foot),[225] to get up [and] walk (or) to stand, it is called *šadānu*; "touch" of Marduk and [Ninurta].[226]

3.227 DIŠ GIG GAR-*šú* GIN$_7$ NA$_4$ *da-an lu ina* GÚ-*šú lu ina su-*⌈*ḫa*⌉*-ti-šú lu ina re-bi-ti-šú* GAR *ana* U$_4$.3.KAM [GAM ...] MU.[NI] (DPS XXXIII:32 [AOAT 43.355])

**If the nature of his sore is that it is hard as a rock (and) it is located either on his neck or on his armpit or on the side of his abdomen (and he has been sick) for three days, [he will die]; [it] is called [. . .][227]

3.228 DIŠ GIG GAR-*šú* GIN_7 NA_4.ZÚ TA* GÚ-*su* NIGIN-*me ša-da-nu* M[U.NI] (DPS XXXIII:28 [AOAT 43.354])

**If the nature of his sore is that it is like obsidian[228] (and) goes around his neck, [it] ⌜is called⌝ *šadānu*.

3.229 DIŠ GIG GAR-*šú ana* TAG *da-an ti-ik-pi* SA_5.MEŠ DIRI *šá-da-nu* M[U.NI] (DPS XXXIII:29 [AOAT 43.354])[229]

**If the nature of his sore is that it is hard to the touch (and) he is full of red spots, [it] ⌜is called⌝ *šadānu*.

The two references below may also be describing the bubonic form of plague since the involved nodes and overlying skin may become dark from necrosis. However, since the masses or nodes are not mentioned, the diagnosis is less certain, as would be expected in references whose primary purpose was prognostic (see Chapter 20).

3.230 ⌜DIŠ SA *šá-pu-li-šu*⌝ *šá* 15 ZI.MEŠ *u* GI_6.MEŠ *ana* U_4.2.KAM BA.ÚŠ (DPS XIV A_2 i 17//C_2 i 7 = *TDP* 132 i 68)

**If the blood vessel(s) of his left inguinal region (feel like they are) pulsating and they are dark (and he has been sick) for two (var. C: three) days, he will die.

3.231 [DIŠ SA] ⌜*šá-pu-li-šu*⌝ *šá* 150 ZI.MEŠ *u* GI_6.MEŠ *ár-hiš* BA.ÚŠ (DPS XIV A_2 i 18//C_2 i 8 = *TDP* 132 i 69)

**If the blood vessel(s) of his right inguinal region (feel like they are) pulsating and they are dark, he will speedily die.

Viral Infections

Many texts from ancient Mesopotamia describe diseases that are probably caused by viruses. It is understood that all pathogenic microorganisms including viruses are in a dynamic and changing relationship with their human hosts, and the diseases of the past would certainly have had some differences from those seen today. Some viral diseases, however, were probably stable over long periods and it is likely that some of the viruses circulating today were present in the past. We have attempted to identify these viruses, although some uncertainties will unfortunately always remain.

VARICELLA VIRUS INFECTIONS

The most common disease caused by the *Varicella zoster* virus (VZV; *Herpes zoster*) is chickenpox. This is a generalized infection with fever and variable numbers of small blisters (vesicles) that can occur on any skin surface. Chickenpox seems to have been included in the syndrome of *ašû* (see Chapter 10). Mothers who develop chickenpox during pregnancy may transmit the infection to their fetuses. In mid-pregnancy, the fetus may develop local dermal scars (pockmarks). Transmission of the virus from mother to fetus in early pregnancy may produce congenital defects. In late pregnancy, infection no longer causes congenital defects but it can cause severe illness and death, as well as extensive vesicles that are often hemorrhagic. References to the scars and vesicles that may be seen in congenital varicella are to be found in the birth omens series Šumma Izbu (see 17.155–156).

There is a skin infection caused by the *Herpes zoster* virus that lies dormant in the dermal nerves only to reactivate and cause local skin infection. It characteristically resembles typical chickenpox lesions except that it is a bandlike process affecting only one-half of the body. We believe that it is this infection, commonly known as "shingles," which is described in two references, 19.328 and 19.329. These texts mention pain and a "yoke" around the neck, abdomen, or pelvis.

SMALLPOX, GERMAN MEASLES, AND MEASLES

Examples of these viral diseases may have been included in the syndrome known to the *āšipu* as *ašû*. For more details, see Chapter 10.

HERPES SIMPLEX VIRUS

The characteristic vesicles (*bubuʾtu*) caused by this virus make it possible to identify examples of HSV1 and HSV2 infections.

3.232 DIŠ IGI.MEŠ-*šú* U_4.BU.BU.UL SA_5 DIRI.MEŠ ŠU ^{d}30 DIN (DPS IX A 47//C 15 = *TDP* 74:47)

**If his face is full of red *bubuʾtu*, "hand" of Sîn; he will get well.

3.233 [DIŠ TA SAG.D]U-*šú* EN $GÌR^{II}$-*šú* U_4.BU.BU.UL SA_5 DIRI *u* SU-*šú* BABBAR KI MUNUS *ina* KI.NÁ KUR ŠU 30 (DPS III A r. 8′//C r. 31 = *TDP* 28:91)[230]

**[If from] his ⌜head⌝ to his feet, he is full of red *bubuʾtu* and his skin/body is white, he was "gotten" in bed with a woman; "hand" of Sîn.[231]

For more details on sexually transmitted HSV2, see Chapter 4. Herpetic stomatitis seems to have been one of the diseases included under the ancient syndrome of *buʾšānu* (see above). There is also a reference to what may be a *Herpes simplex* virus-dendritic ulcer (see 9.70).

RABIES

Ancient physicians were aware that victims of dog bite also risked contracting rabies. The following quote is in a poetic passage from an Old Babylonian incantation describing a rabid dog. For more details on rabies, see Chapter 2.

3.234 *ur-ru-uk bi-ir-ki-šu a-ru-uḫ la-sa-ma-am i-iṣ bu-bu-tam et-nu-uš a-ka-lam i-na ši-in-ni-šu e-ʾi-il ni-il-šu a-šar iš-šu-ku ma-ra-šu i-zi-ib* (LB 20001:1–9 [Whiting, *ZA* 75.182–187])

**He is long of leg, quick at running. He is short of sustenance, poor in food. His semen is suspended from his teeth; wherever he bites, he leaves behind his child.

ADENOVIRUS INFECTIONS

Although there are many possible reasons for corneal opacities to develop, one common cause is an adenovirus infection involving the conjunctiva and cornea. Adenovirus types 8 and 19 are the most likely to cause this problem. This highly contagious form of "pink eye" not only inflames the conjunctiva but also the cornea, resulting in corneal clouding. For texts and more details, see Chapter 9 with 9.66–9.68.

VIRAL HEPATITIS

Among the infectious causes of jaundice (see Chapter 6), we have found apparent references to patients with hepatitis A and hepatitis B. There is also one quote that appears to refer to venereally transmitted hepatitis B (see 4.35).

VIRAL ENCEPHALOMYELITIS/ENCEPHALOPATHY

Infections of the brain, spinal cord, or both are called encephalitis, myelitis, or encephalomyelitis, respectively. The cause of these infections is usually a virus, including *Herpes simplex*, *Varicella zoster*, polio virus, and many arthropod-borne viruses. Not infrequently, the virus can be an indirect cause of nervous system disease by triggering an immunological process that usually becomes symptomatic after the acute infection has receded. This is referred to as postinfectious encephalopathy. One text describes photophobia. Three more display other features of encephalomyelitis, including muscle weakness (paralysis), eyes that "shudder" (probably pendular nystagmus), eyes that "stand still" (ocular paralysis), and a mouth that is "too strong for the words" (presumably spasm or weakness of the muscles involved in speech). For more details, see Chapter 13.

HEMORRHAGIC VIRAL INFECTIONS

Certain viral infections can cause significant bleeding problems in addition to involvement of organs such as the brain, liver, and lungs. The infections include Lassa fever, Ebola and Marburg viruses, Crimean-Congo hemorrhagic fever, and yellow fever. In many of these infections, humans do not appear to be the primary host. Other animals, especially primates, are the primary hosts, and often the infections seem to originate in Africa. It is known that monkeys were kept as pets in ancient Mesopotamia.[232] If they were imported from Africa, they could have been the source of the viral infections. These infections are generally quite serious, causing high fever, severe illness, and often death. Other viral diseases with hemorrhagic tendencies could have been present in ancient Mesopotamia that no longer exist today.

The following quotes all refer to patients with bleeding problems. Shock from blood loss is a possible cause of death, but since the blood loss is otherwise unexplained, it is more likely that the infection caused the blood loss and directly contributed to the death. Although other conditions might mimic hemorrhagic viral infections, we believe it likely that viruses were the cause of most of these conditions.

3.235 [. . . *i*]*-na-a-šú da-mu ma-la-a* x x x[233]*-šú da-mu ma-la-a u meš-re-tu-šú ne-ʾ-a mar-ṣa šu-ú ul i-bal-luṭ* (*SpTU* 3.86 obv. 5–6)

**[If . . .] his eyes are full of blood, his nose/mouth is full of blood, and his limbs are turned back, that patient will not get well.

Ancient physicians attributed this type of illness to different gods/goddesses or spirits, and some are listed below. The symptoms described differ somewhat, and it is possible that the *āšipu* thought that different spirits were at work because there were clinical characteristics that were suggesting varying etiologies. Unfortunately, there is insufficient information to establish different causes.

"HAND" OF THE SIBITTI (PLEIDES)

3.236 DIŠ *ina* GIG-*šú* IGI^{II}-*šú* NU ÍL-*ši ina* IGI^{II}-*šú* KIR$_{4}$-*šú* KA-*šú* GEŠTU^{II}-*šú u* GÌŠ-*šú* MÚD TÉŠ.BI È.ME-*a* ŠU ^{d}7-*bi*: U$_{4}$.31.KÁM ŠU ^{d}MAŠ.TAB.BA (DPS XVII:25–26 [AOAT 43.197])

**If during his illness, he does not raise his eyes (and) blood comes out of his eyes, his nose, his mouth, his ears, and his penis all at the same time, "hand" of the Sibitti. (If he has been sick for) thirty-one days (when this happens), "hand" of the twin gods.

"HAND" OF THE GOD MARDUK

3.237 DIŠ GABA-*su* DU$_{8}$.MEŠ-*át* SAG.KI-*šú* ŠUB-*ut* MÚD *ina* KA-*šú pi-qam la p*[*i-qa*]*m* ⌜DU⌝-*k*[*a*] ŠÀ-*šú pi-qam la pi-qam* MUD-*ud* ŠU ^{d}AMAR.UTU *a-dir-ma* BA.ÚŠ (DPS XII A 2–3 = *TDP* 100 i 2–3)

**If his chest is clear,[234] (the blood vessels of) his temple have collapsed,[235] blood incessantly flows from his mouth/nose, (and) his heart incessantly shudders, "hand" of Marduk; he will be worried and die.

3.238 DIŠ UB.MEŠ-*š*[*ú*] ⌜DU$_{8}$⌝.MEŠ SAG ŠÀ-*šú di-ik-*⌜*šá* TUKU⌝ *pi-qa la pi-qa* MÚD *ina* KA-*šú* DU-*ku* Á^{II}-*šú* SIG.MEŠ NÍG.ZI.[IR] ŠUB.ŠUB-*su* IGI^{II}-*šú* MÚD *šu-un-nu-ʾ-a* ŠU ^{d}AMAR.UTU *a-dir-ma* GAM / DIŠ UB.MEŠ-*š*[*ú* DU$_{8}$].MEŠ SAG.KI^{II}-*šú* ŠUB-*ta*$_{5}$ *gir-ra-šú šu-uḫ-ḫu-ṭa* ŠÀ^{II}-*šú it-te-nen-bi-ṭu kal* U[$_{4}$] *u kal* GI$_{6}$ GIG ŠU ^{d}AMAR.UTU *a-dir-ma* GAM (DPS XXII:34–37 [AOAT 43.254])

**If his limbs are supple, his upper abdomen (epigastrium) ⌜has a needling pain⌝, blood incessantly flows from his mouth/nose, his arms are continually weak, ⌜depression⌝ continually falls upon him, (and) his eyes are suffused with blood, "hand" of Marduk; he will be worried and die. If his limbs [are supple], (the blood vessels of) his temples have collapsed, his throat (looks) skinned, his insides are continually cramped, (and) he is sick all ⌜day⌝ and all night, "hand" of Marduk; he will be worried and die.[236]

"HAND" OF THE GODDESS GULA

3.239 DIŠ *ina* KIR$_4$-*šú* IGI^{II}-*šú u* GEŠTU [^{II}-*šú* MÚD] 1-*niš* DU-*ku* ŠU ^{d}ME.ME SÌG-*su* KI-*šú nit-ta-at* GAM (DPS VI A obv. 19//C i 2–3//D 2 = *TDP* 56:19)

**If [blood] flows from his nose, his eyes and [his] ears all at the same time, "hand" of Gula has struck him and . . . with him; he will die.[237]

Actinomycosis

Actinomycosis is caused by an unusual bacterium, rather than by a fungus as the name implies. The most typical clinical presentation is a chronic infection that develops below the patient's jaw, leading to its common name, "lumpy jaw." The lumps eventually drain a watery material that contains granules (called sulfur granules because of their yellow color). These granules are actually clumps of bacteria. We believe that the sequence of references below describes actinomycosis, and that what the *āšipu* called "silt" is what the modern physician calls "sulfur granules."

3.240 DIŠ GIG GAR-*šú* GIN$_7$ ^{IM}⌜*ṭe*⌝-*ru-ti-šú* NIGIN.ME? *u ti-ik-ka-šú* DIB [*kir-ba-nu*] MU.NI / DIŠ GIG GAR-*šú da-an pa-an* UZU.MEŠ GAR *u* [KÚ]M.KÚM-*im kir*-⌜*ba*⌝-*nu* MU.NI (DPS XXXIII:38–39 [AOAT 43.355]; cf. *BAM* 583 i 3′–5′)

**If the nature of the sore is that it is surrounded by what looks like its silt and it "seizes" his neck, it is called ["lump"]. If the nature of the sore is that it is hard, it is placed on the surface of the flesh and he is continually hot, it is called "lump."

Fungal Infections[238]

MYCETOMA

Ancient Mesopotamian physicians described an illness that they called *muruṣ kabbarti*[239] which appears to be the same condition that modern physicians call mycetoma, or Madura foot.[240] This is a chronic fungal or actinomycotic infection that primarily involves the feet of people living in tropical or subtropical regions who work in the soil without shoes, conditions that must have existed in ancient Mesopotamia. It is caused by trauma to the feet (scratches and puncture wounds) and contamination of the wound with soil containing the organisms. It is a slowly progressive process, often painless, with destruction of the skin, subcutaneous tissue, muscle, and bone. If untreated, it can cause loss of function of the foot and frequent secondary bacterial infections that can lead to even more serious morbidity and mortality. As the disease progresses, the foot and ankle become swollen, the skin becomes thickened, the joint loses mobility, muscles are damaged, and multiple sinus tracts drain pus containing granules that are small colonies of the organisms that are causing the infection. These granules are colored white, black, yellow, pink, or red, depending on the causative organism. Modern physicians recognize other chronic fungal foot infections, including chromomycosis and common athlete's foot (tinea pedis), but neither of these conditions leads to destruction of the bone and muscle, a common problem in mycetoma and described by the *āšipu*.

3.241 DIŠ NA GIG *ka-bar-tim* GIG-*ma eq-ba-šu* MÚ.MÚ-*ḫu* SA.MEŠ GÌR^{II}-*šú kab-ba-ru-ma i-tal-lu-ka la i-le-ʾi ana* TI-*šú* . . . (*BAM* 124 i 8–9//*AMT* 73/1+ i 15–16)[241]

**If a person is sick with *muruṣ kabbarti* and his heels are swollen, the muscles of his feet are so thickened that he cannot walk, to cure him . . .

3.242 DIŠ NA GIG *ka-bar-ti* GIG-*ma* SA GÌR^{II}-*šú sàk-gu* . . . (*BAM* 124 i 28//*AMT* 73/1 i 31+*AMT* 18/5 i 5)

**If a person is sick with *muruṣ kabbarti* so that the muscles of his feet are stiff . . .

3.243 DIŠ NA GIG *ka-bar-ti a-tal-lu-ka la i-le-ʾ-i* . . . (*BAM* 124 i 31//*AMT* 73/1 i 33+*AMT* 18/5 i 7)

**If a person has *muruṣ kabbarti* (and) he cannot walk . . .

3.244 DIŠ NA GIG *ka-*[*bar-t*]*i*⸢*tu*⸣*-ḫar eq-bi-šu* GI[G . . .] (*BAM* 124 ii 2)

**If a person has *muruṣ* ⸢*kabbarti*⸣ (and) his Achilles tendons are ⸢sore⸣ . . .

3.245 DIŠ NA GIG *ka-bar-ti* GIG EN GÌR.PAD.DU *i*[*r-te-ḫi*] GIG *il-ta-za-az ina* SU-*šú* NU DU$_8$ . . . (*BAM* 124 ii 6–7)[242]

**If a person is sick with *muruṣ kabbarti* and it ⸢pentrates⸣ as far as the bone (and) the soreness stays continuously and cannot be dispelled from his body . . .

The three references listed below describe wounds with a black appearance. They might be describing black granules coming from the wound. Necrotic tissue surrounding the wound, however, could also look black.

3.246 [DIŠ N]A GIG *ka-bar-tim* GIG-*ma ši-kìn* UZU.MEŠ-*šú* BABBAR GI$_6$ ŠUB GIG BI *ir-te-ḫi* . . . (*BAM* 124 i 1–2//*AMT* 73/1 i 11+*AMT* 15/3 i 21)[243]

** [If] a ⸢person⸣ is sick with *muruṣ kabbarti* and the appearance of his flesh is white dotted with black, that illness has penetrated . . .

3.247 DIŠ NA GIG *ka-bar-ti ši-kìn* GIG-*šú* GI$_6$ . . . (*BAM* 124 i 33)[244]

**If a person has *muruṣ kabbarti* (and) the appearance of his sore spot is black . . .

3.248 DIŠ NA GIG *ka-bar-ti* GIG EN *kin-ṣi-šú* E$_{11}$*-a ši-kìn* U[ZU-*šú* . . .] *tu-ri-iḫ* IGI GIG-*šú* GI$_6$ GIG.BI *ina na-aṣ-ma-ti* [. . .] *ul i-tel-li* . . . (*BAM* 124 ii 11–13)

**If a person has *muruṣ kabbarti* (and) the soreness extends as far as his shins, the appearance of [his] ⸢flesh⸣ rapidly [changes (for the worse)?], the surface of his sore spot looks black, (and) that illness does not let up despite the use of bandages [and . . .] . . .

The two references below indicate that the ancient physician had some understanding of the cause of this illness. Dirty bath water certainly could contain the infecting organisms and also suggestive of some type of injury is the idea of accidentally stepping on a *barasigû* (a low platform set upon the roof as an emplacement for rituals).

3.249 [DIŠ NA G]IG *ka-[bar-ti]m ša* A.TU$_5$ *ik-bu-us* . . . (*AMT* 100/3+ i 8)[245]

**[If a person has] ⌜*muruṣ kabbarti*⌝ from stepping in (dirty) bath water . . .

3.250 DIŠ NA GIG *ka-bar-tim šá* BÁRA.SI.GA *ik-bu-us* . . . (*AMT* 100/3+ i 15)

**If a person has *muruṣ kabbarti* from stepping on a *barasigû* . . .

Secondary bacterial infection is likely to be the reason for the more serious nature of the problems listed below.

3.251 DIŠ NA GIG *ka-bar-ti* GIG-*ma* SA MUD (*eq-bi*)-*šu* IM *ma-lu-ú ana šu-ṣi-i* . . . (*BAM* 124 i 12–13//*AMT* 73/1+ i 18)

**If a person is sick with *muruṣ kabbarti* and his Achilles tendon(s) are full of "clay," to make it go out . . .[246]

3.252 DIŠ NA GIG *ka-bar-ti ma-gal* NAM.ÉRIM DIB-*su i-pa-šaḫ ana* EGIR U$_4$-*me* BA.ÚŠ (*BAM* 124 ii 34//*AMT* 73/1 ii 10)

**If a person has *muruṣ kabbarti* (and) the curse greatly afflicts him, he will find relief but later he will die.

3.253 DIŠ GIG *ka-bar-ti ru-šum-tú/ ru-ṭib-ta ib-ta-ni* BA.ÚŠ (*BAM* 124 ii 35//*AMT* 74/1 ii 11)

**If a person has *muruṣ kabbarti* (and) there is oozing[247]/*ruṭibtu*, he will die.

DERMATOPHYTOSES (ATHLETE'S FOOT, CROTCH ITCH, AND RINGWORM)

Athlete's foot is the most common of the superficial fungal infections (dermatophytoses). Other areas frequently involved include the groin (crotch itch; tinea cruris) and scalp (ringworm). These infections are caused by many different dermatophytes that can be transmitted from person to person, and from animals to humans. Since the organisms only invade the upper layers of the skin and nails, they are not serious infections, but at times the fungus-infected skin can lead to more serious secondary bacterial infections. These superficial fungal infections occur in all parts of the world, but in tropical areas they are the most common cause of skin disease. Involved skin usually has intense itching, and generally is red and scaling with fissures that may be painful. The following references are likely to be describing athlete's foot (tinea pedis) and crotch itch (tinea cruris).

3.254 DIŠ NA GÌR^{II}-*šú* KÚM TUKU.TUKU-*a i-raš-šá-šú-ma ik-ki-k*[*a*] ⌜*la*⌝ *i-kal-la* GIG.MEŠ DIRI-*a mu-ne-e* GI[G] . . . (*BAM* 120 iii 8–9)

**If a person's feet continually have fever, they are reddish and he cannot stop scratching, (and) they are full of sore spots,[248] he is ⌜sick⌝ with *munû*-lesions . . .

3.255 DIŠ NA GÌR^{II}-*šú um-ma ú-kal-la-ma mu-né-e* D[IRI] . . . (*BAM* 120 iii 1)[249]

**If fever grips a person's feet and they are ⌜full⌝ of *munû*-lesions . . .

3.256 [DIŠ NA *šá-ḫu*]*-ri-šú ri-šu-tú* DIRI . . . *šá-ḫu-ri-šú šá ri-šu-tú ma-lu-ú* . . . (*BAM* 383:1, 13)

**[If a man]'s ⌜sole⌝ (of the foot) is full of redness . . . his sole (of the foot) which is full of redness . . .

3.257 DIŠ GIG *ina* GÌR NA *lu ina* ŠIR NA E_{11}*-ma i-raš-šá-šum-ma ug-gag ru-ṭib-tum qí-lu-tum* MU.[NI] *ana* TI-*šú* . . . (*AMT* 74/1 ii 32–33; cf. DPS XXXIII:22 [AOAT 43.354])

**If a sore comes out on a person's foot or on his scrotum and it is reddish and he scratches, it is called "burning oozing,"[250] to cure him . . .

When a superficial fungal infection involves the scalp, it usually spreads to form a solid lesion that heals first in the center. This causes a ring to develop on the scalp, hence the name *ringworm.* The *āšipu* clearly noted these curious shapes, which he referred to by the term *kurāru*, a word that is related to *garāru*: "to turn, roll over." Another term, *kuraštu/ kurartu*, probably referred to the early, solid lesion, *kibšu* to honey-colored crusts developing around hair follicles, and *kiṣṣatu* to patchy hair loss. For more details, see Chapter 10.

3.258 DIŠ NA SAG.DU-*su* PEŠ.GIG DIB-*it* . . . (*BAM* 3 i 44)[251]

**If a person's head is afflicted by *kurāru* . . .

3.259 DIŠ NA SAG.DU-*su* ⌜*kib*⌝*-šá gi-iṣ-ṣa-tú gu-reš-tú*[252] DIRI . . . (Labat, *RA* 53.10–11 obv. 30)

**If a person's head is full of *kibšu, kiṣṣatu,* (and) *kureštu* . . .

Worms

One disease that both modern and ancient physicians can identify without detailed signs and symptoms or special tests are worms that are large enough to be seen with the naked eye. Some adult worms are a meter (40 inches) long. Some patients can pass or vomit balls of wriggling worms, some 20 centimeters (8 inches) long. The *āšipu* described worm infestations and the clinical problems that worms induced. Unfortunately, the morphology of the worms was poorly described, leaving, in some cases, uncertainty about the specific worm involved. One worm not included in this chapter is *Schistosomiasis hematobium.* It will be found in the chapter on genitourinary tract diseases (Chapter 5). Listed below are three categories used by the *āšipu* in which worms were seen and related to a specific syndrome.

QUQĀNU

3.260 [DIŠ NA IGI]^{II}*-šú qu-qa-ni* DIRI.MEŠ . . . (*BAM* 515 i 27)

**[If a person]'s ⌜eyes⌝ are full of *quqānu*-worms . . .

3.261 [DIŠ NA IGI^{II}]-⌜*šú*⌝ *i-ši-*[*t*]*ú bir-ra-tú u qú-qa-na ú-kal-la* . . . (BM 54641+BM 54826 r. 11)[253]

**[If a person]'s [eyes] contain ⌜confusion of vision⌝, dimness, and *quqānu*-worms . . .

The references above describe both dimmed and blurred vision, and the presence of *quqānu*-worms[254] in the eyes. The Sumerogram for *quqānu*, IGI.GU.LÁ, describes it as a "thread" (GU) that extends (LÁ), across the eye (IGI). This description is quite compatible with the loa-loa worm (*Filaria loa*), a roundworm that is currently restricted to Africa.[255] The worm can be readily seen under the skin and the conjunctival lining of the eyes (2–3 centimeters; 1 inch). What can be seen crawling across the eye is the adult form; the larvae enter the patient via the bite of a "deerfly" (genus *Chrysops*).[256] Fever and visual and systemic complaints may occur, but some patients tolerate the infestation with few symptoms. Although the loa-loa worm is not currently endemic in the Middle East, worms visible in the eye are so characteristic of this disease as to strongly suggest its presence in antiquity.

A final text below lists intestinal worms, *quqānu*-worms, and eggs in the stomach. This is an unusual location for loa-loa worms. We believe the term *quqānu* may have meant worms of a small size rather a specific type. However, when a small worm is seen on the surface of the eye, loa-loa is the most likely cause.

3.262 DIŠ NA ŠÀ-*šú ur-ba-tu qu-qa-nu u pi-lu-u* DIB-*it*... (*BAM* 159 ii 43–44)

**If a person's stomach is afflicted by intestinal worms, *quqānu*-worms and eggs ...

MIQQĀNU

Miqqānu is known from an ancient dictionary to be a small type of worm (*BAM* 401:22–23). We believe that *miqqānu* is pinworm (*Enterobius vermicularis*) infestation, a common childhood problem in the modern era. It generally causes anal burning and itching. For more references to anal burning and itching, see the chapter on gastrointestinal diseases (Chapter 6).

3.263 Ú DÚR *šá mi-qa-na* AL.DIB ... (*BAM* 380:46)

**Plant for anus containing *miqqānu*-worms ...

3.264 Ú DÚR *ḫa-am-ṭí*! *mi-qa-na* DIB-*al*... (*BAM* 1 iii 17)

**Plant for burning sensation in an anus containing *miqqānu*-worms ...

URBATU

3.265 Ú *ur-ba-tu* ŠUB-*e*... (*BAM* 380:59//*BAM* 381 iv 14; cf. *BAM* 421 i′ 20′)[257]

**Plant for expelling *urbatu*-worms ...

3.266 DIŠ NA ŠÀ.MEŠ-*šú* MÚ.MEŠ-*ḫu* IM *ina* ŠÀ-*šú uš-tar-a*ʾ*-ab* ŠÀ-*šú* DIB.DIB-*su-ma rit-ta-šú ina* ŠÀ-*šú e-ta-nab-bal* NA BI *ur-ba-tu* GIG *ana* TI-*šú*... (*BAM* 159 ii 20–22; cf. *BAM* 73 ii 1–3)[258]

**If a person's insides are continually bloated, "wind" rumbles in his stomach, his stomach continually afflicts him, (and) he continually brings his hand to his stomach, that person is sick with *urbatu*-worms, to cure him ...

The Sumerograms for the Akkadian term *urbatu*, MAR, MAR.GAL, and MAR.ŠUR mean "worm," "large worm," and "squashed worm," respectively. The worms varied in color from white to brown.[259] The quotes above indicate the presence of worms in the intestines, and symptoms associated with gastrointestinal disease, namely, bloating, "wind," rumbling stomach, and pain or discomfort. Of the intestinal worms, *Ascaris lumbracoides* is the most likely to produce such symptoms. The adult ascaris usually vary in size from 10 to 20 centimeters (4–8 inches), are brown in color, are round, and exist entirely within the gastrointestinal tract. Patients may be unaware of their existence, but often have gastrointestinal complaints such as those described above. In some situations, the worms can be vomited up or crawl out through the patient's anus, nose, or mouth.[260]

Adult tapeworms (pork, beef, or fish) also reside in the gastrointestinal tract, are flat, are white, and vary in length from 30 to 120 centimeters (1–4 feet). Gastrointestinal complaints are much less common, but nutritional and caloric deficiencies can result from their presence (see Chapter 7). If the pork tapeworm (*Taeniasis solium*) was present in ancient Mesopotamia, it was likely to have caused not only the adult worm infestation of the GI tract, but larval encystment in tissues. This develops when the defecated eggs contaminate food and are subsequently ingested. These eggs hatch in the intestines, penetrate the intestinal lining, and enter the circulation. They lodge in tissues throughout the body and remain in a dormant stage. If the involved tissue is eaten by a carnivore, the encysted parasite then matures in the intestines to the adult egg-laying worm.

This encysted form of pork tapeworm disease is called cysticercosis. It is most serious when it involves the brain, causing a variety of neurological abnormalities, especially seizures. It is likely that some of the seizures described in the neurology chapter (Chapter 13) were due to this disease.

BENNU

The ancient Mesopotamian physician had a term, *bennu*, which was applied to seizures that were thought to be acquired or infectious.[261] We believe that this term includes cysticercosis, but since some references mention cold sensation, a sign that seldom occurs with cysticercosis, it may also include other infections that trigger seizures (see Chapter 13).[262]

3.267 DIŠ NA *ina* KI.NÁ LUḪ-*ut* UZU.MEŠ-*šú* [. . . ^{d}]30 UGU-*šú* GÁL-*ši a-na* BÚR-*ri* . . . (*STT* 95 i 35–36, cf. 41)

**If a person jerks in the bed (and) his flesh [itches,[263] "hand" of *bennu*, deputy] of Sîn is upon him, to dispel it . . .

3.268 DIŠ [N]A *ina* KI.NÁ-*šú* LUḪ.⌜LUḪ⌝-*ut* GIN$_7$ GÙ ÙZ GÙ-*si i-ram-mu-um i-par-ru-ud ma-gal* GÙ.GÙ-*si*/DUG$_4$.DUG$_4$-*ub* ŠU^{II} *be-en-ni* ^{d}[ÀL]AD *šá-né-e* ^{d}30 *ana* TI-*šú* . . . (*BAM* 311:51′–53′//*BAM* 202 r. 5′–7′)

**If a ⌜person⌝ continually jerks in his bed, he cries like a goat, he drones, he shudders, (and) he talks/cries out a lot, "hand" of *bennu*, a *šedû* deputized by Sîn; to cure him . . .[264]

3.269 [DIŠ ŠUB-*ti* ŠUB-*su-ma* U$_4$ ŠUB-*š*]*ú an-nu-ú šu-ú i-qab-bi be-en-nu ṣa-i-du* DIB-*su uš-t*[*e*]-⌜*zeb*⌝ (DPS XXVI:4′ [AOAT 43.278])[265]

** [If a falling spell falls upon him and when it falls upon] ⌜him⌝, he says "This is it," spinning *bennu* afflicts him; he will come through.

3.270 NA$_4$.MEŠ *be-en-nu u šu-ru-up-pu-ú ana* LÚ NU TE-*e* . . . (*STT* 273 iii 6′–7′//*BAM* 358 ii 17′–18′; cf. *SpTU* 4.129 ii 10–11, iii 21, 34, iv 13–14)[266]

**Stones so that *bennu* with cold sensation[267] may not approach a man . . .

When you purchased a slave in ancient Mesopotamia, he came with a thirty- to hundred-day warranty against *bennu*. Should the slave develop *bennu*-seizures within that time period, you were entitled to return the defective slave for a refund of your money.[268] It is likely that a slave working in fields fertilized with animal dung or swimming in irrigation canals contaminated with field runoff or taking his meals in his master's courtyard or standing guard with a dog at the entrance of his house would have occasionally eaten fruit or vegetables contaminated by pork tapeworm eggs. Slaves would, therefore, have been at high risk of developing cysticercosis, as would small children playing in the courtyard or in the river (and using them as impromptu toilet facilities).

3.271 DIŠ GABA.MEŠ-*šú* KÚ.MEŠ-*šú ma-gal* ⌜KÚ⌝-*ma ma-gal* NAG-*ti ik-ta-na-la ma-gal it*!-*ta-na-al ig-ta-na-lut ù ip-ta-na-*⌜*ru*⌝-*ud* LÚ BI *be-en-nu* DIB-*su* LÚ BI *lu ina* ⌜KÁ⌝ *lu-u ina* TÙR *lu ina* ÍD DIB-*su* (*STT* 89:192–195 [Stol, *Epilepsy* 97])[269]

**If his breasts continually hurt him, he stops eating and drinking a lot, (and) he lies down a lot,[270] he continually jerks and shudders, *bennu* afflicts that person. It afflicted him either in the door or in the courtyard or at the river.[271]

3.272 [DIŠ *ṣi*]-*bit be-en-nim šá ina* MU.7.KÁM Ù.TU IGI *ia-a-az-za i-ta-na-šá-áš ina* ŠUB-*šú* ŠU^{II}-*šú ana* EGIR-*šú* NIGIN-*mi* (K 3628+4009+Sm. 1315 r. 18′–19′)

**⌜Affliction⌝ of *bennu* that is observed in the seventh year (after) birth: he makes senseless noises, (his stomach) is continually upset, (and) during his falling spell he winds his hands behind him.

Since the cysts of central nervous system cysticercosis can occur almost anywhere in the brain, many other neurological abnormalities can be seen. Common findings include impaired memory, confusion, agitation, dementia, and hallucinations. Some patients may appear to have a psychiatric illness, as in the following references. The second is drawn from a letter that gleefully reports on the misfortunes of a personal enemy of the recipient for whose demise he has prayed to his god. The mutilation, attributed to the god, was presumably self-inflicted.

3.273 DIŠ *ina* GIG-*šú* MU[D].MUD-*ud u* GIŠ.KUN.ME-*šú* ÍL.MEŠ *ù* KI.SIKIL.LÍL.LÁ.EN.NA *in*[*a* . . .] x TAG-*ma be-en-nu* (DPS XXVI:84′ [AOAT 43.285])

**If during his illness, he continually shudders and he raises his pelvis, and (if) *ardat lilî* (a psychiatric disorder; see Chapter 19) "touches" (him) during [the night(?) . . .], *bennu*.

3.274 *ú-ba-na-ti-ša ú*-[*ka-aṣ*]-*ṣí-is-s*[*i-im*] *ù bi-in-nu-um e-li-ša im-ta-na-aq*-[*qú-ut*] (*ARM* 26/1.312:38′–39′)

**The god ⌜mutilates⌝ her fingers[272] and *bennu* keeps ⌜falling⌝ on her.

GUINEA WORM (*NILUGU*)[273]

We believe that *nilugu* is the guinea worm (*Dracunculus medinensis*). This is a roundworm that is acquired through drinking water contaminated with the immature form of the parasite. The larval form of the parasite penetrates the gut and enters the soft tissues, especially of the lower extremities. The worm enlarges to as long as one meter (40 inches), but it is only about 0.5 centimeters in diameter. The worm usually extends from the thigh through the lymphatic vessels to the foot. When it reaches maturity, it usually forms a painful blister on the foot or ankle which eventually opens. The worm then deposits immature worms from this site into water, thereby completing its life cycle.

3.275 DIŠ GIG *ina* SU NA È GIN$_7$ *i-ba-ri* È-*su ana* ⸢TAG⸣ [DAG]AL-*ma* ⸢GIN$_7$⸣ TAG-*su-ma i-ṣi-tu*[*m*] È SU-*šú tu*-NIGIN *ina ša-nu-ti-šú ina* UZU.ÚR ⸢*e*⸣-*la-a ana* KI *šá-nim-ma ul i-*[*li*] *ana* KI *šá-nim-ma* ⸢DAGAL⸣ x [. . .] x x ṣa *ni-lu-gu*$_4$ MU-*šú ana* ZI-*šú* . . . (*BAM* 417 r. 9′–11′)

**If a sore comes out on a person's body like an *ibaru*-lesion (see Chapter 10), what it produces ⸢grows larger⸣ to the touch, and when he touches it, a wheal (blister) comes out; it goes round his body (and) comes once again up to the thighs;[274] it does not ⸢go up⸣ to another location (but) it may grow larger there [. . .], it is called *nilugu*, to remove it . . .

3.276 [DIŠ GIG] *ina* SU NA ⸢È⸣ SA$_5$ BABBAR KÚ-*šú* A NU TUKU *na-pí-iḫ ana la-pa-t*[*i*!] *i-*[*rap-pu*]*-uš ni-lu-gu*$_4$ MU.NI (*BAM* 417 obv. 25–26//DPS XXXIII:59 [AOAT 43.356])

**[If a sore] comes out on a person's body (and it is) red (or) white (and) it hurts him, there is no fluid (in it but) it is swollen (and) it ⸢grows larger⸣ to the touch, it is called *nilugu*.

The references above describe a lesion that is compatible with the site of egg deposition, and there is also a lesion tracking up the leg and thigh that almost certainly represents the entire extended length of the worm and the inflammation and swelling that typically surrounds it. The reference below mentions something that comes though the skin and is cut off. This is likely to be the worm penetrating the skin. Rather than cutting off the worm and leaving a portion of it within the patient, it is preferable to remove the whole worm by slowly rolling it up on a stick.

3.277 DIŠ GIG *ina* SU NA È GIN$_7$ *i-ba-ri* È *lu* IGI UZU-*šú-ma pa*?-*še-er u na-kis ni-lu-gu*$_4$ MU.NI ŠU ^{d}NIN.GAL *qí-ba* GAR-*an ana* ZI-*šú* . . . (*BAM* 417 obv. 14–15)

**If a sore comes out on a person's body (and) it comes out like an *ibaru*-lesion or it comes through(?) his skin and is cut off, its name is *nilugu*; "hand" of Ningal. You may make a (favorable) prognosis; to remove it . . .

The final text, which appears in the diagnostic/prognostic handbook in sequence with one of the preceding references, describes a sore that produces something called "the scoundrel" (*guzallu*). It seems likely that this was a worm protruding from the wound.

3.278 [DIŠ GIG GAR]-*šú* TAG-*su-ma i-rap-pu-*[*uš*] È-*su* GÚ.ZAL M[U.NI] (DPS XXXIII:60 [AOAT 43.356])

**[If the nature of the sore is that] (if) he touches it, it ⌜grows larger⌝, what it produces ⌜is called⌝ *guzallu* ("the scoundrel").

With the current practice of filtering drinking water through a fine mesh cloth strainer that removes the immature worms, guinea worm infection is beginning to disappear from the Middle East.

ONCHOCERCIASIS

River blindness, or onchocerciasis, is caused by a roundworm that uses human beings as its natural host. The worms, *Onchocerca volvulas*, are transmitted to humans by the bite of black flies that breed along river banks in Africa, South America, and the Middle East.

The commonest signs and symptoms of this disease are itching of the skin and blindness. The skin lesions are often nodules that are full of worms as long as 5 centimeters (2 inches) and their microfilaria. A strong immune response on the part of the host can result in a localized area of intense itching that is darkened, swollen, and scaly. Today, these areas are called "sowda," which is Arabic for black or dark. Blindness may result from scarring of the cornea as well as from atrophy of the optic nerve and chorioretinitis. The Akkadian name for this disease may have been *ḫarāsu*, which literally means "itchies."

3.279 DIŠ IGI^{II}-*šú a-ši-a bir-d*[*u* . . .] (DPS V C ii 5′//E ii 5′ = *TDP* 48 D ii 5)

**If his eyes are "confused" (and) ⌜*birdu*⌝-nodules [. . .].

3.280 DIŠ GIG GAR-*šú* GI_6 *ḫa-ra-su* MU.NI . . . (*BAM* 409 obv. 18′; cf. DPS XXXIII:20 [AOAT 43.354])

**If the appearance of the sore is black, it is called *ḫarāsu* . . .

3.281 DIŠ SU LÚ *bir-di* DIRI.MEŠ-*ma* ⌜UZU.MEŠ⌝-*šú ú-zaq-*⌜*qa-tu*⌝-*šu u ri-šu-ta* ŠUB.ŠUB-*su ḫa-ra-su* MU.NI . . . (*BAM* 409 obv. 19′–20′; cf. DPS XXXIII:21 [AOAT 43.354])

**If a person's body is full of *birdu*-nodules and his flesh stings him and redness continually falls on him, it is called *ḫarāsu* . . .

The failure to mention blindness associated with the skin problems in the last two references might have been due to a time lapse between the skin and (separately treated) eye problems, and a failure to relate them to a single cause. Alternatively, we may be wrong, and another disease may be causing the skin lesions and itching.

Summary

Trying to diagnose infections that occurred three to four millennia ago is like trying to hit a moving target. There is no question that both microorganisms and humans have changed, and there is little chance that we will ever be able to determine for certain exactly which organisms were and were not present, their levels of pathogenicity, and how humans reacted to them. It is clear, however, that infectious disease patterns that bear striking similarity to modern diseases running the gamut of microorganisms from bacteria and viruses to fungi and parasites were already well established in ancient Mesopotamia.

The *āšipu* must have spent a major portion of his professional time in diagnosing and treating infectious diseases, as is still the case for physicians in tropical countries today. What is more important than knowing whether our diagnoses are correct is the realization that physicians of that place and time, despite the absence of modern diagnostic tests, had an understanding of infectious disease syndromes, the nature of contagion, and disease patterns and characteristics. This demonstrates a level of sophistication that would not be seen again in the Western world until the late nineteenth century of the Common Era.

CHAPTER 4

Sexually Transmitted Disease (STDs)

[If from] his ⌜head⌝ to his feet, he is full of red *bubuʾtu* (vesicles, small blisters) and his skin/body is white, he was "gotten" in bed with a woman; "hand" of Sîn.[1]
—DPS III A r. 8′//C r. 31 = *TDP* 28:91

Information is available from sources outside the medical texts about sexual mores and practices in Mesopotamia. This allows for some speculation as to their influence on the incidence and spread of sexually transmitted diseases. It is known that women were expected to be virgins at first marriage, that adultery (intercourse between a married woman and a male to whom she was not married) was punishable by the death of both parties, and that homosexual relationships were not encouraged. Divorce, however, was common, and men were allowed to take slave concubines in addition to their wives.

Prostitution was also tolerated, if not a fully respectable profession.[2] Both female and male prostitutes were available for hire, and it was socially acceptable even for married men to frequent them. Men with barren wives who had children by prostitutes could legally make these children their heirs. Some prostitutes walked the streets, charging set fees for each different position or activity. A hymn to Ištar, divine patroness of prostitutes, mentions the fees charged for standing against a wall or bending over for a prospective customer. Other prostitutes worked out of tavern-brothels, typically managed by women. Rectal intercourse was an acceptable method of birth control. No Victorian fussiness affected sexuality within its accepted limits; a Sumerian poem sings of a beloved's vulva that tastes like fine beer. In this environment, it appears likely that sexually transmitted diseases would have been a significant medical problem.

With some of the conditions described below, we cannot be certain in all cases that they were sexually transmitted, but in many examples it is clear from the quotes that the physician believed them to be. They may have reached this conclusion from patient histories, or from past clinical experience and associations. Another clue for us that a disease was associated with sexual intercourse was when the physician attributed the problem to the "hand" of Ištar. Ištar was the goddess of sexual love, much like Venus in Roman mythology, and she was often cited as the cause of the illness when sexual intercourse appeared to the physician to be a significant preceding event.

4.1 DIŠ *mu-šar-šú u* ŠIR^{II}-*šú nap-ḫu* ŠU ^{d}*Dil-bat ina* KI.NÁ-*šú* KUR-*su* (DPS XIV A ii 38//C ii 12//F 4 = *TDP* 134 ii 38)

**If his penis and his testicles are swollen, "hand" of Dilbat (Ištar) has gotten him in his bed.

Urethritis

Inflammation or infection of the urethra (which drains urine from the bladder) is commonly caused by venereal contact, and in the current era *Neisseria gonorrhea* (gonorrhea), *Chlamydia trachomatis*, and *Herpes simplex* virus type 2 (HSV2, genital herpes) are the main organisms responsible. It is not possible to be certain that these same organisms were present in ancient Mesopotamia, but the descriptions in some cases appear to fit, especially HSV2 because of its characteristic skin lesions.

There are many references to the discharge of semen at times unassociated with ejaculation.[3] We believe that this was a misinterpretation on the part of the *āšipu*, with the discharge actually consisting of pus secondary to urethral infection or inflammation, and not semen. Even twentieth-century physicians until the 1940s believed that whitish discharge from the urethra could be semen and applied the term *spermatorrhea* to it (see Chapter 5). Women were also described with discharge of "semen" from their vagina. The appearance of the discharge must have resembled the penile discharge of pus in men.

GONORRHEAL URETHRITIS

The sexually transmitted diseases caused by *Neisseria gonorrhea* primarily involve the male urethra and the female vagina and urethra. The symptoms and signs are urethral and vaginal discharge of pus and pain on urination. The infection may spread to other parts of the body, especially the joints. Serious eye infections in newborns can occur when the fetus travels through an infected vagina. In addition to painful urination and the discharge of pus, the following references also mention impotence.[4]

4.2 [DIŠ N]A GÌŠ-*šú ú-zaq-qa-su* U$_4$-*ma* KÀŠ.MEŠ-*šú i-šá-ti-nu re-ḫu-su* ŠUB-*a* [*ni-iš*] ŠÀ-*šú ṣa-bit-ma ana* MUNUS DU-*ka* LAL ÚŠ BABBAR *gi-na-a ina* GÌŠ-*šú* DU-*ak* NA.BI *mu-ṣa* GIG *ana* TI-*šú* . . . (*BAM* 112 i 17′–19′//*AMT* 58/6:2–3; *BAM* 112 i 34′–36′)

**[If] a ⌜person⌝'s penis stings him, he lets his semen fall when he urinates he is ⌜impotent⌝ and his going to a woman is diminished (and) pus continually flows from his penis, that person is sick with *mūṣu*,[5] to cure him . . .

4.3 *lu* NITA *lu* MUNUS *su-u*ʾ*-us re-ḫu-su-nu* [*m*]*a-a*ʾ*-da*! DU-*ak lu ina* K[ÀŠ].MEŠ-*šú-nu* [B]IR.[BIR . . .] (*BAM* 205:40′–42′)[6]

**(If) either a man or a woman's semen flows copiously or they ⌜spill⌝ it when they ⌜urinate⌝...

Since complications of gonorrheal urethritis include bloody urine (hematuria) and urethral narrowing (stenosis or stricture), the following may represent conditions secondary to gonorrhea; however, *Schistosomiasis hematobium,* a nonsexually transmitted infection, may also cause similar problems (see Chapter 5).

4.4 DIŠ *ina mu-šar-ri-šú* MÚD SUR ŠU ^{d}UTU MU KI.NU.GI GAM (DPS XIV A ii 37//C ii 12//F 3 = *TDP* 134 ii 37)

**If blood drips from his penis, "hand" of Šamaš on account of sexual intercourse with a woman;[7] he will die.

4.5 DIŠ NA GÌŠ-*šú ú-kàs-sa ḫi-níq-ti* x[...] *ana* TI-*šú*... (*BAM* 182 obv. 3′–4′)

**If a person's penis binds up, constriction [...], to cure him...

Some references describe patients with urethritis as well as other more serious systemic complaints. It is difficult to know if these cases represent advanced forms of the original sexually transmitted disease or some other complication.

4.6 *šum-ma* LÚ *mi-na-tu-šú* GIN$_{7}$ *mar-ṣi* D[U]B.MEŠ-*ka* [...] x GÌR^{II}-*šú pit-ru-šú ra-mu-ú i-qab-bi-ma la i-kaš-šad ni-iš* ŠÀ-*šú e-ṭi-ir* ŠÀ-*šú il-te-nem-mèn lu-u ina* KÀŠ-*šú lu-u ka-am-ma re-ḫu-ut-su ki-ma ša* KI MUNUS *uš-ta-ḫu-u*$_{16}$ ŠUB-*su* LÚ.BI *ul e-el* DINGIR *ù* ^{d}*Iš-tar suḫ*$_{4}$*-ḫu-ru-šu* DUG$_{4}$.GA.BI *ul ma-ag-rat* // [*ana*] LÚ.BI *ep-šu ana* IGI ^{d}*Iš-tar u* ^{d}*Dumu-zi ep-šu-šu* [A]LAM.MEŠ-*šú i-na qab-ri-im šu-nu-lu* LÚ.BI *a-na pa-ṭa-ri-im-ma i-na* ŠU^{II} ZI.KU$_{5}$.RU.DA KAR-*šu* KI DINGIR *u* LÚ *šul-lu-mi-šu k*[*i*]*-mil-ti* DINGIR *u* ^{d}*Eš*$_{4}$*-dar* DU$_{8}$*-ri-im-m*[*a*] *i-piš* MUNUS *i-pu-šú-šú šup-šu-ri-im-m*[*a* TI-*šú*]... U$_{4}$*-um re-ḫu-su i-ṣar-ru-ru*... (W. Farber, *BID* 227–234:1–14, 84′)

**If a person's limbs are tense[8] like one who is ill [...] his feet, his internal organs are relaxed, he says (he will do something) and then does not achieve it, his potency is taken away, he continually gets angry, his semen falls like one who has sexual intercourse with a woman either when he urinates or spontaneously,[9] that man is impure... a ritual has been performed against him before Ištar and Dumuzi. His figurines have been made to lie in a grave. To release that man and to save him from the "hand" of ZI.KU$_{5}$.RU.DA ... to dispel the ritual that a woman performed against him and [to cure him] ... the day his semen flows...

4.7 DIŠ NA *ina* KI.NÁ-*šú* LUḪ.LUḪ-*ut* ŠÀ-*šú e-šu-u ina* KI.NÁ-*šú re-ḫu-su* DU-*ak* NA BI DIB-*ti* ^{d}AMAR.UTU *u* ^{d}*Eš*$_{4}$*-dar* UGU-*šú* GÁL-*ši ana* TI-*šú*... (*STT* 95:16–18//*STT* 280 ii 1–3//*BAM* 205:19′–21′)

**If a person continually jerks in his bed, his heart (beat) is confused,[10] (and) his semen flows in his bed, the anger of Marduk and Ištar is upon that person; to cure him...

One quote describes urethritis with subsequent death of the patient. Gonococcal urethritis may occasionally develop into a disseminated infection that could result in death; however, other nonsexually transmitted infections might also have the same outcome.

4.8 [DIŠ KÀ]Š.MEŠ-*šu u* A.RI.A-*su* DU-*ak* GAM (DPS XIV A ii 45//C ii 17 = *TDP* 136 ii 45)

**[If] his ⌜urine⌝ or his semen continually flows, he will die.

A common complication is gonococcal arthritis. This topic is discussed in Chapter 11.

CHLAMYDIA URETHRITIS

Although less well known than gonorrhea, *Chlamydia trachomatis* is, in the modern era, a common cause of urethritis in both sexes and cervical infection in women. It causes painful urination, as does gonorrhea, but urethral discharge is much less prominent. The following quotes could be cases of *Chlamydia* urethritis, but clear separation from other causes is impossible. The first reference below appears in a therapeutic text next to a possible example of gonorrheal urethritis quoted above.

4.9 DIŠ NA GÌŠ-*šú ú-zaq-qa-ta-šú* . . . (*BAM* 182 obv. 2′, 5′)

**If a person's penis stings him . . .

4.10 MUNUS *ta-ti-ka-at ú-ri-ša* GIG . . . (*BAM* 241 ii 12′)

**(If) a woman is sick with dribbling from her vulva . . .

Other secondary infections and complications can also occur, such as pelvic inflammatory disease in women and reactive arthritis. Here we are on much more secure ground, since a number of references describe arthritis associated with urethritis and skin lesions (tense flesh; induration). For a review of reactive arthritis, see Chapter 11.

HERPES SIMPLEX TYPE 2 (HSV2) URETHRITIS

HSV2 is a viral infection that is spread primarily by venereal contact or via the birth canal of an infected mother. The initial infection in adults occurs five to seven days after exposure, and the first manifestations are small water-filled lesions (vesicles) with surrounding redness that are usually present in the genital area. The first attack is usually the most severe, associated with much pain, fever, and often headache and urinary incontinence. The genital vesicular lesions frequently recur from two to fifteen times per year for many years, if not for life. We believe that the Mesopotamian physician referred to vesicles as *bubuʾtu*, and the following reference provides their description.

4.11 [DIŠ G]IG GAR-*šú* GIN$_7$ TAB KÚM-*ma* A *ú-kal* [*bu*]-*bu-ʾ-tu*$_4$ MU.NI (DPS XXXIII:14 [AOAT 43.353])

**[If] the nature of the ⌜sore⌝ is that it is hot like a burn and contains fluid, it is called *bubuʾtu*.

A term that is sometimes associated with *bubuʾtu* on the genitals is "wind blasting." It is interesting to speculate as to the source of this term. Our guess is that it might refer to redness and irritation of the skin that would result from sand striking the skin during a severe windstorm (see Chapter 10).[11]

4.12 DIŠ GIG GAR-*šú* GIN_7 Ù.[BU].BU.UL *pa-gar-šú* DIRI *ši-biṭ* IM [MU.NI] (DPS XXXIII:26 [AOAT 43.354]//K 3526 r. 8; cf. *BAM* 580 vi 8′)[12]

**If the appearance of the sore is like a *bubu'tu* (and) his body is full (of them), ⌜it is called⌝ "wind blasting."

4.13 DIŠ NA GÌŠ-*šú* IM *iš-biṭ* [. . .] U_4.BÚ.BÚ.UL! DIRI . . . (*BAM* 112 ii 11′–12′)

**If "wind" has blasted a person's penis [. . .] it is full of *bubu'tu* . . .

In some references, "wind blasting" is mentioned without *bubu'tu*. If the skin involved is genital in location, it is still likely to be describing a venereal infection, possibly HSV2 prior to the development of vesicles.

4.14 DIŠ NA [GÌ]Š-*šú* IM *iš-biṭ* . . . (*BAM* 112 ii 8′)

**If "wind" has blasted a person's ⌜penis⌝ . . .

4.15 DIŠ MUNUS IM *iš-biṭ-ma ma-lit ù* SU-*šá* KÚR.KÚR *ana* TI-*šá* . . . (*BAM* 240:20′)

**If "wind" blasts a woman and she is about to give birth and (the appearance of) her skin/body continually changes (for the worse), to cure her . . .

Vesicular lesions may be caused by other viruses such as the cold sore virus (*Herpes simplex* type 1), chickenpox virus (*Varicella* virus), and smallpox virus (*Variola* virus).

Herpes simplex type 1 (HSV1) characteristically produces *bubu'tu* (vesicles) on the face and mouth. Therefore, the following quotes are likely to be illnesses caused by nonvenereal mechanisms. (For more details on herpetic stomatitis, see Chapter 3.)

4.16 DIŠ IGI.MEŠ-*šú* BU.BU.UL SA_5 DIRI.MEŠ ŠU ^{d}30 DIN (DPS IX A 47//C 15 = *TDP* 74:47)

**If his face is full of red *bubu'tu*, "hand" of Sîn; he will get well.

4.17 DIŠ KA-*šú* U_4.BU.BU.UL DIRI *u il-la-tu-šú* [DU-*ka* . . .] (DPS VII B obv. 4′ = TDP 64:43′; cf. DPS XXXIII:87 [AOAT 43.357])

**If a man's mouth is full of *bubu'tu* and his saliva [flows, *bu'sānu* . . .].[13]

However, when the Mesopotamian physician describes vesicles, and he suspects sexual contact to be a significant factor, then it is quite likely that HSV2 is the cause.

4.18 [DIŠ TA SAG.D]U-*šú* EN $GÌR^{II}$-*šú* U_4.BU.BU.UL SA_5 DIRI *u* SU-*šú* BABBAR KI MUNUS *ina* KI.NÁ KUR ŠU 30 (DPS III A r. 8′//C r. 31 = *TDP* 28:91)[14]

**[If from] his ⌜head⌝ to his feet, he is full of red *bubu'tu* and his skin/body is white, he was "gotten" in bed with a woman; "hand" of Sîn.[15]

The preceding quote describes the *bubu'tu* (vesicles) as covering the entire body. In the modern era, HSV2 rarely causes generalized vesicles either in the primary episode or in recurring episodes. The reference above, however, so strongly emphasizes the role of sexual contact that HSV2 appears the likely cause. None of the other common causes of STDs including syphilis, gonorrhea, and *Chlamydia* produce vesicles. It is possible that this is an agent that is no longer a human pathogen, or that HSV2 in an earlier relationship with humans was capable of presenting in this fashion. For further discussion, see Chapter 10.

The following references appear to be citing cases of HSV2 urethritis with associated genital vesicles,[16] but since HSV2 usually does not cause significant urethral discharge of pus it is likely that the patients had a mixed STD such as HSV2 and gonorrhea or HSV2 and *Chlamydia.*

4.19 [DIŠ NA] *re-ḫu-su* DU-*ma* NU ZU *ka-la ú-ri-šú* [... U_4.B]Ú.BÚ.UL TUR.MEŠ DIRI ... (*AMT* 61/1:9′–10′)

**[If a person]'s semen flows and he does not know (it), (and) his whole pubic region is full of [...] (and) small ⸢*bubuʾtu*⸣ ...

4.20 DIŠ NA *i-na-aṭ-ma i-na* DU-*šu re-ḫu-us-su* DU-*ma* NU ZU GIN_7 *šá ana* MUNUS DU *ma-aṣ-ra-aḫ* ⸢KÀŠ⸣-*šu* Ù.BU.BU.UL SIG-*ta* DIRI ... (*BAM* 396 iv 6–8//*AMT* 61/1:5′–6′)

**If a person has a condition of discharge[17] so that when he walks his semen flows and he does not know (it) like one who goes to a woman (and) the "duct of his urine" (urethra) is full of narrow (i.e., small) *bubuʾtu* (vesicles) ...

An interesting aspect of the second quote above is that blisters (vesicles) were seen within the urethra. Since the *āšipu* would have lacked the instruments with the lighting necessary to see farther into the urethra, he must have spread the opening of the urethra and described the appearance of the terminal portion of this structure.

Vaginitis

Infection of the vagina can be due to a sexually transmitted disease such as gonorrhea, *Trichomonas,* or *Chlamydia,* or to non-STD-related organisms such as yeast (*Candida*) and bacterial vaginosis. Vaginal discharge is a common presenting complaint.

4.21 DIŠ MUNUS Ú.ḪI.A *ze-ru-te šu-ku-ul* A.MEŠ *ina* ŠÀ GAL_4.LA-*šá ma-gal* DU-*ku* [...] TUKU-*ú ana* ⸢*ša*⸣ GIG-*ša* NU GÍD.DA ... (*BAM* 237 iv 29–30)

**If a woman has been given plants of hatred to eat (and) much fluid runs from her vagina (and) it has [...] in order that her illness not be prolonged ...

4.22 [KA.INIM.MA DIŠ MUNUS A].MEŠ *ina* ŠÀ GAL_4.LA-*šá* DU-[*ku*] ... (*BAM* 237 iv 44)

**[Recitation for cases where] ⸢fluid⸣ runs from a [woman]'s vagina ...

Syphilis

The origin and spread of syphilis remains a debated topic, with some arguing that it evolved in the New World and was brought to Europe on Columbus's ships. It is also possible that it existed throughout the world,[18] but that the Columbian expedition imported a particularly virulent strain. Although we do not believe that the following quotes are strong evidence for the existence of syphilis in the ancient Near East, they do contain some features that are compatible with that disease.

CONGENITAL SYPHILIS

The first reference below describes an infant with uneven yellow skin color, a rash that can be seen in congenital syphilis. Swollen hands and fingers are common features of this disease. We know that *liʾbu* indicates fever with a rash (see Chapter 3), and the "sick lungs" could be describing the pneumonia that may occur with congenital syphilis. There are a variety of neurologic changes in this condition, including seizures and pupillary changes, especially constriction of the pupils, which may be what is being described in the second reference below.

4.23 DIŠ LÚ.TUR UZU.MEŠ-*šú* SIG$_7$ ŠUB-*ú* ŠÀ.MEŠ-*šú eb-ṭu* ŠU^{II}-*šú* GÌR-*šú nap-ḫa li-ʾ-ba ma-gal* TUKU *ḫa-še-e* GIG ŠU DINGIR TI (DPS XL A 29 = *TDP* 220:29)

**If an infant's flesh is unevenly colored with yellow, his insides are cramped, his hands (and) feet are swollen, he has lots of *liʾbu*, and the lungs are sick, "hand" of god; he will get well.[19]

4.24 DIŠ LÚ.TUR ŠU^{II}-*šú u* GÌR^{II}-*šú it-ta-na-an-pa-ḫa* IGI^{II}-*šú uz-za-na-qap* ^{GIŠ}GIDRU ^{d}30 *u* ^{d}15 (DPS XL A 56 = *TDP* 224:56)

**If an infant's hands and feet are continually swollen (and) he continually constricts (the pupils of) his eyes, scepter of Sîn or Ištar.[20]

PRIMARY SYPHILIS

The first physical finding in patients with syphilis is usually a solitary, firm (indurated), raised, and painless ulcer (chancre) located generally on the penis or vulva. It begins two or three weeks after exposure and, even if untreated, it heals in three to eight weeks. Similar to, and often confused with, syphilitic lesions, are chancroidal ulcers (see below). These are also sexually transmitted, but are painful and soft rather than indurated. The following reference may be describing the chancre of primary syphilis.

4.25 DIŠ GIG MIN *ul* KÚ-*šú* IGI UZU.MEŠ-*šú-ma* GAR-*in* MÚD-*šú-ma* MÚD.[BABBAR] *šur-du-ma* DU-*ak lam-ṣa-at ḫi-la-a-te* MUNUS MU.NI IM *iš-*[*biṭ-su-ma*] *si-ḫi-ip-ti* ^{d}MAŠ.TAB.BA *qí-ba* GAR-*an ana* ZI-*šú* . . . (*BAM* 580 iii 20′–22′)

**If a sore (comes out on a person's body), it does not hurt him, it is placed only on the surface of his flesh, (and) its blood (and) pus flows freely, it is called a female suppurating *lamṣātu*-ulcer . . .[21] You may make a (favorable) prognosis. To remove it . . .[22]

SECONDARY SYPHILIS

After the primary chancre resolves, most patients develop a generalized macular (flat, red) rash that signals the secondary stage of syphilis. Some patients will experience hair loss.

Fever is either low-grade or absent. Some patients develop a transient meningitis with stiff neck and variable neurological abnormalities that are usually reversible.

There are four references (4.26, 4.29–31, cf. 19.24–25) that appear to constitute a single ancient syndrome attributed to the *lilû* family of demons (including also *lilītu* and *ardāt lilî*; see Chapter 12). The reference listed below may be describing secondary syphilis.

4.26 DIŠ SAG.KI-*šú* SAG ŠÀ-*šú* NA₄KIŠIB GÚ-*šú* DIB.DIB-*su* KÚM *la ḫa-aḫ-ḫaš u* IR NU TUKU *ina ma-rak* U_4-*mi* SÍG *šá-pu-li-šú i-šaḫ-ḫu-uḫ* ŠU KI.SIKIL.LÍL.LÁ.EN.NA *la-ʾ-bi* (DPS IV B obv. 20-21 = *TDP* 34:20-21)

**If his temples, his upper abdomen (epigastrium), (and) the vertebrae of his neck continually afflict him, his temperature is lukewarm, and he does not sweat (but) over a long period of time[23] the hair of his inguinal region[24] falls out, infectious "hand" of *ardat lilî*.[25]

Syphilis and the virus causing genital warts (papilloma virus) characteristically cause multiple white-colored genital lesions called condylomata. The following references may be describing patients with these lesions. There is not enough information to suggest whether syphilis or papilloma virus was the causative organism. For more references to these and other skin lesions that may be venereal, see Chapter 10.

4.27 DIŠ MUNUS Ù.TU-*ma* SU-*šá bir-di* DIRI DÚR-*šá ma-qit* . . . (*BAM* 240:29′)

**If a woman gives birth and subsequently her body is full of *birdu*-nodules (and) her anus has prolapsed . . .

4.28 DIŠ ŠIR^{II}-*šú* MÚ.MEŠ-*ḫa* GÌŠ-*šú sik-ka-ta*₅ DIRI *ana* N[IN.DINGIR.RA DINGIR-*šú* TE-*ḫi*] (DPS XIV A_2 ii 16//C ii 30 = *TDP* 136 ii 66)

**If his testicles are continually swollen[26] (and) his penis is full of *sikkatu* (peg-shaped lesions), [he approached] the ⌜*ēntu*⌝ [of his god].

TERTIARY SYPHILIS

The secondary stage resolves with or without treatment. If untreated with antibiotics, tertiary syphilis may develop. Some of its manifestations are possibly described in the references below.

GENERAL PARESIS OF SYPHILIS (brain damage that causes emotional lability, paranoia, delusions, hallucinations, and decreased cognitive ability)

4.29 ⌜DIŠ⌝ U_4 LÁ-*šú* UB.NÍGIN.NA-*šú i-šam-ma-ma-šú i-re-eḫ-ḫi-šum-ma* NI-*šú i-maš-ši* U_4 *ir-te-ḫu-šú* IGI^{II}-*šú* SAR-*ṭa* IGI.MEŠ-*šú* SA₅ : *suḫ*₄-*ḫu-ru* SA.MEŠ-*šú* ZI.MEŠ *u i-leb-bu ap-pat* U.MEŠ ŠU^{II}-*šú u* GÌR^{II}-*šú ka-ṣa-a* GIG BI MAŠ.MAŠ *ú-šad-bab-šú-ma ša ú-šad-ba-bu-šú i-qab-bi* U_4 *un-deš-ši-ru-šú šá id-bu-bu* NU ZU ŠU LÍL.LÁ.EN.NA *la-ʾi-bi* (DPS XXVI:22′–25′ [AOAT 43.280])

**If when (a confusional state) comes over him, his limbs go numb, as it flows over him he forgets himself, when it has flowed over him, his eyes (look) "(wind) blasted,"[27] his face flushes (var. he turns away), his blood vessels (feel like they) are pulsating and he groans, the tips of his fingers and toes are cold, (and) the *āšipu* makes that patient say (something) and (the patient) says what (the *āšipu*) has him say (but) when (the confusional state) has left him, (the patient) does not know what he said, infectious "hand" of *lilû*.[28]

TABIES DORSALIS (syphilis-induced spinal cord disease causing an unsteady wide-based, foot-slapping gait, and severe shooting pain in the back and legs)

4.30 ⌜DIŠ GÚ⌝-*su i-tar-rak* SAG.DU-*su* ŠUB.ŠUB-*ut* ŠU^{II}-*šú u* GÌR^{II}-*šú it-ta-na-aš-gag-gu u ana qaq-qa-ru ú-ḫa-an-na-aṣ* KI.SIKIL.LÍL.LÁ DIB-*su* (DPS X A obv. 12–13//B obv. 12–13 = *TDP* 80:12–13)

**If his neck throbs, his head continually falls (i.e., he lets it drop), his hands and feet are continually stiff, and he rubs (them) on the ground, *ardat lilî* afflicts him.

4.31 DIŠ *la-ma* DIB-*šú* IGI.⌜MEŠ⌝-[*šú* . . .]-*su ne-ḫu* ŠU^{II}-*šú u* GÌR^{II}-*šú am-šá mi-na-tu-šú i-ṭa-ma-a* [. . . ŠU LÍL.LÁ.EN.N]A *la-ʾi-bi šum-ma* U_4 DIB-*š*[*ú* . . .]-*ku* [. . .] G[IG.BI . . .] (DPS XXVI:53′–55′ [AOAT 43.283])

**If, before it afflicts ⌜him⌝, [his] face [. . .], his [. . .] is calm, his hands and his feet are immobilized, his limbs twist [. . .], infectious ["hand" of *lilû*]. If when it ⌜afflicts him⌝ [. . ., that] ⌜patient⌝ [will not live].

Chancroid

The ulcers of chancroid are soft yet painful. Uncircumcised males are more susceptible to chancroid. Prostitution plays a major role in transmission, and among merchant seamen and military troops whose sexual contacts are prostitutes, chancroid is more common than syphilis. The classic chancroidal ulcer is superficial, ranging in size from a few millimeters to several centimeters in diameter. The ulcers are often multiple and may merge to form giant or serpiginous ulcers. The following reference, which appears in sequence in a therapeutic text with the putative syphilitic chancre quoted (4.25) above, may be describing chancroidal ulcers.

4.32 DIŠ GIG MIN *ul-la-nu-ma ḫa-ri-is* ŠÀ-*ba-šu* KAK.MEŠ DIRI KAK.MEŠ-*šú* BAD KÚ[M] *u* DU-*ak lam-ṣa-at ḫi-la-a-ti* NÍTA MU.NI IM *iš-biṭ-su-ma si-ḫi-*[*ip-ti*] ^{d}PA.BIL.SAG DUG_4.GA GAR-*an ana* ZI-*šú* . . . (*BAM* 580 iii 15′–17′)

**If a sore (comes out on a person's body), it has been itching for a long time, the inside of it is full of *sikkatu* (peg-shaped lesions), it encloses its *sikkatu*, it is hot and it flows, it is called a male suppurating *lamṣātu*-ulcer . . .[29] You may make a (favorable) prognosis. To remove it . . .[30]

Fitz-Hugh Curtis Syndrome

Gonorrhea and chlamydial urethritis occasionally spread to the abdomen to infect the capsule of the liver (perihepatitis). These organisms cause not only painful urination and urethral discharge, but also abdominal pain in the area of the liver. This problem is most common in women but can also occur in men. This reference may be describing patients with this syndrome.

4.34 DIŠ NA GÌŠ-*šú u* SAG ŠÀ-*šú* KÚM *ṣar-ḫa ú-kal* TÙN ŠÀ-*šú* KÚ-*šú u* ŠÀ-*šú ma-ḫu* Á^{II}-*šú* GÌR^{II}-*šú u* ŠÀ-*šú* KÚM-*em* NA BI GIG *na-a-ki* GIG ŠU ^{d}15 (DPS XXII:14–15 [AOAT 43.252]; cf. DPS XIV A ii 34–36//C ii 10–11 = *TDP* 134 ii 34–36)

**If a person's penis and his upper abdomen (epigastrium) hold burning fever, his liver[31] hurts him and his stomach goes crazy, (and) his arms, his feet, and his stomach are hot, that person is sick with a disease of sexual intercourse; "hand" of Ištar.

Hepatitis

We do not usually think of hepatitis as a sexually transmitted disease, but some types can be spread in this fashion. It is well documented that the hepatitis B virus may be spread between sexual partners. The illness described below is likely to be hepatitis, and clearly the physician believed that sexual contact was playing a role in its spread.

4.35 DIŠ NA SAG ŠÀ-*šú i-ḫa-am-maṭ-su u* KÚM-*em* NINDA KÚ-*ma* UGU-*šú* NU DU-*ak* A NAG-*ma* UGU-*šú* NU DÙG.GA *u* SU-*šú* SIG$_7$ NA BI GIG *na-a-ki* GIG (DPS XXII:12–13 [AOAT 43.252]; cf. DPS XIII B i 5′–6′ = *TDP* 110 i 9′–10′)

**If his upper abdomen (epigastrium) gives him a burning pain and he is feverish, he eats bread and it does not agree with him, he drinks water and it does not taste good to him, and his body is yellow, that person is sick with a disease of intercourse.

Summary

The sexual mores of ancient Mesopotamia, although in some regards Victorian, still allowed for a wide variety of sexual partners, so it comes as no surprise that STDs were common problems then as now. The *āšipu* appears to have understood that STDs were associated with sexual activity. He used medicines to treat these illnesses, but there is no evidence of public health measures used to deal with this problem. It seems likely that some of the same causative organisms present now were also causing STDs in ancient Mesopotamia, but as with other types of infections there may have been changes in patient response to individual organisms, the loss of some pathogens, and the acquisition of new pathogens.

CHAPTER 5

Genitourinary Tract Diseases[1]

If his penis is blocked off, he will die.

—DPS XIV A ii 32//C ii 9 = *TDP* 134 ii 32

Much of ancient Mesopotamia was dry and hot with little shade. These conditions placed the inhabitants at greater risk of dehydration and concentrated urine, and the potential for developing kidney stones. Another factor is the likely presence of *Schistosomiasis hematobium* in ancient Mesopotamia. We cannot be certain that this infection was present at the time, but it is certainly widespread in the modern Near East. This organism requires an intermediate snail host (*Bulinus truncatus*), which is known to have existed along the banks of the Tigris and Euphrates rivers and their irrigation canals, as was demonstrated by the discovery of *Bulinus* shells embedded in the bricks used to construct the walls of Babylon and the ziggurat at Dur Kurigalzu (modern ʿAqar Quf).[2] In addition, the eggs of *Schistosomiasis hematobium* have been found in Egyptian mummies dating to 1250 B.C.E.[3]

The parasite is released from the snail during the daylight and can penetrate the intact skin of anyone in the water. Since the irrigation canals required constant maintenance by workmen, and the river was probably used for recreation and relief from the heat by adults and children, there would have been ample opportunity for exposure to this infectious organism. The other information that supports the presence of *Schistosomiasis hematobium* in Mesopotamia is the frequent description of signs and symptoms compatible with this illness such as bloody urine (hematuria) and urinary tract obstruction (see below).

Examination of Urine

The ancient Mesopotamian physician observed and recorded most of the important physical characteristics of urine in evaluating his patients. When the patient's urine looked entirely normal, it suggested to the *āšipu* that the patient's illness was not severe, and that the prognosis was good.[4]

5.1 DIŠ KÀŠ.MEŠ-*šú taq-na* [DIN][5] (DPS XIV A_2 ii 1//C ii 20 = *TDP* 136 ii 51)

**If his urine is normal, [he will get well].

COLOR AND CONSISTENCY

Many urine colors and tones are described in the texts, including white, red, wine, dark or greenish-yellow, black, and dark.

WHITE This term was probably not applied to clear, colorless urine, but to cloudy (milky white) urine (see below).

RED Free hemoglobin from broken-down (lysed) red blood cells secondary to a condition such as trauma or tumor may cause red urine. Some foods such as beets may also produce this color.

5.2 DIŠ KÀŠ.MEŠ-*šú* SA_5.MEŠ ŠU DINGIR-*šú* DIN (DPS XIV A ii 39//C ii 14 = *TDP* 134 ii 39)

**If his urine is reddish, "hand" of his god; he will get well.

WINE One form of porphyria, a group of inherited metabolic diseases, may produce "port wine" colored-urine.[6] Also associated with this disease are episodes of severe pain and skin abnormalities. These episodes may improve, but the patients often die in middle age of kidney and liver disease. For more information on this and other metabolic disorders, see Chapter 7.

5.3 DIŠ KÀŠ.MEŠ-*šu* GIN_7 GEŠTIN GIG-*su* DUGUD-*ma* DIN (DPS XIV A ii 49//C ii 19 = *TDP* 136 ii 49)

**If his urine is like wine, his illness may be difficult,[7] (but) he will get well.

GREENISH-YELLOW Bile byproducts in urine due to biliary tract obstruction or severe liver disease will produce this color. The statement in the following reference that the disease will be prolonged suggests a serious illness, which is compatible with the nature of these problems.[8] Urinary tract infection may occasionally cause green-colored urine.

5.4 DIŠ KÀŠ.MEŠ-*šú* SIG_7.MEŠ GIG-*su* GÍD (DPS XIV A ii 40 = *TDP* 136 ii 40)[9]

**If his urine is (greenish) yellow, his illness will be prolonged.

BLACK The following reference describes black urine and predicts the death of the patient. In spite of the minimal data provided, there is a good possibility that this represents hemoglobinuria secondary to massive breakdown of red blood cells in patients with falciparum malaria (see Chapter 3). Reduced hemoglobin in urine may appear dark brown to black and, when caused by malaria, it is often called "blackwater fever." Death in this clinical setting is common. Alkaptonuria, an inherited metabolic disease, and malignant melanoma are uncommon causes of black urine. Alkaptonuria causes arthritis, but death is an unusual consequence; however, death from untreated malignant melanoma is almost inevitable.

5.5 [DIŠ K]ÀŠ.MEŠ-*šú* GI$_6$.MEŠ TAG ÚŠ TAG-*it* GAM (DPS XIV A ii 41 = *TDP* 136 ii 41)

**[If] his ⌜urine⌝ is black, he was touched with the touch of death; he will die.

DARK/THICK VERSUS WATERY Watery urine could be dilute urine caused by malfunctioning kidneys that are unable to concentrate the urine.[10] Dark or thick urine could be very concentrated because of heat-related dehydration, or excess fluid loss from a gastrointestinal problem such as vomiting or diarrhea. Other possible causes of dark urine are listed above, under black urine.

5.6 [DIŠ K]ÀŠ.MEŠ-*šu* GIN$_7$ A.MEŠ GIG-*su* GÍD-*ma* DIN (DPS XIV A ii 47//C ii 18 = *TDP* 136 ii 47)

**[If] his ⌜urine⌝ is watery, his illness may be prolonged, (but) he will get well.

5.7 DIŠ KÀŠ.MEŠ-*šú tar-ka* GAM (DPS XIV A ii 42//C ii 15 = *TDP* 136 ii 42)

**If his urine is dark, he will die.

5.8 [. . .] GÌŠ-*šú eb-bu* . . . (*AMT* 39/9:6′)

**[If the liquid from][11] his penis becomes thick . . .

As modern physicians are prone to do, ancient physicians used analogous foods or substances to describe the appearance of urine. For example, in the references below urine was described as looking like *kasû* juice or light varnish. Since we cannot be sure what these fluids looked like, we are unable to use this information to help us determine the nature of the disease causing this change.

5.9 DIŠ KÀŠ.MEŠ-*šu* GIN$_7$ A GAZI$^{\text{[SAR]}}$ KI.MIN (DPS XIV A ii 48//C ii 18 = *TDP* 136 ii 48)[12]

**If his urine is like ⌜*kasû*⌝ juice, (his illness may be prolonged, but he will get well).

5.10 [DIŠ NA] KÀŠ.MEŠ-*šú* GIN$_7$ ŠE.GÍN *ḫi-li-ti* NA BI *mu-ṣa* GI[G] . . . (*BAM* 112 i 16′; *BAM* 114:4)

**[If a person]'s urine is like light-colored varnish, that person is ⌜sick⌝ with *mūṣu* (discharge; see below) . . .

Where we have some idea what the substance would have looked like (e.g., milk or leather), the description provides useful information.

MILK This is consistent with the appearance of urine from some patients with a parasitic disease, namely, *Wuchereria bancrofti.* This form of filariasis can cause obstruction of deep peritoneal lymphatics leading to the diversion of fat absorbed from the intestines into the urine. This fat typically gives the urine a milky (chylous) appearance. Occasionally very high-fat meals in normal individuals will produce milky urine.

5.11 DIŠ NA KÀŠ.MEŠ-*šu* GIN_7 GA DIN (DPS XIV A ii 50//C ii 19 = *TDP* 136 ii 50)[13]

**If a person's urine is like milk, he will get well.

Another cause of white or milky urine is the presence of calcium phosphate (apatite) crystals, which usually form in alkaline urine. This material seldom reaches a size capable of blocking the urinary tract or causing the pain associated with larger kidney stones. The reference below is compatible with this condition.

5.12 [*šu*]*m*$_4$-*ma* KÀŠ-*šú* BABBAR-*ma e-ba-a* NA BI NA_4 *šá-ḫi-ḫ*[*u*] GIG . . . (*BAM* 114:7 //*BAM* 161 iv 1′–2′//*AMT* 58/4:3′)

**⌜If⌝ his urine is white and thick, that person is sick with ⌜excreted⌝[14] stones . . .

DŪŠU LEATHER/STONE There are two clues in the following quote. The patient was observed to have stones, and the urine or the stones in it have the appearance of *dūšu* stones or the similarly colored tanned leather.[15] The color of tanned leather is orange/brown, the color of uric acid stones in the presence of uracil. Patients with gout commonly have urinary tract stones of this type and color.

5.13 *šum*$_4$-*ma* KÀŠ-*šú* GIN_7 ^{KUŠ}/^{NA_4}*du*$_8$-*ši-e* NA BI NA_4 G[IG] . . . (*BAM* 114:8//*BAM* 161 iv 2′–3′//*AMT* 58/4:4′)

**If his urine is like *dūšu* leather/(colored) stone, that person is ⌜sick⌝ with stones . . .

BEER/WINE DREGS The consistency of urine could be characterized as resembling beer or wine dregs, which probably means that it had a large amount of sediment. This material could be amorphous calcium phosphate (apatite) crystals described above, but pigmented by contaminating material such as red or white blood cells. Cellular debris by itself may also collect in urine to form a sediment.

5.14 [DIŠ NA] KÀŠ.MEŠ-*šú* GIN_7 *šur-šum-me* KAŠ NA BI *mu-ṣa* G[IG] . . . (*BAM* 112 i 14′; *BAM* 114:2; *AMT* 66/7:4)

**[If a person]'s urine is like beer dregs, that person is ⌜sick⌝ with *mūṣu*[16] . . .

5.15 [DIŠ NA] KÀŠ.MEŠ-*šú* GIN_7 *šur-šum-me* GEŠTIN NA BI *mu-ṣa* GI[G] . . . (*BAM* 112 i 15′; *BAM* 114:3)

**[If a person]'s urine is like wine dregs, that person is ⌜sick⌝ with *mūṣu* . . .

HEMATURIA

Hematuria (bloody urine) was frequently mentioned, and could have been due to schistosomiasis, kidney stones, urinary tract cancer, trauma, and other causes.

5.16 DIŠ NA *mi-na-tu-šú* DUB.DUB GABA-*su u* SA.SAL.MEŠ-*šú* KÚ.MEŠ-*šú* Á^{II}-*šú* x [. . .] KÚ.MEŠ-*šú bir-bir-ki-šú lu šá* 15 *lu šá* 150 SÌG-*su-ma ina múš-tin-*[*ni*]-*šú* MÚD *ú-kal-lam* NA

BI *ḫi-niq-ti* DÚR GIG GIG *ana* TI-*šú* . . . (*AMT* 40/5 iii 14–16//*AMT* 56/1 obv. 1–3//*BAM* 88:1′–2′)

**If his limbs are continually tense,[17] his breast and his back continually hurt him, his arms [and legs?] continually hurt him, his loins[18] either on the left or right side give him a jabbing pain, and from his ⌜urethra⌝ he shows blood,[19] that person is sick with the constriction of DÚR.GIG,[20] to cure him . . .

5.17 DIŠ NA *ina* GÌŠ-*šu* MÚD *ú-tab-ba-ka* GIN$_7$ MUNUS ^{GIŠ}TUKUL *ma-ḫi-iṣ ana* TI-*šú* . . . (*BAM* 159 i 9–10//*BAM* 182 obv. 6′//*BAM* 396 iv 3)[21]

**If a person pours blood from his penis[22] like a (menstruating) woman, he was wounded with a weapon, to cure him . . .

5.18 DIŠ *ina mu-šar-ri-šú* MÚD SUR ŠU ^{d}UTU MU KI.NU.GI GAM (DPS XIV A ii 37//C ii 12//F 3 = *TDP* 134 ii 37)

**If blood drips from his penis, "hand" of Šamaš on account of sexual intercourse with a woman;[23] he will die.

5.19 DIŠ KI.MIN-[*m*]*a ina* KÀŠ-*šú* MÚD *iš-tin ana* KI GIG GAM (DPS XVI:7 [AOAT 43.172])[24]

**If (it is the first day he is sick) ⌜and⌝ he urinates blood in his urine, he is at an acute stage of the illness;[25] he will die.

The following text describes urine that was initially free of blood and with either a deep yellow color (donkey urine) or light (almost colorless: white), but became bloody at the end of urination. This type of terminal hematuria has been described in schistosomiasis, although it can occur in other conditions as well. It is due to bleeding near the base of the bladder (trigone).

5.20 DIŠ NA UZU.ÉLLAG-*su* KÚ-*šu* MURUB$_4$-*šú* TAG.TAG-*šú ù* KÀŠ-*šú* GIN$_7$ KÀŠ ANŠE BABBAR-*a* EGIR KÀŠ-*šu* MÚD *ú-kal-lam* NA BI *mu-ṣa-am* GIG . . . (*BAM* 396 i 23′–24′//*AMT* 66/7:18–19)

**If a person's kidney hurts him,[26] his pelvic region continually hurts him intensely, and his urine is like the urine of a donkey[27] (or) it is white (and) after his urine he shows blood, that person is sick with *mūṣu*[28] . . .

"SEMEN"

There are numerous references to semen appearing in the urine or coming from the penis when the individual had not ejaculated. The likely explanation is that the ancient Mesopotamian physician was confusing semen with the whitish discharge (pus) seen in patients with urethral infection or inflammation. Even twentieth-century C.E. physicians until the 1940s believed that whitish discharge from the urethra could be semen and applied the term *spermatorrhea* to it. Closer examination has shown that this nonejaculatory discharge consists primarily of inflammatory cells (pus) and very few sperm.

5.21 *lu* NITA *lu* MUNUS *su-u*ʾ*-us re-ḫu-su-nu* [*m*]*a-a*ʾ*-da*! DU-*ak lu ina* K[ÀŠ].MEŠ-*šú-nu* [B]IR.[BIR . . .] (*BAM* 205:40′–42′)

**(If) either a man or a woman's semen flows ⌜copiously⌝ in his bed or they ⌜spill⌝ it when they ⌜urinate⌝ . . .

5.22 [DIŠ N]A GÌŠ-*šú ú-zaq-qa-su* U_4-*ma* KÀŠ.MEŠ-*šú i-šá-ti-nu re-ḫu-su* ŠUB-*a* [*ni-iš*] ŠÀ-*šú ṣa-bit-ma ana* MUNUS DU-*ka* LAL MÚD.BABBAR *gi-na-a ina* GÌŠ-*šú* DU-*ak* NA.BI *mu-ṣa* GIG *ana* TI-*šú* . . . (*BAM* 112 i 17′–19′//*AMT* 58/6:2–3; *BAM* 112 i 34′–36′)

**[If] a ⌜person⌝'s penis stings him, he lets his semen fall when he urinates,[29] he is ⌜impotent⌝ and his sexual appetite is diminished, (and) pus continually flows from his penis,[30] that person is sick with *mūṣu*,[31] to cure him . . .

STINK

The odor of urine is described in the quote below as "stinking" in a patient with kidney stones. We know that kidney stones are commonly associated with infection of the urinary tract, since kidney stones can be both the cause and consequence of some infections. The infection may cause the urine to smell bad, especially if the infecting bacteria are members of the genus *Proteus*. Kidney stones (struvite stones) are more likely to form as a consequence of *Proteus* infections than with other organisms infecting the urinary tract.

5.23 KI.5-*ma ù* KÀŠ-*šú ú-ṣa-nu* . . . (*BAM* 396 ii 19′)

**If (a person is sick with stones)[32] and his urine also stinks . . .

MŪṢU

The ancient physician often used the term *mūṣu* to identify any abnormal-looking material coming from the urethra. This word is a noun probably derived from a verb (*waṣû*) which means to "come out," but it was only applied to urine, and only to urine of unusual color or consistency, suggesting to the ancient physician the presence of a discharge.[33]

5.24 [DIŠ NA] KÀŠ.MEŠ-*šú* GIN_7 KÀŠ ANŠE NA.BI *mu-ṣa* G[IG / DIŠ NA] KÀŠ.MEŠ-*šú* GIN_7 *šur-šum-me* KAŠ NA.BI *mu-ṣa* G[IG / DIŠ NA] KÀŠ.MEŠ-*šú* GIN_7 *šur-šum-me* GEŠTIN NA.BI *mu-ṣa* GI[G / DIŠ NA] KÀŠ.MEŠ-*šú* GIN_7 ŠE.GÍN *ḫi-li-ti* NA.BI *mu-ṣa* GI[G] (*BAM* 112 i 13′–16′; *BAM* 114:1–4; cf. *AMT* 66/7:4)

**[If a person]'s urine is like the urine of a donkey, that person is ⌜sick⌝ with *mūṣu*. [If a person]'s urine is like beer dregs, that person is ⌜sick⌝ with *mūṣu*. [If a person]'s urine is like wine dregs, that person is ⌜sick⌝ with *mūṣu*. [If a person]'s urine is like light-colored varnish, that person is ⌜sick⌝ with *mūṣu*.

SOLIDS

Solid material was also noted in the urine. Ancient physicians were well aware of kidney stones and their association with pain and hematuria, and they observed that the stones were frequently passed into the urine. The climate in Mesopotamia would have increased the likelihood of dehydration, and the increased concentration of urine raises the potential for kidney stones to develop. This condition continues to be a common problem in the present era. Kidney stones are also a common complication of schistosomiasis.

5.25 [DIŠ NA *ina* G]ÌŠ-*šú* NA_4 ŠUB-*a* NA.BI [NA_4] GIG *ana* TI-*šú* . . . (*BAM* 111 iii 15′–16′//*AMT* 66/11:16)[34]

**[If a person] produces a stone [from] his ⌜penis⌝, that person is sick with [stones], to cure him . . .

5.26 Ú NA_4 *kaṣ-ri* . . . (*BAM* 380:55//*BAM* 381 iv 10)[35]

**Plant for concentrated stones . . .

The *āšipu* also described fleshy material in the urine. This material is probably necrotic tissue from the drainage structure of the kidney (papillary necrosis) that is likely to occur in infected and obstructed kidneys and in patients with diabetes. See Chapter 7 with 7.29–7.30 for a discussion of "touched in the steppe."

5.27 DIŠ KÀŠ.MEŠ-*šu* IGI-*ma* UZU.MEŠ-*šú* È.MEŠ-*ni ina* EDIN T[AG] (DPS XIV A_2 ii 3//C ii 22 = *TDP* 136 ii 53)[36]

**If you look at his urine and (bits of) his flesh come out of it, he was ⌜"touched"⌝ in the steppe.

Urine Flow

When a patient's urine output is noted to decrease markedly or stop completely, modern physicians recognize three general causes of this problem. Severe dehydration will reduce and eventually stop urine production. Mechanical obstruction to urine flow anywhere along the drainage system including the ureters, bladder, and urethra can occur. Primary kidney diseases can slowly or rapidly cause urine production to decrease and eventually stop.

Physicians of ancient Mesopotamia knew the location of the kidneys, and there is indirect evidence that they understood their role in the production of urine.[37] The importance of this process seems to have been recognized since the *āšipu* usually expressed a grim prognosis when urine flow ceased (see below).

As medical texts below indicate, ancient physicians understood the problem of obstruction and possibly dehydration. Stones were treated by medicines (see below), and urethral obstructions could have been treated with the same copper and bronze tubes that were used to infuse medicines into the bladder.[38] Their understanding of kidney disease is less clear, although they spoke of "sick kidneys."[39]

DEHYDRATION

The quantity of urine produced by an individual would be reduced by heat-induced dehydration or water loss from enteritis causing vomiting and diarrhea.

5.28 DIŠ ŠÀ.MEŠ-*šú iṣ-ṣa-na-pu-ú* KÀŠ.MEŠ-*šú ta-ba-ka* NU ZU-*e* ŠU⸢d⸣[. . .] (DPS XIII G_2 13 = *TDP* 124 iii 20)

**If his insides are continually purged[40] (but) he is not able to pour out his urine, "hand" of [. . .]

5.29 DIŠ NA NINDA KÚ KAŠ NAG-*ma* ŠÀ.ME[Š]-*šú in-nim-me-ru* KÀŠ.[MEŠ]-*šú* DIB.DIB-*at* UD.DA SÁ.SÁ (*AMT* 48/1:10′ + 78/3:7′)

**If a person eats bread (and) drinks beer and subsequently his stomach is colicky (and) he continually holds in his urine, *ṣētu* (enteric fever; see Chapter 3) has "gotten" him.

OBSTRUCTION

Scar tissue surrounding the urethra can narrow and obstruct the canal, resulting in slowed urine flow and eventually kidney failure. The causes are multiple including trauma, gonorrhea, and schistosomiasis (see below). An enlarged prostate, commonly seen in older men, may produce similar problems. Kidney stones may cause rapid cessation of urine flow.

URETHRAL CONSTRICTION

5.30 DIŠ NA DÚR-*šú* [. . .] x-*su* KÀŠ.MEŠ-*šú* DIB.DIB x [. . .] NA.BI DÚR.GIG.GA.KÁM GIG . . . (*BAM* 94 r. 2′–3′)[41]

**If a person's anus [. . .] him and he continually holds in his urine [. . .] that person is sick with DÚR.GIG[42] . . .

5.31 [DIŠ] NA MAŠ.SÌLA^{II}-*šú* KÚ.MEŠ-*šú i-ta-an-na-aḫ im-ta-na-aš-ši im-te-en* x [. . .] [MAŠ].GI$_6$!.MEŠ-*šú par-da* SÍG UGU-*šú* GUB.GUB-*az* ŠÀ-*šú pi-qám!*[43] NU *pi-qám! i-par-*x [. . .] [U$_4$-*r*] *a u* GI$_6$ *la i-ṣal-lal* NA BI *ḫi-niq-ti* BUN GIG *ana* TI-*šú* . . . (*AMT* 31/1+:3–5)[44]

**[If] a person's shoulders continually hurt him, he is continually tired, he continually forgets things, he continually [. . .] his ⸢dreams⸣ are troubled, the hair of his scalp continually stands on end, he vomits incessantly, [. . .] (and) he cannot sleep ⸢day⸣ or night, that person is sick with constriction of the urethra, to cure him . . .

5.32 DIŠ NA GÌŠ-*šú ú-kàs-sa ḫi-níq-ti* x [. . .] *ana* TI-*šú* . . . (*BAM* 182 obv. 3′–4′)

**If a person's penis binds up, constriction [. . .], to cure him . . .

5.33 DIŠ NA *ḫi-niq-ti* BUN GIG . . . (*AMT* 59/1 i 16, 33, 35; *BAM* 168:45; cf. *AMT* 53/8:4′; *AMT* 60/1 ii 3)[45]

**If a person is sick with constriction of the urethra . . .

OBSTRUCTION FROM STONES

5.34 [. . .] ⸢3⸣ U$_4$-*me* DIŠ NA$_4$ *muš-tin-ni* GAR-*šú* DIŠ NA BI KAŠ NAG [NA$_4$.BI *i-š*] *aḫ-ḫu-uḫ* NA BI KAŠ NU NAG-*ma* A UL$_4$.GAL NAG *ana* NAM-*šú* GAR-*šú* (DPS XVIII:40′–41′ [AOAT 43.219])

**[If . . . he has been sick for] three days. If he has a stone in the urethra, if that person drinks beer, [that stone] ⸢will fall out (or dissolve)⸣.[46] (If) that person does not drink beer but drinks a lot of water, he will certainly die.[47]

The reason for the success of beer in treating urethral stones, as described above, is uncertain, but could either be due to change in urine acidity causing the stone to dissolve, or to the anesthetic effect of alcohol leading to relaxation of muscle spasm. Drinking excess water if the patient's urinary tract is obstructed could hasten kidney failure and death.

Whatever the cause of urinary obstruction, it was clear to the ancient physician that failure to solve the problem led to death of the patient, and if urine flowed, the patient's prognosis improved.[48]

5.35 DIŠ GÌŠ-*šú is-se-kir* GAM (DPS XIV A ii 32//C ii 9 = *TDP* 134 ii 32)[49]

**If his penis is blocked off, he will die.

5.36 [DIŠ KÀ]Š.MEŠ-*šú it-te-né-es-ki-ra* GAM (DPS XIV A ii 43//C ii 16 = *TDP* 136 ii 43)

** [If] his ⌜urine⌝ is continually blocked off, he will die.

5.37 [DIŠ DIB-*su-ma* ŠÈ-*šú i*]*z-zi ana* TI.BI GAR-*šú* / DIB-*su-*⌜*ma*⌝ KÀŠ-*šú* SUR *ana* TI.⌜BI⌝ [GAR-*š*]*ú* (DPS XIX/XX:107′ [AOAT 43.232])

** [If it afflicts him and he] excretes [his excrement], it is a sign that he will live. If it afflicts him and his urine flows, [it is a sign] that he will live.

KIDNEY FAILURE AND OTHER CAUSES OF BODY SWELLING

There are many diseases that can directly attack the kidneys and eventually lead to decrease or cessation of urine production. Secondary kidney failure will also occur as a consequence of urinary tract obstruction. Some of the signs and symptoms of kidney failure include swelling of body tissues (anasarca) including the hands, feet, and face as fluid is retained, vomiting, intestinal colic, and mental status changes. In the following quote, the patient appears to have kidney failure as a consequence of urinary tract obstruction caused by trauma.

5.38 DIŠ IGI.MEŠ-*šú u* IGI^{II}-*šú* MÚ.MEŠ KI.A IGI^{II}-*šú* SA$_5$ IM KIR$_4$-*šú* KÚM : *ṣa-bit* ⌜KÀŠ⌝.MEŠ-*šú ta-ba-ka* NU ZU-*e* GABA.RI SÌG-*iṣ* ŠU ^{d}MAŠ (DPS IX A 69–70//B r. 15–16 = *TDP* 78:69–70)

**If his face and his eyes are swollen, the rims of his eyes are red, the breath of his nose is hot (var. seized) (and) he is not able to pour out his urine,[50] he was wounded on the front side; "hand" of Ninurta.[51]

Another cause of body swelling is the nephrotic syndrome, a group of kidney diseases that leads to protein loss in the urine. The underlying causes of this syndrome are many, and include diabetes, systemic lupus erythematosus, vasculitic-immunologic diseases such as polyarteritis, infections, and certain medicines. The protein loss in the urine causes reduced urine output and secondary swelling.

Congestive heart failure (see Chapter 8) and liver failure (see Chapter 6) can also cause body swelling (anasarca). The patient in the following quote has body swelling that could be due to any of the above conditions, but the nephrotic syndrome seems the most likely possibility.

5.39 DIŠ NA SAG.DU-*su* *pa-nu-šú* IGI^{II}-*šú* G[Ì]R^{II}-*šú* NUNDUN-*šú* MÚ.MEŠ-*ḫu* S[AG.DU-*su*] *ana* IGI-*šú* GÍD.DA-*su* ŠU^{II}-*šú u* GÌR^{II}-*šú* KÚ-*šú mi-na-tu-šú tab-ka* SU-*šu šim-*[*m*]*a-tú* TUKU.MEŠ *ana* TI-*šú* . . . (Jastrow, *TCPP* 399 obv. 35–37//*BAM* 480 iv 32–33; cf. *AMT* 1/3:16′–17′)[52]

**If a person's head, his face, his eyes, his feet, (and) his lips are swollen, [his] ⌜head⌝ (feels like it) draws him forward,[53] his hands and his feet hurt him, his limbs are tense,[54] (and) his body continually has numbness, to cure him . . .

BLADDER PARALYSIS

Certain battle injuries can lead to bladder paralysis with the inability to urinate. Spinal injury was a known cause of failure to urinate, presumably secondary to bladder paralysis from cord injury. Many patients with bladder paralysis due to cord injury, however, will develop reflex involuntary voiding so that urinary obstruction is not permanent.

5.40 DIŠ *ina* GÚ.MURGU-*šú* SÌG-*ma* BAD-*ma* KI.GUB-*šu* NU È-*a* ŠU GU$_4$ *šag-ga-ši* [GAM] (DPS XII D iii 35//E iii 38–39 = *TDP* 106 iii 35; cf. DPS XV:46 [AOAT 43.152])

**If he was wounded on his spine and, as a consequence, he is stopped up so that his excrement cannot come out,[55] "hand" of a murderous ghost; [he will die].

5.41 DIŠ KI.MIN-*ma* GU.DU.MEŠ-*šú* GI$_6$.MEŠ-*ma* KI.GUB-*su* NU È-*a u* A NU *ú-še-rid* EGIR-*ta*$_5$ SÌG-*iṣ* GAM (DPS XV:51 [AOAT 43.153]; cf. DPS XIV A$_2$ i 8–9//D obv. 5 = *TDP* 132 i 60)

**If (it is the first day he is sick) and his buttocks are dark so that his excrement cannot come out and he cannot pass water, he was wounded on the back side;[56] he will die.

URINARY INCONTINENCE

Urinary incontinence is caused by a variety of neurological conditions that paralyze the muscle (sphincter) that closes the urethral opening. Also some anatomical changes in the bladder and urethra can cause incontinence. The first reference below indicates that the *āšipu* was aware of the social implications of this problem.

5.42 DIŠ NA KI DAM-*šú ina* É.ÉŠ.DAM KÀŠ.MEŠ-*šú iz-zi* (*CT* 39.45:22 [Šumma Alu])[57]

**If a person voids his urine when he is in a tavern with his wife.

5.43 [KÀŠ].MEŠ-*ku-nu ki-ma ti*!-*ki ana qaq-qar lit-ta-tuk*! (Parpola and Watanabe, SAA 2 no. 6:470–471 [a curse])

**May your [urine] dribble to the ground like raindrops!

5.44 DIŠ NA GÌŠ-*šú* DIB.MEŠ-*at* KÀŠ.MEŠ-*šú ut-ta-na-t*[*ak* . . . *t*]*a-ma*!-*ḫar*[58] *tam-mar ina* ŠU.SI-*ka* [. . . N]A.BI *ḫi-niq* BÚN GIG . . . (*AMT* 63/1:14)[59]

**If a person's penis is continually "seized" (and) he continually ⌜dribbles⌝ his urine, you ⌜collect⌝ [the urine(?)]. You examine (it). You [. . .] with your finger. [If . . .], that ⌜person⌝ is sick with constriction of the urethra . . .[60]

The problem described below could represent a patient with urinary incontinence plus the commonly observed complication, secondary urinary tract infection.

5.45 DIŠ NA KÀŠ.MEŠ-*šú ut-ta-na-tak ka-la-a la i-la-ʾi* ^{UZU}BUN-*šu ḫe-sa-at* IM DIRI-*ma ma-as-la-aḫ* KÀŠ.MEŠ-*šú i-bi-ta* DIRI *ana* TI-*šú* . . . (*BAM* 111 ii 21′–24′)

**If a person continually dribbles his urine (and) cannot hold it back,[61] his urethra is pressured (and) full of "clay," and the urinary tract[62] is full of thick matter, to cure him . . .

BED WETTING

Bed wetting (enuresis) is a common problem of childhood. Emotional disturbances can delay the child's ability to achieve this control. There are also anatomical and neurological causes of this condition, but they are uncommon.

5.46 DIŠ NA *ina ṣa-la-li-šú* KÀŠ-*šú iš-tin* [. . .] (*AMT* 65/4:8′; cf. *CT* 28.41 [K 8821]:11′)

**If a person urinates in his sleep . . .

5.47 DIŠ NA *ina* KI.NÁ-*šú* KÀŠ *iš-tin* ŠU ^{d}NIN.M[AḪ]/^{d}*Be-lit*-DINGIR.MEŠ (*STT* 238:1; *BAM* 115 obv. 14′)

**If a person urinates in his bed, "hand" of Belit-ili.

Urinary Tract Infections

Urinary tract infections are usually caused by bacteria that often infect the kidneys, ureters (tubes transporting urine from the kidneys to the bladder), bladder, and urethra (the structure that drains the bladder). Common signs and symptoms include fever, pain over the kidneys and bladder, and painful urination. This infection is more likely to occur when the urinary tract is abnormal, especially with stones or partial obstruction of the ureters or urethra. The patient's urine is often cloudy during the infection. It is possible that the following references are examples of urinary tract infections. Sexually transmitted infections are also a frequent cause of urethritis with painful urination (see Chapter 4).

5.48 DIŠ NA GÌŠ SÌG.SÌG-*šú i-te-e*[*b*]-*bi* KI A-*šú* MURUB$_4$.MEŠ-*šú* KÚ.MEŠ-*šú šá* NA BI ⸢xx⸣ *ki-mil-ti* ^{d}UTU UGU-*šú* GÁL-*ši* . . . (*STT* 95 i 42–43)

**If a person's penis continually gives him a jabbing pain, he gets up (to urinate and) with his water his pelvic region hurts him, that person [. . .] the anger of Šamaš is upon him . . .

5.49 DIŠ NA MURUB$_4$.MEŠ-*šú lu ina* DU-*šú lu ina* KI.NÁ-*šú* TAG.GA.MEŠ-*šú* ni [. . . G]ÍR.GÍR-*su ú-ḫa-ma-aṭ-su i-tar-rak-šú* EGIR KÀŠ.MEŠ-*šú iš-t*[*in* . . .] (*AMT* 60/1 ii 22′–23′)[63]

**If his pelvic region hurts him intensely either when he walks or when he sleeps, [. . .] stings him, burns him, throbs, after he ⸢urinates⸣ [. . .]

5.50 KI.5-*ma ù* KÀŠ-*šú ú-ṣa-nu* . . . (*BAM* 396 ii 19′)

**If (a person is sick with stones) and his urine also stinks . . .

5.51 *šum-ma* LÚ *ḫi-níq-ti* GIG ÉLLAG.ME GIG DÚR.GIG MIN TAB UD.DA MIN *um-ma* DIB.DIB-*su* . . . (BM 78963:66)

**If a person is sick with stricture (or) sick kidneys (or) DÚR.GIG[64] (or) burning of *ṣētu* (or) if fever continually afflicts him . . .

SCHISTOSOMIASIS HEMATOBIUM

As described in the introduction to this chapter, *Schistosomiasis hematobium* is a parasitic infection with a predilection for urinary tract involvement. A person infected with *Schistosomiasis hematobium* harbors the organism in his or her urinary tract, especially the bladder. The infection can have both acute and chronic manifestations. In addition to hematuria and urinary tract obstruction, the signs and symptoms include lower abdominal and pelvic pain, decreased urine flow and dribbling, painful urination secondary to bacterial infection or kidney stones, sexual impotence, persistent penile erection (priapism), and nocturnal and premature ejaculations. Bladder cancer is a frequent and fatal complication of schistosomiasis if untreated, and complete urinary tract obstruction is also fatal.

The references below have been cited elsewhere in this chapter, and are likely to be describing patients with this parasitic disease.

5.52 DIŠ KI.MIN-[*m*]*a ina* KÀŠ-*šú* MÚD *iš-tin ana* KI GIG GAM (DPS XVI:7 [AOAT 43.172])

**If (it is the first day he is sick) ⌜and⌝ he urinates blood in his urine, he is at an acute stage of the illness;[65] he will die.

5.53 DIŠ NA *mi-na-tu-šú* DUB.DUB GABA-*su u* SA.SAL.MEŠ-*šú* KÚ.MEŠ-*šú* Á^{II}-*šú* x [. . .] KÚ.MEŠ-*šú bir-bir-ki-šú lu šá* 15 *lu šá* 150 SÌG-*su-ma ina múš-tin-*[*ni*]-*šú* MÚD *ú-kal-lam* NA.BI *ḫi-niq-ti* DÚR GIG GIG *ana* TI-*šú* . . . (*AMT* 40/5 iii 14–16; *AMT* 56/1 obv. 1–3//*BAM* 88:1′–2′)[66]

**If his limbs are continually tense,[67] his breast and his back continually hurt him, his arms [and legs?] continually hurt him, his loins either on the left or right side give him a jabbing pain, and from his ⌜urethra⌝ he shows blood, that person is sick with the constriction of DÚR.GIG, to cure him . . .

5.54 DIŠ NA UZU.ÉLLAG-*su* KÚ-*šu* MURUB$_4$-*šú* TAG.TAG-*šú ù* KÀŠ-*šú* GIN$_7$ KÀŠ ANŠE BABBAR-*a* EGIR KÀŠ-*šú* MÚD *ú-kal-lam* NA.BI *mu-ṣa-am* GIG . . . (*BAM* 396 i 23′–24′//*AMT* 66/7:18–19)

**If a person's kidney hurts him, his pelvic region continually hurts him intensely, and his urine is like the urine of a donkey (or) it is white (and) after his urine he shows blood, that person is sick with *mūṣu*[68] . . .

The second reference above (see also below) links generalized complaints with urethral constriction and hematuria. The generalized complaints probably result from progressive kidney failure due to the same condition that is causing urethral constriction and hematuria. Although *Schistosomiasis hematobium* is a likely cause, other conditions are possible such as kidney stones leading to urethral injury and stricture.

5.55 DIŠ NA *mi-na-tu-šú* DUB.DUB GABA-*su u* SA.SAL.MEŠ-*šú* KÚ.MEŠ-*šú* Á^{II}-*šú* x [...] KÚ.MEŠ-*šú bir-bir-ki-šú lu šá* 15 *lu šá* 150 SÌG-*su-ma ina múš-tin-*[*ni*]*-šú* MÚD *ú-kal-lam* NA.BI *ḫi-niq-ti* DÚR GIG GIG *ana* TI-*šú* . . . (*AMT* 40/5 iii 14–16; *AMT* 56/1 obv. 1–3//*BAM* 88:1′–2′)

**If his limbs are continually tense,[69] his breast and his back continually hurt him, his arms [and legs] continually hurt him, his loins[70] either on the left or right side give him a jabbing pain, and from his ⌜urethra⌝ he shows blood, that person is sick with the constriction of DÚR.GIG, to cure him . . .

BACK PAIN

The *āšipu* made numerous references to pain in the part of the back over the kidneys, and this complaint could be a bad prognostic sign, especially if it was so severe that the patient could not lie on his back. In this case the patient generally did not survive. There is no way to determine the cause of this pain but Mujais suggests, and we concur, that unilateral pain with a good prognosis may represent kidney stones (nephrolithiasis) and bilateral pain with a bad prognosis may represent bilateral kidney infection (pyelonephritis) with or without papillary necrosis.[71] Pancreatitis and paravertebral abscesses are other possible causes of severe life-threatening back pain.

5.56 DIŠ ÉLLAG 15-*šú* KÚ-*šú-ma ina* UGU-*šá* NU NÁ-*al ina* U$_4$.7.KÁM GAM (DPS XII D iii 16 = *TDP* 104 iii 16)[72]

**If his left kidney hurts him so that he cannot lie on it, on the seventh day, he will die.

5.57 DIŠ ÉLLAG 150-*šú* KÚ-*šú-ma ina* UGU-*šú* NÁ-*al* GÍD-*ma* DIN (DPS XII D iii 14 = *TDP* 104 iii 14)[73]

**If his right kidney hurts him but he can lie on it, it may be prolonged, (but) he will get well.

Sexual Dysfunction

Sexual dysfunctions that were described include priapism (persistent unwanted erection, often painful), nocturnal and premature ejaculations, and impotence (inability to achieve an erection).

PRIAPISM

In addition to the pain and embarrassment[74] caused by priapism, it can impede although not completely obstruct urination. The second reference below might be describing priapism in a patient with sickle cell disease (see Chapter 19 with 19.316–19.318), although the details are not sufficiently complete to permit a firm conclusion.

5.58 DIŠ NA *ana* KÀŠ.MEŠ-*šú ma-gal* ZI.ZI-*bi* . . . (*BAM* 116 r. 8′ // *BAM* 164:20; *BAM* 161 v 15)[75]

**If a person continually has an erection when he tries to urinate . . .

5.59 DIŠ *su-ḫar* GÌR[II]-*šú* ŠED$_7$ KI.A IGI[II]-*šú nu-up-pu-ḫa* GÌŠ-*šú aš-ṭa-at* LI.DUR-*su* DU$_8$-*át* ŠU NAM.ÉRIM.MA *ú-zab-bal-ma* GAM (DPS XIV A iv 17–18 = *TDP* 144 iv 52′–53′)

**If the soles of his feet are cold, the rims of his eyes are swollen, his penis is stiff and hard, (and) his navel is supple, "hand" of curse; (if) he lingers, he will die.

NOCTURNAL EMISSION

Ejaculation during sleep is a common and benign condition, occurring primarily in teenage boys. The following are drawn from the omen series *Šumma ālu*.

5.60 DIŠ NA *ina* GI$_6$ TE-*ma ina* MÁŠ.GI$_6$-*šú ni-il-šú bul-lul* . . . (*CT* 39.44:9)

**If a person approaches (a woman) at night and subsequently in his dream, he is spattered with his semen . . .

5.61 DIŠ NA TE-*ma u ina* GI$_6$-*šú ig-luṭ* . . . DIŠ NA *ina* MÁŠ.GI$_6$-*šú* MIN-*ma ni-il-šú bul-lul* . . . (*CT* 39.45:25, 26)

**If a person approaches (a woman) and also subsequently he ejaculates in his sleep . . . If a person (ejaculates) during his dream and is spattered with his semen . . .

PREMATURE EJACULATION

Premature ejaculation is commonly caused by stress or psychological problems. The reference below, also drawn from *Šumma ālu*, describes this problem.

5.62 DIŠ NA *ana* MUNUS TE-*ma ig-luṭ-ma* MIN . . . (*CT* 39.44:10)

**If a person approaches a woman and he has an ejaculation and (he is spattered with his semen) . . .

IMPOTENCE

5.63 [DIŠ NA] *ka-šip-ma mun-ga* TUKU-*ši bir-ka-šú ga-an-na k*[*a*]-*la-tu-šú* DU x [. . .] x-*ma ana e-peš* Á.ÁŠ NU ÍL-*šú ni-i*[*š* ŠÀ-*šú*] DIB-*ma ana* MUNUS D[U-*ka* LAL ŠÀ-*šú* MUNUS *ḫa-ši*]*ḫ-ma* MUNUS IGI-*ma* ŠÀ-*šú* GUR-*ra* NA.BI [*re-ḫu-s*]*u* KI LÚ.Ú[Š *šu-nu-lat*] . . . (*SpTU* 1.9:19′–21′)[76]

**[If a person] is hexed so that he has *mungu*[77] and his knees are bent(?), his kidneys [. . .] so that (his heart) does not rise in him to do what he wants,[78] he is ⌜impotent⌝ so that his ⌜desire to go⌝ to a woman [is diminished, his heart desires a woman] and then when he sees a woman, his heart turns away, that person's [semen has been made to lie] with a ⌜corpse⌝ . . .

5.64 Ú SU.DAR KÚ ŠÀ.ZI.GA *ú-maṭ-ṭa*! (*BAM* 1 iii 34//*CT* 14.43 [S. 60]:10′)

**If he eats SU(MUN).DAR-vegetable,[79] his ability to have an erection will diminish.

5.65 KA.INIM.MA ŠÀ.ZI.GA (*LKA* 95 r. 18; *STT* 280 iv 20; *LKA* 102 obv. 13; *LKA* 99c:10 [Biggs, ŠÀ.ZI.GA, pp. 17, 21, 22, 23–24]; *SpTU* 1.10:17′)

**Recitation for ability to have an erection.

5.66 [DIŠ N]A ÍL ŠÀ-*šú* DIB-*ma ana* MUNUS-*šú u ana* MUNUS BAR-*ti* ŠÀ-*šú* NU ÍL-*šú* . . . (*SpTU* 1.9:17′; Biggs, ŠÀ.ZI.GA no. 11:18)[80]

**[If] a ⌜person⌝ is impotent so that he cannot get an erection[81] (either) for his woman or for a strange woman . . .

It seems clear from the above quote that the physician is trying to rule out boredom with the patient's regular partner as the cause of impotence, by indicating that a new partner did not solve the patient's problem. Whether the physician provided a new partner as a diagnostic test or the patient tried it on his own initiative is unknown.

Both impotence and priapism can have multiple causes but *Schistosomiasis hematobium* is capable of causing both of them. The ancient Mesopotamian physician recognized that impotence commonly occurs with sexually transmitted diseases (see Chapter 4) and advanced age, and that back or abdominal injuries could also have this effect.

5.67 [DIŠ NA] *lu-u ina* ⌜ŠU⌝.GI.MEŠ *lu-ú ina* ^{GIŠ}GIDRU *lu-u ina ḫi-miṭ* UD.DA [*lu*]-*ú ina ni-ḫi-is* ^{GIŠ}GIGIR *a-na* MUNUS *a-la-ka mu-uṭ-ṭu-ṭú a-na* ŠÀ.ZI.GA *šur-ši-šu-ma ana* MUNUS DU-*šu* . . . (*AMT* 88/3:1–3 [see Biggs, ŠÀ.ZI.GA, p. 52])

**[If a person], either as a result of being in his eighties,[82] or burning pain[83] or burning of *ṣētu* ⌜or⌝ jostling by a chariot has diminished desire for a woman, to cause him to have an erection and to let him go to a woman . . .

5.68 DIŠ *ina* GÚ-*šú* SÌG-*iṣ-ma u du-us-su* KAR-*et* ŠU ^{d}15 GAM (DPS X A obv. 18//B obv. 20 = *TDP* 82:18)

**If he was wounded on his neck and his virility is taken away, "hand" of Ištar; he will die.

5.69 DIŠ *ina em-ši-šú* SÌG-*iṣ-ma u du-u*[*s-su* KAR-*et* ŠU ^{d}15 . . .] (DPS XIII D r. 4 = *TDP* 126 iv 13′)

**If he was wounded on his lower abdomen and [his] ⌜virility⌝ [is taken away, "hand" of Ištar . . .].

What we might consider to be the psychological causes of impotence were recognized, at least on an empirical level, by ancient physicians.[84] One type of treatment required the *āšipu* to rub salves containing magnetic hematite (for "magnetic" attraction) on the male partner's penis and the female partner's vagina while reciting sexually explicit poetry.[85]

Male infertility was also recognized as a possibility, as in the following curse, and there were plants recommended to treat it.

5.70 GIN$_7$ *šu-ut re-e-ši la a-li-di ni-il-ka li-bal* (*CT* 23.10:14)

**May your semen dry up like that of a barren eunuch!

5.71 Ú NUMUN TUKU . . . (*BAM* 1 i 18–19; *BAM* 380:25–26)

**Plant to have seed[86] . . .

Eunuchs (castrated males: *ša rēši*) were a feature of the Neo-Assyrian court alongside "those with beards" (*ša ziqni*).[87] Being unable to have children, they made ideal provincial governors. Less pleasantly, being transformed into a eunuch (i.e., being castrated) was the punishment reserved in the Middle Assyrian Laws for a man who was caught *in flagrante* with another man's wife as an alternative to being killed.[88]

Loss of sexual desire (libido) was a frequently listed symptom, but is likely in most of these cases to be due only to the debilitating nature of the underlying disease.

5.72 [DIŠ NA . . .] *pit-ru-šú ir-ta-nam-mu-u šit-tú ir-te-né-ḫi-šú* [. . .] KÚM ŠÀ TUKU-*ši* A.MEŠ *iṣ-ṣa-nam-ma* NINDA.MEŠ *u* KAŠ SAG LAL *bir-di im-ta-na-al-la* [. . .] *ik-ka-šú ik-ta-na-ru* GAZ ŠÀ-*bi* TUKU.MEŠ *ana* MUNUS DU-*ka* LAL [. . . ŠU] ⌜NAM⌝.ÉRIM DIB-*su ana* TI-*šú* . . . (K 2426 i 9′–12′)

**[If a person] . . . his internal organs are consistently relaxed, sleep keeps flowing over him . . . he has internal fever, he is continually thirsty for water (but) his appetite for bread and beer is diminished, he is continually full of *birdu*-nodules[89] . . . he is continually short of breath, he continually has a crushing sensation in his chest, his desire to go to a woman is diminished . . . ["hand"] of curse afflicts him, to cure him . . .

Scrotum and Penis

Complaints and physical findings relative to the patient's external genitalia received considerable attention from the ancient Mesopotamian physician. Painful and swollen penis and testicles were described, as well as infection with the production of pus.

5.73 DIŠ NA *ina* LÍL-*šú* KÚM *ina* GÌŠ-*šú ip-pu-uš* . . . (*BAM* 3 iv 10)

**If during the course of a person's illness, fever/inflammation spreads to his penis . . .

5.74 DIŠ GÌŠ-*šú nap-ḫat na-ḫi-iṭ* (DPS XIV A ii 28//C ii 7 = *TDP* 134 ii 28)

**If his penis is swollen, it is worrisome.

5.75 [DIŠ NA] *tas-li-a-te-šú* TAG.GA-*šú* KÀŠ.MEŠ-*šu* DIB.MEŠ [. . .] (*AMT* 61/1:14′)

**[If a person]'s sprinklings hurt him intensely, he continually holds in his urine [. . .]

5.76 DIŠ *mu-šar-šú u* ŠIR^{II}-*šú nap-ḫu* ŠU ^{d}*Dil-bat ina* KI.NÁ-*šú* KUR-*su* (DPS XIV A ii 38//C ii 13//F 4 = *TDP* 134 ii 38)[90]

**If his penis and his testicles[91] are swollen, "hand" of Dilbat (Ištar) has gotten him in his bed.

5.77 DIŠ NA ŠIR-*šú* GIG . . . (*BAM* 396 iv 13)

**If a person's testicle is sore . . .

5.78 DIŠ NA ŠIR-*šú* MÚD.BABBAR *ú-kal* . . . (*AMT* 61/5:6)

**If a person's testicle contains pus . . .

Another bit of evidence that ancient physical examinations were thorough is the fact that physicians recognized unilateral testicular abnormalities. Only careful scrotal examination would permit these observations.

5.79 BE *iz-bu* ŠIR-*šú šá* 15/150 *re-qat* . . . (*CT* 28.7:5–6)

**If the left/right testicle of the malformed fetus is empty . . . (it is a bad sign).

5.80 DIŠ ⸢NA TAB? ŠIR DILI⸣ . . . (*BAM* 396 iv 15)

**If a person has a burning sensation(?) in one testicle . . .

Some of these unilateral cases might have been due to mumps orchitis since this infection often causes only one-sided testicular disease with pain and swelling followed by testicular atrophy. Other illnesses may present in a similar fashion. The absence of a testicle in the scrotum may also be due to an undescended testicle that remains in the abdominal cavity.

The reference below describes "stiffness" of a man's testicles. This suggests that there is some abnormal mass in the scrotum. A fluid-filled sack (hydrocele) within the scrotum is a common, benign condition. They are usually painless and generally cause no particular problem. Other masses such as tumors and abscesses may occur within the scrotum. However, with no additional information, we cannot identify the underlying cause.

5.81 [DIŠ N]A ŠIR-*šú mun-ga* DIB . . . (*AMT* 61/5:5)

**[If] stiffness seizes a ⸢person⸣'s testicle . . .

The following quote describes a patient with a scrotal sack containing atrophied testicles. He apparently lacks normal male secondary sexual characteristics, which would be expected if both testicles are atrophied (see Chapter 7).

5.82 DIŠ LÚ *tu-ka-na-at iš-ki-šu ra-ab-bi-a ù iš-ka-šu na-ša-al-lu-la a-na sí-in-ni-iš-tim qí-ru-ub* (Köcher and Oppenheim, *AfO* 18.64 i 23–25 [physiognomic omens])

**If the sack of his testicles is large but his testicles slither about (in it), he is close to (being) a woman.

Torsion or twisting of the testicles was also recognized to be a painful and sometimes dangerous problem, possibly leading to testicular necrosis, as suggested by the black testicles in the second reference.

5.83 DIŠ ŠIR^{II}-*šú ze-ra* GAM : *ana* NIN.DINGIR.RA [DINGIR-*šú* TE-*ḫi*] (DPS XIV A_2 ii 12//C ii 27 = *TDP* 136 ii 62; cf. DPS XXI:19 [AOAT 43.247])

**If his testicles are twisted, he will die (var. [he approached] the *ēntu* [of his god]).[92]

5.84 DIŠ ŠIR^{II}-*šú* SA$_5$.MEŠ DIN . . . DIŠ ŠIR^{II}-*šú* GI$_6$.MEŠ GAM (DPS XIV A$_2$ ii 4, 6//C ii 23, 24 = *TDP* 136 ii 54, 56)

**If his testicles are red, he will get well . . . If his testicles are black, he will die.

Scrotal injuries, acquired in war (or during quarrels with Assyrian women), were identified.

5.85 *šum-ma* MUNUS *i-na ṣa-al-te iš-ka ša* LÚ *ta-aḫ-te-pi* . . . *ù šum-ma* ^{LÚ}A.ZU *ur-tak-ki-is-ma iš-ku ša-ni-tu il-te-ša-ma ta-at-ta-al-pa-at* [*e*]*-ri-im-ma tar-ti-i-ši* [*ù*] *lu-ú i-na ṣa-al-te* [*iš*]*-ka ša-ni-ta taḫ-te-pi* . . . (Middle Assyrian Laws A § 8)

**If a woman crushes a person's testicle in a quarrel . . . and if the *asû* bandages it up and subsequently the other testicle becomes affected from it and gets an *erimu*-mark or if she crushed the other ⸢testicle⸣ in the quarrel . . .

5.86 DIŠ ÉLLAG *zi-kar-ti-šu* GAZ-*át pa-pa-a*[*n* ŠÀ-*šú* . . .] KÀŠ.MEŠ-*šú* DIB.DI[B . . .] (DPS XIV A$_2$ ii 19-20//C ii 33 = *TDP* 138 ii 69–70)[93]

**If his testicle was crushed, [his] ⸢umbilical area⸣ [. . .] he ⸢continually⸣ holds in his urine [. . .]

5.87 DIŠ *ina* ŠIR^{II}-*šú* SÌG-*iṣ ana* NIN.DINGIR.RA DINGIR-*šú* TE-*ḫi* : [. . .] (DPS XIV A$_2$ ii 17//C ii 31 = *TDP* 138 ii 67)[94]

**If he was wounded in his testicles, he approached the *ēntu* of his god.

Summary

The genitourinary system is clearly vital to life. The connection between its function and the health of the patient was easier for the *āšipu* to evaluate than most other organs with the possible exception of the lungs. Failure to breathe in good air rapidly leads to illness and death. Similarly, the amount and appearance of an individual's urine is easily monitored. Therefore, important correlations were made between changes in the patient's urine and changes in his or her health. Additionally, many other genitourinary tract diseases were recognized by the *āšipu* that were caused by infections, trauma, and developmental abnormalities. There is nothing to indicate that the ancient Mesopotamian physicians understood the exact nature of kidney function, but they knew that life stopped when urine production stopped.

CHAPTER 6

Gastrointestinal Diseases

If after falling ill he vomits and flies will not come near his vomitus, he will die.

—DPS XVII:60 [AOAT 43.201]; cf. StBoT 36.60:9

Intestinal Tract

The *āšipu* had an excellent understanding of the anatomy of the intestinal tract as well as a good grasp of many of the common gastrointestinal diseases. A specialized vocabulary was used to describe gastrointestinal diseases, a good indication of the sophistication and precision of the *āšipu*'s observations.

The entire gastrointestinal tract was known collectively as the *libbu.*[1] In the recitation cited below not only are the individual portions of the tract listed (stomach [*karšu*], small intestine [*irrû*], and colon [*riqītu*]), but there is a clear description of the greater and lesser omentum and the mesenteries ("eyes" of the *libbu*), the thin membrane that supports these structures. We believe that they were called the "eyes" of the *libbu* for two reasons: because the greater and lesser omentum constitute a pair like the eyes, and because the membranes are transparent, allowing the *libbu* to see through them, as it were.[2] Also mentioned are the blood vessels that traverse the omentum and mesenteries to provide circulation to the intestinal tract.

6.1 *da-an lìb-bu qar-rad lìb-bu šá lìb-bi ar-ra-qa* IGI^{II}-*šú pur-si-it* MÚD *na-ši-ma ir-ru sa-ḫ̮i-ru-ti ul-lu-lu ina a-ḫ̮i-šú e ta-lak lìb-bu e ta-tu-ra* MIN *ana* GURUŠ *dam-qí ana* KI.SIKIL *da-me-eq-tu*$_4$ *uš-šir* GURUŠ-*ma* É *li-pu-uš uš-šir* KI.SIKIL *qin-na liq-nun ir-ru saḫ̮-ḫ̮u-ru zi-ir kar-šum ù ši-i ri-qí-tú bu-up-pa-ni-šá saḫ̮-pat liš-lim kar-šum ir-ri-šú lì!*[3]*-ši-ru-ma ri-qí-tum lit-ru-uṣ* GIN$_7$ IM *ina šu-bur-ri* GIN$_7$ *ge-šu-ti ina na-piš-ti li-ṣa-a* (*BAM* 574 iv 17–22; cf. iv 24–29, 34–35)

**Mighty is the *libbu* . . . the "eyes" of the *libbu* are elongated;[4] it carries blood vessels[5] and the convoluted intestines hang down[6] . . . The intestines are tangled; the stomach is twisted and as for the colon, it has fallen on its face.[7] May the stomach finish its task; may it go straight through his intestines and may the colon point the way (out). May it come out like wind from the anus, like a belch from the throat.

The *āšipu*'s knowledge of the anatomy of the human intestinal tract probably came from a combination of observations of war wounds and autopsies (see below). Additional information was presumably obtained from his colleague, the *barû* (diviner). In the course of the practice of extispicy (taking omens from the organs of sacrificial animals), the diviner obtained a remarkable amount of information about animal anatomy.[8] For example, the names given to the right and left hepatic bile ducts (*malāk mārti*: "channel of the gallbladder") and to the sphincter of Oddi that controls the flow of bile (*isilti mārti*: "contracting muscle of the gall bladder") show that the diviner was not only familiar with these structures, but recognized their function.[9] If the sphincter of Oddi was relaxed and dilated, the diviner made a note of it, as also with the anal sphincter, as described in the following reference.

6.2 BE *iz-bu i-si-il-ta-šú* DU$_8$-*a*[*t*] ... (Šumma Izbu XVII 48′ [Leichty, *Izbu* 169])

**If the sphincter of the malformed (lamb) fetus is relaxed and dilated...

Combining this store of information with his own observations, the *āšipu* was able to describe accurately the digestive flow in sheep, a process to which analogy is drawn in the following charming spell.

6.3 *im-mer* U$_4$-*ma i-ʾa-ra* [...] *pu-u a-na kar-ši kar-ši a-na ri-q*[*í-tú*] *ri-qí-tu a-na ár-qat i-nam-*[*din*] *i-ma-qut* A.GAR.GAR-*ma* ^{Ú}KI.KAL *i-*⌜*ma-ḫar*⌝ ^{Ú}KI.KAL *ma-ḫi-rat kal lum-ni muḫ-ri-in-ni-ma* ^{Ú}KI.KAL *lum-ni tab-li* (*KAR* 165 obv. 9–14; cf. Moran, *JCS* 21.178–182)

**The sheep, when it vomits up [the grass], the mouth ⌜gives⌝ (it) to the (first and second) stomach, the (first and second) stomach to the third (and fourth) stomach, the third (and fourth) stomach to the rear; it falls as mere dung (and) the grass ⌜receives⌝ [(it)]. Grass that receives every evil receive (mine) from me and, grass, carry off my evil!

The following recitation is a fascinating combination of the description of intestinal physiology and malfunction with the clinical description of a patient with intestinal bloating with gas. For anyone who has directly observed animal or human intestinal movement (peristalsis), the description given in this text ("intestines knotted"; "stomach twisted"; "wriggles like a fish"; "makes itself bigger like a snake") is quite clear and recognizable. For the "eyes" of the *libbu* (i.e., the greater and lesser omentum), see above. We are uncertain what part of the gastrointestinal tract the "lips" are supposed to represent, but the outer edge of the rectal opening is a possibility.

6.4 [ÉN ... *it-ta*]-*nap-šá-ru zi-ir kar-ši* ŠÀ.NIGIN *ku-uṣ-ṣu-*⌜*ru*⌝ [...] x *ek-le-ta ki-i me-e ḫi-ri-ti a-la-pa-a na-du-ú* IGI.MEŠ-*šú* [IM] EDIN *e-di-ip na-di i-ta-nag-gi*$_5$-*šu* EDIN *ma-la-a* IGI.MEŠ-*šú e-t*[*a-n*]*a-ba-la ša-pa-tu-šú i-ta-na-pa-aṣ ki-ma* KU$_6$.MEŠ *it-ta-nak-bir ki-ma* MUŠ *e-*[*nu-m*]*a* ^{d}*Gu-la na-di-na-at ba-la-ṭi* NAM.LÚ.U$_{18}$.LU *ina* É ^{d}ASAL.LÚ.ḪI *ú-bil eṭ-lu* ^{d}[AMAR.UTU] *re-mi-nu-u ip-pa-lis-su-ma gi-ša-ma* TI-*uṭ eṭ-lu šum*$_4$-*ma* IM *ina* DÚR *lu-ṣi šum*$_4$-*ma gi-ša-tu ina nap-šá-ti li-še-ṣi* TU$_6$ ÉN (*BAM* 574 ii 21–27)

**The [. . . are continually] loosened; the stomach is twisted; intestines are knotted [. . .] the darkness. (The *libbu*)'s eyes are like ditch water covered with algae. [Wind] from the steppe blows in, is put down, and roams the steppe. Its eyes are full; its "lips" continually ⌜dry out⌝. It wriggles like a fish and makes itself bigger like a snake. ⌜When⌝ Gula, giver of life, brought mankind to the temple of Asalluḫi, merciful Marduk looked upon the young man and he belched and the young man got well. Either let the wind come out of the anus, or let it send out a belch from the throat.

How was the *āšipu* able to observe peristalsis? One possibility might be war wounds that opened the abdomen, allowing for direct observation of the human intestinal tract, knowledge of which was then applied to the patient with intestinal gas. Another possibility might be observation of intestinal movement in connection with the sacrifice of sheep. Finally, since sheep can have a potentially fatal disease involving large accumulations of intestinal gas that is usually relieved by cutting open the sheep to allow the gas to escape, intestinal movement in sheep may have been observed in the course of veterinary diagnosis or treatment.

EXAMINATION OF VOMITUS

The *āšipu*, lacking our sophisticated x-ray scanning and blood testing techniques, observed what was available to him, namely, vomitus and stool, and even performed some (by our standards) crude tests of the gastrointestinal tract. His observations on the appearance of vomitus provided information about the source of this material.[10] Red vomitus indicates fresh bleeding, while black (dark brown) vomitus is caused by the interaction of blood and stomach acid that results in partial breakdown of hemoglobin.[11] This material resembles, and is called, "coffee grounds" by modern physicians.[12] (Coffee is native to Yemen. It was first drunk outside of its homeland by Sufi mystics to aid in their devotions, and reached Europe from the Ottoman Empire. It was unknown in ancient Mesopotamia.) The *āšipu* recognized red and black vomitus as indicating the presence of blood, and yellowish material that of gall bladder bile.

BLOODY VOMITUS AND BILE Dark or bright red blood can be caused by many diseases, but the most common are peptic ulcer disease and cancer of the stomach.[13] Bile in vomitus comes from the liver and gall bladder. Since bile normally enters the upper small intestine (duodenum), vomited bile usually indicates severe or protracted vomiting rather than a specific disease.

6.5 DIŠ *ina* GIG-*šú* 1-*šú* 2-*šú* *ina* IGI ZÉ *i-ḫa-ḫu* EGIR-*nu* MÚD *i-ḫa-ḫu* GAM (DPS XVII:27 [AOAT 43.197])

**If once or twice during (the course of) his illness, he first vomits bile and afterward vomits blood, he will die.

6.6 ⌜DIŠ⌝ NA KA-*šú* MÚD ḪAL . . . (BM 78963:79)

**If a person's mouth vomits blood . . .

6.7 DIŠ *ina* ŠÀ-*šú* Á 15-*šú u* 150-*šú di-ik-šú u* ^{GIŠ}GIDRU GAR-*nu-šum-ma* MÚD MUD ŠUB.ŠUB GAM (DPS XIII B ii 32 = *TDP* 120 ii 32)

**If a needling pain or burning pain[14] is firmly established in his abdomen on the left or right side and he continually produces dark blood, he will die.

MUCUS The *āšipu* also described mucus present in the upper gastrointestinal tract.[15] Mucus is a nonspecific finding and is produced by cells lining the gastrointestinal tract. The final reference attributes the presence of mucus to "sorcery" (*kišpu*); for more on *kišpu*, see Chapter 15. Although not stated, it is likely that some of the mucus was vomited up, or the *āšipu* would not have been aware of it.

6.8 DIŠ NA ŠÀ.MEŠ-*šú nap-ḫ*[*u*] SAG ŠÀ-*šú ru-pu-ul-ta* TUKU.MEŠ-*ši ana* TI-*šú* . . . (*BAM* 575 ii 45)

**If a person's insides are bloated (and) his upper abdomen (epigastrium) continually has mucus,[16] to cure him . . .

6.9 DIŠ [N]A ŠÀ-*šú ḫa-aḫ-ḫa* DIRI *ana* TI-*šú* . . . (*BAM* 575 iii 18)

**If a ⌜person's⌝ insides are full of *ḫaḫḫu* (bloody mucus), to cure him . . .

6.10 DIŠ SAG ŠÀ-*šú ru-púl-ta* TUKU.MEŠ-*ši* SAG ŠÀ-*šú ú-ṣa-rap-šú ur-ra u* GI_6 *la i-ṣal-lal* NINDA *u* A LAL UZU^{II}-*šú tab-ku* NA.BI *kiš-pi* KÚ *u* NAG *a-na šup-šu-ri* . . . (*AMT* 48/2:1–3)[17]

**If his upper abdomen (epigastrium) continually has mucus, his epigastrium burns him hotly, he cannot sleep day or night, he loses his appetite for bread and water, (and) his flesh is tense,[18] that person has eaten or drunk *kišpu*, to dispel it . . .

In the following reference, it appears that the vomitus was allowed to settle, permitting the *āšipu* to recognize that it contained both bile and "thick sputum" (probably mucus).

6.11 *ina* UGU *mar-ti šá* LUGAL *be-lí iš-pur-an-ni ma-a iq-ṭi-a pa-šu-ut-tu*! *ši-i ka-ṣir-tú iq-ṭi-a mar-tu ana šap-liš it-tu-šib* (*ABL* 363 obv. 8–15 [Parpola, *SAA* 10.217])

**As for the bile that the king my lord wrote me about, saying "It came up." It is *pašittu* (cholecystitis; see below). The thick sputum came up; the gall settled down below.

THE FLY TEST Another curious reference observes that in certain cases the vomitus failed to attract flies.

6.12 DIŠ TA GIG *ip-ru-ma ana ḫu-ḫa-ti-šú* NIM *la* TE-*ḫi* GAM (DPS XVII:60 [AOAT 43.201]; cf. StBoT 36.60:9)[19]

**If after falling ill he vomits and flies will not come near his vomitus, he will die.

This test is not likely to become popular with modern physicians, but ancient physicians were undoubtedly recognizing that some substance in the vomitus was repelling the flies. Unfortunately, it is impossible to determine what this substance was, and whether it was the cause or the effect of the illness.

EXAMINATION OF STOOLS

Stool color and consistency were also recorded. Again, a red color probably means fresh bleeding, while black stools are caused by bleeding higher up in the gastrointestinal tract. This finding carries a grave risk of death.

RED OR BLACK STOOLS Black stools might be due to a bleeding stomach or duodenal peptic ulcer. Bright red blood in stools can have many causes, including bleeding hemorrhoids and colon cancer.

6.13 DIŠ ŠÈ-*šú* SA$_5$.MEŠ DIN . . . DIŠ ŠÈ-*šú* [GI$_6$].MEŠ GAM / DIŠ ŠÈ-*šú du-ʾ-ú-*[*um* . . .] (DPS XIV A ii 16, 18–19//E 3′, 4′ = *TDP* 134 ii 16, 18–19)

**If his excrement is red, he will get well . . . If his excrement is [black], he will die. If his excrement is ⸢dark red⸣ [. . .].

6.14 ⸢DIŠ *ina* DÚR-*šú* A⸣.M[EŠ] ⸢SA$_5$.MEŠ DU-*ku* GIG-*su* GÍD⸣ (DPS XIV C$_2$ i 11a = *TDP* 132 ii 2)

**If red liquid flows from his anus, his illness will be prolonged.

6.15 ⸢DIŠ *ina* DÚR-*šú* ZÉ⸣ [S]A$_5$ ⸢DU-*ak* GÍD-*ma* DIN⸣ (DPS XIV C$_2$ i 12a = *TDP* 132 ii 4)

**If ⸢red⸣ bile flows from his anus, (his illness) may be prolonged, but he will get well.

6.16 DIŠ *ina* DÚR-*šú* MÚD *it-*⸢*te*⸣*-eṣ-ṣí* ŠU [. . .] / DIŠ *ina* DÚR-*šú* MÚD MUD *it-te-eṣ-ṣi* Š[U . . .] / DIŠ *ina* DÚR-*šú* MÚD *u* MÚD.BABBAR *it-te-eṣ-ṣi* ŠU ^{d}[. . .] (DPS XIV A ii 12-14//E 1′–2′ = *TDP* 132 ii 12–14)[20]

**If he excretes blood from his anus, "hand" of [. . .]. If he excretes dark blood from his anus, ⸢"hand"⸣ [of . . .]. If he excretes blood and pus from his anus, "hand" of [. . .].

6.17 DIŠ KI.MIN-*ma* MÚD MUD *iz-zi* GAM : *ana* GAL$_5$.LÁ ÚŠ *pa-qid* GAM (DPS XVI:10 [AOAT 43.172])

**If (it is the first day he is sick) and he excretes dark blood, he will die (var. he was entrusted to a *gallû* of death; he will die).

6.18 ⸢DIŠ *ina* DÚR-*šú* ZÉ⸣ G[I$_6$ D]U-⸢*ak* GAM⸣ (DPS XIV A ii 6//C$_2$ i 13a = *TDP* 132 ii 6)

**If ⸢black⸣ bile ⸢flows⸣ from his anus, he will die.

The text below mentions "flesh" coming from the anus. It seems likely that the "flesh" is actually blood clots that formed in the colon and were subsequently expelled from the anus.

6.19 DIŠ *ina* DÚR-*šú* ⸢UZU ŠUB.ŠUB⸣-[*a* . . .] (DPS XIV A ii 9//C$_2$ i 14b = *TDP* 132 ii 9)[21]

**If he continually produces flesh from his anus, [. . .].

YELLOW OR LIGHT-COLORED STOOLS Yellow (or light-colored) stools could have been caused by common bile duct obstruction, usually due to a bile duct stone, since bile is the major substance giving the stool its normal brown color. Diarrhea also tends in general to lighten stool color.[22]

6.20 DIŠ ŠÈ-*šú* SIG_7.[MEŠ . . .] (DPS XIV A ii 17 = *TDP* 134 ii 17)[23]

**If his excrement is yellow [. . .].

6.21 ⌜DIŠ⌝ [*ina* DÚR]-⌜*šú*⌝ [A].⌜MEŠ SIG_7.MEŠ DU-*ku* NA⌝.B[I . . .] (DPS XIV C_2 i 11b = *TDP* 132 ii 3)

**If yellow liquid flows [from] his [anus], ⌜that person⌝ [. . .].

6.22 ⌜DIŠ⌝ [*ina*] ⌜DÚR-*šú*⌝ [Z]É ⌜SIG_7⌝ DU-*ak* k[a]? lu? mir-riš BA.ÚŠ[24] (DPS XIV C_2 i 12b = *TDP* 132 ii 5)

**If yellow ⌜bile⌝ flows [from his anus] . . . he will die.

FATTY STOOLS A common cause of fatty stools (steatorrhea) is pancreatic failure due to chronic pancreatitis (see below).

6.23 DIŠ *ina* DÚR-*šú* ⌜Ì ŠÀ-*šú* DU-*ku* GAM⌝ (DPS XIV A ii 7//C_2 i 13b = *TDP* 132 ii 7)

**If his body fat flows from his anus, he will die.

6.24 DIŠ KI.MIN-*ma* ŠÈ *ma-ru-ti-šú iz-zi* GAM (DPS XVI:6 [AOAT 43.172])[25]

**If (it is the first day he is sick) and he excretes the excrement of his body fat,[26] he will die.

6.25 DIŠ U_4.MEŠ-*šú* GÍD.DA.MEŠ-*ma* ŠÈ *ma-ru-ti-šú iz-zi* GAM (DPS XVI:90′ [AOAT 43.180])

**If he is in his seventies[27] and he excretes the excrement of his body fat, he will die.

QERBĒNU GIG ("SICK INSIDES")

Patients who were observed to have blood or bile in their vomitus or stools were said to have *qerbēnu* GIG ("sick insides"). We believe that *qerbēnu* GIG was not considered to be a single disease or syndrome, but was applied to any disease where it was appropriate.

6.26 DIŠ NA SAG ŠÀ-*šú* KÚ-*šú ina ge-ši-šu* ZÉ *im-ta-na-*ʾ NA.BI *qer-bé-na* GIG SUM^{SAR} $GA.RAS^{SAR}$ UZU GU_4 UZU ŠAḪ KAŠ LÚ.KÚRUN.NA NU *uš-ta-maḫ-ḫar ana* TI-*šú* . . . (*BAM* 578 i 1–2)

**If a person's upper abdomen (epigastrium) hurts him and when he belches, he continually produces bile, that person has *qerbēnu* GIG. He is continually unable to keep down garlic, leeks, beef, pork, or *kurunnu*-beer; to cure him . . .

The preceding reference is likely to be an upper intestinal problem, probably gall bladder disease, especially cholecystitis. The following reference clearly involves the colon with significant anal bleeding. Active bleeding from the anus can have many causes, including hemorrhoids, colon cancer, and blood vessel (arteriovenous) malformation.

6.27 DIŠ NA *ina* DÚR-*šú* MÚD *ú-tab-ba-ka* NA.BI *qer-bé-nu* GIG *ana* GIG-*šú* NU GÍD.DA . . . (*BAM* 152 iii 11–12//*BAM* 99:30–31)[28]

**If a person pours blood out of his anus, that person has *qerbēnu* GIG, in order that his illness not be prolonged . . .

SIGNS AND SYMPTOMS OF GASTROINTESTINAL ILLNESS

The *āšipu* used five different words to describe vomiting, not counting an equivalent of our "to produce" (*nadû*). Of these, several appear to have specialized meanings: *arû* refers to any type of vomiting, whereas *parû* is often used specifically to mean "to vomit the contents of a full stomach," *gâšu* to mean "to vomit the contents of an empty stomach (dry heaves)," *ḫaḫû* to mean "to vomit blood," and *mâʾu* or *wâʾu* to mean "to vomit bile."

6.28 DIŠ SAG.KI-*šú* DIB-*su-ma* KI.MIN *ma-gal i*$_{16}$*-à-ru u* NÁ NU ÍL ŠU GIDIM$_7$ GAM (DPS IV B obv. 11 = *TDP* 32:11)[29]

**If his temple afflicts him and (he keeps crying out: "my insides, my insides"), he vomits (*arû*) a lot and cannot stand the bed, "hand" of ghost; he will die.

6.29 DIŠ NA NINDA KÚ-⌈*ma*⌉ *i-par-ru* ⌈KAŠ⌉ NAG-*ma* [. . .] NA BI DÚR.GIG *ana* TI-*šu* . . . (*AMT* 56/3+84/7:3–4)[30]

**If a person eats bread and then vomits the contents of his stomach (*parû*), he drinks beer and then [. . .] that person (has) DÚR.GIG, to cure him . . .

6.30 DIŠ NA *du-ga-nu* DIB-*su* SAG ⌈ŠÀ-*šú*⌉ *ú-ṣa-rap-šú* NU *pa-tan ú-ga-áš* NA BI KA *kar-še* GIG *ana* TI-*šú* . . . (*STT* 96:9–10)

**If *tugānu* (peptic ulcer; see below) afflicts a person, his upper abdomen (epigastrium) burns him hotly, (and) he vomits without having eaten (*gâšu*), that person (has) sick mouth of the stomach, to cure him . . .

6.31 DIŠ *ina* SAG.DU-*šú* SÌG-*iṣ-ma u* MÚD *i-*⌈*ḫa*⌉*-ḫu* ŠU ^{d}MAŠ.TAB.BA GAM (DPS III C r. 19//E$_2$ r. 16 = *TDP* 26:79)

**If he was wounded on his head and vomits blood (*ḫaḫû*), "hand" of the twin gods; he will die.

6.32 DIŠ *ina* KA-*šú* ZÉ BABBAR *i-ú-a ana* U$_4$.⌈3⌉.[KÁM . . .][31] (DPS VII B obv. 13′ = *TDP* 64:52′)

**If he vomits white bile (*wâʾu*) from his mouth (and he has been sick) for three days [. . .]

Other signs and symptoms of gastrointestinal illness mentioned in medical texts include abdominal bloating/protrusion, presence or absence of abdominal rigidity, intestinal gas, loud noise, rumbling and "wind," colic-cramping or spasmodic intestinal pain, loss of appetite, nausea/vomiting, constipation, diarrhea, pain—focal or general (also described as burning, gnawing, jabbing, stinging, and stabbing or needling; see Chapter 13), and upper abdominal (epigastric)/internal fever.

ABDOMINAL BLOATING/PROTRUSION When the abdomen protrudes due to an acute illness rather than obesity it is usually due to intestinal gas or abdominal fluid (ascites). Ascites can be caused by cirrhosis, the nephrotic syndrome (see Chapter 5), or heart failure,[32] while ileus (see below) and intestinal obstruction can lead to excess intestinal gas. There are two verbs, in addition to the neutral *distended* and *protruding*, which were used to describe swollen abdomens. The verb (Sumerian: MÚ; Akkadian: *napāḫu*), which is used in two of the references below and translated as "bloated," is otherwise used to describe the action of a bellows. It can, therefore, imply the presence of air or gas in the cavity and is used in contexts where intestinal gas is clearly meant.

6.33 DIŠ SAG ŠÀ-*šú* MÚ.MEŠ DIB GIDIM$_7$ (DPS XIII B i 14′ = *TDP* 112 i 18′; cf. StBoT 36.41 r. 8′–9′)[33]

**If his upper abdomen (epigastrium) is continually bloated, affliction by a ghost.

6.34 DIŠ NA Ú NAG-*ma la i-ár-ru ṣe-me-er* . . . (*BAM* 575 iii 42)[34]

**If a person drinks a plant and does not vomit (but) is distended . . .

6.35 [DIŠ N]A ŠÀ-*šú it-ta-na-az-qáp* ŠÀ.MEŠ-*šú* MÚ.MÚ *šá* KA-*šú* GUR.GUR *mim-ma* KÚ-*ma* UGU-*šú* NU DÙG.GA NA BI *ki-ṣir-te* ḪAR.MEŠ GIG *ana* TI-*šú* . . . (*BAM* 556 ii 70′–71′)

**[If] a ⌜person's⌝ abdomen continually protrudes,[35] his insides are continually bloated, he continually returns (food) to his mouth, whatever he eats does not agree with him, that person is sick with thick sputum in the lungs, to cure him . . .

There is a second verb (Sumerian ÍL; Akkadian: *našû*), which we have consistently translated "puffed up" and which means literally "to raise, lift." Since this verb is used in diseases where increased abdominal fluid is likely to occur, we believe that it refers to abdominal distention due to increased abdominal fluid, as in the following references.

6.36 DIŠ SAG ŠÀ-*šú* ÍL-*ma* IGI.MEŠ-*šú* MÚ.MEŠ-*ḫu ina* IGI^{II}-*šú* ÍR DU GÍD-*ma* GAM (DPS XIII B i 18′ = *TDP* 112 i 22′; cf. DPS XV:34 [AOAT 43.152])

**If his upper abdomen (epigastrium) is puffed up and his face is swollen (and) tears flow from his eyes, (if) it is prolonged, he will die.

6.37 DIŠ ⌜NA SAG.ŠÀ-*šú*⌝ *na-ši* MURUB$_4$.MEŠ-*šú mi-na-tu-šú* KÚ.MEŠ-*šú* . . . (*BAM* 579 iv 44; *AMT* 43/6:1)[36]

**If a person's upper abdomen (epigastrium) is puffed up (and) his hips and limbs continually hurt him . . .

6.38 DIŠ NA ŠÀ.MEŠ-*šú* ÍL-*ú* [. . .] ⌜TÙN⌝.ŠÀ-*šú* DIB.DIB-*su* [. . .] (*BAM* 84:5′–6′)

**If a person's insides are puffed up [. . .] and his liver[37] continually afflicts him [. . .]

6.39 DIŠ NA *aḫ-ḫa-zu* IGI^{II}-*šú* E$_{11}$-*a-ma* IGI^{II}-*šú* GU.MEŠ SIG$_7$.MEŠ [*u*]*d-du-ḫa* ŠÀ.MEŠ-*šú na-šu-ú* NINDA *u* KAŠ *ú-tar-ra* NA BI *ú-za-bal-ma* ⌜BA.ÚŠ⌝ (*BAM* 578 iv 43–44)[38]

**If *aḫḫāzu*-jaundice rises to a person's eyes so that his eyes are ⌜covered⌝ with a network of yellow threads, his insides are puffed up (and) return bread and beer (to his mouth), (if) that person lingers, he will die.

PRESENCE OF ABDOMINAL RIGIDITY Hardness or rigidity of the abdominal wall is usually due to spasm of the abdominal muscles. Infection of the abdominal cavity is usually the cause, and is called peritonitis (see Chapter 3). Both of the following references mention a "puffed up" upper abdomen, indicating the presence of fluid (ascites). Abdominal fluid alone is not indicative of peritonitis in the absence of rigidity and pain. The Mesopotamian physician could have understood the significance of these medical signs only by long experience in observing and palpating the abdomens of his patients.

6.40 DIŠ SAG.DU-*su u* ŠÀ-*šú* KÚM-*im* SA SAG.KI^{II}-*šú* ŠU^{II}-⌜*šú u*⌝ [GÌR^{II}-*šú* 1-*niš* ZI.MEŠ] SAG ŠÀ-*šú na-ši* ḪÁŠ-*su* ⌜*da*⌝-*an* ŠE [D$_7$ . . .] (DPS III C obv. 57–58 = *TDP* 24:57–58)

**If his head and his abdomen are hot (and) the blood vessel(s) of his temples, his hands and [his feet all seem to pulsate together], his upper abdomen (epigastrium) is puffed up, his lower abdomen (hypogastric region)[39] is hard, he has ⌜chills⌝ [. . .].

6.41 DIŠ SAG ŠÀ-*šú* ÍL-*ma* ḪÁŠ-*su da-an* KÚM *u* ŠED$_7$ *ana* NIN.DINGIR DINGIR-*šú* TE-*ḫi ana* U$_4$.31.KÁM BÚR-*ma* DIN (DPS XIII B i 20′–21′ = *TDP* 112 i 24′–25′)[40]

**If his upper abdomen (epigastrium) is puffed up and his lower abdomen (hypogastric region) is hard (and) he is hot and then cold, he has approached the *ēntu* priestess of his god.[41] (If) it lets up within thirty-one days, he will get well.

ABSENCE OF ABDOMINAL RIGIDITY The reference below is mentioned in footnote 110 in our discussion of cholera (Chapter 3). It describes the abdomen as "soft." This is quite compatible with the clinical description of cholera, since it is a purely toxin-related disease that causes excess fluid loss without irritating the intestines or abdomen.

6.42 DIŠ ŠÀ-*šú* DIG-*ub* A UL$_4$-*gal* APIN-*eš* KÚM-*šú mit-ḫar* TA *taš-ri-ti* EN SAG GI$_6$ / DIŠ GIG-*su id-da-lip* SÌG-*iṣ* MAŠKIM : GIDIM SÌG-*iṣ* GAM (DPS XIII B ii 13–14 = *TDP* 118 ii 13–14)[42]

**If his abdomen is soft,[43] he asks for a lot of water (but) his temperature is normal, (and) if his illness has kept him awake from the beginning to the middle of the night, he was stricken with the blow of a *rābiṣu*-demon (var. ghost); he will die.

INTESTINAL GAS

6.43 *ša-ru-um-mi šá-ru šá-ru-ma* (coll.) DINGIR.MEŠ *at-ta*$_5$ *ša-ru ša bi-rit ze-e u ši-na-a-ti at-ta*$_5$ *tu-ṣi-a-ma it-ti* DINGIR.MEŠ ŠEŠ.MEŠ-*ka na-di-a-at* ^{GIŠ}GU.ZA-*ka* (*BAM* 574 iii 56–57)

**O Wind, wind, you are the wind of the gods; you are the wind that is between the shit and the urine. (If) you come out, your throne will be set down with the gods your brothers.

LOUD NOISE, RUMBLING, AND "WIND" Loud intestinal noise and rumbling can be caused by increased intestinal mobility such as is seen with infectious diarrhea. Partial intestinal obstruction can also cause noise as gas is forced through a narrowed intestine.

6.44 DIŠ NA ŠÀ.MEŠ-*šú* MÚ.MEŠ-*ḫu ir-ru-šú i-ár-ru-ru ir-ru-šú* GÙ.GÙ-*ú* IM *ina* ŠÀ-*šú i-le-eb-bu ina* DÚR![44] -*šú ú-na-kap* NA BI *nik-ma-ti* GIG *ana* TI-*šú* . . . (*BAM* 159 v 48–50)

**If a person's insides are continually bloated, his intestines rumble,[45] his intestines continually make a loud noise, "wind" groans in his stomach (and) "butts" into his anus, that person is sick with pent-up (wind),[46] to cure him . . .

6.45 DIŠ NA ŠÀ.MEŠ-*šú* MÚ.MEŠ-*ḫu ir-ru-šú* GIN_7 *šá* MAR.GAL *ma-gal* GÙ.GÙ-*ú* NA BI *ni-kim-ti* IM *u* UD.DA GIG KIN-*šú i-la-bir-ma* ŠU.GIDIM.MA *ana* TI-*šú* . . . (*BAM* 52:66–67//*BAM* 471 ii 3′–4′//*BAM* 88:17′–20′//*BAM* 168:1–3; *AMT* 52/4:2′–4′)[47]

**If a person's insides are continually bloated (and) his intestines continually make a (loud) noise like an *iššqippu*-bird, that person is sick with pent-up "wind" (and) *ṣētu* (enteric fever). If his attack is prolonged, "hand" of ghost, to cure him . . .

COLIC-CRAMPING, SPASMODIC INTESTINAL PAIN (see chapter 13) Any irritation of the intestines can cause colic, including infectious diarrhea and peptic ulcer disease.

6.46 DIŠ NA ŠÀ.MEŠ-*šú* MÚ.MÚ *it-ta-ni-bi-ṭu* ŠÀ-*šu ana pa-re-e e-ta-ne-pa-áš ana* TI-*šú* . . . (*BAM* 575 ii 17)[48]

**If a person's insides are continually bloated (and) cramped (and) his stomach continually makes as if to vomit, to cure him . . .

6.47 [DIŠ NA] NINDA KÚ KAŠ NAG-*ma* ŠÀ-*šú in-nen-me-er nap-ḫu* A *ma-gal* NAG UD.DA SÁ.SÁ . . . (*AMT* 48/3:8+*AMT* 23/5:7+*AMT* 48/1:1; *AMT* 48/1:7+*AMT* 78/3:4)[49]

[If a person] eats bread (and) drinks beer and subsequently his stomach is colicky and bloated (and he drinks a lot of water, *ṣētu* (enteric fever) has "gotten" him . . .

"RELAXED" INSIDES This term probably indicates an abdomen free of abdominal wall spasm, retching from vomiting, and the noise of prominent bowel sounds that can be heard in diarrhea and vomiting.

6.48 DIŠ *ina* GIG-*šú pa-su-šú ir-*⌜*mu*⌝-*ú u* ZI.IR.MEŠ GIG-*su* TAG_4-*šú* (DPS XVII:29 [AOAT 43.197])

**If during (the course of) his illness, his insides[50] are (alternatively) relaxed and upset, his illness is leaving him.

LOSS OF APPETITE

6.49 DIŠ LÚ.TUR *ina te-ni-qí-šú* UZU.MEŠ *i-šaḫ-ḫu-ḫu u mu-še-niq-ta-šú* UBUR SIG-*at* UBUR ÍL-*šum-ma* NU KÚ UBUR *šú-ú mur-ra i-šú ana* UBUR *eš-ši tu-na-kar-šú-ma* TI (DPS XL A 36–37 = *TDP* 220/222:36–37)

**If an infant's flesh wastes away while he is nursing and his wetnurse's breast is weak (and if) you raise the breast to him he will not eat,[51] that breast has a bitter taste. (If) you move him to a new breast, he will get well.

6.50 DIŠ GIG-*ma ina* GIG-*šú* GIN$_7$ *šá* DIN-*šú* KI DAM-*šú* DUMU-*šú* DUMU.MUNUS-*šú* SIG$_5$-*iš i-ta-mu* NINDA NU KÚ *di-ḫu* D[IN] (DPS XVII:41–42 [AOAT 43.199]; cf. Labat, *Syria* 33.121–126 obv. 15)

**If he is sick and, during his sickness, he speaks in a friendly way with his wife, son, (and) daughter just as if he were feeling well (but) he will not eat bread,[52] it is *diʾu* (enteric fever without dehydration; see Chapter 3); he will get ⌜well⌝.

In the following references, "it doesn't agree ('go') with him" probably means that the patient is complaining that the food does not taste good, whereas "his appetite is diminished" means that he has been observed to eat less than usual.

6.51 DIŠ NA ŠÀ.MEŠ-*šú* MÚ.MEŠ-*ḫu ir-ru-šú i-ár-ru-ru* IGI.MEŠ-*šú* NIGIN.MEŠ-*du* [SA].MEŠ-*šú tab-ka-ma* TA! GÌR^{II}-*šu* <EN> MURUB$_4$.MEŠ-*šú* ZI-*ma kin-ṣa-a-šú* KÚ.MEŠ-*šú* [*mim-ma*] KÚ *u* NAG UGU-*šú* NU DU-*ak* NA.BI GIG *di-ʾu* GIG ⌜*šum-ma*⌝ NA.BI TI.LA *ḫa-ši-iḫ ana* TI-*šú*... (*BAM* 106 obv. 1–4//*BAM* 108 r. 2′–8′//*AMT* 39/4 r. 3′–5′//*BAM* 52:101; BM 42298:23–25 [Finkel, *Fs. Lambert* 181])

**If a person's insides are continually bloated, his intestines rumble, his face seems continually to spin, his [blood vessels] are tense and pulsate from his feet <to> his hip region and consequently his legs continually hurt him, (and) [whatever] he eats and drinks does not agree with him,[53] that person is sick with *diʾu*; if that person wants to live, to cure him . . .

6.52 DIŠ LÚ.TUR *ú-nap-paq* KÚM DIB.DIB-*su* UBUR *muṭ-ṭú* NAM.ÉRIM DIB-*su* (DPS XL A 119 = *TDP* 230:119)

**If an infant chokes, fever continually afflicts him, (and) his appetite for the breast is diminished, a curse afflicts him.

6.53 DIŠ NA ŠÀ.MEŠ-*šú nap-ḫu gu-ḫa u* ÚḪ TUKU.MEŠ-*ši* NINDA *u* KAŠ LAL *ana* TI-*šú*... (*BAM* 575 ii 43)[54]

**If a person's insides are bloated, he continually has *guḫḫu* cough and phlegm, (and) his appetite for bread and beer is diminished,[55] to cure him . . .

NAUSEA/VOMITING

6.54 DIŠ NA KÚM *ma-dam* TUKU-*ma* NU *i-na-aḫ ú-na-ḫaṭ u i-sa-ul u* ŠÀ-*šú a-na a-re-e i-ta-na-šá-a* NAM.ÉRIM GIG (DPS XXII:26–27 [AOAT 43.253/254])[56]

**If a person is very feverish and cannot find rest, he breathes deeply[57] and coughs, and his stomach is continually nauseous to the point of vomiting, he is sick with a curse.

6.55 DIŠ NA MIN (UD.DA KUR-*id*) NINDA *u* KAŠ NU *i-le-em ana* TI.BI . . . (*BAM* 66 r. 8′//*AMT* 14/7:5)[58]

**If *ṣētu* (enteric fever) has "gotten" a person (and his insides) cannot take bread or beer, to cure him . . .

In the following references, the observation that the stomach "will not accept bread and beer" probably means that the patient is nauseated but not vomiting while the phrase "returns bread to the mouth" means actual vomiting.

6.56 DIŠ [ŠÀ]-*šú e-ta-na-šá-áš* NINDA *u* KAŠ *la i-maḫ-ḫar* MAŠ.$SÌLA^{II}$-*šú* KÚ.MEŠ-*šú* . . . (*BAM* 574 ii 29//*BAM* 575 iii 16)

**If his [stomach] is continually upset (and) will not accept bread and beer[59] (and) his shoulders continually hurt him . . .

6.57 ⸢DIŠ⸣ NA ŠÀ.MEŠ-*šú ma-gal nap-ḫu* ⸢NINDA⸣.MEŠ KAŠ.MEŠ *ina* KA-*šú* GUR.GUR-*ra* . . . (*BAM* 575 ii 35)[60]

**If a person's insides are greatly bloated (and) continually return bread and beer to his mouth . . .[61]

6.58 DIŠ LÚ.TUR *i-mi-iš-ti* ŠÀ-*bi i-šu* KA-*šú* BAD.BAD-*te ma-la* KÚ *ut-ta-nar-ra* ŠU DINGIR.MAḪ : ŠU DINGIR TI (DPS XL A 50//B 49 = *TDP* 222:50)

**If an infant has intestinal colic, he continually opens his mouth and as much as he eats continually returns,[62] "hand" of Dingirmaḫ (var. "hand" of god); he will get well.

The *āšipu* also noted situations in which some foods, but not others, produced nausea and vomiting. In the first reference below, the length of time the patient has been sick is inferred from the severity of his nausea and, in the second, a patient with esophageal reflux (see below) is observed to be unable to digest certain specified foods.

6.59 DIŠ KI.MIN *ka-la* U_4-*mi u* GI_6 *i-le-eb-bu-ma la i-ṣal-lal* [NINDA] *u* KAŠ (coll.) *la i-maḫ-ḫar* GURUN KÚ *u* A NAG NA.BI ITI.1.KÁM GIG [*ana*] GIG-*su* NU GÍD.DA . . . (DPS XXXI:52′–54′ [AOAT 43.344])[63]

**If (*ṣētu* [enteric fever] burns him and) he groans all day and all night so that he cannot sleep, (his insides) do not accept [bread] and beer (but) he can eat fruit and drink water, that person has been sick for a month; in order for his illness not to be prolonged . . .

6.60 DIŠ NA *di-ik-šu ina* GABA-*šú* TAG.TAG-*su-ma* GIN_7 *ši-ni-ʾ-ti* SAḪAR *i-šá-an-na-ʾ-šu ina g*[*e-ši-šú*] ZÉ *i-par-ru ina da-ba-bi-šú ik-ka-šu ik-te-*[*ne*]*r-ru* NA <BI> *bi-rit* ŠÀ-*bi* GIG KU_6 SUM^{SAR} UZU ⸢GU_4⸣ [UZU.ŠAḪ] *u* KAŠ LÚ.KÚRUN.NA *la uš-ta-maḫ-ḫar ut-ta-šar* . . . (*BAM* 575 iii 65–67)[64]

**If a needling pain continually hurts a person intensely in his breast and something like suffusions of dirt[65] suffuse him, when [he] ⸢belches⸣ he vomits bile (and), when he talks, he is [continually] short of breath, <that> person is sick inside his abdomen. He cannot keep down fish, garlic, beef, [pork], or *kurunnu*-beer but releases it . . .

The *āšipu* knew that vomiting had potential for both good and bad. Severe unremitting vomiting, in an era before the availability of intravenous fluids, could result in death, and physicians had medicine aimed at stopping it.

6.61 DIŠ GIG-*ma* NINDA *šá* KÚ *ina* ŠÀ-*šú* NU *i-kal-la-ma bal-ṭa ina* KA-*šú* NU GIN-*an ina* KA-*šú* ŠUB-*a* GAM (DPS XVII:52–53 [AOAT 43.200])

**If he is sick and he cannot retain the food that he eats in his stomach[66] and he cannot (even) put anything raw into his mouth (but) he produces it from his mouth, he will die.

6.62 DIŠ GIG-*šú* DU_8-*ma* $BURU_8$ NU KUD-*us* GAM (DPS XVII:33 [AOAT 43.198])[67]

**If his illness lets up (but) he cannot stop vomiting, he will die.

6.63 *ana a-ra-a* TAR-*si* . . . (K 2426 iv 7; BM 78963:17)[68]

**(If you want) to stop vomiting . . .

Vomiting, however, can remove poisons and other toxins from the stomach before they can be absorbed, and the *āšipu* had methods to induce vomiting.

6.64 *šum-ma* LÚ *ana* ḪAL-*šú* . . . (BM 78963:7)

**If you want to make a person vomit . . .

6.65 Ú *a-re-e* . . . (*BAM* 579 i 38)

**Plant(s) to cause vomiting . . .

6.66 DIŠ LÚ.TUR *šá* GA *in-ni*-[. . .] *a-na šu-up-ri-i* . . . (BM 54914:17–18)

**If a suckling infant is [. . .] to get him to vomit . . .

CONSTIPATION The second text below is a lyrical and fanciful approach to constipation which makes clear the distress that this problem can cause and the relief that successful treatment can bring.

6.67 Ú DÚR *es-lim* . . . (*BAM* 380:48–49)[69]

**Plant for constipated anus . . .

6.68 [*man*]-*nu lu-uš-pur a-na* GÚ.GAL ŠÀ-*bi-ka liš-šá-a* ^{GIŠ}MAR.MEŠ *šá* KÙ.BABBAR *u gi-dim-me-ti šá* KÙ.SIG_{17} *li-pat-ta-a* ÍD.MEŠ *li-pat-ta-a a-tap-pa-ti li-par-ši-du-ni lu-ṣu-ú-ni zu-ú-šú a-šam-šu-tu šá* ŠÀ-*bi-šú li-ṣa-a-ma* ^{d}UTU *li-mur* (*BAM* 508 ii 4′–8′//*AMT* 45/5 obv. 2′–7′//*BAM* 509 i 2′–6′//*BAM* 577:1′–4′)[70]

**⌜Whom⌝ should I send to the canal inspector of your *libbu* (gastrointestinal tract)? Let (the helpful goddesses) bring up silver spades and golden shovels! Let them open up rivers (and) branch canals! Let his excrement escape (and) come out! Let the whirlwind in his *libbu* come out and see the light of day!

DIARRHEA Ancient physicians distinguished two different types of diarrhea: "loose bowels" (painless diarrhea) and "flowing of the bowels" (diarrhea with cramping, blood, and pus). For more details, see Chapter 3.

6.69 DIŠ NA ŠÀ SI.SÁ TUKU-*ma* NU TAR-*as* . . . (BM 59623:1 [Leichty, *Mem. Sachs* 263–264])[71]

**If a person's bowels are loose and will not stop . . .

6.70 [DIŠ N]A NINDA KÚ KAŠ NAG-*ma* ŠÀ-*šú in-nim-me-ru in-ne*-[*e*]*n-bi-ṭú re-du-ut ir-ri* TUKU UD.DA SÁ.SÁ . . . (*AMT* 48/1:12+*AMT* 78/3:9; *AMT* 44/6:1–2)[72]

**[If] a ⌜person⌝ eats bread (and) drinks beer and subsequently his stomach is colicky, he has ⌜cramps⌝ (and) he has a "flowing of the bowels," *ṣētu* has "gotten" him . . .

Particularly loose bowel movements were sometimes graphically described.

6.71 [DIŠ N]A NAM.ÉRIM *šaḫ-[ḫi]-ḫu* GIG *mim-mu-u i-lem-mu*⸢*ina*⸣ ŠÀ-*šú la i-na-aḫ*⸢*bal*⸣-*ṭam*!-*ma*[73] *ana* DÚR-*šú ú-tab-bak* NINDA NU KÚ NA.BI GÍD-*ma* ÚŠ *ana maš-taq-ti-šú u bul-lu-ṭí-šú* . . . (*BAM* 156:1–3)[74]

**[If a] ⸢person⸣ is sick with a ⸢wasting⸣ curse, whatever he eats does not rest easy in his stomach[75] but he pours (it) raw into his anus (and) he cannot eat bread, if that person lingers, he will die; for his splitting off and to cure him . . .

6.72 DIŠ NA NU *pa-tan* ŠÀ-*šú ana pa-re-e e-te-né-la-a* ÚḪ *ma-gal* SUB.MEŠ A.MEŠ *ina* KA-*šú mál-da-riš* DU-*ku pa-nu-šú iṣ-ṣa-nu-du* ŠÀ.MEŠ-*šú* MÚ.MÚ-*ḫu* MURUB$_4^{II}$-*šú kin-ṣa-šú* TAG.GA.MEŠ-*šú* KÚM ŠED$_7$ IR TUKU.MEŠ-*ši* NINDA *u* KAŠ LAL A ŠED$_7$ *ma-gal* NAG *i-par-ru ina* DÚR-*šú* GÌŠ-*šú* SIG$_7$ *ú-tab-ba-kam* MÙŠ.MEŠ-*šú i-te-nen-nu-u* UZU.MEŠ-*šu tab-ku mìm-ma* KÚ-*ma* UGU-*šú ul* DÙG.GA NA BI ZÉ *saḫ-pa-su ana* TI-*šú* . . . (*BAM* 578 i 27–30)[76]

**If . . . his insides are continually bloated . . . his appetite for bread and beer is diminished . . . he pours yellow/green (matter) from his anus (and) his penis . . . (and) whatever he eats does not agree with him, the gall bladder has turned over on that person, to cure him . . .

UPPER ABDOMINAL (EPIGASTRIC) FEVER/INTERNAL FEVER There are numerous references in ancient Mesopotamian medical texts that identify fever in the abdominal region. A specific location is indicated by the use of the term *epigastrium*, namely, that part of the abdomen below the chest and above the navel, whereas "internal fever" appears to be referring to the entire abdomen.

6.73 DIŠ NA SAG ŠÀ-*šú um-ma-am* TUKU-*ši a-na* KÚM *šá ina* [SAG Š]À-*šú šá-ḫa-ṭi* . . . (*BAM* 579 i 22)[77]

**If a person's upper abdomen (epigastrium) has fever, to strip off the fever that is in his ⸢upper abdomen (epigastrium)⸣ . . .

6.74 *ana* NA *ṣi-ri-iḫ-ti* KÚM ŠÀ ZI-*ḫi* . . . (*BAM* 579 i 34//*BAM* 174 r. 1)[78]

**(If you want) to remove a person('s) burning internal fever . . .

In analyzing the texts that contain these terms, it is clear that they are being applied to many diseases with widely different signs and symptoms. In most cases, however, the references include findings localized to the upper abdomen or to the abdomen in general, as in the following references, which mention upper abdominal pain (gnawing), bloating, active bowel sounds (wind), and vomiting.

6.75 [DIŠ NA *ina*] DIB ŠU.GIDIM.MA SAG ŠÀ-*šú* KÚM-*im* KÚM ŠÀ TUKU-*ši* SAG ŠÀ-*šú* [*i-k*]*a-as-sa-su* . . . (*AMT* 76/1:11–12)

**[If, as the result of] affliction by "hand" of ghost, [a person]'s upper abdomen (epigastrium) is hot; he has internal fever (and) his upper abdomen (epigastrium) gnaws at him . . .

6.76 DIŠ NA SAG ŠÀ-*šú* KÚM ŠÀ-*šú* MÚ.MÚ-*ḫu ana* TI-*šú* . . . (*BAM* 575 ii 31; *BAM* 579 i 4)[79]

**If his upper abdomen (epigastrium) is hot and his insides are continually bloated, to cure him . . .

6.77 DIŠ NA SAG ŠÀ-*šú* KÚM TUKU.MEŠ-*ši* ŠÀ-*šú* GIG NINDA *u* A.MEŠ ŠÀ-*šú* NU IGI-*šú* GABA.MEŠ-*šú* *ir-te-nem-mu-u* ŠÀ-*šú* *ina pi-qi ana* ḪAL-*e* DÙ.DÙ-*uš* NU *i-par*$_5$*-ru* IM *ina* ŠÀ-*šú* *i-sa-na-ḫur i-le-eb-bu* ŠÀ.MEŠ-*šú* *eb-ṭù* NA BI ^{d}ŠU.NAM.ÉRIM DIB-*su ana* TI-*šú* . . . (*BAM* 49:9–14′//*BAM* 50 obv. 11–15//*BAM* 51:1′–3′)[80]

**If a person's upper abdomen (epigastrium) continually has fever, his stomach is sick, his stomach will not accept bread and water,[81] both sides of his chest are continually relaxed, his stomach suddenly makes as if to vomit but he cannot throw up, the "wind" in his stomach continually roils (and) groans, (and) his insides are cramped, "hand" of curse afflicts that person, to cure him . . .

6.78 DIŠ MUNUS Ù.TU-*ma* KÚM *ir-ri* TUKU.[TUKU]-*ši i-ár-ru* ŠÀ *ši* [. . .] MÚD *ḫa-riš-ti-šá ina* ŠÀ-*šá it-t*[*e-es*]-*ki-ru* MUNUS BI *ina* Ù.TU-*š*[*á* . . .] . . . (*BAM* 240:39′–40′)

**If a woman gives birth and subsequently she [continually] has internal fever, she vomits [. . .] the blood of her confinement has been ⌜locked up⌝ inside her; that woman, while giving birth [. . .] . . .

What, then, is the significance of these terms? We believe that, when a patient presented with upper abdominal or abdominal complaints, the *āšipu* would examine the involved area with his hands, paying careful attention to the temperature of the abdominal surface. If he sensed an elevated temperature, it was described as upper abdominal or internal (abdominal) fever. References quoted elsewhere (Chapter 3 with 3.1–3.2) would seem to suggest that the *āšipu*'s special interest in surface temperature also applied to other body sites with associated signs and symptoms.

The observation of upper abdominal or internal fever does not necessarily mean that the upper abdomen or abdomen was hot, while the head, chest, back, legs, and so on, were normal or cool. Regional differences in surface temperature may occur, but there is nothing in these references to suggest that only the upper abdomen or abdomen was hot. On the contrary, the following references mention pulsating blood vessels in the rest of the body or copious sweating, suggesting the presence of a generalized elevation in surface temperature.

6.79 DIŠ SAG ŠÀ-*šú* KÚM-*ma* SA SAG.KI^{II}-*šú* ŠU^{II}-*šú u* GÌR^{II}-*šú* ZI.ME IGI^{II}-*šú* DUGUD-*šú* (DPS XIII B i 27′ = *TDP* 112 i 31′)[82]

**If his upper abdomen (epigastrium) is hot and the blood vessels of his temples, his hands, and his feet continually (feel like they) are pulsating, (and) his eyes bother him.

6.80 DIŠ ŠÀ-*šú* KÚM IR GIN$_7$ *lu-ba-ṭi* ŠUB.ŠUB-*su u* ZI.IR.MEŠ ŠU 20 MAŠ.MAŠ-*su* DÙ-*uš u* ŠU.⌜ÚR⌝-*šú-ma* DIN (DPS XIII B ii 5–6 = *TDP* 116 ii 5–6)[83]

**If his abdomen is hot, sweat keeps falling upon him as in *lubāṭu*, and (his stomach) is continually upset, "hand" of Šamaš. (If) you do his treatment and you continually wipe him off, he will get well.

MISCELLANEOUS On a less serious note, there are some gastrointestinal complaints that can be caused by dietary indiscretion and emotional upheaval. The following three quotes describe problems that most of us in the modern era can understand and probably recall.

6.81 SUM.SIKIL.SAR NU KÚ *ṣu-ru-up* ŠÀ-*bi* TUKU-*ši* (Labat, *Hémérologies* 168:12–13, 170:40–41, 176:2–3; ND 5545:7, 24 [Hulin, *Iraq* 21.46–53])

**He should not eat onions (or else) he will have heartburn.

6.82 ^{Ú}LU.ÚB^{SAR} ^{Ú}<LÚ>.U$_{19}$.LU^{SAR} *šá* ŠÀ-*šú* GIG NU KÚ (*BAM* 1 iii 39; cf. *BAM* 318 iii 25)

**Whoever's stomach is sick[84] should not eat ^{Ú}LU.ÚB^{SAR}-vegetable (and) ^{Ú}<LÚ>.U$_{19}$.LU^{SAR}-vegetable.

6.83 DIŠ NÍG.ZI.IR ŠUB.ŠUB-*su* ZI.MEŠ-*šú* LUGUD.MEŠ NINDA KÚ A/KAŠ NAG-*ma* UGU-*šú* NU DU-*ak*ʾ*ú-a* ŠÀ-*bi i-qab-bi u uš-tan-na-aḫ* NA BI GIG *ra-mi* GIG *ana* NÍTA *u* MUNUS 1-*ma* (DPS XXII:8–9 [AOAT 43.252])[85]

**If depression continually falls upon him, his breath is continually short, he eats bread (and) drinks water/beer but it does not agree with him, he says "Ua my heart" and he is dejected, that person is sick with love-sickness; it is the same for a man and a woman.

KĪS LIBBI OR *KIṢIR LIBBI*

These terms mean literally "binding"[86] or "knotting" of the *libbu* (intestinal tract). The ancient Mesopotamian physician used them to describe similar and overlapping syndromes with complaints that include the inability to keep food down, right upper quadrant abdominal pain, bloating, flatulence, and abdominal cramping. There is no indication that these were serious problems; they were probably similar to what we call indigestion.

6.84 DIŠ NA *ki-is* [ŠÀ GIG NINDA *u* KAŠ] ŠÀ-*šú* NU IGI-*ḫar-šú ina* KA-*šú* GUR.GUR-*ra* TÙN-*šú ú-sa-ḫal-šú ip-ta-na-ru* [UZU.MEŠ-*šú ir-t*]*a-nam-mu-ú* IM *ina* DÚR-*šú* NIGIN ŠÀ.MEŠ-*šú eb-ṭù ana* TI-*šú* . . . (*BAM* 574 i 26–27)[87]

**If a person [is sick with] *kīs* [*libbi*], his insides will not accept [bread and beer] but it keeps returning to his mouth, his liver[88] gives him a stabbing pain, he continually vomits, [his flesh] is continually ⌜limp⌝,[89] "wind" roils about in his anus, and his insides are cramped, to cure him . . .

6.85 DIŠ NA *ki-is* ŠÀ GIG ŠÀ.MEŠ-*šú ma-*⌜*gal* MÚ⌝.MÚ-*ḫu* mu še er? [. . .] . . . (*BAM* 574 i 21)[90]

**If a person is sick with *kīs libbi* (and) his insides are continually bloated a lot [. . .] . . .

6.86 [DIŠ NA] *ki-ṣir* ŠÀ-*bi* GIG NINDA *u* KAŠ ŠÀ-*šú* NU IGI-*šú ina* KA-*šú* GUR.GUR *ip-te-né-ru ana* TI-*šú* . . . (*BAM* 575 iv 43)[91]

**[If a person] is sick with *kiṣir libbi* and his insides will not accept bread and beer but continually return it to his mouth (and) he continually vomits, to cure him . . .

Similar problems occurring in animals were recognized and treated.

6.87 Ú *ki-is* ŠÀ-*bi šá* ANŠE.KUR.RA . . . (*BAM* 159 v 35–36)

**Plants for *kīs libbi* affecting horses . . .

ENTERITIS

Soldiers on campaign, men called up and shipped to distant parts of the Assyrian empire to perform their labor service, and merchants on business had little choice but to travel, and traveler's diarrhea was doubtless as common in ancient Mesopotamia as it is today. One ancient text, already quoted above (3.115), consists of a prescription for a tried and true remedy for cases where "a person's bowels are loose and will not stop." The small size and conveniently portable shape of the text suggest that this (and similar tablets) were intended to be carried with a traveler for use during a trip.[92] Other aspects of infections of the gastrointestinal tract (enteritis) were extensively discussed by the *āšipu*, and are covered in Chapter 3.

ESOPHAGEAL REFLUX

Esophageal reflux is a common condition caused by acid from the stomach entering the esophagus from below. If this condition occurs over a long enough period of time, the esophagus becomes irritated and inflamed, leading to "heartburn." The quote below seems to be describing this condition, although a less common problem, diaphragmatic hernia, as well as gall bladder disease could also cause similar symptoms. The text mentions "dirt" as part of this syndrome. It seems likely that the "dirt" was dark material found in vomited gastric contents. Since bleeding commonly occurs in esophageal reflux, and since gastric acid will cause blood to look like dark brown particles, this material must have looked like "dirt" to the *āšipu*. Modern physicians use the term *coffee ground emesis* to define this phenomenon, but coffee was unknown in ancient Mesopotamia (see above).

6.88 DIŠ NA *di-ik-šu ina* GABA-*šú* TAG.TAG-*su-ma* GIN$_7$ *ši-ni-ʾ-ti* SAḪAR *i-šá-an-na-ʾ-šu ina g*[*e-ši-šú*] ZÉ *i-par-ru ina da-ba-bi-šú ik-ka-šu ik-te-*[*ne*]*r-ru* NA <BI> *bi-rit* ŠÀ-*bi* GIG KU$_6$ SUM^{SAR} UZU ⌜GU$_4$⌝ [UZU.ŠAḪ] *u* KAŠ LÚ.KÚRUN.NA *la uš-ta-maḫ-ḫar ut-ta-šar* . . . (*BAM* 575 iii 65–67)[93]

**If a needling pain continually hurts a person intensely in his breast and something like suffusions of dirt suffuses him, when [he] ⌜belches⌝ he vomits bile (and), when he talks, he is [continually] short of breath, <that> person is sick inside his abdomen. He cannot keep down fish, garlic, beef, [pork], or *kurunnu*-beer but releases it . . .[94]

OBSTRUCTION

The *āšipu* appears to have recognized that any blockage of the gastrointestinal tract if unrelieved would lead to death, whatever the underlying cause.

6.89 ⌜DIŠ DÚR-*šú* BAD.BAD-*ir*⌝ GAM (DPS XIV A$_2$ i 21//C$_2$ i 10a = *TDP* 132 i 72)[95]

**If his anus is continually blocked off,[96] he will die.

6.90 DIŠ NA NINDA KÚ KAŠ NAG-*ma i-ši-bi* ŠÀ-*šú ik-ta-na-su-šú* DIB.MEŠ-*su* ŠÀ.MEŠ-*šú* MÚ.MÚ *u i-sil* ŠÀ-*šú* MU.ŠE KIN.NIM GIG *ana* TI-*šú* . . . (*BAM* 574 ii 17–18)

**If a person eats bread and drinks beer until he is satisfied and his stomach continually "binds" him (see above) and afflicts him and his insides are bloated and he is constipated, his stomach is sick with MU.ŠE KIN.NIM, to cure him . . .

6.91 DIŠ *ina* SAG ŠÀ-*šú di-i*[*k-š*]*ú* [*u* ^{GIŠ}NÍG.GIDRU GAR-*nu*]-*šum-ma e-sil* GAM (DPS XIII B i 40′ = *TDP* 114 i 44′)

**If a ⌜needling⌝ pain [or burning pain[97] is firmly established] in his upper abdomen (epigastrium) and he is constipated, he will die.

PEPTIC ULCER DISEASE

Peptic ulcer disease is the result of a specific type of infection caused by the bacterium, *Helicobacter pylori.* It results in damage and ulceration of the lining of the stomach and upper small intestine (duodenum). Its signs and symptoms include upper abdominal pain, bleeding, and in some cases intestinal obstruction. Obstruction can occur when the duodenum is ulcerated and swollen. The following references are likely to be describing peptic ulcer disease.

6.92 DIŠ NA KA *kar-ši* GIG ⌜SAG⌝ ŠÀ-*šú ú-*⌜*ḫa*⌝*-maṭ-su ú-ṣar-rap-su ú-zaq-*⌜*qat*⌝*-šú u* KÚ.MEŠ-*su* x x ku ni *u* DÚR.GIG ⌜*ana* TI⌝*-šú* . . . (*STT* 96:20–21)

**If the mouth of a person's stomach is sick (and) his upper abdomen (epigastrium) burns him, burns him hotly, stings him and continually hurts him, ?? or DÚR.GIG, to cure him . . .

6.93 DIŠ *ina* SAG ŠÀ-*šú* ^{GIŠ}NÍG.GIDRU GAR-*su-ma u* MÚD MUD ŠUB.ŠUB-*a* GAM (DPS XIII B i 36′ = *TDP* 114 i 40′)[98]

**If a burning pain[99] is firmly established in his upper abdomen (epigastrium) and he continually produces dark blood, he will die.

6.94 DIŠ *ina* SAG ŠÀ-*šú di-ik-šú u* ^{GIŠ}NÍG.GIDRU GAR-*nu-šum-ma* MÚD *i-te-zi* GAM (DPS XIII B i 38′ = *TDP* 114 i 42′)

**If a needling pain or burning pain is firmly established in his upper abdomen (epigastrium) and he excretes blood, he will die.[100]

6.95 DIŠ *ina* SAG ŠÀ-*šú di-ik-šú u* ^{GIŠ}NÍG.GIDRU GAR-*nu-šum-ma* MÚD *i-ḫa-ḫu ana* U_4.2.KÁM *ana* U_4.3.KÁM GAM (DPS XIII B i 39′ = *TDP* 114 i 43′)[101]

**If a needling pain or burning pain is firmly established in his upper abdomen (epigastrium) and he vomits blood (and he has been sick) for two or three days, he will die.

The cause of death described in three of the references above, if the underlying problem was peptic ulcer disease, could be either blood loss or intestinal perforation with death caused by secondary peritonitis. The Sumerian term A.GA.ZI[102] and the Akkadian term *tugānu* were used for complaints that appear to be compatible with peptic ulcer diseases.[103] We believe that the terms are interchangeable.

6.96 DIŠ NA NU *pa-tan* SAG ŠÀ-*šu i-kaṣ-ṣa-as-su* KÚM ŠÀ TUKU.MEŠ *ina ge-ši-šu* ZÉ *i-ár-rù* NA.BI *pa-šit-tu tu-ga-na* GIG *ana* TI-*šú* . . . (*BAM* 578 ii 20–21)[104]

**If, before he has eaten, a person's upper abdomen (epigastrium) gnaws at him, he continually has internal fever, and, when he belches, he vomits bile, that person is sick with *pašittu* (gall bladder disease; see below) (or) *tugānu*, to cure him . . .

6.97 [DIŠ] ⌜NA⌝ [SAG ŠÀ?]-*šú ú-ḫa-*[*ma-su ú-ma*]-*ḫa-su ú-za-qat-su ú* KÚ-*šú* NA.BI A.[GA.ZI G]IG *ana* TI-*šú* . . . (*BAM* 75:1–2)[105]

**[If] a person's [upper abdomen (epigastrium)?] ⌜burns⌝, [gives him a] ⌜jabbing⌝ pain, stings, and hurts him, that person is ⌜sick⌝ with A.[GA.ZI], to cure him . . .

The references below make it clear that the *āšipu* paid attention to whether the patient was eating and if the food was helpful in relieving the pain. Although, in general, food tends to relieve the pain associated with duodenal ulcers and does not relieve the pain in gastric (nonduodenal) ulcers, these findings are not always consistent, particularly if there is gastric outlet obstruction.

6.98 DIŠ NA *du-ga-nu* DIB-*su* SAG ⌜ŠÀ-*šú*⌝ *ú-ṣa-rap-šú* NU *pa-tan ú-ga-áš* NA BI KA *kar-še* GIG *ana* TI-*šú* . . . (*STT* 96:9–10)[106]

**If *tugānu* afflicts a person, his upper abdomen (epigastrium) burns him hotly, (and) he vomits without having eaten, that person (has) sick mouth of the stomach, to cure him . . .

6.99 DIŠ NA NU *pa-tan* SAG ŠÀ-*šu i-kaṣ-ṣa-as-su* KÚM ŠÀ TUKU.MEŠ *ina ge-ši-šu* ZÉ *i-ár-rù* NA.BI *pa-šit-tu tu-ga-na* GIG *ana* TI-*šú* . . . (*BAM* 578 ii 20–21)

**If, before he has eaten, a person's upper abdomen (epigastrium) gnaws at him, he continually has internal fever, and, when he belches, he vomits bile, that person is sick with *pašittu* (gall bladder disease; see below) (or) *tugānu*, to cure him . . .

6.100 DIŠ NA SAG ŠÀ-*bi-šú ú-ṣar-rap-šú ú-zaq-qat*!-*su* KÚ.MEŠ-*šú* IM [*ina* ŠÀ-*šú*] ⌜*i*⌝-*li-ib-bi ana* DÚR-*šú ú-na-kap-šú* ŠÀ.M[EŠ-*šú* MÚ].MEŠ *ma-du* NU KÚ *m*[*a*]-*du* NU NAG NA.BI KA *kar-šú* GIG *a-na* DIN-*šú* . . . (BM 42406+43507+43544:3–7 [Finkel, *Fs. Lambert* 208])[107]

**If a person's epigastrium burns him hotly, stings him, (and) continually hurts him, "wind" groans [in his stomach] (and) "butts" into his anus, his insides [are bloated] (and) he does not eat a lot or drink a lot, that person has sick mouth of the stomach, to cure him . . .

An interesting aspect of some of the texts that appear to be describing peptic ulcers are references to "sick mouth of the stomach."

6.101 DIŠ NA *du-*[*ga-nu*] ⌜*sa*⌝-«x»-*aḫ-ḫu* TUKU-*ši* NA BI [K]A *kar-še* GIG *ana* TI-[-*šú*] . . . (*STT* 96:5)[108]

**If a person has ⌜*tugānu*⌝ (with) ⌜*saḫḫu*⌝,[109] that person (has) sick ⌜mouth⌝ of the stomach, to cure him . . .

6.102 DIŠ NA *du-ga-nu* DIB-*su* SAG ⸢ŠÀ-*šú*⸣ *ú-ṣa-rap-šú* NU *pa-tan ú-ga-áš* NA BI KA *kar-še* GIG *ana* TI-*šú* . . . (*STT* 96:9–10)[110]

**If *tugānu* afflicts a person, his upper abdomen (epigastrium) burns him hotly, (and) he vomits without having eaten, that person (has) sick mouth of the stomach, to cure him . . .

6.103 DIŠ NA NINDA KÚ KAŠ NAG-*ma saḫ-ḫa* ŠUB.MEŠ *pi-qam* NU *pi-qam saḫ-ḫa ip-te-né-ru s*[*aḫ-ḫa u* M]ÚD GI$_6$ *ú-kal-lam ḫi-niq-te* KA *kar-ši u* [SAG ŠÀ?] *ú-ḫa-ma-s*[*u*] *ú-ṣa-rap-šú* GÍR.GÍR-*su u* KÚ-*šu* NA BI A.GA.ZI GIG *ana* TI-[*šú*] . . . (*BAM* 75:5–9)

**If a person eats bread (and) drinks beer and then he continually produces *saḫḫu*,[111] he incessantly vomits *saḫḫu*, he shows ⸢*saḫḫu*⸣ [and] black ⸢blood⸣, he has constriction of the mouth of the stomach, and his [upper abdomen (epigastrium)?] burns, burns hotly, stings, and hurts him, that person is sick with A.GA.ZI, to cure [him] . . .

Some of the texts only indicate that the mouth of the stomach was sick, while the last reference describes constriction. We have concluded that the "mouth" of the stomach is the gastroduodenal junction (the lower portion of the stomach that connects to the small intestine) rather than the gastroesophageal junction for the following reasons. We know from other contexts that the nipple was considered the "mouth" of the breast, the entrance to the uterus the "mouth" of the womb, and the anus the "mouth" of the buttocks.[112] If the same principle was used for the stomach, then the "mouth" of the stomach was the gastroduodenal junction. This fits very well with the pathology commonly seen in peptic ulcer disease. Ulcers, swelling, and obstruction (constriction) are commonly found in that region. In support of this possibility is the fact that, in ancient Mesopotamian enumerations of animal parts, the "mouth of the stomach" (*pî karši*) is listed after the rumen (*karšu*) and before the omasum or third stomach (*riqītu*). If, as has been argued by Moran,[113] the "mouth" refers to the lower, ruminoreticular orifice and not the upper junction with the esophagus, this animals' "mouth of the stomach" would correspond to the gastroduodenal junction in humans.[114]

Most interesting is the question of how the *āšipu* knew that the mouth of the stomach was "sick" and even "constricted." There is no way to see this region in an intact patient, and feeling the abdomen is likely to detect only upper abdominal tenderness. It seems likely to us that autopsies were performed on patients who died, possibly from a bleeding ulcer, and the *āšipu* found the ulcers and constriction near the gastroduodenal junction.

ENLARGED SPLEEN (SPLENOMEGALY)

There are a number of references in ancient Mesopotamian medical texts to an organ called the *tulīmu*, which was said to hurt or to "stand up." This is conventionally translated as "spleen" on etymological grounds, and the references are not inconsistent with disorders of that organ. It is probable that a spleen that "stands up" was enlarged and palpable when the *āšipu* examined the abdomen. Malaria, a disease that we believe to have been common in ancient Mesopotamia (see Chapter 3), often causes an enlarged spleen.

6.104 DIŠ NA *tu-lim-šú* ⸢KÚ⸣-*šú* U$_4$ *u* GI$_6$ *la i-ṣal-lal pa-gar-šú* KÚM *ú-*[*kal*] . . . (*BAM* 77:20′//*BAM* 78:1–2)

**If a person's *tulīmu* hurts him, he cannot sleep day and night (and) fever ⌜grips⌝ his body . . .

6.105 [DIŠ NA *tu-lim-šú*] ⌜KÚ⌝-*šú u* GUB.GUB-*az* . . . (*BAM* 77:28′)

**[If a person's *tulīmu*] hurts him and continually "stands up" . . .

6.106 DIŠ NA *tu-lim-šú* GUB.GUB-⌜*az*⌝ . . . (*BAM* 77:30′; cf. *BAM* 77:33′, 39′)[115]

**If a person's *tulīmu* continually "stands up" . . .

GALL BLADDER DISEASE

Whether by animal or human autopsy, *āšipus* were aware of the existence of the gall bladder. Two of the references below indicate that the gall bladder was responsible for the observed symptoms. There is no indication of how the *āšipu* reached this conclusion. Was the gall bladder enlarged or tender? In spite of this uncertainty, many of the complaints, namely, vomiting, intolerance of fatty and rich foods, bloating, and altered appetite, can be found with gall bladder stones and/or inflammation (cholecystitis). Yellow/green stools may be due to stones blocking the common bile duct (see above). Spinning (lightheadedness or vertigo) was probably secondary to vomiting and diarrhea.

Patients with gall bladder disease often have secondary infections of the gall bladder and the biliary tree. This condition, ascending cholangitis, usually is accompanied by fever, and may have associated reactive arthritis (see Chapter 11). The last reference below, which mentions fever and joint pains, may be a case of ascending cholangitis.

6.107 DIŠ NA SAG ŠÀ-*šú* KÚ-*šú ina ge-ši-šu* ZÉ *im-ta-na-ʾ* NA BI *qer-be-na* GIG SUM^{SAR} GA.RAS^{SAR} UZU GU$_4$ UZU ŠAḪ KAŠ LÚ.KÚRUN.NA NU *uš-ta-maḫ-ḫar ana* TI-*šú* . . . (*BAM* 578 i 1–2)

**If a person's upper abdomen (epigastrium) hurts him and when he belches, he continually produces bile, that person has *qerbēnu* GIG ("sick insides"). He is continually unable to keep down garlic, leeks, beef, pork, or *kurunnu*-beer; to cure him . . .

6.108 DIŠ NA NINDA KÚ KAŠ NAG-*ma ú-nap-paq u* IGI.MEŠ-*šú* NIGIN.MEŠ-*du* NA BI GIG ZÉ GIG *ana* TI-*šú* . . . (*BAM* 578 i 38//*BAM* 159 i 29–30//*BAM* 60:7′–8′)[116]

**If a person eats bread and drinks beer and then chokes and his face seems to be spinning, that person is sick with a sickness of the gall bladder, to cure him . . .

6.109 DIŠ NA NU *pa-tan* ŠÀ-*šú ana pa-re-e e-te-né-la-a* ÚḪ *ma-gal* ŠUB.MEŠ A.MEŠ *ina* KA-*šú mál-da-riš* DU-*ku pa-nu-šú iṣ-ṣa-nu-du* ŠÀ.MEŠ-*šú* MÚ.MÚ-*ḫu* MURUB$_4$^{II}-*šú kin-ṣa-šú* TAG.GA.MEŠ-*šú* KÚM ŠED$_7$ IR TUKU.MEŠ-*ši* NINDA *u* KAŠ LAL A ŠED$_7$ *ma-gal* NAG *i-par-ru ina* DÚR-*šú* GÌŠ-*šú* SIG$_7$ *ú-tab-ba-kam* MÙŠ.MEŠ-*šú i-te-nen-nu-u* UZU.MEŠ-*šu tab-ku mìm-ma* KÚ-*ma* UGU-*šú ul* DÙG.GA NA BI ZÉ *saḫ-pa-su ana* TI-*šú* . . . (*BAM* 578 i 27–30)[117]

**If a person, (despite) not having eaten, his stomach continually rises up to vomit, he continually produces a lot of phlegm, liquid continuously flows from his mouth, his face continually (feels like it) is spinning, his insides are continually bloated, his hips (and) his shins continually hurt him intensely, he is hot and then cold, he continually has sweat, his appetite for bread and beer is diminished, he drinks a great deal of cold water (and then) vomits, he pours yellow/green (matter) from his anus (and) his penis, his appearance continually changes (for the worse), his flesh is tense,[118] (and) whatever he eats does not agree with him, the gall bladder has turned over on that person, to cure him . . .

The Akkadian term for cholecystitis appears to have been *pašittu. Pašittu* is lexically equated with bile, and the Sumerogram (ZÚ.MUŠ.Ì.KÚ.E) indicates an associated severe pain.[119] In the following reference, *pašittu* is given as an alternative diagnosis to *tugānu* (peptic ulcer; see above), which is still included in the differential diagnosis for chronic cholecystitis.

6.110 DIŠ NA NU *pa-tan* SAG ŠÀ-*šu i-kaṣ-ṣa-as-su* KÚM ŠÀ TUKU.MEŠ *ina ge-ši-šu* ZÉ *i-ár-rù* NA BI *pa-šit-tu tu-ga-na* GIG *ana* TI-*šú* . . . (*BAM* 578 ii 20–21)[120]

**If, before he has eaten, a person's upper abdomen (epigastrium) gnaws at him, he continually has internal fever, and, when he belches, he vomits bile, that person is sick with *pašittu* (or) *tugānu*, to cure him . . .

In a picturesque recitation, the illness threatens the patient with intolerance of rich foods and flatulence.

6.111 *mar-tu mar-tu mar-tu* ⌜*pa-šit*⌝-[*tu-ma*] *mar-tu* GIN$_7$ KI.SAG.SAL^{MUŠEN} SIG$_7$ *it-ta-na-al-lak*⌜*a-lak*?-[*ta*] *it-ta-na-za-az ina gi-šal-li ša* BÀD *i-da-gal a-ki-lum ak-li i-da-gal šá-tu-ú ku-ru-un-ni ki-i tak-ka-la ak-la ki-i ta-ša-ta-a ku-ru-un-ni a-ma-qú-tak-ku-nu-šim-ma tu-ga-ša-a ki-i* GU$_4$ TU$_6$ ÉN (*BAM* 578 ii 39–44)[121]

**Bile, bile, bile, ⌜*pašittu*⌝. Bile goes about in the form of a yellow heron standing on the parapet of a wall. He sees the one who eats bread; he sees the one who drinks *kurunnu*-beer, (saying) "When you eat bread, when you drink *kurunnu*-beer, I will fall upon you and you will belch like a bull!"—healing spell.

In the reference below, the patient with *pašittu* has severe vomiting and diarrhea accompanied by fever. Vomiting bile is not necessarily a sign of gall bladder disease since this can occur in other conditions. The presence of fever suggests either a primary infectious cause or a secondary infection such as may occur in cholecystitis.

6.112 *ina* UGU *mar-ti šá* LUGAL *be-lí iš-pur-an-ni ma-a iq-ṭi-a pa-šu-ut-tu*! *ši-i ka-ṣir-tú iq-ṭi-a mar-tu ana šap-liš it-tu-šib* GAR-*šú an-nu-ú la de-iq šá a-na e-liš a-na šap-liš ú-še-šir-u-ni* 2 U$_4$.MEŠ *zu-ú-tú ik-tar-ra* DI-*mu šu-ú* (*ABL* 363 obv. 8-r. 8 [S. Parpola, *SAA* 10 no. 217])

**As for the bile that the king my lord wrote me about, saying "It came up." It is *pašittu*. The thick sputum came up; the gall settled down below (see above). This is not a good sign that he has been sending (the food) straight through (both) upward (and) downward. (However), he produced sweat for (only) two days. That is good.[122]

The text below refers to gall bladder disease and teeth oozing blood. It is possible that the gall bladder disease has caused chronic biliary tree obstruction. This is known to lead to vitamin K deficiency and subsequent bleeding, including bleeding from the gums. The reason for the patient's difficulty in opening his mouth is unclear. The *āšipu*'s apparent association of gall bladder disease and bleeding gums suggest a sophisticated level of observation and interpretation.

6.113 DIŠ NA GABA-*su u šá-šal-la-šú* KÚM.MEŠ ZÚ.MEŠ-*šú i-ḫi-la e-piš* KA-*šú* DUGUD NA BI ZÉ GIG *ana* TI-*šú* . . . (*BAM* 578 i 50//*BAM* 159 i 38–39)[123]

**If a person's breast and back are warm and his teeth ooze blood and opening his mouth is difficult, that person (has) gall bladder disease, to cure him . . .

LIVER DISEASE

Liver disease (TÙN.GIG)[124] was recognized by ancient physicians.[125] They were also alert to the importance of jaundice, of which they distinguished several types, mentioned together with treatments for the condition. When the term *aḫḫāzu*: "gall" is used, it appears to mean simply "jaundice," whereas *amurriqānu* appears to mean "jaundice and bloating or wasting" (see below). As Haussperger points out,[126] in the recent past, modern physicians also used a clinical finding to categorize subtypes of liver disease. This was not, however, the presence or absence of wasting as used by the *āšipu*, but the presence or absence of pain and colic. Pain and colic are characteristic of gall stone obstruction of the biliary tree, but not of hepatitis or cirrhosis.[127]

6.114 *mar-ḫa-ṣu* ⸢*an*⸣-[*n*]*u*-[*u*] *ana aḫ-ḫa-zi u a-mur-ri-q*[*a-ni*] *da-mi-iq lat-ku* (*BAM* 186: 10–12)[128]

**⸢This⸣ lower-body bath is good for *aḫḫāzu* or ⸢*amurriqānu*⸣; tested.

6.115 Ú.ḪI.A *mar-rat ša* SIG$_7$ *aḫ-ḫa-za u* ZÉ^{II} SIG$_5$ . . . (*BAM* 52:96)

**Plants, bitters good for *amurriqānu*, *aḫḫāzu*, and "gall" . . .

Of these types of jaundice one, *aḫḫāzu*, was clearly associated with the liver. The bleeding that is associated with liver disease occurs in advanced liver injury when the clotting factors normally produced by the liver are no longer available in adequate quantities. If scarring (cirrhosis) involves the liver, bleeding could be secondary to esophageal varices (see below).

6.116 DIŠ NA TÙN.GIG TÙN ŠÀ-*šú* BAL-*ma* IGI^{II}-*šú aḫ-ḫa-za* ⸢DIRI⸣ MÚD *ina* KA-*šú ina pi-qí* NU [*pi-q*]*í* DU-*ku ana* TI-*šú* . . . (*BAM* 92 iii 10–13)[129]

**If a person (has) TÙN.GIG ("sick liver" and) his liver[130] (feels like it is) turning over, his eyes are full of *aḫḫāzu*-jaundice, (and) blood ⸢incessantly⸣ comes to his mouth, to cure him . . .

Jaundice is due to elevated levels of bilirubin (a byproduct of broken-down hemoglobin) which can occur with liver injury or obstruction of the common bile duct usually with gall stones. This yellow color is most easily recognized in fair-skinned individuals. In heavily pigmented individuals, modern physicians know that jaundice can most readily be identified by examining the "whites" of the eyes and the base of the tongue. From the reference below, it is clear that ancient Mesopotamian physicians knew this as well.

6.117 DIŠ IGI.MEŠ-*šú* SIG_7.MEŠ ŠÀ IGI^{II}-*šú* SIG_7.MEŠ SUḪUŠ EME GI_6 *aḫ-ḫa-zu* (DPS IX A 13//B obv. 12 = *TDP* 72:13; cf. DPS XXXIII:93 [AOAT 43.357])[131]

**If his face is yellow and the inner part of his eyes is yellow, (and) the base of the tongue is dark, *aḫḫāzu*.

6.118 DIŠ NA *aḫ-ḫa-zu* IGI^{II}-*šú* E_{11}*-a-ma* IGI^{II}-*šú* GU.MEŠ SIG_7.MEŠ [*u*]*d-du-ḫa* ŠÀ.MEŠ-*šú na-šu-ú* NINDA *u* KAŠ *ú-tar-ra* NA BI *ú-za-bal-ma* ⌜BA.ÚŠ⌝ (*BAM* 578 iv 43–44)

**If *aḫḫāzu* rises to a person's eyes so that his eyes are ⌜covered⌝ with a network of yellow threads, his insides are puffed up (and) return bread and beer (to his mouth), (if) that person lingers, he will die.

Bloating is likely to be due to fluid filling the abdominal cavity (ascites), a condition that occurs when the liver becomes scarred (cirrhosis—see below). The wasting that was noted in patients with *amurriqānu*-jaundice might best be explained by two diseases. Patients with advanced chronic liver disease such as cirrhosis (due to alcohol or hepatitis) frequently have both jaundice and marked wasting. Not infrequently, cirrhotic patients appear to have obese abdomens because of the fluid retention (ascites), while the rest of their bodies show marked muscle and soft tissue loss. The second condition that may show this combination of signs is cancer that involves and destroys most of the normal liver tissue.

6.119 DIŠ NA *lu* ZÉ *lu aḫ-ḫa-zu lu a-mur-ri-qa-nu* GIG *ana* TI-*šú* . . . (*BAM* 188:1–2)[132]

**If a person is sick either with "gall" or *aḫḫazu* or *amurriqānu*, to cure him . . .

6.120 DIŠ NA SU-*šu* SIG_7 *pa-nu-šú* SIG_7 *ši-ḫat* UZU TUKU*-a a-mur-ri-qa-nu* MU.NI (*BAM* 578 iii 7)

**If a person's body is yellow,[133] his face is yellow, (and) he has wasting of the flesh, it is called *amurriqānu*.

6.121 [DIŠ SU-*šu* S]IG_7 IGI^{II}-*šú* SIG_7.MEŠ *šiḫ-ḫat* UZU TUKU.MEŠ *a-mur-ri-qa-nu* (DPS XVIII:24 [AOAT 43.219]; cf. DPS XXXIII:92 [AOAT 43.357])[134]

**[If a person's body] ⌜is yellow⌝, his eyes are yellow, (and) he has wasting of the flesh, *amurriqānu*.

6.122 DIŠ NA IGI.[S]IG_7.SIG_7 GIG*-ma* GIG*-su ana* ŠÀ IGI^{II}-*šú* E_{11}*-a* ŠÀ IGI.MEŠ-*šú* GU.MEŠ SIG_7.MEŠ *ud-du-ḫu* ŠÀ.MEŠ-*š*[*ú n*]*a-šu-u* NINDA *u* KAŠ *ú-tar-ra* NA BI IM DÙ.A.BI GIG *ú-za-bal-ma* BA.ÚŠ (*BAM* 578 iii 4–5)[135]

**If a person is sick with *amurriqānu* and his illness rises to his eyes, the inside of his eyes is covered with a network of yellow threads, ⌜his⌝ insides are ⌜puffed⌝ up (and) return bread and beer (to his mouth), (and) that person is sick with any sort of "wind," (if) he lingers, he will die.

The uneven yellow color or yellow spots in the following references are probably not due to jaundice, since jaundice tends to be evenly distributed. The yellow color may be caused by subcutaneous bleeding (ecchymosis), which is initially red or purple but eventually fades to a yellow color.[136] This sort of bleeding can be secondary to liver disease, but other bleeding problems can be the cause. Suggestive of liver disease are the eyes "full of blood" or "unevenly colored with red," a condition probably caused by inadequate levels of clotting factors.

6.123 DIŠ U_4.5.KÁM GIG-*ma* UZU.MEŠ-*šu* SIG_7 ŠUB-*ú* IGI^{II}-*šú* MÚD DIRI.MEŠ GAM (DPS XVI:47′ [AOAT 43.176])[137]

**If he has been sick for five days and his flesh is unevenly colored with yellow (and) his eyes are full of blood, he will die.

6.124 DIŠ KI.MIN-*ma* UZU.MEŠ-*šú ur-qá it-ta-du-ni* IGI^{II}-*šú* SA_5 ŠUB.MEŠ NU DIN (DPS XVI:86′ [AOAT 43.179])

**If (he has been sick for a long time) and his flesh is unevenly colored with yellow (and) his eyes are unevenly colored with red, he will not get well.[138]

6.125 [DIŠ . . . S]IG_7 DIRI IGI^{II}-*šú* MÚD DIRI.MEŠ NINDA *šá* KÚ *ina* ŠÀ-*šú* NU *ina-aḫ is-ḫur-ma* DUB-*ka* GAM (DPS XVIII:42′ [AOAT 43.219])[139]

**[If his flesh?] is full of ⸢yellow⸣ (spots),[140] his eyes are full of blood, the bread that he eats does not rest easy in his stomach but it turns about and pours (it) out, he will die.

INFECTIOUS CAUSES OF JAUNDICE

The following references describe jaundice along with other signs and symptoms that suggest infectious etiologies.[141]

HEPATITIS The reference below mentions both yellow eyes and right-sided abdominal pain. The pain is likely to be due to the rapid enlargement of the liver, causing stretching of the liver capsule, and by this means causing pain (see Liver Pain, below).

6.126 DIŠ *ina* ŠÀ-*šú* Á 150-*šú* ^{GIŠ}GIDRU GAR-*su-ma* IGI^{II}-*šú* GU.MEŠ SIG_7.MEŠ DIRI.MEŠ ŠU ^{d}15 GAM (DPS XIII B ii 29–30 = *TDP* 120 ii 29–30)[142]

**If a burning pain[143] is firmly established in his abdomen on the right side and his eyes are full of yellow threads, "hand" of Ištar; he will die.

HEPATITIS A The etiology of the disease described in the following reference is likely to be hepatitis given the jaundice and fever. Since hepatitis A is spread by ingesting the virus in food or water, and the quote suggests that food contamination was involved, we favor hepatitis A as the cause.

6.127 DIŠ *ina taš-rit* GIG-*šú* KÚM ÚḪ NINDA KAŠ GURUN *ma-da* KÚ *ina* ŠÀ-*šú* NU ḪUN DUB-*ka* U-*šú* LAL-*aṣ* IGI^{II}-*šú* BAD.BAD-*te ana* ⸢AKKIL⸣ *i-qal* NÍ-*šú ú-dam-ma-aq* ZI.IR.MEŠ *u* IGI^{II}-*šú i-ta-nar-ri-qu* MAŠKIM SÌG-*su* TA TAG-*ma* KI-*šú* [K]EŠDA *ina* NINDA *ik-ka-lu* KÚ *ina* A NAG-*ú* NAG NA BI *ana* U_4.5.KÁM : *ana* U_4.7.KÁM DIN (DPS XVII:10–13 [AOAT 43.195/196])

**If at the beginning of his illness he burns with fever,[144] he eats a lot of bread, beer, and fruit (but) it does not rest easy in his stomach (and) he pours it out, he can straighten out his finger,[145] he continually opens his eyes, at a mournful cry, he is silent,[146] he treats himself well, (his stomach) is continually upset, and his eyes continually turn yellow, a *rābiṣu* has struck him (and) after it touched him, it was ⸢bound⸣ with him (or) he ate it with the bread he ate (or) drank it with the water he drank; (if he is sick) for five (var. seven) days, he will get well.

HEPATITIS B Since arthritis and skin lesions are commonly seen in hepatitis B, we believe that references below are describing that disease. It is well documented that the hepatitis B virus may be spread between sexual partners and by exposure to infected blood. For a possible reference to venereally transmitted hepatitis B,[147] see 4.35.

6.128 [DIŠ N]A TÙN.GIG *bur-ka-šu* TÙN ŠÀ-*šú*- «*šú*» [U]ZU.SA.SAL^{II}-*šú* KÚ-*šú* . . . (*BAM* 92 iii 38′–39′)[148]

**[If] a ⸢person⸣ (has) TÙN.GIG ("sick liver" and) his knees, his liver,[149] (and) his back hurt him . . .

6.129 DIŠ NA [TÙN] ŠÀ-*šú* DIB-*s*[*u* . . .] *di-kiš* ŠÀ GIG ŠÀ-*šú* KÚ-*šú* ŠÀ-*šú ru-uq-šú* ŠÀ-*šú i-sa-bu-u*ʾ DÙ UZU.MEŠ-*šú tab-ku ni-kim-tú* ŠÀ-*bi* TUKU-*ši na-aš-pa-ak bir-ki u a-ḫi* GIG NA BI TÙN.GIG *ana* TI-*šú* . . . (*BAM* 87:1–5)

**If a person's ⸢liver⸣[150] afflicts ⸢him⸣ [. . .] he is sick with a needling pain in the abdomen, his abdomen hurts him, his heart is distant from him, his stomach churns, all of his flesh is tense,[151] he has bloated stomach, (and) he is sick with tenseness[152] in the arms and legs, that person (has) TÙN.GIG ("sick liver"), to cure him . . .

RELAPSING FEVER AND LEPTOSPIROSIS Relapsing fever and leptospirosis, relapsing or biphasic febrile illnesses (see Chapter 3), are caused by spirochetes. These diseases have frequent liver involvement with jaundice (*aḫḫāzu*). The texts listed below may be describing patients with one of these diseases.

6.130 [DIŠ *i-na*] SAG.DU-*šú* KÚM *ṣa-ri-iḫ* U[$_4$.1.KÁM TAK$_4$-*šum-ma* U$_4$.2.KÁM] DUGUD-*su i-re-<eḫ-ḫi>-šu-ma* KI.TA [GÌR^{II}-*šú* ŠED$_7$ *ina* BAR-*šú*] ŠU^{II}-*šú u* GÌR^{II}-*šú* KÚM-*ma* GIN$_7$ DIB-*it* GI[DIM ^{d}DÌM.ME.LAGAB] (*KAR* 211 obv. 4–6 [restored from DPS III C r. 10–11//E$_1$ r. 11–12+E$_2$ r. 7–8 = *TDP* 26:70–71])

**[If in] his head he burns with fever [(and) over the course of a day it leaves him and then (later)] it overpowers him (and) flows over him [for two days] and the bottom (plantar) surfaces[153] of [his feet (feel) cold, (and) when (the fever) releases him], his hands and feet are hot as in affliction by a ⸢ghost⸣, [*aḫḫāzu*].

6.131 DIŠ U$_4$.1.KÁM TAG$_4$-*šú-ma* U$_4$.1.KÁM LÁ-*šú* NÍG.KÚ ^{d}DÌM.ME.LAGAB ŠU DINGIR.GAL.MEŠ GAM (DPS XVI:12 [AOAT 43.173])

**If over the course of a day it leaves him and then later (febrile seizures) come over him for one day, "eating" of *aḫḫāzu*; "hand" of the great gods, he will die.

6.132 DIŠ U$_4$.4.KÁM U$_4$.5.KÁM GIG-*ma* IR ŠUB.ŠUB-*su* DU$_8$-*ár* GIG / DIŠ U$_4$.4.KÁM U$_4$.5.KÁM GIG-*aṣ* ŠU DÌM.ME.LAGAB (DPS XVI:44′–45′ [AOAT 43.176])

**If he is sick for four or five days and subsequently sweat continually falls upon him, letting up of the illness. If he has been sick for four or five days, "hand" of *aḫḫāzu.*

WINTER LIVER PROBLEMS

6.133 Ú TÙN.MEŠ *šá* EN.TE.NA . . . (*BAM* 161 vii 18–19)

**Plant for the liver[154] for the cold season . . .

6.134 [. . .] *ina* DÚR-*šú* [. . .] x *pa-nu-š*[*u* . . .] SIG_7 NA BI TÙ[N.GIG *š*]*a* EN.TE.NA . . . (*BAM* 92 i 1′–4′)

**[If . . .] from his anus [. . .] ⌜his⌝ face [and . . . are] yellow, that person (has) winter TÙ[N.GIG] ("sick liver") . . .

We are unable to identify with certainty an infectious liver disease that has a predominantly winter incidence. One possible, but somewhat remote, explanation is that the liver disease is secondary to pneumonia, a condition that has a winter predominance. Bacteria or viruses might spread from the lungs to the liver. However, it is surprising that in the "winter liver" references quoted above, the *āšipu* would not have observed or described signs or symptoms related to the lungs, as in the following reference.

6.135 [. . .] ⌜ḪAR⌝.MEŠ GIG-*ma* GIG-*su ana* TÙN-*šu* x [. . .] (*AMT* 55/4:9′)

**[If . . .] (he has) "sick lungs" and his illness [spreads?] to his liver[155] [. . .]

Another possibility for "winter liver" might be Q fever (*Coxiella burnetii*). This is a rickettsial infection of sheep that can be spread through the air or by drinking infected milk. It can affect many organs in humans but especially the lungs and liver. This disease might have had a predominantly winter incidence in ancient Mesopotamia, though it does not in modern times. Sheep-herding nomadic pastoralists regularly wintered in the ancient Mesopotamian flood plain, spending the summer in the Zagros mountains. This meant that meat and milk from sheep were more readily available in the winter. Cooking would have prevented sheep meat from spreading the disease, but unpasteurized milk would have been a likely source of infection.

Whatever the actual cause or causes of "winter liver," these texts further illustrate the fact that the ancient Mesopotamian physicians were attempting to make associations and connections that could ultimately be helpful in understanding, diagnosing, and treating disease.

JAUNDICE IN THE ELDERLY

The cause of the hepatitis in the following quote is unclear, but the description suggests that advanced age was a risk factor for a fatal outcome. This is certainly true in the current era.

6.136 DIŠ KI.MIN IGI^{II}.MEŠ-*šú* GIN_7 *si-ka-a-ti ana* $GA.RAŠ^{SAR}$ SIG_7.ME GAM (DPS XVI:91′ [AOAT 43.180])

**If (he is in his seventies and) his eyes are as yellow as the "peg"[156] on a leek, he will die.

LIVER PAIN

In the reference below, the *āšipu* made the association between vigorous movement and the development of abdominal and specifically liver pain. It is likely that the patient had an underlying liver abnormality such as enlargement due to hepatitis, congestive heart failure, or liver abscess (see above). In congestive heart failure, because of a weak heart, blood backs up and causes swelling of the liver. Stretching of the liver capsule by acute liver enlargement due to any cause can produce pain, and movement certainly has the potential of aggravating this problem.

6.137 [DIŠ NA] *di-kiš* ^{GIŠ}GIGIR GIG-*ma* ŠÀ-*šú u* TÙN-*šú* KÚ.MEŠ-*šú* . . . (*AMT* 96/1:17, cf. 20)[157]

**[If a person] is sick with needling pain after (riding in) a chariot and his abdomen and liver[158] continually hurt him . . .

LIVER FAILURE

Liver failure can occur secondary to severe hepatitis, cirrhosis (see below), or liver poisons (hepatotoxins). In the absence of liver transplantation technology, patients with liver failure would be almost certain to die with bleeding problems, altered mental status (hepatic encephalopathy), and generalized body swelling (anasarca). The following quotes are likely to be descriptions of patients with hepatic failure.

6.138 DIŠ IGI.MEŠ-*šú* KÚR.KÚR-*ru* EME-*šú* SIG$_7$: SU-*šú* SIG$_7$ TÙN.GIG *ana* U$_4$.3.KÁM GAM (DPS IX A 31 = *TDP* 74:31)[159]

**If his face continually alters (and) his tongue is yellow (var. his body is yellow), TÙN.GIG ("sick liver");[160] (if he has been sick) for three days, he will die.

6.139 DIŠ NA *aḫ-ḫa-zu* GIG SAG.DU-*su pa-nu-šu* SU-*šú ka-la-šú ù* SUḪUŠ E [ME-*šú ṣa-bit*] *ana* GIG *šu-a-tu* ^{LÚ}A.ZU ŠU-*su* NU *ub-bal* NA BI ÚŠ NU [TI.LA] (*BAM* 578 iv 45–46)

**If a person is sick with *aḫḫāzu* (jaundice without wasting) and his head, his face, his whole body, and the base of his ⌜tongue⌝ [are affected], the *asû* (pharmacist) is not to lay his hands on that patient (to treat him); that person will die; he will not [live].

6.140 DIŠ ⌜KA⌝-[*šú*] ⌜KÚR⌝.KÚ[R-*ir u*] SIG$_7$.MEŠ *i-ár-ru u* UZU.MEŠ-*šú* SIG$_7$.MEŠ *ana* U$_4$.3.K[ÁM . . .] (DPS VII B r. 5 = *TDP* 64:61′)

**If [his] words are ⌜unintelligible⌝ [and] he vomits yellow stuff and his flesh is yellow (and he has been sick) for three days [. . .].

6.141 DIŠ KA-*šú* KÚR.[KÚR-*i*]*r* MÚD *ina* KA-*šú* ŠUB.ŠUB-*a u* ŠÀ.MEŠ-*šú* ÍL-*ú ana* U$_4$.10.[KÁM . . .] (DPS VII B r. 10 = *TDP* 66:66′)[161]

**If his words are ⌜unintelligible⌝, he continually produces blood from his mouth, his insides are puffed up, (and he has been sick) for ten days [. . .].

A common sign of advanced liver failure is "liver flap" (asterixis). This is best demonstrated by asking the patient to raise his hand up at the wrist and hold this position for a minute or two. A patient with liver failure is often unable to hold this position and will intermittently jerk his hand downward as if waving good-bye. It appears likely that the patient in the text below has liver failure and the "shuddering" described represents liver flap.

6.142 [DIŠ NA] TÙN-*šú* TAG.TAG-*su* [. . .] x-*šú* [NINDA] *u* KAŠ LAL [. . .] x-nam-mu *pi-qam la pi-qam i-par-ru-ud* [ŠÀ-*šú*] *i-sa-bu-u*ʾ ŠÀ-*šú* [. . .] *pit-ru-šú* DÙ-*šú-nu* [. . .]-*šú* NA BI TÙN.GI [G GIG ŠU N]AM.ÉRIM KUR-*su* . . . (*BAM* 87:14–17)

**[If a person]'s liver[162] continually hurts him intensely, [. . .] he loses his appetite for [bread] and beer, [. . .] he shudders incessantly,[163] [his stomach] churns, (and) his entire abdomen(?) [. . .] him, that person [is sick] with ⌜"sick liver"⌝; ["hand"] of ⌜curse⌝ has "gotten" him . . .

The following reference indicates that the patient's face has a variable color. It seems likely that this is the facial pigmentation (chloasma) that can be seen in pregnancy (see Chapter 12) as well as in patients with chronic liver failure.

6.143 DIŠ U_4.4.KÁM GIG-*ma* ŠU^{II}-*šú ina* ŠÀ-*šú* GAR.GAR-*an* IGI.MEŠ-*šú* SIG_7 ŠUB-*ú* GAM (DPS XVI:43′ [AOAT 43.176])

**If he has been sick for four days and his hands are continually placed on his abdomen (and) his face is unevenly colored with (tannish) yellow,[164] he will die.

Also similar to pregnancy, when the abdomen is distended with fluid in a patient with cirrhosis and liver failure (see below), stretch marks (stria) may develop that can become pigmented. The texts below appear to be describing this condition.

6.144 DIŠ ŠÀ.MEŠ-*šú nap-ḫu-ma* SA.MEŠ ŠÀ-*šú šu-ud-du-du* SIG_7 ŠUB-*ú* KÚM *mit-ḫar ana mál-[da-riš]* GUR-*šum-ma* GAM (DPS XIII B ii 47–48//G_2 38+G_1 21 = *TDP* 120 ii 47–48)

**If his insides are bloated and the muscles of his abdomen are stretched taut (and) unevenly colored with (tannish) yellow[165] (and) his temperature is normal, (if) it keeps coming back, he will die.

6.145 DIŠ KI.MIN SU-*šú* GIN_7 KI.MIN SIG_7 ŠÀ.MEŠ-*šú nap-ḫu* SA ŠÀ-*šú* SIG_7 GIL.ME GAM (DPS XVI:92′ [AOAT 43.180])

**If (he is in his seventies[166]) and his body is as yellow as (the "peg" on a leek), his insides are bloated, (and tannish) yellow crosses the muscles of his abdomen, he will die.

The following contrasting references (see Preface) appear to be describing another type of skin color change that is often seen in chronic liver failure of almost any cause. Patients with this condition often have very red palms (palmar erythema) as in the first reference below. Patients with acute-onset jaundice from acute hepatitis, liver poisoning, or bile duct obstruction, by contrast, are likely to have palms the same color as the rest of the skin surface, as in the second reference below.

6.146 DIŠ ŠU^{II}-*šú* SA_5.MEŠ *u* UZU.MEŠ-*šú* S[IG_7 . . .] (DPS XI B 9 = *SpTU* 1.34:9)

**If his hands are red and his flesh is ⌜yellow⌝ [. . .].

6.147 DIŠ ŠU^{II}-*šú* SIG$_7$.MEŠ *u* UZU.MEŠ-*šú* SIG$_7$.MEŠ [. . .] (DPS XI A obv. 11//B 10 = *TDP* 90:11//*SpTU* 1.34:10)

**If his hands are yellow and his flesh is yellow [. . .].

The exact diagnosis of the following set of references is much less certain, but they may also be describing liver failure ending in death. Fincke's[167] suggestion of Parkinson's disease seems less likely, since the patient dies.[168] An interesting third alternative is Wilson's disease, which combines the neurologic symptoms of Parkinson's with hepatic insufficiency and which can terminate in liver failure and death. Wilson's disease is a rare abnormality of copper metabolism, but other equally rare conditions ending in fatality are described in the diagnostic and prognostic handbook.

6.148 DIŠ IGI.MEŠ-*šú* IM.GÁ.LI ŠUB-*ú* NUNDUN.MEŠ-*šú ši-ši-tú* DIRI.MEŠ IGI^{II}-*šú* SIG$_7$ ŠUB.ŠUB⌜-*a*⌝ *u* IGI-*šú šá* 15 *i-ṣa-par* GAM (DPS IX A 29//B obv. 27–28 = *TDP* 74:29)

**If his face is unevenly colored with *kalû*-clay yellow, his lips are full of glaze,[169] his eyes are continually colored with yellow, (and) his left eye flutters, he will die.

6.149 DIŠ IGI.MEŠ-*šú* BABBAR *u* SIG$_7$ ŠUB.ŠUB-*ú* KA-*šú* NUNDUN.ME-*šú ši-ši-tu* IGI-*šú šá* 150 *i-ṣap-par* GAM (DPS IX A 8–9 = *TDP* 72:8–9)

**If his face is unevenly colored with white and yellow, his mouth (and) his lips (have) a glaze, (and) his right eye flutters, he will die.

The fluttering eye could be associated with hepatic encephalopathy. Alternatively, the reference could be to Myerson's sign. In Parkinson's, eye blinking is lost or diminished, but blepharospasm can readily be induced by tapping the frontalis muscle. Parkinson's patients also have a tendency to seborrheic dermatitis, which could account for the yellowish spots on the face. Alternatively, the uneven (tannish) yellow color could be chloasma due to chronic liver failure (see above).

The glaze present on the patient's lips could be dried saliva or mucus that a comatose patient is unable to wipe off. Another possible cause, if there was concomitant kidney failure, is uremic frost. Patients with advanced kidney failure (see Chapter 5) have high levels of urea in their blood, which becomes deposited as a powdery white "frost" on the patient's lips and face.

Uneven yellow coloring in the eyes is probably not due to jaundice, since this typically produces a uniform yellow color. It might, however, represent the late stages of conjuntival bleeding in patients with the clotting abnormalities of liver failure. Alternatively, if this is Wilson's disease, the reference could be to a Kayser-Fleischer ring, a golden-brown or greenish-brown deposit of copper at the limbus that encircles the iris.

CIRRHOSIS

Scarring of the liver is called cirrhosis, and it can be caused by a number of diseases, most commonly by chronic and excessive alcohol intake. It can lead to liver failure, as described above, but the scarring can also cause blockage of blood flow through the liver. This causes the veins of the esophagus to dilate and to become engorged with blood and fluid to collect in the abdomen (ascites). If the esophageal veins rupture, the patient may vomit blood and die of blood loss. Swelling of other parts of the body (the face in the first text) can occur when the malfunctioning liver produces too little protein, especially albumin, causing retention of fluid within the circulatory system and tissues (edema).

6.150 DIŠ IGI.MEŠ-*šú u* ⸢ŠÀ⸣.MEŠ-*šú* MÚ.ME-*ḫu* TÙN.GIG *ana* U$_4$.3.KÁM GAM (DPS IX A 67//B r. 13 = *TDP* 78:67)[170]

**If his face and his insides are continually swollen, TÙN.GIG ("sick liver");[171] (if he has been sick) for three days, he will die.

6.151 DIŠ NA TÙN ŠÀ-*šú* DIB.DIB-*su gi-na-a* MÚD *ina* KA-*šú* DU-*ku* MÚ.MÚ-*aḫ u in-ne-sil* NA BI DÚR.GIG *ana* TI-*šú* . . . (*BAM* 159 i 21–23)

**If a person's liver[172] continually afflicts him, blood comes constantly from his mouth/nose, he is continually bloated and constipated, that person (has) DÚR.GIG, to cure him . . .

The final reference above suggests that DÚR.GIG is the underlying cause of the problem. We believe that the liver disease in this situation might be related to ulcerative colitis. To understand our reasons for considering this possibility, see DÚR.GIG below.

The following reference describes "dripping blood," which could be due to bleeding esophageal varices in cirrhosis. In advanced cirrhosis, the liver is usually small, scarred, and generally without pain. However, when a patient has acute liver toxicity due to alcohol or some other poison, this can cause an acutely enlarged and tender liver, as well as bleeding from clotting factor deficiency.

6.152 DIŠ *ina* ŠÀ-*šú* Á 150-*šú* ^{GIŠ}GIDRU GAR-*su-ma u* MÚD SUR ŠU ^{d}IM GAM (DPS XIII B ii 28//G$_2$ 26+G$_1$ 9 = *TDP* 120 ii 28)

**If a burning pain[173] is firmly established in his abdomen on the right side and he drips blood, "hand" of Adad; he will die.

The sequence of references below mentions small webs on the patient's temples, nose/mouth, abdomen, and hands. In one case, the prognosis is bad, and in another it is good. This sounds like a description of spider angiomas. These are small arteries that appear on the surface of the skin and radiate from a central point in a sunburst pattern that ranges from the size of a dime to a quarter.

The *āšipu* apparently visualized this pattern as a spider web. The origin of the modern term is uncertain, possibly also referring to a spider's web or to the legs of the spider radiating out from its body. These lesions commonly occur in end-stage liver disease such as advanced cirrhosis, in which case the prognosis would be poor. They may also be seen in pregnancy or in perfectly healthy individuals, where naturally the prognosis is good. The reason for the attribution of this phenomenon to the sun-god Šamaš is unclear, but may refer to the fact that the spider pattern also resembles a sunburst.

6.153 DIŠ *ina* SAG.KI-*šú* [. . .-*šú*] GU.MEŠ TU[R.MEŠ . . .] TI-*uṭ* / DIŠ *ina* SAG.KI-*šú* KIR$_4$-*šú* ŠÀ-*šú* GU.MEŠ TU[R.MEŠ . . .] ⸢^{d}⸣UTU / DIŠ *ina* SAG.KI-*šú u pu-ti-šú* ŠU^{II}-[*šú* . . .] x DU GAM (DPS IV A obv. 49–51//F 10–12 = *TDP* 36:49–51//*LKU* 77:10–12)

**If ⌜small⌝ webs [. . .] on his temple (and) [his . . .], he will get well. If ⌜small⌝ webs [. . .] on his temple, his nose/mouth, (and) his abdomen, ["hand" of] Šamaš. "If [small webs . . .] on his temple and his frontside, [his] hands [. . .], he will die.

ILEUS

The loss of intestinal motility (ileus) can occur in patients with abdominal cavity infection (peritonitis) and is associated with abdominal and spinal cord injuries. The following appear to describe patients with ileus.

6.154 ⌜DIŠ DÚR-*šú* GUB-*iz* GAM⌝ (DPS XIV A_2 i 19//C_2 i 9a = *TDP* 132 i 70)[174]

**If his anus stands still, he will die.

6.155 DIŠ KI.MIN-*ma ina* GÚ.SIG_4-*šú* SÌG BAD-*ir-ma* KI.GUB-*šú* NU ⌜È⌝-*a* ŠU $GIDIM_7$ *šag-ga-ši* GAM (DPS XV:46 [AOAT 43.152]; cf. DPS XII D iii 35//E iii 38–39 = *TDP* 106 iii 35)

**If (it is the first day he is sick) and he was wounded on his spine and he is stopped up so that his excrement cannot come out,[175] "hand" of a murderous ghost; he will die.

6.156 DIŠ *ina ri-biti-šú* SÌG-*iṣ-ma* DÚR-*šú* BAD.BAD-*ir* ŠU ^{d}*Nin-giz-zi-da* (DPS XIV A iii 18 = *TDP* 140 iii 52′)[176]

**If he was wounded on the side of his abdomen and consequently his anus is continually stopped up, "hand" of Ningišzida.

Signs and Symptoms Localized to the Anus

Listed below are findings reported by ancient Mesopotamian physicians that were localized to the anus.

ITCHING AND BURNING

Burning and itching in the anal region can be caused by pinworm (*miqqānu*, the roundworm, *Enterobius vermicularis*; see Chapter 3). Although small, the adult worm may be seen near the anus.

6.157 Ú DÚR *šá mi-qa-na* AL.DIB . . . (*BAM* 380:46)

**Plant for anus containing pinworm (*miqqānu*) . . .

6.158 Ú DÚR *ḫa-am-ṭí*! *mi-qa-na* DIB-*al* . . . (*BAM* 1 iii 17)

**Plant for burning sensation in an anus containing pinworm (*miqqānu*) . . .

Another cause of intense rectal itching, burning, and redness is the same superficial fungal infection that causes athlete's foot. The patient noted below might have this fungal infection as the cause of his or her itching.

6.159 Ú DÚR TAB . . . (*BAM* 1 iii 15; *BAM* 380:47)

**Plant for burning sensation in the anus . . .

6.160 Ú DÚR *šá i-ra-šu-ú* . . . (*BAM* 380:50//*BAM* 381 iv 2)[177]

**Plant for anus that is reddish . . .

ANAL SPHINCTER

The muscle (sphincter) that controls the anal opening is important in preventing stool incontinence. The references below are describing patients with either normal anal sphincter tone ("anal opening is continually constricted") or a nonfunctioning anal sphincter ("anal opening is continually open"). There are potentially fatal neurological diseases that can cause anal sphincter paralysis, and sphincter relaxation can be seen premortem in a dying patient. It is understandable, therefore, that a relaxed anal sphincter would be viewed as a sign of impending death.

6.161 DIŠ *pu-qa-a-šú it-ta-na-az-qa-pa* DIN (DPS XIV C_2 iii 17//F 5//J 5 = *TDP* 142 iii 62′)

**If his anal opening[178] is continually constricted, he will live.

6.162 DIŠ *pu-qa-a-šú it-te-né-ep-ta-a* GAM (DPS XIV C_2 iii 16//F 4//J 4 = *TDP* 142 iii 61′)

**If his anal opening is continually opened, he will die.

With trauma or inflammation of the rectum, the muscles of the anal sphincter can go into spasm. The patient may consequently experience tenesmus, or painful, protracted, straining at stool.

6.163 DIŠ NA ka x [. . .] MÚ.MÚ-*ḫu ú-na-baq qer-bé-nu* GIG *um-ṣa-tum* . . . (*BAM* 96 iii 2′–3′//*BAM* 104:42)

**If a person's [. . .] are bloated and (his anus) chokes due to *qerbēnu* GIG and *umṣātu* . . .

The reference above mentions *qerbēnu* GIG and *umṣātu*. As described earlier, *qerbēnu* GIG in this context probably means rectal bleeding. *Umṣātu* (see below) is quite likely to mean hemorrhoids. Thrombosed and bleeding hemorrhoids are a very painful condition and typically cause tenesmus or "choking" of the anus.

6.164 DIŠ NA DÚR.GIG GIG-*ma i-te-nek-ki-*[*i*]*k* IM *ina* DÚR-*šú ú-kal ú-na-paq* . . . (*AMT* 58/1+*AMT* 56/5:8)

**If a person is sick with DÚR.GIG and he continually scratches, he holds "wind" in his anus (and it) chokes . . .[179]

6.165 [DIŠ NA DÚR].GIG GIG-*ma e-sil ù ú-nap-paq* i-x [. . .] (*AMT* 43/5:13)

** [If a person] is sick with [DÚR].GIG and he is constipated and (his anus) chokes [. . .]

6.166 DIŠ NA DÚR.GIG GIG MÚD *i-te-ez-zi qé-reb* DÚR-*šú ú-ḫa-áš ana* [TI-*šú*] . . . (*BAM* 99:25//*BAM* 95:27)[180]

**If a person is sick with DÚR.GIG and he excretes blood and within his anus he trembles . . .

The three references above are to a condition called DÚR.GIG. An analysis of all the DÚR.GIG texts is found later in this chapter, where we conclude that this diagnosis probably covered a number of diseases including hemorrhoids and ulcerative colitis that may produce rectal inflammation, bleeding, and severe rectal pain. Tenesmus is also a common complaint in patients with ulcerative colitis involving the rectum, since rectal pain often is associated with sphincter spasm. In two of the references, the anus is said to "choke" and in the third to "tremble," probably a reference to a fluctuation in the level of sphincter spasm.

Modern physicians normally examine for rectal pathology by inserting a finger into the rectum to evaluate for bleeding, tenderness, sphincter tone, and abnormal masses. Since rectal sphincter spasm and "trembling" would not be readily visible, it appears likely that the *āšipu* performed a rectal exam with his finger in order to make this observation as well as to look for blood.

RECTAL PROLAPSE

Protrusion of rectal tissue through the anus is called rectal prolapse. It occurs more frequently with advanced age and following traumatic injury. In children, it can occur as a complication of pinworm infestation. A further possibility is that the sphincter and rectal walls have been weakened by receptive anal intercourse.

6.167 DIŠ NA *mi-qit ir-ri* TUKU . . . (*AMT* 61/5:7//*AMT* 62/1 i 2)

**If a person has a rectal prolapse[181] . . .

6.168 DIŠ LÚ.TUR *šá* SAL NU ZU *mi-qit ir-ri* TUKU . . . (*AMT* 61/5:12//*AMT* 62/1 i 7)

**If a virgin boy has a rectal prolapse . . .[182]

HEMORRHOIDS

Other conditions affecting the rectum were *baṣkiltu*, *uršu*, and *umṣātu* lesions. All three could be easily seen by the *āšipu* protruding from the anus. The latter two terms were often used together, and were associated with rectal bleeding, constipation, tenesmus, and anal obstruction (see below). It seems very probable that all of these terms mean "hemorrhoids."

UMṢĀTU

6.169 DIŠ KI.MIN *šum-ma* DÚR-*šú il-ta-p*[*a-a*]*t* . . . (*BAM* 96 iii 6′//*AMT* 53/1 iv 4)[183]

**If (a person's anus chokes due to an *umṣātu*-lesion and) if it ⌜touches⌝ his anus . . .

6.170 DIŠ NA DÚR-*šú um-ṣa-*⌜*ti*⌝ [DIRI] KÁ-*šú* BAD-*ḫi ana um-ṣa-t*[*i*] *qut-tu-pi* . . . (*STT* 97 iii 19)[184]

**If a person's anus [is full of] *umṣātu*-lesions (and) his (anal) opening is closed off, to remove the *umṣātu*-lesions . . .

6.171 *ana* NA *ur-še* GAZ.MEŠ-*e um-ṣa-a-ti qut-tu-pi* KÁ MUD-*šú mu-uṣ-*[*ṣ*]*i-i* . . . (*BAM* 95:12//*STT* 97 iii 10)[185]

**If (you want) to annihilate *uršus*, remove *umṣātu*-lesions (and) ⌜widen⌝ his anal opening . . .

Umṣātu was also used in association with nosebleeds.

6.172 DIŠ NA *na-ḫi-ri-šú um-ṣa-at ḫi-li it-tab-ši* . . . (*SpTU* 1.44:34)

**If there is an exuding *umṣātu*-lesion in a person's nostrils . . .

Since nasal turbinates could be easily seen by the *āšipu*, he might have thought them to be analogous to hemorrhoids when they enlarge and bleed.

BAṢKILTU Since the term *baṣkiltu* was also applied to a portion of sheep lung described as the "middle finger,"[186] we presume that it is a pink or flesh-colored projection. In the text below, the lesion is seen coming out of the anus, suggesting that in this context *baṣkiltu* is an internal hemorrhoid that has prolapsed during defecation.

6.173 *šum-ma* LÚ *i-na pí-i qí-in-na-ti-šu ba-aṣ-ki-il-tum it-ta-ṣi-a-am* . . . (*YOS* 11.29:8; *YOS* 11.28:3)

**If a *baṣkiltu*-lesion comes out at the mouth of a person's anus . . .

URŠU *Uršu* is related to a verb that means "to be dirty"[187] and should therefore be darker in color than the *umṣātu*. This would seem to suggest that an *uršu* was the bluish lump produced by thrombosis of a hemorrhoid.

6.174 DIŠ NA *ina* DÚR-*šú* MÚD *i-te-ez-zi ur-ši ina* x [. . .] (*BAM* 152 iii 16//*BAM* 182 r. 4')

**If a person excretes blood from his anus (and) there is an *uršu*-lesion [. . .]

6.175 DIŠ NA *ur-šu dan-nu* KA MUD-*šú* DIB-*ma* KA MUD BAD-*ḫi* . . . (*BAM* 95:10//*STT* 97 iii 1)

**If a large *uršu* "seizes" his anal opening so that it closes the anal opening . . .

DÚR.GIG

In the use of the phrase DÚR.GIG as found in forty-five references, the *āšipu* appears to have considered it to define a particular syndrome, and we have reviewed these references to determine whether they might indeed constitute a single disease or group of similar diseases. In translation, GIG means "sick" and DÚR means either "crotch," "buttocks," or "perineum." It is clear from the nature of the references that diseases involving both the urethra and anus were included, but close scrutiny shows that DÚR.GIG was not used for all illnesses affecting these structures. This term appears to have been reserved for chronic conditions that blocked or retarded the passage of urine or stool. It is clear that more than one disease was included under this rubric, but it is not known whether the *āšipu* recognized this fact.

Of the quotes dealing with urethral problems, six of the eight specify retained urine or urethral constriction as important aspects of the syndrome. There is no mention of frequent urination or fever; other signs and symptoms that are listed included bloating, loss of appetite, bloody urine (hematuria), stones, incontinence, pain, and "sick" kidney.

6.176 DIŠ NA *mi-na-tu-šú* DUB.DUB GABA-*su u* SA.SAL.MEŠ-*šú* KÚ.MEŠ-*šú* Á^{II}-*šú* x [. . .] KÚ.MEŠ-*šú bir-bir-ki-šú lu šá* 15 *lu šá* 150 SÍG-*su-ma ina mùš-tin-*[*ni*]-*šú* MÚD *ú-kal-lam* NA BI *ḫi-niq-ti* DÚR.GIG GIG *ana* TI-*šú* . . . (*AMT* 40/5 iii 14–16; *AMT* 56/1 obv. 1–3//*BAM* 88:1′–2′)

**If a person's limbs are continually tense,[188] his breast and his back continually hurt him, his arms [and legs?] continually hurt him, his loins[189] either on the left or on the right give him a jabbing pain and from his ⌜urethra⌝ he shows blood, that person is sick with the constriction of DÚR.GIG,[190] to cure him . . .

6.177 *šum*$_4$-*ma* KÀŠ-*šú* GIN$_7$ *šá gi-na-a* MURUB$_4$.MEŠ-*šú u* SAG ŠÀ-*šú* KÚ.[MEŠ-*šú*] NA BI *ḫi-niq-ti* DÚR/BÚN GIG *ana* TI-*šú* . . . (*BAM* 114:9–10//*BAM* 161 iv 4′–7′//*AMT* 58/4:5′–6′)[191]

**If his urine is like that of one whose pelvic region and upper abdomen (epigastrium) [continually] hurt [him], that person (has) the constriction of DÚR.GIG (var. is sick with constriction of the urethra), to cure him . . .

The above references do not provide sufficient information to positively identify a specific modern disease as the cause of the "constriction of DÚR.GIG"; however, the bloody urine and urethral constriction could be due to *Schistosomiasis hematobium* (see Chapter 5). Urethritis caused by some of the sexually transmitted diseases, especially gonorrhea, may also lead to urethral constriction; there is, however, no indication that ancient physicians regarded DÚR.GIG as a "disease of intercourse" (see Chapter 4).

Kidney stones (and the obstruction caused by them) were recognized as a separate syndrome (see Chapter 5). Other conditions, including bladder cancer and prostate enlargement which also produce similar symptoms may, however, have been included in this clinical category.

There are twenty-eight references dealing with gastrointestinal problems, and eighteen of them have constipation or the inability to pass gas as part of the syndrome. Neither diarrhea nor fever is listed in any of the twenty-eight gastrointestinal quotes, although pain, bloody stools, bloating, vomiting, insomnia, weight loss, colic, itching, discharge of pus from the rectum, and hemorrhoids are described.

6.178 DIŠ NA [*it-te-n*]*en-me-er i-te-nek-*[*ki-ik* I]M *ina* DÚR-*šú ú-kal* NINDA *u* A *tur-ra i-sil-ti* DÚR.GIG DIRI *us-su-ul la-ma* DUGUD-*šú-ma* . . . (*AMT* 58/1+*AMT* 56/5:1–2)[192]

**If a person [continually] has colic, he continually ⌜scratches⌝, he holds ⌜wind⌝ in his anus,[193] (and) bread and water come back up (on him), he is full of constipation due to DÚR.GIG; he is completely constipated; before it becomes difficult for him . . .

6.179 DIŠ NA *ina-aṭ-ma lu ni-ṭa lu* MÚD.BABBAR *lu nik-ma-tu* ⌜*šá* DÚR⌝.GIG *ú-tab-ba-ka ana* TI-*šú* . . . (*BAM* 159 ii 49–50)[194]

**If a person has a condition of discharge[195] so that he pours out bloody excrement[196] or pus[197] or the pent-up (wind) of DÚR.GIG, to cure him . . .

6.180 [DIŠ NA DÚ]R.GIG GIG-*ma* DÚR-*šú* GÍR.GÍR-*su* . . . (*AMT* 56/1 obv. 10//*BAM* 88:10′)[198]

**[If a person] is sick with ⸢DÚR.GIG⸣ and his anus continually stings him . . .

6.181 DIŠ SA DÚR-*šú* ZI.ZI-*šú* DÚR.GIG GIG (Böck, *Morphoskopie* 266:25)

**If the blood vessel(s) of his anal region continually (seem) to pulsate, he is sick with DÚR.GIG.

6.182 [DIŠ NA D]ÚR.GIG-*ma um-ṣa-ti* ŠU.TI . . . *ur-še* GAZ.MEŠ *um-ṣa-a-ti uq-*[*ta-ta-pa*] (*BAM* 182 r. 7′–8′)

**[If a person (has) D]ÚR.GIG and so acquires *umṣātu* (hemorrhoids) . . . the *uršu* will be annihilated (and) the *umṣātu* ⸢removed⸣.

As with the urethral component of DÚR.GIG, the above quotes do not by themselves allow for a definite diagnosis in modern terms. The first reference above could apply equally well to any of the many causes of constipation, since all of the complaints are likely to be direct complications of the constipation itself. The next two references mention rectal pain and a rectal discharge of blood and pus. Some of the conditions suggested by these observations include rectal cancer and ulcerative colitis with a predominant rectal involvement. Since the last reference above mentions that *uršu* and *umṣātu* lesions were seen in association with DÚR.GIG, we are fairly certain that hemorrhoids fell under the general DÚR.GIG category, at least when constipation was also seen.

There are eight other references where DÚR.GIG was used, two that are associated with apparent liver problems and six with arthritis. One of the liver quotes cites liver pain, bleeding from the nose and mouth, and constipation. The second quote refers to swollen eyes and jaundice.

6.183 DIŠ NA TÙN ŠÀ-*šú* DIB.DIB-*su gi-na-a* MÚD *ina* KA-*šú* DU-*ku* MÚ.MÚ-*aḫ u in-né-sil* NA BI DÚR.GIG *ana* TI-*šú* . . . (*BAM* 159 i 21–23)[199]

**If a person's liver[200] continually afflicts him, blood comes constantly from his mouth/nose, he is continually bloated and constipated, that person (has) DÚR.GIG, to cure him . . .

6.184 [DIŠ NA . . .].ME-*šú* SIG$_7$ IGI^{II}-*šú* MÚ.MÚ NA BI DÚR.⸢GIG⸣ . . . (*STT* 97 iv 12)

**[If a person]'s [. . .] are yellow, his eyes are continually swollen, that person (has) DÚR.GIG . . .

Both of these patients appear to have advanced liver failure, and one was constipated. There are many conditions affecting the anus or rectum that could have associated liver problems, including rectal cancer that has spread to the liver and ulcerative colitis. In favor of the latter possibility is the fact that DÚR.GIG was considered by ancient physicians to be a treatable condition.

The remaining quotes all mention arthritis and/or bone pain.

6.185 DIŠ NA *ki-ṣal-la-la-šú* KÚ.ME [. . .] DÚR.GIG GIG . . . (*AMT* 53/1 iii 6′–7′, cf. 4′)

**If a person's ankles continually hurt [. . .] he is sick with DÚR.GIG . . .

6.186 DIŠ NA MURUB$_4$.MEŠ-*šú* K[Ú.MEŠ-*š*]*ú iš-tu-šú* ⌜DU$_8$.DU$_8$?⌝ [. . . NA B]I DÚR. GIG . . . (*BAM* 96 ii 14)

**If a person's hips [continually] ⌜hurt him⌝ (but) continue to be supple[201] afterward, that person (has) DÚR.GIG . . .

In two cases, the descriptions appear to be either juvenile rheumatoid arthritis or arthritis occurring in young adults.

6.187 DIŠ NA *ina la si-ma-ni-šú* MURUB$_4$.MEŠ-*šú* KÚ.MEŠ-*šú* (GÌR^{II}.MEŠ-*šú i-ta-n*[*a-aḫ*]) *kim-ṣa-a-šú* (*i-za-qat-šu* ÚR.MEŠ-*šú i-tan-na-aḫ bur-ka-šu*) *i-kaṣ-ṣa-a-šú* NA.BI *ina meṣ-ḫi-ru-ti-šú* DÚR.GIG GIG *ana* TI-*šú* . . . (*BAM* 168:70–72//*AMT* 43/1 i 1–3//*BAM* 95:16–17)[202]

**If a person's hips hurt him before (the age when) this would be expected, his feet are continually [tired], his legs sting him, his thighs are continually tired, and his knees give him a gnawing pain, that person was sick with DÚR.GIG in his childhood, to cure him . . .

Although none of these references (as preserved) mention genitourinary or gastrointestinal problems, it is possible that they were present and understood by the physician to be part of the syndrome. If so, then the arthritis may have been that associated with ulcerative colitis. Another possibility is that some of the arthritis is "reactive" arthritis triggered by a salmonella infection that commonly complicates *Schistosomiasis hematobium* (at least in modern times). One of the texts above (*BAM* 96 ii 14) suggests that the joint stiffness was reversible. This supports the possibility that "reactive" arthritis was the cause.

It is our conclusion that ancient physicians tended to use DÚR.GIG for patients with diseases where urethral or rectal excretion was impeded, and especially where these problems tended to be relatively chronic and afebrile. It seems unlikely that a single disease explains everything, although *Schistosomiasis hematobium* or bladder cancer may well be included in the "constriction of DÚR.GIG" and hemorrhoids, rectal cancer, and ulcerative colitis in the rest of the syndrome.

The clear reference to a retrospective diagnosis[203] suggests that ancient physicians not only observed their patients with care but also kept records of particular patients over time. As to why they chose to include liver and arthritis symptoms under DÚR.GIG, the obvious possibility is that they observed a significant number of patients diagnosed with DÚR.GIG to develop liver and joint findings of the type described. As noted above, the liver problems are consistent with complications of rectal cancer or ulcerative colitis and the arthritis with either ulcerative colitis or a salmonella infection complicating *Schistosomiasis hematobium.*

Summary

Gastrointestinal diseases formed a large part of the practice of the ancient Mesopotamian physician. As with other organ systems, his powers of observation were excellent, and his clinical observations were surprisingly complete and lucid, and used precise terminology. Most impressive of all, however, was the description of peptic ulcer disease. Not only did the *āšipu* know that the condition he called A.GA.ZI/*tugānu* caused upper abdominal pain, bleeding, and obstruction of the gastrointestinal tract, but he also identified the internal anatomical location of the disease. There is also indirect evidence to suggest that the *āšipu* performed digital rectal examinations. Diagnostic skill at this level of sophistication seems amazing in such an early culture, and reflects the *āšipu*'s intellectual curiosity and understanding.

CHAPTER 7

Metabolic and Nutritional Diseases

If he chews his fingers and eats his own lips [. . .]

—DPS XI A r. 52 = *TDP* 98 r. 52

Abnormalities in growth, development, and energy production can be caused by acquired or inherited defects in biochemical pathways and by nutritional deficiencies. Hormonal (endocrine) abnormalities may also play a role in growth and development. The signs and symptoms produced by these diseases often do not identify a specific condition, and modern laboratory techniques may be required to establish the diagnoses. There are, however, some metabolic diseases that can be identified with some degree of confidence from the signs and symptoms that they produce.

Nutritional Deficiencies[1]

PROTEIN MALNUTRITION

When individuals have an adequate calorie intake, but inadequate protein intake, they develop protein malnutrition, sometimes called kwashiorkor. Growing children are especially prone to develop this condition. We have found sixteen references (not including duplicates) describing changes in the hair of the patient's head. Twelve of these include the phrase "touched in the steppe." Two quotes state only that the hair was abnormal, while the others describe hair that is brittle, stands on end, trembles (possibly meaning thin or with loss of substance), is frizzed, can be easily pulled out, and has changed color to red.

ABNORMAL

7.1 DIŠ SÍG SAG.DU-*šú is-sa-na-la-*ʾ *ina* EDIN TAG KI.MIN (DPS III A r. 22′b//C r. 47 = *TDP* 30:107)[2]

**If the hair of his head continually becomes abnormal, he was "touched in the steppe;" (it is worrisome).

BRITTLE

7.2 DIŠ SÍG SAG.DU-*šú is-se-ni-ip-pi ina* EDIN TAG-*it na-*ʾ*-id* (DPS III A r. 22′a//C r. 46 = *TDP* 30:106)[3]

**If the hair of his head continually becomes brittle,[4] he was "touched in the steppe"; it is worrisome.

7.3 DIŠ SÍG S[AG].⌜DU⌝-*šú ḫa-šat* DIN / DIŠ SÍG SAG.DU-*šú sa-pat* GAM (DPS III A r. 21′//C r. 45 = *TDP* 30:105)

**If the hair of his ⌜head⌝ is chopped-looking, he will live. If the hair of his head is brittle, he will die.

STANDS ON END

7.4 DIŠ SÍG SAG.DU-*šú zuq-qú-pat ina* EDIN TAG-*it* [KI.MIN] (DPS III A r. 23′//C r. 48 = *TDP* 30:108)[5]

**If the hair of his head seems to stand on end, he was "touched in the steppe"; [(it is worrisome)].

TREMBLES

7.5 DIŠ *b*[*i-rit*] SAG.DU-*šú i-sal-li-iḫ ina* EDIN TAG (DPS III A r. 19′//C r. 43 = *TDP* 30:103)

**If the (hair on the) ⌜central area of⌝ his head trembles, he was "touched in the steppe."

FRIZZED

7.6 DIŠ *kal-li* SAG.DU-*šú sa-ḫir* : *is-saḫ-ḫar* GAM (DPS III A obv. 33//C obv. 23a = *TDP* 20:23a)[6]

**If the (hair on the) crown of his head frizzes, he will die.

EASILY PULLED OUT

7.7 DIŠ SÍG S[AG.DU]-*šú i-na* x x a ZI-*at* GAM (DPS III A r. 26′//C r. 51//G 7a = *TDP* 30:110)

**If the hair of his ⌜head⌝ [. . .] is (easily) pulled out, he will die.

CHANGED TO RED

7.8 DIŠ *bi-rit* SAG.DU-*šú sa-mi ina* [EDIN TAG-*it*] (DPS III C obv. 23b = *TDP* 20:23b)

**If the (hair on the) central area of his head is red,[7] [he was touched] in [the steppe].

7.9 DIŠ SÍG S[AG.DU-*šú*] SA$_5$ GAM / DIŠ SÍG SAG.DU-*šú* SA$_5$ *u saḫ-*[*rat* GAM] (DPS III A r. 28′//C r. 53//G 8 = *TDP* 30:112; cf. Labat, *Syria* 33.125 r. 2–3)[8]

**If the hair of [his] ⸢head⸣ is red, he will die. If the hair of his head is red and ⸢frizzes⸣, [he will die].

These references indicate that the hair changes are associated with a very poor prognosis (worrisome) or a fatal outcome. Another "touched in the steppe" reference does not mention hair abnormalities but describes changes in the patient's face that clearly indicate a wasted or cadaveric appearance. This patient also will have had a fatal outcome.

7.10 DIŠ A.SAG-*šú* ŠÚ-*ip ina* EDIN TAG-*it* GAM (DPS IX A 79//B r. 26 = *TDP* 78:79)

**If (his face) falls flat against his skull, he was "touched in the steppe"; he will die.

These findings are all highly compatible with protein malnutrition, or kwashiorkor, a condition with a poor prognosis. Current medical texts describe patients with this condition having thin, brittle hair that can be pulled out in bunches and that has changed to a red color.[9] Certainly the wasted, cadaveric-looking face of starvation victims is well known to everyone.

It is clear that ancient Mesopotamian physicians recognized many of the findings that diagnose protein deficiency. However, it is not known whether they understood the cause. They would not have known what protein was since it was not described until modern times, but they may have known that their patients were starving. Even the phrase "touched in the steppe" carried some significance for the physician. The term here translated "steppe" (*ṣēru*) included agricultural or grazing lands of limited productivity, and was proverbial as the habitat of wild animals such as lions and gazelles as well as of nomads, runaways, and demons.[10]

Such an area, during periods of drought or other distress, might quickly cause its inhabitants to develop kwashiorkor. Bēl-ibni, governor of the Sealand for the Assyrian king Aššurbanipal, reports that, as a result of famine, neighboring tribesmen were attempting to live on a sort of bread made from an unappetizing mix of bitter herbs and seeds of a plant otherwise eaten only by wild asses. This permitted his arch enemy Nabû-bēl-šumāte ("whose hide the god Nabû will offer for sale") to hire himself a tribal army for a paltry ten GUR of dates and two slaves.[11] Starvation also occurred when a city was cut off from the outside world during a protracted siege, and people had to resort to cannibalism to survive.[12]

CALORIC DEFICIENCY

When a person's diet is properly balanced, but with inadequate calories, the individual loses energy and weight. Ultimately, severe wasting and death will result. Both inadequate intake of food and gastrointestinal abnormalities that interfere with absorption of food can be responsible for this problem. The texts below appear to be describing this condition.

7.11 *la a-ka-lu la šá-tu-u ṭè-e-mu ú-šá-šá mur-ṣu ú-rad* (*ABL* 5 r. 16–18 [Parpola, *SAA* 10.196])

**Not eating or drinking confuses the mind, brings on sickness.

7.12 DIŠ NA *ḫu-šaḫ-ḫu* DIB-*su* . . . (*BAM* 575 iii 39)

**If famine afflicts a person . . .

7.13 DIŠ LÚ.TUR *ina te-ni-qí-šú* UZU.MEŠ *i-šaḫ-ḫu-ḫu u mu-še-niq-ta-šú* UBUR SIG-*at* UBUR ÍL-*šum-ma* NU KÚ UBUR *šú-ú mur-ra i-šú ana* UBUR *eš-ši tu-na-kar-šú-ma* TI (DPS XL A 36–37 = *TDP* 220/222:36–37)

**If an infant's flesh wastes away while he is nursing and his wetnurse's breast is weak, (and if) you raise the breast to him he will not eat, that breast has a bitter taste. (If) you move him to a new breast, he will get well.

7.14 [DIŠ N]A NAM.ÉRIM *šaḫ-*[*ḫi*]*-ḫu* GIG *mim-mu-u i-lem-mu* ⌜*ina*⌝ ŠÀ-*šú la i-na-aḫ bal-ṭam*!*-ma*[13] *ana* DÚR-*šú ú-tab-bak* NINDA NU KÚ NA BI GÍD-*ma* ÚŠ *ana maš-taq-ti-šú u bul-lu-ṭí-šú* . . . (*BAM* 156:1–3)[14]

** [If a] ⌜person⌝ is sick with a wasting curse, everything he eats does not rest easy in his stomach but he pours (it) raw into his anus, (and) he cannot eat bread, if that person lingers he will die; for his splitting off and to cure him . . .

7.15 DIŠ NA SAG ŠÀ-*šú* GIN$_7$ *ša* ^{d}NAM.ÉRIM *i-ka-su-šú* DIŠ GIG-*šú* GUR.GUR IM *ina* ŠÀ-*šú* GIN$_7$ *ša* DÚR.GIG *uš-tar-ʾ-ab* DÙ UZU.MEŠ-*šú šaḫ-ḫu/šá-pik* ŠÀ-*šú ru-uq-šú ana* TI-*šú* . . . (*BAM* 49:32′–34′//*BAM* 579 iv 33–35//*BAM* 50 r. 7–10)

**If a person's upper abdomen (epigastrium) binds him like a case of curse (and) if his illness keeps coming back, "wind" in his stomach rumbles like a case of DÚR.GIG (see Chapter 6), all his flesh wastes away/is tense,[15] his heart is distant from him, to cure him . . .

The ancient physician also recognized that low body weight was not always a sign of disease, but could be a normal variant, as the following reference indicates.

7.16 DIŠ ŠÀ.MEŠ-*šú raq-qu* PA NU TUKU (DPS XIII B ii 42 = *TDP* 120 ii 42)

**If his chest and abdomen are flat, it is of no consequence.[16]

VITAMIN A DEFICIENCY

This deficiency is due to inadequate intake of green leafy vegetables, and is characterized by dry eyes, thickening of the skin around hair follicles, and poor vision at night (night blindness). The latter symptom is described in 9.58 (see Chapter 9), where the *āšipu* recommends eating liver, a known source of high levels of vitamin A.[17] If treated early enough with vitamin A, the visual loss is reversible, but prolonged deficiency leads to irreversible damage to the retinas and corneas.

STRACHAN'S SYNDROME

This syndrome is caused by vitamin B deficiency, and its abnormalities include vision loss, painful neuropathy (paralysis and decreased sensation), and dermatitis involving the mouth and groin. Since the references below contain all of these features except vision loss, it seems likely that they are describing this syndrome.

7.17 [DIŠ UGU-*š*]*ú* ⸢GAZ.ME⸣ *ḫi-ḫi-en* KIR$_4$/KA-*šú i-raš-ši-šú* SÍG GAL$_4$.LA-*šú* TAB-*su* ŠU-*šú* BAR.ME-*šu* [U] GU-⸢*šú* NU⸣ [ŠUB-*ma*] *sú-ḫur*? *ina* GI$_6$ DIB.DIB-*su u* NUN.MEŠ ŠU *Úr-bi-li-ti* (DPS III A obv. 15–16//C obv. 6–7 = *TDP* 18:6–7)

**[If the top] of ⸢his⸣ head continually feels as if split in two, the soft parts of his nose/mouth are reddish, the hair of his pubic region burns him, his hand continually hangs down limply, he does not [lay himself down] ⸢on top of⸣ (a woman),[18] but turns away, it continually afflicts him in the night, and he continually trembles, "hand" of Ištar of Arbela.[19]

7.18 DIŠ SAG.DU-*su* 1-*niš* TUK$_4$-*aš ḫi-ḫi-en* KIR$_4$/KA-*šú i-raš-ši-šum-ma* TAB-*su tu-*⸢*gu-un*⸣-*šú* TAB-*su* K[I.NÁ[20] NU ÍL . . .] (DPS III C obv. 24 = *TDP* 20:24)

**If his head shakes all over, the soft parts of his nose/mouth are reddish and burn him, his turban? burns him, [he cannot stand] the ⸢bed⸣ [. . .]

VITAMIN C DEFICIENCY (SCURVY)

Scurvy is the result of a diet deficient in citrus fruit and vegetables.[21] Its signs and symptoms include hemorrhage into muscles, under the skin, and from the gums. The gums become swollen and teeth loosen. The following references describe a patient with either scurvy or severe periodontitis (see Chapter 18).

7.19 DIŠ NA ZÚ.MEŠ-*šú en-šá lu* MÚD *i-ḫi-il-la* [. . .] MÚD *i-ḫa-al ana* TI-*šú* . . . (*BAM* 543 i 13–14)

**If a person's teeth are wobbly or ooze blood [. . .] oozes blood, to cure him . . .

7.20 DIŠ NA ZÚ.MEŠ-*šú nu-uš-šá-ma* MÚD *i-ḫi-il-la ana* TI-*šú* . . . (*STT* 279:1//*BAM* 543 i 17)

**If a person's teeth move and ooze blood, to cure him . . .

CELIAC DISEASE (GLUTEN ENTEROPATHY)

This condition is caused by hypersensitivity to a component of wheat flour, gluten. It is a relatively common condition in populations that use wheat flour in cooking, which includes ancient Mesopotamia. The nutritional deficiency is caused by poor absorption of nutrients due to bowel changes that develop in reaction to wheat gluten. Primary symptoms include large, bulky, foul-smelling stools, abdominal distention, loud bowel sounds, and abdominal cramps. The secondary problems that develop as the bowel pathology worsens include deficiencies in iron, folic acid, calcium, and vitamin B12, resulting in weight loss, weakness, mental changes, and abnormal growth in children. A reference that describes chronic wasting and diarrhea is shown below. There is insufficient information to reach a firm conclusion regarding this diagnosis, but we suspect that it may have been celiac disease.

7.21 [DIŠ N]A NAM.ÉRIM *šaḫ-[ḫi]-ḫu* GIG *mim-mu-u i-lem-mu ina* ŠÀ-*šú la i-na-aḫ* ⌜*bal*⌝-*ṭam!-ma ana* DÚR-*šú ú-tab-bak* NINDA NU KÚ NA BI GÍD-*ma* ÚŠ *ana maš-taq-ti-šú u bul-lu-ṭí-šú* . . . (*BAM* 156:1–3)

**[If] ⌜a person⌝ is sick with a wasting curse, everything he eats does not rest easy in his stomach but he pours (it) raw into his anus (and) he cannot eat bread, if that person lingers he will die; for splitting (him) off (from the illness) and to cure him . . .

Endocrine Diseases

We believe that we have identified references that are compatible with two different types of hormone (endocrine) deficiencies plus one with excess hormone production.

PRIMARY ADRENOCORTICAL DEFICIENCY (ADDISON'S DISEASE)

Destruction of the adrenal glands by invading malignancies or infectious diseases (especially tuberculosis) is the most common cause of this disease. It leads to deficiency in adrenocortical hormones. The signs and symptoms include fatigibility, weakness, loss of appetite, nausea and vomiting, weight loss, increased skin pigmentation, and low blood pressure. The reference below has many of the characteristics of adrenal insufficiency.

7.22 DIŠ NA KÚ NAG-*ma ana* UZU.BI NU *i-te-eḫ-ḫi za-mar* SIG_7 *za-mar* SA_5 *za-mar pa-nu-šú iṣ-ṣa-na-al-li-mu ú-ta-ad-dar* ⌜*uš-ta*⌝-*na-aḫ ana da-ba-bi* ŠÀ-*šú* [. . .] *qá-ad-di-iš* [. . .] *ma-a-a-al-šú* [. . .] LÚ.BI $LÚ.UŠ_{11}$ [. . .] (*AMT* 86/1 ii 12–18)

**If a person eats and drinks (but) does not put on weight,[22] he is sometimes flushed, sometimes pale, his face is continually turning black, he is continually depressed (and) tired, [his] heart [is too low] for him to speak [. . .] hunched over [. . .] his bed [. . .] that person, a sorcerer [. . .].

TESTOSTERONE DEFICIENCY

Testosterone is produced primarily in the testicles and is responsible for developing and maintaining male secondary sex characteristics such as facial hair, penis, and prostate. If testosterone deficiency occurs before puberty, the effect on male secondary sex characteristics is the greatest. A quote (5.82) refers to someone with atrophied testicles and absence of normal male sexual characteristics. There is no way to determine which disease was responsible for testicular atrophy, although mumps involving the testicles (mumps orchitis) is a frequent cause. As also mentioned in Chapter 5, castration was practiced in ancient Mesopotamia, and it is clear from the following reference that they understood that it caused sterility.

7.23 GIN$_7$ *šu-ut re-e-ši la a-li-di ni-il-ka li-bal* (*CT* 23.10:14)

**May your semen dry up like that of a barren eunuch!

GRAVES' DISEASE

This disease is caused primarily by the excess production of thyroid hormone, but there are other features that are probably autoimmune in nature. It is characterized by nervousness, agitation, rapid heart rate, heat intolerance, frequent bowel movements, weight loss, diffuse itching, and neck swelling caused by an enlarged thyroid.[23] The patient's eyes are often prominent, with a widened distance between the upper and lower eyelids (exophthalmos; see last reference below). Legs are often swollen (edematous) and the skin is warm and often thickened with raised, firm nodules that are pink to purple-brown in color.

The texts below are suggestive of Graves' disease since they indicate weight loss, eye and skin changes, itching, and compatible mental changes. The "troubled heart" is likely to mean rapid heart rate (see Chapter 8).

7.24 DIŠ NA Á^{II}-*šú ina* UGU SAG.DU-[*šú* GAR.GAR-*an*] Á.MEŠ-*šú* [. . .] GÌR^{II}-*šú mu-ne-e* ŠUB.ŠUB UZU.MEŠ-*šú* [. . .] *ana* MUNUS *a-la-ka mu-uṭ-ṭù* NINDA KÚ-*ma* [. . .] IGI^{II}-*šú it-ta-na-za-za* IGI [. . .] *i-te-ki-ik* DUG$_4$-*šú* LÙ.MEŠ [. . . *qí-bit* KA-*šú*] *i-ma-aš-ši* ŠÀ-*šú it-ta-na-a*[*d-la-aḫ* . . .] ALAM^{II}-*šú šá* Ì.UDU DIB-*šu-m*[*a*] ⸢UR.GI$_7$⸣ *šu-k*[*u-lu* . . .] *ana* ^{d}*Bil-gi paq-du-u na-áš*!-[*pa-r*]*a-at* ZI.KU$_5$.RU.D[A . . .] NA.BI EN UR.GI$_7$ GAR *ina* [. . .] ⸢*i*⸣-*ku-lu* TI.LA UR.[GI$_7$ . . .] *la-me* TE-*šu-ma* BA.[ÚŠ] . . . (K 2351+:6′–15′//*BAM* 467 ii 5′–11′)

**If a person [continually puts] his arms over [his] head, his arms [. . .], his feet (look like they) are spotted with *munû*-lesions (see Chapter 10), his flesh [wastes away?], his going to a woman is diminished, he eats bread and then [pours it out?], his eyes continually stand still [. . .], he scratches himself, his words are troubled [. . .], he forgets [what he has said], his heart is continually ⸢troubled⸣ [. . .] figurines of him were taken of tallow and fed to a dog; [figurines of him were taken of wax? and] entrusted to Bilgi (the fire god, i.e., he appears to melt away), machinations of *zikurudû* . . . before it approaches him and he ⸢dies⸣ . . .

7.25 DIŠ IGI.MEŠ-*šú* KÚM.MEŠ IGI^{II}-*šú um-mu-ra ina ú-kul-ti* : *ina qú-ul-ti* SÌG-*iṣ* GAM (DPS IX A 35 = *TDP* 74:35)

**If his face is continually warm (and) his eyes are prominent,[24] he was stricken in the dead of night; he will die.[25]

Fincke suggests[26] that the following reference, drawn from the physiognomic omens, is describing exophthalmos, an eye condition associated with hyperthyroidism, and we concur. It mentions eyes that are open and showing more conjunctival surface than normal (whites are "too big"), a picture that is compatible with exophthalmos. The phrase "the lower part of her eyes turns" could be referring to chemosis, an inflammatory complication of exophthalmos. The patient's inappropriate speech could be due to the emotional lability that is commonly seen with hyperthyroidism, a condition that is more common in women than in men.

7.26 DIŠ MUNUS INIM-*šá* NÍG.GIG BABBAR IGI^II-*šú ma-ʾ-ad* KAR [. . .] KI.TA IGI^II-*šá* NIGIN-*ú* . . . (Kraus, *TBP* no. 25 r. 4–5)

**If a woman says things she shouldn't,[27] the whites of her! eyes are (too) big [. . .], (and) the lower part of her eyes turns . . .[28]

In patients over forty, cardiovascular and myopathic symptoms dominate the clinical picture. In addition to velvety skin, silky hair, excessive sweating, and heat intolerance, patients experience rapid heart rate (sinus tachychardia; "pulsating temporal blood vessels"), heart murmurs, and, at times, overt heart failure ("protruding epigastrium" due to the accumulation of abdominal fluid). Some of these symptoms appear to be described in the following references.

7.27 DIŠ *ú-ru-uḫ* SAG.KI-*šú šá* 15 *bé-e-er* SA.MEŠ-*šú šá* 150 ZI.MEŠ DIB-*it* ŠÀ TUKU *u* SAG ŠÀ-*šú i-ru-ur* SÌG-*iṣ* ⌜MAŠKIM⌝ GAM (DPS IV B r. 20//E iv 4 = *TDP* 42 r. 41–42//*SpTU* 3.88 iv 4)

**If the hair of his left temple is fine (lit. "select"),[29] his blood vessels, the ones on the right (feel like they) are pulsating (i.e. the fine head hair and pulsating temporal blood vessels appeared simultaneously), he has affliction of the abdomen and his upper abdomen (epigastrium) rumbles, blow of a *rābiṣu*; he will die.

7.28 DIŠ ⌜*ú*⌝-*r*[*u*]-*uḫ* SA SAG.KI-*šú šá* ZAG *bé-e-*[*e*]*r* [. . .] SAG ŠÀ-*šú za-qir* SÌG-*iṣ* MAŠKIM SÌG-[*iṣ* GAM] (Ni. 470:3–4 [Kraus, *ZA* 77.197])

**If the hair of his left temple is fine (lit. "select") [. . .], (and) his upper abdomen (epigastrium) protrudes, he was stricken with the blow of a *rābiṣu*; [he will die].

Other Metabolic Diseases

As in the modern era, there were probably many patients in ancient Mesopotamia who had inherited defects in metabolic pathways. Unfortunately, relatively few of these diseases have sufficiently unique signs or symptoms that they can be identified many centuries later.

DIABETES MELLITUS

Diabetes is a disease caused by difficulty in getting glucose into cells of the body to be used as a source of energy. Insulin is the hormone that is necessary to accomplish this process. When it has difficulty getting into cells, glucose tends to build up high levels in the blood. Acutely, this causes the patient to have marked thirst (polydypsia) and hunger (polyphagia), and increased urinary frequency (polyuria). There are many other secondary problems that develop if high levels of blood glucose persist.

As discussed above, most of the references that include the phrase "touched in the steppe" describe symptoms that are compatible with protein malnutrition or kwashiorkor. In addition, there are several "touched in the steppe" quotes that do not seem to fit this diagnosis. One of them describes fleshy material and another a membranous substance called *lipištu*,[30] both of which were observed by the *āšipu* in the patient's urine.

7.29 DIŠ KÀŠ.MEŠ-*šú* IGI-*ma* UZU.ME-*šú* È.MEŠ-*ni ina* EDIN T[AG] (DPS XIV A_2 ii 3//C ii 22 = *TDP* 136 ii 53)

**If you look at his urine and (bits of) his flesh come out of it, he was ⌜touched⌝ in the steppe.

7.30 DIŠ KÀŠ.MEŠ-*šú* IGI-*ma li-piš-tú* È.MEŠ-*ni ina* EDIN TA[G] (DPS XIV A_2 ii 2//C ii 21 = *TDP* 136 ii 52)

**If you look at his urine and *lipištu* comes out of it, he was ⌜touched⌝ in the steppe.

The fleshy material in the urine could either be blood clots or tissue from papillary necrosis, but neither condition is known to be a common complication of kwashiorkor. Since diabetes is a known cause of papillary necrosis, and since untreated diabetes commonly causes severe wasting that can mimic protein malnutrition, the *āšipu* may have included cases of untreated diabetes in his syndrome "touched in the steppe." The increased thirst and hunger (polydypsia and polyphagia) that accompanies some forms of diabetes would certainly be appropriate to a condition associated with the barren and waterless steppe.

LESCH-NYHAN SYNDROME

This rare disease is caused by an inherited deficiency of the enzyme hypoxanthine-guanine phosphoribosyl transferase. Its clinical characteristics include a neurologic syndrome consisting of spasticity, irregular and jerky movements of hands and feet, occasionally mental retardation, and a striking behavioral disturbance, namely, self-mutilation. These patients have episodes of agitation and anxiety, and finger and lip biting. If unrestrained, they can destroy their fingers and seriously deform their lips. Since self-mutilation is such an uncommon medical phenomenon, and the translation below leaves almost no alternative to self-mutilation, we believe that this may be Lesch-Nyhan syndrome.

7.31 DIŠ U.MEŠ-*šú i-la-am-ma-am u* NUNDUN NÍ-*šú* KÚ [. . .] (DPS XI A r. 52 = *TDP* 98 r. 52)

**If he chews his fingers and eats his own lips [. . .].

PORPHYRIA

This is a group of diseases that have in common abnormalities of the porphyrin molecule. This molecule plus iron comprises hemoglobin, the oxygen-carrying unit of red blood cells. One form of this disease causes acute gastrointestinal disturbances, muscle paralysis, and psychiatric problems. A unique feature is the production of dark "port wine" urine, that further darkens when exposed to light. The color change is due to excess excretion of porphyrin precursors. In Chapter 5 there is a reference (5.3) to wine-colored urine that may be an example of this condition. However, there are other conditions that may mimic the appearance of urine in porphyria.

ALKAPTONURIA

This disease is one of the causes of black urine (see Chapter 5). This is a rare inherited disorder caused by decreased amounts of the enzyme homogentisate oxidase. The pigmented material causes ochronosis, a disease of cartilage and joints.

7.32 [DIŠ K]ÀŠ.MEŠ-*šú* GI_6.MEŠ TAG ÚŠ TAG-*it* GAM (DPS XIV A ii 41 = *TDP* 136 ii 41)

**[If] his ⌜urine⌝ is black, he was touched with the touch of death; he will die.

Since the reference only lists the black urine, we cannot be certain that alkaptonuria is the cause. Another more common possible cause is hemoglobinuria secondary to massive breakdown of red blood cells in patients with falciparum malaria (see Chapter 3). A third but rare cause of black urine is malignant melanoma.

Summary

Wasting from starvation and chronic disease is an obvious deviation from health that the *āšipu* described in many references. However, more subtle clinical abnormalities, such as changes in the texture and color of hair, were noted and were recognized to be signs of a grave prognosis which we know is caused by protein deficiency. Abnormalities caused by vitamin deficiencies were also noted. Although the *āšipu* could not have known the true nature of these diseases, his trial-and-error approach to therapy seems to have provided some success in treatment, as in the prescription of liver for night blindness (see above).

There are references that describe diseases that seem to be recognizable hormonal (endocrine) and congenital metabolic abnormalities. These conditions, however, would have been much less amenable to treatment in ancient Mesopotamia.

CHAPTER 8

Heart, Circulatory System, and Lungs

If a person continually has a crushing sensation
in his chest.
—*BAM* 317 r. 10; *BAM* 444 r. 14′; *BAM* 445:1

The physicians of ancient Mesopotamia were aware that the heart has a rhythmic movement and that there are structures throughout the body that contain blood. They sometimes referred to these structures literally as "vessels with blood," but more typically in medical texts, muscles, veins, and arteries are all referred to by a single term SA/*šer*ʾ*ānu*, leaving the exact translation to be derived from context (see below).[1] It is unclear whether they knew that blood was circulated through the blood vessels by the heart, or that arteries carry the blood away from the heart and veins are responsible for returning it. It was known that the heart contained blood, and that when life ceased, this blood was "extinguished." Cessation of the heart's pulse was also equated with death.[2]

The *āšipu* paid close attention to the movement of the heart, the pulse rate and strength, and whether the veins were engorged with blood or empty and collapsed. He knew that blood vessels were located in the hands, feet, temples, breast, and abdominal wall.[3] Recitations also describe blood vessels in the intestinal omentum (see 6.1). Ancient Mesopotamian physicians have been criticized for observing the pulse but not counting it.[4] However, since it is not possible to count the pulse without a short-interval timer, such as a wristwatch, the *āšipu* can hardly be faulted for this "failure." What he could, and did do, was to observe the force of pulsation, its rhythm, and to evaluate the patient's pulse rate by comparing it to his own (see below).

The Heart

HEART RATE AND RHYTHM

Two terms applied to the heart are *ešû* ("to be confused") and *dalāḫu* ("to be troubled"). These terms were also used in relation to visual disturbances (see Chapter 9), and we interpreted them to mean differing degrees of visual loss, with *dalāḫu* indicating the more marked loss. The references below that use these terms appear to be complicated clinical syndromes of multiple etiologies. We believe that *ešû* and *dalāḫu* mean an irregular heart rate, with the latter term indicating the more marked irregularity. There are many causes and types of irregular heart rate. The underlying diseases in the three references below may be disseminated gonococcal infection, (meningo)encephalitis, and Ménières disease, respectively, and are discussed in Chapters 9, 11, and 13.

8.1 DIŠ NA *ina* KI.NÁ-*šú* LUḪ.LUḪ-*ut* ŠÀ-*šú e-šu-u*^{5} *ina* KI.NÁ-*šú re-ḫu-su* DU-*ak* NA BI DIB-*ti* ^{d}AMAR.UTU *u* $^{\ulcorner d \urcorner}$EŠ$_4$.DAR UGU-*šú* GÁL-*ši ana* TI-*šú*... (*BAM* 205:19′–21′//*STT* 95:16–18//*STT* 280 ii 1–3)

**If a person continually jerks in his bed, his heart(beat) is confused (*e-šu-u*), (and) his semen flows in his bed, the anger of Marduk and Ištar is upon that person, to cure him...

8.2 DIŠ NA SAG.KI.DIB.BA TUKU.TUKU-*ši* GEŠTU^{II}-*šú i-šag-gu-ma* IGI^{II}-*šú i-bar-ru-ra* SA.GÚ-*šú* KÚ.MEŠ-*šu* Á^{II}-*šú šim-ma-tum* TUKU.TUKU-*ši* ÉLLAG-*su ú-maḫ-ḫa-as-su* ŠÀ-*šú da-li-iḫ* GÌR^{II}-*šú ri-mu-tú* TUKU.TUKU-*ši* NA BI GIDIM *ri-da-ti* ÚS.MEŠ-*šú ana* TI.LA-*šu* ... (*BAM* 323:89–92//*BAM* 228:23–27//*BAM* 229 obv. 17′–21′)

**If a person continually has headaches, his ears roar, his eyes become dimmed, his neck muscles continually hurt him, his arm(s) are continually numb, his kidney gives him a jabbing pain, his heart is troubled (*da-li-iḫ*), his feet are continually limp, a pursuing ghost continually pursues that person, to cure him...

8.3 *šum*$_4$*-ma* NA IGI.MEŠ-*šú* NIGIN.DU-*šú* GEŠTU.MEŠ-*šú i-šá-gu-ma* UZU.MEŠ-*šú šim-ma-ta* TUKU.TUKU-*ú* ŠÀ-*šú it-ta-na-ad-láḫ* GAR-*in* GIG-*šú* NU ZU.ZU NA BI *ka-šip* NU.MEŠ-*šú* DÙ.MEŠ-*ma ina* KI GUL.MEŠ *ana* ^{d}EREŠ.KI.GAL *pa-aq-du* (*BAM* 214 i 1–9)

**If a person's face seems continually to be spinning, his ears roar, his flesh is continually numb, his heart is continually troubled (*it-ta-na-ad-láḫ*), (and) the appearance of his illness is mysterious, that person is hexed, figurines of him were manufactured and in a place of desolation they were entrusted to Ereškigal.

A cardiac term of uncertain meaning describes the heart as being "awake" (*êru*). The two texts below are describing seizure activity in a patient (see Chapter 13). The outcome appears to have been determined by whether the patient's heart was awake, with a good outcome found when it was. It is possible that the patient whose heart was not awake had suffered cardiac arrest. Since low blood oxygen levels, as occur in cardiac arrest, can trigger tonic seizures, there is a logical association between these two medical conditions.

8.4 [DIŠ U$_4$] DIB-*šú* GIN$_7$ *áš-bu-ma* IGI-*šú i-ṣap-par* NUNDUN-*su ip-paṭ-ṭar* ÚḪ *ina* KA-*šú* ⌜DU⌝-*ak* ŠU-*su* GÌR-*šú ta-lam-ma-šú šá* 150 GIN$_7$ UDU.NÍTA *ṭa-ab-ḫi i-nap-pa-aṣ* AN.TA.ŠUB.B[A] *šum-ma* U$_4$ DIB-*šú* ŠÀ-*šú e-er* ZI-*aḫ šum-ma* U$_4$ DIB-*šú* ŠÀ-*šú* NU *e-er* NU ZI-*aḫ* (DPS XXVI:62′–63′ [AOAT 43.283])

**[If when] it afflicts him, as he is sitting, his eye flutters, his lips come apart, his spittle flows from his mouth, his hand, his foot, (and) his right buttock thrash around like (those of) a slaughtered sheep, ⌜AN.TA.ŠUB.BA⌝ (seizure). If, when it afflicts him, his heart is awake (*e-er*), it can be removed; if, when it afflicts him, his heart is not awake (NU *e-er*), it cannot be removed.[6]

8.5 DIŠ GIG GÚ-*su ana* 15 NIGIN.ME ŠU^{II}-*šú u* GÌR^{II}-*šú am-šá* IGI^{II}-*šú* DUL-*ma* BAL-⌜*ma*⌝ *ina* KA-*šú* ÚḪ DU-*ak i-ḫar-ru-ur* AN.TA.ŠUB.BA *šum-ma e-nu-ma* DIB-*šú* ŠÀ-*šú e-er* ZI *šum-ma e-nu-ma* DIB-*šú* NÍ-*šú* NU ZU-*e* NU ZI (DPS X A obv. 1–3//B obv. 1–3//DPS IX A 80//B r. 27 = *TDP* 80:1–3//*TDP* 78:80)

**If the patient continually turns his head to the left, his hands and his feet are immobilized, he closes and rolls his eyes and spittle flows from his mouth (and) he makes rumbling noises, AN.TA.ŠUB.BA (seizure). If when it afflicts him, his heart is awake (*e-er*), it can be removed. If when it afflicts him, he does not know who he is, it cannot be removed.[7]

A rapid fluttering heart rate was described by the *āšipu* as a "shudder" (MUD/*parādu*) of the heart (ŠÀ/*libbu*), as in the following examples.

8.6 DIŠ GABA-*šú* DU$_8$.MEŠ-*át* SAG.KI-*šú* ŠUB-*ut* MÚD *ina* KA-*šú pi-qam la p*[*i-qa*]*m* ⌜DU⌝-*k*[*a*] ŠÀ-*šú pi-qam la pi-qam* MUD-*ud* ŠU ^{d}AMAR.UTU *a-dir-ma* BA.ÚŠ (DPS XII A 2–3 = *TDP* 100 i 2–3)

**If his chest is clear,[8] (the blood vessels of) his temple have collapsed, blood incessantly flows from his nose/mouth, (and) his heart shudders (MUD-*ud*) incessantly, "hand" of Marduk; he will be worried and die. (viral hemorrhagic fever; see Chapter 3)

8.7 [DIŠ L]Ú TÙN.ŠÀ DIB.DIB-*su bir-ka-šú i-ta-na-na-ḫa* x x šú *ù ša-sal-la-šú* KÚ.KÚ-*šú ú-man-ga-ag in-ne-eṣ-ṣil* [*i*]*l-la-ta-šú* ZAG *u* GÙB *il-la-ka* KÚM ŠÀ-*šu* TUKU-*ši* ŠÀ-*šu pi-qa la pi-qa* MUD-*ud* LÚ.BI *ka-šip a-na* TI-*šu* . . . (*BAM* 397:33–37)

**If his liver[9] continually afflicts him, his knees continually become tired, his [. . .] and his back continually hurt him, he is stiff and sluggish, his ⌜spittle⌝ flows left and right, he has internal fever, (and) his heart shudders (MUD-*ud*) incessantly, that person is hexed, to cure him . . . (poisoning; see Chapter 15)

8.8 DIŠ NA ŠÀ-*šú* GAZ.MEŠ-*šú pi-qam* NU *pi-qam i-par-ru-ud* NA BI DIB-*ti* DINGIR *u* ^{d}*Eš$_4$-dar* UGU-*šú* GAL-*ši* DINGIR-*šú* KI-*šú ze-ni ana* BÚR . . . (*BAM* 316 iii 8′–10′//*BAM* 317 r. 13–14)

**If his heart continually crushes him (and) shudders (*i-par-ru-ud*) incessantly, the anger of god and goddess is upon him, to loosen the god who is angry with him . . .

The first text below mentions a rapid upper abdominal pulse. The examiner was undoubtedly feeling this rapid pulse by pressing down in the upper abdomen and feeling the pulsating aorta. A patient's heart rate may suddenly jump from a normal rate to a flutter (125 to 200 beats per minute) as was noted in the second reference below.

8.9 DIŠ ŠÀ-*šú* MUD.MUD-*ud* SAG ŠÀ-*šú* GU$_4$.UD.MEŠ IGI^{II}-*šú ana e-ṭú-ti* NIR.NIR-*aṣ* ŠU GIDIM$_7$ (DPS XIII B ii 15–16 = *TDP* 118 ii 15–16)

**If his heart flutters, his upper abdomen (epigastrium) pulses rapidly,[10] (and) he stretches out his eyes toward the darkness (photophobia), "hand" of ghost.

8.10 DIŠ Á^{II}-*šú bir-ka-šú i-ta-na-na-ḫa ina pi-qam* ŠÀ-*šú* MUD-*ud ina* KI.N [Á-*š*] *ú il-la-tu-šú* DU-*ak pi-qam la pi-qam in-né-ṣil* KÚM ŠÀ-*šú* TUKU.MEŠ NA BI ÚḪ DIB-*su* KI.MIN GIDIM$_7$ DIB-*su* (DPS X B r. 8–10 = *TDP* 88 r. 8–10)

**If his arms and knees continually become tired, all at once his heart flutters suddenly, his spittle flows (when he is) in ⌜his bed⌝, he is incessantly sluggish, (and) he continually has internal fever, sorcerous spittle afflicts that person (or) a ghost afflicts him.

CARDIAC BLOOD SUPPLY

The heart muscle receives its blood supply from the coronary arteries. When a branch of the coronary artery is partially blocked, and the amount of blood supplied to the heart muscle is significantly reduced, the patient may experience chest pain (angina).[11] If the blood supply is reduced too much, a portion of the heart muscle dies (myocardial infarction). Chest pain is also associated with an infarction. In the quote below, there is mention of both heart flutter and crushing chest pain. The chest pain could be due to either angina or infarction. The relationship between the pain and flutter is unclear. Heart flutter caused by some other mechanism could produce angina or infarction in a patient with diseased and narrowed coronary arteries. However, heart flutter can also be caused by myocardial infarction.

8.11 DIŠ NA IGI.MEŠ-*šú* NIGIN-*du*.ME GÌR^{II}.MEŠ-*šú* DUB.DUB-*ka ḫu-uṣ-ṣa* GAZ [ŠÀ] *pi-rit-tum* TUKU.TUKU-*ši* ŠU.NAM.LÚ.U$_{18}$.LU UGU-*šú* GÁL (*BAM* 317 r. 24–25)

**If a person's face seems continually to be spinning, his feet are continually tense,[12] he continually has a crushing sensation in his heart and fluttering, "hand" of mankind is upon him.

We have found many references to crushing chest pain, and suspect that angina and myocardial infarction due to coronary artery disease may have been common problems.

8.12 DIŠ NA *ḫu-uṣ-ṣa* GAZ ŠÀ-*bi* TUKU.TUKU-*ši* . . . (*BAM* 317 r. 10; *BAM* 444 r. 14′; *BAM* 445:1)[13]

**If a person continually has a crushing sensation in his chest . . .[14]

8.13 *qù-taru šá* GAZ ŠÀ-*bi* . . . (*BAM* 388 i′ 6//*TCL* 6.34 iii 5; *BAM* 388 i′ 7//*TCL* 6.34 iii 6; BM 92494 [jar label, Walker, *Iraq* 42.84])[15]

**Fumigants for crushing sensation in the chest . . .

8.14 Ú *ḫu-ṣa* GAZ ŠÀ-*bi* TUKU.MEŠ-*ši* . . . (*BAM* 159 iii 29//BM 78693:84)[16]

**Plants (for cases where a person) continually has a crushing sensation in his chest . . .

One particularly interesting text indicates that eating and emotional upheaval were recognized then, as now, to be triggers of anginal pain.

8.15 DIŠ NA *ina ma-ka-li-šú* ŠÀ-*šú* GAZ.MEŠ-*šú ina* É *ṣal-te ina* SILA *pu-úḫ-pu-ḫu-u* GAR-*šú šá* NA BI *ki-mil-ti* ᵈAMAR.UTU UGU-*šú* GÁL-*ši* DIB-*ti* ᵈAMAR.UTU *ana* BÚR-*ri* . . . (*STT* 95 i 7–8//*BAM* 317 r. 27–28//*AMT* 40/2:4′–6′)[17]

**If when a person eats, his heart continually crushes him, (and) in the house quarrel and in the street disturbance are inflicted upon him, the anger of Marduk is upon that person, to loosen the anger of Marduk . . .

Note the contrast with the following examples, where the emotional problems follow (and presumably result from) the chest pain.

8.16 DIŠ NA *ḫu-uṣ-ṣa* GAZ ŠÀ-*bi u* SAG.PA.KIL TUKU.MEŠ-*ši nu-ul-la-ti* ŠÀ-*šú i-ta-mu* . . . (*BAM* 316 iii 23′–24′)[18]

**If a person continually has a crushing sensation in his chest and depression (and) his heart ponders untruths . . .

8.17 DIŠ NA GAZ ŠÀ-*bi* TUKU.TUKU-*ši ur-ra u* GI_6 *pu-luḫ-tú*/[*pi*]-*rit-tú* TUKU-*ši* DINGIR-*šú* KI-*šú ze-ni* DINGIR-*šú* KI-*šú ana* SILIM-*me* . . . (*BAM* 316 iii 13′–14′//*BAM* 317 r. 16–17//*STT* 95 iv 145//*BAM* 447:4′)

**If a person continually has crushing of the chest (and) day and night he has fearfulness/shuddering, his god is angry with him, in order to make his god at peace with him . . .

CONGESTIVE HEART FAILURE

Congestive heart failure occurs when the heart muscle weakens from some disease to the point where blood circulation becomes inadequate. The most common cause in the modern era is coronary artery disease leading to death of a portion of the heart muscle (myocardial infarction). There are many other causes of congestive heart failure. Signs and symptoms of failure include shortness of breath especially with exertion, moist crackles during breathing (heard with a stethoscope), enlarged heart or liver, and fluid accumulation (edema) in the feet and legs, abdomen (ascites), and generalized swelling (anasarca). It is certain that heart failure would have been seen in ancient Mesopotamia, especially in older patients; however, we failed to find any references that provide a convincing description of that condition. This is probably due to the limited physical signs that would have been apparent in that era. Shortness of breath and swelling (edema) would have been the major signs that the *āšipu* would have recognized (see below), but unfortunately there are other causes, and we are unable to differentiate.

8.18 DIŠ ZI-*šú* GU_4.UD.ME *u* ŠÀ.MEŠ-*šú it-te-nen-bi-ṭu* GAM (DPS X A obv. 30//B obv. 34 = *TDP* 84:30)

**If his breath becomes rapid[19] and his insides are continually cramped, he will die.

8.19 DIŠ ZI-*šú* GU_4.UD.ME *u* SA.MEŠ-*šú šap-ku* GAM / DIŠ ZI-*šú i-tar-rak-ma qit-ru-bat* [G]AM (DPS X A obv. 31//B obv. 35–36 = *TDP* 84:31)

**If his breath becomes rapid[20] and his muscles are tense,[21] he will die. If his breath throbs and comes closely spaced, ⌜he will die⌝.

8.20 DIŠ ZI-*šú ú-šel-li* NU DIN (DPS X A obv. 32a = *TDP* 84:32a)

**If he makes his breath go up, he will not get well.

Swelling (edema) was generally referred to by the *āšipu* as "puffing up" (see 6.36–6.39) or by a term A.GA.NU.TIL.LA/ *aganutillû*, which lexical texts explain as "full of water."

8.21 DIŠ SAG ŠÀ-*šú* ÍL-*ma* IGI.MEŠ-*šú* MÚ.MEŠ-*ḫu ina* IGI^{II}-*šú* ÍR DU GÍD-*ma* GAM (DPS XIII B i 18′ = *TDP* 112 i 22′; cf. DPS XV:34 [AOAT 43.152])

**If his upper abdomen (epigastrium) is puffed up and his face is swollen (and) tears flow from his eyes, (if) it is prolonged, he will die.

8.22 DIŠ SAG ŠÀ-*šú za-qir* KÚM NU TUKU UŠ$_4$-*šú* KÚR.KÚR ŠÚ.ŠÚ A.GA.NU.TIL-*le-e* SI-*šum-ma ina* U$_4$-*um* BI.IZ AN-*e* GAM (DPS XIII B i 16′–17′ = *TDP* 112 i 20′–21′)[22]

**If his upper abdomen (epigastrium) protrudes (but) he does not have a fever (and) his mentation is altered, overwhelming of *aganutillû* (edema). (If) it increases, he will die on a day when it is hailing.[23]

8.23 [DIŠ N]A A.GA.NU.TIL.LA GIG . . . (*BAM* 174 r. 33)

** [If] a ⸢man⸣ is sick with *aganutillû* (edema) . . .

8.24 DIŠ IGI.MEŠ-*šú* ⸢*nap*⸣-*ḫu u* IGI^{II}-*šú* ⸢MÚ⸣.ME GAM / DIŠ IGI.ME-*šú nap-ḫu u* ŠÀ.ME-*šú* MÚ.MEŠ GAM (DPS IX A 66//B r. 11–12 = *TDP* 76:66)

**If his face is swollen and his eyes are swollen, he will die. If his face is swollen and his insides are bloated, he will die.

When a patient develops swelling of the ankles and feet due to fluid accumulation (ankle edema), congestive heart failure is a common cause. The following references appear to describe ankle edema. We believe that the use of "wind" in these texts is to illustrate the balloon-like appearance of edematous ankles.[24]

8.25 DIŠ NA GÌR^{II}-*šú* MÚ.MÚ . . . (*BAM* 121:12)[25]

**If a person's feet are continually swollen . . .

8.26 DIŠ *šap-la-tu-šú nap-ḫ*[*a* . . .] (DPS XIV A$_2$ ii 21//G iii 1′ = *TDP* 138 ii 71)

**If the lower parts (of his body) are swollen [. . .]

8.27 ⸢*maš*⸣-*ši-ti šá* [GÌR^{II}] *šá* IM *id*-⸢*pi*⸣-*t*[*u*] *ù šá-ag-gi a-na lu-ub-bu-k*[*i*] 4 *maš-šá-a-ti šá lu-ub-bu-k*[*i*] . . . (*BAM* 303:20′–23′, cf. 7′)

**Set of ingredients to lubricate [feet] that (look) inflated with "wind" and are stiff; four sets of ingredients for lubricating . . .

The following reference is possibly the most suggestive of heart failure. It mentions heart pain (possibly indicating coronary artery disease), protruding upper abdomen (abdominal fluid; ascites), and varying weight ("now fat, now thin"; suggesting shifts in fluid retention). The shortness of breath followed by the statement that the patient "cannot stand the bed" may be referring to one or both of the classic signs of congestive heart failure:

orthopnea or paroxysmal nocturnal dyspnea. With orthopnea, the patient cannot lie flat in bed because this position increases shortness of breath. Patients with paroxysmal nocturnal dyspnea may be able to fall asleep, but frequently wake up suddenly with a sense of apprehension and rapid breathing.

There are other signs that fit congestive heart failure, such as weakness (sluggishness), but others that do not, such as chills. The patient described may have been emotionally depressed, judging from the loss of appetite and the statement that "his heart is [too low] for (him) to speak." Depression may be a consequence of many diseases, including congestive heart failure. However, appetite can also be decreased due to intestinal edema in heart failure, and the "low" heart may be referring to some physical change in heart function.

8.28 [DIŠ NA *a-ka-li*]-*šú muṭ-ṭu ana da-ba-bi* ŠÀ-*šú* x [*ša-pil ḫu-u*] *ṣ* GAZ ŠÀ TUKU.MEŠ-*ši mi-na-ti-šu it*-[*ta-na-áš-pa-ka* EME-*šú*] *it-te-nen-bi-iṭ* NUNDUN[26].MEŠ-*šú ú-na-áš-šak* GEŠTU^{II}-*šú* G[Ú.GÚ-*a*] ŠU^{II}-*šú i-šam-ma-ma-šú bir-ka-šú kin-ṣa-šú i-kas-s*[*a-sa-šú*] SAG ŠÀ-*šú it-ta-na-áš-qàr ana* MUNUS DU-*ka mu*[*ṭ-ṭu*] *ana* MUNUS ŠÀ-*šú* NU ÍL-*šú ḫur-ba-šu* ŠUB.ŠUB-[*su*] *i-kab-bir i-ba-aḫ-ḫu* ÚḪ *ana* KA-*šú it-ta-na*-[*at-la-ak*] *ik-ka-šú* LÚGUD.DA.MEŠ KI.NÁ NU ÍL x *pi-qa la pi-qa ú-ta-ṣal* NA BI *ka*-[*šip*] NU.MEŠ-*šú* DÙ-*ma ina* ÚR LÚ.ÚŠ *šu-nu*-[*lu*] . . . (*BAM* 438 obv. 5–14)[27]

**[If a person]'s [appetite] is diminished, his heart is [too low] for (him) to speak, he continually has a crushing sensation in his heart, his limbs are continually [tense,[28] his tongue] is continually cramped, he bites his lips, his ears [continually] ⌜ring⌝, his hands go numb, his knees (and) his shins give him a gnawing pain, his upper abdomen (epigastrium) continually protrudes, his desire to go to a woman ⌜is diminished⌝, (and) he cannot get an erection for a woman, chills keep falling on [him], he is now fat (and now) thin, spittle continually ⌜comes⌝ to his mouth, his breath is continually short, he cannot stand the bed, (and) he is incessantly sluggish, that person is ⌜hexed⌝; figurines of him were manufactured and made to ⌜lie⌝ in the lap of a corpse . . .

The following references describe patients displaying symptoms that possibly relate to the heart. The emotional distress ("changes of mood") of the first quote would be appropriate to a patient with heart problems, and the "dark" hands and feet and a preference for a squatting position after exertion are suggestive of congenital heart disease with cyanosis (underoxygenated blood causing blue skin color). Less clear are the "shuddering" and "jerking" of the second quote, unless these refer to convulsions brought on by a sudden increase in cyanosis due to a reduction in pulmonary blood flow. If so, the dismal prognosis would be appropriate.

8.29 [DIŠ ŠU^{II}-*šú* I]GI.BAR.MEŠ BAL.BAL Z[I]-*bi u* DU$_{10}$.GAM *ina* SAG [GI$_6$ TAG-*it* . . .] [DIŠ ŠU^{II}-*šú u* G]ÌR^{II}-*šú* GI$_6$.MEŠ *uš-ta-nab-lak-kát* ZI-*bi u* D[U$_{10}$.GAM . . .] (DPS XI A obv. 38–39 = *TDP* 92:38–39)[29]

**[If] he continually ⌜gazes⌝ at [his hands], he has changes of mood, he ⌜gets up⌝ and (has to) squat down, (and) [he is particularly affected] at the beginning of [the night . . .] [If his hands and] his ⌜feet⌝ are dark, he has changes of mood (and) he gets up and ⌜(has to) squat down⌝ [. . .]

8.30 DIŠ *ina* GIG-*šú pa-rid* ZI-*bi u* DU_{10}.GAM-*is* GAM / DIŠ *ina* GIG-*šú* LUḪ.LUḪ-*uṭ* ZI-*bi u* TUŠ-*ab* NINDA KÚ A NAG ŠUK *qu-bu-ri-šú il-qí* GAM (DPS XVII:23–24 [AOAT 43.197])

**If during his illness he shudders (and) he gets up and (has to) squat down, he will die. If during his illness he continually jerks, he gets up and (has to) sit down (and) he eats bread (and) drinks water, he has eaten provisions for his grave; he will die.

The Circulatory System

As mentioned above, muscles, veins, and arteries are usually referred to by a single term, SA/*šerʾānu*, leaving the exact translation to be derived from context. Muscles are described as hurting or going numb, thickening, and becoming tense or stiff (see Chapter 11). Blood vessels are said to "jump" (GU_4.UD/*šaḫāṭu*), to "rise," that is, pulsate (ZI/*tebû*), to be "calm/still" (*nēḫu*), to be "established/present" (GAR/*šaknu*), "to go" (DU.MEŠ/*alāku*), and "to continually stand up" (GUB.GUB/*itazzuzu*).

Of these terms, there is one that we feel certain is describing veins and not arteries. In the following references, the blood vessels "stand up" on the patient's ankle. We believe that this is referring to varicose veins in their most common location. Also tending to confirm this conclusion is the nature of the treatment offered for this condition. Wrapping stones strung like beads on a string around the extremity could very logically have been used to place pressure on the venous varicosities to cause them to collapse, such as when we use elastic stockings today.

8.31 NA_4.MEŠ SA MUD-*šú* GUB.GUB-*az* . . . (*AMT* 58/7 i 6′; *BAM* 354 iii 18//Sm. 1948:5′)

**Stones (for cases where) the blood vessels of a person's heel continually stand up . . .

8.32 DIŠ NA SA MUD-*šú* GUB.GUB-*az* SA MAŠ.DÀ NU.NU È ⌜3⌝ KA.KEŠDA KEŠDA [É]N *ka-ra-ra-tum* [ŠID-*n*]*u ina* GÌR-*šú* KEŠDA (*BAM* 194 ii 6–10; cf. *BAM* 354 iii 14–16//*AMT* 70/5 ii 4′–7′; *AMT* 69/9:4′–6′)

**If the blood vessels of a person's heel continually stand up, you twine gazelle tendon (and) thread (the stones on it). You tie three knots. You recite the ⌜recitation⌝ "*kararatu.*" You tie it to his foot (var.[30] heel).

The text below is also describing veins engorged with blood, but since the hands are involved the cause is not likely to be varicosities. A more likely possibility is that the engorgement is due to congestive heart failure.

8.33 [DIŠ SA.MEŠ $ŠU^{II}$]-*šú* MÚD *il-te-qu-ú* [. . .] (DPS XI A r. 8 = *TDP* 94 r. 8)

**[If the blood vessels] of his [hands][31] take up blood [. . .]

Conversely, blood vessels that are said to "jump" (GU_4.UD/*šaḫāṭu*) or to "rise," i.e., pulsate (ZI/*tebû*) must be arteries. A physiognomic omen text (part of a series predicting the future on the basis of a person's appearance) describes the following "pulsating" blood vessels.[32] These blood vessel locations correspond closely to the known arteries of the face.

The pulses of these arteries can be palpated on the surface of the face, but it is difficult because of their small size. It must have taken great care and patience to find them. Below, we suggest the modern names of these arteries based on their described locations.

8.34 SA SAG.KI 15-*šu*/150-*šu* (*AMT* 61/8:1–2)

**blood vessel of his left/right temple (left/right temporal artery)

8.35 SA TE.MURUB$_4$ 15-*šu*/150-*šu* (*AMT* 61/8:3–4)

**blood vessel of his left/right cheek middle (left/right transverse facial artery)

8.36 SA TE 15-*šu*/150-*šu* (*AMT* 61/8:5–6)

**blood vessel of his left/right cheek (left/right facial artery)

8.37 SA GEŠTU 15-*šu*/150-*šu* (*AMT* 61/8:7–8)

**blood vessel of his left/right ear (left/right external carotid artery)

8.38 SA AN.TA IGI 15-*šu*/150-*šu* (*AMT* 61/8:9, 11)

**blood vessel above his left/right eye (left/right anterior superficial temporal artery)

8.39 SA KI.TA IGI 15-*šu*/150-*šu* (*AMT* 61/8:10, 12)

**blood vessel below his left/right eye (left/right transverse facial artery)

8.40 SA KA-*šu* 15/150 (*AMT* 61/8:13–14)

**the blood vessel of his left/right mouth (left/right superior labial artery)

Ancient Mesopotamian physicians were quite interested in patients' pulses, which were palpated in the arms, legs, and especially the temples. An upper abdominal (aortic) pulse was also noted (see 8.9), but this pulse is difficult to feel, especially in obese or heavily muscled patients. Physicians were also aware that the pulses were roughly synchronous, which shows that they felt the pulses at two places at once.

8.41 DIŠ SAG.DU-*su* KÚM-*im* SA SAG.KI^{II}-*šú* ŠU^{II}-*šú* *u* GÌR^{II}-*šú* 1-*niš* ZI.MEŠ SA$_5$ *u i-mim* ŠU [DINGIR DIN] (DPS III C obv. 55 = *TDP* 24:55)

**If his head is hot (and) the blood vessel(s) of his temples, his hands, and his feet all (feel like they) are pulsating together[33] (and) he is flushed and feverish, "hand" of [god; he will get well].

8.42 DIŠ SAG ŠÀ-*šú* KÚM-*ma* SA SAG.KI^{II}-*šú* ŠU^{II}-*šú* *u* GÌR^{II}-*šú* ZI.ME IGI^{II}-*šú* DUGUD-*šú* (DPS XIII B i 27′ = *TDP* 112 i 31′)[34]

**If his upper abdomen (epigastrium) is hot and the blood vessels of his temples, his hands, and his feet continually (feel like they) are pulsating (and) his eyes bother him.

The patient described below has a head wound that is probably infected, a condition likely to cause a rapid bounding pulse that would be easy to detect.

8.43 DIŠ *ina* SAG.DU-*šú* SÌG-*iṣ-ma* SA SAG.KI-*šú* ŠU[^{II}]-*šú* *u* [GÌ]R^{II}-*šú* 1-*niš* ZI.MEŠ ⸢SA$_5$⸣ *u*⸢*i-mim* ŠU DINGIR⸣ TI (DPS III C r. 21 = *TDP* 26:81)[35]

**If he was wounded on his head and the blood vessel(s) of his temple, his ⌜hands⌝ and his ⌜feet⌝ all seem to pulsate together, (and) he is flushed and feverish, "hand" of god; he will get well.

Another infection, namely, *ṣētu* (see enteric fever, Chapter 3), was also noted to cause bounding pulses that the patient could feel.

8.45 DIŠ NA UD.DA KUR-*id* ZI SAG.KI [TUKU *ina lam* DUGUD-*šú*] . . . (*BAM* 66 r. 4′//*AMT* 14/7:1)[36]

**If *ṣētu* has "gotten" a person (and) he [experiences] pulsating of the temples, [before it becomes difficult for him] . . .

8.46 DIŠ NA SAG.DU-*su* UD.DA TAB-*ma* SÍG SAG.DU-*šú*/UGU-*šú* *i-šaḫ-ḫu-uḫ* ZI SAG.KI TUKU.TUKU-*ši* . . . (*BAM* 3 ii 27–28//*BAM* 480 iii 8//*BAM* 9:23–24)

**If a person's head is burned by *ṣētu* so that the hair of his head/scalp falls out, (and) he continually experiences pulsating of the temples . . .

Also described is a migraine headache, which often causes pain in the temples that coincides with the pulse rate. This "pounding headache" is common in migraine and is often unilateral. The pulse described in this case was probably related by the patient to the physician rather than detected by the physician's examination.

8.47 DIŠ LÚ ZI-*ib* SAG.KI TUKU . . . (*BAM* 11:16)[37]

**If a person experiences pulsating of the temples . . .[38]

8.48 DIŠ NA SA SAG.KI 15/150-*šú* ZI-*ma* IGI 15/150-*šú* ÍR *ú-kal* . . . (*BAM* 3 iii 20//*BAM* 35 iv 1′//*AMT* 20/1 ii! 13′; *BAM* 3 iii 24//*BAM* 35 iv 4′//*AMT* 20/1 ii! 15′; *BAM* 6:1–2, 7–8)[39]

**If the blood vessels of a person's left/right temple (feel like they) are pulsating and his left/right eye contains tears . . .

The remaining terms used to describe blood vessels are: "calm/still" (*nēḫu*), "established/present" (GAR/*šaknu*), and "to go" (DU.MEŠ/*alāku*). In principle "calm/still" (*nēḫu*) should refer to a slow pulse and "established, present" (GAR/*šaknu*) to a normal pulse and/or normally engorged veins. The difficulty lies with the remaining term *go*.[40] When a blood vessel "goes," it could mean either that the normal pulsation is lost because it was weak or that it was very rapid, making it difficult to discern. Rapid pulse rate that the physician could still detect would probably be called "flutter."

Arterial disease such as atherosclerosis could cause weak or absent pulses. In the following reference the vessel was alternatively described as tense and "going." An artery with atherosclerosis can feel very hard or "tense" to the examining physician's fingers, and the pulse may be weak or absent. A patient in vascular collapse due to shock would also have weak pulses.

8.49 [DIŠ SA.MEŠ Š]U^{II}-*šú tab-ku šá* GÌR^{II}-*šú* ZI.MEŠ IGI^{II}-*š*[*ú* . . .] [DIŠ SA.MEŠ Š]U^{II}-*šú šá* 15 *tab-ku-ma* : DU-*ku-ma ù* [. . .] (DPS XI A r. 13–14 = *TDP* 94 r. 13–14)

**[If the blood vessels] of his ⌜hands⌝ are tense[41] (and) those of his feet (feel like they are) pulsating, ⌜his⌝ eyes [. . .]. [If the blood vessels] of his ⌜hands⌝, the ones on the left are tense (var. "go") and [the ones on the right . . .]

Another explanation, however, could be that the blood vessels to which the *āšipu* was applying this term were superficial veins. The following references we believe are describing patients with severe dehydration due to diarrhea (in the first case probably cholera—see Chapter 3). The *āšipu* notes that the blood vessels of the patient's hands "go." In severe dehydration, the normally engorged veins of the hands would eventually collapse and "go." It is also true, however, that severe untreated diarrhea can lead to shock and vascular collapse, causing the normal pulse of the arteries to weaken and disappear.

8.50 DIŠ *uṣ-ṣu-ub* A.MEŠ APIN.MEŠ-*iš* KÚM *mit-ḫar* SA.MEŠ ŠU^{II}-*šú* DU-*k*[*a*] TA *taš-rit* GI$_6$ EN SA$_9$ EN.NUN *i-leb-bu* ŠU GIDIM$_7$ (DPS XXVII:27–28 [AOAT 43.299])

**If he keeps asking for more and more water (but) his temperature is normal, the blood vessels of his hands "go," (and) he groans from the beginning of the night until the middle of the watch, "hand" of ghost.

8.51 [DIŠ SA.MEŠ ŠU^{II}-*š*] *ú u* GÌR^{II}-*šú* 1-*niš* DU.MEŠ KÚM ÚḪ *u* SAG-*š*[*ú* . . .] (DPS XI A r. 25 = *TDP* 96 r. 25)[42]

**[If the blood vessels] of ⌜his⌝ [hands] and his feet "go" at the same time, he burns with fever, and ⌜his⌝ head [. . .].

8.52 [DIŠ SA.MEŠ Š] U^{II}-*šú u* GÌR^{II}-*šú* 1-*niš* DU.MEŠ KÚM ÚḪ *ina* SU-*šú* [. . .] (DPS XI A r. 27 = *TDP* 96 r. 27)[43]

**[If the blood vessels] of his ⌜hands⌝ and his feet "go" at the same time, he burns with fever, (and) in his body [. . .].

The following reference tends to eliminate a rapid pulse as the meaning of "go," since different pulse rates between the hands and feet would be impossible. The "go" in this case means either a pulse sufficiently weak that the *āšipu* is having difficulty finding it or collapsed veins.

8.53 [DIŠ] SA GÌR^{II}-*šú* DU-*ku-ma šá* ŠU^{II}-*šú ne-e-ḫu ár-ḫiš* ÚŠ : AL.TI (DPS XIV A iv 23 = *TDP* 144 iv 58')[44]

**[If] the blood vessel(s) of his feet "go" and those of his hands are slow, he will speedily die (var. he will get well).

8.54 ⌜DIŠ SA⌝ GÌR^{II}-*šú* DU-*ku-ma šá* ŠU^{II}-*šú* GAR-*nu* KI.TA-*nu* GIG KU$_4$-*šú* NÍG.GIG IGI-*ma* DI[N] (DPS XIV A iv 24–25 = *TDP* 144 iv 59′–60′)[45]

**If the blood vessel(s) of his feet "go" and those of his hands are present,[46] his illness has entered him from below; he may have a difficult time of it (but) ⌜he will get well⌝.

The following clinical descriptions are not sufficiently complete to differentiate among septic shock, heart failure, and cardiovascular collapse due to hemorrhage. Also, the vessels that "go" could either be collapsed veins or arteries with weak pulse.

8.55 [DIŠ SA S]AG.KI^{II}-*šú* ŠU^{II}-*šú u* GÌR^{II}-*šú it-ta-*[*na*]-⸢*lak*⸣-*ku* GAM (DPS IV A$_2$ r. 29+A$_5$ r. 13//B r. 9 = *TDP* 42 r. 29)

**[If the blood vessel(s)] of his ⸢temples⸣, his hands, and his feet continually "go," he will die.

8.56 DIŠ SA SAG.KI^{II}-*šú* ŠU^{II}-*šú* GÌR^{II}-*šú* GÚ-*šú u* SAG ŠÀ-*šú* DU.MEŠ U$_4$.7.KÁM SAL.KALAG.GA ⸢IGI-*ma*⸣ <NU> DIN (DPS IV A$_2$ r. 33//B r. 13 = *TDP* 42 r. 33)

**If the blood vessel(s) of his temples, his hands, his feet, his neck, and his upper abdomen (epigastrium) "go," (if) he has a very hard time of it for seven days, he will <not> get well.

8.57 DIŠ SA SAG.KI^{II}-*šú* ŠU^{II}-*šú* GÌR^{II}-*šú* GÚ-*šú pa-pan* ŠÀ-*šú* DU.MEŠ *u* SU-*šú* ŠED$_7$ *za-mar* IGI DU$_8$ DUL-*ma ni-š*[*i*] (DPS IV A r. 1//B r. 14 = *TDP* 42 r. 34)

**If the blood vessels of his temples, his hands and his feet, his neck, and his umbilical area[47] "go" and his body is cold,[48] (if) he occasionally opens and closes his eyes, there may be a recovery.

The references below describe blood vessels that "go" in the right or left temple. Since this finding is the result of a wound, it is likely that head trauma either interrupted the arterial blood flow, or tissue swelling from the injury made it difficult to feel the pulse. The reason for loss of pulse on the left side when the individual was wounded from in front, and on the right when he was wounded from behind is explained in Chapter 13.

These references also clarify the meaning of "go." Since the veins of the temples are rarely prominent or engorged, it can be reasonably concluded that "go" does not mean venous collapse. This term, therefore, must have been used by the *āšipu* to mean a very weak or absent arterial pulse. In the references below, the loss of pulse was due to trauma. Other causes of weak pulse include a rigid arterial wall from atherosclerosis, shock with low blood pressure, or a very rapid pulse making detection difficult. Since ancient Mesopotamian physicians did not have the technical knowledge to measure blood pressure or arterial wall elasticity, they would have been unable to separate these possibilities.

8.58 [DIŠ SA SAG.K]I^{II}-*šú šá* [15 DU.D]U-*ma šá* 150 GAR-*nu* GAB[A.RI] SÌG-*iṣ* GIG-*su* DUGUD-*ma* GAM (DPS IV A$_2$ r. 5+A$_6$ r. 9//G r. 4 = *TDP* 40 r. 5//*LKU* 94 r. 4)

**[If the blood vessel(s) of] his ⸢temples⸣, the ones on [the left continually] ⸢"go"⸣ and the ones on the right are present, he was wounded ⸢from in front⸣; (if) he has a difficult time of it, he will die.

8.59 [DIŠ SA SAG.KI^{II}]-*šú šá* ⸢150 DU-*ku-ma*⸣ *šá* 15 GAR-*nu* GABA.RI SÌG-*iṣ* DIN (DPS IV A$_2$ r. 6+A$_6$ r. 10//G r. 5 = *TDP* 40 r. 6//*LKU* 94 r. 5)

**[If the blood vessel(s) of] his [temples], the ones on the right "go" and the ones on the left are present, he was wounded from behind(!);[49] he will get well.

RAYNAUD'S PHENOMENON

This condition is caused by transient spasm of the arteries supplying the hands and feet. Attacks are usually brought on by exposure to cold air or water. In its first phase when the arterial spasm is strongest, the fingers and/or toes become white. As the spasm abates, the involved digits become blue (cyanotic), then bright red. There is accompanying pain and tingling.

The four quotes below constitute a short series that suggests that the *āšipu* considered them to be the same disease. The statement that the hands or feet were full of blood probably refers to a bright (blood) red color. The restriction of this condition to hands or feet, plus the presence of pain, further supports the diagnosis of Raynaud's phenomenon. The failure to mention white fingers or toes weakens this diagnosis; however, since the pallor represents an early phase of the process, the *āšipu* may have been less aware of its existence. Cellulitis can also produce red, painful hands or feet, but it would be very unlikely that two or even four extremities would develop cellulitis at the same time. On the other hand, it would be quite common for Raynaud's phenomenon to have this distribution.

8.60 DIŠ U.MEŠ ŠU^{II}-*šú šá* 15 MÚD DIRI.MEŠ-*ma* KÚ.MEŠ-*šú* [. . .] (DPS XI A r. 37 = *TDP* 98 r. 37)

**If the fingers of his hands, the ones on the left are full of blood and continually hurt him, [. . .]

8.61 DIŠ U.MEŠ ŠU^{II}-*šú šá* 150 MÚD DIRI.MEŠ-*ma* KÚ.MEŠ-*šú* [. . .] (DPS XI A r. 38 = *TDP* 98 r. 38)

**If the fingers of his hands, the ones on the right are full of blood and continually hurt him, [. . .]

8.62 DIŠ U.MEŠ ŠU^{II}-*šú šá* 15 *u* 150 MÚD DIRI.MEŠ-*ma* KÚ.MEŠ-*šú* [. . .] (DPS XI A r. 39 = *TDP* 98 r. 39)

**If the fingers of his hands, the ones on the left and right are full of blood and continually hurt him, [. . .]

8.63 DIŠ U.MEŠ ŠU^{II}-*šú u* GÌR^{II}-*šú šá* 15 *u* 150 MÚD DIRI.MEŠ-*ma* KÚ.MEŠ-*šú* [. . .] (DPS XI A r. 40 = *TDP* 98 r. 40)

**If the digits of his hands and his feet, the ones on the left and right are full of blood and continually hurt him, [. . .]

The Lungs

Lung anatomy in sheep was well known due to the importance of the lungs in extispicy.[50] The major causes of lung disease are infections (see Chapter 3) and pollution. Pollution would not have been as great a problem in ancient Mesopotamia as in the modern era, because smoking did not exist and industrial air pollution would have been minimal. However, smoke from cooking fires and smelting or bread ovens could still have been sufficiently irritating to cause chronic lung disease or lung cancer. Cough, breathing difficulty, abnormal breath sounds, choking, and cyanosis (bluish-tinged skin due to low levels of blood oxygen) are the signs and symptoms that the ancient Mesopotamian physician would have observed.

COUGH

8.64 ÉN *su-alu su-alu su-alu da-ni ṣi-b*[*it-su*] *ina bi-rit ḫa-še-e it-ta-di* ^{GIŠ}GU.ZA-*šú at-lak su-alu ul šu-bat-*[*ka*] *šá ki-ṣir-ti gu-uḫ-ḫi u su-alu* ^{d}*Gu-la be-lit* TI.LA *lul-li/ li-še-lu šur*!*-ši-šú* TU$_6$ ÉN / KA.INIM.MA *ana* UGU GABA-*šú* ŠID-*nu* . . . (*BAM* 549 iv 6–10//*ABRT* 2.11 obv.! ii! 21–26//*BAM* 553 obv. 1′–4′)

***Su*ʾ*ālu* (cough; see below), *su*ʾ*ālu*, *su*ʾ*ālu*, mighty is [its] ⸢grip⸣. It set up its throne between the lungs. Go away, *su*ʾ*ālu*; that is not [your] seat. May Gula, mistress of life, remove the root of thick sputum, *guḫḫu*, and *su*ʾ*ālu*: healing spell— Recitation to be recited over the breast . . .

Cough is in most cases a sign of lung or airway (trachea/bronchi) disease. Infection is a common cause of cough (see Chapter 3), but there are other causes including allergies and lung tumors. The *āšipu* described coughs of various types and severity, including productive and dry coughs. He divided cough into two major categories, *su*ʾ*ālu*-cough and *guḫḫu*-cough. We suspect, on the basis of the fact that the term *su*ʾ*ālu* seems to be used to describe pertussis (see Chapter 3 with 3.97–3.98), that this was a barking cough and that the *guḫḫu* was a brassy cough.

BARKING COUGH (*SU*ʾ*ĀLU*-COUGH)[51]

8.65 DIŠ NA *su-alu šá ši-ḫi* GIG-*ma* GI.GÍD ḪAR.MEŠ-*šú* IM DIRI *ú-sa-al ú-gan-na-aḫ* ÚḪ TUKU-*ši* . . . (Labat and Tournay, *RA* 40.116 obv. 8–9)

**If a person is sick with wheezing *su*ʾ*ālu*-cough so that the windpipe (trachea and/or bronchi) is full of wind, he *su*ʾ*ālu*-coughs (and) *guḫḫu*-coughs (and) has phlegm . . .

8.66 DIŠ NA KÚM *ma-dam* TUKU-*ma la i-na-aḫ ú-na-ḫaṭ u i-sa-ul u* ŠÀ-*šú ana a-re-e i-ta-na-šá-a* NAM.ÉRIM GIG (DPS XXII:26–27 [AOAT 43.253/254])[52]

**If a person is very feverish and cannot find rest, he breathes deeply[53] and *su*ʾ*ālu*-coughs[54] and his stomach is nauseous to the point of vomiting, he is sick with a curse.

BRASSY COUGH (*GUḪḪU*-COUGH)[55]

8.67 [DIŠ NA] SAG ŠÀ-*šú* M[AŠ.SÌ]LA.MEŠ-*šú* KÚ.MEŠ-*šú ú-gan-na-aḫ* [NA B]I ḪAR.MEŠ G[I]G UD.DA SÁ.SÁ *ana* TI-*šú* . . . (*BAM* 564 ii 14′–15′)

**[If a person]'s upper abdomen (epigastrium) (and) his ⸢shoulders⸣ continually hurt him (and) he *guḫḫu*-coughs, ⸢that⸣ [person] has sick lungs; he was "gotten" by *ṣētu* (enteric fever; see Chapter 3), to cure him . . .

8.68 [DIŠ] NA GABA-*su* SAG ⸢ŠÀ⸣ MAŠ.SÌLA.MEŠ-*šú* KÚ.MEŠ-*šú* [UD].DA SÁ.SÁ *šum*$_4$-*ma ú-ga-*⸢*na*⸣*-aḫ* [ḪAR].ME GIG . . . (*CTN* 4.114 r. 7′–9′)

**[If] a person's breast, upper abdomen (epigastrium), (and) shoulders continually hurt him, he was "gotten" by *ṣētu* (enteric fever). If he *guḫḫu*-coughs, (he has) sick ⸢lungs⸣ . . .

8.69 DIŠ NA *g*[*i-na-a*] ḪAR.MEŠ GIG-*ma ú-gan-na-aḫ* ⸢*ul*⸣*-tú* ÚḪ-*šú* MÚD ŠUB-*a* . . . (*BAM* 44:16′)[56]

**If a person ⌜constantly⌝ has sick lungs so that he *guḫḫu*-coughs (and) produces blood with his spittle . . .

DRY COUGH

8.70 DIŠ NA *ta-bi-lam ú-sa-al ul* ŠUB-*a el-la-tú* [. . .] *ana* TI-*šú* . . . (*BAM* 549 iv 4–5//*AMT* 81/1 iii 22′//*BAM* 551 iii 6′)[57]

**If a person coughs a dry *suʾālu*-cough and does not produce phlegm [. . .], to cure him . . .

PRODUCTIVE COUGH

8.71 DIŠ NA *su-a-lam u* ÚḪ [TUKU-*ši*] . . . (*BAM* 549 iv 12; *AMT* 81/1 iii 17′–18′//*BAM* 551 iii 2′)

**If a person [has] *suʾālu*-cough with phlegm . . .

8.72 DIŠ NA KI.MIN *su-a-lam* BABBAR ŠUB.MEŠ-*a* [. . .] *ana* TI-*šú* . . . (*AMT* 50/3:1–2)[58]

**If . . . a person continually produces white *suʾālu*-cough (phlegm) [. . .], to cure him . . .

8.73 DIŠ NA *su-a-lam ḫa-ḫa u ki-ṣir-tú* Ḫ[AR.MEŠ GIG] . . . (*BAM* 548 iv 14′)[59]

**If a person [is sick with] *suʾālu*-cough, *ḫaḫḫu* (bloody phlegm), and thick sputum in the ⌜lungs⌝ . . .

SHORTNESS OF BREATH (DYSPNEA)

When a patient's lungs are sufficiently damaged that they are unable to absorb adequate amounts of oxygen into the blood, the patient attempts to compensate by increasing the rate of respiration. This symptom is not only seen in primary lung diseases, but also in other conditions such as congestive heart failure. Shortness of breath can become so severe that it makes normal speech difficult, as noted in the first reference below.

8.74 DIŠ NA GABA-*su* GIG-*ma* GIN_7 *ši-né-e-ti* SAḪAR TUKU.TUKU-*ši ina da-ba-bi-šú ik-ka-šú ik-ta-nar-ru ù* ZÉ *ip-te-nar-ru* NA BI *bi-rit* ŠÀ GIG *ana* TI-*šú* . . . (*BAM* 575 iii 55–56)[60]

**If a person's breast is sore and he continually has something like suffusions of dirt, when he talks, he is continually short of breath and he continually vomits bile, that person is sick inside his abdomen, to cure him . . .

8.75 DIŠ NA GABA-*su u* MAŠ.SÌLA.MEŠ-*šú* KÚ.MEŠ x [. . . *na-p*]*iš* KA-*šú* DUGUD . . . (*AMT* 51/2:7–8)

**If a person's breast and shoulders continually hurt [. . .] his ⌜breathing⌝ is difficult . . .

8.76 [DIŠ NA] *na-piš* KA-*šú* DUGUD . . . (*BAM* 566 i 6′)

**[If a person]'s breathing is difficult . . .

8.77 DIŠ ZI-*šú* GIN$_7$ *šá* TA A E$_{11}$-*a* LÚGUD.MEŠ ŠU ^{d}[. . .][61] : ŠU ^{d}*Nin-giz-zi-da* : ŠU GIDIM$_4$ *šá ina* A [ÚŠ DIB-*šú*] (DPS X A obv. 32b–33 = *TDP* 84:32b–33)[62]

**If his breath is short like one who has just come up from the water, "hand" of [. . .], "hand" of Ningišzida, or "hand" of the ghost of one who [died] in the water [afflicts him].

8.78 DIŠ IGI.MEŠ-*šú* NIGIN.MEŠ ZI.ME-*šú* LÚGUD.MEŠ ZI-*šú* GIN$_7$ *šá* A *ṣa-mu-ú i-te-ner-ru-ub* ŠU GIDIM$_7$ *mur-tap-pi-di ina* EDIN DIB-*su* (DPS IX A 62//B r. 6–7 = *TDP* 76:62)[63]

**If his face seems continually to spin (and) his breaths have become short[64] (and) his breath constantly enters his throat as if he were thirsting for water, "hand" of a ghost roving in the steppe afflicts him.

RESPIRATORY DISTRESS

If oxygen deficiency is severe, it leads to a breathing pattern referred to as respiratory distress. In infants and young children, this type of breathing has certain characteristics. The diaphragm moves rapidly and deeply. Since the ribs of infants tend to be very flexible and the tissues between the ribs are thin and plastic, the force of the diaphragm tends to suck in the tissues between the ribs during inspiration. This is called "rib retraction," a poor term since it is the tissues between the ribs that are being retracted. The reference below is likely to be describing respiratory distress in an infant. The phrase "goring by Sîn" may be referring to rib retraction, since the depression of the interrib tissue may have been seen as caused by the invisible horn of the moon-god.

8.79 DIŠ LÚ.TUR *ina ni-kip-ti* ^{d}30 ŠÀ.MEŠ-*šú pur-ru-du u qa-tu-um-ma i-qat-ti ana* TI-*šú* . . . (DPS XL A 42//B 42 = *TDP* 222:42)

**If an infant's chest and abdomen shudder as a result of goring by Sîn and likewise it is (about to) perish, to cure him . . .

ABNORMAL BREATH SOUNDS

Lung sounds that are mentioned include wheezing, gurgling, growling noises, "a mouth that roars," gasping respiration, and deep breathing. It is not known whether the physician listened to these breath sounds from the bedside, or actually put his ear to the patient's chest.[65] However, it seems likely that the more impressive sounds such as gasping respiration, deep breathing, and "a mouth that roars" were heard at the bedside, whereas the wheezing and gurgling sounds were noted by putting an ear to the patient's chest.

The first reference below is probably describing fluid in the tracheobronchial tree, or pulmonary edema. The second text is describing the high-pitched expiratory noises found in asthma. References 3 and 4 are louder sounds, possibly caused by a severe tracheo-bronchitis. These loud sounds could also be deep or severe coughing, although in that case one would expect one of the terms for cough to have been employed.

8.80 [DIŠ NA GIN$_7$] *a-ge-e ša* ÍD *i-ḫab-bu-ub* x [. . . *s*]*u ana šib-sat* ^{d}INNIN GUR-*šú ana* KAR-*šú* . . . (*AMT* 15/5:5′–6′)

**[If a person] gurgles like the waves of a canal [. . .] it will turn into anger of goddess; to save him . . .

8.81 DIŠ NA *su-alu šá ši-ḫi* GIG-*ma* GI.GÍD ḪAR.MEŠ-*šú* IM DIRI *ú-sa-al ú-gan-na-aḫ* ÚḪ TUKU-*ši* . . . (Labat and Tournay, *RA* 40.116 obv. 8–9)

**If a person is sick with wheezing *suʾālu*-cough so that his windpipe (trachea and/or bronchi) is full of wind, he *suʾālu*-coughs (and) *guḫḫu*-coughs (and) has phlegm . . .

8.82 DIŠ KI.MIN (NA *mu-kil* SAG HUL-*tim* DIB-*su*) KÚM *ina* SU-*šú la-zi-iz-ma u ma-gal i-le-ḫi-ib* NA BI *bit-qu*$_{5}$ [. . .] *u* IR TUKU . . . (*BAM* 520 ii 9′–10′; *BAM* 39:2′//*AMT* 49/4 r. 1)[66]

**If (a *mukīl rēš lemutti*-headache afflicts a person and) fever persists in his body and he makes a loud growling noise, that person has a "cleft" (empyema; see Chapter 3) [. . .] and sweat . . .

8.83 DIŠ *ta-bi*: SA ZI.IN.GI-*šú* KÚM TUKU ⸢ḪAR⸣.MEŠ-*š*[*ú* GIG].MEŠ *u* KA-*šú i-šag-gúm* TI-*uṭ šum*$_{4}$-*ma* GIG-*su* ⸢GÍD⸣-*ma* GAM (DPS XIV A iv 29–30//C$_{2}$ iv 22–23 = *TDP* 146 iv 64′–65′)

**If it (that is) a blood vessel (in his feet) (feels like it) is pulsating, his ankles are hot, ⸢his⸣ lungs are continually [sick], and his mouth roars, he will get well. If his illness is prolonged, he will die.

8.84 DIŠ U$_{4}$.5.KÁM U$_{4}$.10.KÁM GIG-*ma uš-tar-di-ma ḫu-qu ka-a-a-man-šú* GAM (DPS XVI:49′ [AOAT 43.176])[67]

**If he has been sick for five or ten days and gasping respiration[68] persists in being continuous for him, he will die.

NORMAL BREATH SOUNDS

The *āšipu* also noted when the lungs were "clear" (*paṭru*)[69] or "relaxed" (*ramû*).[70] These expressions presumably mean that there was steady, symmetrical, unlabored breathing without wheezing or other abnormal breath sounds.

8.85 DIŠ NA GABA-*šú paṭ-rat-ma ú-sa-ʾ*-[*al* . . .] (*AMT* 51/1:10)

**If a person's chest is clear (but) he ⸢*suʾālu*-coughs⸣ [. . .]

8.86 DIŠ NA SAG ŠÀ-*šú* KÚM TUKU.MEŠ-*ši* ŠÀ.MEŠ-*šú* MÚ.MEŠ-*ḫu* [. . .] x ṣa nam x x *ik-ka-šú ik-ta-nar-ru* [. . .]. MEŠ-*šú* DU$_{8}$.MEŠ NA BI NAM.ÉRIM [. . . *ana* T]I-*šú* . . . (*BAM* 49:21′–24′)

**If a person's upper abdomen (epigastrium) continually has fever, his insides are continually bloated [. . .], he is continually short of breath, (and) both sides of his [chest] are clear, a curse [afflicts] that person, [to] ⸢cure⸣ him . . .

8.87 DIŠ NA SAG ŠÀ-*šú* KÚM TUKU.MEŠ-*ši* ŠÀ-*šú* GIG NINDA *u* A.MEŠ ŠÀ-*šú* NU IGI-*šú* GABA.MEŠ-*šú ir-te-nem-mu-u* ŠÀ-*šú ina pi-qi ana* ḪAL-*e* DÙ.DÙ-*uš* NU *i-par*$_{5}$-*ru* IM *ina* ŠÀ-*šú i-sa-na-ḫur i-le-eb-bu* ŠÀ.MEŠ-*šú eb-ṭù* NA BI ^{d}ŠU.NAM.ÉRIM DIB-*su ana* TI-*šú* . . . (*BAM* 49:9–14′//*BAM* 50 obv. 11–15//*BAM* 51:2′–3′)

**If a person's upper abdomen (epigastrium) continually has fever, his stomach is sick, his stomach will not accept bread and water, both sides of his chest are continually relaxed, his stomach suddenly makes as if to vomit but he cannot throw up, the "wind" in his stomach continually roils (and) groans, (and) his insides are cramped, "hand" of curse afflicts that person, to cure him . . .

CHOKING

Patients may choke when they aspirate either liquids or solids of any kind. The critical issue is the volume of liquid and the size and shape of the solid material aspirated. Liquid even in small amounts can cause the upper airway to go into spasm (laryngospasm) which if severe enough can obstruct the airway. Although this is a frightening experience, the outcome is typically benign. The reason for this is that even if the spasm is severe enough to prevent breathing, the worst consequence is that the patient will lose consciousness, at which point the laryngospasm relaxes and breathing is again possible. In the reference below, the patient is likely to have aspirated a small volume of fluid, because the prognosis is favorable.

8.88 DIŠ GÚ.MUR-*su ḫa-niq* NÍG.GIG DINGIR-*šú* KÚ : *uš-te-zeb* (DPS X A obv. 28//B obv. 32 = *TDP* 84:28)

**If his larynx is constricted, he ate something offensive to his god (var. he will get through).

Large volume aspiration of any fluid (blood, vomitus, sea water, beer, etc.) can result in death from drowning. Aspiration of a solid has the potential of completely blocking the airway and causing rapid anoxia and death. Trying to swallow large pieces of meat is a common cause of this problem. The reference below may be describing this type of occurrence, but laryngeal edema secondary to food allergy is also possible.

8.89 DIŠ KI.MIN-⌜*ma*⌝ G[Ú.MUR-*s*]*u* ⌜*ḫa-niq* NÍG.GIG DINGIR-*šú*⌝ KÚ ŠU DINGIR-*šú* GA[M] (DPS XV:7 [AOAT 43.150])

**If (it is the first day he is sick) and ⌜his larynx⌝ is constricted, he ate something offensive to his god; "hand" of his god; he will ⌜die⌝.

The text below appears to be describing a choking patient who vomits blood. It is likely that the patient has cancer of the throat or neck, eventually causing airway obstruction and death. Another condition that could explain these findings is an abscess of the throat or neck.

8.90 DIŠ IGI.MEŠ-*šú* GIN$_7$ *ḫi-in-qí* UDU.NITÁ GÁL-*ú ú-šam-šá u* MÚD *i-ḫa-ḫu* GAM (DPS IX A 74 = *TDP* 78:74)

**If his face looks like that of a strangled sheep, it keeps him up all night, and he vomits blood, he will die.

CYANOSIS

The cause of the cyanosis in the reference below is likely to be laryngeal obstruction secondary to a severe allergic reaction, as suggested by the thickened lips (see Chapter 18) and changing (edematous?) face. Another possible cause is hereditary angioneurotic edema. This is a rare cause of skin swelling and laryngeal edema, but it is inherited and the last sentence of the text suggests a familial or inherited condition.

8.91 DIŠ IGI.MEŠ-*šú* GI$_6$.MEŠ-*ma* GIN$_7$ *šá-lam-ti ib-šu-ú* IGI.MEŠ-*šú i-te-eb-ṭú* NUNDUN.MEŠ-*šú ma-diš ik-tab-ra* IGI.MEŠ-*šú iš-ta-na-an-nu-ú mu-du-šú ul* GIG-*ma i-qab-bi* ÚŠ *ug-ga-ti* GAM EGIR-*su na-ʾ-da-at* É-*su* BIR-*aḫ* (DPS IX A 21–24//B obv. 20–22 = *TDP* 72:21–24)

**If his face turns dark and becomes like (that of) a corpse, his face is continually frowning, his lips are very much thickened, his face keeps changing (and) one who knows him says: "Is he not sick?"[71] death from (divine) anger; he will die. His inheritance will be in danger; his house will be scattered.

The patient in the following reference appears to have been wounded on the throat, producing cyanosis. Depending on the location of the wound, trauma to the throat could cause airway obstruction directly. Alternatively, in view of the observed vomiting, the patient could be choking on aspirated blood (see above).

8.92 DIŠ IGI.MEŠ-*šú* GI$_6$.MEŠ-*ma* MÚD *i-par$_5$-ri*[72] GABA.RI SÌG-*iṣ* GAM (DPS IX A 20 = *TDP* 72:20; cf. DPS XV:5 [AOAT 43.150])

**If his face is dark and he vomits blood, he was wounded on the front side; he will die.

PULMONARY EDEMA

When the air sacs (alveoli) of the lungs contain fluid rather than air, the condition is known as pulmonary edema. The breath sounds in this condition have a moist, crackling character but would probably not have been heard unless the physician put his ear to the patient's chest. The patient essentially drowns to death when enough of the alveoli are filled with fluid. There are many causes of pulmonary edema, including heart, liver, kidney, and lung failure. We believe that the *āšipu* used the term *saḫḫu*, as in the references below, to indicate fluid in the lungs (pulmonary edema). The primary meaning of the word is "marsh," which correlates well with the nature of the breath sounds.

8.93 [. . .] ⌜ŠÀ⌝(?)-*šú* KÚM TUKU.TUKU *di-kiš* ⌜GABA GIG⌝ [. . .]-*ḫa-ru sa-ḫa ḫa-aḫ-ḫa ši-ḫat* UZU.ME [. . .]-*aḫ-ḫa* DIB.MEŠ-*su ú-sa-al ina su-a-*[*li-šú* . . .] x-*šú nu-pu-ḫa ina lam* DUGUD-*šú* NA BI x x [. . .] TÙM ^{LÚ}ḪAL *qí-ba la* GAR-*a*[*n*] (*AMT* 51/2:2–6)

**[If . . .] his abdomen(?) is continually feverish, he is sick with needling pain in the chest [. . .] *saḫḫu*, *ḫaḫḫu* (bloody sputum), wasting away of the flesh [. . .] continually afflicts him, he coughs (and) when [he] ⌜coughs⌝ [. . .] are bloated, before it becomes difficult for him, that person [. . . If . . .], the diviner should not make a (favorable) prognosis [. . .]

8.94 DIŠ ḪAR *sa-ḫi* [. . .] x SIG_5*-iq* (*BAM* 42:33–34)

**If the lung [has] *saḫḫu* [of the lungs . . .] (the remedy) is good.

8.95 Ú NA *šá saḫ-ḫa* GIG . . . (*BAM* 1 ii 41)[73]

**Plant for a person who is sick with *saḫḫu* . . .

ASTHMA

Some individuals are prone to narrowing of the small airways because of muscle spasm and increased mucus production, a condition known as asthma. Allergy to inhaled substances such as pollen, and increased sensitivity to dust and pollutants may be partially responsible for this disease. The narrowed airways make it difficult to exhale, causing a high-pitched wheezing sound. Cough and thick phlegm are commonly present. When this occurs, the patient develops increasing shortness of breath and wheezing in the chest that the patient can usually hear, and often can be heard by the physician at the bedside even without a stethoscope. Secondary bronchitis and pneumonia are common, and can cause an exacerbation of the problem. The following texts are clearly describing asthma.

8.96 DIŠ NA *su-alu šá ši-ḫi* GIG-*ma* GI.GÍD ḪAR.MEŠ-*šú* IM DIRI *ú-sa-al ú-gan-na-aḫ* ÚḪ TUKU-*ši* . . . (Labat and Tournay, *RA* 40.116 obv. 8–9)

**If a person is sick with wheezing *su'ālu*-cough so that his windpipe (trachea and/or bronchi) is full of wind, he *su'ālu*-coughs (and) *guḫḫu*-coughs (and) has phlegm . . .

8.97 Ú ḪAR.MEŠ *šá še-ḫa za-am-ru* . . . (*BAM* 1 ii 26; *CT* 14.31 [D.T. 136]:6)

**Plant for lungs that sing with wheezing . . .

8.98 DIŠ NAM.KALAG DIB-*su-ma a-ka-la muṭ-ṭu ḫa-šu-šu i-ḫal-lu-la* U_4*-mu-us-su* KÚM DIB.DIB-*su ina ku-uṣ-ṣi* GAM (DPS XXII:71–72 [AOAT 43.257])

**If a mighty illness afflicts him so that he has a reduced appetite for bread, his lungs sing like a reed flute, (and) fever continually afflicts him daily in winter, he will die.[74]

The final reference in this group states that the prognosis for the patient is bad in winter. Cold air is a well known trigger of bronchospasm and wheezing, and can contribute to death in patients with asthma.

Summary

Although the nature of the cardiopulmonary system was not completely understood by the *āšipu*, there was a realization that heart beat and pulse were important indicators of health and life. Breathing and lung function were also known to be vital bodily activities that required prompt attention from the physician in the event of disease.

Eyes, Ears, and Nose

If a person [sees] flashes in his eyes [. . .] a ⌜roving?⌝ ghost
of the wastes [afflicts him].
—*AMT* 85/2:4–5

Eye Diseases

The importance of good vision to an individual's activities and his or her functioning within society caused the *āšipu* to be acutely aware of the signs and symptoms of eye diseases (IGI.GIG).[1] He also devised a series of technical terms to describe various degrees and types of vision loss in his patients. It would appear that there were three similar but distinguishable types of vision loss: "clouding," "confusion," and "dimness," and that these were further subdivided into patients experiencing a simple diminution versus those having serious difficulty seeing. Frequently, the minimal vision loss words appear together, which might imply that whatever difference there was did not always matter when it came to treating the eyes.

APÛ VERSUS *ERĒPU*

Apû is related to a word for a type of cloud;[2] *erēpu* is related to another word for a type of cloud[3] (the kind that forms into shapes and delivers rain, i.e., cumulus). In principle, then, *erēpu* should indicate a more severe degree of "clouding" than *apû* and what the *āšipu* apparently wanted to know was whether the patient's vision was merely "clouded" (*apû*) or "heavily clouded" (*erēpu*).

9.1 KA.INIM.MA IGI^{II} *a-pa-ti* IGI.MEŠ [. . .] (*BAM* 516 i 55′)[4]

**Recitation for *apû*'d eyes, [. . .] face . . .

9.2 DIŠ *ina* SAG.DU-*šú* SÌG-*ṣi-ma* IGI^{II}-*šú ur-ru-pa* ŠU ^{d}N[IN].GÍR.SU (DPS III C r. 15 = *TDP* 26:75)[5]

**If he was wounded on his head and consequently his eyes are *erēpu*'d, "hand" of ⌜Ningirsu⌝.

AŠÛ VERSUS *DALĀḪU*

Ašû literally means "to confuse";[6] *dalāḫu* means "to trouble" (as in troubled waters). Here, what the *āšipu* apparently wanted to know was the degree of the eye problem, namely, whether the patient's vision was merely "confused" (*ašû*) or actually "troubled" (*dalāḫu*). The nature of the eye problem is uncertain, but could be referring to visual changes or degrees of irritation.

9.3 DIŠ NA *i*[*na* UGU I]GI^{II}-*šú* SÍG *a-ṣa-at u* IGI^{II}-*šú a-šá-a* . . . (*BAM* 515 i 17)

**If a hair grows ⌜toward⌝ a person's ⌜eyes⌝ and his eyes are *ašû*'d . . .

9.4 [DIŠ NA I]GI^{II}-*šú* MÚD *ṭi-ri* LÙ.MEŠ . . . (*BAM* 522:6′)[7]

** [If a person]'s ⌜eyes⌝ are *dalāḫu*'d with penetrating blood . . .

BARĀRU VERSUS *EṬÛ*

Barāru is related to a word for (the dim light) of evening;[8] *eṭû* means "to darken." In principle, *eṭû* should indicate a more severe degree of "darkening" than *barāru*, and what the *āšipu* apparently wanted to know was whether the patient's vision was merely "dimmed" (*barāru*) or actually "darkened" (*eṭû*).

9.5 DIŠ NA IGI^{II}-*šú i-bar-ru-ra* . . . (*BAM* 159 iv 26′; *SpTU* 2.50:15//BM 54641+BM 54826 obv. 18′; *SpTU* 2.50:20)[9]

**If a person's eyes become *barāru*'d . . .

9.6 DIŠ *i-na* IGI[^{II}-*šú* . . .]x *i-te-ni-ṭa-a* NA BI KIN-*šú* SUMUN-*ma* IGI^{II}-*šú ip-pa-a ana* TI-*šú* . . . (*BAM* 515 i 54′–55′; cf. *BAM* 22:1′)

**If (there are) [. . .] in [his] eye[s], they continually are *eṭû*'d (and if) that person's work is prolonged,[10] his eyes become *apû*'d, to cure him . . .

Fincke[11] gives an alternative explanation for *barāru*, suggesting that the patient is squinting to reduce scattered light (as from a scarred cornea or a lens with a cataract) to thereby improve clarity of vision.

LAL/*MAṬÛ* VERSUS DUGUD/*KABĀTU*

"Eyesight" (*diglu*) is said "to diminish" (LAL/*maṭû*) or "to be difficult/heavy" (DUGUD/*kabātu*). Frequently, *apû*, *ašû*, and *barāru* (the minimal vision loss words) appear together, which might imply that the significant difference was between "diminished" and "difficult" vision.

9.7 DIŠ NA *di-gi-il* IGI^{II}-*šú ma-a-ṭi* . . . (*BAM* 516 ii 8′)

**If a person's eyesight is diminished . . .

9.8 DIŠ NA IGI^{II}-*šú* [. . .]x *di-gal-šu* DUGUD... (*BAM* 515 ii 54)

**If a person's eyes [. . .] (and) seeing is difficult for him . . .

As might be expected, tears, worms, hairs, redness, and pink eye are used with the words for minimal vision loss whereas corneal opacities, membranes, and penetrating blood are used with words for severe vision loss.

9.9 DIŠ NA UGU-*šú* KÚM *ú-kal* SA ZI SAG.KI TUKU-*ma* IGI^{II}-*šú i*-BÁR IGI^{II}-*šú bir-ra-tú i-pi-tú i-ši-tú mur-din-na qu-qa-na a-šá-a ù* ÍR ŠUB.ŠUB-*a* [. . .] (*BAM* 480 i 1–3//*BAM* 3 i 1–3)

**If fever grips the top of a person's head, he experiences pulsating of the temporal blood vessels, and his eyes flutter[12] (and) his eyes (have) dimness, clouding, "confusion" of vision, *amurdinnu* (pink eye), *quqānu*-worms, (or) are "confused" or continually tear . . .[13]

9.10 DIŠ NA IGI^{II}-*šú* GIG-*ma ši-ši-tú* UGU ^{d}L[AMMA IGI . . .]-*šú-ma* DUGUD *ana* TI-*šú* . . . DIŠ NA IGI^{II}-*šú* MÚ-*aḫ* GIŠ.MI *ša* 7 ITU 18 ITU *ṣí-ḫa-ti* (*BAM* 23:1–3//*BAM* 515 ii 65–66)

**If a person's eyes are sore and there is a membrane over the ⌜cornea⌝ [. . .] and it is difficult [for him to see], to cure him . . . If the person's eyes are swollen, there will be an opaque spot for seven months and *ṣiḫḫu*'s (corneal ulcers) for eighteen months.

FLASHES (PHOTOPSIA)

The impression of flashing lights[14] can be produced by diseases of the retina such as detached retina,[15] physical force to the eye or brain, migraine headaches,[16] and some brain diseases.[17] The ancient Mesopotamian physician called these flashes *birṣu* or *burṣu*.[18] Because of the unusual nature of this sign it is not surprising that the *āšipu* attributed it to ghosts.

9.11 *e-nu-ma* IGI^{II}-*šú bu-ur-ṣa id-da-nag-ga-la* ŠU.G[IDIM.MA . . .] ⌜*ana*⌝ [T]I-*šú* . . . (*BAM* 516 i 2–3; cf. *AMT* 85/2:12)[19]

**When his eyes continually see flashes, "hand" [of ghost (or). . .], to cure him . . .

9.12 DIŠ NA *ina* IGI.MEŠ-*šú bir-ṣi* x[. . .] GIDIM *ḫur-ba-ti mu-u*[*š*-. . .] (*AMT* 85/2:4–5)

**If a person [sees] flashes in his eyes [. . .] a ⌜roving?⌝ ghost of the wastes [afflicts him] . . .

9.13 NA_4.MEŠ DIŠ NA *bir-ṣu* IGI.MEŠ . . . (*SpTU* 4.129 i 12//*STT* 111:18′(!)//*SpTU* 2.22 i 11+*SpTU* 3.85 i 16)[20]

**Stones (for cases) where a person continually sees flashes . . .

9.14 DIŠ NA ŠU.GIDIM$_4$.MA DIB-*su-ma ina* IGI^{II}.MEŠ-*šú* GIN$_7$ [*nu-ri*] *lu-u* GIN$_7$ NIM.GÍR x[. . .] ⌜*lu*⌝-*u* GIN$_7$ [. . .] *lu-u* GIN$_7$ ÙZ [GAR].⌜GAR-*an* NA.BI⌝ ŠU. GIDI[M$_4$.MA . . .] i-kal [. . .] IGI^{II}.MEŠ-*šú* [. . .] § *ana* ZI-*šú*... (*BAM* 209 r. 19′–23′)[21]

**If "hand" of ghost afflicts a person so that in his eyes (something that looks) like [a light] or like lightning [. . .] or like [. . .] or like a goat [is continually established, that person] "hand" of ⌜ghost⌝ [. . .] his eyes [. . .] to remove it . . .

The last reference mentions an object shaped like a goat. We interpret this to mean that it was an amorphous shape produced by distorted light perception. Retinal detachment can produce such an amorphous shape, as well as the flashes described above. Migraine headaches (a condition caused by ghosts; see Chapter 13) may also cause flashes but not the amorphous objects.

PHOTOPHOBIA

Painful sensitivity to light can occur in eye infections (see Adenovirus below). Photophobia can also be found in more serious problems such as encephalitis. The phrase in the references below "stretches out his eyes toward the darkness" means photophobia.[22]

9.15 DIŠ ŠÀ-*šú* MUD.MUD-*ud* SAG ŠÀ-*šú* GU$_4$.UD.MEŠ IGI^{II}-*šú ana e-ṭú-ti* NIR.NIR-*aṣ* ŠU GIDIM$_7$ (DPS XIII B ii 15–16 = *TDP* 118 ii 15–16)

**If his heart flutters, his upper abdomen (epigastrium) pulses rapidly, (and) he stretches out his eyes toward the darkness, "hand" of ghost.

9.16 DIŠ SAG.KI^{II}-*šú ma-aq-ta$_5$* IGI^{II}-*šú ú-tar-ra-aṣ* TU.RA BI NU DIN (DPS IV A obv. 68+A$_6$ obv. 3//E ii 12 = *TDP* 38:68//*SpTU* 3.88 ii 12)

**If (the blood vessels of) his temples have collapsed (and) he stretches out his eyes (toward the darkness), he will not recover from that illness.

Eye diseases may be divided into three categories: external eye diseases, corneal diseases, and internal eye diseases.

External Eye Diseases

ABNORMAL REDNESS AND BLEEDING

Abnormal redness and bleeding in the outer eye may be due to a number of causes: dilated conjunctival blood vessels, conjunctiva suffused with blood, periorbital ecchymosis (black eye), bleeding from the eye, and conjunctivitis.

DILATED CONJUNCTIVAL BLOOD VESSELS When the blood vessels on the surface of the eye (white of the eye; conjunctiva) become dilated, we describe the eye as being "bloodshot." This finding may occur with irritation due to dust or pollution, following an alcoholic binge (hangover), and associated with some infections and fevers, as well as glaucoma.[23] The first reference below describes the dilated vessels as "red threads," and in this case it appears to be due to an infection.

9.17 DIŠ *kal* U$_4$*-mi* ŠED$_7$*-ma ḫur-ba-šú* ŠUB.ŠUB-*su* IGI^{II}-*šú* GU.MEŠ SA$_5$.MEŠ ⸢DIRI⸣[24] [. . .] (DPS XVII:77 [AOAT 43.202])

**If he is cold all day and chills continually fall upon him (and) his eyes are full of red threads [. . .][25]

9.18 IGI^{II} *a-pa-tu* IGI^{II} *a-ša-tu* IGI^{II} *pur-sit* MÚD *šu-te-eṣ-li-pa-a-tu am-mìn tap-pá-a am-mìn taš-šá-a* . . . (*BAM* 514 iii 14–15//*BAM* 510 iii 9–10; cf. *BAM* 510 iii 9–10; Nougayrol, *Ugaritica* 5 no. 19:2, 4–5)

**Clouded eyes, "confused" eyes, eyes crisscrossed with blood vessels, why are you clouded; why are you "confused"? . . .

When this condition is due to irritation from dust, wind, smoke, or sun exposure, there usually is accompanying soreness and burning, as in the following references.[26]

9.19 DIŠ NA IGI^{II}-*šú* GIG-*ma u ḫa-an-ṭa* . . . (*AMT* 20/2:7′)[27]

**If a person's eyes are sore and also burn . . .

9.20 DIŠ NA IGI^{II}-*šú ta-bi-lam* GIG . . . (BAM 513 i 11′//*BAM* 510 i 21′)

**If a person's eyes are sore with dryness . . .

In the reference below, it appears that one eye is irritated, possibly from a foreign body or trauma, and the eye is fluttering or blinking in response to the irritation.

9.21 [DIŠ NA IGI] ZAG/[G]ÙB-*šú i*-BÀR SA *ta-mar-ma ma-gal* SA$_5$ . . . (*STT* 105:16′, 18′)

**[If a person]'s left/⸢right⸣ eye flutters[28] (and if) you look at the blood vessel, it is very red . . .[29]

CONJUNCTIVA SUFFUSED WITH BLOOD The blood vessels of the conjunctiva may bleed into the conjunctival tissue and turn the white of the eye a solid red color. This may occur as a result of trauma or clotting abnormalities such as those that may occur with overwhelming infections. The third reference below appears to be due to hemorrhagic viral infections (see Chapter 3).

9.22 DIŠ NA IGI^{II}-*šú* MÚD *šu-un-nu-ʾ* . . . (BAM 514 i 43′//*BAM* 510 i 35′//*BAM* 513 i 26′)

**If a person's eyes are suffused with blood . . .

9.23 IGI^{II} GIN$_7$ *nik-si* UDU.NÍTA MÚD *še-en-a* . . . (*BAM* 510 ii 28′//*BAM* 513 ii [43′] (= BM 98942 obv. 4)[30]//*BAM* 514 ii 39′ [W. Farber, *Fs. Borger* 65])[31]

**. . . eyes suffused with blood like a sheep with its throat cut . . .[32]

9.24 DIŠ UB.MEŠ-⸢*šú* DU$_8$⸣.MEŠ SAG ŠÀ-*šú di-ik*-⸢*šá* TUKU⸣ *pi-qam la pi-qam*[33] MÚD *ina* KA/KIR$_4$-*šú* DU-*ku* Á^{II}-*šú* SIG.MEŠ NÍG.ZI.[IR] ŠUB.ŠUB-*su* IGI^{II}-*šú* MÚD *šu-un-nu-ʾ-a* ŠU ^{d}AMAR.UTU *a-dir-ma* GAM (DPS XXII:34–35 [AOAT 43.254])[34]

**If his limbs are supple, his upper abdomen (epigastrium) has a needling pain, blood incessantly flows from his mouth/nose, his arms are continually weak, ⌜depression⌝ continually falls upon him, (and) his eyes are suffused with blood, "hand" of Marduk; he will be worried and die.

PERIORBITAL ECCHYMOSIS (BLACK EYE) The ancient Mesopotamian physician described a dark eye that in some cases the patient could not open. This might have been the result of trauma (like getting punched in the eye), but a similar appearance can be due to periorbital infection, especially from an underlying sinusitis.

9.25 ⌜DIŠ IGI 15⌝-*šú tar-kàt-ma* NU BAD *qu-t*[*u* . . .] (DPS V A 15′ = *TDP* 46 B 15)[35]

**If his left eye is dark and he cannot open (it) [. . .]

BLEEDING FROM THE EYE Blood coming out of the eyes is an uncommon clinical finding. It is more likely to be seen when severe clotting abnormalities occur, especially in patients with hemorrhagic viral infections (see Chapter 3).

9.26 DIŠ *ina* GIG-*šú* IGI^{II}-*šú* NU ÍL-*ši ina* IGI^{II}-*šú* KIR$_4$-*šú* KA-*šú* GEŠTU^{II}-*šú u* GÌŠ-*šú* MÚD TÉŠ.BI È.ME-*a* ŠU ^{d}7-*bi*: U$_4$.31.KÁM ŠU ^{d}MAŠ.TAB.BA (DPS XVII:25–26 [AOAT 43.197])

**If during his illness, he does not raise his eyes (and) blood comes out of his eyes, his nose, his mouth, his ears, and his penis all at the same time, "hand" of the Sibitti. (If he has been sick for) thirty-one days (when this happens), "hand" of the twin gods.

CONJUNCTIVITIS (INFLAMMATION) Ancient Mesopotamian physicians described "redness" in the eye and used the term *amurdinnu* or *murdinnu*, literally meaning "rose eye,"[36] when the patient had conjunctival inflammation or what we commonly call "pink eye."[37] There are many causes of this condition, but viruses are frequently responsible, especially adenovirus (see below for additional references to adenovirus).

9.27 [DIŠ NA IGI]^{II}-*šú ri-šu-tú* DIRI.MEŠ . . . (BM 54641+BM 54826 r. 10)

**[If a person]'s ⌜eyes⌝ are full of redness . . .

9.28 DIŠ NA IGI^{II}-*šú mur-din-ni* DIRI . . . (*BAM* 510 iv 47; *BAM* 515 i 1)[38]

**If a person's eyes are full of *murdinnu* . . .

9.29 *zaq-ta-a-ti* IGI^{II}-*a mur-din-ni* . . . (K 6461:4)[39]

**My eyes stinging with *murdinnu* . . .

Measles (rubeola) rash can involve the entire body, but it tends to affect the head first, causing red, swollen eyes with conjunctivitis. The following references appear to be descriptions of the measles rash (see Chapter 10).

9.30 DIŠ GIG *ina* SU NA È-*ma pa-nu-šú u* IGI^{II}-*šú* MÚ.MEŠ-*ḫ*[*u di-ig-la ka-bit*] *ù* SA$_5$ *a-šu-*⌜*ú*⌝ [MU.NI] . . . (Labat, *RA* 53.12–13 r. 8//*AMT* 84/6 ii 5′–6′)

**If a sore comes out on a person's body and, consequently, his face and his eyes are swollen, [(and) his sight is difficult], and (his eye is) red, [it is called] *ašû*...

9.31 [DIŠ *pa*]*-nu-šú u* IGI^{II}*-šú* MÚ.MEŠ*-ḫa di-ig-la ka-bit u* SA$_5$[40] *a-šu-ú* MU.⌜NI⌝ (DPS XXXIII:4 [AOAT 43.353])

**[If] his ⌜face⌝ and his eyes are swollen (and) his sight is difficult and (his eye is) red, ⌜it⌝ is called *ašû* (generalized body rash; see Chapter 10).

"EYES FULL OF/CONTAINING BLOOD" The *āšipu* also used these rather non-specific terms to describe anything from pink eye to bleeding from the eye, as judged from the other signs and symptoms listed in the references. Below are some examples of the broad use of these terms.[41]

9.32 [DIŠ NA U]GU*-šú* UD.DA TAB*-ma* [IGI^{II}*-šú i-bar-r*]*u-ra ù* MÚD DIRI*-a*... (*BAM* 480 ii 21)[42]

**[If a person]'s ⌜skull⌝ is burned by *ṣētu* (enteric fever)[43] so that [his eyes become] ⌜dimmed⌝ and are full of blood...

9.33 [DIŠ NA SAG.DU*-s*]*u* KÚM TUKU*-ma* IGI^{II}*-šú i-bar-ru-ra* MÚD *ú-kal-la*... (*BAM* 480 ii 12//*AMT* 5/3 i 4′)

**[If a person]'s [head] is feverish so that his eyes become dimmed (and) contain blood...

9.34 DIŠ U$_4$*-ma* UD.DU*-šú* IGI*-šú šá* 150 GIN$_7$ ^{GIŠ}BA[L *i-lam-mi*] IGI*-šú šá* ZAG MÚD DIRI*-at* KA*-šú* [BAD.BAD*-te* EME*-šu*] *ú-na-šak* ^{d}LUGAL.GÌR.RA D[IB*-su*...] ÚS.ÚS [...] (*STT* 89:109–112 [Stol, *Epilepsy* 92])[44]

**If when it comes over him, his right eye (bobs) like when a spindle ⌜whorl⌝ [spins] (and) his left eye is full of blood, [he continually opens] his mouth (and) he chews [his tongue], ^{d}LUGAL.GÌR.RA ⌜afflicts⌝ [him...] continually pursues [him...].

9.35 DIŠ NA SA SAG.KI*-šú* DIB*-su-ma* IGI^{II}*-šú* MÚD *ú-kal-la*... (*BAM* 3 iii 15)[45]

**If the blood vessels of a person's temple afflict him and his eyes contain blood...

9.36 DIŠ U$_4$.5.KÁM GIG*-ma* UZU.MEŠ*-šu* SIG$_7$ ŠUB*-ú* IGI^{II}*-šú* MÚD DIRI.MEŠ GAM (DPS XVI:47′ [AOAT 43.176])[46]

**If he has been sick for five days and his flesh is unevenly colored yellow (and) his eyes are full of blood, he will die.

CONJUNCTIVAL JAUNDICE

When the normally white portion of the eye (conjunctiva) becomes yellow, it is usually due to elevated serum bilirubin, a breakdown product of hemoglobin. A healthy liver excretes the bilirubin into the gall bladder, and subsequently into the intestines. A diseased liver or biliary tree obstruction permits the buildup of bilirubin, and causes yellow (jaundiced) conjunctiva as well as yellow skin (see Chapter 6).[47]

9.37 DIŠ *ina* ŠÀ-*šú ši-qu ina* ŠÀ IGI^{II}-*šú* GU.MEŠ SIG$_7$.MEŠ *ip-ri-ku* GAM (DPS XIII B ii 34 = *TDP* 120 ii 34)

**If there is *šīqu* (colored phlegm) in his abdomen (and) yellow threads cross in his eyes, he will die.

9.38 DIŠ *ina* ŠÀ-*šú* Á 150-*šú* ^{GIŠ}GIDRU GAR-*su-ma* IGI^{II}-*šú* GU.MEŠ SIG$_7$.MEŠ DIRI. MEŠ ŠU ^{d}15 GAM (DPS XIII B ii 29–30 = *TDP* 120 ii 29–30)

**If a burning pain is firmly established in his abdomen on the right side and his eyes are full of yellow threads, "hand" of Ištar; he will die.

9.39 DIŠ NA *aḫ-ḫa-zu* IGI^{II}-*šú* E$_{11}$-*a-ma* IGI^{II}-*šú* GU.MEŠ SIG$_7$.MEŠ [*u*]*d-du-ḫa* ŠÀ.MEŠ-*šú na-šu-ú* NINDA *u* KAŠ *ú-tar-ra* NA BI *ú-za-bal-ma* ⸢BA.ÚŠ⸣ (*BAM* 578 iv 43–44)[48]

**If *aḫḫāzu* (jaundice)[49] rises to a person's eyes so that his eyes are ⸢covered⸣ with a network of yellow threads, his insides are puffed up (ascites) (and) return bread and beer (to his mouth), (if) that person lingers, he will die.

9.40 DIŠ NA IGI^{II}-*šú a-mur-ri-qa-nu* DIRI . . . (*BAM* 578 iv 17)[50]

**If a person's eyes are full of *amurriqānu* (jaundice with wasting)[51] . . .

PINGUECULA

Older individuals often develop pingueculae, triangular yellow plaques on the white of the eye on either or both sides of the pupil. These lesions are completely benign and require no treatment. The text below might be describing this condition.

9.41 DIŠ IGI^{II}-*šú* IM.GÁ.LI ŠUB.MEŠ [. . .] (DPS V A 11′ = *TDP* 46 B 11)[52]

**If (both) his eyes are unevenly colored with *kalû*-clay yellow [. . .]

Other possibilities include conjunctivitis with pus of a yellow color, and the late phase of conjunctival hemorrhage.[53]

TEARING

Tearing is due to excess production of tears, generally occurring when the eye is irritated or when the lacrimal duct that drains the tears from the eye is obstructed. The texts below that mention diminished or blurred vision are likely to be in patients with sufficient irritation to the eye to cloud the cornea. If the Ḫammurapi of the third reference is, as seems probable, the king of that name who reigned from 1792 to 1750 B.C.E.,[54] then the treatment dates (or at least claims to date) from the Old Babylonian period.

9.42 DIŠ NA IGI^{II}-*šú* ÍR ŠUB.MEŠ-*a* . . . (*BAM* 22:23′)[55]

**If a person's eyes continually shed tears . . .

9.43 DIŠ NA IGI^{II}-*šú* ÍR *lu-ḫa-a* ŠUB.MEŠ . . . (*BAM* 159 v 3; BM 54641+BM 54826 r. 8)

**If a person's eyes continually shed dirty tears . . .

9.44 DIŠ NA IGI^{II}-*šú a-pa-a a-šá-a u* ÍR ŠUB.ŠUB-*a na-ṭa-la mu-uṭ-ṭu ana* TI-*šú . . . te-qit* IGI^{II}.MEŠ *šá* ^{m}*Ḫa-am-mu-ra-pí lat-ku* (see *BAM* 159 iv 16′–17′, 22′//*AMT* 18/4:1′; *BAM* 521:10′)[56]

**If a person's eyes are clouded, "confused," and continually shed tears (and his) eyesight is diminished, to cure him . . . eye daub of Ḫammurapi; tested.

9.45 DIŠ NA IGI^{II}-*šú bar-ra u* ÍR *ú-kal-la . . .* (*BAM* 159 iv 28′; *SpTU* 2.50:18//BM 54641+BM 54826 r. 4)[57]

**If a person's eyes are/become dimmed and contain tears . . .

FOREIGN BODY IN THE EYE[58]

9.46 *at-*[*ta*] ⸢*i*⸣*-n*[*u-ú*] *pur-*⸢*si*⸣*-*[*m*]*i-it* MÚD *šu-ḫur-ra-tú am-mi-ni ta-aš-ša-ni ḫa-ma ḫa-an-d*[*a-aš-pi-r*]*a šu-ur-šu-ra e-la*!*-pa-a ša* ÍD *ina* SILA.MEŠ *kir-ba-ni ina tub-kí*[*n-na*]*-a-te ḫu-ṣa-a-ba am-mi-ni taš-ša-ni zu-un-na-ni* GIN$_7$ MUL *mi-ta-qu-*⸢*ta*⸣*-ni* GIN$_7$ *nab-li la-am ik-šu-du-ki-na-ši ṣur-ru nag-la-bu šá* ^{d}*Gu-la* . . . § KA.INIM.MA *ḫa-a-mu ḫu-ṣa-ba u mìm-ma ša* IGI^{II} *šu-li-i* (*BAM* 510 iv 34–40//*BAM* 514 iv 39–45)[59]

**⸢You, eyes⸣ covered with ⸢blood vessels⸣ as with a net, why did you carry off chaff, thorns, sharp bits, (and) river algae? Why did you carry off clods from the street (and) litter from the ⸢garbage dumps⸣? Rain down like a star; fall down like ball lightning before the obsidian knife and razor of Gula get you![60] . . . Recitation to remove litter, chaff, or anything else from the eyes.

9.47 IGI^{II} *a-pa-tu* IGI^{II} *a-ša-tu* IGI^{II} *pur-sit* MÚD *šu-te-eṣ-li-pa-a-tu am-mìn tap-pá-a am-mìn taš-šá-a am-ma-ni ik-kal-ki-na-ši ba-a-ṣu ša na-a-ri tal-tal-lu-ú šá* ^{GIŠ}GIŠIMMAR *šá ti-it-tu ni-iq-qa-šá šá za-ri-i* IN.NU-*šu* (*BAM* 514 iii 14′–17′//*BAM* 513 iii 11′–12′//*BAM* 510 iii 9–12)

**"Clouded" eyes, "confused" eyes, eyes crisscrossed with blood vessels, why are you clouded; why are you "confused"? Why do the river's sand, the date palm and the fig tree's pollen, and the winnower's straw hurt you?

9.48 DIŠ N[A IGI]^{II}-*šú* IM *ud-du-pa-a-ma a-pá-a a-š*[*a*]*-*⸢*a*⸣ *u* ÍR ŠUB.ŠUB-*a* . . . (*BAM* 159 iv 11′–12′; *BAM* 518:9′)[61]

**If a ⸢person's eyes⸣ have been blown into by the wind so that they are clouded, ⸢"confused"⸣, and continually shed tears . . .

INGROWN EYELASH

Some eye conditions, especially Hansen's disease (see Chapter 3) and trachoma (*Chlamydia trachomatis*),[62] can cause scarring and distortion of the eyelid. This often causes the eyelashes to grow toward the conjunctiva, resulting in mechanical irritation of the eye.[63] The following quote does not provide enough information to determine the primary cause of this problem.

9.49 DIŠ NA [*ina* UGU I]GI^{II}-*šú* SÍG *a-ṣa-at u* IGI^{II}-*šú a-šá-a* . . . (*BAM* 515 i 17)

**If a hair grows [toward] a person's ⸢eyes⸣ and his eyes are "confused" . . .

STY (HORDEOLUM)

There are glands on the eyelid that may become infected and enlarged to produce a sty. This irritating but benign condition was observed by the *āšipu.*

9.50 KA.INIM.MA *mi-ir-ḫu ša* ŠÀ IGI^{II} *š*[*u-li-i*] . . . (*BAM* 510 iv 46)

**Recitation to ⌜remove⌝ a sty[64] from the eyes . . .

ECTROPION

There are numerous inflammatory conditions of the eyelids that can cause the lids to roll back or retract. This results in exposure of more of the conjunctiva than normal and an inability to close the eye completely. Fincke suggests[65] that the following text may be describing this condition.

9.51 DIŠ IGI^{II}-*šú be-e-r*[*a* . . .] (DPS V F 14 = *TDP* 50 F 14)

**If his eyes leave a space between (the lids)[66] [. . .].

EXTRAOCULAR MUSCLES

The muscles that move the eyeball may be subject to inflammation and paralysis. The texts below suggest the presence of inflammation of the extraocular muscles and the muscles of the neck. Viral and parasitic infections such as influenza and trichinosis are possible causes in these cases.

9.52 DIŠ SAG.KI-*šú* KÚ-*šú ú-maḫ-ḫa-ṣa-šú* SA.MEŠ IGI^{II}-*šú ú-z*[*aq-qa-tu*]-*šú* SA GÚ KÚ.MEŠ-*šú* ŠU GIDIM$_7$ (DPS IV B obv. 34//E i 14–15 = *TDP* 36:35–36//*SpTU* 3.88 i 14–15)[67]

**If his temple hurts him and gives him jabbing pains, his eye muscles ⌜sting⌝ him, (and his) neck muscles hurt him, "hand" of ghost.

9.53 [DIŠ N]A *ina* DIB-*it* ŠU.GIDIM.MA SAG.KI^{II}-*šú* ŠÀ-*ba-šú* IGI.MEŠ-*šú* [*im*]-*maḫ-ḫa-ḫu ú-zaq-qa-ta-šú ù* GÚ-*su* KÚ-*šú* [*ana* T]I-*šú* . . . (*BAM* 216:12′–14′)

** [If], as a result of affliction by "hand" of ghost, a ⌜person⌝'s temples, his abdomen, (and) his eyes [are] "soaked" (and) sting him and his neck hurts him, [to] ⌜cure⌝ him . . .[68]

PERIORBITAL CELLULITIS

Infection of the soft tissues surrounding the eye is a relatively common problem that is often secondary to a sinus infection. The references below could be describing this condition.

9.54 DIŠ NA SAG.KI ZAG/GÙB-*šú* KÚ-*šú-ma* IGI ZAG/150-*šú nap-ḫat ù* ÍR BAL-*qí* ŠU.GIDIM.MA *šá-né* ^{d}EŠ$_4$.DAR *ana* TI-*šú* . . . (*BAM* 482 ii 62′–63′; *AMT* 18/3:6–7)[69]

**If a person's left/right temple hurts him and his left/right eye is swollen and sheds tears, "hand" of ghost, deputy of Ištar; to cure him . . .[70]

9.55 DIŠ SA SAG.KI-*šú šá* 15/150 *ka-bar ma-mál-li-šú* IGI *šá* 15/150 ŠU GIDIM$_7$ (DPS IV E ii 27–28//H 1–2 = *SpTU* 3.88 ii 27–28)

**If the muscle(s) of his left/right temple are evenly thickened (around) the left/right eye, "hand" of ghost.

The quote below could be bilateral periorbital cellulitis, but nonspecific periorbital swelling can occur in many generalized infections.

9.56 DIŠ NA SAG.KI DIB-*su-ma i-mim i-kaṣ-ṣa* IGI^{II}-*šú nu-up-pu-ḫa* ŠU.GIDIM.MA . . . (*BAM* 482 iii 5)[71]

**If a person's temples afflict him and he becomes hot (and then) cold (and) his eyes are swollen, "hand" of ghost . . .

ANKYLOBLEPHARON

For a possible reference to fusion of the eyelids (ankyloblepharon), see Chapter 17.

Corneal Diseases

The cornea is critical in transmitting and focusing light on the retina. Injury or inflammation of the cornea can cause diminished or blurred vision.

SINLURMA

Two opposite problems were included under the term *Sinlurma*.[72] The first, and probably most common condition, is what we call "night blindness." The usual cause is vitamin A deficiency, which can affect both the cornea and retina. This explains why the *āšipu* prescribed eating liver,[73] which has high levels of vitamin A (see also Chapter 7).

9.57 DIŠ NA U$_4$ DÙ.A.BI IGI.DU$_8$ GI$_6$ DÙ.A.BI NU IGI.DU$_8$ ^{d}30-*lu-ur-ma-a* (*BAM* 516 ii 31′)

**If a person can see all day (but) he cannot see all night, *Sinlurma*.

9.58 DIŠ NA IGI^{II}-*šú si-lu-ur-ma-a* . . . *ma-ku-ut ga-bi-di ta-ḫar-ra-aṣ* KÚ . . . (*BAM* 516 ii 32′, iii 1–2//*BAM* 25:4′, 9′)

**If a person's eyes (have) *Sinlurma* . . . you cut off a chunk of liver (and) he eats (it) . . .

The second condition causes reduced vision during the day, but more normal vision at night.[74]

9.59 DIŠ NA U$_4$ DÙ.A.BI NU IGI.DU$_8$ GI$_6$ DÙ.A.BI IGI.DU$_8$ ^{d}30-*lu-ur-ma-a* (*BAM* 516 ii 30′)

**If a person cannot see all day (but) he can see all night, *Sinlurma*.

We believe that this condition is due to corneal scars from past trauma or corneal infection. The reduced daylight vision is due to refraction and distortion of the higher light levels in daytime compared to night. Rare inherited retinal abnormalities can also cause these symptoms.

CORNEAL OPACITIES

Ancient Mesopotamian physicians recognized four different pathological states that were able to distort the normally transparent cornea: *šišītu*, *ṣillu*, *ṣiḫḫu*, and *šīlu*.

ŠIŠĪTU *Šišītu* means "membrane"[75] and represents tissue that grows out over the surface of the cornea.[76] This condition is frequently due to a chronic infection (see below).

9.60 DIŠ NA IGI^{II}-*šú ši-ši-tú* DIRI . . . (*BAM* 23:4//*BAM* 515 ii 67; *BAM* 23:5)[77]

**If a person's eyes are full of membrane . . .

9.61 *ši-ši-tú* ZI-*aḫ* (*BAM* 578 iv 15)

**(If the treatment is performed), the membrane will be removed.

ṢILLU GISSU/*ṣillu* literally means "shadow."[78] In most of the references, this "shadow" is described as a lesion that the *āšipu* could actually see in the patient's eyes. In these cases, the term was probably applied to swelling or inflammation of the external surface of the cornea (see adenovirus and trachoma, below).[79] It may also have been used for deeper, intrinsic scarring of the cornea from trauma or invasive infection.

9.62 *ki-ma* DUG A.GEŠTIN.NA ŠUB-*a ṣil-la* . . . (*BAM* 510 ii 29′//*BAM* 513 ii 44′ (= BM 98942 obv. 5)[80] //*BAM* 514 ii 40′)[81]

**(Eyes) spotted with opaque spots like a pot of vinegar . . .

PTERYGIUM Another type of superficial corneal membrane is a pterygium. This is a membrane that grows on the corneal surface but infrequently crosses the pupil and therefore usually does not affect the patient's vision. It is probably caused by chronic corneal irritation, since it commonly occurs in hot, dry, and sunny environments such as exist in Mesopotamia. It is opaque and varies in color from white to tan or, if irritated, bright red. The reference below may be describing a patient with a pterygium.[82]

9.63 DIŠ NA IGI^{II}-*šú* GISSU KALAG.GA *ina* ŠU^{II} ^{LÚ}A.ZU NU DU$_8$ GUR.GUR-*šú* . . . (*BAM* 22:12′–13′)[83]

**If there is a strong opaque spot that does not go away despite treatment by the *asû* (pharmacist) but keeps coming back . . .

Another "shadow" that the *āšipu* may have seen in a patient's eyes were cataracts. This abnormality does not involve the cornea, but is due to reduced light transmission of the more internally located lens. It is quite likely that cataracts were found in ancient Mesopotamia, especially in older patients, but the *āšipu* might not have understood the anatomical differences between the lens and cornea. It is quite possible that some of the shadows described in the references were due to cataracts.

ṢIḪḪU[84] AND *ŠĪLU* *Ṣiḫḫu* is an indentation or ulcer (see below) and *šīlu* an actual hole in the eye.[85] The texts below do not indicate the location of the *šīlu*. Fincke[86] suggests that they are specifically describing a hole in the iris (coloboma) that will cause a distortion of the pupil.[87] Alternatively, the perforation could be in the cornea, which might also cause an abnormal shape of the pupil (iris prolapse). Perforation of the cornea is a much more serious condition than a corneal ulcer, since it permits the fluid in the anterior chamber to escape and also to become secondarily infected. A corneal perforation, if untreated, may lead to adherence of the iris to the cornea (anterior synechia—possibly the "drawing taut" of the second reference). Perforation may be caused by trauma or an aggressive eye infection.

9.64 DIŠ NA IGI^{II}-*šú* GIG-*ma ši-lu* DUL . . . (*BAM* 513 i 6′)

**If a person's eyes are sore and a perforation closes (them) . . .

9.65 DIŠ NA *ši-li* IGI^{II}-*šú šad-du-ma* KI.NÁ NU ÍL . . . (*BAM* 516 ii 27′)

**If a perforation draws a person's eyes taut so that he cannot stand the bed . . .[88]

INFECTIOUS CAUSES OF CORNEAL OPACITIES

Although there are many possible reasons for corneal opacities to develop, one common cause is an adenovirus infection involving the conjunctiva and cornea.

ADENOVIRUS Adenovirus types 8 and 19 are the most likely to cause this problem. This highly contagious form of "pink eye" not only inflames the conjunctiva but also the cornea, resulting in corneal clouding. Photophobia and pain are common symptoms. The blurred and distorted vision may take months to return to normal. Another infectious cause is *Chlamydia trachomatis*, but the corneal opacities produced by trachoma are not likely to be reversible.

9.66 DIŠ NA IGI^{II}-*šú a-šá-a bir-ra-tú u ri-šu-t*[*ú*] *ú-kal-la* . . . (*BAM* 159 v 7–8)

**If a person's eyes are "confused" and contain dimness and redness . . .

9.67 DIŠ NA IGI^{II}-*šú* GIG-*ma* MÚD DIRI ^{ŠEM}BULUḪ.ḪI.A BAD *ul-ta-ta-ni-ʾ* BAD ÍR *ina* ŠÀ IGI^{II}-*šú* È-*a* GISSU ^{d}LAMMA IGI^{II}-*šú ú-na-kap a-ši-tu ana* GISSU GUR *di-kal*[89] DUGUD-*šú* . . . (BAM 514 ii 27′–28′ // *BAM* 510 ii 16′–17′ // *BAM* 513 ii 31′)

**If a person's eyes are sore and full of blood (and) either[90] he has been continually suffusing (them) with *baluḫḫu,* or tears come from his eyes, an opaque spot abuts his cornea,[91] "confusion" of vision turns into opaque spots (and) seeing is difficult for him . . .

9.68 DIŠ NA IGI^{II}-*šú* GIG-*ma* U$_4$.MEŠ *ma-ʾ-du-ti* NU BAD-*te ina* KÚM SAG.DU-*šú* IGI^{II}-*šú* GISSU DIRI . . . (*BAM* 159 iv 2′–3′//*BAM* 510 i 18′//*BAM* 513 i 8′//*BAM* 515 ii 45–46//*BAM* 20:11′–13′)

**If a person's eyes are so sore that he does not open them for many days (and) during a fever in his head his eyes fill with opaque spots . . .

CHLAMYDIA TRACHOMATIS The corneal membrane damage in the reference below is likely to be due to *Chlamydia trachomatis.* This type of lesion usually does not resolve spontaneously.

9.69 DIŠ N[A IGI^{II}]-*šú* GIG-*ma ši-ši-tu* UGU ^{d}LAMMA IGI^{II}-*šú* ⌜x x⌝ ÍR.ḪI.A DU-*ak* IGI^{II}-*šú* GISSU DIRI . . . (*BAM* 515 ii 49)[92]

**If a ⌜person's⌝ [eyes] are sore and there is a membrane over his corneas [. . .] tears flow (and) his eyes are full of opaque spots . . .

HERPES SIMPLEX VIRUS DENDRITIC ULCER HSV1 can cause a chronic corneal ulcer with visual distortion. We believe that the following text describes such a case.

9.70 DIŠ NA IGI^{II}-*šú* GIG-*ma ši-ši-tú* UGU ^{d}L[AMMA IGI . . .] *šú-ma* DUGUD *ana* TI-*šú* . . . DIŠ NA IGI^{II}-*šú* MÚ-*aḫ* GISSU *ša* 7 ITU 18 ITU *ṣi-ḫa-ti* . . . (*BAM* 23:1–3//*BAM* 515 ii 65–66)

**If a person's eyes are sore and there is a membrane over the ⌜cornea⌝ [. . .] and it is difficult [for him to see], to cure him . . . If the person's eyes are swollen, there will be an opaque spot for seven months and *ṣiḫḫus* (corneal ulcers) for eighteen months . . .

OPHTHALMIA NEONATORUM For possible examples of this superficial eye infection that is acquired by the newborn from the mother's birth canal during delivery and that can cause scarring, membrane formation, and blindness, see Chapter 17.

Internal Eye Problems

IRIS — COLOR CHANGES

The references below describe changes in the color of the iris in one or both eyes.[93] Black and dark colors in this location can be caused by melanoma involving the iris or by a benign nevus that forms on the iris.[94]

9.71 DIŠ SA *kak-kul-ti* IGI 15/150-*šú* GI$_6$.MEŠ [. . .] (DPS V G 14–15 = *TDP* 52 G 14–15)[95]

**If the muscle(s) of the iris[96] of his left/right eye are black [. . .].

9.72 DIŠ SA *kak-kul-ti* IGI 15/150-*šú tar-ku* [. . .] (DPS V G 17–18 = *TDP* 52 G 17–18)

**If the muscle(s) of the iris of his left/right eye are dark [. . .].

IRITIS

Fincke[97] suggests that the following text may be referring to iritis, since the blood vessels in this condition radiate out from the center of the cornea in a fashion suggestive of a spider's web. Iritis is an inflammatory condition of the iris and surrounding structures that can be caused by many infections and immunologic processes.

9.73 DIŠ SA IGI^{II}-*šú* GIN$_7$ *ši-te-e* [. . .] ŠU DINGIR-*šú lu* ŠU DINGIR UR[U-*šú*][98] (DPS V G 11–12 = *TDP* 52 G 11–12)

**If the blood vessel(s) of his eyes are [. . .] like a spider's web, "hand" of his god or "hand" of the god of [his] ⌜city⌝.

ANNULAR POSTERIOR SYNECHIA

Fincke[99] interprets the following text to represent annular posterior synechia, and we concur. This is a condition where the iris is adherent and fixed to the lens.[100] Glaucoma (see below) and blindness are likely outcomes if the condition is left untreated. The "grapes of the eyes pulled taut" mentioned in the references below are almost certainly describing the increased tension within the eye caused by glaucoma. This can be determined by the physician's thumb pressing on the eye.

9.74 DIŠ KI.MIN-*ma ka-ra-an* IGI^{II}-*šú* *š*[*ád*(?)-*du* . . .][101] (DPS XXI:3 [AOAT 43.246])

**If (his blood vessels are healthy) but the "grape(s)" of his eyes are pulled taut [. . .].

9.75 *ka-ra-an* IGI^{II}-*šú šad-du* [. . .] *šá kak-kul-tu*$_4$ *i-ni-šú a-na bi-ta-nu i-ru-*[*bu*] (Leichty, *AfO* 24.82-86:3–4)

**The "grapes" of his eyes are pulled taut. [. . .] (That means that) his irises go inside.

9.76 *ka-ra-an* IGI^{II}-*šú šad-du šá kak-kul-tu*$_4$ *i-ni-šú ú-ṣa-a* : ÚR-*šú ta-a-ka šá ana da-ke-e u šá-ka-nu dan-na niš-šú šá ši-kin-ni là iš-nu-ú* (*SpTU* 1.40 obv. 8–11 [commentary to DPS XXI:3 [AOAT 43.246])

**The "grape(s)" of his eyes are pulled taut. (That means that) his iris sticks out (and) its "lap" is . . .[102] (It means an iris) that is (too) thick/hard for lifting up and putting down (and) that (when) he looks (at something) it does not change shape.

The reference to "lifting up and putting down" in the preceding quote indicates that the *āšipu* was aware that the iris dilates and constricts the pupil. The iris accomplishes this by virtue of two muscles. It is perhaps these muscles to which the expression SA.MEŠ *kak-kul-ti* IGI: "muscles of the iris of the eye" refers.[103]

XANTHOGRANULOMA OF THE IRIS

The following reference mentions a *pindû* of the iris. In references to *pindû* of the skin (see Chapter 10 with 10.126), we suggest that these raised, red, granular lesions might be cavernous hemangiomas. When *pindû*-lesions occur on the iris, Fincke[104] gives a tentative diagnosis of xanthogranuloma. It is probable that other diseases such as syphilis and tuberculosis could cause similar lesions.[105]

9.77 DIŠ (*pi-in-du*) *ina ka-kul-ti* IGI-*šú* ZAG/GÙB GAR . . . (Böck, *Morphoskopie* 196:14–15)

**If there is a *pindû* on the iris of his left/right eye . . .

ANTERIOR CHAMBER

The *āšipu* would not have been able to see behind the iris, but the anterior chamber of the eye (between the cornea and the iris) is normally filled with clear, colorless fluid that can be easily seen with the naked eye.

FLOATERS If the anterior chamber fluid gets contaminated with red or white blood cells or other debris, they can float in the fluid and be seen as spots moving over the field of vision. The texts below describe floaters.

9.78 DIŠ NA [IGI^{II}]-*šú* UZU *a-li-kam* DIRI-*a* . . . (*BAM* 515 i 19)[106]

**If a person's [eyes] are full of moving tissue . . .

9.79 DIŠ NA IGI^{II}-*šú* UZU DU-*kam* DIRI-*ma u* DU-*ak ana* TI-*šú* . . . (*BAM* 515 i 22//*BAM* 22:4′)

**If a person's eyes are full of moving tissue and it moves, to cure him . . .[107]

9.80 DIŠ NA IGI^{II}-*šú* UZU *u* MÚD DIRI.MEŠ . . . (*BAM* 515 i 25//*BAM* 22:9′)

**If a person's eyes are full of tissue and blood . . .

9.81 DIŠ NA *ina* ŠÀ IGI^{II}-*šú* GISSU *lu* U[ZU] DU-*ku* GAR-*ma da-ga-šu* NU KAL . . . (*BAM* 22:16′–17′)

**If there is an opaque spot or moving ⌜tissue⌝ in a person's eye but the stinging? is not fierce . . .

BLOOD AND SEDIMENT IN THE ANTERIOR CHAMBER There are texts (see below) that mention blood and sediment in the eye. It seems very likely that the *āšipu* was describing blood, white blood cells, or debris that was of sufficient amount that it could be seen layering out or filling the anterior chamber. If the anterior chamber is filled with blood or pus, the patient's vision will be severely distorted or even lost.

9.82 DIŠ NA IGI^{II}-*šú* MÚD *iṭ-ri* . . . (*BAM* 22:25′)[108]

**If blood penetrates a person's eyes . . .[109]

9.83 DIŠ NA IGI^{II}-*šú šik-na šá* MÚD *šak-na* . . . (*BAM* 22:27′)

**If a person's eyes have blood clots in them . . .

9.84 DIŠ NA IGI^{II}-*šú* MÚD DIRI-*ma ur-ra u* GI$_6$ *la i-ṣal-*[*lal la i-na*]*-ṭal šum*$_4$*-ma* ŠÀ IGI^{II}-*šú* SA$_5$ IGI^{II}-*šú* DUL-*ma* . . . (*BAM* 510 i 31′–32′//*BAM* 514 i 38′–39′)[110]

**If a person's eyes are full of blood and he cannot ⸢sleep⸣ day or night [(and) he cannot] ⸢see?⸣, if the inside of his eyes is red (and) he also closes his eyes . . .

The sedimentation of these cells in the anterior chamber is suggestive of layers of silt, which may be why the pus is referred to as "fine clay" in the following references. In the first reference below, the cause was clearly trauma, but infection can also fill the chamber with pus.

9.85 DIŠ IGI^{II}-*šú pa-ʾa-ṣa-ma* IM.G[Ú DIRI . . .] (DPS V A 8′ = *TDP* 46 B 8)[111]

**If his eyes were smashed and [are full] of "⸢fine clay⸣" [. . .]

9.86 DIŠ U$_4$.6.KÁM GIG-⸢*ma ina* U$_4$.7⸣.[KÁM DIN GIG TI U$_4$-*ma* TI GIG IGI]⸢II⸣-*šú* IM.GÚ DIRI.DIRI.MEŠ MÚD *ina* KIR$_4$-*šú* DU-*ku-ma* DIN (DPS XVI:72′ [AOAT 43.178])[112]

**If he has been sick for six days and on the seventh, [he gets well (and) he recovers from the illness (but) when he has recovered, he gets sick (again and)] his ⸢eyes⸣ are continually full of "fine clay," (if) blood flows from his nose, he will get well.

9.87 *e-na-a-šu qá-du-ti sà-a-mi ma-a-li* [. . .] (StBoT 36.23 r. 5′b)

**(If) his eyes are full of "fine red clay" [. . .]

GLAUCOMA

Fincke suggests[113] that the "beautiful eye" mentioned in the following reference is buphthalmos, a form of glaucoma that is congenital or occurs in early infancy. It often leads to blindness, but it also produces very large eyes that many people find attractive (as in the English expression "cow-eyed beauty").[114]

9.88 BAD MUNUS *dam-qá-mi-nam* Ù.TU . . . (Šumma Izbu I 75 [Leichty, *Izbu* 38])

**If a woman gives birth to a "beautiful-eye". . . [115]

One of the commentaries[116] equates this "beautiful eye" with *ṣuḫḫutu*, which means "squeezed" or "pressed." In the following reference, drawn from a therapeutic text, an adult patient is also described as having "squeezed" eyes.

9.89 DIŠ NA IGI^{II}-*šú ṣu-uḫ-ḫu-ta* . . . (*BAM* 515 i 63′)

**If a person's eyes (feel) squeezed . . .

Since the eyeball in glaucoma is under greater pressure than a normal eye, and since it is possible for a practiced physician to detect this difference by feeling the eyeball, it is conceivable that the *āšipu* was describing patients with glaucoma when he spoke of "squeezed" eyes.

OPTIC NEUROPATHY

In the following references, the eye is said to "make" or "cause" a *ṣillu*: "shadow" (see above). What is probably being described is some form of transient monocular blindness or retrobulbar optic neuropathy. The former is often described by patients as a "shade" that falls smoothly and painlessly over the field of vision and the latter as a "veil" or "haze" covering every object seen.

9.90 DIŠ U_4.2.KÁM GIG-*ma* SAG.KI-*šú šá* 15 KÚ-*šú* IGI-*šú šá* 15 GISSU DÙ ŠU ^{d}UD.AL.TAR BÚR-*ma* DIN / DIŠ U_4.2.KÁM GIG-*ma* SAG.KI-*šú šá* 150 KÚ-*šú* IGI-*šú šá* 150 GISSU DÙ ŠU ^{d}UD.AL.TAR BÚR-*ma* DIN (DPS XVI:21–22 [AOAT 43.174])[117]

**If he has been sick for two days and his left/right temple hurts him and his left/right eye makes a "shadow," "hand" of Dapinu. (If) it goes away, he will get well.

9.91 DIŠ SAG.KI-*šú šá* 15 *u* 150 KÚ.MEŠ-*šú* IGI^{II}-*šú šá* 15 *u* 150 GISSU DÙ-*a* LÚ.BI DINGIR-*šú u* DINGIR URU-*šú iz-zur ik-ri-ba*! *ana* DINGIR-*šú iq-bi* BÚR-*ma* DIN (DPS IV B obv. 29//E i 9 = *TDP* 36:29–30//*SpTU* 3.88 i 9)[118]

**If his left and right temple hurt him and his left and right eye make a "shadow," he cursed his god and the god of his city; he made a vow to his god. (If) it goes away, he will get well.

VISION

Many texts mention reduced or distorted vision, but there is one reference that documents farsightedness or excellent long-distance vision. Modern distance equivalents are based on the calculations of Powell.[119]

9.92 DIŠ LÚ *iš-tu* 1 UŠ *ana* 30 GAR LÚ *ú-we-ed-di* (Köcher and Oppenheim, *AfO* 18.65 ii 14 [physiognomic omens])

**If a person recognizes (another) person from a distance of 1 UŠ (356 m) to 30 GAR (178 m).

Ear Diseases

The most common ear problems in ancient Mesopotamia appear to have been due to trauma and infection. Abnormal sound perception and deafness were frequent outcomes, and serious illness and death were not unusual, due in large part to the proximity of the ear to the brain.

TRAUMA

A head wound can cause hearing loss by either ear damage or brain injury. The text below that ends in death more than likely represents a brain injury. The quote that mentions bleeding from the ears could be due to trauma or to some clotting problems.

9.93 DIŠ *ina* U[G]U-*šú* SÌG-*ma* GEŠTU^{II}-*šú* NU ŠE.GA-*a* ŠU ^{d}15 *ana* AŠ-*tim* (DPS III A obv. 19//C obv. 10 = *TDP* 18:10; cf. StBoT 36.35 r. 1//StBoT 36.57 r. 8′)

**If he was wounded on his ⸢skull⸣ and consequently his ears do not hear, "hand" of Ištar . . .

9.94 DIŠ *ina* SAG.DU-*šú* SÌG-*iṣ-ma ḫa-si-si-šú* ⸢*kùd*?-*du*?[120]⸣-*ta-at* ⸢GEŠTU^{II}? xxxxxxxx ŠU⸣ DINGIR *šag-gaš-šú na-kud* GAM (DPS III C r. 20 = *TDP* 26:80)

**If he was wounded on his head and, as a consequence, his hearing is low (and) his ears [. . .], "hand" of a murderous god; it is serious; he will die.

9.95 DIŠ GEŠTU^{II}-*šú* DU$_8$.DU$_8$-*ra* GAM (DPS VIII 7b = *TDP* 68:7b)[121]

**If (both) his ears were (broken) open, he will die.

9.96 DIŠ NA *ana* ŠÀ GEŠTU^{II}-*šú* MÚD DU-*ak*/MÚD *ina* GEŠTU-*šú* DU-*ak* . . . (*BAM* 3 iv 23//*CTN* 4.113 ii 21)

**If blood runs from(!) inside a person's ears . . .

"WIND BLASTING"

As stated earlier (Chapter 4), the term *wind blasting* is often associated with the presence of small water blisters (vesicles). The presence of these lesions on one ear is compatible with the recurrent form of chickenpox (*Varicella zoster*) virus, which is usually called shingles.

9.97 DIŠ NA GEŠTU^{II} ZAG-*šú* IM *iš-biṭ-ma* DUGUD *ana* T[I-*šú*] . . . (Labat, *RSO* 32.112 iv 6′)

**If "wind" blasts his left ear and, as a consequence, it (feels) heavy, to ⸢cure him⸣ . . .[122]

EAR WAX

Excessive buildup of ear wax can lead to obstruction of the ear canal, discomfort, and decreased hearing ability. The Akkadian term for ear wax was literally "ear shit" (*zê uzni*). One mystical miscellany, which describes various parts of a god by equating them with actual plants or objects, compares his beard to a palm frond, his penis to a snake, his heart to a kettledrum, his fingers to reeds, his irises to grapes, and his "ear shit" to lead.[123]

9.98 GEŠTU^{II}-*a-a šá uṭ-ṭa-am-mi-ma us-sa-ki-ka ḫa-šik-kiš it-bal a-mi-ra-šin ip-te-ti neš-ma-a* (Lambert, *BWL* 52:18–19)

**My ears that were clogged and obstructed like (those of) a deaf person, he removed their obstruction (and) opened up my hearing.

9.99 *a-me-ra ze-e uz-ni* (Ludlul Commentary to *BWL* 52:19)

**Obstruction (means) ear wax.

9.100 U$_4$ GIG GEŠTU.MEŠ-*šu sú-uk-ku-ka-ma la i-še-em-ma-a* . . . (*MDP* 57.11 vi 7′–8′)[124]

**If the patient's ears are stopped up so that he cannot hear . . .

OTITIS EXTERNA

The ear canal that leads from the outside to the eardrum can become infected. This infection may cause obstruction of the ear canal, reduced hearing, and if persistent may lead to meningitis or brain abscess (see Chapter 13). When a central nervous system infection occurs, without antibiotic therapy, death would be likely. In some of the references below we cannot be certain that the patient did not have otitis media (middle ear infection) rather than otitis externa.

9.101 DIŠ NA *ina* ŠÀ GEŠTU-*šú lu* A.MEŠ *lu* MÚD *lu* MÚD.BABBAR DU-*ak* . . . (*BAM* 503 iii 42′)

**If either liquid or blood or pus flows from a person's ear . . .

9.102 DIŠ NA GEŠTU ZAG-*šú* TAG-*su* IM DIRI-*at u* MÚ.MEŠ . . . (*AMT* 105/1 iv 7//Labat, *RSO* 32.112 v 18′)[125]

**If a person's left ear hurts him intensely, is full of "clay" (thick pus), and is swollen . . .

9.103 DIŠ GIG *mar-ṣu ina* U$_4$-*mi šá* GIG-*su* Ú.ḪÚB-*ma* SU-*šú* K[Ú-*šú* . . .] (Labat, *Syria* 33.124 obv. 20)

**If a patient is sick (and) on the day he becomes ill (his ears) are obstructed and his body ⌜hurts⌝ [him . . .].

OTITIS MEDIA

When the middle ear (the portion of the ear within the eardrum and adjacent to the inner ear) becomes infected, it causes pain, hearing loss, and general signs of infection. It can cause rupture of the eardrum with drainage of pus from the ear. This problem is seen most commonly in early childhood, but can occur in adults.[126]

9.104 DI[Š N]A KÚM *ana* ŠÀ GEŠTU^{II}-*šú i-pu-uš-ma neš-mu-šú* DUGUD *ù lu* IR *ú-kal*... (*BAM* 503 ii 58′)[127]

**⌜If⌝ fever spreads into a ⌜person's⌝ ears and, as a consequence, his hearing (feels) heavy or (his ears) contain sweat . . .

9.105 DIŠ NA GEŠTU^{II}-*šú* KÚ.MEŠ-*šú neš-ma-a ḫe-e-si* . . . (Labat, *RSO* 32.112 ii 11)[128]

**If a person's ears continually hurt him (and) his hearing is pressured . . .

9.106 DIŠ NA GEŠTU^{II}-*šú* GIN$_7$ ŠU.GIDIM.MA KÚ.MEŠ-*šú ù* SÌG.SÌG-*su* . . . (*BAM* 3 iv 12//*BAM* 503 ii 63′//Labat, *RA* 53.12–13 r. 18; cf. *RA* 53.12–13 r. 22)

**If inside a person's ears it continually hurts him and continually gives him a jabbing pain like (an attack) of "hand" of ghost . . .

9.107 [DIŠ NA GEŠTU ZA]G/GÙB-*šú* IR *ana qer-bi-nu ip-ḫur-⌜ma⌝* MÚD.BABBAR ŠUB-*ni* . . . (*BAM* 503 iii 72′, 75′)[129]

**[If a person]'s ⌜left⌝/right [ear] collects sweat on the inside and produces pus . . .

9.108 ⌜DIŠ⌝ NA MÚD.BABBAR *ina* ŠÀ GEŠTU^{II}-*šú* DU-*ak* . . . (*BAM* 503 iii 39′, cf. ii 72′)[130]

**If pus flows from a person's ears . . .

9.109 DIŠ NA GEŠTU^{II}-*šú* MÚD.BABBAR *ú-kal-la ana* TI-*šú* . . . (*BAM* 3 iv 20//*BAM* 410 obv. 5′//Labat, *RA* 53.12–13 r. 25//*CTN* 4.113 ii 16; Labat, *RSO* 32.112 ii 8)

**If a person's ears contain pus, to cure him . . .

9.110 *lip-pi šá* GEŠTU^{II} *šá* MÚD.BABBAR . . . (BM 59593:18)[131]

**Tampon for the ears for pus . . .

Some texts mention ear infections that have pus that "stinks." These are likely to be infections with anaerobic bacteria.

9.111 DIŠ NA GEŠTU^{II}-*šú* GIG-*ma* ŠÀ GEŠTU^{II}-*šú bi-iš* SÌG.SÌG-*su u* KÚ-*šú-ma la* NÁ-*lal* . . . (*BAM* 3 iv 14)[132]

**If a person's ears are sore[133] and the inside of his ears stinks (and) it continually gives him a jabbing pain and hurts him so badly that he cannot sleep . . .

MASTOIDITIS

The bone behind the ears is normally full of air-containing chambers. Chronic middle ear infection may cause infection and swelling of the mastoid with bone infection and fluid (pus) filling the air chambers. This typically causes the external ear to be pushed forward. We suspect that the *āšipu* was describing mastoiditis in the following quote.

9.112 DIŠ GEŠTU^{II}-*šú it-ta-na-az-qa-pa* ŠU GÍDIM (DPS VIII 17a = *TDP* 70:17a)

**If his ears continually stand up, "hand" of ghost.

ABNORMAL OR DISTORTED HEARING

EUSTACHIAN TUBE INFLAMMATION OR OBSTRUCTION When the tube that leads from the throat to the middle ear (eustachian tube) becomes inflamed and swollen due to a throat infection or allergy, the air pressure in the middle ear can vary rapidly, causing popping or crackling noises. The unexplained nature of these sounds caused the *āšipu* to attribute the phenomenon to ghosts.

9.113 [DI]Š GEŠTU^{II}-*šú i-az-za-za* ŠU GÍDIM (DPS VIII 17b = *TDP* 70:17b)[134]

**⌜If⌝ his ears make strange noises, "hand" of ghost.

TINNITUS (RINGING IN THE EARS) A spontaneous and often persistent ringing in one or both ears is a common complaint. This usually occurs in older adults and can be caused by a tumor of the eighth nerve (acoustic neuroma). More commonly, however, it is idiopathic and benign. The *āšipu* used two different terms, *šagāmu* and *šasû*, to describe ringing in the ears. As with terms used to describe loss of vision (see above), this pair of terms probably reflects a difference in the severity of ringing experienced by the patient.

9.114 DIŠ NA GEŠTU^{II}-*šú i-šag-gu-ma* . . . (*BAM* 503 i 38′, 40′; *BAM* 506:31′; *AMT* 37/8:4′)[135]

**If a person's ears roar . . .[136]

9.115 GEŠTU^{II}-*šú iš-ta-na-as-sà*! ŠU.GIDIM.MA (*SpTU* 3.100:13, cf. 12; *SpTU* 1.49:34)

** (If) his ears continually ring,[137] "hand" of ghost.

9.116 DIŠ GEŠTU^{II}-*šú* GÙ.GÙ.MEŠ GIG-*su* DUGUD (DPS VIII 9 = *TDP* 68:9)[138]

**If (both) his ears continually ring, his illness will be difficult.

MÉNIÈRE'S SYNDROME In the inner ear, sound is converted to nervous impulses that are then transmitted to the brain. The inner ear is also important in maintaining balance. Patients with Ménière's syndrome have an inner ear disease that causes acute attacks of ringing and roaring in the ears, hearing loss, and severe vertigo (dizziness). This condition, although not fatal, can be extremely distressing to the patient. Below is a reference to patients who are likely to have had Ménière's syndrome because they have both "roaring in the ears" and "spinning" (vertigo).

9.117 *šum$_4$-ma* NA IGI.MEŠ-*šú* NIGIN.DU-*šú* GEŠTU.MEŠ-*šú i-šá-gu-ma* UZU.MEŠ-*šú šim-ma-ta* TUKU.TUKU-*ú* ŠÀ-*šú it-ta-na-ad-láḫ* GAR-*in* GIG-*šú* NU ZU.ZU NA BI *ka-šip* NU.MEŠ-*šú* DÙ.MEŠ-*ma ina* KI GUL.MEŠ *ana* ^{d}EREŠ.KI.GAL *pa-aq-du* . . . (*BAM* 214 i 1–9)

**If a person's face seems continually to be spinning, his ears roar, his flesh is continually numb, his heart is continually troubled, (and) the appearance of his illness is mysterious, that person is hexed, figurines of him were manufactured and in a place of desolation they were entrusted to Ereškigal . . .

ENCEPHALITIS Distorted hearing may be associated with more serious problems. For a discussion of (meningo)encephalitis, see Chapter 13.

Diseases of the Nose

Many of the illnesses that affect the nose are systemic problems that are discussed in other chapters. The conditions to be considered here are common colds, allergies, and simple nosebleeds. Various treatments were available for the ubiquitous stuffed-up, "heavy" nose or head.

9.118 DIŠ NA KIR$_4$/KA-*šú* DUGUD . . . (BAM 547 iv 14′; *BAM* 543 iv 59′; *BAM* 548 iv 13'; cf. *AMT* 49/1 iv 12′)[139]

**If a person's nose/mouth (feels) heavy . . .[140]

9.119 DIŠ NA SAG.DU-*su* DUGUD *ana* DIN-*šú* . . . (*BAM* 3 ii 43//*BAM* 480 iv 23)[141]

**If a person's head (feels like it) is heavy, to cure him . . .

9.120 DIŠ *na-ḫi-ra-šú* DIB.DIB-ta_5 [. . .] (DPS VI B_4 r. 1//C ii 11 = *TDP* 58 r. 1)[142]

**If his nostrils are continually stopped up [. . .].

Nosebleeds are common in the current era and were likely to have been common in ancient Mesopotamia as well. They are due to multiple etiologies including trauma, dry air causing the nasal lining to crack and bleed, and inflammation of the nasal lining from colds and allergies. In the first reference below, the patient's nose is not simply bleeding profusely or blocked with blood clots, but also swollen, possibly due to trauma.

9.121 [DIŠ NA B]ÀD KIR_4-*šú nu-up-pu-uḫ* [xxx] MÚD *i-ḫa-ḫum lu-ú i-pu-qu ana* TI.LA-*šú* . . . (BM 55352:1–3)

**[If] the ⌜side⌝ of [a person's] nose is all swollen (and) [his nostrils?] discharge blood or have become solid(?), to cure him . . .

9.122 KA.INIM MÚD *ina* KIR_4-*šú šur-du-ma* DU-*ku*! . . . (*SpTU* 4.129 vi 28)[143]

**Recitation (for cases where) blood flows freely from his nose . . .

9.123 MÚD KIR_4 KUD-*su* . . . SA KIR_4 TÉŠ *ka-ṣir-ma* [. . .] (*BAM* 524 ii 4′, 6′)[144]

**(You perform such and such a treatment and) the blood from the nose will be cut off . . . the blood vessel of his nose will be knotted together so that [blood no longer flows].

The term *umṣātu*-lesion was used primarily for hemorrhoids (see Chapter 6). However, in the reference below, it was also used to identify something in the nose that is exuding some substance.

9.124 DIŠ NA *na-ḫi-ri-šú um-ṣa-at ḫi-li it-tab-ši* . . . (*SpTU* 1.44:34)

**If there is an exuding *umṣātu*-lesion in a person's nostrils . . .

The *umṣātu* in the nostrils was probably a nasal turbinate. Nasal turbinates normally serve to warm inhaled air. In allergies due to inhaled substances such as pollen, however, the turbinates may become enlarged and covered with mucus. It seems likely that the *āšipu* saw a resemblance between the appearance of hemorrhoids and enlarged nasal turbinates. In some allergic conditions, nasal polyps may enlarge and have an appearance similar to hemorrhoidal tissue.

Summary

The eyes, ears, and nose are important and sensitive structures that are also very vulnerable to trauma and infections. The dry, hot, and windy conditions that prevailed in much of ancient Mesopotamia would have been additional factors contributing to eye, ear, and nose problems. The physicians of this period displayed an extensive experience with these diseases.

CHAPTER 10

Skin and Hair

If a person's head is feverish and the ⌜hair⌝ of his head
falls out, to [remove] the fever of his head and to make the hair,
which is going, stand firm . . .
—*BAM* 480 iii 22

Skin

Modern physicians consider the skin to be the window of the body because so many diseases leave important clues on its surface. It is clear from reviewing ancient Mesopotamian medical literature that *āšipu*s had reached the same conclusion. The number and variety of signs and symptoms relating to the skin that they described exceed those assigned to any other organ.

The population of ancient Mesopotamia was a mixed one, including by the first millennium B.C.E. not only Sumerians and Akkadians but also Hurrians, Arameans, and a host of other population groups including some Indo-Europeans. The origin of the Sumerians is hotly disputed, but if they were Dravidians from the Indus valley, as some scholars have argued, then they would have been black-skinned. Since the inhabitants of southern Mesopotamia in the early periods seem to have shaved off their beards and head hair (see below), the expression "black-headed people" which the Mesopotamians used to describe themselves may originally have referred to dark skin color. Akkadians and Arameans came from the homeland of Semitic peoples (usually placed in the Syrian desert). They were presumably of medium complexion with dark hair and brown eyes, like modern Arabs. Texts dealing with nutritional deficiencies speak of the hair turning red (see 7.8–7.9), a good indication that black was the normal hair color. Physiognomic omens describe persons with a variety of possible skin and hair colors. For example, *burruqu* (attested also as a nickname) meant a person with a reddish face and thick red hair.[1]

Sumerian dress, if accurately represented in statuary, wall plaques, and the Ur Standard, left a great deal of the male torso exposed to sun and wind. Later fashions seem to have corrected this tendency; Assyrian reliefs show soldiers with all but their lower arms and legs covered by their tunics. Still, sun and wind must have taken their tolls on ancient skins; soldiers boasted of braving mountain roads "where the body of him who passes along is blasted by the fierce wind and his flesh is burned by the cold."[2] Ancient bodies itched with lice (see Chapter 2) and ancient scribes catalogued at least five types of flies[3] in addition to a wide variety of other insects.

To protect themselves, ancient Mesopotamians wielded fly whisks and rubbed themselves with "oil, the pride of mankind, which soothes the muscles."[4] The wild man, Enkidu, who had to be taught the ways of civilization, "rubbed himself with oil and turned into a human being."[5] This was often just vegetable oil, but ancient Mesopotamians knew how to make oils perfumed with cedar, myrtle, and other aromatics. Sorcerers were reputed to take advantage of this habit by adding poison to the oil, which was then absorbed through the victim's skin (see Chapter 15).

Included in the following references are over fifty terms for different types of skin lesions and skin conditions. There was also a general term for abnormalities in the skin, GIG/*simmu*, which was used with nonspecific treatments for skin conditions.[6]

10.1 Ú GIG DÙ.A.BI SIG . . . (*BAM* 380:8//*STT* 92 iii 23′; *STT* 92 iii 18′)[7]

**Plant good for any kind of sore . . .

SKIN ABNORMALITIES

Some terms, such as *rišiktu*, *ruṭibtu*, *rišūtu*, *munû*, *šibiṭ šāri*, *ripḫu*, *tabku*, *ramû*, *kiṣṣatu*, and *ekketu*, appear to describe the texture or appearance of the affected area. Was it dry or oozing, red or swollen, indurated (hard) or relaxed, or sweaty? Had the hair fallen out? Had the patient been scratching it?

RIŠIKTU (DRYNESS) Skin with dry patches[8] and scaling was called *rišiktu*. Psoriasis is one of many possible causes.

10.2 [DIŠ GIG GA]R-*šú* GIN_7 BAR KU_6 SU-*šú* DIRI *u a-dan-na* TUKU *ri-*[*šik-t*]*um*[9] MU.NI (DPS XXXIII:11 [AOAT 43.353])

**[If the] ⌜nature⌝ of the [sore] is that his body is full of what look like fish scales and it has a predictable course, it is called ⌜*rišiktu*⌝.

10.3 Ú UZU.MEŠ *ša ri-šik-ta* TUKU.MEŠ . . . (*BAM* 1 iii 30//*CT* 14.43 [S. 60]:7′)[10]

**Plant for flesh that continually has *rišiktu* . . .

In the following reference, *rišiktu* is associated with *kurāru* (ringworm; see below). This may refer to a dry form of the infection, without pus (suppuration). Alternatively, the patient may have had two concomitant skin conditions.

10.4 DIŠ NA SAG.DU-*su ku-ra-ra*/PEŠ.GIG *u ri-šik-ta* GIG . . . (*BAM* 3 i 49//*BAM* 152 i 14)

**If a person's head is sore with *kurāru* and *rišiktu* . . .

RUṬIBTU (OOZING) When a skin lesion oozes fluid (probably more serum-like fluid rather than thick pus) this is called *ruṭibtu* ("dampness").[11]

10.5 DIŠ GIG GAR-*šú* GIN$_7$ *um-me-di ig-gig*[12] *i-na* [. . .] A DU.MEŠ *ru-ṭib-tum* MU.[NI] (DPS XXXIII:18 [AOAT 43.354])

**If the nature of the sore is that it is clustered, he scratches, (and) fluid flows from [. . .], [it] is called *ruṭibtu.*

10.6 DIŠ GIG GAR-*šú* SA$_5$ BABBAR KÚ-*šú u* A *ú-*[*k*]*al ru-ṭib-tum* MU.[NI] (DPS XXXIII:19 [AOAT 43.354])

**If the nature of the sore is that it is red (or) white, it hurts him, and it contains fluid, [it] is called *ruṭibtu.*

The term can be applied to some stages of superficial fungal skin infections (tinea; see Chapter 3), as in the following reference.

10.7 DIŠ GIG *ina* GÌR NA *lu ina* ŠIR NA E$_{11}$-*ma i-raš-šá-šum-ma ug-gag ru-ṭib-tum qí-lu-tum* MU.[NI] *ana* TI-*šú* . . . (*AMT* 74/1 ii 32–33; cf. DPS XXXIII:22 [AOAT 43.354])

**If a sore comes out on a person's foot or on his scrotum and it is reddish, and he scratches, it is called "burning *ruṭibtu*," to cure him . . .

Ruṭibtu may also be used to describe deeper fungal infections with secondary bacterial infection (mycetoma; see Chapter 3), as in the following reference.

10.8 DIŠ GIG *ka-bar-ti ru-šum-tú*/*ru-ṭib-ta ib-ta-ni* BA.ÚŠ (*BAM* 124 ii 35//*AMT* 74/1 ii 11)

**If a person has *muruṣ kabbarti* (mycetoma and) there is oozing[13]/*ruṭibtu*, he will die.

A completely benign form of oozing, described in the following reference, is seborrhea (oily skin):

10.9 DIŠ IGI.MEŠ-*šú* GIN$_7$ Ì.GIŠ È-*ú* DIN (DPS IX A 42//C 10b = *TDP* 74:42)

**If his face exudes something like oil,[14] he will get well.

RIŠŪTU (REDNESS) This term means "redness," and is derived from the verb *râšu*, "to turn red."[15] Lexical texts group *rišūtu* with *ekketu* (scratchiness) and *ḫarāsu* (itching, see below) and equate it with the colorful Sumerogram SA UMBIN.AK.AK: "to continually fingernail the muscle."[16] The implication is that the redness that is being described is expected to lead to continual scratching of the affected area with the fingernails. There are many possible causes of skin redness, including local contact dermatitis (allergy), athlete's foot (tinea pedis; see Chapter 3), thermal burns, and sunburns.[17]

10.10 [DIŠ GIG GA]R-*šú* GIN$_7$ TAB KÚM-*ma* ⸢x x⸣ GIG *ri-*[*šu-t*]*um* MU.NI (DPS XXXIII:12 [AOAT 43.353])

**[If the] ⸢nature⸣ of the [sore] is that it (feels) hot like a burn and . . . , the sore is called ⸢redness⸣.

10.11 *a-na su-um-mu ri-šu-tu šá* A.MEŠ *na-du-ú* SIG$_5$ (BM 43171+:15–16 [Finkel, *Fs. Lambert* 152])

**(The salve) is good for red spots (and) redness that produce fluid.

10.12 [DIŠ NA *šá-ḫu*]*-ri-šú ri-šu-tú* DIRI . . . *šá-ḫu-ri-šú šá ri-šu-tú ma-lu-ú* . . . (*BAM* 383:1, 13)

**[If a man]'s ⸢sole⸣ (of the foot) is full of redness . . . his sole (of the foot) that is full of redness . . .

10.13 DIŠ IGI.MEŠ-*šú ri-šu-tú* DIRI.ME DIN (DPS IX A 52a//B obv. 51 = *TDP* 76:52a)

**If his face is full of redness, he will get well.

10.14 *nap-šá-al-tum šá ra-šu-tu* . . . (*BAM* 391:7–8)[18]

**Salve for redness . . .

MUNÛ This term is used to describe athlete's foot (tinea pedis; see Chapter 3) and scurvy or trench mouth (Vincent's stomatitis; see Chapter 3) as well as the peau d'orange skin of Grave's disease (see Chapter 7). Other conditions may also be included.

10.15 DIŠ NA GÌR^{II}-*šú* KÚM TUKU.TUKU-*a i-raš-šá-šu-ma ik-ki-k*[*a*] ⸢*la*⸣ *i-kal-la* GIG.MEŠ DIRI-*a mu-ne-e* GI[G] . . . (*BAM* 120 iii 8–9)[19]

**If a person's feet continually have fever, they are reddish and he cannot stop scratching (and) they are full of sores, he is ⸢sick⸣ with *munû* . . .

10.16 DIŠ NA ZÚ.MEŠ-*šú mu-nu u bu-uʾ-šá-nu* (*ḫe-pi eš-šú*) <DIB>-*al ina* DAL.BA.AN.NA ZÚ.MEŠ-*šú* MÚD È.MEŠ-*ni* . . . (*SpTU* 1.44:80–81)

**If *munû* and *buʾšānu* (see Chapter 3) grip a person's teeth (and) blood comes out between his teeth . . .

ŠIBIṬ ŠĀRI The term means literally "wind blasting" and presumably designates areas of the body that look or feel as if they had suffered wind burn. It is used to describe infected ears (see Chapter 9) and genitals (see Chapter 4). It is often accompanied by *bubuʾtu* (vesicles; see below).

10.17 DIŠ GIG GAR-*šú* GIN$_7$ Ù.[BU].BU.UL *pa-gar-šú* DIRI *ši-biṭ* IM [MU.NI] (DPS XXXIII:26 [AOAT 43.354]//K 3526 r. 8)[20]

**If the appearance of the sore is like a *bubuʾtu* (and) his body is full (of them), ⸢it is called⸣ *šibiṭ šāri*.

RIPḪU (SWOLLEN) These lesions are swellings.[21] The text below describes swellings and lesions on a patient's face that might be due to acne or to many other possible causes.

10.18 DIŠ NA *rip-ḫi* UGU.MURUB$_4$.LÚ IGI.MEŠ-*šú* DIRI . . . (*BAM* 35 i 25′)

**If a person's face is full of swellings (and) UGU.MURUB$_4$.LÚ (see below) . . .

TABKU (INDURATED) The term means literally "poured out" or "heaped up." To judge from its use to describe limbs affected by stroke (see Chapter 13), it is best understood as "bunched up" or "tense." When applied to flesh, we believe it refers to thickened (indurated) skin, that is, skin lesions detected by feel rather than by sight.

10.19 Ú UZU.MEŠ *tab-ku-te* . . . (*BAM* 1 iii 32//*CT* 14.43:8′ [S. 60]; cf. *BAM* 421 i′ 23′)

**Plant for tense flesh . . .

Since arthritis and skin lesions are commonly seen in hepatitis B, we believe that the following reference is describing that virus (see Chapter 6).

10.20 DIŠ NA [TÙN] ŠÀ-*šú* DIB-*s*[*u* o o] *di-kiš* ŠÀ GIG ŠÀ-*šú* KÚ-*šú* ŠÀ-*šú ru-uq-šú* ŠÀ.MEŠ-*šú i-sa-bu-ú*ʾ DÙ UZU.MEŠ-*šú tab-ku ni-kim-tú* ŠÀ-*bi* TUKU-*ši na-aš-pa-ak bir-ki u a-ḫi* GIG NA BI TÙN.GIG *ana* TI-*šú* . . . (*BAM* 87:1–5)[22]

**If a person's ⌜liver⌝ afflicts ⌜him⌝ [. . .] he is sick with a needling pain in the abdomen, his abdomen hurts him, his heart is distant from him, his stomach churns, all of his flesh is tense, he has bloated stomach, (and) he is sick with tenseness in the arms and legs, that person (has) TÙN.GIG ("sick liver"), to cure him . . .

The references below describe urethritis and arthritis associated with skin lesions (tense flesh; induration). We believe that reactive arthritis is the likely diagnosis (see Chapter 11).

10.21 [DIŠ NA] *ka-šip-ma* UZU.MEŠ-*šú tab-ku lu ina* DU-*šú lu-u ina i-šu-zi-šu* [*lu-u ina*] *i-tul-i-šu lu-u e-nu-ma* KÀŠ.MEŠ *i-šá-ti-nu re-ḫu-su* DU-*ak* GIN$_7$ MUNUS *su*ʾ*-su* NU *e-el* NA BI *re-ḫu-su* KI LÚ.ÚŠ *ina* KI *šu-nu-lat ana* TI-*šú* . . . (W. Farber, *BID* 234–235:*23–*26)

**If a person is hexed so that his flesh is tense, either when he walks or when he stands still [or when] he lies down or when he urinates, his semen flows, (and) his bed is impure like a (menstruating) woman, that person's semen has been made to lie in the earth with a corpse, to cure him . . .

10.22 DIŠ NA *ka-šip-ma* UZU.MEŠ-*šú tab-ku mun-ga* TU [KU-*šú*] *u bir-ka-šú ga-an-na* ŠÀ-*šú* MUNUS *ḫa-šiḫ-*[*ma*] MUNUS IGI.BAR-*ma* ŠÀ-*šú* GUR NA BI *re-ḫu-su* KI LÚ.ÚŠ *šu-nu-*[*lat*] *ana* TI-*šú* . . . (*BAM* 205:7′–10′//Biggs, *ŠÀ.ZI.GA* 68–69:9′–13′)

**If a person is hexed so that his flesh is tense, he has stiffness and his knees are bent, his heart desires a woman [and then] when he sees a woman, his heart turns away, that person's semen has been made to ⌜lie⌝ with a corpse, to cure him . . .

RAMÛ (RELAXED) This term seems to have been used to describe flesh that was "limp" rather than "tense." This may imply that there was no muscle tension or spasm. In the final reference below, the *āšipu* may have been expecting "tense flesh" in view of the pain in the vicinity of the liver (see above).

10.23 [DIŠ NA NI]NDA *u* KAŠ ŠÀ-*šú* NU IGI-*šú* UZU.MEŠ-*šú ir-ta-nam-mu* IM *ina* DÚR-*šú* NIGIN-*úr ana* TI-*šú* . . . (*BAM* 575 iv 48)

**[If a person]'s insides will not accept ⸢bread⸣ and beer, his flesh is continually limp, and "wind" roils about in his anus, to cure him . . .

10.24 DIŠ N[A . . .] kun UZU.MEŠ-*šú šim-⸢ma⸣-tú u ri-mu-tú* TUKU.MEŠ *u ši-ḫat* UZU.MEŠ [TUKU-*ši*] *ana* TI-*šú* . . . (*AMT* 52/5 obv. 4–5//*BAM* 139 obv. 1′–3′)

**If a ⸢person's⸣ [. . .] his flesh is continually numb and limp and he also [has] wasting of the flesh, to cure him . . .

10.25 DIŠ NA *ki-iṣ* [ŠÀ TUKU NINDA *u* KAŠ] ŠÀ-*šú* NU IGI-*ḫar-šú ina* KA-*šú* GUR.GUR-*ra* TÙN-*šú ú-sa-ḫal-šú ip-ta-na-ru* [UZU.MEŠ-*šú ir-t*]*a-nam-mu-ú* IM *ina* DÚR-*šú* NIGIN ŠÀ.MEŠ-*šú eb-ṭú ana* TI-*šú* . . . (*BAM* 574 i 26–27)

**If a person [has] *kīs* [*libbi*] (indigestion), his insides will not accept [bread and beer] but it keeps returning to his mouth, his liver gives him a stabbing pain, he continually vomits, [his flesh] is continually ⸢limp⸣, "wind" roils about in his anus, and his insides are cramped, to cure him . . .

LUBĀṬU (SWEATY) The *āšipu* seems to have used the term *lubāṭu* to describe excessive sweating, as in the following reference.

10.26 DIŠ ŠÀ-*šú* KÚM-*ma* IR GIN$_7$ *lu-ba-ṭi* ŠUB.ŠUB-*su u* ZI.IR.MEŠ-*aš* ⸢ŠÀ-*šú*⸣ KÚM ÚḪ U.MEŠ GÌR^{II}-*šú* ŠED$_7$.MEŠ U$_4$.3.KÁM ZAL-*ma* DIN (DPS XIII B ii 7–8 = *TDP* 116 ii 7–8)[23]

**If his abdomen is hot, sweat keeps falling upon him as in *lubāṭu* and (his stomach) is continually upset, [his] abdomen burns with fever (and) his toes are cold, (if) he lingers for three days, he will get well.

KIṢṢATU (HAIRLESS) If ancient etymologies may be trusted, the term refers to areas of skin that look as if they have been shorn with a razor as one might shear a goat (i.e., hairless but also red and irritated-looking).[24]

10.27 *gi-iṣ-ṣa-tú* : *ana* UGU *ga-za-az šá* SÍG ÙZ (*SpTU* 1.51:3)

***Kiṣṣatu* is related to (the verb) "to shear," said of goat's hair.

Kiṣṣatu is used to describe lesions on the head and feet, as well as loss of hair in the region of the eyes (eyebrows/eyelashes). Dermatomycosis (i.e., ringworm) can cause hair loss and red, inflamed skin. In the so-called endothrix infection, the hair shaft breaks off at the skin surface, leaving hairs visible as black dots in the scalp. For the loss of eyelashes/eyebrows, Hansen's disease is a possible cause. Hypothyroidism can also cause loss of eyebrows, but redness and inflammation are not seen with this disease.

10.28 DIŠ NA SAG.DU-*su* ⸢*kib*⸣-*šá gi-iṣ-ṣa-tú gu-reš-tú*[25] DIRI . . . (Labat, *RA* 53.10–11 obv. 30)[26]

**If a person's head is full of *kibšu, kiṣṣatu,* (and) *kureštu* . . .

10.29 DIŠ NA GÌR^{II}-*šú ki-iṣ-ṣa-tú* DIRI . . . (*AMT* 69/5:1)

**If a person's feet are full of *kiṣṣatu* . . .[27]

10.30 DIŠ *a-na* IGI^{II}.MEŠ *ki-ṣa-a-ti bul-lu-ṭi u kap-pi* IGI^{II}-*šú šu-ṣi-i* . . . (*BAM* 22:32′–33′)

**If you want to cure eyes with *kiṣṣatu* and to make his eyelashes/eyebrows sprout . . .

10.31 PA IGI^{II}-*šú* GÁL-*ši* (*BAM* 515 ii 25)

**(After treatment) he will have eyelashes/eyebrows.

EKKETU (EVIDENCE OF SCRATCHING) *Ekketu* literally means "scratchies," and refers to severe itching leading to scratching and secondary sores.[28] Potential causes of severe itching range from allergies to mosquito bites. In the last reference below, the patient may have sat down in the wrong place.

10.32 DIŠ NA *ek-ke-tú* GIG . . . (*BAM* 3 ii 5//Beckman and Foster, *Mem. Sachs* 19 no. 18:6′)[29]

**If a person is sick/sore with *ekketu* . . .

10.33 DIŠ NA SAG.DU-*su ek-ke-tú u ri-šu-tú* DIRI . . . (BAM 3 ii 3//*BAM* 494 i 33′; cf. *BAM* 33:19)

**If a person's head is full of *ekketu* and redness . . .

10.34 [DIŠ GIG GA]R-*šú* GIN$_7$ *um-me-di* MURUB$_4$.MEŠ-*šú* NIGIN-*mi ek-*[*ke-t*]*um* MU.NI (DPS XXXIII:10 [AOAT 43.353])

**[If the] ⌜nature⌝ of the [sore] is that it is clustered (and) it goes round the hips, its name is ⌜*ekketu*⌝.

The *āšipu* was well aware that the patient's continual scratching was aggravating the problem.

10.35 [DIŠ . . .]-ši NA GIG *e-gig-ma* DÙG.GA-*šú e-gig-ma* x [. . .] xx GIG BI ŠÀ-*bi-nu-ma* ⌜DU⌝-*ak ana* ZI-*šú* . . . (*CTN* 4.116 obv. 23–24)

**[If . . .] (and) a person scratches the sore and it feels good to him, he scratches it and [. . .], that sore is going down inside him, to remove it . . .

ABNORMAL COLORATION OF THE SKIN

The color of the patient's skin was also noted and commented upon (see Chapter 20). For yellow (jaundiced) patients, see Chapter 6.

GI$_6$ = *TARKU* (DARK) OR *ṢALMU* (BLACK) Sumerian GI$_6$ has two Akkadian equivalents, *tarku*: "dark" and *ṣalmu*: "black." Both terms are used to describe pathological colors of the skin, often in a context of trauma. In the following quote, we believe that the patient was run through with the shaft of a spear or arrow passing through the back with the point emerging from the rib cage. The black color was likely to be due to subcutaneous bleeding (ecchymosis).

10.36 DIŠ KI.MIN-*ma* TI-*šú šá* 15 GI_6 KA-*šú* ḪÁD.MEŠ *u it-ta-nag-ra-ár* ŠU ᵈ*Da-mu ina* ÉLLAG-*šú* SÌG-*iṣ* GAM (DPS XV:42 [AOAT 43.152])[30]

**If (it is the first day he is sick) and his left rib is dark, his mouth is continually dry, and he rolls over and over, "hand" of Damu. He was wounded on his kidney; he will die.

In the following text, the periorbital ecchymosis (black eye) was probably the result of trauma or periorbital infection, possibly from an underlying sinusitis (see Chapter 9).

10.37 ⌜DIŠ IGI 15⌝-*šú tar-kàt-ma* NU BAD qu x [. . .] (DPS V A 15′ = *TDP* 46 B 15)[31]

**If his left eye is dark and he cannot open (it) [. . .]

Tarku or *ṣalmu* also describes septic shock gangrene (see Chapter 14) and cyanosis (see Chapter 8), as in the following examples.

10.38 DIŠ IGI.MEŠ-*šú* GI_6.MEŠ-*ma* GIN_7 *šá-lam-ti ib-šu-ú* IGI.MEŠ-*šú i-te-eb-ṭú* NUNDUN.MEŠ-*šú ma-diš ik-tab-ra* IGI.MEŠ-*šú iš-ta-na-an-nu-ú mu-du-šú ul* GIG-*ma i-qab-bi* ÚŠ *ug-ga-ti* GAM EGIR-*su na-ʾ-da-at* É-*su* BIR-*aḫ* (DPS IX A 21–24//B obv. 20–22 = *TDP* 72:21–24)

**If his face turns black and becomes like (that of) a corpse, his face is continually frowning, his lips are very much thickened, his face keeps changing, (and) one who knows him says: "Is he not sick?" death from (divine) anger; he will die. His inheritance will be in danger; his house will be scattered.

10.39 [DIŠ ŠU^{II}-*šú u* G]ÌR^{II}-*šú* GI_6.MEŠ *uš-ta-nab-lak-kát* ZI-*bi u* D[U_{10}.GAM . . .] (DPS XI A obv. 39 = *TDP* 92:39)

**[If his hands and] his ⌜feet⌝ are dark, he has changes of mood (and) gets up and ⌜(has to) squat down⌝ [. . .]

THERMAL BURNS

TAB/*ḪIMṬI* The word is from the verb *ḫamāṭu*: "to burn" and probably refers to thermal burns.

10.40 Ú TAB IZI . . . (*STT* 92 iii 13′, 14′)

**Plant for the burning of fire . . .

10.41 Ú *ḫi-im-ṭi* . . . (*STT* 92 iii 15′)

**Plant for a burn . . .

The reference below describes a facial burn that appears to have produced scar tissue resulting in a narrowing of the ocular opening.[32]

10.42 DIŠ MIN-*ma* (*pa-nu-šu ḫa-an-ṭù*) IGI-*šú šá* ZAG/GÙB *pi-qat* (Böck, *Morphoskopie* 112:76–77)

**If his face has been burned and, as a result, his left/right eye is narrowed.

BRUISES

MIQTU This term, derived from the verb *maqātu*: "to fall" is generally used to describe seizures (see Chapter 13). In a few cases, however, it refers not to a "falling spell" but to skin lesions with variable characteristics.[33]

10.43 DIŠ *i-na zu-mu-ur* LÚ *mi-iq-tum it-ta-ṣi-a-ma* . . . (BM 113970++ ii 3–4; *YOS* 11.29:1)

**If a *miqtu* has come out on a person's body . . .

10.44 *si-im-ma ak-ṣa la-az-za mi-iq-ta la ta-ba-a i-na zu-um-ri-šu li-še-ṣi* (*MDP* 6 pl. 11 iv 6–9)

**May (Gula) cause to come out on his body a dangerous and persistent sore, a *miqtu* that will not let up![34] [a curse]

These lesions are possibly to be connected with a usage of the verb from which *miqtu* comes, *maqātu* or *muqqutu* (its D-stem form), (usually in the stative) to describe the skin of patients and/or the condition of various body parts.

10.45 [DIŠ Ú]R.KUN-*šú* SA$_5$-*át* DIN / [DIŠ] ÚR.KUN-*šú* SIG$_7$-*át* GIG-*su* MAN-*ni* / [DIŠ Ú]R.KUN-*šú* GI$_6$-*át* GAM / [DIŠ Ú]R.KUN-*šú tar-kát na-ḫi-id* / [DIŠ ÚR].KUN-*šú du-ʾ-ú-mat* GIG-*su* MAN-*ni* / [DIŠ ÚR].KUN-*šú nap-ḫat* GIG-*su* DUGUD / [DIŠ ÚR].KUN-*šú muq-qú-ta-át* PA NU TUKU / DIŠ ÚR.KUN-*šú šu-uḫ-ḫu-ṭa-át na-kid* / DIŠ ÚR.KUN-*šú pu-uṭ-ṭu-rat* GAM (DPS XII D iv 7–15//E iv 14–22//G$_2$ iv 5–13 = *TDP* 108 iv 7–15)

**[If] his ⌜coccyx⌝[35] is red, he will get well. [If] his coccyx is yellow, his illness will alter (for the worse). [If] his ⌜coccyx⌝ is black, he will die. [If] his ⌜coccyx⌝ is dark, it is worrisome. [If] his ⌜coccyx⌝ is dark red, his illness will alter (for the worse). [If] his ⌜coccyx⌝ is swollen, his illness will be difficult. [If] his ⌜coccyx⌝ was *muqqutu*'d, it is of no consequence.[36] If his coccyx was skinned, it is worrisome. If his coccyx was (cut) open, he will die.

This type of sequence appears over and over again in the diagnostic series referring to different parts of the body.[37] Given that being "skinned" and "(cut) open" are included in the list, the most likely explanation for the swelling and the observed pathological colors is wound healing (or failure to heal). If so, then *muqqutu* should also refer to some sort of trauma, and minor trauma at that, given the relative lack of concern displayed by the *āšipu*.

10.46 [DIŠ ÚR].KUN-*šú muq-qú-ta-át* PA NU TUKU (DPS XII D iv 13//G$_2$ iv 11 = *TDP* 108 iv 13)

**[If] his ⌜coccyx⌝ was *muqqutu*'d, it is of no consequence.[38]

Muqqutu could conceivably mean literally "attacked" or "fallen upon." A commentary to Tablet XIV of the diagnostic series explains *muq-qú-tú* as *šá-pil*: "dented,"[39] and *tarku*: "dark (blue)" is sometimes given as a supplemental symptom to *muqqutu* or used in identical contexts. This suggests that *muqqutu* refers to bruising and the related term *miqtu* to a bruise. Since a bruise is a common consequence of a fall, this interpretation would appear to link the two meanings of this root.

SPOTS

DIRI/*MALÛ* One way in which the *āšipu* indicated uneven coloration was to use the verb DIRI/*malû*: "to be full of (spots)", as in the following examples.

Yellowish spots (SIG_7)

10.47 [BE MUNUS Ù.TU]-*ma* MIN-*ma* SIG_7 *ma-li* . . . (Šumma Izbu IV 5 [Leichty, *Izbu* 66])

**[If a woman gives birth] and (from the beginning the child) is full of yellowish (spots) . . .

Ancient Mesopotamian color terminology is somewhat limited, which sometimes makes it difficult to determine exactly which color was meant. Since, however, cats, dogs, cows, sheep, and goats were described as "yellow,"[40] the range is likely to have included a cream or light brown color, as in the English "yellow Gypsy." Flat areas of increased pigmentation that vary in color from brown to black may be referred to as café-au-lait spots by modern physicians. These lesions may be isolated findings or associated with other syndromes, especially neurofibromatosis and tuberous sclerosis.

Black spots (GI_6)

10.48 [BE MUNUS Ù.TU]-*ma* MIN-*ma* GI_6 *ma-li* . . . (Šumma Izbu IV 6 [Leichty, *Izbu* 66])[41]

**[If a woman gives birth] and (from the beginning the child) is full of black (spots) . . .

This quote is probably describing nevuses or dark café-au-lait spots. Nevuses are black to brown pigmented areas that may be flat or elevated.

ŠUB/*NADÛ* The verb means to "pour out" or "to color." It seems likely that the use of the expression with color terms implies an uneven pattern of color, that is, spots or streaks.

10.49 DIŠ IGI.MEŠ-*šú* BABBAR GI_6 SA_5 *u* SIG_7 ŠUB : *ú-kal-lu* GIG-*su* GÍD-*ma* DIN (DPS IX A 10 = *TDP* 72:10)

**If his face is unevenly colored with (var. contains) white, black, red, and yellow (spots), his illness may be prolonged, (but) he will get well.

10.50 DIŠ NA ŠÀ-*šú* GIG-*ma* ŠÀ GÌR.PAD.DA-*šú* SIG_7 ŠUB-*a* ŠÀ-*šú* [G]IG.MEŠ DIRI NA BI UD.DA SÁ.SÁ (BAM 52:63–64//*BAM* 575 i 21)[42]

**If a person's stomach is sick and (the area) along his bones is unevenly colored with yellow, (and) his abdomen is full of ⌜sore⌝ spots, that person was "gotten" by *ṣētu* (enteric fever; see Chapter 3).

Deep red spots ($IM.SIG_7.SIG_7$)

10.51 DIŠ NUNDUN [. . .] x GAM / DIŠ NUNDUN.MEŠ-*šú* IM $SIG_7.SIG_7$ Š[UB . . .] (DPS VI B_5 r. 3//E_2 8+E_1 4//F 4 = *TDP* 58 r. 16′+22′)

**If his lip(s) [. . .], he will die. If his lips are ⌜unevenly colored⌝ with deep red colored spots [. . .]

The reference above might be referring to an inherited condition called Osler-Rendu-Weber syndrome. It is characterized by blood vessel abnormalities affecting especially the gastrointestinal tract causing acute or chronic bleeding and frequently death. The abnormal blood vessels commonly involve the lips, producing red spots.

TARĀPU Another less commonly used verb that apparently refers to a sprinkling of color is *tarāpu.* If these "sprinklings" of color were very small, some of the red or dark spots described in the following references could be the petechial skin lesions seen in patients with heart valve infections (endocarditis). This would explain the fatal outcome in some of the references, since endocarditis is always fatal in the absence of antibiotic therapy.

10.52 DIŠ GEŠTU 15-*šú* [*t*] *ur-ru-pat* GIG-*su* GÍD-*ma* DIN / DIŠ GEŠTU 150-*šú tur-ru-pat na-kud* / DIŠ GEŠTU^{II}-*šú tur-ru-pa* GAM (DPS VIII 4–6a = *TDP* 68:4–6a)

**If the patient's left ear ⌜looks sprinkled⌝, his illness may be prolonged (but) he will get well. If his right ear looks sprinkled, it is worrisome. If (both) his ears looks sprinkled, he will die.

10.53 DIŠ *kar-ši* U.MEŠ-*šú* GI$_6$ *tur-ru-pa* GAM (DPS XI A r. 56 = *TDP* 98 r.56)

**If the undersides of his fingers are sprinkled with dark (spots), he will die.

There were a number of specific terms (*pūṣu, sūmu, ṣiriptu, terku*) to describe individual white, red, or dark spots. There was also a word that meant simply "spot" (*tikpu*) and another (*miqtu*) that may have referred to a bruise. There were also two terms that seem to have referred to generalized red or dark spots (*kullāru* and *ziʾpu*).

PŪṢU (WHITE SPOTS) This term literally means "white spot." Kinnier-Wilson has suggested that the third quote below is a reference to the lesions of tuberculoid leprosy (Hansen's disease).[43] These white spots are caused by loss of normal skin pigmentation, and are associated with reduced pain and touch sensations. There are, however, many causes of skin depigmentation, and some are benign conditions. The reaction of gods and men mentioned in that reference indicates that whatever the problem, it was socially stigmatizing, which is consistent with the almost universal tendency of societies to shun and isolate patients with Hansen's disease.

10.54 DIŠ ŠU^{II}-*šú* SIG$_7$.MEŠ *u* U.MEŠ-*šú pu-ṣa* ŠUB [. . .] (DPS XI A obv. 12 = *TDP* 90:12)

**If his hands are yellow and his fingers are unevenly colored with white spots [. . .].

10.55 DIŠ ŠU^{II}-*šú* SIG$_7$.MEŠ IGI^{II}-*šú pu-ṣa* ŠU [B . . .] (DPS XI B 11 = *SpTU* 1.34:11)

**If his hands are yellow (and) his eyes are ⌜unevenly colored⌝ with white spots [. . .].

10.56 DIŠ LÚ *pa-ga-ar ši-ru-šu pu-ṣa-am ku-ul-lu-u*[*m*]*-ma ù nu-uq-di i-ta-ad-du* LÚ *šu-ú it-ti i-lí-šu sà-ki-ip it-ti a-wi-l*[*u-t*] *i sà-ki-ip* (Köcher and Oppenheim, *AfO* 18.66 ii 42–45 [physiognomic omens])

**If a person's body (and) his flesh contain white spots and are spotted with "points," that man is rejected by his god; he is rejected by mankind.

SŪMU (RED SPOTS) This term literally means "red spot."

10.57 *a-na su-um-mu ra-šá-na* SIG_5*-iq* (BM 79244:19–20 [Finkel, *Fs. Lambert* 150 (with parallels)])

**(The salve) is good for red spots (and) hair fall.

10.58 *a-na su-um-mu ri-šu-tu šá* A.MEŠ *na-du-ú* SIG_5*-iq* (BM 43171+:15–16 [Finkel, *Fs. Lambert* 152])

**(The salve) is good for red spots (and) redness that produce fluid.

ṢIRIPTU (BRIGHT RED SPOTS) This term is from a verb that means "to dye (leather) red" and literally means "spot (that looks like) red-dyed (leather)." The leather in question, known to us as "Cordoba" leather (and still manufactured in Morocco), is a bright fire-engine red. In the first reference below *ṣiriptu* appears to be describing the skin lesions of scarlet fever (see Chapter 3 with 3.52).[44]

10.59 DIŠ *gir-ra-a-šú šu-uḫ-ḫu-ṭa u* UZU.ME-*šú* ŠUB-*tu u ṣi-rip-tu* ŠUB.ŠUB-*a* [KI.MI]N (DPS X A obv. 52/D 12 = *TDP* 86:52)

**If both sides of his throat (look) skinned and his flesh (looks) terrible[45] and is unevenly colored with red dye spots, ⸢(it is worrisome)⸣.

10.60 DIŠ *ṣi-rip-ta-šu id-⸢di⸣-a-am-ma ù ṣi-rip-ta-*[*šu* . . .] (*PBS* 2/2.104:11)[46]

**If he is colored with red dye spots and his red dye spots [. . .].

TERKU (DARK SPOTS) This term means "dark spot." In the reference below, the dark spots may be caused by subcutaneous bleeding (ecchymosis). In other contexts, the dark spots may have other etiologies.[47]

10.61 DIŠ MUNUS MIN-*ma* KÚM *li-ʾ-ba u ter-ku ina* UZU.MEŠ-*šá u* SA.MEŠ-*šá* KAB.M[EŠ] *qer-bi-nu* MÚD.BABBAR *ú-kal* . . . (*BAM* 240:59′–60′)

**If a woman (gives birth) and subsequently she (has) fever (and) *liʾbu* (see Chapter 3) and dark spots accumulate(?) on her flesh and her blood vessels (and) inside she contains pus . . .

TIKPU (SPOTS, ANY COLOR) The term means "spot."[48]

10.62 ⸢DIŠ⸣ MUNUS *ti-ik-pi ina* ARḪUŠ-*šá i-tak-kip* . . . (*SpTU* 5.253 r. 1)

**If a woman becomes spotted with spots on her womb (cervix) . . .

NUQDU (PINPOINT SPOTS) The Arabic cognate of this word is used to describe the dots used in Arabic script to distinguish similar letters from one another. What is being described are probably pinpoint (punctate) lesions.

10.63 DIŠ LÚ *pa-ga-ar ši-ru-šu pu-ṣa-am ku-ul-lu-u*[*m*]*-ma ù nu-uq-di i-ta-ad-du* LÚ *šu-ú it-ti i-lí-šu sà-ki-ip it-ti a-wi-l*[*u-t*] *i sà-ki-ip* (Köcher and Oppenheim, *AfO* 18.66 ii 42–45 [physiognomic omens])

**If a person's body (and) his flesh contain white spots and are spotted with *nuqdu*, that man is rejected by his god; he is rejected by mankind.

KULLĀRU (GENERALIZED DARK SPOTS) This type of lesion is characterized as being dark (possibly dark red or purple), flat (i.e., macular), dry (i.e., not a vesicle), and itching (pruritic). The first reference below indicates that the patient's body was full of them. One likely cause is an allergic reaction. The substance causing this reaction could be from food, or a medicine administered by the *āšipu*. A particular type of *kullāru* was known as the *kullāru* of *ašû* (see below).

10.64 [DIŠ] GIG GAR-*šú* GIN_7 *ter-ke-e-ti kal* SU LÚ DIRI *kul-la-ri* MU.NI (DPS XXXIII:7 [AOAT 43.353])

**[If] the nature of the sore is that it is like dark spots (*terku*; see above) and the person's entire body is full (of them), it is called *kullāru*.

10.65 [DIŠ] ⌜GIG GAR⌝-*šú* GI_6 *ri-šik i-raš-ši-šum-ma ug-gag kul-la-ri* MU.NI (DPS XXXIII:8 [AOAT 43.353])

**[If] the appearance of the sore is dark (and) dry (and) (his skin) is reddish and he scratches, it is called *kullāru*.

ZIʾPU (GENERALIZED RED SPOTS) Lexical equations associate this term with *liʾbu*-fever (see Chapter 3) and with *šīpu*.

10.66 *li-ʾ-bu : zi-i-pi / ši-i-pu* : MIN (*CT* 18.31 r. 15–16//*STT* 394:161–162; cf. *SpTU* 1.38:10)[49]

***Liʾbu* (and) *šīpu* are equivalent to *ziʾpu*.

Šīpu is known from the commentaries to astronomical omens, where it is explained as being a red spot.

10.67 *ši-pa tak-pat . . . ši-pa* : SA_5 (Virolleaud, *ACh* Ištar 6:24, 26; *ACh* Supp. 2.56 K 2153:11)[50]

**It is spotted with *šīpu* . . . *šīpu* (means) "red (spot)."

It would seem from these references that *ziʾpu* was a generalized flat (macular), (febrile) rash.

CATEGORIES OF SKIN LESION WITH MODERN EQUIVALENTS

Modern physicians distinguish between macules (see above), scales, wheals, nodules, vesicles, pustules, and ulcers, and so did the *āšipu*. Following are the ancient Mesopotamian terms that we believe correspond to these types of lesions as well as some of the other skin lesions and syndromes that they help to define.

BAR/*QULIPTU* (SCALE) *Quliptu* is a scale,[51] or the shedding of sheets of skin (desquamation). Causes of desquamation are many, but include severe sunburn and allergic reactions.

10.68 *šum*$_4$*-ma* SU NA GIG [. . .] *u qu-lip-ta* ŠUB-*di* . . . (*BAM* 35 i 38′–39′)[52]

**If a man's body is [spotted with] sore(s) and sheds scales . . .

(*I*)*ṢĪTU* (WHEAL) This term is derived from a verb that means "to come out."[53] Given the context of the first reference below, which we believe to refer to infection with a guinea worm (see Chapter 3), "wheal" seems a likely translation. The wheal (local swelling or edema) probably represents a secondary bacterial cellulitis from organisms entering at the *ibaru*-lesion and tracking up the lymphatics along the path of the worm.

10.69 DIŠ GIG *ina* SU NA È GIN$_7$ *i-ba-ri* È-*su ana* ⌜TAG⌝ [DAG]AL-*ma* ⌜GIN$_7$⌝ TAG-*su-ma i-ṣi-tu*[*m*] È SU-*šú tu*-NIGIN *ina ša-nu-ti-šú ina* UZU.ÚR ⌜*e*⌝*-la-a ana* KI *šá-nim-ma ul i*-[*li*] *ana* KI *šá-nim-ma* ⌜DAGAL⌝ x [. . .] x x ṣa *ni-lu-gu*$_4$ MU-*šú ana* ZI-*šú* . . . (*BAM* 417 r. 9′–11′)

**If a sore comes out on a person's body like an *ibaru*-lesion, what it produces ⌜grows larger⌝ to the touch, and when he touches it, a wheal (blister) comes out; it goes round his body (and) comes once again up to the thighs;[54] it does not ⌜go up⌝ to another location (but) it may grow larger there [. . .], it is called *nilugu*, to remove it . . .

10.70 DIŠ LÚ *ṣi-i-ta* GIG . . . (*CT* 44.36:1)

**If a person is sore with a wheal . . .

10.71 LÚ.TUR *ša ma-aḫ-ri-ia ma-ru-uṣ ša-ap-la-nu-um* [*u*]*z-ni-šu ṣi-tum ú-ṣí-im* (*ARM* 14.3 [Finet, *AIPHOS* 14 pl. 2]:5–8)

**The boy who is with me is sick. A wheal came out below his ear.[55]

BIRDU (NODULE) *Birdu* appears to mean a raised, solid skin lesion (nodule or papule).[56] Unlike flat (macular) lesions such as *kullāru*, *birdu* are not described as "spots" (flat); neither, in contrast to vesicular lesions such as *bubuʾtu*, are they described as having fluid. Harmless accumulations of *birdu* on the face are mentioned in the diagnostic series.

10.72 DIŠ IGI.MEŠ-*šú bir-di* DIRI.ME ŠU DINGIR-*šú* DIN (DPS IX A 50a//B obv. 49a = *TDP* 76:50a)

**If his face is full of *birdu*, "hand" of his god; he will get well.

References suggest that the term was used to describe venereal warts or condyloma (see Chapter 4).

10.73 DIŠ MUNUS Ù.TU-*ma* SU-*šá bir-di* DIRI DÚR-*šá ma-qit* . . . (*BAM* 240:29′)

**If a woman gives birth and subsequently her body is full of *birdu*-nodules (and) her anus has prolapsed . . .[57]

Red *birdu* also appear, alongside *kullāru* (macular lesions), *bubuʾtu* (vesicles), and reddish or clustered sores, as possible lesions of *ašû* (see below). Black *birdu* were the characteristic lesions of *ḫarāsu.*

ḪARĀSU (DARK NODULE)

10.74 DIŠ GIG GAR-*šú* GI_6 *ḫa-ra-su* MU.[NI] (DPS XXXIII:20 [AOAT 43.354]; cf. *BAM* 409 obv. 18′)

**If the appearance of the sore is black, [it] is called *ḫarāsu.*

10.75 DIŠ SU LÚ *bir-di* DIRI UZU.MEŠ-*šú ú-zaq-qa-t*[*u-š*]*ú u ri-šu-tum* ŠUB.ŠUB-*su ḫa-ra-su* M[U.NI] (DPS XXXIII:21 [AOAT 43.354]; cf. *BAM* 409 obv. 19′–20′)

**If a person's body is full of *birdu* and his flesh ⌜stings him⌝ and redness continually falls on him, [it] ⌜is called⌝ *ḫarāsu.*

There are probably many causes of pigmented nodular skin lesions but, in the reference below, there is an associated decrease or blurring of vision. One possible etiology for *ḫarāsu* is the microfilarial infestation, onchocerciasis (see Chapter 3). That disease produces skin nodules that itch, and it leads to blindness.

10.76 DIŠ IGI^{II}-*šú a-ši-a bir-d*[*u* . . .] (DPS V C ii 5′//E 5′ = *TDP* 48 D ii 5)

**If his eyes are "confused" (and) ⌜*birdu*⌝ [. . .].

U_4.BÚ.BÚ.UL/*BUBUʾTU* (VESICLE)

Bubuʾtus are clearly described as small water blisters (vesicles) that often have surrounding redness.[58] The term is used to describe fever blisters (cold sores), and the last reference below may be describing this viral (HSV1) infection.[59]

10.77 [DIŠ G]IG GAR-*šú* GIN_7 TAB KÚM-*ma* A *ú-kal* [*bu*]*-bu-ʾ-tum* MU.NI (DPS XXXIII:14 [AOAT 43.353])

**[If] the nature of the ⌜sore⌝ is that it is hot like a burn and contains fluid, it is called *bubuʾtu.*

10.78 *bu-bu-ʾ-tu šá a-ṣu-šu la ṭa-a-bu* . . . (Lugale V 32 [description of Asakku], apud *CAD* B 300a)

***bubuʾtu* whose outpouring (liquid) is not good . . .

10.79 DIŠ *ina* SAG GIG-*šú* IR *bu-úḫ-bu-úḫ-ta*[60] TUKU-*ma* IR *ši-i* TA *kin-ṣi-šú* EN ZI.IN.GI-*šú u* KI.TA $GÌR^{II}$-*šú* NU KUR-*ád* GIG.BI LÍL-*ti* U_4.2.KÁM U_4.3.KÁM LÍL-*ma* DIN (DPS XVII:1–3 [AOAT 43.195]); cf. DPS XVI:103′ [AOAT 43.180])[61]

**If at the beginning of his illness, he has sweat (and) *bubuʾtu*[62] and that sweat does not reach from his shins to his ankles and the soles of his feet, that sickness is an illness of two days. (If) he is ill for three days, he will get well.

The best known causes of vesicles are chickenpox (*Varicella zoster* virus; VZV), *Herpes simplex* viruses 1 and 2 (HSV1 and HSV2), and smallpox virus (*Variola*). Vesicles occurring on the genitals were diagnosed by ancient physicians as "wind blasting" (genital herpes; see Chapter 4).

10.80 DIŠ NA GÌŠ-*šú* IM *iš-biṭ* [. . .] U$_4$.BÚ.BÚ.UL! DIRI . . . (*BAM* 112 ii 11′–12′)[63]

**If "wind" has blasted a person's penis [. . .] it is full of *bubuʾtu* . . .

Vesicles in the mouth were *buʾšānu* (herpetic stomatitis; see Chapter 3).

10.81 [DIŠ KA-*šú bu-bu-ʾ*]-*ta* DIRI *u il-la-tu-šú il-la-ka bu-ʾ-šá-nu* MU.[NI] (DPS XXXIII: 87 [AOAT 43.357]; cf. DPS VII B obv. 4′ = *TDP* 64:43′)[64]

**[If his mouth] is full of ⌜*bubuʾtu*⌝ and his saliva flows, [it] is called *buʾšānu.*

Vesicles on the face were attributed to the "hands" of various gods/goddesses depending on the color of the lesion and the potential for fatality.

10.82 DIŠ IGI.MEŠ-*šú* U$_4$.BU.BU.UL SA$_5$ DIRI.MEŠ ŠU ^{d}30 DIN (DPS IX A 47//C 15 = *TDP* 74:47)

**If his face is full of red *bubuʾtu*, "hand" of Sîn; he will get well.

10.83 DIŠ IGI.MEŠ-*šú* U$_4$.BU.BU.UL BABBAR DIRI.MEŠ ŠU ^{d}UTU DIN (DPS IX A 48//B obv. 47//C 16 = *TDP* 74:48)

**If his face is full of white *bubuʾtu*, "hand" of Šamaš; he will get well.

10.84 DIŠ IGI.MEŠ-*šú* BU.BU.UL GI$_6$ DIRI.MEŠ ŠU ^{d}15 GAM (DPS IX A 49//B obv. 48 = *TDP* 74:49)[65]

**If his face is full of black *bubuʾtu*, "hand" of Ištar; he will die.

The first reference above is likely to be due to *Herpes simplex* type 1 (HSV1; see Chapter 4). The other two references do not contain enough information to suggest an etiology. However, we believe that the black *bubuʾtus* are caused by subcutaneous hemorrhage (ecchymosis) that becomes black as the trapped blood ages.[66] Hemorrhage occurs in more serious infections, which explains the expectation of patient death. The "red" *bubuʾtu* is presumably a vesicle with surrounding inflamed skin.[67]

Generalized vesicles that could be traced to venereal contact were also attributed to the "hands" of various gods/goddesses depending on the color of the lesion and the color of the surrounding skin.[68] *Herpes simplex* type 2 (HSV2; see Chapter 4) is the vesicular infection most closely associated with venereal contact. Genital distribution of lesions is the common appearance in modern humans, but the presentation of this disease in previous populations could have been different. Jaundice noted in the second text is probably due to HSV2 hepatitis.

10.85 [DIŠ TA SAG.D]U-*šú* EN GÌR^{II}-*šú* U$_4$.BU.BU.UL SA$_5$ DIRI *u* SU-*šú* BABBAR/GI$_6$ KI MUNUS *ina* KI.NÁ KUR ŠU 30 (DPS III A r. 8′–9′//C r. 31–32 = *TDP* 28:91–92)[69]

**[If from] his ⸢head⸣ to his feet, he is full of red *bubu'tu* and his skin/body is white/dark, he was "gotten" in bed with a woman; "hand" of Sîn.

10.86 [DIŠ T]A SAG.DU-*šú* EN GÌR^{II}-*š*[*ú*] U_4.BU.BU.UL DIRI *u* SU-*šú* SIG_7 KI.MIN ŠU ^{d}15 (DPS III A r. 10′//C r. 33 = *TDP* 28:93)[70]

**[If] ⸢from⸣ his head to his feet, he is full of (red) *bubu'tu* and his skin/body is yellow, (he was "gotten" in bed with a woman), "hand" of Ištar.

10.87 [DIŠ T]A SAG.DU-*šú* EN [GÌR^{II}-*šú* U]$_4$.BU.BU.UL BABBAR/GI_6 DIRI *u* SU-*šú* GI_6/SA_5 KI.MIN ŠU ^{d}UTU (DPS III A r. 11′–12′//C r. 34–35 = *TDP* 28:94–95)[71]

**[If] ⸢from⸣ his head to [his feet], he is full of white/dark *bubu'tu* and his skin/body is dark/red, (he was "gotten" in bed with a woman), "hand" of Šamaš.

Some river toxins were also capable of producing blisters (see Chapter 15).

10.88 ⸢DIŠ NA⸣ ŠUB-*ta ina* A ÍL-*ši* UZU.MEŠ-*šú ut-tap-pa-ḫ*[*u* . . . U_4.B]Ú.[B]Ú.UL *ina* U_4.BÚ.BÚ.UL *ina* SU-*šú* E_{11}-*a* [. . .] (*BAM* 568:1–2)

**If a falling spell comes upon a ⸢person⸣ in the water, his flesh is made to swell [. . .] (and) ⸢*bubu'tu*⸣ rides on top of *bubu'tu* in his body [. . .]

AŠÛ Patients with generalized red vesicles appear to have been diagnosed with *ašû*. Other diffuse lesions including nodules (*birdu*) and macular rashes (*kullāru*) were also associated with *ašû*. Having analyzed all of the texts in which *ašû*[72] appears as a diagnosis, it is our conclusion that the term was applied to any skin condition of nonvenereal origin that covers the entire body with characteristic lesions. It is clear from the signs and symptoms listed in the references below that a number of different diseases were included under this rubric.

Lesions associated with *ašû* include those that were reddish and clustered. Many infections can cause a generalized red rash, including measles, German measles, and scarlet fever. The last two references below might be describing severe allergic reactions.

10.89 [DIŠ GIG] GAR-*šú* GIN_7 *um-me-di a-šu-ú* MU.N[I] (DPS XXXIII:1 [AOAT 43.353])

**[If] the nature of the [sore] is that it is clustered, it is called *ašû*.

10.90 [DIŠ G]IG GAR-*šú* GIN_7 *um-me-di i-raš-ši-šum-ma ug-gag* IGI GIG A ŠUB [. . .] *a-šu-ú* MU.N[I] (DPS XXXIII:2 [AOAT 43.353])

**[If] the nature of the ⸢sore⸣ is that it is clustered, (his body) is reddish, and he scratches (and) the top of the sore produces fluid[73] [. . .], it is called *ašû*.

10.91 [DIŠ G]IG GAR-*šú* GIN_7 *um-me-di u* È-*su e-mid*[74] SU-*šú i-raš-ši-šum-ma* EN ⸢x⸣ [. . .] ⸢x⸣ TE GIG *ug-dal-lab a-šu-ú* MU.N[I] (DPS XXXIII:3 [AOAT 43.353])

**[If] the nature of the ⸢sore⸣ is that it is clustered and what comes out of it clings (to it), his body is reddish, and the side of the sore has been scraped until [it bleeds], ⸢it⸣ is called *ašû*.

Lesions associated with *ašû* are also described as consisting of *birdu*, *bubu'tu*, or *kullāru*.

With birdu *(nodules)*

10.92 [DIŠ *p*] *a-nu-šú* MÚ.MEŠ-*ḫu di-gíl-šú ma-ṭi* SU-*šú bir-di ma-lu u* ŠÀ-*šú* [D]IB-*su a-šu-ú* MU.NI (DPS XXXIII:5 [AOAT 43.353]; cf. *AMT* 84/6 ii 8′–9′)

**[If] his ⸢face⸣ is swollen, his eyesight is diminished, his body is full of *birdu*, and his abdomen ⸢afflicts⸣ him, it is called *ašû*.

Nodular lesions and decreasing vision, as noted in the reference above, suggest onchocerciasis. Another possibility are the calabar swellings of loiasis, a parasitic infection that may also affect the eyes (see Chapter 3). Finally, this reference could be describing erythema nodosum, a hypersensitivity reaction that can occur in response to drugs including salicylic acid (available to ancient Mesopotamians in the form of willow bark) or may be produced by a variety of diseases including tuberculosis, Hansen's disease, syphilis, and measles.

With bubuʾtu *(vesicles)*

10.93 U.BU.BU.UL SA$_5$ *ina* SU NA GÁL-*ši a-ša-⸢a⸣* [. . .] ŠU ^{d}30 NAM.ÉRIM DIB-*su* ŠU ^{d}INNIN . . . (*BAM* 584 ii 25′–26′)

**(If) there are red *bubuʾtu* in a person's body, it is *ašû* (or) [. . .] (or) "hand" of Sîn (or) "hand" of curse afflicts him (or) "hand" of Ištar . . .

When the *ašû* consisted of *bubuʾtu* (vesicles), the most likely cause of infection is chickenpox (primary VZV infection).[75] Smallpox (variola) also causes a generalized vesicular rash, but it is such a severe and sporadic problem that the *āšipu* probably had more experience with chickenpox.[76]

With kullāru *(dark, flat [macular], dry, and itching [pruritic] lesions)*

10.94 [DIŠ GIG GA]R-*šú* IGI.MEŠ-*šú šag-gu*$_5$ *i-ta-ti-⸢šú⸣ um-me-di* DIRI *u i-*[. . .]*-un kul-la-ár a-ši-i* MU.NI (DPS XXXIII:9 [AOAT 43.353])

**[If] the ⸢nature⸣ [of the sore] is that its surface is stiff, the area around it is full of clusters (and) [. . .], it is called the *kullāru* of *ašû*.

The text above could be describing an allergic reaction or resolving crusted chickenpox, but there are many skin conditions that can also have this appearance.

Although generalized, the rash of *ašû* particularly affected the patient's head and eyes. Measles (rubeola) rash can involve the entire body, but it tends to affect the head first, causing red, swollen eyes with conjunctivitis (pink eye; see Chapter 9).

10.95 DIŠ GIG *ina* SU NA È-*ma pa-nu-šú u* IGI^{II}-*šú* MÚ.MEŠ-*ḫ*[*u di-ig-la ka-bit*] *ù* SA$_5$ *a-šu-⸢ú⸣* [MU.NI] . . . (Labat, *RA* 53.12–13 r. 8//*AMT* 84/6 ii 5′–6′)

**If a sore comes out on a person's body and consequently, his face and his eyes are swollen, [(and) his sight is difficult], and (his eye is) red, [it is called] *ašû* . . .

10.96 [DIŠ *pa*]*-nu-šú u* IGI^{II}*-šú* MÚ.MEŠ*-ḫa di-ig-la ka-bit u* SA$_5$[77] *a-šu-ú* MU.N[I] (DPS XXXIII:4 [AOAT 43.353])

**[If] his ⌜face⌝ and his eyes are swollen (and) his sight is difficult and (his eye is) red, ⌜it⌝ is called *ašû*.

10.97 DIŠ NA SAG.DU*-su a-šá-a a-ḫi-iz* . . . (*BAM* 481 obv. 10′)[78]

**If a person's head is gripped by *ašû* . . .

In addition to the rash, *ašû* caused headache and runny nose (rhinorrhea). These symptoms are compatible with an allergic reaction. The headache could be due to allergy-triggered sinusitis, and a runny nose is a common complaint in allergies. However, measles and other viral diseases also have a prodrome consisting of febrile headaches with or without nasal discharge.

10.98 [K]A.INIM.MA *a-šu-ú* DIB*-su-ma* A.MEŠ *ina nap-pa-še-šú* D[U*-ak* . . . SÌ]G*-as-su u* SAG.KI.MEŠ*-šú* KÚ.[MEŠ*-šú* . . .] (*AMT* 16/4:8′–9′//*BAM* 494 ii 49)

**⌜Recitation⌝ (for cases where) *ašû* afflicts him so that fluid ⌜flows⌝ from his nostrils, [. . .] gives him a ⌜sharp⌝ pain and his temples [continually] hurt [him] . . .

In addition, *ašû* sometimes produced seizures. In the text below, there is not enough information available to suggest a specific cause, but some viral infections that may produce generalized rashes (e.g., measles and chickenpox) can also cause encephalitis or postinfectious encephalopathy with seizures.

10.99 DIŠ NA *a-šu-ú u* ŠUB*-tu* DIB*-su* . . . (*BAM* 497 ii 17′//*BAM* 494 ii 14; *BAM* 494 ii 16//*BAM* 498 iv 2)

**If *ašû* with seizures afflicts a person . . .

Some forms of *ašû* were considerably less serious than others. It was, however, possible to die with *ašû*. Among the conditions referred to as *ašû*, smallpox and measles would be high on the list of those causing death. In the second reference below, the cause of the problem might in fact be louse bites, but other diseases are also possible.

10.100 ÚŠ *a-ši-i* (Böck, *Morphoskopie* 94:105)

**Death from *ašû*.

10.101 [DIŠ] GIG GAR*-šú* GIN$_7$ *ni-šik* UḪ*-ma pa-gar-šú* DIRI *a-šu-ú m*[*ut-ta*]*p-ri-šú* MU.NI (DPS XXXIII:6 [AOAT 43.353])[79]

**[If] the nature of the sore is that it is like the bite of a louse (i.e., red, dry, and itching) and his body is full (of them), it is called ⌜"fleeting"⌝ *ašû*.

NĪRU The term literally means "yoke," and refers to a lesion that curves round the pelvis, neck, or abdomen, forming a yokelike (i.e., semicircular) pattern.

10.102 DIŠ ⌜ÚR⌝.KUN*-šú* KÚ*-šú* ŠU ^{d}*Gu-la* DIŠ *ni-ri* ÍL*-ma* NIGIN*-šú* (DPS XII D iv 16//G$_2$ iv 14 = *TDP* 108 iv 16)

**If his coccyx hurts him, "hand" of Gula. If a yoke-shaped lesion rises and curves round, ("hand" of Gula).

10.103 [DIŠ] ŠÀ-*šú* DIB-[*-su-ma ú-a* D]UG$_4$.GA ŠU ^{d}ME.ME DIŠ *ni-ri ina* GÚ-*šú* GAR-*ma* NIGIN (DPS XIII B i 51′//F 10//G$_2$ 1 = *TDP* 116 i 55′)

**[If] his abdomen afflicts [him so that] he ⸢says⸣ [wah!], "hand" of Gula. If a yoke-shaped lesion is established on his neck and curves round, ("hand" of Gula).

The association of "hand" of Gula with *samānu* (cellulitis; see Chapter 3) and *ašû* (see above)[80] suggests that the yoke was reddish and consisted of a macular, papular, or vesicular eruption. This is likely to be describing the characteristic lesions of shingles (see Chapter 19 with 19.328–19.329), caused by reactivation of the *Varicella zoster* virus present in the dermal nerves. Typically, the skin lesions resemble chickenpox, but they form a bandlike structure around half of the body at any level from the head to the lower extremities.

SAGBĀNU If a patient had blister-like lesions that itched, the term *sagbānu* was used.[81] The following reference localizes the lesions to the patient's foot. One form of athlete's foot (tinea pedis) is associated with reddening of the skin, bacterial superinfection, and occasional blisters.

10.104 DIŠ GIG *ina* GÌR NA È-*ma* GIN$_7$ BU.BU.UL-*te i-ḫar-ra-aṣ sàg-ba-nu* MU.NE (*AMT* 74/1 iii 13)[82]

**If a sore comes out on a person's foot and it itches like a *bubuʾtu* (blister), it is called *sagbānu*.

BÙR/*PILŠU* (POCKMARKS) This term means "bored through." and is thought to represent pockmarks or depressed scars that can be seen with acne, smallpox, and occasionally chickenpox. It appears only in physiognomic omens.

10.105 DIŠ [SAG.K]I LÚ BÙR.MEŠ DIRI.M[EŠ] . . . (Böck, *Morphoskopie* 88:170)

**If a person's ⸢forehead⸣ is full of pockmarks . . .

IBĀRU (EVOLVING LESIONS) Since it is etymologically related to Hebrew and Arabic words for welts and scars, an *ibāru* was presumably a raised lesion.[83] Connections of the word with paint (or brand marks) also suggest that its color differed from that of the surrounding skin.[84] Physiognomic omens describe *ibāru*-lesions as covering the face or as located on the cheeks, throat, or arms.[85] One suggestion for such lesions would be acne with pimples, boils, and ultimately scars.[86]

10.106 DIŠ *i-ba-ru ina* ÚNU ZAG GAR . . . *ina* GÙB GAR . . . *ina* TE ZAG GAR . . . *ina* GÙB GAR . . . *ina gir-ri* ZAG GAR . . . *ina* GÙB [GAR] . . . *ina a-ḫi* ZA[G GAR] . . . *ina* G[ÙB GAR] . . . (Böck, *Morphoskopie* 210:5–12)[87]

**If there is an *ibāru*-lesion on the left cheekbone . . . on the right (cheekbone) . . . on the left cheek . . . on the right (cheek) . . . on the left side of the throat . . . on the right (side of throat) . . . on the ⸢left⸣ arm . . . on the ⸢right⸣ (arm) . . .

NILUGU[88] This term is further discussed in Chapter 3. The *ibāru*-like lesion in this case would be the papule, blister, and ultimately ulcer that forms when the end of the guinea worm penetrates the skin to release immature organisms.

10.107 DIŠ GIG *ina* SU NA È GIN$_7$ *i-ba-ri* È *lu* IGI UZU-*šú-ma pa?-še-er u na-kis ni-lu-gu*$_4$ MU.NI ŠU ^{d}NIN.GAL *qí-ba* GAR-*an ana* ZI-*šú*... (*BAM* 417 obv. 14–15)[89]

**If a sore comes out on a person's body (and) it comes out like an *ibāru*-lesion or it comes through(?) his skin and is cut off, its name is *nilugu*; "hand" of Ningal. You may make a (favorable) prognosis; to remove it...

ZIQTU (WHITEHEAD)[90] This lesion is small and raised like an *ibāru*-lesion, with a white spot on top. This is in all likelihood a whitehead. The white material is lipid, which accumulates in the sebaceous glands of the skin. When the lipid becomes oxidized on the surface, it turns black, becoming a blackhead.

10.108 D[IŠ] GIG GAR-*šú kup-pu-ut u* UGU/KIR$_4$-*šú ḫu-un-du-ud zi-iq-tum* MU.NI / DIŠ [GIG] GAR-*šú* GIN$_7$ *i-bar-⌜rim-ma⌝* KIR$_4$-*šú* BABBAR [Š]UB *zi-iq-tum* MU.NI / [DIŠ GIG] GAR-*šú* SA$_5$ BABBAR TUR *u* KÚ-*šú zi-iq-tum* MU.NI (DPS XXXIII:40–42 [AOAT 43.355]; cf. *AMT* 30/2:9–11)

**⌜If⌝ the nature of the sore is that it is compact and the upper part/tip[91] is deeply incised, it is called *ziqtu*. If the nature of the [sore] is that it is like an *ibāru*-lesion and its tip[92] is dotted with white, it is called *ziqtu*. [If] the nature of the [sore] is that it is red, white, (and) small[93] and it hurts him, it is called *ziqtu*.

10.109 DIŠ IGI.MEŠ-*šú ziq-ti* DIRI.MEŠ ŠU ^{d}AMAR.UTU DIN KI.MIN ŠU ^{d}IM (DPS IX A 51//B obv. 50 = *TDP* 76:51)

**If his face is full of *ziqtu*, "hand" of Marduk; he will get well. Alternatively, "hand" of Adad.

LAMṢĀTU (ULCER) This is an ulcerated lesion that is variously described as nonsuppurating, male suppurating, or female suppurating. Another use of the term was as a name for a horse, *lamṣatānu*: "(covered with) ulcers"[94] or perhaps better "(covered with saddle) sores." Also mentioned is a *lamṣātu*-insect, whose Sumerian name NIM.SAḪAR.RA means literally "sandfly."[95] If this is the same as our "sandfly" (*Phlebotomus papatasii*), the bite of an infected fly can indeed cause an ulcer.[96] The resulting disease can either be just the local ulcer (oriental or tropical ulcer), or the ulcer with a systemic infection, visceral leishmaniasis. This would also apply to the nonsuppurating ulcers of the first reference below. Other diseases may produce suppurating or nonsuppurating lesions.

10.110 [Ú] *šá-mi lam-ṣa-te*... (*BAM* 422 ii 1′)[97]

**[Plant] for (nonsuppurating) *lamṣātu*-lesions...

10.111 DIŠ NA *lam-ṣa-at ḫi-la-a-ti* GIG-*ma ma-gal a-li-kat ana* ZI-*šú*... (*BAM* 580 iii 26′)

**If a person is sick with suppurating *lamṣātu*-lesions and they flow a lot, to extricate him...

It is one author's guess that female suppurating *lamṣātu*-lesions are ulcers on an elevated base from which pus is draining. This would give the lesion a breastlike configuration with milk (pus) coming from the ulcer at the apex. A male suppurating lesion would be similar except for the absence of an elevated base. Alternatively, it is the male lesion that hurts.

10.112 DIŠ GIG MIN *ul-la-nu-ma ḫa-ri-is* ŠÀ-*ba-šu* KAK.MEŠ DIRI KAK.MEŠ-*šú* BAD KÚ[M] *u* DU-*ak lam-ṣa-at ḫi-la-a-ti* NÍTA MU.NI IM *iš-biṭ-su-ma si-ḫi-*[*ip-ti*] ^{d}PA.BIL.SAG DUG_4.GA GAR-*an ana* TI-*šú* . . . (*BAM* 580 iii 15′–17′)

**If a sore (comes out on a person's body), it has been itching for a long time, the inside of it is full of *sikkatu* (see below), it encloses its *sikkatu*, it is hot and it flows, it is called a male suppurating *lamṣātu*-lesion . . .[98] You may make a (favorable) prognosis. To cure him . . .[99]

10.113 DIŠ GIG MIN *ul* KÚ-*šú* IGI UZU.MEŠ-*šú-ma* GAR-*in* MÚD-*šú-ma* MÚD.[BABBAR] *šur-du-ma* DU-*ak lam-ṣa-at ḫi-la-a-te* SAL MU.NI IM *iš-*[*biṭ-su-ma*] *si-ḫi-ip-ti* ^{d}MAŠ.TAB.BA *qí-ba* GAR-*an ana* ZI-*šú* . . . (*BAM* 580 iii 20′–22′)

**If a sore (comes out on a person's body), it does not hurt him, it is placed only on the surface of his flesh, (and) its blood (and) pus flow freely, it is called a female suppurating *lamṣātu*-lesion . . .[100] You may make a (favorable) prognosis. To remove it . . .[101]

Since the "male suppurating" *lamṣātu*-lesions are painful and the "female suppurating" *lamṣātu*-lesions painless, they are likely to be chancroidal ulcers and the chancre of primary syphilis, respectively (see Chapter 4).

OTHER CATEGORIES OF SKIN LESIONS

The ancient physician also had terms for categories of skin lesions that do not readily translate into modern equivalents. For example, a distinction seems to have been made between isolated and clustered lesions (*ṣennītu*; *ummedu*).

AŠ. (GI_6) / *ṢENNĪTU* The Sumerogram means literally "individual (black) lesion." The term is primarily known from omen texts and lists of diseases.[102] We believe that the term is intended to describe isolated as opposed to clustered lesions.[103]

10.114 *ṣe-en-ni-tum šá ina ap-pi a-ṣ*[*u-š*]*u la dam-qu* (Lugale V 33 [description of Asakku], apud *CAD* Ṣ 127b)

***Ṣennītu* whose eruption on the nose is not good.

10.115 [DIŠ MUNUS] Ù.TU-*ma* LÚ.TUR *ṣi-in-ni-tam* DIRI . . . (Šumma Izbu IV 10 [Leichty, *Izbu* 67])

**[If a woman] gives birth and the infant is full of *ṣennītu* . . .

UMMEDU The exact meaning of this term is uncertain, but if it is related to the verb *emēdu*, as it would appear to be, it should mean lesions that are joined, come together, or meet, in other words, a cluster.[104] Rashes associated with a number of conditions, including *ašû* (see above), are described as being *ummedu*-like.[105]

10.116 Ú *um-me-di* ZI-*ḫi* . . . (*STT* 92 iii 16′; cf. 17′)

**Plant to remove clusters (of lesions) . . .

10.117 DIŠ GIG *ina* SU NA È GIN$_7$ *um-*[*me-di* . . .] (*AMT* 52/3:12′)

**If a sore comes out on a person's body and it is ⌜clustered⌝ [. . .]

Another ancient Mesopotamian term used for a type of skin lesion was *umṣātu*. Following are the references to these lesions as well as to some of the other skin lesions and syndromes that they help to define.

UMṢĀTU This, along with *uršu* and *baṣkiltu* (see below), are the three terms used to describe hemorrhoids (see Chapter 6). Physiognomic omens mention *umṣātu* almost anywhere on the body including the under part of the nose, the ears, and at the opening of the penis.[106] Birth omens indicate that such lesions were already present in newborn infants.[107] Medical texts use the term *umṣātu* for a mass or tissue enlargement located in or near a body opening (orifice).[108]

10.118 DIŠ NA DÚR-*šú um-ṣa-ti* ⌜DIRI⌝ KÁ-*šú* BAD-*ḫi ana um-ṣa-t*[*i*] *qut-tu-pi* . . . (*STT* 97 iii 19)[109]

**If a person's anus is full of *umṣātu*-lesions (and) his (anal) opening is closed off, to remove the *umṣātu*-lesions . . .

Besides hemorrhoids, *umṣātu* is also used to describe nasal turbinates (see Chapter 9) and swellings within the areolar tissue of the breasts of pregnant women. The breast lesions are normal enlargements of sebaceous (oil) glands, and are called Montgomery's tubercles.[110]

10.119 DIŠ NA *na-ḫi-ri-šú um-ṣa-at ḫi-li it-tab-ši* . . . (*SpTU* 1.44:34)

**If there is an exuding *umṣātu*-lesion in a person's nostrils . . .

10.120 DIŠ SAMAG.MEŠ BABBAR.MEŠ DIRI SI.SÁ PEŠ$_4$-*át* (DPS XXXVI A 33 = *TDP* 202:33)

**If (the tip of a woman of childbearing age's breast) is full of white *umṣatus*, the delivery will be easy.[111]

10.121 DIŠ SAMAG.MEŠ SA$_5$.MEŠ DIRI NU SI.SÁ PEŠ$_4$-*át* (DPS XXXVI A 34 = *TDP* 202:34)[112]

**If (the tip of a woman of childbearing age's breast) is full of reddish *umṣātus*, the delivery will not be easy.[113]

URŠU AND *BAṢKILTU* In contrast to *umṣātu*, these terms seem to be used exclusively to describe hemorrhoids (see Chapter 6).

10.122 DIŠ NA *ur-šu dan-nu* KÁ MUD-*šú* DIB-*ma* KÁ MUD BAD-*ḫi* . . . (*BAM* 95:10// *STT* 97 iii 1)[114]

**If a large *uršu* "seizes" his anal opening so that it closes the anal opening . . .

10.123 *šum-ma* LÚ *i-na pí-i qí-in-na-ti-šu ba-aṣ-ki-il-tum it-ta-ṣi-a-am* . . . (*YOS* 11.29:8; *YOS* 11.28:3)

**If a *baṣkiltu*-lesion comes out at the mouth of a person's anus . . .

The term *umṣātu* is also used to describe other similar lesions such as *ḫalû* and *pindû*.[115]

ḪALÛ This lesion is primarily known from physiognomic omens, which describe faces, chests, and bodies full of *ḫalû*-lesions, usually described as black. Birth omens indicate that such lesions were already present in newborn infants;[116] commentaries to the texts explain *ḫalû*-lesions as being "black *umṣātu*." The term is also used to describe a rust or other fungus appearing on harvested grain.[117] It is likely that the *āšipu* was describing pedunculated or raised sessile black moles (pigmented nevus).[118] One text prescribes a treatment for them.

10.124 DIŠ NA *ḫa-le-e* IGI.MEŠ [DIRI] . . . (*BAM* 35 i 4′)

**If a person's face [is full of] *ḫalû* . . .

Two fragmentary entries in Tablet XXXIII, the section of the diagnostic/prognostic series describing skin lesions, appear to make reference to hairs growing from a nevus (hairy nevus).

10.125 [. . .] ŠÀ-*šú* SÍG GI_6 È-⌜*a* x⌝ [. . .] / [. . .] ŠÀ-*šú* SÍG BABBAR È-*a* NU ⌜x⌝ (DPS XXXIII:85–86 [AOAT 43.357])

**[If . . .] (and) a black hair grows out of it [. . .]. [If . . .] (and) a white hair grows out of it [. . .]

PINDÛ *Pindû*-lesions are known primarily from physiognomic omens, where they are described as occurring on the head, body, and penis.[119] Birth omens indicate that such lesions were already present in newborn infants;[120] commentaries to the texts explain *pindû*-lesions as being "red *umṣātu*."[121] Red swellings at birth especially on the head and trunk are quite likely to be cavernous hemangiomas.[122] This birth mark can be unsightly and disfiguring but usually resolves spontaneously during childhood.

Pindû is also the name of a stone that is described as being granulated like mottled barley or cucumber seeds.[123] The granular nature of the lesion would seem to be confirmed by the phrase "it holds all of them" in the following reference.

10.126 DIŠ GIG GAR-*šú* GIN_7 x SA_5 x x.MEŠ *ka-li-šú-nu* DIB *pi-en-du₄* (DPS XXXIII:27 [AOAT 43.354])

**If the appearance of the sore is that it is as red as [. . .] (and) it holds the [. . .], all of them, [it] ⌜is called⌝ *pindû*.

GARĀBU Although *pindû*-lesions were red, there was a similar-looking (i.e., granular) lesion that was white and called *garābu*. *Garābu*-lesions appeared on people with *saḫaršubbû* (see below) and were known to be infectious.

10.127 *šum₄-ma ina* SU NA *pi-in-du-ú* BABBAR *ša ga-ra-bu i-qab-bu* . . . (*BAM* 580 v 17′)

**If (there are) white *pindû* on a man's body which they call *garābu* . . .[124]

10.128 Ú *ga-ra-bi* . . . (*STT* 92 iii 7′)

**Plant for *garābu* . . .

10.129 *ga-ra-bu gara-bu li-ʾ-bu* (Meissner, *Supp*. pl. 7 K 4166 ii 8; apud *CAD* L 181a)

***Garābu* is infectious (*liʾbu*).

A number of conditions suggest themselves for this lesion in humans.[125] One is condylomata (see Chapter 4). Another is lichen planus, a benign skin and mouth condition of unknown etiology with raised, white, and sometimes scaly lesions. A final possibility is the lesion of lepromatous leprosy (see Chapter 3).[126]

In addition to human beings, *garābu*-lesions were also observed in sheep. The term for sheep with *garābu*-lesions was *girriṣānu*.[127] Sheep, cattle, and horses are not subject to Hansen's disease (leprosy). There are, however, many chronic skin conditions in large animals caused by bacteria, fungi, and parasites that can mimic lesions seen in leprosy.[128]

EPQU This condition appeared in newborn children and adults. Some forms were considered to be contagious.[129] There is also a related word *epqēnu* ("*epqu*-like") which indicates a similar yet somehow different skin problem.[130] If, as seems probable, the term is related to the verb *uppuqu*, it should imply a thickening or solidification of the skin.[131] *Epqu*-like lesions came in a variety of colors, as in the following reference.

10.130 Ú.MEŠ *ša ep-qa-an-ni* . . . *šum-ma pé-ṣú-ú* . . . *šum-ma pa-ni sí-im-mi-šu mi-it-ḫu-ru-ma sà-a-mu* . . . (Tsukimoto, *Priests and Officials* 199–200:72, 74, 79–80)

**Plants for a person with *epqu*-like lesions . . . if they are white . . . if the faces of his lesions are uniform and red . . .

SAḪARŠUBBÛ An adult who was covered with *epqu* was said to have *saḫaršubbû*.

10.131 LÚ.SAḪAR.ŠUB.BA = *ša e-ep-qá-am ma-lu-ú* (OB LÚ A 274, apud *CAD* E 246a)

**The person with *saḫaršubbû* means somebody who is full of *epqu*.

10.132 DIŠ *ina* SU [N]A *saḫar-šub-bu-u it-tab-ši* . . . (*BAM* 35 ii 5′)

**If *saḫaršubbû* has appeared on a ⸢person's⸣ body . . .[132]

Saḫaršubbû is also lexically equated with *garābu* (see above), which indicates that the victim of this disease was expected to display hypopigmented (white) granular lesions (*garābu*) and variously colored thickenings of the skin (*epqu*). At least some of these lesions were expected to respond to treatment.[133]

10.133 BAD LÚ SAḪAR.ŠUB.BA BABBAR *ina* IM.TE-*šú* GÁL . . . KI.MIN SIG_7 *ina* IM.TE-*šú* GÁL . . . KI.MIN SA_5 *u* GI_6 *ina* IM.TE-*šú* GÁL . . . (Tsukimoto, *Priests and Officials* 199-200:53, 55, 56)

**If a person has white *saḫaršubbû* on his body . . . (if he has) yellow ones on his body . . . (if he has) red or dark ones on his body . . .

Saḫaršubbû was thought to be infectious, and covered the body "like a garment," as may be seen in the following curses.

10.134 SAḪAR.ŠUB.BA-*a šèr-ti* DINGIR *ka-bit-ta zu-mur-šu lil-la-ib-ma* (*MDP* 6 pl. 10 vi 14–15)

**May his body be infected (*la'ābu*)[134] with *saḫaršubbû*, the severe punishment of the god!

10.135 SAḪAR.ŠUB.BA-*a pa-gar-šu ki-ma ṣu-ba-ti lik-tu-um* (Borger, *AfO* 23.3 iii 2–3)[135]

**May (the god)[136] cover his body with *saḫaršubbû* as with a garment!

The victim of *saḫaršubbû* was disqualified from becoming a diviner, and was imagined as inhabiting a separate part of the netherworld after death.[137] It may, therefore, be this particular infectious disease (*li'bu*) that is referred to in the Laws of Ḫammurapi (see Chapter 2 with 2.13).[138]

10.136 **If a man marries a wife and *li'bu* afflicts her (and) he sets his mind on marrying another wife, he may marry her (but) he may not divorce his wife whom *li'bu* afflicts; she shall live in a house that he builds (for her) and as long as she lives he shall support her. (Laws of Ḫammurapi § 148)

It has long been suggested[139] (and hotly denied), on etymological and other grounds,[140] that *saḫaršubbû* represents the skin manifestations of leprosy (Hansen's disease; see Chapter 3).[141]

INDIVIDUAL LESIONS WITH DESCRIPTIVE NAMES

Lesions with a distinctive appearance attracted specific descriptive names: "rolled up" (*kurāru*); "strawberry" (*girgiššu*); "fungus/mold" (*kibšu*); "lump" (*kirbānu*); "peg" (*sikkatu*); "branching" (*ṣiršu*); "grain (of barley)" (ŠE or *uṭṭeṭu*); "on a person's trunk" (UGU.MURUB$_4$.LÚ).

PEŠ.GIG; *G/KURĀRU* *Kurāru* is conventionally translated as "carbuncle" because it is supposed that "soup cooked over *gurāru*" refers specifically to embers.[142] However, the term appears to be related to *garāru*: "to turn, roll over," which suggests that the *kurāru* over which the soup was cooked was some sort of (heated) ring of stones or pottery cylinder. It is probably not irrelevant that several treatments for this condition involve the magical use of gold rings.[143] In view of the shape and the common location of this lesion on the head,[144] it seems likely that the following references are to the common scalp dermatophytosis, ringworm.[145]

10.137 DIŠ NA SAG.DU-*su* PEŠ.GIG DIB-*it* . . . (*BAM* 3 i 44)[146]

**If a person's head is afflicted by *kurāru* . . .

10.138 DIŠ NA PEŠ.GIG/*ku-ra-ra* GIG . . . (*BAM* 3 i 48; Labat, *RA* 53.10–11 obv. 42)[147]

**If a person is sick/sore with *kurāru* . . .

10.139 Ú *šá-mi ku-ra-ri* ZI . . . (*BAM* 422 ii 12′)[148]

**Plant for removing *kurāru* . . .

G/KURAŠTU *Kuraštu/kurartu* is conventionally translated as "eczema,"[149] but the available references do not fit very well with this diagnosis. The term is the feminine of *kurāru*, which should imply that the two are at least similar to, if not by-forms of, one another, with some difference in size and/or appearance. Ringworm begins as a solid lesion; the characteristic ring forms as a result of the more rapid healing of the central portions of the lesion. One possibility, then, is that *kuraštu* was meant to describe the early solid lesion.

10.140 DIŠ NA Ì *la-ta-ki* ŠÉŠ-*ma* SAG.DU-*su gu-*[*raš-tu* . . .] (*AMT* 5/2:5)

**If a person rubs on an oil to be tested and as a result his head [is afflicted] with ⌜*guraštu*⌝ . . .

10.141 DIŠ NA *gu-raš-tu* DIRI . . . SÍG È (*BAM* 494 iii 1)[150]

**If a person is full of *guraštu* . . . (after treatment) the hair will sprout.

It seems likely that the references above are describing dermatophytosis (ringworm) or contact dermatitis.

GIRGIŠŠU This lesion is an elevated red nodule that resembles a strawberry. *Girgiššu* literally means "strawberry plant."

10.142 [DIŠ GIG G]AR-*šú* GIN_7 TAB KÚM-*ma* du ⌜x⌝ A NU *ú-kal* G[IG . . .] TUKU *gir-giš-šum* MU.NI (DPS XXXIII:13 [AOAT 43.353])

**[If the] ⌜nature⌝ of the [sore] is that it is hot like a burn [. . .] does not contain fluid and the ⌜sore⌝ has a [. . .], its name is *girgiššu*.

10.143 6,40[151] *a-wi-lum gi-ir-gi-ša-am ma-li* . . . (*BAM* 393 obv. 14)[152]

**If a man is full of *girgiššu* . . .

10.144 *gir-giš-šum* ŠU ^{d}UTU (DPS XXXIII:110 [AOAT 43.358])[153]

***Girgiššu*, "hand" of Šamaš.

Raised, red, hot, fluidless, and painful skin infections can be caused by group A streptococci (erysipelas).[154] The commonest site of involvement is the face, which may account for the attribution of this lesion to Šamaš, god of the sun.[155]

KIBŠU The term is used to describe galls for tanning and growths on jars used to contain ointment[156] as well as a type of skin lesion associated with *kureštu* (ringworm; see above) and *kiṣṣatu* (hair loss; also see above).

10.145 DIŠ NA SAG.DU-*su* ⸢*kib*⸣-*šá gi-iṣ-ṣa-tú gu-reš-tú*[157] DIRI . . . (Labat, *RA* 53.10–11 obv. 30)

**If a person's head is full of *kibšu*, *giṣṣatu*, (and) *kureštu* . . .

The references above might be describing a chronic form of dermatophytosis called favus. This disease usually involves the scalp, causing honey-colored crusts to develop around hair follicles. Hair loss occurs, with thickening of the scalp and eventually scarring. The yellowish color of tanning galls (*kibšu*) provides a logical association with the color of this fungal infection of the skin.

KIRBĀNU This skin lesion is raised to form a larger mass ("lump"). The description of the "silt" and the location of this lesion on the neck suggest that this is what we call "lumpy jaw" (actinomycosis; see Chapter 3).

10.146 DIŠ GIG GAR-*šú* GIN$_7$ ^{IM}⸢*ṭe*$_4$⸣-*ru-ti-šú* NIGIN.ME? *u ti-ik-ka-šú* DIB [*kir-ba-nu*] MU.NI / DIŠ GIG GAR-*šú da-an pa-an* UZU.MEŠ-*šú* GAR *u* [KÚ]M.KÚM-*im kir*-⸢*ba*⸣-*nu* MU.NI (DPS XXXIII:38–39 [AOAT 43.355]; cf. *BAM* 583 i 3′–5′)

**If the nature of the sore is that it is surrounded by what looks like its silt and it "seizes" his neck, it is called ["lump"]. If the nature of the sore is that it is hard, it is placed on the surface of his flesh, and he is continually hot, it is called "lump."

UZU.GAG.MEŠ / *SIKKATU* The term, which literally means "peg," is used to describe broad roundish, that is, peg-shaped, lesions of various types. In some cases, the lesions appear to have ulcerated, producing a peg-shaped concavity (i.e., a hole into which a peg might be placed or from which a peg had been removed). In others, large, raised lesions were called *sikkatu*, presumably because they resembled pegs that were in place. Included in the references are at least five different diseases or skin conditions.

10.147 GAG.MEŠ *ina* SU NA *id-*[*d*]*a-a-ki-a it-ta-ši-na* [. . .] BABBAR.MEŠ GAL.MEŠ *e-la-a ana* ZI.MEŠ-*ši-na* . . . (*BAM* 268 iii 6′–7′ // *BAM* 582 i 3′–4′)

**(If) *sikkatu* are transferred to the body of a person (and) their characteristic feature (is that they are) [. . .], white, large, (and) they come up; to remove them . . .

10.148 *sí-ik-ka-tum im-ta-qú-ut e-li ka-li bu-li-im úḫ-ta-am-mi-iṭ la-a-le-e ka-lu-mi ù ṣé-eḫ-ḫe-ru-tim i-na bu*-⸢*ú*⸣-*ud ta-ri-i-tim* . . . KA.INIM.MA UDU.GAG.ŠUB.BA . . . (*YOS* 11.7:3–7, 17)

**The *sikkatu* fell on all the herds; it made the kids, lambs, and babies in the arms of the nurse burn (with fever) . . . recitation for *sikkatu* falling on sheep . . .

The two references above appear compatible with the viral infection orf (see Chapter 2).[158] Either condylomata lata or condylomata accuminata (both sexually transmitted diseases; see Chapter 4) may have caused the condition discussed below.

10.149 DIŠ ŠIR^{II}-*šú* MÚ.MEŠ-*ḫa* GÌŠ-*šú sik-ka-ta*$_5$ DIRI *ana* N[IN.DINGIR.RA DINGIR-*šú* TE-*ḫi*] (DPS XIV A$_2$ ii 16 // C ii 30 = *TDP* 136 ii 66)

**If his testicles are continually swollen (and) his penis is full of *sikkatu*, [he approached] the ⌜*ēntu*⌝ [of his god]).

In the two references below, *sikkatu* is used to describe lesions that appear in wounds or insect bites. The first quote is difficult to explain, but may represent areas of abscess formation or necrosis present within larger wounds. The black color in the second reference could be related to bleeding into the lesions, possibly secondary to scratching, or in the case of more toxic insects and spiders, tissue necrosis.

10.150 *šum*$_4$*-ma ina* ŠÀ GIG UZU.GAG.MEŠ È . . . (*BAM* 32:13′//*BAM* 417 obv. 11)

**If *sikkatu* come out in the middle of the wound . . .

10.151 DIŠ GAG.MEŠ GI$_6$.MEŠ *ma-li* MU.⌜BI⌝ *ut-ta-aš-ši-ik-m*[*a* . . .] (*PBS* 2/2.104:10)

**If he is full of black *sikkatus*, that is because he has been bitten all over and [. . .]

For *sikkatu* as part of the description of the chancroid ulcer, see above under *lamṣātu*. Finally, there is a quote that associates *sikkatu* in the mouth with fever and *bu*ʾ*šānu*. This is probably a reference to the ulceration of the intraoral vesicles of herpetic stomatitis, which we believe was included under the term *bu*ʾ*šānu* (see Chapter 3).

10.152 ZI-*iḫ šá* KIR$_4$/KA-*šú um-mu sik-ka-tum la-ba-ṭu u bu-u*ʾ*-šá-nu* (*SpTU* 1.44:74// *BAM* 28 r. 11′//*BAM* 29 r. 31′–32′//*BAM* 533:89//*AMT* 54/3 ii 6′–7′//*BAM* 543 iv 1–2 [W. Farber, *JNES* 49.315])

**May fever, *sikkatu*, *lubaṭu*-fever, and/or *bu*ʾ*šānu* be removed from his nose/mouth.

ṢIRŠU The term is related to a verb, *ṣurrušu*, which means "to grow shoots, branches" and which refers to the branching of trees or the formation of starlike shapes of oil in water. This would seem to indicate that the lesion had radiating lines (presumably small blood vessels) making it sound like a spider angioma (telangiectasis).[159] Lesions of this type are commonly associated with advanced liver cirrhosis, and are most frequently found on the face, neck, and upper torso. For other possible references to spiders (described as "webs"), see Chapter 6 with 6.153.

10.153 DIŠ NA *ṣir-ši* IGI.MEŠ-*šú* [. . .] (*BAM* 35 i 7′)

**If a person's face [is full of] *ṣiršu* [. . .]

UṬṬEṬU This term means "grain (of barley)" and the lesion usually seems to be red.[160] Since it is often described as being present on the forehead of pregnant women, "grains" may be pimples or folliculitis.[161]

10.154 DIŠ *uṭ-ṭe-ṭì* DIRI *šà*-ŠÀ-*šà* NITA : NÍG.TUKU (DPS XXXVI A 6 = *TDP* 200:6)

**If (the top of the forehead of a woman of childbearing age) is full of "grains," her fetus is male (var. richness [plenty of fat]).

10.155 DIŠ *uṭ-ṭe-ṭì* SA$_5$.MEŠ DIRI *šà*-ŠÀ-*šà*[162] *i*$_{11}$*-šár-rù* (DPS XXXVI A 7 = *TDP* 200:7)

**If it is full of red "grains," her fetus will become rich (i.e., fat).

UGU.MURUB$_4$.LÚ These lesions, which appear alongside swellings in the first reference below were, if the name is correctly read, located "on a person's trunk" as well as on the face. The color given in the second reference is black.

10.156 DIŠ NA *rip-ḫi* UGU.MURUB$_4$.LÚ IGI.MEŠ-*šú* DIRI . . . (*BAM* 35 i 25′)

**If a person's face is full of swellings (and) UGU.MURUB$_4$.LÚ . . .

10.157 DIŠ NA UGU.MURUB$_4$.LÚ GI$_6$.MEŠ IGI.MEŠ-*šú* DIRI . . . (*BAM* 35 i 14′)[163]

**If a person's face is full of black UGU.MURUB$_4$.LÚ . . .

Two possible explanations come to mind. The black lesions could be blackheads and the swelling could be oil accumulated within the oil glands that constitute the basic source of the blackheads. The second possibility is that the lesions are pigmented nevi (moles), which may be elevated structures. In favor of the first possibility is the fact that there is another word *ḫalû* (see above) which also describes raised nevi.

MYSTERY LESIONS

The remaining words for skin lesion are not well enough attested or described to attempt an identification. We include them here in the hope that future discoveries will make it possible ultimately to identify them.

ERIMU This lesion is primarily known from physiognomic omens, although there are treatments for it.[164]

10.158 *a-na e-ri-mu ma-gal na-gul* x [. . .] (*BAM* 582 ii 8′, 10′)

**To [. . .] an *erimu* (which is) very shiny(?) [. . .]

10.159 *ana* GIG.MEŠ *e-r*[*ìm*? S]IG$_5$ . . . (*STT* 93:61′)

**(The plant) is good for *erimu*-lesions . . .

Physiognomic omens describe faces spotted with white, yellow, red, or black *erimu*-lesions, and other similar lesions are mentioned on the lips, back, and chest.[165] Lexical equations indicate that the primary color of the lesion was red.[166] The text below describes an *erimu*-lesion on the scrotum following an injury.[167] Without a better understanding of the nature of this lesion it is difficult to interpret the pathology. It could represent redness and swelling[168] due to trauma, but necrosis due to compromised blood supply, or secondary infection are other possibilities.

10.160 *šum-ma* MUNUS *i-na ṣa-al-te iš-ka ša* LÚ *ta-aḫ-te-pi* . . . *ù šum-ma* ^{LÚ}A.ZU *ur-tak-ki-is-ma iš-ku ša-ni-tu il-te-ša-ma ta-at-ta-al-pa-at* [*e*]*-ri-im-ma tar-ti-i-ši* [*ù*] *lu-ú i-na ṣa-al-te* [*iš*]-*ka ša-ni-ta taḫ-te-pi* . . . (Middle Assyrian Laws A § 8)

**If a woman crushes a person's testicle in a quarrel . . . and if the *asû* (pharmacist) bandages it up and subsequently the other testicle becomes affected from it and gets an *erimu*-lesion or if she crushed the other ⌜testicle⌝ in the quarrel . . .

Ḫ̬ÁD.A/*RAMĪṬU* The meaning of Akkadian *ramīṭu* is uncertain since the root does not appear in Hebrew, Aramaic, or Arabic. However, there are two roots in Arabic (*rmḍ* and *rmd*) which, while not proper matches, are close enough to be possible cognates. The first should mean "excessively hot" or "sun baked,"[169] which might suggest a lesion resulting from overexposure to the sun. This would not be inappropriate in view of the fact that *ramīṭu*-lesions are usually described as appearing on the face. The second root is a color term, meaning "ashen" (i.e., pale or grayish, "of a dusty color in which is a duskiness or dinginess").[170] The concern of the *āšipu* in these cases was to distinguish harmful from harmless lesions.

10.161 DIŠ IGI.M[EŠ-*šú*] Ḫ̬ÁD.A SA$_5$.MEŠ DIRI.MEŠ GIG-*su* GÍD-*ma* DIN (DPS IX A 43//C 11 = *TDP* 74:43)

**If [his] face is full of red *ramīṭu*-lesions, his illness may be prolonged, (but) he will get well.

10.162 DIŠ IGI.MEŠ-*šú* Ḫ̬ÁD.A BABBAR.MEŠ DIRI.MEŠ DIN (DPS IX A 44//C 12 = *TDP* 74:44)

**If his face is full of white *ramīṭu*-lesions, he will get well.

10.163 DIŠ IGI.MEŠ-*šú* Ḫ̬ÁD.A SIG$_7$.MEŠ DIRI.MEŠ ŠU ^{d}BAD DIN (DPS IX A 45//C 13 = *TDP* 74:45)

**If his face is full of yellow *ramīṭu*-lesions, "hand" of Bēl; he will get well.

10.164 DIŠ IGI.MEŠ-*šú* Ḫ̬ÁD.A GI$_6$.MEŠ DIRI.MEŠ GAM (DPS IX A 46//C 14 = *TDP* 74:46)[171]

**If his face is full of black *ramīṭu*-lesions, he will die.

Overexposure to the sun can cause actinic keratosis, a benign but precancerous condition. Squamous cell skin cancer and malignant melanomas (bluish-black lesions with irregular borders) are also much more common in skin with prolonged sun exposure. The large numbers of ancient Mesopotamians employed as farmers and shepherds should have provided the *āšipu* with a great deal of experience with squamous cell carcinoma. Skin cancer is an easily controlled disease if removed early, but can become invasive and fatal if ignored. Malignant melanoma is the most dangerous, and still the leading cause of death from all diseases arising in the skin. Certain locations on the face were considered to worsen the prognosis.

10.165 DIŠ *ina* SAG KIR$_4$-*šú* Ḫ̬ÁD.A SA$_5$ *u* BABBAR *it-tab-šu-ú* PA NU TUKU (DPS VI A obv. 28//C i 14 = *TDP* 56:28)[172]

**If there are red or white *ramīṭu*-lesions on the bulb of a man's nose, it is of no consequence.[173]

10.166 DIŠ *ina* SAG IGI.MEŠ-*šú* Ḫ̬ÁD.A.MEŠ SA$_5$.MEŠ È.MEŠ GAM/DIN (DPS IX A 77//B r. 24 = *TDP* 78:77)

**If red *ramīṭu*-lesions erupt on the upper part of his face, he will die (var. B: he will live).

10.167 DIŠ *ina* SAG IGI.MEŠ-*šú* ḪÁD.A.MEŠ GI_6.MEŠ È.MEŠ GAM (DPS IX A 78//B r. 25 = *TDP* 78:78)

**If black *ramīṭu*-lesions erupt on the upper part of his face, he will die.

Primary tumor site can be important in the outcome of skin cancers. Black *ramīṭu*-lesions were also observed on the tongue, and preexistent black lesions were associated with a vaguely described (and fatal) systemic illness. Although there is not much to go on in these references, malignant melanoma could be the underlying disease.

10.168 DIŠ EME-*šú* ḪÁD.A GI_6.MEŠ [D]IRI ⸢x⸣ [. . .] (DPS VII A obv. 10 = *TDP* 62:10)

**If his tongue is ⸢full⸣ of black *ramīṭu*-lesions [. . .]

10.169 DIŠ *ina* SAG KIR_4-*šú* ḪÁD.A GI_6.MEŠ *it-tab-šu-ú ana* U_4.3.KÁM GAM (DPS VI A obv. 29//C i 15 = *TDP* 56:29)

**If there are preexistent black *ramīṭu*-lesions on the bulb of a man's nose (and he has been sick) for three days, he will die.[174]

10.170 DIŠ *ina* SAG KIR_4-*šú* ḪÁD.A GI_6.MEŠ *it-tab-šu-ú u* IGI^{II}-*šú* MÚD DIRI.MEŠ GAM (DPS VI A obv. 30//C i 16 = *TDP* 56:30)

**If there are preexistent black *ramīṭu*-lesions on the bulb of a man's nose and his eyes are continually full of blood, he will die.

The reference below describes a chronic bleeding lesion of unspecified type. Skin cancer, either basal cell or squamous cell varieties, typically have these characteristics, and may therefore be described in this text. There are, however, other chronic skin lesions that can bleed.

10.171 DIŠ GIG *ina* SU NA È MÚD.MEŠ *uš-te-né-ṣa-a* . . . (*BAM* 580 iii 29′)

**If a sore comes out on a person's body (and) it continually makes blood come out of it . . .

IZI/*IŠĀTU* A series of Middle Babylonian letters from a physician to the king describes an outbreak of a contagious disease involving at least ten palace women and one man.[175] The patients had common findings of fever and the presence of small numbers (two to three) of lesions (*išātu*) on the chest and ribs. Some patients also had pneumonia. The lesions lingered, "sweated" (i.e., produced serum or pus), and become spotted with red spots (*šīpu*) before being finally cured. The condition does not appear to have caused any fatalities, and had a duration of five to ten days. We have been unable to think of a modern disease that fits this description. The word *išātu* literally means "fire," presumably a reference to the vivid red color and/or warmth of the lesion.[176]

10.172 ⸢DIŠ KI.MIN SA_5⸣ KÚ-*šú u* [. . .] GIG BI IZI MU.NI *ana* ZI-*šú* . . . (Labat, *RA* 53.12–13 r. 15)

**If (a sore comes out on a person's body and) it is red (and) it hurts him and [. . .], that sore is called "fire," to remove it . . .

IŠĪTU This lesion is described as being warm, solid (without fluid), but with small water blisters on the surface.

10.173 [DIŠ] GIG GAR-*šú* GIN_7 TAB KÚM-*ma* A NU *ú-kal* Ù.BU.[BU].UL TUR.MEŠ DIRI *i-ši-tum* MU.[NI] (DPS XXXIII:15 [AOAT 43.354]; cf. Labat, *RA* 53.12–13 r. 10)[177]

**[If] the nature of the sore is that it is hot like a burn and does not contain fluid (and) is full of little ⌜*bubuʾtu*⌝, [it] is called *išītu*.[178]

10.174 DIŠ IGI.MEŠ-*šú i-ši-tú* DIRI.MEŠ DIN (DPS IX A 52b = *TDP* 76:52b)

**If his face is full of *išītu*, he will get well.

KU_7.KU_7 / *MATQŪTI* The term means "sweet," but it is unclear how this applies to skin lesions. It is unlikely that the *āšipu* was so foolhardy as to actually taste fluids coming out of a skin lesion.[179] Since fresh milk and other foods were considered "sweet" and spoiled milk "sour," the *āšipu* might have classified uninfected or minimally infected serum coming from a wound to be "sweet." When the exuded material becomes thick and foul-smelling it is no longer "sweet."

10.175 DIŠ NA SAG.DU-*su* GIG.MEŠ KU_7.KU_7 DIRI.MEŠ . . . (BAM 3 ii 9//*CT* 23.50:12; *BAM* 3 ii 12//*BAM* 155 iii 9′)[180]

**If a person's head is full of "sweet" sores . . .[181]

10.176 DIŠ NA SAG.DU-*su kal-ma-tú ma-tuq-tú* DIRI . . . (Labat, *RA* 53.10–11 obv. 35; *BAM* 494 i 30′; cf. *SpTU* 1.51:1)

**If a person's head is full of "sweet" louse bites . . .[182]

LIPTU This lesion is thus far only attested in physiognomic omens[183] and extispicy. *Liptu*-lesions are described everywhere on the body; they can be bright red or black, and can have a single hair growing in the center.[184]

LUḪIGĀTU Even the reading of the name of these lesions is uncertain,[185] but hair loss seems to be involved.

10.177 DIŠ *lu-ḫi-ga-tú ina* SU NA GÁL *ana lu-ḫi-ga-ti šu-le-e* . . . SÍG *e-la-a* (Labat, *RA* 53.10–11 obv. 39//*BAM* 497 ii 7′, 8′//*AMT* 1/3:3′)

**If there are *luḫigātu* on a person's body, to remove the *luḫigātu* . . . (after treatment) hair will sprout.

NAḪRU Presumably the term is related to a verb *nuḫḫuru*, which is used to describe injured bones.

10.178 Ú GIG *na-aḫ-ri* . . . (*CT* 14.43 [S. 60]:2′//*BAM* 1 iii 25)

**Plant for *naḫru*-sore . . .

10.179 [. . . *ma-ḫi*] *r-ta-šú nu-uḫ-ḫu-ra-at-ma* . . . (*AMT* 75/1 iii 28)

**(If) . . . and his ⌜fibula⌝ is *nuḫḫuru*'d . . .

10.180 NÍG.LAL GÌR *nu-uḫ-ḫur-*[*ti*] . . . (*BAM* 124 iii 19)[186]

**Bandage for *nuḫḫuru*'d foot . . .

NIPIŠTU

10.181 DIŠ GIG GAR-*šú* GIN$_7$ TAB KÚM-*ma um-me-di* DIRI *ri-šu-tam* TUKU *ni-piš-tum* MU.[NI] (DPS XXXIII:16 [AOAT 43.354])

**If the nature of the sore is that it is hot like a burn and is full of clusters (and) has redness, [it] is called *nipištu*.

10.182 DIŠ GIG GAR-*šú* GIN$_7$ *um-me-di u* DIŠ È-*su* SAMAG DIB-*bat ni-piš-tum* MU.NI (DPS XXXIII:17 [AOAT 43.354])

**[If] the nature of the sore is that it is clustered and if a swelling blocks its exit, it is called *nipištu*.

ŠARŪRU

10.183 Ú GIG *šá-a-ru-ru-u* . . . (*BAM* 380:11//*STT* 92 iii 27′)

**Plant for *šarūru* sore . . .

ŠE/KITTABRU This term appears only in physiognomic omens, often as multiple lesions and usually somewhere on the head: on top of the ear, on the upper or lower eyelid, in the corner of the eye, on the palate, on the upper or lower lip.[187] It shares a common Sumerogram with three other lesions, *ḫalû*, *umṣātu*, and *pindû*. All three are raised lesions, *ḫalû* being defined as a "black *umṣātu*" and *pindû* as a "red *umṣātu*-lesion. This might indicate that *kittabru* was also a raised lesion, possibly a "yellow" or "white *umṣātu*."[188]

ŠIKṢU This term is lexically equated with "sore." In addition to its use to describe a lesion on newborn babies, this is attested only as a mark that can be white on internal organs.[189]

10.184 BE MUNUS Ù.TU-*ma* MIN-*ma šik-ṣi* DIRI . . . (Šumma Izbu IV 11 [Leichty, *Izbu* 67])

**If a woman gives birth and (from the beginning the child) is full of *šikṣu* . . .

URĀŠU This lesion is only attested in the physiognomic omens.[190] Von Soden[191] suggests that the reference is to a low (depressed), impure mark. These lesions tend to be multiple, since the term *nadû* (see above) is used to describe them.[192]

Last, and certainly least, are two terms that are attested only in Tablet XXXIII of the diagnostic/prognostic series in fragmentary and difficult context. Of these, all we know is that one (*abābu*?)[193] did not hurt and that the other *abiktu*[194] hurt so badly that the victim could not sleep.

Hair

HAIR STANDING ON END

There are many texts that refer to the patient's hair standing on end or standing up. There are two possible explanations for this observation. There is a mechanism by which hair can literally stand up, and this is due to a muscle that is attached to the base of the hair follicle, the erector pili muscle. The conditions that can cause this muscle to contract are a sense of fear and patients who are cold or chilled, as in the following reference.

10.185 DIŠ NA MURUB$_4$ UGU-*šú* ⸢SAG⸣.KI.MEŠ-*šú* TAG.TAG-*s*[*u*] GEŠTU^{II}-*šú i-šag-gu-ma liq pi-šú i-ta-na-b*[*al*] *šim-ma-tú ri-mu-tú* TUKU.TUKU-*ši* GABA.MEŠ-*šú* KÚ.MEŠ-⸢*šú*⸣ ZI-*šú ik-ta-nàr-rù* SÍG UGU-*šú* GUB.GUB-*az ḫur-ba-šú* ŠUB.ŠUB-*su mi-na-tu-šú i-šam-ma-ma-šú ḫu-uṣ* GAZ ŠÀ-*bi* TUKU.TUKU-*ši a-šu-uš-tum* ŠUB.ŠUB-*su bi-bil* ŠÀ-*bi* TUKU-⸢*ma*⸣ NU KÚ ⸢*la*⸣ *ina-aḫ* [*ur-r*]*a u* [GI$_6$ *i*]-*ár-ru* LÚ BI GID[IM *m*]*ur-tap-pi-du* DIB-*su ù lu-ba-ṭù* ⸢ŠU^{II}⸣ ^{d}AMAR.UT[U] *ana* KAR-*šú* . . . (*LKA* 88 obv. 1–9//*LKA* 87 obv. 1′–10′)

**If the middle of a person's scalp (and) his temples continually hurt ⸢him⸣ intensely, his ears roar, his palate keeps getting ⸢dry⸣, he continually has numbness and paralysis, his breasts keep hurting him, he is continually short of breath, the hair of his scalp continually stands on end, chills keep attacking him, his limbs go numb, he continually has a crushing sensation in the chest, depression continually falls on him, he has an appetite but then cannot eat, without relief he ⸢vomits day⸣ and [night], a roving ghost has seized that man or *lubāṭu*, "hand" of ⸢Marduk⸣; to save him . . .

The text below describes delirium tremens (DTs). The hallucinations that occur in that condition are likely to cause intense fear with stimulation of the erector pili muscles (see Chapter 15).

10.186 DIŠ *tu-gu-un-šú ú-zaq-qat-su* GEŠTU^{II}-*šú* GÙ.DÉ.MEŠ SÍG SU-*šú* GUB.GUB-⸢*az*⸣ *kal* LÚ.AD$_6$-*šú* GIN$_7$ *kal-ma-tum i-ba-šú-ú i-nam-muš u* ŠU-*su ub-bal-ma la i-ba-áš-šú* : *la ig-gi-ig* ⸢ŠU⸣ GIDIM$_7$ . . . (DPS XXVII:32–34 [AOAT 43.300])

**If (the skin under) his headband stings him, his ears roar, the hair of his body continually stands on end, his whole body crawls as if there were lice but when he brings his hand up, there is nothing to scratch, "hand" of ghost . . .

In addition to elevating the hair, the erector pili muscle also causes the skin around the hair follicle to become raised. This, of course, is a "goosebump." Patients with infections or fevers are likely to have goosebumps and raised hair when they become chilled at the beginning of a temperature elevation. However, there may be another explanation for raised hair in such cases. A patient who has been sick enough to spend much time in bed may have hair that stands up simply due to the time in bed and lack of attention to personal hygiene.

10.187 [DIŠ NA U]D.DA TAB.B[A]-*ma* SÍG SAG.DU-*šú* GUB.GUB-*az* IGI.MEŠ-*šú* NIGIN.MEŠ-*du-šú-*[*ma*] *it-ta-na-aṣ-ra-ḫu* . . . NA BI UD.DA.TAB.BA *ana* TI-*šú* . . . (*BAM* 145:1-17//*BAM* 146:29′–38′)

**[If] *ṣētu* (enteric fever; see Chapter 3) burns [a person] so that the hair of his head continually stands on end,[195] his face seems continually to spin, [and] he continually feels burning hot . . . that person is burned by *ṣētu*, to cure him . . .

10.188 [DIŠ] NA MAŠ.SÌLA^{II}-*šú* KÚ.MEŠ-*šú i-ta-an-na-aḫ im-ta-na-aš-ši im-te-en*[. . .] [MAŠ].GI$_6$.MEŠ-*šú par-da* SÍG UGU-*šú* GUB.GUB-*az* ŠÀ-*šú pi-ḫi* NU *pi-ḫi i-par*[*-ru* . . .] [U$_4$-*r*]*a u* GI$_6$ *la i-ṣal-lal* NA BI *ḫi-niq-ti* BUN GIG *ana* TI-*šú* . . . (*AMT* 31/1:3–5)

**[If] a person's shoulders continually hurt him, he is continually tired, he continually forgets things, he continually [. . .] his ⌜dreams⌝ are troubled, the hair of his scalp continually stands on end, he ⌜vomits⌝ incessantly, [. . .] (and) he cannot sleep ⌜day⌝ or night, that person is sick with constriction of the urethra, to cure him . . .

In some of the descriptions of hair changes in protein malnutrition discussed in Chapter 7[196] and in the following reference, the patient's hair standing on end is of uncertain cause. The patient did not have any obvious signs of fever (the pulse rate was normal), and nothing indicates that the patient was bedridden.

10.189 [DIŠ GIG NIGI]N SA.MEŠ-*šú šal-mu-ma* SÍG S[AG.DU-*šú in*]*a* GEŠTU-*šú zaq-pat* GAM (DPS XXI:1//DPS XIX/XX:125′ [AOAT 43.233 (catchline)])

**[If the patient]'s blood vessels are normal but the hair of [his] ⌜head⌝ stands on end ⌜at⌝ his ear, he will die.

HAIR LOSS

There are references to hair loss that probably represent cases of "normal" male pattern hair loss.[197] Providing or attempting to provide treatments for balding heads appealed to the vanity of the patient as it does in the modern era.

10.190 KA.INIM.MA SÍG SAG.D[U] NÍG.GUB.BA KÉŠ.DA.KÁM . . . (*BAM* 480 iii 28; cf. iii 45, 56)

**Recitation to bind in the hair of the ⌜head⌝ and make it stand firm . . .

10.191 [DIŠ NA SA]G.DU-*su gu-ub-bu-uḫ* . . . (*BAM* 3 i 54)

**[If a person]'s ⌜head⌝ is going bald . . .

Hair loss in women, then as now, was probably less common.

10.192 [KA.INIM.MA SÍ]G SAG.DU MUNUS *ka-le-e* . . . SÍG *a-lik-tum ik-kal-la* (*BAM* 499 ii 16′, 20′//*BAM* 497 ii 3′; cf. *BAM* 491:4′)

**[Recitation] to retain the ⌜hair⌝ of a woman's head . . . the "going" hair will be retained.

10.193 KA.INIM.MA SÍG SAG.DU MUNUS *i-šaḫ-ḫu-uḫ* . . . (*BAM* 499 ii 7′; *BAM* 498 iii 1)

**Recitation for (cases where) the hair of a woman's head falls out . . .

The verb used to describe balding in women (*šaḫāḫu*) differs from the adjective used to describe "normal" balding in men (*gubbuḫu*; see above) but is the same as that used for hair falling out due to fever, as in the following reference.

10.194 DIŠ NA SAG.DU-*su* KÚM-*ma* SÍ[G] SAG.DU-*šú i-šaḫ-ḫu-uḫ ana* KÚM SAG.DU [ZI-*ḫi*] *u* SÍG DU-*tú* GUB-*zi*... (*BAM* 480 iii 22)[198]

**If a person's head is feverish and the ⌜hair⌝ of his head falls out, to [remove] the fever of his head and to make the hair that is going stand firm...

The text below refers to hair "falling out in tufts" (the specific image is of an oxhide that has been treated with depilatories; see Chapter 12 with 12.65–12.66). Physiognomic omens describe this happening to the middle part of a man's head.[199] As with more normal patterns of male baldness, those with rapidly thinning manes had to put up with nicknames calling specific attention to their problem. Mr. Bald and Mr. Dehaired make an occasional appearance in private contracts, alongside even unkinder sobriquets such as Mr. Cripple, Mr. Squint, and Mr. Blockhead.[200] This type of accelerated hair loss may follow severe infections with high fever, or an idiopathic condition called alopecia areata. Cancer chemotherapy in the current era may also cause rapid hair loss.

10.195 DIŠ NA SAG.DU-*su qur-ru-ud*... (*BAM* 3 ii 32//*BAM* 34:12′)[201]

**If a person's head hair falls out in tufts...

Loss of beard hair is not part of male pattern baldness, and is an uncommon problem. It is seen in secondary syphilis, a condition whose existence in ancient Mesopotamia is uncertain. It can also occur as part of the condition, alopecia areata (mentioned above), and with some chronic fungal infections of the skin.

In relief representations and statuary, the inhabitants of the southern part of the ancient Mesopotamian flood plain are generally shown as beardless and with shaved heads.[202] Their northern neighbors, by contrast, are typically represented as having shoulder-length hair and beards.[203] Body hair seems to have been plentiful, not only on the chin but also on the chest and in the armpits from which it was collected for use in magical rites.[204] Assyrian courtiers sported magnificently curly square-cut full beards unless they happened to be one of the palace eunuchs (castrati),[205] a comparison that doubtless added a certain level of anxiety to the prospect of losing one's beard hair.

10.196 DIŠ NA SÍG TE.MEŠ-*šú ma-gal i-šaḫ-ḫu-uḫ* NA BI DINGIR-*šú* ^{d}EŠ$_4$.DAR-*šú* KI-*šú ze-nu-u*... (*BAM* 480 iii 48)

**If the hair on a person's cheeks falls out a lot, his god and goddess are angry with that person...

Ancient physicians recognized a syndrome, *raʾšānu*, which "afflicted" cattle, sheep, and goats[206] as well as producing loss of head and facial hair in humans. Dermatophytosis (fungus infecting skin and hair) is known to cause hair loss in animals, and this infection can spread to humans. It is likely that the *āšipu* recognized the association between hair loss in animals and their human caretakers.[207]

10.197 Ú *šá-mi ra-sa-n*[*i*] . . . (*BAM* 421 i′ 22′)

**Plant for *raʾšānu* . . .

10.198 DIŠ NA SAG.DU-*su ra-ʾ-šá-nu* ⌜DIB⌝-*it* . . . (*BAM* 3 i 31)

**If a person's head is afflicted by *raʾšānu* . . .

10.199 DIŠ NA *ra-ʾ-šá-nu* DIB-*su* SAG.DU-*su pa-nu-šú* SU_6.MEŠ-*šú* [*gu-ub*]-*bu-ḫa* . . . (*BAM* 3 i 26–27)

**If *raʾšānu* afflicts a person (and) his head, his face, (and) his beard are going bald . . .[208]

10.200 *a-na su-um-mu ra-šá-nu* SIG_5-*iq* . . . (BM 79244:18–19 [Finkel, *Fs. Lambert* 150])

**It is good for red spots and *raʾšānu* . . .

GRAY HAIR

Another vanity issue was graying hair, especially if it occurred prematurely. The *āšipu* had a variety of treatments for this condition. Some treatments, such as rubbing the hair with a specially manufactured charcoal mixed with oil, were presumably intended simply to dye the whitened hair. Others, however, involve rubbing medicaments on the scalp and may have been intended to cause the normal hair color to return.

10.201 DIŠ NA *ina* TUR-*šú* SAG.DU-*su še-bi-tú* DIRI *ana* SÍG GI_6 . . . (*AMT* 5/1:5′)[209]

**If a person's head is full of gray hair while he is still young, to make the hair turn black . . .

10.202 *ana šib-tum* NU GÁL . . . (*AMT* 3/6 ii 7′)[210]

**In order for there not to be any gray hair . . .

10.203 SÍG BABBAR GI_6 (AMT 76/6:11′, 13′; *BAM* 499 iii 6′)[211]

**The white hair will turn black.

"TOUCHED IN THE STEPPE"

A syndrome with the above name was discussed in detail in Chapter 7. Some of the most important features of this condition involved changes in the patient's hair, including thinning of the hair shaft, brittleness, and altered hair color including a red color in some cases. These changes in the character of the patient's hair plus other signs and symptoms are essentially diagnostic for protein-deficient malnutrition.

Nails

YELLOW NAIL SYNDROME

The texts below contain little information except for the color of the patient's nails (yellow or red) and the fatal outcome associated with yellow nails. Since yellow toenails are an uncommon physical finding, it seems possible that the patient had the yellow nail syndrome. Patients with this rare disease often have swelling (edema) of the extremities due to underdeveloped (hypoplastic) lymphatic vessels. The lymphatic abnormalities are the proximate cause of the yellow nails. Other common problems include fluid around the lungs, and other lung abnormalities. Patients may die from infections or malignancies that are frequent complications of this condition.

10.204 DIŠ UMBIN U.MEŠ GÌR^{II}-*šú* SIG$_7$.M[EŠ] GAM (DPS XIV A iv 12//K 6 = *TDP* 144 iv 47′)

**If his toenails are continually yellow, he will die.

10.205 DIŠ UMBIN U.MEŠ GÌR^{II}-*šú* SA$_5$.MEŠ *i-šar-*[*r*]*ù* : DIN (DPS XIV A iv 13//K 7 = *TDP* 144 iv 48′)

**If his toenails are continually red, he will get rich (var. he will get well).

Summary

Although this chapter does not describe many texts that have definitive diagnostic information, it does demonstrate an impressive interest by the *āšipu* in the nature of skin and hair abnormalities. These skin changes with their many identifying names clearly demonstrate that the *āšipu* understood their importance. The attention he paid to nomenclature and detail indicate his recognition that these distinctions were important in determining the optimal treatment.

CHAPTER 11

Bones and Joints

If you want to lubricate stiff hips . . .

—*AMT* 56/1 r. 5′//*AMT* 69/8:11

Fractures

Modern people tend to think of broken bones (fractures) as less serious medical problems because of our facility in stabilizing the broken bone until it fully heals. Fractures in early humans must have been life-threatening problems. Without stabilizing the bone in the correct position, the fracture might never heal or could knit in a configuration that would be detrimental to function. This could markedly interfere with the individual's ability to compete in a hostile environment. Other more immediate problems associated with fractures include secondary infections and blood clots.

Ancient Mesopotamians recognized the potential problems associated with fractures. Legal codes specified penalties for deliberately breaking the bones of another individual.[1] One text even provided a penalty for causing a hired ox to break its leg. There are also letters that refer to various accidents resulting in broken bones. Two are particularly noteworthy: "a pig crossed (in front of) me so that I fell and broke my foot"[2] and "Two slaves fell into a well. One of them broke a collar bone and the other broke his hip."[3]

The *āšipu* had methods for the treatment of fractures that included stabilization of the broken bone and plant medicines to prevent infection. The second text below seems to indicate that physicians were aware of the importance of proper alignment of the broken bone for a successful outcome.

11.1 *ana ši-me-er-te ka-li-šu šu-ṣe-e* LÚ TI . . . (*BAM* 158 iv 26–27//*BAM* 171:44′; *AMT* 82/1:10′)

**To make any kind of fracture go away (and) to cure the man . . .

11.2 *še-bir-tú ana ke-ši-ru* . . . (BM 30918:32//*BAM* 124 iii 57//*BAM* 125:28//*BAM* 413 obv. 1′–2′)

**To straighten up fractures . . .

We have from another reference the ingredients for the material used to make a fracture-stabilizing cast. Physicians called this "a bandage to make (limbs) go straight" (*BAM* 181:7). It included crushing together a mixture of reeds and cuttings (probably used to strengthen the cement), plaster of Paris (*gaṣṣu*), wheat and barley flour, gums, malt, gazelle dung, and oven slag, and boiling it in beer to form a medicated cement. Boiling would sterilize the ingredients, especially the dung. Unfortunately, there is no information about how the cast was put on, or how long it was left in place.

Joints

The mechanical ability to manipulate our environment depends on muscles attached to intact stable bones, as well as joints that permit movement when the muscles contract. If our joints were to freeze up, we would end up in the same predicament as the tin woodsman in the *Wizard of Oz*. Ancient Mesopotamian physicians knew that smooth, free movement of joints was important.

11.3 DIŠ *a-na* MURUB$_4$ *áš-ṭa-a-te lu-ub-bu-ka* . . . (*AMT* 56/1 r. 5′//*AMT* 69/8 obv. 11)[4]

**If you want to lubricate stiff hips . . .

Ancient physicians distinguished three different varieties/grades of joint immobility and change. The term *ašṭu*, which also means "hard" and is used to describe the impenetrable qualities of stone walls, mountain passes, and the cuneiform script,[5] was applied to joints with severe stiffness. As one might suppose from this, affected limbs were not merely stiff but also hard and might actually be immobilized, as in the last reference.

11.4 [DI]Š NA GÚ-*su uš-šu-uṭ* . . . (*SpTU* 3.100:1)[6]

**⌜If⌝ a person's neck is stiff all over . . .

11.5 Ú.MEŠ MURUB$_4$ *áš-ṭa-te* . . . (*BAM* 80:9; *BAM* 380:12//*STT* 92 iii 28′; *BAM* 327 i 10′)[7]

**Plants for stiff hips . . .

11.6 DIŠ U$_4$.5.KÁM U$_4$.10.KÁM U$_4$.15.KÁM U$_4$.20.KÁM U.MEŠ ŠU^{II}-*šú u* GÌR^{II}-*šú am-šá aš-ṭa-a-ma* BAD-*a u* GUB-*za* NU ZU-*e*ŠU ^{d}15 *uš-šar-ma* : *iš-šìr-ma* DIN (DPS XVI:59′–60′ [AOAT 43.177])[8]

**If he has been sick for five, ten, fifteen, (and then) twenty days (and) the digits of his hands and his feet are immobilized (and) so stiff that he cannot open (them) or stand (on them), "hand" of Ištar. (If) it leaves him (var. he comes through), he will get well.

The second category of joint stiffness, *šaggu* or *šiggatu*,[9] was used to refer to stiff necks, feet, and hands. It was specifically used to describe a sensation of stiffness in the muscles surrounding the inflamed joint. There was also a difference in the degree of immobilization between *šaggu* and *ašṭu*. The victim of *šaggu* foot stiffness was unable to walk, in contrast to the victim of *ašṭu*, who might not even be able to stand.

11.7 DIŠ NA SA GÌR^{II}-*šú ša-ag-gu-ma a-tál-lu-ka la i-le-ʾi ana* SA.MEŠ GÌR^{II}-*šú pu-uš-šu-ḫi* . . . (*BAM* 122 r. 2′–4′//*AMT* 68/1 r. 8–9)[10]

**If the muscles of a person's feet are so stiff that he cannot walk, to relax the muscles of his feet . . .

11.8 [DIŠ] NA GIDIM DIB-*su* MUD-*su šá-gi-ig* [SA] MUD-*šú u* SA.SAL-*šú šu-u*[*p*]-*šu-ḫi* . . . (Scheil, *RA* 14.88 i 3′–4′)

**[If] a ghost afflicts a person (and) his heel is stiff, in order to relax the muscles of his heel and Achilles tendon . . .

11.9 NÍG.LÁL *šig-ga-ti šá* EN.TE.NA . . . (AMT 32/5 iv! 13+*AMT* 43/3 iv 2′//*BAM* 124 iii 8//*BAM* 131 r. 3′)[11]

**Bandage for winter stiffness . . .[12]

A third type of stiffness was referred to as *mungu*. *Mungu* is used to refer to stiff knees and hips, as in the first two references below. The term comes from a verb (*magāgu*) that means "to stretch out" (as in a gesture of begging). *Mungu* need not, however, imply that the affected limb was in a stretched position—on the contrary, the victim in the third reference below is described as keeping his knees bent. What may be implied is stretching of the skin and muscles around the joint through swelling. At least that would explain how *mungu* comes to be used to describe a pointing abscess (see 3.187) and hydrocele (see 5.81). Swelling may also be implied in the use of the verb *magāgu* to exhort a flaccid penis to potency, as in the last reference.

11.10 DIŠ NA *bur-ka-šú mun-ga* DIRI . . . (*AMT* 43/3 iv 7′//*BAM* 131 r. 9′)

**If a person's knees are full of stiffness . . .

11.11 DIŠ NA MURUB$_4$ *u* ^{UZU}ÚR GIG *mun-ga* TU[KU] . . . (*AMT* 69/3:6′+*AMT* 26/5:2′; *AMT* 61/2:2′)

**If a person's hip and thigh ⌜have⌝ stiffness . . .

11.12 DIŠ NA *ka-šip-ma* UZU.MEŠ-*šú tab-ku mun-ga* TU[KU-*šú*] *ù bir-ka-a-šú ga-an-na* ŠÀ-*šú* MUNUS *ḫa-šiḫ*-[*ma*] MUNUS IGI.BAR-*ma* ŠÀ-*šú* GUR NA BI *re-ḫu-su* KI LÚ.ÚŠ *šu-nu*-[*lat*] *ana* TI-*šú* . . . (Biggs, *ŠÀ.ZI.GA* 68-69:9′–13′//*BAM* 205:7′–10′)[13]

**If a person is hexed so that his flesh is tense, he has stiffness and his knees are bent, his heart desires a woman [and then] when he sees a woman, his heart turns away, that person's sperm has been made to ⌜lie⌝ with a corpse, to cure him . . .

11.13 *lim-gu-ug* ANŠE-*ma* SAL.ANŠE *li-ir-kab* (Biggs, *ŠÀ.ZI.GA* 33:3)

**Let (the penis of the) donkey stiffen (*lim-gu-ug*); let him mount the jenny!

Mungu could make riding over an unpaved road in a springless chariot a miserable experience.

11.14 [DIŠ NA] MURUB$_4$ *u* ÚR GIG *mun-ga* TU [KU *u*] *ni-ḫi-is* ^{GIŠ}GIGIR *a-ni-iḫ ana* TI-[*šú*] . . . (*AMT* 69/3:6′–7′+*AMT* 26/5:2′–3′)

**[If a person's] hip and thigh ⸢have⸣ stiffness [and] he is tired (after) jostling in a chariot, to cure [him] . . .

Arthritis

Joint disease (arthritis) was identified by physical signs that included stiffness, pain, swelling, sluggishness (impaired movement), and shrinking (possibly permanent deformity).

11.15 [DIŠ ŠU^{II}-*š*] *ú it-ta-na-aš-gag-ga* [. . .] (DPS XI A obv. 33//B 32 = *TDP* 92:33//*SpTU* 1.34:32)[14]

**[If his hands] continually become stiff, [. . .].

11.16 [DIŠ ŠU^{II}-*šú*] ⸢*ú*⸣-*ta-ṣa-la* : *ú-ta-ka-ṣa ut-tap-pa-ḫ*[*a* . . .] (DPS XI A obv. 35//B 34 = TDP 92:35//*SpTU* 1.34:34)

**If his hands become sluggish (var. become stiff[15] and) become swollen, [. . .]

11.17 [DI]Š *bir-ka-šú* KÚ.MEŠ-*šú* AZAG ^{d}UTU KÚ (DPS XIV A iii 24//F 2//J 2 = *TDP* 140 iii 58′)[16]

**⸢If⸣ his knees continually hurt him, he has done something offensive to Šamaš.

11.18 DIŠ NA MURUB$_4$-*šú* GIG MÚ.MÚ . . . (*BAM* 56 obv. 8′)[17]

**If a person's hip is sore (and) swollen . . .

11.19 DIŠ U.MEŠ ŠU^{II}-*šú it-te-nen-ṣi-la-šú* [. . .] (DPS XI A r. 35 = *TDP* 96 r. 35)[18]

**If his fingers are continually sluggish, [. . .].

11.20 DIŠ GÌR^{II} [-*šú i*]*k-te-ner-ra-a* ⸢ŠU DINGIR ḪUL DIB-*su*⸣ (DPS XIV A$_2$ iv 8′//C$_2$ iii 33b = TDP 142 iv 8′)[19]

**If (both) [his] feet become shrunken,[20] "hand" of an evil god afflicts him.

11.21 DIŠ GÌR^{II}-*šú it-t*[*e*]-⸢*nin*⸣-*gi-ra* ⸢ŠU ^{d}⸣UTU (DPS XIV A$_2$ iv 12′//C$_2$ iii 37//G iv 2′ = *TDP* 142 iv 12′)

**If his feet are ⸢continually twisted⸣, "hand" of Šamaš.

Arthritic involvement of most joints was cited including the fingers, toes, feet, hips, elbows, knees, neck (cervical vertebrae), and back (thoracic, lumbar, and sacral vertebrae). There are many specific causes of arthritis as well as specific clinical syndromes that include arthritis but lack a known cause. Listed below are ancient Mesopotamian texts that appear to be describing types of arthritis that are recognized by modern physicians.

EFFECTS OF ARTHRITIS ON JOINT FUNCTION

BACK

11.22 DIŠ NA GÚ-*su* UZU.SA.SAL^{II}-*šú áš-ṭa* . . . (*BAM* 415 r. 7)[21]

**If a person's neck (and) back are stiff . . .

11.23 DIŠ GÚ.MURGU-*šú qa-nin na-ḫi-id* (DPS XII D iii 32 = *TDP* 104 iii 32)

**If his spine is curved, it is worrisome.

11.24 DIŠ GÚ.MURGU-*šú* GAM-*ma* LAL NU ZU-*e* GÍD-*ma* GAM (DPS XII D iii 33 = *TDP* 106 iii 33; cf. DPS XV:47 [AOAT 43.153])

**If his spine is curved so that he cannot straighten it out, (if) it is prolonged, he will die.

11.25 DIŠ GÚ.MURGU-*šú* GAM-*ma* LAL NU ZU-*e* UŠ$_4$-*šú* NU DIB GÍD-*ma* GAM (DPS XII D iii 34 = *TDP* 106 iii 34)

**If his spine is curved so that he cannot straighten it out (and) he is not in full possession of his faculties, (if) it is prolonged, he will die.

A form of chronic arthritis that predominantly affects the spine (vertebrae) is called spondylitis. Lacking in the first quote above is any indication of chronicity, but spondylitis is the probable diagnosis. The remaining references are a clear description of the long-term consequence of spondylitis, namely, the fusion of vertebrae in a curved configuration. This generally leaves the patient permanently bent over, unable to look forward or move in a smooth, coordinated fashion.

SHOULDER JOINTS With severe shoulder arthritis, the patient may be unable to bring his hand to his mouth.

11.26 DIŠ ŠU-*su šá* 15 *ana* KA-*šú tur-ra* NU ZU-*e šá* 150 *ana tur-ra aš-*⸢*ṭa*⸣-[*át*. . .] / DIŠ ŠU-*su šá* 150 *ana* KA-*šú tur-ra* NU ZU-*e šá* 15 *ana tur-ra aš-ṭa-át* KI.[MIN] (DPS XI A obv. 7–8//B 6–7 = *TDP* 90:7–8//*SpTU* 1.34:6–7)

**If he is unable to turn his left hand to his mouth (and) his right turns ⸢stiffly⸣ [. . .]. If he is unable to turn his right hand to his mouth (and) his left turns stiffly, (the diagnosis) is the ⸢same⸣.

FINGERS AND TOES

11.27 DIŠ U.MEŠ ŠU^{II}-*šú u* GÌR^{II}-*šú* KÚ.MEŠ-*šú* [. . .] (DPS XI A r. 43 = *TDP* 98 r. 43)

**If the digits of his hands and his feet continually hurt him, [. . .].

11.28 DIŠ U.MEŠ ŠU^{II}-*šú u* GÌR^{II}-*šú* MÚ.MEŠ-*ḫa* [. . .] (DPS XI A r. 44 = *TDP* 98 r. 44)

**If the digits of his hands and his feet are continually swollen, [. . .].

11.29 DIŠ U.MEŠ ŠU^{II}-*šú u* GÌR^{II}-*šú it-te-nen-ṣi-la-šú* [. . .] (DPS XI A r. 45 = *TDP* 98 r. 45)

**If the digits of his hands and his feet are continually sluggish, [. . .].

The references above were listed sequentially by the *āšipu*, and are therefore likely to be related conditions. They describe pain, swelling, and impaired mobility (sluggishness) of both feet and hands. Symmetrical joint involvement (both right and left sides) as well as the joints described strongly suggest that the cause was rheumatoid arthritis. There is, however, insufficient information to exclude other causes such as reactive arthritis (see below).

ARTHRITIS AFFECTING SPECIFIC AGE GROUPS

OLD PATIENTS

11.30 DIŠ KI.MIN ŠU^{II}-*šú u* GÌR^{II}-*šú ik-tap-pá* GIG-*su* KÚR-*šum-ma* UGU-*šú* KI.MIN DIN (DPS XVI:94′ [AOAT 43.180])

**If (he is in his seventies and) his hands and feet have become bent, (even if) his illness changes so that they (beat their breasts) over him, he will get well.

11.31 DIŠ KI.MIN ŠU^{II}-*šú u* GÌR^{II}-*šú ik-ra-a* GIG-*su* KÚR-*šum-ma* UGU-*šú* KI.MIN DIN (DPS XVI:95′ [AOAT 43.180])

**If (he is in his seventies) and his hands and feet become shrunken,[22] (even if) his illness changes so that they (beat their breasts) over him, he will get well.

Osteoarthritis is predominantly a disease of older individuals. It can be deforming and painful, but it seldom has nonarthritic complications as is commonly the case with rheumatoid arthritis. Death from osteoarthritis is rare. The texts above seem to be describing elderly patients with this disease.

YOUNG PATIENTS

11.32 [DIŠ NA] *ina la si-ma-ni-šú* MURUB$_4$.MEŠ-*šú* KÚ.MEŠ-*šú* [*kim-ṣa*]-*a-šú i-za-qat-šú* ÚR.MEŠ-*šu* [*i-tan-na*]-*aḫ bur-ka-šú i-kaṣ-ṣa-ṣa-šú* [NA BI *ina*] *meṣ-ḫi-ru-te-šú* DÚR.GIG GIG . . . (*BAM* 108 obv. 15–18)

**[If] a⌜person's⌝hips hurt him before (the age when) this would be expected, his⌜legs⌝ sting him, his thighs [are continually] ⌜tired⌝, and his knees give him a gnawing pain, [that person] was sick with DÚR.GIG (see below) [in] his youth . . .

11.33 DIŠ NA *ina la si-ma-ni-šú* MURUB$_4$.MEŠ-*šú* KÚ.MEŠ-*šú* (C adds: GÌR^{II}.MEŠ-*šú i-ta-n*[*a-aḫ*]) *kim-ṣa-a-šú i-za-qat-šu* ÚR.MEŠ *i-tan-na-aḫ bur-ka-šu i-kaṣ-ṣa-a-šú* NA BI *ina meṣ-ḫi-ru-ti-šú* DÚR.GIG GIG *ana* TI-*šú* . . . (*BAM* 168:70–72; *AMT* 43/1 i 1–3; *BAM* 95:16–17)

**If a person's hips hurt him before (the age when) this would be expected, (C adds: his feet are continually [tired]), his legs sting him, his thighs are continually tired, and his knees give him a gnawing pain, that person was sick with DÚR.GIG (see below) in his childhood, to cure him . . .

The references above describe arthritis that occurs at an early age. This is probably juvenile rheumatoid arthritis.

DÚR.GIG

11.34 DIŠ NA *a-ḫa-šú kìn-ṣa-šú ki-sàl-la-šú* [KÚ-*šú*] NA BI *qé-reb* DÚR.GIG . . . (*BAM* 89:8–9)[23]

**If a person's arms, his legs, (and) his ankles [hurt him], that person is in the midst of DÚR.GIG . . .

11.35 DIŠ NA MURUB$_4$.MEŠ-*šú* ⌜KÚ.MEŠ-*šú*⌝ *iš-tu-šú* ⌜DU$_8$.DU$_8$?⌝ [. . . NA B]I DÚR.GIG . . . (*BAM* 96 ii 14)

**If a person's hips [continually] hurt [him] (but) afterward continually (feel) supple,[24] that person (has) DÚR.GIG . . .

11.36 DIŠ NA *kim-ṣa-*⌜*a*⌝-[*šú* KÚ.MEŠ-*šú* . . .]-zi *e-ṣil ši-ḫat* UZU TUKU-*ši* MÚD DUB.MEŠ NA BI DÚR.GIG ŠU ^{d}NAM.ÉRIM *ana* TI-*šú* . . . (*BAM* 95:19–20//*AMT* 53/9:5′–6′)

**If a person['s] legs [hurt him . . .] he is sluggish, he has wasting away of the flesh and pours out blood, that person (has) DÚR.GIG (or) "hand" of curse, to cure him . . .

11.37 DIŠ NA *mi-na-tu-šú* DUB.DUB GABA-*su u* SA.SAL.MEŠ-*šú* KÚ.MEŠ-*šú* Á^{II}-*šú* x [. . .] KÚ.MEŠ-*šú bir-bir-ki-šú lu šá* 15 *lu šá* 150 SÌG-*su-ma ina múš-tin-*[*ni*]-*šú* MÚD *ú-kal-lam* NA BI *ḫi-niq-ti* DÚR.GIG GIG *ana* TI-*šú* . . . (*AMT* 40/5 iii 14–16//*AMT* 56/1 obv. 1–3//*BAM* 88:1′–2′)

**If his limbs are continually tense,[25] his breast and his back continually hurt him, his arms [and legs?] continually hurt him, his loins[26] either on the left or right side give him a jabbing pain, and from his ⌜urethra⌝ he shows blood, that person is sick with the constriction of DÚR.GIG, to cure him . . .

We believe that patients described as having DÚR.GIG and joint pain were suffering either from arthritis associated with ulcerative colitis or from "reactive" arthritis triggered by a salmonella infection that commonly complicates *Schistosomiasis hematobium.* See Chapter 6 for a more complete discussion.

ARTHRITIS WITH A SORE THROAT

11.38 DIŠ GEŠTU^{II}-*šú kir-ra-šu u ki-ṣir* 1.KÙŠ.M[EŠ-*š*]*ú* TA GIG-*su* TAK$_4$-⌜*šu*⌝ 1-*niš*! KÚ.MEŠ-*šú ki-*⌜*ma* DU$_8$?-*ra*⌝ GIG-[*su* GUR-*m*]*a ana* É.MEŠ GUR-*šú-ma* GIG SAL. KALAG.GA IGI-*ma* DIN [o o o o] DIŠ ŠU^{II}-*šú u* GÌR^{II}-*šú ana* x-x[. . .] GIG.BI *šum$_4$-ma* É.MEŠ [. . .] (DPS VIII 18–21 = *TDP* 70:18–21)

**If after his illness has left him his ears, his throat, and his elbows all hurt him at the same time (and) after it has let up, [his] illness [returns] ⌜and⌝ comes back inside him so that he gets sick (again), he may have a difficult time of it, but he will get well. [. . .] If his hands and feet [. . .]. If his illness [comes back] inside him [a third time . . .]

11.39 *e-na-a-šu bur-kà-a-šu ke-er-ra-a-šu k*[*i . . . mì-i*]*t-ḫa-ri-iš ik-kà-la-a-šu ul-tu mu-ra-sú it-ta-*⌜*ab*⌝!-*šu a-na* [. . .] x *ti$_7$-ik ša-me-e* BA.Ú[Š] (StBoT 36.23 r. 6′-8′)[27]

**(If) his eyes, his knees, his throat, (and) [his] ⌜legs?⌝ all hurt him at once (and) after his illness? comes about [it turns] into [*aganutillû* (edema)], he will ⌜die⌝ [on a day] when it is hailing.[28]

Both of the above references mention throat pain as well as arthritis. We believe that the throat pain could be due to streptococcal infection (see Chapter 3). The second text also mentions *aganutillû*, which means generalized swelling or edema (anasarca). The most likely explanation is that the streptococcal infection resulted in the complication, rheumatic fever. Arthritis is a frequent problem in rheumatic fever.[29] The most feared complication of rheumatic fever is heart involvement which, if severe, can cause congestive heart failure. Edema or fluid collection is frequently seen in patients with congestive heart failure.

RĀBIṢU

A human *rābiṣu* was a person commissioned by another individual to act as complainant in a legal case, or someone dispatched by the palace on a similar errand.[30] On the divine plane, the *rābiṣu* was a demon dispatched by a god to punish an erring human being. Like all demons, *rābiṣu*s often free-lanced, attacking persons whom they had not been ordered to punish. The *rābiṣu* of the river was a hazard to swimmers, causing them to have seizures (see Chapter 15 with 15.27–15.28). Hardly less fortunate were those who fell afoul of the *rābiṣu* of the lavatory, who caused strokes affecting one side of the body (see Chapter 13). Any contact with such a demon was ill advised; eating the same food or drinking the same water would give you a disease that we believe to be hepatitis A (see Chapter 6). What happened to the victim in the text below was that he inadvertently stepped into the tracks left by a *rābiṣu* and soon felt the effects.

11.40 DIŠ GÌR^{II}-*šú it-t*[*a-n*]*a-aš-gag-ga ina* KI.ÚS MAŠKIM GUB-*iz* DIN (DPS XIV A_2 iv 15′//G iv 5′ = *TDP* 142 iv 15′)

**If his feet ⌜continually⌝ become stiff, he stood in the footsteps of a *rābiṣu*; he will get well.

11.41 DIŠ NA GÌR^{II}-*šú* GIG-*ma te-ba-a u ú-zu-za la i-*[*le-ʾ-i*] *ù* ŠU^{II}-*šú* GÌR^{II}-*šú i-ra-ʾ-*⌜*u*⌝*-ba* NA BI KI.GUB/*man-za-az* MAŠKIM [. . .] ⌜*ana*⌝ GÌR^{II}-*šú bul-lu-ṭi* . . . (*AMT* 69/2:2–4// *BAM* 152 iv 1–3; restored from *AMT* 70/7 i 9′)

**If a person's feet are so sore that he ⌜can⌝ not get up and stand and his hands and feet tremble, that person [trod(?) on] the emplacement of a *rābiṣu*; to cure his feet . . .

These references do not provide much information other than the fact that the patient is undergoing severe foot pain, yet the condition is not life-threatening. Gout is a form of arthritis that can affect many joints, but the foot is commonly involved and the pain often is quite severe. The most common form of gout is an inherited condition that occurs because of difficulty excreting uric acid. Crystals of uric acid develop in the joints, which triggers acute arthritis. There is too little data provided to have more than just a suspicion that gout is the disease described. (For an alternative suggestion see p. 451.)

"HAND" OF ŠAMAŠ

We know from other references (DPS XXXIII:112 [AOAT 43.358]) that "hand" of Šamaš is associated with scales. It seems possible that the scales (*quliptu*; see Chapter 10) are due to psoriasis, a skin condition that is often associated with arthritis. The texts below may, therefore, be describing patients with psoriatic arthritis.

11.42 DIŠ GÚ-*su* KÚ-*su* ŠU DINGIR-*šú* : ŠU ^{d}UTU *ana* ŠÙD *qí-bit* KA-*šú* DIN (DPS X A obv. 7//B obv. 7 = *TDP* 80:7)[31]

**If his neck hurts him, "hand" of his god (var. "hand" of Šamaš on account of a vow promised by him); he will get well.

11.43 DIŠ KÙŠ.MEŠ-*šú kin-ṣi-šú u* GÌR^{II}-*šú* KÚ.MEŠ-*šú* ŠU ^{d}UTU (DPS X B r. 16 = *TDP* 88 r. 16)

**If his forearms, his legs, and his feet continually hurt him, "hand" of Šamaš.

11.44 DIŠ GIG *rit-ta-šú šá* 15 KÚ-*šú* ŠU ^{d}UTU *ana ik-rib qí-bit* KA-*šú* DIN (DPS XI A obv. 1//B 1//DPS X B r. 19 = *TDP* 88 obv. 1//*SpTU* 1.34:1//*TDP* 88 r. 19)[32]

**If the patient's left hand hurts him, "hand" of Šamaš for a vow that he promised; he will get well.

11.45 DIŠ *bir-ka-a-šú u* $MURUB_4$.MEŠ-*šú ina* GI_6 KÚ.ME-*šú* SU-*šú* KÚM NU TUKU ⸢AZAG⸣ <d>UTU DIB-[*su*] (DPS XIV A iii 25–26//C_2 iii 15//F 3//J 3 = *TDP* 142 iii 59′–60′)[33]

**If his knees and his hips continually hurt him in the night (and) his body has no fever, an offense against Šamaš afflicts [him].

11.46 DIŠ *kin-ṣa-a-šú* KÚ.MEŠ-*šú* ŠU ^{d}UTU MU KÙ.BABBAR ZAG.10.MEŠ D[IN] (DPS XIV C_2 iii 22//F 10)

**If his legs continually hurt him, "hand" of Šamaš on account of the silver for a tithe; he will ⸢get well⸣.

11.47 DIŠ $MURUB_4$.ME-*šú* KÚ.ME-*šú* ŠU ^{d}UTU BÚR-*ma* [DIN] (DPS XII D iii 36 = *TDP* 106 iii 36)

**If his hips continually hurt him, "hand" of Šamaš; (if) it goes away, [he will get well].

11.48 DIŠ GÌR^{II}-*šú it-t*[*e*]-⸢*nen*⸣-*gi-ra* ⸢ŠU ^{d}⸣UTU (DPS XIV A_2 iv 12′//C_2 iii 37//G iv 2′ = *TDP* 142 iv 12′)

**If his feet are ⸢continually twisted⸣, "hand" of Šamaš.

"HAND" OF IŠTAR

There are many texts (see below) that refer to arthritis, especially of the feet, hands, and hips, which attribute that disease to "hand" of Ištar. As described in Chapter 4, Ištar is often associated with venereal diseases, especially urethritis, since she is the goddess of sexual love. Gonococcal urethritis, one of the most common venereal diseases in the current era, often leads to gonococcal arthritis, and it seems likely that the following references are describing this condition. Reactive arthritis (see below) is another possible cause.

11.49 DIŠ U_4.5.KÁM U_4.10.KÁM U_4.15.KÁM U_4.20.KÁM U.MEŠ $ŠU^{II}$-*šú u* $GÌR^{II}$-*šú am-šá aš-ṭa-a-ma* BAD-*a u* GUB-*za* NU ZU-*e* ŠU ^{d}15 *uš-šar-ma*: *iš-šir-ma* DIN (DPS XVI:59′–60′ [AOAT 43.177])[34]

**If he has been sick for five, ten, fifteen, (and then) twenty days (and) the digits of his hands and his feet are immobilized (and) so stiff that he cannot open (them) or stand (on them), "hand" of Ištar. (If) it leaves him (var. he comes through), he will get well.

11.50 DIŠ GÌR-*šu šá* 15 KÚ-*šu* ŠU $^{d}EŠ_4$.DAR / DIŠ $GÌR^{II}$-*šu šá* 1[50 KÚ-*šu* . . .] / DIŠ $GÌR^{II}$-*šu* KÚ.MEŠ-*šu* [. . . -*s*]*u* DIN (DPS XIV A_2 iv 1′–2′//C_2 iii 28–29 = TDP 142 iv 1′–2′)

**If his left foot hurts him, "hand" of Ištar. If his ⸢right⸣ foot [hurts him . . .] If both his feet continually hurt him [. . .] he will get well.

11.51 DIŠ GÌR⸣-*šu*⸣ *šá* 15 *ik-te-ner-ru* ŠU ^{d}15 . . . / [DIŠ GÌR-*šu*] ⸢*šá* 150⸣ *ik-te-ner-ru* ŠU ^{d}15 (DPS XIV A_2 iv 6′–7′//C_2 iii 32–33 = TDP 142 iv 6′–7′)[35]

**If his left/right foot becomes shrunken,[36] "hand" of Ištar.

11.52 DIŠ KÙŠ.MEŠ-*šú* $MURUB_4$.ME-*šú u* $GÌR^{II}$-*šú* 1-*niš* KÚ.MEŠ-*šú* ŠU ^{d}15 MU TAG TE (DPS X A r. 3//B r. 17 = *TDP* 88 r. 17)[37]

**If his forearms, his hips, and his feet all continually hurt him at the same time, "hand" of Ištar on account of touching the cheek.[38]

11.53 DIŠ *ki-is-su šá* 15 KÚ-*šú* KÚM-*šú mit-ḫar* ŠU $^{d}EŠ_4$-DAR MU [. . .] (DPS XIV C_2 iii 18//F 6//J 6 = *TDP* 142 iii 63′)

**If his left leg hurts him (and) his temperature is normal, "hand" of Ištar on account of [. . .].

REACTIVE ARTHRITIS[39]

Reactive arthritis typically includes arthritis, urethritis, conjunctivitis, and skin lesions, especially on the feet. The infections that may trigger this process include sexually transmitted urethritis or bowel infections (enteritis).

Although infections appear necessary to initiate reactive arthritis, it is believed that an immunologic process causes the arthritis. The references below describe arthritis associated with urethritis and skin lesions (tense flesh; induration). Although there is no mention of conjunctivitis, this feature of reactive arthritis may be minimal and occasionally absent.[40] We believe that reactive arthritis is the likely diagnosis.

11.54 [DIŠ NA] *ka-šip-ma* UZU.MEŠ-*šú tab-ku lu ina* DU-*šú lu-u ina i-šu-zi-šu* [*lu-u ina*] *i-tul-i-šu lu-u e-nu-ma* KÀŠ.MEŠ *i-šá-ti-nu re-ḫu-su* DU-*ak* GIN_7 MUNUS *su-ʾ-su* NU *e-el* NA BI *re-ḫu-su* KI LÚ.ÚŠ *ina* KI *šu-nu-lat ana* TI-*šú* . . . (W. Farber, *BID* 234–235:*23–*26//BM 68033:9′–10′).

**If a person is hexed so that his flesh is tense, either when he walks or when he stands still [or when] he lies down or when he urinates, his semen flows, (and) his bed is impure like a (menstruating) woman, that person's semen has been made to lie in the earth with a corpse, to cure him . . .

11.55 [DIŠ NA] *ka-šip-ma mun-ga* TUKU-*ši bir-ka-šú ga-an-na k*[*a*]-*la-tu-šú* DU x[. . .]x-*ma ana e-peš* Á.ÁŠ NU ÍL-*šú ni-i*[*š* ŠÀ-*šú*] DIB-*ma ana* MUNUS D[U-*ka* LAL ŠÀ-*šú* MUNUS *ḫa-ši*]*ḫ-ma* MUNUS IGI-*ma* ŠÀ-*šú* GUR-*ra* NA BI [*re-ḫu-s*]*u* KI LÚ.Ú[Š *šu-nu-lat*] . . . (*SpTU* 1.9:19′–21′)

**[If a person] is hexed so that he has *mungu* (stiffness with swelling) and his knees are bent, his kidneys [. . .] so that (his heart) does not rise in him to do what he wants, he is ⌜impotent⌝ so that his ⌜going⌝ to a woman [is diminished, his heart desires a woman] and then when he sees a woman, his heart turns away, that person's [semen has been made to lie] with a corpse . . .

11.56 DIŠ NA *ka-šip-ma* UZU.MEŠ-*šú tab-ku mun-ga* TU[KU-*šú*] *ù bir-ka-a-šú ga-an-na* ŠÀ-*šú* MUNUS *ḫa-šiḫ-*[*ma*] MUNUS IGI.BAR-*ma* ŠÀ-*šú* GUR NA BI *re-ḫu-su* KI LÚ.ÚŠ *šu-nu-*[*lat*] *ana* TI-*šú* . . . (Biggs, *ŠÀ.ZI.GA* 68–69:9′–13′//*BAM* 205:7′–10′)

**If a person is hexed so that his flesh is tense, he has *mungu* (stiffness with swelling) and his knees are bent, his heart desires a woman [and then] when he sees a woman, his heart turns away, that person's semen has been made to ⌜lie⌝ with a corpse; to cure him . . .

Low Back Pain

Low back pain is a common complaint, especially with increasing age. There are many causes including vertebral arthritis, slipped disk, and muscle strain. The texts below make it clear that many ancient Mesopotamians suffered from this condition, referred to by the *āšipu* as SA.GIG/*maškādu*[41] or SA.GAL/*sagallu*,[42] depending on the severity of the pain.[43] Those references that emphasize pain radiating from the back down one leg are likely to be due to a slipped intervertebral disk, putting pressure on nerves to one or both legs.

11.57 DIŠ NA SA ÚR-*šú ka-la-šu-ma tab-ku* ZI-*a a-tál-lu-ka la i-le-ʾi sa-gal-lum* DIB-*s*[*u*] . . . (*BAM* 130:19–21)

**If all of the muscles of a person's thigh are so tense that he cannot stand up (or) walk about, *sagallu* afflicts ⌜him⌝ . . .[44]

11.58 [DIŠ SA.M]EŠ ^{UZU}ÚR-*šú* 1-*niš* KÚ.MEŠ-*šú* ZI-*a u* DU.MEŠ-*ka la i-le-ʾ-e* SA.GAL [MU.NI] (DPS XXXIII:98 [AOAT 43.357]; cf. *AMT* 42/6:1; *CT* 23.1–2:1; DPS XIV A iii 5 = *TDP* 140 iii 39′)

**[If the muscle(s)] of his thigh all hurt at once (and) he cannot stand up or walk about, [it is called] *sagallu.*

11.59 [DIŠ ^{UZU}]ÚR-*šú* TA *giš-ši-šú* EN *ki-ṣal-li-šú* KÚ-*šú* ZI-*bi u* DU-[*a*]*k maš-ka-d*[*ù* MU.NI] (DPS XXXIII:99 [AOAT 43.357]; cf. *AMT* 69/9:2′; DPS XIV A iii 3–4 = *TDP* 140 iii 37′–38′)

**[If] his thigh hurts him from his hips to his ankles (but) he can stand and walk, [it is called] ⌜*maškādu*⌝.

11.60 [DIŠ TA] ^{UZU}GIŠ.KUN-*šú* EN ŠU.SI.MEŠ GÌR^{II}-*šú* SA.MEŠ-*šú* KÚ.MEŠ-*šú maš-ka-d*[*ù* MU.NI] (DPS XXXIII:100 [AOAT 43.357]; cf. *AMT* 69/9:3′; DPS XII D iv 18 = *TDP* 108 iv 18)

**[If from] his coccyx to his toes his muscles continually hurt him, [it is called] ⌜*maškādu*⌝.

11.61 DIŠ NA *di-ik-šá* TUKU-*ma ki-ma ṣil-le-e ú-dàk-ka*[*s-su*] ŠU.GIDIM.MA *ana* TI-*šú* . . . (*BAM* 216:29′–30′)[45]

**If a person has a stabbing pain[46] and it ⌜stabs him⌝ like a thorn, "hand" of ghost, to cure him . . .

11.62 DIŠ *na-aṣ-mad di-ik-ši lu šá* 15/ZAG *lu šá* 150/GÙB . . . (*BAM* 3 iv 35//*AMT* 96/1:1//*BAM* 217:5//*BAM* 564 iii 6; cf. BM 42298:4 [Finkel, *Fs. Lambert* 181])[47]

**If (you want) a bandage for stabbing pain either of the left or of the right (side of the body) . . .

An Old Babylonian recitation gives a picturesque description of the pain produced by a slipped intervertebral disk or sciatica. The "bite of a wolf" refers to the severity of the pain, the "leap of the Elamite dog" to the shooting nature of the pain, and the entering and leaving "like a wild animal" suggest the sudden onset and departure of the pain. We believe the mention of the flint knife and razor to have been an idle threat, since the modern surgical procedure used to treat slipped disks would have been far too complicated and risky to perform in that era.

11.63 *na-ša-ak ba-ar-ba-ri-im i-na-aš-ša-ak ša-ḫa-aṭ kal-bi-im e-la-m*[*i* . . . *i*]*-ša-ḫi-iṭ* ⌜*e*⌝*-re-eb bu-lim i-*⌜*ru*⌝*-u*[*b w*] *a-ṣe-e bu-lim uṣ-*⌜*ṣi*⌝ [*ṣ*]*i-i ma-aš-ka-*[*du*]*-*⌜*um la*⌝*-a-ma* ⌜*ik*⌝*-šu-du-ka ṣú-ur-ru na-ag-la-b*[*u ša* ^{d}] *Gu-la* (*YOS* 11.14 r. 3–5)

**It bites with the bite of a wolf; it leaps with the leap of an ⌜Elamite⌝ dog. [. . .] It ⌜enters⌝ and leaves as wild animals enter and ⌜leave⌝. ⌜Go out⌝, ⌜*maškādu*⌝, before the flint knife (and) razor [of] Gula get you!

Summary

Bones and joints play a critical role in manipulating our environment, and ancient Mesopotamian physicians understood their importance. Fractures of bones during work, play, and warfare must have constituted an important part of the *asû*'s practice (see Chapter 1). Arthritis caused by infection and immunologic mechanisms is common now, and it appears to have been common in ancient Mesopotamia. Arthritis is often a chronic process that responds poorly to treatment, and it must therefore have been a source of considerable morbidity and loss of function.

CHAPTER 12

Obstetrics and Gynecology

If (in) a woman of childbearing age, pus is continually produced from (the womb)'s mouth, she will die together with her fetus.

—DPS XXXVI A 83 = *TDP* 208:83

Women's illnesses, including gynecological and obstetrical problems, received considerable attention from ancient Mesopotamian physicians. Treatments were prescribed for most of them, and the patients were followed as closely as their male counterparts. Judging from the clinical texts, there did not appear to be any reluctance on the part of the patient to be examined by the physician, including palpation of the abdomen during pregnancy to ascertain the size of the uterus (and therefore the fetus). The external genitalia also were examined and described. Although the *āšipu* is unlikely to have performed a regular pelvic (vaginal) exam in pregnant or nonpregnant women, he apparently had an instrument to spread the vagina open in order to see the cervix. We have this impression because in the references below there are what appear to be descriptions of the cervix.

12.1 DIŠ MUNUS *ti-ik-pi ina* ARḪUŠ-*šá i-tak-kip* . . . (*SpTU* 5.253 r. 1)

**If a woman becomes spotted with spots on her womb (cervix) . . .

12.2 DIŠ TU ŠÀ.SUR$_{11}$-*sa sa-a-mu/pe-lu-ú* NITA *ir-ḫi* (DPS XXXVI A 100–101 = *TDP* 210:100–101)

**If a woman of childbearing age's womb(?)[1] is red/bright red, she was impregnated with a male.

12.3 DIŠ TU ŠÀ.SUR$_{11}$-*sa nam-ru* NU SI.SÁ *ir-ḫi* (DPS XXXVI A 102 = *TDP* 210:102)

**If a woman of childbearing age's womb(?) is shining, she was impregnated with a child that will not do well.

Gynecology

AMENORRHEA (ABSENCE OF MENSTRUATION)

The references listed below document amenorrhea and recommend treatment, but there is no information available to determine a cause. The second reference is curious because it appears to consider both the absence and the presence of menstruation to be a "trouble." The ancient physician was certainly aware that menstruation was a normal process.

12.4 DIŠ MUNUS MÚD-*šá* TAR-*ma* MÚD-*šá* NU [IGI] ... (*SpTU* 1.59:14′)

**If a woman's blood is cut off so that her blood is not [seen] ...

12.5 NÍG GIG NÍG NU *im-mar ana šá* GIG *šá i*[*m*]-*mar*... (*SpTU* 1.59:12′)

**[To turn?] trouble that one does not see into trouble that one sees ...

MENHORRHAGIA (EXCESSIVE MENSTRUATION)

Irregular bleeding (*naḫšātu*)[2] was known to be a problem. Blood loss would have been an obvious concern in ancient Mesopotamia. Again, there is no information available to determine the cause.

12.6 *maš-qit šá* MÚD MUNUS TAR-*si*... (*SpTU* 4.153:17)[3]

**Potion to stop a woman from bleeding ...

12.7 DIŠ MUNUS MÚD.MEŠ-*šú* DU.MEŠ-*ma la ip-par-ra-su ana pa-ra-si* . . . (*SpTU* 4.153:1)

**If a woman's blood flows and does not stop, to stop it ...

12.8 Ú MUNUS *šá na-aḫ-šá-a-ti* GIG ... (*BAM* 381 iii 24)[4]

**Plant for a woman who is sick with *naḫšātu* (menorrhagia) ...

INFERTILITY

Female infertility has many causes, among them advancing age. A letter sent by Ramses II to Ḫattušili III in the mid-second millennium B.C.E. chides the Hittites for supposing that Egyptians had some sort of "miracle cure" that would enable a sixty-year-old woman to have children.[5] Medicines, recitations, and charms were available to treat infertile women.

12.9 (DIŠ) MUNUS *a-la-da* TAR-*sà*-[*at*] ... (*BAM* 241 iii 3′; *BAM* 243:5′)

**(If) a woman is past childbearing age ...

12.10 Ú MUNUS NU Ù.TU ... (*BAM* 381 iii 20//*BAM* 380:27; cf. *BAM* 421 i′ 25′)[6]

**Plant for a woman who is unable to give birth ...

12.11 NA_4.MEŠ MUNUS NU $PEŠ_4$ *ana* $PEŠ_4$ . . . (*BAM* 250:3–4)[7]

**Stones to enable a woman who is not pregnant to get pregnant . . .

Although it was realized that infertility could be the man's fault (see Chapter 5), we are probably safe in presuming that the solution to a childless marriage was first to treat the woman for barrenness, then to have the man try other partners, and only when that failed would the *āšipu* worry about the man's infertility. A section of Ḫammurapi's laws deals with the tricky situations that could arise when men took secondary wives or concubines to produce the children denied them by wives who were either barren or priestesses not allowed to have intercourse.[8]

BIRTH CONTROL

At the opposite extreme, it is apparent that ancient Mesopotamian physicians were consulted for treatment to prevent pregnancy and for methods to abort an established pregnancy.[9]

12.12 Ú MUNUS NU $PEŠ_4$ . . . (*BAM* 381 iii 21–22//*BAM* 380:28–29; cf. BM 51246+53217+53744 r. 12′)

**Plant for a woman not to get pregnant . . .

12.13 Ú *šá-mi* ARḪUŠ ŠUB-*e* . . . (*BAM* 422 iii 5)[10]

**Plant to make the fetus drop . . .

The reasons to prevent and abort pregnancies were undoubtedly multiple, but one is illustrated by a passage in the omen literature: "the man's wife will become pregnant by another man and she will constantly pray to Ištar (saying) while looking at her husband: 'I want to make my fetus look like him.'"[11] Another reason for an abortion would have been that the baby had died (i.e., was immobile) in the womb, as in the following letter.

12.14 ITI.7.KAM *an-nu-um ši-ru-um ina li-bi-ia iš-tu* ITI.1.KAM *ši-ru-um ina li-bi-ia mi-it-ma* (al-Zeebari, *ABIM* 15:7–10)

**For these seven months, there has been an infant in my womb (but), for a month now, the infant in my womb has been dead.

Ancient Mesopotamians were also aware that abstinence and anal intercourse were effective means of preventing pregnancies.

12.15 "Can she be pregnant without having had sexual intercourse? Can she get fat without eating?" (Lambert, *BWL* 241 ii 40–42)

12.16 "The *ēntu*-priestess will have (her illicit lover) perform anal intercourse in order not to get pregnant." (*BRM* 4.12:32; cf. *CT* 31.44 obv! 10)

PREGNANCY TESTING

The text below describes a test for pregnancy. It sounds remarkably similar to many modern medical tests that are determined by color changes. It is impossible at the present time to know how sensitive or specific it might have been, but if future research can determine the nature of the ingredients employed in such tests, it might be possible to learn their reliability. It is known that there are changes in the vaginal secretions of a pregnant woman that could have been the basis for this test. For example, there are changes in vaginal acidity and salt, as well as the levels of estrogen and progesterone.

12.17 [. . .] 1/2 GÍN Ú.BABBAR 4-*tú* NA$_4$ *gab-u* [. . . *ana* ŠÀ.T]ÙR-*šá* GAR-*an mu-šú gab-bi* [. . .]x-*nu-tú* LUḪ-*si ki-*⸢*i* SÍG⸣.ÀKA SA$_5$-*at lu* MÚD *ul-lu-ḫa-tú* [MUNUS BI PEŠ$_4$] *ki-i* SÍG.ÀKA *ši-i* SIG$_7$-*at* MUNUS BI NU PEŠ$_4$ (*UET* 7.123:1–4 [Reiner, *ZA* 72.134])

**You [wrap] one half shekel "white plant," a quarter shekel alum, and [. . . in a tuft of wool]. You put it [into] her ⸢vagina⸣. [She keeps it in place] all night. [The next morning . . .] you wash it. If the tuft of wool is red or streaked with blood red, [that woman is pregnant]. If that tuft of wool is green, that woman is not pregnant.

12.18 *ana maš-*⸢*ši*⸣*-ti* ⸢*ù* [ooooo] 1 GÍN ^{Ú}*tar-muš* 1/2 [GÍN Ú.BABBAR] 1 GÍN NA$_4$ *ga-bu-ú ina* SÍG.ÀKA NIGIN-*mi* [*ana* ŠÀ.TÙR-*šú* GAR] -*ma kal* U$_4$-*mu ú-*[*kal tu-še-e*] *l-lam-ma ina* A LUḪ-*si šum$_4$-ma* [SIG$_7$ MUNUS BI *la*] *e-ri* : NU [PEŠ$_4$ *šà-*ŠÀ-*šà*] ŠUB : *šum$_4$-ma* SÍG.ÀKA SA$_5$-*at* [*lu* MÚD *ul*]-*lu-ḫat u* ŠÀ.TUR-*šú* UD-*ma* [MUN]US BI *er-ri* (BM 42313+43174 r. 29–32)

**For a tampon and [. . .]. You wrap one shekel *tarmuš*, one half [shekel "white plant"], (and) a shekel alum in a tuft of wool. [You put it into her vagina] and she [keeps it in place] all day. [You] ⸢take it out⸣ and wash it with water. If [it is green, that woman is not] pregnant (var. will lose [her fetus]). / If the tuft of wool is red [or] ⸢streaked⸣ [with blood red] and her womb is white/dry, that ⸢woman⸣ will remain pregnant.

UTERINE PROLAPSE

The uterus, especially following many pregnancies, may lose its normal support and sag into the vagina. It may progress to the point that it protrudes from the vagina. This phenomenon was noted and treated by ancient Mesopotamian physicians. It appears unlikely that a medicinal plant (see below) would have affected this condition. Possibly it was intended to treat one of the complications of uterine prolapse such as a urinary tract infection.

12.19 Ú *mi-qít* ŠÀ . . . (*BAM* 380:66, 67, 72//*BAM* 381 iv 22, 23, 30; cf. *BAM* 422 iii 31′, 32′)[12]

**Plant for the falling out of the womb . . .

VAGINAL INFECTIONS

These infections are discussed in the chapter on sexually transmitted diseases (Chapter 4). Genital crabs are discussed in Chapter 2 with 2.25.

Obstetrics

MIDWIVES

The birth of a child[13] was attended by a ritual which, according to myth, commemorated the first creation of mankind by the goddess Bēlet-ilī. Men seem, as a rule, to have been banned from the birth room.[14] Childbirth took place in the home and was normally attended by a midwife (*šabsūtu*) and/or *qadištu* (or other holy woman with similar responsibilities). As the woman neared time for the birth,[15] the midwife covered her head and girded her loins. While reciting blessings with a beaming, joyful face, she drew a circle on the floor with flour and laid an unbaked brick within it.[16] If all went well, the baby would be safely delivered by her skill alone; if there were complications, the *āšipu* would have to be called in.[17]

The midwife's duties were hardly completed by the safe delivery of the baby. Much care was taken in severing the baby's umbilical cord. The cutting was done either with a knife[18] or with a sharp sliver of reed.[19]

12.20 "The reed is what cuts the umbilical cord" (11N-T3:12–13 [Civil, *JNES* 33.332]).

12.21 "She (Nintu) took out the reed-sliver (taken from) the canebrake, severer of the umbilical cord" (Atraḫasīs S iii 7 [Jacobsen, *OrNS* 42.291 n. 67]).

The use of a reed may sound strange, but since reeds were cheap and readily available, a separate reed could have been used for every patient which might, like our own disposable scalpel blades, have presented considerably less danger of infection to the patient than the physician's knife. It would appear that, in at least some cases, a reed was filled with salve and was broken over the baby's navel,[20] presumably to soothe the wound.

According to the Sumerian composition "Enki and the World Order," the umbilical cord when cut was treated with *immanakku*-stone (in this case perhaps coarse sand)[21] and by a leek to stop the bleeding.[22] Also listed in "Enki and the World Order" was a water pail, probably used for cleaning the blood from mother and baby.[23] A recitation presumably meant to be recited at this point in the birth ritual reads: "She (the midwife) rubs (the newborn's) breast with oil. She inserts her finger into his mouth. He (the baby) will put down the amniotic fluid(?)."[24] A similar practice of clearing the newborn's mouth with a finger is found in modern Iran.[25]

The Ninisinna hymn also describes midwifely duties to include "to make the son of a man, once he has been caught by the thighs, to scream loudly; to put his abdomen toward the ground (i.e., to turn him over) (and) to make (him) exchange places with (his) head (i.e., to turn him upside down)."[26] One thinks immediately of the modern practice of dangling the child upside down and smacking it on the bottom to make it gasp and cry to clear its lungs.

The final duty of the midwife was to take care of the afterbirth (placenta). Another piece of equipment used by the midwife and mentioned in the hymn to Ninisinna[27] was the "vessel in which the afterbirth is placed,"[28] presumably for ultimate disposal.[29]

GROWTH OF THE FETUS

The ancient Mesopotamian physician was aware of the normal growth and enlargement of the fetus, as demonstrated by the reference below, and this provided the *āšipu* with the information that he needed to recognize signs of abnormal development.

12.22 LÚ.TUR U_4-*mu šá ina* ŠÀ AMA!-*šú* DÙ-*ú* 1/2 ŠE *šú-ú i-na* 2-*i* U_4-*mu* ŠE *šú-ú i-na šal-šú* U_4-*mu* ŠE 1/2 ŠE *šú-ú ina* 4-*i* U_4-*mu* 2 ŠE *šú-ú i-na* 5-*šú* U_4-*mu* 2 1/2 ŠE *šú-ú ina* 6!-*šú* U_4-*mu* 3 ŠE *šú-ú i-na* 7-*i* U_4-*mu* 3 1/2 ŠE *šú-ú ina* 8-*i* U_4-*mu* 4 ŠE *šú-ú i-na* 9-*i* U_4-*mu* 4 1/2 ŠE *šú-ú ina* 10-*i* U_4-*mu* 5 ŠE *šú-ú i-na* ITI U_4.MEŠ 3 ŠU.SI *šú!-ú i-na* 10 ITI.MEŠ 1 KÙŠ *šú-ú* (*SpTU* 4.173 ii 2–9, apud Hunger, *NABU* 1994 no. 34)[30]

**An infant is a half grain the day it is created in the womb of his mother. On the second day, it is a grain.[31] On the third day, it is a grain and a half. On the fourth day, it is two grains. On the fifth day, it is two and a half grains. On the sixth day, it is three grains. On the seventh day, it is three and a half grains. On the eighth day, it is four grains. On the ninth day, it is four and a half grains. On the tenth day, it is five grains. In a full month, it is three fingers. In ten months, it is a cubit (distance from the elbow to the extended middle finger).

PREPARTUM CARE

The *āšipu* was aware that a pregnant woman's activities would influence her health and the outcome of labor.

12.23 DIŠ ⸢TU *m*⸣*i-ra-a pal-ḫat ina šà*-ŠÀ-*šà i-šal-lim* (DPS XXXVI A 103 = *TDP* 210:103)

**If a woman of childbearing age is properly respectful of pregnancy, she will get well from her being with child.

12.24 DIŠ T[U *mi*]*-ra-a še-la-at ina šà*-ŠÀ-*šà* ÚŠ (DPS XXXVI A 104 = *TDP* 210:104)

**If a ⸢woman of childbearing age⸣ is careless of ⸢pregnancy⸣,[32] she will die from her being with child.

The woman's appearance also suggested her state of health and the likelihood of survival.

12.25 DIŠ TU IGI.MEŠ-*šá ik-ki-ru ina šà*-ŠÀ-*šà* ÚŠ (DPS XXXVI A 77 = *TDP* 206:77)

**If the face of a woman of childbearing age changes (for the worse), she will die as a result of her being with child.[33]

12.26 DIŠ TU IGI.MEŠ-*šá ne-e-ḫu ina šà*-ŠÀ-*šà ú-šal-lam* (DPS XXXVI A 78 = *TDP* 206:78)

**If the face of a woman of childbearing age is calm, she will bring the fetus to term as a result of her being with child.

The ancient physician also evaluated specific parts of the woman's body to predict the success of the pregnancy. Logically, the health of the woman's breasts would be important for fetal survival. The following references illustrate this concern. It is likely that the first text describes inverted nipples, a condition that could interfere with an infant's ability to nurse.

12.27 DIŠ TU *ap-pa* UBUR-*šá zi-i-ir*$_9$ *šà*-ŠÀ-*šà* NU SI.SÁ (DPS XXXVI A 26 = *TDP* 202:26)

**If the tip of a woman of childbearing age's breast is twisted (shut), her fetus will not do well.

12.28 DIŠ *pa-ṭi-ir*$_9$ *šà*-ŠÀ-*šà* SI.SÁ (DPS XXXVI A 27 = *TDP* 202:27)

**If (the tip of a woman of childbearing age's breast) is open, her fetus will do well.

In the following references, an "unraveled" navel probably describes one that is protruding. Since naval protrusion develops in most pregnancies as the uterus enlarges, an "unraveled" navel would be evidence of normal fetal development. Failure of the navel to protrude indicates retarded fetal development and a high probability of fetal death.

12.29 DIŠ TU SAG *a-bu-un-na-ti-šá pa-ši-ir šá*-ŠÀ-*šà ú-šal-lam* (DPS XXXVI A 85 = *TDP* 208:85)

**If the head of the navel of a woman of childbearing age is unraveled, she will bring her fetus to term.

12.30 DIŠ *zi-ir*$_9$ <NU> *pa-ši-ir šá*-ŠÀ-*šà* NU DIN (DPS XXXVI A 86 = *TDP* 208:86)

**If (the head of the navel of a woman of childbearing age) is twisted <and not> unraveled, her fetus will not live.

In particular, the *āšipu* worried about the continuation of a pregnant woman's sexual relations, identified in the following references as "approaching" her. It is possible that the circumlocution represents a prudishness that occasionally surfaces in the texts. For example, hemerologies refer to a sexual taboo in force during the New Year's Festival as follows: "He should not 'approach' a woman; he should sleep in a secluded room."[34] Alternatively, the expression was intended to also cover the insertion of objects other than a penis into the vagina. Treatments for various gynecological problems involve the use of vaginal suppositories, and it would have been possible to probe the vagina with the bronze or copper tubes used to infuse medicines into the womb (compare probing the urethra with tubes used to infuse medicines into the bladder—see Chapter 5).

Up to a point, the reasoning behind the recommendations is clear. Sexual intercourse too early in the pregnancy was not contemplated, doubtless due to the danger of miscarriage. In the third month,[35] however, the *āšipu* was of the opinion that sexual intercourse or a vaginal exam was safe, even if the patient was still exhibiting signs of morning sickness.

12.31 DIŠ MUNUS.PEŠ$_4$ GIG-*ma šum-ma šá* ITI.3.KÁM *ir-tu-bu-niš-ši* : *iq-ru-bu-niš-ši* MUNUS BI AL.TI (DPS XXXVII A obv. 1 = *TDP* 212:1)

**If a pregnant woman is ill and if when she is in the third month they continue to approach her, that woman will live.

12.32 *šum-ma šá* ITI.4.KÁM *ir-tu-bu-niš-ši* MUNUS BI AL.TI (DPS XXXVII A obv. 2 = *TDP* 212:2)

**If when she is in the fourth month they continue, that woman will live.

The following reference describes the results of a vaginal exam carried out in the third month of pregnancy.

12.33 DIŠ MUNUS *šá* 3 ITI MÚD.MEŠ DU-*ak* DIŠ *šà*-ŠÀ-*šà* [. . .] *si-lit tak-pat u šá-lat* . . . (BM 42313+ r. 12–13)

**If (in) a woman three months (pregnant) the blood flows, if the fetus [. . .] (and) the womb (cervix) is spotted and sprinkled . . .

More mysterious are the *āšipu*'s concerns about the middle term of pregnancy. The parallel section of the diagnostic/prognostic handbook (see below) indicates that the worry was that a woman who had intercourse (or a vaginal exam) in these months would have an episode of bleeding that might lead to a miscarriage. It is unclear how the *āšipu* reached this conclusion.

12.34 *šum-ma šá* ITI.5.KÁM *ir-tu-bu-niš-ši* MUNUS BI *na-ʾ-da-át* (DPS XXXVII A obv. 3 = *TDP* 212:3)

**If when she is in the fifth month they continue, that woman is a cause for worry.

12.35 *šum-ma šá* ITI.6.KÁM *ir-tu-bu-niš-ši* MUNUS BI *na-ʾ-da-át* (DPS XXXVII A obv. 4 = *TDP* 212:4)

**If when she is in the sixth month they continue, that woman is a cause for worry.

The *āšipu* was of the opinion that intercourse was safe in the seventh month, but began to be worried again in the eighth month, and positively forbade it in the last two (lunar) months of pregnancy.

12.36 *šum-ma šá* ITI.7.KÁM *ir-tu-bu-niš-ši* MUNUS BI AL.TI (DPS XXXVII A obv. 5 = *TDP* 212:5)

**If when she is in the seventh month they continue, that woman will live.

12.37 *šum-ma šá* ITI.8.KÁM *ir-tu-bu-niš-ši* MUNUS BI TI-*uṭ* : *ma-mit* AD-*šú* DIB-*si* (DPS XXXVII A obv. 6 = *TDP* 212:6)

**If when she is in the eighth month they continue, that woman will live (var. the curse of her father will afflict her).

12.38 *šum-ma šá* ITI.9.KÁM *ù* ITI.10.KÁM *ir-tu-bu-niš-ši* MUNUS BI *ul* <<NIN>> TI-*uṭ* : *ul* TU (DPS XXXVII A obv. 7 = *TDP* 212:7)

**If when she is in the ninth or tenth month[36] they continue, that woman will not live (var. she will not give birth).

One of the references above indicates that a woman engaging in sexual intercourse too late during the pregnancy runs the risk of being "afflicted," presumably with a malformed or dead baby, but it also mentions "the curse of her father." This "curse" could simply refer to inherited defects. To note, however, is that fetal abnormalities and death are much more common in consanguineous relationships.

A separate section of the diagnostic handbook gives more details on the problematic fifth month of pregnancy, providing day by day prognoses from the third to the tenth days.

These references look suspiciously like they were generated by more general notions of "good" and "bad" days. We know enough, however, about ancient Mesopotamian hemerological speculations to prove that this is not the case. What is a good day for what sort of activity varies somewhat from month to month, but one invariable regularity is that the seventh day of the month is a bad day, and the seventh day of the seventh month particularly so.[37] Despite or perhaps because of the frequent use of the number 7 and multiples of 7 in magical rites, 7 was an unlucky number. If this sort of speculation was generating these recommendations, the *āšipu* would not have failed to predict death on the seventh day. However, this is not the *āšipu*'s prediction in this case.

12.39 DIŠ TU PEŠ$_4$-*ma ša* ITI 7 U$_4$-*mi iq-ri-bu-niš-ši* NAM.TI.[LA] (DPS XXXVI A 110// D 7 = *TDP* 210:110)

**If a woman of childbearing age is pregnant and at (five) months (and) seven days (they approach her), life.[38]

As to what *was* generating the speculation, there is one obvious suggestion. The count of days begins with the third (good). The fourth is also good, but the fifth and sixth are problematic. The seventh is good again; the eighth foresees problems with "father's evil"—see above. The ninth is bad and the tenth (and last day) is good again.

12.40 DIŠ T[U PEŠ$_4$-*ma š*]*a* 5 ITI 3 U$_4$-*mi iq-ri-bu-niš-šú* NAM.TI.[LA] (DPS XXXVI A 106 = *TDP* 210:106)[39]

**If a woman of ⌜childbearing age⌝ [is pregnant and] ⌜at⌝ five months (and) three days they approach her, life.

12.41 DIŠ TU ⌜PEŠ$_4$⌝-*ma ša* ITI 5 U$_4$-*mi iq-ri-bu-niš-ši ša na-aḫ-šá-ti* G[IG][40] (DPS XXXVI A 108//B 40'//D 5 = *TDP* 210:108)[41]

**If a woman of childbearing age is pregnant and at (five) months (and) five days they approach her, she ⌜will be sick⌝ with irregular bleeding.

12.42 DIŠ TU PEŠ$_4$-*ma ša* ITI 8 U$_4$-*mi iq-ri-bu-niš-ši* ḪUL *a-bi* NAM.ÉRIM DIB-*su* (DPS XXXVI A 111//D 8 = *TDP* 210:111)

**If a woman of childbearing age is pregnant and at (five) months (and) eight days they approach her, father's evil; a curse will afflict her.

12.43 DIŠ TU PEŠ$_4$-*ma ša* ITI 9 U$_4$-*mi iq-ri-bu-niš-ši* BA.ÚŠ (DPS XXXVI A 112//D 9 = *TDP* 210:112)

**If a woman of childbearing age is pregnant and at (five) months (and) nine days they approach her, she will die.

This corresponds exactly to the pattern of months in which the *āšipu* considered it safe to have intercourse (assuming, of course, that the intercourse in the tenth month was taken to be after the birth). No statement is made about days after the tenth. Since lunar months have twenty-nine or thirty days, however, it is conceivable that the sequence was understood to repeat. It appears that in this case the *āšipu* was making logical, if not necessarily correct, assumptions.

BLEEDING

Uterine bleeding during pregnancy was noted to be a serious problem by the ancient physicians.

12.44 *šá* MUNUS.PEŠ$_4$ *šá* 3 4 ITI.MEŠ-*šú u* MÚD *i-ta-nam-ma-ru* . . . (*SpTU* 4.153:8)

**For a pregnant woman who is three or four months along and blood is continually seen . . .

12.45 MUNUS *šá* 1 U$_4$-*mu* 2 U$_4$-*mu i-ḫi-lu* [. . .] (*SpTU* 4.153:19)

**A woman who oozes blood for one or two days [. . .]

12.46 DIŠ MUNUS PEŠ$_4$-*ma* ⌜ŠÀ.MEŠ⌝ [. . .] . . . *za-mar* ⌜xx⌝ *ši-i* SA$_5$ *i-tab-ba-ka* . . . (*BAM* 240:4′, 8′)

**If a woman is pregnant and her insides [. . .] suddenly [. . .] pours out red . . .

ENDOMETRITIS (INTRAUTERINE INFECTION)

Another series of quotes describes pregnant women with dark blood or pus coming from the mouth of the uterus (cervix). The cause of the bleeding is unknown, but heavy uterine bleeding is commonly associated with a poor outcome. Similarly, pus from the cervix is a very serious sign that usually leads to fetal death and, in the absence of antibiotics, maternal death as well.

12.47 DIŠ TU MÚD *ina* KA-*šú* DU-*ku ina* PEŠ$_4$-*šú* NU DIN (DPS XXXVI A 82 = *TDP* 208:82)[42]

**If (in) a woman of childbearing age, dark blood flows from (the womb)'s[43] mouth, she will not get well from her pregnancy.

12.48 DIŠ TU MÚD.BABBAR *ina* KA-*šú* ŠUB.ŠUB-*a qá-du šà*-ŠÀ-*šà* GAM (DPS XXXVI A 83 = *TDP* 208:83)

**If (in) a woman of childbearing age, pus is continually produced from (the womb)'s mouth, she will die together with her fetus.

MISCARRIAGES

A number of texts suggest treatments to prevent miscarriages.

12.49 DIŠ MUNUS *lu* [1 IT]U *lu* 2 ITU [*l*]*u* 3 ITU *šà*-ŠÀ-*šà* [Š]UB.ŠUB-*a* . . . (BM 42333+:1–2//BM 42313+ r. 9 [Finkel, *Fs. Lambert* 171–172])

**If a woman is pregnant for [one] ⌜month⌝ or two months ⌜or⌝ three months and continually aborts her fetuses . . .

12.50 *šum$_4$-ma er-ri u* A.MEŠ ŠUB.ŠUB-*ma* . . . (BM 42333+:11//BM 42313+ r. 36[44] [Finkel, *Fs. Lambert* 171–172]; cf. BM 51246+53217+ r. 13′–14′)

**Also if she gets pregnant but she continually puts down (her) waters . . .[45]

12.51 DIŠ MUNUS *ina* ŠÀ TUKU-*at ka-la-a la i-le-ʾ-e ana* MUNUS *nu-uḫ-ḫi* . . . (*BAM* 240:71′)

**If a woman is not able to retain what she has in her womb, to calm the woman . . .

12.52 DIŠ [MUNUS].PEŠ$_4$ UŠ$_{11}$.ZU NU TE-*ma ša*-ŠÀ-*šá* NU [ŠUB?] . . . (BM 51246+ 53217+ obv. 1)

**If you want sorcery not to approach a pregnant [woman] and for her not to [abort?] her fetus . . .

As the last reference indicates, malicious sorcery (practiced against the victim by other women) was suspected in cases of miscarriage. It must be remembered that the pregnant woman in question would have been a firm believer in sorcery, which made her susceptible to a hysterical (and dangerous) reaction if she found something nasty that a jealous neighbor had left at her door.[46] Although the *āšipu* also believed in sorcery, he was not unaware of the positive psychological effects of amulets: "A bandage for releasing a pregnant woman or a woman in confinement to whom something (evil) was shown. If you put it on her neck, they can show (it) to her (all they want) and it will not affect her."[47] In other words, armed with an appropriate magical protection, the expectant mother would not be frightened into having a miscarriage.

INCONTINENCE IN PREGNANCY

The enlarged uterus of pregnancy puts pressure on the urinary bladder. This may lead to incontinence, as described in the text below. Painful urination with an overfull bladder, as also mentioned in this reference, is something that most of us have experienced.

12.53 DIŠ MUNUS *ina ṣal-lu-ti-šú* KÀŠ-*šú ina* ^{GIŠ}NÁ-*šú iš-tin* ŠÀ KÀŠ.MEŠ *ma-a-du-ti* MUNUS KÚ-*šú-ma* MUNUS.BI KÀŠ *ši-ti* BÚR (BM 42313+ r. 7–8)

**If a woman urinates her[48] urine in her sleep (and) during (the urination) of large amounts of urine, it hurts her, that woman (has) escaping urine; it will go away (by itself).

URINARY TRACT INFECTION

The following reference describes a pregnant woman who appears to have difficulty voiding, presumably due to a urinary tract infection.

12.54 DIŠ MUNUS ŠUB DIB KÀŠ GIG-*at* . . . (BM 42313+ r. 6)

**If a woman is sick with "letting fall" (and) "holding in" of urine . . .

GASTROINTESTINAL PROBLEMS

Vomiting is a common problem in pregnancy. Often called morning sickness, it usually diminishes by the twelfth to fourteenth week of pregnancy. Severe, persistent, and frequent vomiting sometimes occurs, which can lead to dehydration and starvation. Without fluid replacement, death of the woman and/or fetus is likely.

12.55 DIŠ TU *ip-ta-na-ar-ru ul ú-šal-lam* (DPS XXXVI A 81 = *TDP* 208:81)

**If a woman of childbearing age continually vomits, she will not bring (her fetus) to term.[49]

12.56 DIŠ T[U . . .] *-šá i-ta-na-aš-šá-šu šà*-ŠÀ-*šà* ÚŠ (DPS XXXVI A 105 = *TDP* 210:105)

**If a woman of ⌜childbearing⌝ age's [stomach?] is continually upset, her fetus will die.

Constipation due in part to blockage of the colon by the enlarged uterus could be a problem.

12.57 Ú *šá-mi ud-du e-sil* . . . (*BAM* 421 i′ 26′)

**"Plant for a pregnant woman(?) who is constipated . . .

Diarrhea was also noted and treated.

12.58 ⌜DIŠ [SAL]⌝*ḫa-riš-tú* ŠÀ.SI.SÁ DIB-*si* . . . (*BAM* 240:36′)

**If diarrhea afflicts a woman in confinement . . .

SMALL PELVIS OR LARGE BABY

Difficult births due to a woman's small pelvis or to a large baby could present serious problems.[50] We are unaware of instruments (i.e., forceps) that were used to assist delivery. It was proposed by A. L. Oppenheim that an expression which appears in adoption contracts, *šilip rēmim*: lit. "slipped from the womb," was meant to designate infants not born in the usual way (for which other expressions were used) but taken from the mother's womb by Caesarean section.[51] If Caesarean sections were indeed performed, it would have been only to benefit the fetus. Survival of the mother from this type of surgery at the time would have been almost impossible.

12.59 DIŠ MUNUS Ù.TU-*ma* (*ina* Ù.TU) *uš-tap-šiq* . . . (*AMT* 67/1 iv 6//*BAM* 248 iv 13//*BAM* 249 i 8′; *BAM* 249 i 11′; cf. Šumma Izbu IV 45 [Leichty, *Izbu* 70])

**If a woman is too narrow to give birth . . .

12.60 [KA.INIM.MA MUNUS] *šup-šu-qat a-la-da* . . . (K 8210 i 9′//*BAM* 248 i 36)[52]

**[Recitation for a woman] who is too narrow to give birth . . .

12.61 [DIŠ] ITI *šá* Ù.TU-*šú iq-ri-ba-am-ma la ú-[la-ad]* . . . (*SpTU* 4.153:21)

**[If] the month for her to give birth approaches and she does not ⌜give birth⌝ . . .

12.62 *a-na* MUNUS *šá tu-lu-di ta-kul-lu-ú ik-kal-lu-ši* SIG_5 (BM 43229 r. 3′–6′ [Finkel, *Fs. Lambert* 158])

**It is good for a woman for whom giving birth and birth pangs are delayed.[53]

12.63 qu_5*-taru* MUNUS NU SI.SÁ . . . (*STT* 281 i 11)[54]

**Fumigants for a woman who does not give birth right away . . .

12.64 Ú MUNUS.LA.RA.AḪ . . . (*BAM* 379 iii 9, 14; *BAM* 380:36//*BAM* 381 iii 31; *BAM* 380:31//*BAM* 381 iii 25; *KADP* 1 v 8)[55]

**Plant for a woman having difficulty giving birth . . .

SYSTEMIC LUPUS ERYTHEMATOSIS (SLE) IN PREGNANCY

In a very interesting text, the *āšipu* describes skin lesions on the face of a pregnant woman as resembling KUŠ.TAB. According to Deller,[56] KUŠ.TAB is hide (KUŠ) treated with a depilatory paste (*kurru* of the tanner)[57] with the result that the hair changes consistency (TAB = *sepû*)[58] so that it may easily be removed with a scraper.[59]

12.65 DIŠ TU KUŠ.TAB IGI-*šá ma-lu-ú šà*-ŠÀ-*šà* GAM (DPS XXXVI A 79 = *TDP* 208:79)

**If the face of a woman of childbearing age is full of (patches of what looks like) oxhide treated with depilatories, her fetus will die.

12.66 DIŠ TU KUŠ.TAB IGI-*šá* DIRI-*ú* IGI DIDLI-*šá tur-ru-pa qá-du šà*-ŠÀ-*šà* GAM (DPS XXXVI A 80 = *TDP* 208:80)

**If the face of a woman of childbearing age is full of (patches of what looks like) oxhide treated with depilatories (and) both her eyes are spotted, she will die together with her fetus.[60]

A systemic disease that causes hair loss and skin lesions reminiscent of KUŠ.TAB and is likely to result in the death of both the mother and baby is systemic lupus erythematosis (SLE). The skin lesions are prominent on the cheek bones, but can be seen almost anywhere. The spots on the eyes described by the *āšipu* are of unclear nature when compared with modern descriptions of the disease; however, they may be due to ocular bleeding in those patients with lupus that have poor blood clotting due to low blood platelet levels, a complication of SLE.

Another complication of SLE is increased blood clotting caused by abnormal antibodies such as anticardiolipin. This can result in recurrent abortions, intrauterine fetal death, and intrauterine fetal growth retardation. With modern treatment of this immunologic disease with steroids and other immunosuppressive agents, the outcome is more favorable than it would have been for women in ancient Mesopotamia.

HYSTERIA

This term comes from the Greek word *hysteria*, meaning "uterus," and refers to the frequent psychological problems in pregnant women that result from the mental and physiological stress involved with pregnancy. The problems range from fear and apprehension to depression and psychosis. The references below list some of these presentations.

12.67 BE MUNUS IM *i-ri-ma* IM Ù.TU . . . (Šumma Izbu I 50 [Leichty, *Izbu* 36])[61]

**If a woman becomes pregnant with wind and gives birth to wind . . .

12.68 DIŠ MUNUS *ina* GIG-*šá* ŠÀ-*bi ku-ri i-qab-bi* ŠU ^{d}15 AL.TI (DPS XXXVII A obv. 17 = *TDP* 214:17)

**If a woman during her illness says: "My abdomen is (too) short," (it is) "hand" of Ištar; she will get well.

12.69 DIŠ MUNUS GIG-*ma* DIB-*sa ina* GI_6 DIB.DIB-*si* DIB-*it* LÍL.LÁ.EN.NA (DPS XXXVII A obv. 12 = *TDP* 214:12)[62]

**If a woman is sick and her affliction always afflicts her during the night, it is an affliction of *lilû* (see below).

12.70 DIŠ MUNUS GIG-*ma* DIB-*sa ina* AN.ÚSAN DIB.DIB-*si u* TÚG-*sa* ŠUB.ŠUB-*di* DIB-*it* LÍL.LÁ.EN.NA (DPS XXXVII A obv. 13 = *TDP* 214:13)

**If a woman is sick and her affliction always afflicts her in the evening and she continually takes her clothes off, it is an affliction of *lilû*.

LILÛ

In addition to psychological problems in pregnant women (see above), *lilû*-demons were held responsible for the sort of nervous behavior, fainting spells, and false seizures (see Chapter 19 with 19.18–19.21) which we associate with adolescent girls, and which was also referred to by nineteenth-century physicians as "hysteria."

12.71 DIŠ *ina ṣal-lu-ti-šú* DIB-*su-ma* DIB-*su* IGI.BAR-*as i-re-eḫ-ḫi-šum-ma* NÍ-*šú i-maš-ši* GIN_7 *šá id-ku-šú* MUD-*ud* ZI.ZI-*bé* : U_4 *id-de-ku-šú re-ḫi* ŠU LÍL.LÁ.EN.NA *sar-⌜ru⌝ ana* MUNUS LÍL.LÁ.EN.NA ZI.ZI-*bé* (DPS XXVI:48′–49′ [AOAT 43.282])

**If it afflicts him in his sleep and he gazes at the ones who afflict him, it flows over him and he forgets himself, he shudders like one whom they have awakened (and) he can still get up (var. when they try to wake him, he is groggy), false "hand" of *lilû*. For a woman, (it is) a *lilû*; she can get up (afterward).

12.72 DIŠ *pa-rid-ma it-te-né-et-bi ma-gal* DUG_4.DUG_4-*ub u i*[*g-d*]*a-⌜na⌝-al-lu-u*[*t*] *ana* MUNUS LÍL.L[Á].EN.NA *ana* NITA SAL.LÍL.LÁ.EN.NA ZI.ZI-*bé* (DPS XXVI:82′–83′ [AOAT 43.285])

**If he shudders and he can get up (afterward), he talks a lot and he continually ⌜jerks⌝, for a woman, (it is) a *lilû*, for a man, (it is) a *lilītu*; he can get up (afterward).

In the Hippocratic tradition, this sort of psychiatric problem was supposed to be caused by the woman's uterus wandering from its proper place. Ancient Mesopotamians, on the other hand, attributed this type of illness to a nonsexist class of demons who were also capable of causing genuine seizures, schizophrenia, or the combination of both (see Chapters 13 and 16). Since males were as likely to be victimized as women, this class of demon provided a ready-made explanation for the unhappy lot of the teenage boy.

12.73 [DIŠ UG]U-*šú* [GAZ.ME SA]G.DU-*su* TAB-*su* ŠÀ-*šú i-ta-na-ši* GIN_7 *šá ana* UGU MUNUS ŠUB-*tu* ÍL ŠÀ TUKU-*ši* ŠU KI.SIKIL.LÍL.LÁ.EN.NA (DPS III A obv. 12//C obv. 3 = *TDP* 18:3)

**[If] the ⌜top of his head⌝ [continually feels as if split in two], his ⌜head⌝ burns, he continually has sexual desires,[63] (and) like one who lays himself down on top of a woman, he has an erection, "hand" of *ardat lilî.*

12.74 [DIŠ UGU-*šú*] *ka*[*l* U_4/GI_6 G]AZ.ME ŠÀ-*šú*![64] *i-ta-na-áš-ši-ma* KI.NÁ *it-ta-na-as-ḫar*![65]*-šu* GIN_7 *šá ana* UGU MUNUS ŠUB-*tu* ÍL ŠÀ TUKU-*ši* ŠU K[I.[SIKI]L.LÍL.LÁ.EN.NA (DPS III A obv. 13–14//C obv. 4–5 = *TDP* 18:4–5)

**[If the top of his head] ⌜continually feels as if split in two all⌝ [day/night long], he continually has sexual desires,[66] and the bedding is continually turned around him, (and) like one who lays himself down on top of a woman, he has an erection, "hand" of ⌜*ardat lilî*⌝.

The *lilû*-demons and their female counterparts, the *lilītu* or *ardat lilî*-demons, were hungry for victims because they had once been young men and women who had themselves died young.[67] If a girl or boy had the misfortune of dying before having had the opportunity to marry and have children, it was believed that his or her ghost was forever doomed to prowl the earth.

12.75 ***Ardat-lilî* slips in a man's window; young girl not fated (to be married); young woman who was never impregnated like a woman; young woman who was never deflowered like a woman; young girl who never experienced sexual pleasure in her husband's lap; young girl who never removed a garment in her husband's lap; young woman whose garment-pin a good man never loosened; young woman in whose breasts there never was milk, who cries in pain; young girl who was never filled with sexual pleasure in the lap of a young man, who never had her fill of desire; young girl who never had (her own) women's quarters, whom they did not call by the name: "mother"; young girl who in desolation mistreated (her) cheeks; young girl who never rejoiced with (other) young girls; young girl who was never seen during her(!) city's festival, does not raise her eyes; young girl who was snatched away from a husband in her women's quarters; young girl who never had a husband, never gave birth to a child; young girl who never had a husband, never brought forth a child; young girl who never had a husband, never had a child; young girl who was snatched away from a husband, snatched away from a child; young girl who was driven from her father-in-law's house; *ardat-lilî* who was driven out the window like the wind; *ardat-lilî* whose ghost (when she died) was not in her mouth; *ardat-lilî* whose heartache carried her (down) to the netherworld; *ardat-lilî* whom the "hand" of Ištar mistreated in the (family) nest; *ardat-lilî* who roams outside in the broad steppe . . . (Lackenbacher, *RA* 65.131–132 i 3-ii 4//*SpTU* 2.7 obv. 1′–18′//*SpTU* 2.6:36–45).[68]

Similarly, men who had died young became *lilû*-demons.

12.76 **[Young man] who always sits, silent and ⌜alone⌝, [in] the street; [young] man who cries bitterly in the grip of his death-demon; young man to whose fate silence was attached; young man to whom his mother, crying, gave birth in the street; young man whose body grief has burned; young man whose god has ⌜cruelly bound⌝ him; young man whose goddess has cut him off; young man who never married a wife, never raised a child; young man who never experienced sexual pleasure in his wife's lap; young man who never removed a garment in his wife's lap; young man who was driven out of the house of his father-in-law . . . (Lackenbacher, *RA* 65.124 i 1–22).

Note that the young man's deprivation is not restricted to purely sexual satisfaction. It was presumably because he longed for fulfillment as a father[69] that the *lilû*-demon preyed on suckling children.[70]

PREDICTIONS OF OUTCOME

The *āšipu* was called upon to predict various pregnancy outcomes such as the sex of the baby, health of the mother and baby, and single versus multiple fetuses. It was the *āšipu*'s belief that women also produce "semen."[71] They based this belief on the secretions produced by women during intercourse. Although the *āšipu* is to be commended for not regarding woman as simply the oven in which a man bakes his loaves, we now know that vaginal secretions are for lubrication only and that the woman's real contribution, the egg (ovum), migrates internally. The *āšipu* also apparently believed that male and female "semen" were in competition and that the dominant "semen" determined the sex of the child.[72] In fact, it is the man's semen only that determines sex.

MALE VERSUS FEMALE BABY[73] Traditional methods of predicting the sex of a child are usually inspired by minor variations in normal pregnancies. In many cases, our ignorance of the meaning of technical vocabulary makes it impossible to ascertain what exactly the *āšipu* was trying to describe. If the structure described in the first reference below is, in fact, a blood vessel, the condition being described may be Mondor's disease. This is a superficial inflammation of the veins of the breast (lateral thoracic and thoracoepigastric veins). It is a benign and transient thickening and reddening of the veins.

12.77 DIŠ TU SA UBUR-*šá šú-šú-ru* MUNUS $PEŠ_4$-*at* (DPS XXXVI A 49 = *TDP* 204:49)

**If the muscle(s)/blood vessel(s) of her breast run in a straight line, she is pregnant with a female.

12.78 DIŠ GU.MEŠ DIB.DIB NITA $PEŠ_4$-*at* / DIŠ SA_5 NÍTA $PEŠ_4$-*at* (DPS XXXVI A 50–51 = *TDP* 204:50–51)

**If (the muscles/blood vessels) are held by threads, she is pregnant with a male. If they are red, she is pregnant with a male.

It does not follow that we have no idea what the *āšipu* might have been looking for, or upon what basis he felt able to make prognoses. Universal in sex prediction schemes is a particular interest in variations that can be differentiated along a left-right axis (although individual cultures may differ dramatically as to whether "male" is indicated by left or right). In the case of ancient Mesopotamia (as in the Chinese example quoted below as the first reference), right was female and left was male.

**A male baby shows itself in a stronger left finger pulse and a female in the right. (*The Adventures of Wu* 8).[74]

12.79 DIŠ (TU SA SAG.KI-*šá*) KI.TA-*nu* ZAG *te-bi šà*-ŠÀ-*šà* MUNUS / DIŠ KI.TA-*nu* GÙB *te-bi šà*-ŠÀ-*šà* NITA (DPS XXXVI A 11–12 = *TDP* 200:11–12)

**If (the blood vessels of a woman of childbearing age's temple), the lower ones to the "right" pulsate, her fetus is female. If the lower ones to the "left" pulsate, her fetus is male.

12.80 DIŠ TU SA *k*[*i*]-*ṣil-li-šá* ZAG ZI-*b*[*i*] MUNUS $PEŠ_4$-*at* / DIŠ GÙB ZI-*b*[*i*] NITA $PEŠ_4$-*at* (DPS XXXVI A 90–91//B 25′–26′ = *TDP* 208:90–91)

**If the blood vessel of a woman of childbearing age's "right" ankle pulsates, she is pregnant with a female. If the "left" (one) pulsates,[75] she is pregnant with a male.

On the surface of it, this association of right and left is curious, since Mesopotamian magical rituals generally associate the right hand with maleness and the left with femaleness.

**He raises the male (bird) in his right hand, the female in his left hand (Maul, *Zukunftsbewältigung* 241:66)[76]

The obvious resolution of this problem is to assume that, in magical rituals where instructions are being given to the participants as to what they are to do, "right" and "left" refer to the performer's right and left sides. In the diagnostic handbook, by contrast, where instructions are being given to the physician to aid him in diagnosing an illness, "right" and "left" refer to the *observer*'s right and left sides. Modern physicians use the patient's orientation only and the *āšipu*'s "right" and "left" have accordingly been rendered (when not in quotes as in 12.79–80) left and right in the translation (see Introduction).

Variations in the way in which a child was carried in the womb were divided into male and female along a right-left axis. A baby angled across the abdomen so that (when it was about to be born) its feet were to the left and its head to the right (from the mother's point of view) was presumed to be male. Feet to the right and head to the left (again from the mother's point of view) was female.

12.81 ⌜DIŠ⌝ KI.TA-*nu* 15 ZI-*bi šà*-ŠÀ-*šà* NITA / DIŠ KI.TA-*nu* 150 ZI-*bi šà*-ŠÀ-*šà* MUNUS (DPS XXXVI A 22–23 = *TDP* 202:22–23)

**If (the base? of a woman of childbearing age's "tip") rises from below to the left (= feet to left), her fetus is male. If it rises from below to the right (= feet to right), her fetus is female.

12.82 DIŠ TU SA.MEŠ-*šá ana* SAG ŠÀ-*šá zaq-ru* MUNUS PEŠ-*at* (DPS XXXVI A 73 = *TDP* 206:73)[77]

**If the muscles of a woman of childbearing age point toward her upper abdomen (epigastrium), she is pregnant with a female.

12.83 DIŠ *ana im-ši-šá zaq-ru* NITA PEŠ-*at* (DPS XXXVI A 74 = *TDP* 206:74)[78]

**If they point toward her lower abdomen (hypogastric region), she is pregnant with a male.

A woman with a baby angled across the abdomen might be presumed to list somewhat, and to attempt to compensate for this by favoring the foot on the side opposite from the excess weight. A baby angled downward toward the left (and therefore theoretically female) might be expected to produce excess weight on the left side and should therefore theoretically have induced in the pregnant patient a preference for the right foot and vice versa, as in the following examples.

12.84 DIŠ GÙB ZUKUM-*as* MUNUS PEŠ$_4$-*at* (DPS XXXVI A 95 = *TDP* 208:95)

**If (a woman of childbearing age in the midst of her difficulty) steps to the right, she is pregnant with a female.[79]

12.85 DIŠ TU ZAG ZUKUM-*as u* GÌR-*šá* DUGUD-*at* NITA *u* MUNUS PEŠ$_4$-*at* (DPS XXXVI A 96 = *TDP* 208:96)

**If a woman of childbearing age steps to the left and her foot feels heavy (because it is swollen), she is pregnant with a male or a female.

12.86 DIŠ GÙB ZUKUM-*as u* KI.MIN MUNUS PEŠ$_4$-*at* (DPS XXXVI A 97 = *TDP* 210:97)

**If she steps to the right and (her foot feels heavy because it is swollen), she is pregnant with a female.

In ancient Mesopotamian magical rituals, red and white are frequently used to designate opposites. It is, therefore, hardly surprising that red and white colors in the pregnant woman were taken as prognosticating male and female children, respectively, as in the following examples.

12.87 DIŠ TU S[A].MEŠ SAG.KI-*ša* SA$_5$ DIDLI *šà*-ŠÀ-*šà* NITA (DPS XXXVI A 13 = *TDP* 200:13)[80]

**If the ⸢muscles⸣ of a woman of childbearing age's temple are reddish, her fetus is male.

12.88 DIŠ SAG.KI-*ša* BABBAR DIDLI *šà*-ŠÀ-*šà* ⸢MUNUS⸣ (DPS XXXVI A 14 = *TDP* 200:14)[81]

**If (the muscles of a woman of childbearing age)'s temple are white, her fetus is female.

Less clear is the case of some of the other color contrasts. Predictions that contrast "dark" with "reddish" display an apparently random distribution of prognostics between male and female outcomes, possibly a reflection of the fact that the *āšipu*'s observations were not yielding consistent results and/or that there was a bit of what ancient Mesopotamians called *nipḫāt barîm* (lack of scholarly consensus) on the subject.

A number of prognoses that specifically mention "blood-red" and "bright-red" raise the possibility that apparent inconsistencies involving "red" may be due to the presence of different shades (namely, pink, orange, and brown) in the actual patient. Note the similarity between the following Mesopotamian prognoses and Persian tradition on the subject of the color of the mother's nipples and areola (pigmented area surrounding the nipple).

**If the end of the breast is pink, a boy; if brown, a girl. (Massé, *Persian Beliefs and Customs* 10)

12.89 DIŠ SA$_5$ MUNUS PEŠ$_4$-*at* (DPS XXXVI A 29 = *TDP* 202:29)

**If (the tip of a woman of childbearing age's breast) is reddish, she is pregnant with a female.

12.90 DIŠ GI_6/MÚD![82] SA_5 NITA $PEŠ_4$-*at* (DPS XXXVI A 28, 31//B 15, 18 = *TDP* 202:28, 31)[83]

**If it is dark/blood-red, she is pregnant with a male.

We are on more solid ground with the assignment of "yellow" to males and "(shining) white" to females. Traditional Chinese midwives are of the opinion that pregnancies with male babies are more difficult and male fetuses more demanding, as in the following reference.

**A girl baby makes the expectant mother look particularly charming during pregnancy, while a boy on the other hand, makes the mother look off-color, pale and dryish of skin (*The Adventures of Wu* 8).

Ancient Mesopotamian examples of this principle include the two references below. The first text appears to describe chloasma, a pigmentation of the face and neck that is common during pregnancy, but is fortunately reversible afterward.

12.91 *šum₄-ma* TU $PEŠ_4$-*ma* UGU SAG.KI-*šá* SIG_7 *šà*-ŠÀ-*šà* NITA : *i-kar-ri-iṣ* (DPS XXXVI A 1 = *TDP* 200:1)[84]

**If a woman of childbearing age is pregnant and the top of her forehead is yellow/tan, her fetus is male.

12.92 DIŠ TU *mu-úḫ* SAG.KI-*šá* BABBAR *na-mir šà*-ŠÀ-*šà* MUNUS : *i-šár-rù* (DPS XXXVI A 2 = *TDP* 200:2)[85]

**If the top of the forehead of a woman of childbearing age is white (and) shines, her fetus is female.

Pregnant women with chloasma may also have pigmentation of the abdominal stretch marks (stria) caused by an enlarged uterus. The texts below are likely to be describing this finding.

12.93 DIŠ TU *ina* SAG ŠÀ-*ša* SA.MEŠ SIG_7.MEŠ ŠUB-*ú šà*-ŠÀ-*šà* SI.SÁ (DPS XXXVI A 56 = *TDP* 204:56)

**If on the upper abdomen (epigastrium) of a woman of childbearing age, the muscles are unevenly colored with yellow/tan, her fetus will do well.

12.94 DIŠ SIG_7 ŠUB-*ú šà*-ŠÀ-*šà ú-šak-lal* (DPS XXXVI A 69 = *TDP* 206:69)

**If (the chest and abdomen of a woman of childbearing age) are unevenly colored with yellow/tan, she will completely form her fetus.

The *āšipu* also attributed to male fetuses other signs of comparatively difficult pregnancies, as in the following examples.

12.95 DIŠ TU K[A-š]*á ṣa-pir* : *za-qir* AŠ *šà*-ŠÀ-*šà* NITA [x] (DPS XXXVI A 15 = *TDP* 202:15)

**If a woman of childbearing age's ⌜"tip"⌝ twitches/protrudes, her fetus is male.

12.96 DIŠ TU ŠU^{II}-*šá* ŠÀ.ME-*šá ú-kal-la* NITA PEŠ-*at* (DPS XXXVI A 72 = *TDP* 206:72)[86]

**If a woman of childbearing age holds her insides with her hands, she is pregnant with a male.

12.97 DIŠ TU ŠÀ.MEŠ-*ša pat-tal* NITA PEŠ-*at* (DPS XXXVI A 57 = *TDP* 204:57)

**If a woman of childbearing age's insides feel balled up (?), she is pregnant with a male.

12.98 DIŠ TU ŠÀ.MEŠ-*ša nap-ḫu* NITA PEŠ-*at* (DPS XXXVI A 76 = *TDP* 206:76)

**If the insides of a woman of childbearing age are bloated, she is pregnant with a male.

12.99 DIŠ *eb-ṭù* NITA PEŠ-*at* (DPS XXXVI A 66 = *TDP* 206:66)

**If they are cramped, she is pregnant with a male.

12.100 DIŠ *nap-ḫu* MUNUS PEŠ-*at* (DPS XXXVI A 67 = *TDP* 206:67)

**If they are (merely) bloated, she is pregnant with a female.

Male babies were also supposed to be particularly prone to give their mothers bad skin and varicose veins (normal hazards of pregnancy).

12.101 DIŠ *ut-ṭe-ṭì* DIRI *šà*-ŠÀ-*šà* NITA : NÍG.TUKU (DPS XXXVI A 6 = *TDP* 200:6)

**If (the top of the forehead of a woman of childbearing age) is full of "grains" (raised blemishes), her fetus is male.

12.102 DIŠ TU SA *ki-ṣil-li-šá* MÚD DIRI.MEŠ NITA PEŠ$_4$-*at* (DPS XXXVI A 93 = *TDP* 208:93)

**If the blood vessel of a woman of childbearing age's ankle is continually full of blood (varicose veins), she is pregnant with a male.

Despite (or perhaps because of) these tendencies, male babies were expected to be smaller on average than female babies.

12.103 DIŠ *ma-ʾ-du* MUNUS PEŠ-*at* (DPS XXXVI A 68 = *TDP* 206:68)[87]

**If (a woman of childbearing age's abdomen) is large, she is pregnant with a female.

Babies with a decreased chance of surviving were also generally assumed to be male.

12.104 DIŠ GI$_6$ *šà*-ŠÀ-*šà* MUNUS : SILIM-*im* (DPS XXXVI A 3 = *TDP* 200:3)

**If (the top of the forehead of a woman of childbearing age) is dark, her fetus is female (var. it will be healthy).

12.105 DIŠ SA_5 *šà*-ŠÀ-*šà* NITA : ÚŠ (DPS XXXVI A 4 = *TDP* 200:4)

**If it is reddish, her fetus is male (var. it will die).

12.106 DIŠ *pár-sat šà*-ŠÀ-*šà* NITA (DPS XXXVI A 8 = *TDP* 200:8)

**If she is past (normal childbearing age), her fetus is male.

Persian traditions on the subject of the relative difficulties of pregnancies with male and female fetuses notice these differences but allow sexist attitudes to reverse the prediction. Men are happy and smiling and hard-working; women are bad-tempered and do nothing but eat and sleep; it follows that a woman who is bad-tempered and wants to do nothing but eat and sleep is pregnant with a girl.[88] It is also girls and not boys who are supposed to give their mothers bad complexions.[89] Curiously, however, the tradition on specific food cravings (the first example below) is consistent with that of ancient Mesopotamian references (the second and third examples below).

**If she has an appetite for foods preserved in vinegar it will be a girl; if an appetite for sweets, a boy. (H. Massé, *Persian Beliefs and Customs* 10)

12.107 DIŠ SAG.KI-*su u pa-nu-šú* BABBAR *ina* U_4-*me-šú-ma* A.GEŠTIN.NA APIN-*iš* (DPS IV B r. 25 = *TDP* 44 r. 48)

**If (the patient's) forehead and face are white (according to DPS XXXVI A 2 = *TDP* 200:2 the sign of a female fetus), on that same day, he or she will ask for vinegar.

12.108 DIŠ SAG.KI-*su* SIG_7-*at ina* U_4-*me-šú-ma* ^{GIŠ}NU.ÚR.MA APIN-*iš* (DPS IV B r. 26 = *TDP* 44 r. 49)

**If (the patient's) forehead is yellowish (according to DPS XXXVI A 1 = *TDP* 200:1 the sign of a male fetus), on that same day, he or she will ask for pomegranate.

HEALTHY VERSUS SICKLY FETUSES As noted above, male fetuses were generally not expected to do as well as females (so that fetuses that were not doing well were predicted to be male and vice versa). There are, however, exceptions to the pattern.

12.109 DIŠ *uṭ-ṭe-ṭì* DIRI *šà*-ŠÀ-*šà* NITA : NÍG.TUKU (DPS XXXVI A 6 = *TDP* 200:6)[90]

**If (the top of the forehead of a woman of childbearing age) is full of "grains" (raised blemishes), her fetus is male (var. richness [plenty of fat]).

SINGLE VERSUS MULTIPLE FETUSES In the text below twins are predicted when the uterus is large, and both ankles are swollen. Whatever the merits of other birth prognoses, in this case the signs seem quite logical since in general a uterus with two fetuses would be larger, and swollen ankles might be more prevalent with a larger uterus putting greater pressure on the veins draining the legs.[91]

12.110 DIŠ *ma-ʾ-du* GÌR DIDLI-*ša u* ZI.IN.GI DIDLI-*šá nu-up-pu-ḫa* ZAG *u* GÙB ZUKUM-*as* MAŠ.TAB.BA PEŠ-*at* (DPS XXXVI A 71 = *TDP* 206:71)[92]

**If (the insides of a woman of childbearing age) are large, both her feet and both her ankles are swollen, (and) she steps to left and right, she is pregnant with twins.

DEFECTIVE FETUSES The ancient Mesopotamian physician in his observations of the pregnant uterus reached the conclusion that when the fetus was crammed into the lower part of the abdominal cavity, there was a danger that the child would be born deaf or mentally retarded. There is nothing in the modern medical literature to either support or contradict this association.

12.111 DIŠ *ana im-ši-ša* GAR-*nu suk-ku-ku* Ù.TU (DPS XXXVI A 61 = *TDP* 206:61)

**If (a woman of childbearing age's insides) are packed into her lower abdomen (hypogastric region), she will give birth to a deaf/retarded child.

12.112 DIŠ *ana im-ši-ša* ŠUB-*ú* ŠU.BI.DIL.ÀM (DPS XXXVI A 62 = *TDP* 206:62)

**If they are poured into her lower abdomen (hypogastric region), (she will give birth to a deaf/retarded child).

A baby angled in the womb in such a way as to produce a particular listing gait in the patient (see below) was suspected of more serious defects. Similar results were expected when the pregnant woman had a "multicolored" forehead.

12.113 DIŠ TU *ina* ŠÀ *ma-ru-uš-ti-šá* ZAG ZUKUM-*as* NÁ PEŠ$_4$-*at* (DPS XXXVI A 94 = *TDP* 208:94)

**If a woman of childbearing age in the midst of her difficulty steps to the left, she is pregnant with a child that lies down (see below).[93]

12.114 DIŠ GÙN.A : *ba-ru-um šà*-ŠÀ-*šà* NÁ (DPS XXXVI A 5 = *TDP* 200:5)

**If (the top of the forehead of a woman of childbearing age) is multicolored, the child in her womb will lie down.

The multicolored forehead may be describing some complex skin disease associated with a systemic illness or skin changes connected with some sort of nutritional deficiency. Both prognostic signs indicate that a child will be born that "lies down." It seems likely that the child has a neurological disease that interferes with normal movement and standing. Cerebral palsy (which was known and described by the *āšipu*—see Chapter 13) is a common neurological problem in newborns that could be the condition indicated here.

Neurological problems in the mother, such as the one described below, were known to be dangerous to the fetus.

12.115 DIŠ TU I[GI]^{II}-*šá* BAL.BAL.MEŠ *ar-na-ab-ba* ÍL *šà*-ŠÀ-*šà* GAM (DPS XXXVI A 89 = *TDP* 208:89)

**If a woman of childbearing age continually rolls her ⌜eyes⌝ (and) she carries a hare, her fetus will die.

"The pregnant woman continually rolls her eyes" is probably describing some type of seizure activity. Seizures have many causes, but in pregnancy eclampsia is the most common.[94] The basic problem is hypertension, and death of the woman and/or baby are likely without treatment. The statement that she "carries a hare" is likely to mean that the child has a hare-lip (cleft lip) deformity. Hare-lip deformity is not a consequence of eclampsia, but can be a consequence of epilepsy. There is a two- to threefold higher incidence of fetal malformations, including cleft lip and palate, in offspring of epileptic women. Without surgery, children with hare-lip deformity often die because of a defect in their palates, which leads to ear infections and aspiration pneumonia.

POSTPARTUM COMPLICATIONS

Illnesses suffered by women shortly following delivery include bloating, diarrhea, urinary tract infection, bleeding, uterine atony, and child-bed (puerperal) fever.

BLOATING

12.116 DIŠ MUNUS Ù.TU-*ma ṣi-im-rat u* IM *ud-du-pat* . . . (*BAM* 240:26′)[95]

**If a woman gives birth and subsequently becomes distended and is inflated with "wind" . . .

DIARRHEA

12.117 DIŠ MUNUS MIN-*ma ir-ru-šá* SI.SÁ . . . (*BAM* 240:33′)

**If a woman (gives birth) and subsequently her bowels are loose . . .

12.118 DIŠ MUNUS MIN-*ma re-du-ut ir-ri* TUKU . . . (*BAM* 240:34′)

**If a woman (gives birth) and subsequently she has a flowing of the bowels . . .

"BINDING OF THE URINE" The text below describes a patient with postpartum puerperal fever, but with an additional complication. She has "binding of the urine," meaning difficulty emptying her bladder. The cause could be the partial obstruction of her urethra secondary to trauma during delivery. Another possibility could be a reluctance to empty her bladder secondary to a urinary tract infection. Such infections are common in pregnancy, and when they cause inflammation of the urethra, the pain during urination can be severe.

12.119 DIŠ MUNUS Ì.KÚM *ki-is* KÀŠ GIG-*at* MÚD.MEŠ-*šú ana* ⌜ŠÀ.TUR-*šú*⌝ *šá-ḫir* MUNUS BI Ì.KÚM GIG-*at* . . . (BM 42313+ r. 1–2)

**If a woman is sick with (puerperal) fever[96] and "binding of the urine" (and) her blood has turned back into her womb, that woman is sick with (puerperal) fever . . .

URINARY TRACT INFECTION

12.120 DIŠ MUNUS Ù.TU-*ma e-la-an ú-ri-šá ú-sa-ḫal-lim em-ša-ša* TAG.MEŠ-*ši* MUNUS BI Ì.RA DIB-*si* . . . (*BAM* 240:17′–18′)

**If a woman gives birth and subsequently her pubic region stings (and) her lower abdomen (hypogastric region) continually hurts her intensely, "striking" afflicts that woman . . .

BLEEDING This condition probably resulted most often from a retained placenta, a problem recognized and treated by the *āšipu.*

12.121 MUNUS-*šú* Ù.TU-*ma* MÚD.MEŠ-*šú la ip-par-ra-su* . . . (*SpTU* 4.153:7)

** (If) his wife gives birth and subsequently her blood flows and does not stop . . .

UTERINE ATONY The text below describes one of the complications that can occur after delivering a baby. The woman's uterus has lost its muscle tone (uterine atony) and is filling with blood. This is one reason why her abdomen is distended, but in addition to this, her intestines seem to have lost their normal contraction (ileus; see Chapter 6). This latter condition is the likely cause of her constipation. The primary cause of this obstetric illness is that part or all of the placenta is retained in the uterus.

12.122 MUNUS Ù.TU-*ma em-rat šit-t*[*u* . . .] ŠÀ.MEŠ-*ša es-lu* A.MEŠ-*ša u* MÚD.M[EŠ-*šá* . . .] GUR.MEŠ-*ru ana šup-šu-ri-ša* (Lambert, *Iraq* 31 pl. 5:1–3)

** (If) a woman gives birth and subsequently she is distended, [her] excrement [. . .], her insides are constipated, and her waters and [her] blood have gone back [inside her].

CHILD-BED (PUERPERAL) FEVER Infection of the uterus at the time of delivery is a very serious and often fatal problem in the absence of antibiotic therapy. The *āšipu* described fever, sweating, and the discharge of blood and pus from the uterus. In the last reference below, the dark spots may be subcutaneous bleeding (ecchymosis) due to the sepsis syndrome caused by a severe infection.

12.123 DIŠ MUNUS MIN-*ma* LI.DUR-*sa* DU_8-*at* IR *a-la-ka la i-kal-la* . . . (*BAM* 240:30′)

**If a woman (gives birth) and subsequently her umbilical area (feels) supple (but) she cannot stop the sweat from coming . . .

12.124 DIŠ MUNUS Ù.TU-*ma* KÚM *ir-ri* TUKU.[TUKU]-*ši i-ár-ru* ŠÀ ši [. . .] MÚD *ḫa-riš-ti-šá ina* ŠÀ-*šá it-t*[*e-es*]*-ki-ru* MUNUS BI *ina* Ù.TU-*š*[*á* . . .] (*BAM* 240:39′–40′)

**If a woman gives birth and subsequently she [continually] has internal fever, she vomits [. . .] the blood of her confinement has been ⌜locked up⌝ inside her; that woman, while giving birth [. . .]

12.125 DIŠ MUNUS MIN-*ma* KÚM *li-ʾ-ba u tir-ku ina* UZU.MEŠ-*šá u* SA.MEŠ-*šá* KAB.M[EŠ] *qer-bi-nu* MÚD.BABBAR *ú-kal ana šup-šú-ḫi* . . . (*BAM* 240:59′–60′)[97]

**If a woman (gives birth) and subsequently she (has) *liʾbu*-fever and dark spots accumulate (?) on her flesh and her blood vessels (and) inside she contains pus, to soothe it . . .

Summary

Although normal childbirth took place with the assistance of a female midwife, the *āšipu* seems to have intervened when something went wrong. The fact that there were collections of therapeutic texts devoted exclusively to women's problems also suggests that obstetrics and gynecology may have been a separate subspecialty of ancient Mesopotamian medicine. The *āšipu* devised treatments for amenorrhea, menorrhagia and infertility, uterine prolapse, and vaginal infections. He also provided birth control, and attempted to predict the sex of unborn children. Most important, he attempted to treat uterine bleeding and gastrointestinal problems during pregnancy, prevent miscarriages, and deal with postpartum complications including child-bed (puerperal) fever. The attention paid to maternal health and fetal development reflects both the importance of procreation in maintaining the labor pool for agriculture, manufacturing, and the military and the strong sense, particularly visible in references to the *lilû*-demon, that love, marriage, and children were essential to the happiness and fulfillment of individual men and women.

CHAPTER 13

Neurology

If a man's feet lick the ground . . .

—*BAM* 393 r. 19

The signs and symptoms associated with diseases of the nervous system provide some of the most unique and focused findings. These abnormalities can readily be found by an observant physician, a characteristic that certainly applies to the *āšipu*. Another advantage to the student of neurologic illnesses is that the signs and symptoms described in the past can generally be explained in terms that are understandable today. Pain, paralysis, tremors, and seizures, both focal and generalized, are well described in ancient medical texts. This has resulted in an impressive array of diseases and symptom complexes that can be identified by modern physicians, and they give us a very clear idea of the problems faced by our colleagues in ancient Mesopotamia.

Signs and Symptoms of Neurologic Disorders

PAIN

Pain can be a normal response to a disease such as infection or trauma, but it can also be the result of a disease of the nervous system. As it has been frequently noted with ancient Mesopotamian medical terminology, the *āšipu* distinguished not only different types of pain but also different levels of pain experienced by his patients. Pains in various parts of the body (but particularly the head and internal organs) were described as simply hurting the patient (KÚ/ *akālu*) or actively "afflicting" him (DIB/ *ṣabātu*).

HURTING (KÚ/*AKĀLU*)

13.1 DIŠ NA SAG.KI-*šú* KÚ^{II}-*šú* . . . (*BAM* 482 i 64′)

**If a person's temples continually hurt him...

13.2 DIŠ NA SA GÚ-*šú* KÚ-*šú* ŠU.GIDIM.MA (*AMT* 97/4:18; *BAM* 209 r. 18′; *BAM* 473 iv 16′)

**If the muscles of a person's neck hurt him, "hand" of ghost.

13.3 DIŠ NA *ina* ŠU.GIDIM.MA ŠÀ-*šú* KÚ.MEŠ-*šú* . . . (*BAM* 161 iii 19′)[1]

**If as a result of "hand" of ghost, a person's abdomen continually hurts him . . .

AFFLICTING (DIB/*ṢABĀTU*)

13.4 DIŠ LÚ SA SAG.KI-*šú* DIB-*su-ma* KÚ^{II}-*šú* (*BAM* 482 ii 8)

**If the blood vessels of a person's temple afflict him and continually hurt him.

13.5 DIŠ SAG.DU-*su* DIB.DIB-*su u* KÚM NU TUKU ŠU ⌜d⌝15 (DPS III C obv. 35 = *TDP* 22:35)

**If his head continually afflicts him and he does not have a fever, "hand" of Ištar.

13.6 Ú *šá-mi* DIB-*it* ŠÀ-*bi* . . . (*BAM* 422 iii 29′, 33′; *BAM* 423 i 30′; *STT* 92 ii 31–34; *BAM* 2 r. 6′–11′)[2]

**Plant for affliction of the stomach . . .

Another way of describing pain was to say that a part of the body was "sick," that is, sore (GIG/*marāṣu*) or that it "touched" (TAG/*lapātu*) the patient.

"SICK" (SORE)

13.7 KA.INIM.MA KA.GIG.GA.KÁM . . . (*BAM* 538 iv 49′; *BAM* 538 iii 56′, 62′//*AMT* 24/2:7′, 16′; *BAM* 538 iii 43′, 68′; *AMT* 23/6:6′; *AMT* 25/2:5′)

**Recitation for "sick" (sore) mouth . . .

13.8 DIŠ NA MURUB$_4$-*šú* GIG MÚ.MÚ . . . (*BAM* 56 obv. 8′)

**If a person's hip is "sick" (sore) (and) swollen . . .

13.9 DIŠ NA *kab-bal-ta-šu* GIG . . . (*BAM* 124 ii 47//*AMT* 74/1 ii 20)

**If a person's ankles are "sick" (sore) . . .

TOUCHING (TAG/*LAPĀTU*)

13.10 DIŠ NA GEŠTU ZAG-*šú* TAG-*su* IM DIRI-*at u* MÚ.MEŠ . . . (*AMT* 105/1 iv 7)

**If a person's left ear "touches" him, is full of "clay," and is swollen . . .

13.11 [DIŠ N]A ŠU.⸢GIDIM$_4$⸣.MA DIB-*su-ma* Á GÙB-*šú* TAG.TAG-*su* . . . (*BAM* 197: 8[–9]; *AMT* 97/4:2 [coll.])

**[If] "hand" of ghost afflicts a ⸢person⸣ (so that) his right side continually "touches" him . . .

In light of English "a touch of cold," one might have expected "touching" pain to be less intense than normal, but the opposite conclusion seems to have been reached by the *āšipu*, as may be seen in the following commentary that uses this term to characterize what we call a splitting headache. We consequently have chosen to interpret TAG/*lapātu* as referring to intense pain.

13.12 [*ši-bit*] SAG.DU-*šú paṭ-rat* ÚŠ : SAG.DU-*šú* TAG.MEŠ (*STT* 403:22 [commentary to DPS III A obv. 24//C obv. 15 = *TDP* 20:15])

**[(If) the seam] of his head (feels like it) is open, he will die. (That means) his head continually "touches" him (i.e., hurts him intensely).

VISELIKE (*ḪESÛ*) Pain in the head, jaw, and lower back might also be described as "squeezing," that is, viselike (*ḫesû*).

13.13 DIŠ SAG.KI *ḫe-si-ma* ŠÀ.MEŠ-*šú* AL.DU ŠU ^{d}*Kù-bi* (DPS IV B obv. 2 = *TDP* 32:2)[3]

**If he has a viselike headache and his bowels are loose,[4] "hand" of Kubu.

13.14 DIŠ SAG.KI *ḫe-si-ma* GEŠTU.MEŠ-*šú* NU ŠE.GA-*a* ŠU DINGIR-*šú* UGU-*šú um-mu-da* GAM (DPS IV B obv. 4 = *TDP* 32:4)

**If he has a viselike headache and his ears do not hear, "hand" of his god has been imposed on him; he will die.

13.15 DIŠ ÉLLAG.MEŠ-*šú ḫé-sa$_5$* GAM (DPS XII D iii 9 = *TDP* 102 iii 9)[5]

**If (both) his kidneys have viselike pain, he will die.

"THROBBING" (*TARĀKU*) What we call throbbing pain was rendered by the *āšipu* by using a verb that literally means "to beat" (*tarāku*).

13.16 [DIŠ N]A ŠU.GIDIM$_7$.MA DIB-*su-ma* SAG.KI-*šu i-tar-rak-šú* . . . (*AMT* 14/5:3 //*BAM* 227:4′–5′)

**[If] "hand" of ghost afflicts a ⸢person⸣ (so that) his temple throbs . . .

13.17 DIŠ NA TA GÌR^{II}.MEŠ-*šú a-di* MAŠ.SÌLA.MEŠ-*šú i-tar-rak* NA BI *li-i-bu šá-di-i* DIB-*su* . . . (K 2581 obv. 20′–21′//*AMT* 53/7+K 6732:1)

**If from his feet to his shoulders it throbs, the *liʾbu* of the mountain afflicts that person . . .

There are two terms used to describe abdominal symptoms, *ebēṭu* and *emēru*, which are often interpreted as mere synonyms of *napāḫu*, "to bloat."[6] However, since all three terms appear side by side in medical context, they are unlikely to have exactly the same meaning.

In any case, there was hardly a need for three separate terms (in addition to "wind" and various rumbling noises) to describe abdominal bloating. Since there is independent evidence to connect *emēru* with distention[7] and *ebēṭu* with contraction,[8] we interpret this pair of terms as a reference to colic (intestinal pain)[9] produced by distension and cramping pain produced by contraction of the intestines, respectively (see Chapter 6). Similar cramping pains in other parts of the body are also mentioned.

13.18 DIŠ NA ŠÀ.MEŠ-*šú* MÚ.MÚ-*ḫu* GÌR^{II}-*šú it-te-nen-bi-ṭa* . . . (*BAM* 159 ii 12//*BAM* 160:4′)

**If a person's insides are continually bloated (and) his feet continually have cramps . . .

13.19 DIŠ LÚ ⸢KA-*šú*⸣ MAŠKIM DIB-*it-ma* KA.DIB.BI.DA TUKU.MEŠ-*ši* [EM]E?-*šú e-bíṭ na-piš* KA-*šú* DUGUD-*it* ÚḪ.MEŠ-*šú* DU.MEŠ-*ma la* TAR.MEŠ [Z]Ú.MEŠ-*šú* SIG.MEŠ-*šú ù da-mu i-ḫi-la* . . . (*BAM* 28 obv. 1–3//*BAM* 533:1–3)

**If a *rābiṣu* seizes a person's mouth so that he continually has inability to talk, his ⸢tongue⸣ is cramped, his breathing is difficult, his saliva flows and will not stop, his ⸢teeth⸣ are weak and ooze blood . . .

Nonspasmotic pain in the abdominal or upper abdominal region was described as burning, gnawing (*kasāsu*), jabbing (SÌG/*maḫāṣu*), stinging (GÍR/*zaqātu*), and stabbing or needling.

13.20 DIŠ NA SAG ŠÀ-*šú i-ḫa-mat-su i-dak-ka-su* ÚḪ-*su* x[. . .] UD.DA SÁ.SÁ . . . (*AMT* 45/6:6–7)[10]

**If a person's upper abdomen (epigastrium) burns him (and) gives him a needling pain (and) his spittle [is red/dark?], *ṣētu* (enteric fever) has "gotten" him . . .

13.21 [DIŠ] ⸢NA⸣ [SAG ŠÀ?]-*šú ú-ḫa-*[*ma-su ú-ma*]*-ḫa-su ú-za-qat-su ú* KÚ-*šú* NA BI A.[GA.ZI G]IG *ana* TI-*šú* . . . (*BAM* 75:1–2)

**[If] a person's [upper abdomen (epigastrium)?] ⸢burns⸣, [gives him a] ⸢jabbing⸣ pain, stings, and hurts him, that person is ⸢sick⸣ with ⸢A.GA.ZI⸣ (see Chapter 6), to cure him . . .

13.22 [DI]Š NA *ina* DIB ŠU.GIDIM.MA SAG ŠÀ-*šú i-kàs-sa-su ana* TI-*šú* . . . (*AMT* 76/1:15)[11]

**If, as the result of affliction by "hand" of ghost a person's upper abdomen (epigastrium) gnaws at him, to cure him . . .

Pains in other parts of the body were similarly described.

13.23 DIŠ NA IGI.MEŠ-*šú* GÚ-*su u* NUNDUN-*su šim-mat* TUKU.MEŠ-*a ù ki-ma* IZI *i-ḫa-am-ma-ṭa-šú* NA BI MAŠKIM *mu-sa-a-ti* DIB-*su ana* DIN-*šú* . . . (*SpTU* 1.46:6–8)

**If a person's face, his neck, and his lips are continually numb and it burns him like fire, the *rābiṣu* of the lavatory afflicts him; to cure him . . .

13.24 DIŠ NA GEŠTU^{II}-*šú* GIG-*ma* ŠÀ GEŠTU^{II}-*šú bi-iš* SÌG.SÌG-*su u* KÚ-*šú-ma la* NÁ-*lal* . . . (*BAM* 3 iv 14)

**If a person's ears are sore and the insides of his ears stink, (and) it continually gives him a jabbing pain and hurts him so badly that he cannot sleep . . .

13.25 DIŠ NA KI.TA GÌR^{II}-*šú* GÍR.GÍR-*su* . . . (*AMT* 75/1+ iv 24)[12]

**If the bottoms of his feet continually sting him . . .

13.26 DIŠ NA *ina la si-ma-ni-šú* MURUB$_4$.MEŠ-*šú* KÚ.MEŠ-*šú* (GÌR^{II}.MEŠ-*šú i-ta-n*[*a-aḫ*]) *kim-ṣa-a-šú* (*i-za-qat-šu* ÚR.MEŠ-*šú i-tan-na-aḫ bur-ka-šu*) *i-kaṣ-ṣa-a-šú* NA BI *ina meṣ-ḫi-ru-ti-šú* DÚR.GIG GIG *ana* TI-*šú* . . . (*BAM* 168:70–72//*AMT* 43/1 i 1–3//*BAM* 95:16–17)[13]

**If a person's hips hurt him before (the age when) this would be expected, his feet are continually [tired], his legs sting him, his thighs are continually tired, and his knees give him a gnawing pain, that person was sick with DÚR.GIG (see Chapter 6) in his childhood; to cure him . . .

There were two grades of burning pain in the abdomen: *ḫamāṭu* (just burning) and *ṣarāpu* (burning hotly) and two grades of stabbing or needling pain: *saḫālu* (a brief and relatively mild needling sensation) and *dikšu/ dakāšu* (the same type of pain, only more intense and continuous).[14]

13.27 DIŠ NA SAG ŠÀ-*šú i-ḫa-am-maṭ-su u* KÚM-*em* NINDA KÚ-*ma* UGU-*šú* NU DU-*ak* A NAG-*ma* UGU-*šú* NU DÙG.GA *u* SU-*šú* SIG$_7$ NA BI GIG *na-a-ki* GIG (DPS XXII:12–13 [AOAT 43.252]; cf. DPS XIII B i 5′–6′ = *TDP* 110 i 9′–10′)

**If a person's upper abdomen (epigastrium) gives him a burning pain and he is feverish, he eats bread and it does not agree with him, he drinks water and it does not taste good to him, and his body is yellow, that person is sick with a disease of sexual intercourse.

13.28 [DIŠ N]A SAG ŠÀ-*šú ú-ṣar-rap-šú na-piš* KA-*šú* DUGUD . . . (*AMT* 45/6:5)

**[If a] ⸢person's⸣ upper abdomen (epigastrium) burns him hotly[15] (and) his breathing is difficult . . .

13.29 DIŠ NA *ki-ṣir* ŠÀ GIG NINDA *u* KAŠ ŠÀ-*šú la* IGI-*šú ina* KA-*šú* GUR.GUR TÙN-*šú ú-sa-ḫal-šú ana* TI-[*šú*] . . . (*BAM* 575 iv 37//*BAM* 58:8–9)

**If a person is sick with *kiṣir libbi* (indigestion; see Chapter 6) and his insides will not accept bread and beer, and his liver gives him a needling pain, to cure [him] . . .

13.30 DIŠ NA IM GIN$_7$ *di-ik-ši ina* Š[À]-*šú* TAG.MEŠ-*su* . . . (*BAM* 575 iii 28//*BAM* 54:1)[16]

**If "wind" continually hurts him intensely in his abdomen like an intense stabbing pain . . .

The terms *saḫālu* or *siḫiltu* and *dakāšu* or *dikšu* are also used to describe stabbing or needling pain in other parts of the body,[17] particularly the legs as in sciatica.

13.31 DIŠ NA *di-ik-šá* TUKU*-ma ki-ma ṣil-le-e ú-dàk-k*[*as-su*] ŠU.GIDIM.MA *ana* TI-*šú* . . . (*BAM* 216:29′–30′)

**If a person has an intense stabbing pain and it gives [him] an intense stabbing pain like a thorn, "hand" of ghost, to cure him . . .

13.32 DIŠ *na-aṣ-mad di-ik-ši lu šá* 15/ZAG *lu šá* 150/GÙB . . . (*BAM* 3 iv 35//*AMT* 96/1:1//*BAM* 217:5//*BAM* 564 iii 6)

**If (you want) a bandage for intense stabbing pain on the left or the right (side of the body) . . .[18]

13.33 KA.INIM.MA *ana si-ḫi-il-ti* ⌜GIDIM⌝ . . . (*KAR* 56 r. 1)

**Recitation for needling pain caused by a ghost . . .

13.34 DIŠ NA GÌR^{II}-*šú kin-ṣa-šú* DUGUD-*šú-ma ú-saḫ-ḫa-la-šú* . . . (*BAM* 152 iv 16//*BAM* 158 iii 27′–28′//*AMT* 70/7 i 3; *BAM* 405:14′)

**If a person's feet (and) his legs feel heavy and needle him . . .

LOSS OF SENSATION AND MOVEMENT

With brain or peripheral nerve injury, the patient may experience loss of sensation (pain, heat, cold, and touch), or movement (paralysis).

NUMBNESS (*ŠAMĀMU/ŠIMMATU*) There are some sixty texts that use this verb and the adjective derived from it, and in most of them, the best translation appears to be numbness (i.e., loss of sensation). The parts of the body affected by this finding make more sense as numbness than as paralysis, the conventional translation.[19] For example, involvement of the hands or feet is mentioned in a number of references.

13.35 NA_4.MEŠ *šim-ma-ti šá* ŠU 150 . . . (*BE* 31.60 iii 10//*BAM* 354 iv 22)

**Stones for *šimmatu* of the right hand . . .

13.36 NA_4.MEŠ *šim-ma-ti šá* GÌR 15 . . . (*BE* 31.60 iii 3//*BAM* 354 iv 15)

**Stones for *šimmatu* of the left foot . . .

Isolated paralysis of the hand or foot would be unusual, whereas numbness in such a distribution would be common. One text refers to *šimmatu* following a scorpion bite.

13.37 DIŠ NA *šim-mat* GÍR.TAB GIG . . . (*AMT* 91/1 r. 4)

**If a person is sick with *šimmatu* due to a scorpion bite . . .

Again, this validates the translation of "numbness" for this term, since scorpion bites primarily cause numbness and not paralysis. Finally, the following reference makes an excellent description of trigeminal neuralgia if "numbness" is the correct translation for *šimmatu*.

13.38 DIŠ NA IGI.MEŠ-*šú* GÚ-*su u* NUNDUN-*su šim-mat* TUKU.MEŠ-*a ù ki-ma* IZI *i-ḫa-am-ma-ṭa-šú* NA BI MAŠKIM *mu-sa-a-ti* DIB-*su ana* DIN-*šú* . . . (*SpTU* 1.46:6–8)

**If a person's face, his neck, and his lips continually have *šimmatu* and it burns him like fire, the *rābiṣu* of the lavatory afflicts him; to cure him . . .

PARALYSIS Muscle weakness or paralysis can be caused by nerve injury or disease. Temporary paralysis may also occur following a seizure. A number of terms were used by the *āšipu* to describe these phenomena, including *amāšu, ḫamû* and *ḫamītu,* and *kabālu.* Of these, *ḫamû* and *ḫamītu* seem to have been general, whereas *amāšu* is almost invariably used to describe paralysis of the extremities and *kabālu* paralysis of specific muscles or muscle groups.

Amāšu

13.39 DIŠ LÚ.TUR ŠUB-*tu* ŠUB-*su-ma* ŠU^{II}-*šú u* GÌR^{II}-*šú am-šá* IGI^{II}-*šú maḫ-ḫa ina* GÌR-*šú* É AD-*šú* BIR-*aḫ* (DPS XL A 111 = *TDP* 230:111)

**If falling spells fall on an infant and his hands and feet are immobilized (and) his eyes are "soaked," the house of his father will be scattered at his foot.

13.40 DIŠ U$_4$.5.KÁM U$_4$.10.KÁM U$_4$.15.KÁM U$_4$.20.KÁM U.MEŠ ŠU^{II}-*šú u* GÌR^{II}-*šú am-šá-aš-ṭa-a-ma* BAD-*a u* GUB-*za* NU ZU-*e* ŠU ^{d}15 *uš-šar-ma* : *iš-šir-ma* DIN (DPS XVI:59′–60′ [AOAT 43.177])

**If he has been sick for five, ten, fifteen, (and then) twenty days (and) the digits of his hands and his feet are immobilized (and) so stiff that he cannot open (them) or stand (on them), "hand" of Ištar. (If) it leaves him (var. he comes through), he will get well.

Ḫamû and *Ḫamītu*

13.41 DIŠ TA A.MEŠ *ina* E$_{11}$-*šú* ^{LÚ}AD$_6$-*šú iḫ-mi-šu-ma* NIGIN-*ma* ŠUB-*ut* ⌜MAŠKIM⌝ ÍD SÌG-[*i*]*ṣ* (DPS XXVII:25 [AOAT 43.299]; cf. Ni. 470:11 [Kraus, *ZA* 77.197])

**If when he comes up from the water, his body is paralyzed[20] and he (feels like he) is spinning and falls down, he was struck by the *rābiṣu* of the river (see Chapter 15).

13.42 DIŠ U$_4$ LÁ-*šú* SAG.KI^{II}-*šú* KÚ.MEŠ-*šú* ŠÀ-*šú* GAZ.MEŠ-*šú* EGIR-*nu* ŠU^{II}-*šú u* GÌR^{II}-*šú ú-kap-p*[*ár*] BAL.BAL-*ut* ÚḪ NU TUKU : *it-ta-nag-ra-ár* ŠUB-*tu* : *ḫa-mi-tum* ŠU ^{d}15 ZI-*bé* (DPS XXVI:28′–29′ [AOAT 43.280])

**If when (a confusional state) comes over him, his temples continually hurt him, he continually has a crushing sensation in his heart (and) afterward he ⌜rubs⌝ his hands and his feet, he rolls over and over (but) he does not have any spittle (var. he rolls over and over), falling spell (var. paralysis)[21] of "hand" of Ištar; he can get up (afterward).

Kabālu

13.43 DIŠ NA KA-*šú* NUNDUN-*su ana* ZAG/GÙB *kub-bu-ul-ma da-ba-ba la i-le-*[ʾ*i*] *da-ba-ab-ta-šú tu-ur-ri* . . . (*BAM* 523 iii 3′–4′, 9′–10′ // *BAM* 174 obv. 5′–6′)

**If his mouth (and) his lips are immobilized (*kabālu*) to the left/right so that he ⸢cannot⸣ talk, in order to restore his speech . . .

13.44 [DIŠ N]A ⸢*tu*⸣*-ḫar eq-bi-šu ka-bíl* IGI UZU.MEŠ-*šú* KÚR.KÚR GIG [. . . G]A DUGUD . . . (*BAM* 124 i 50–51)

**[If] a ⸢person's⸣ Achilles tendon (i.e., the calf muscle to which it is attached)[22] is immobilized (and) his flesh looks worse and worse, the illness [. . .] is difficult . . .

Some of these terms, for example, *anāḫu* ("to be tired"), *eṣēlu* ("to be sluggish"), and *kabātu* ("to feel heavy"), refer to a sensation of weakness as perceived by the patient, as in the quotes below.

13.45 DIŠ NA ŠU^{II}-*šú* GÌR^{II}-*šú an-ḫa tab-k*[*a* . . .] (*AMT* 69/1:22′)

**If a person's hands and his feet are tired and tense [. . .].

13.46 DIŠ *ina* GÚ-*šú* SÌG-*iṣ-ma e-lat* IGI^{II}-*šú* KÚ.ME-*šú* MÚD *ina* KA-*šú* ŠUB.ŠUB-*a* ŠU^{II}-*šú u* GÌR^{II}-*šú eṣ-la* NA BI ḪUL DIB-*su* (DPS X A obv. 21//B obv. 23–24 = *TDP* 82:21; cf. *CTN* 4.72 i 15′–19′)

**If he was wounded on his neck and consequently the upper part of his eyes continually hurts him, he continually produces blood from his nose/mouth, (and) his hands and his feet are sluggish, a *gallû* afflicts that person.

13.47 DIŠ NA GÌR^{II}-*šú kin-ṣa-šú* DUGUD-*šú-ma ú-saḫ-ḫa-la-šú* . . . (*BAM* 152 iv 16//*BAM* 158 iii 27′–28′//*AMT* 70/7 i 3; *BAM* 405:14′)

**If a person's feet (and) his shins feel heavy and needle him . . .

Two terms, *nabalkutu* ("to cross over/turn over/shift") and *parāru* ("to become disconnected"), seem to refer to a loss of motor control in the lower extremities and trunk, respectively, as in the following examples.

Nabalkutu

13.48 DIŠ NA GÌR^{II}-*šú šim-ma-tú* TUKU-*a* KÚ.MEŠ-*šú* SA GÌR^{II}-*šú sa-ag-gu-ma* GÌR^{II}-*šú* BAL.BAL.MEŠ-*šu* . . . (*BAM* 122 obv. 8–10//*AMT* 70/7 ii 7′–8′)

**If a person's feet are numb (and) hurt him, the muscles of his feet are stiff, and his feet shift constantly under him . . .

13.49 [DIŠ NA GÌR.MEŠ *i*]*t-ta-na-aq-na-na-šú šá-pu-la-šú* BAL.BAL-*šú* NA BI *a-ri-im* [. . .] *ana* TI-*šú* . . . (*AMT* 70/3 i 3–4)[23]

**[If a person's feet] ⸢continually⸣ become contorted (and) his inguinal regions shift constantly under him,[24] that person is "enveloped" [. . .], to cure him . . .

Parāru

13.50 DIŠ IGI.MEŠ-*šú ṣep-ru ta-lam-ma-šú pur-ru-ur* ŠU-*su šá* 150 *na-šá-a* NU ZU-*e* GÌR^{II}-*šú i-maš-šar* GAM (DPS IX A 71//B r. 17–18 = *TDP* 78:71)

**If his face twitches, his torso is "disconnected," he is unable to lift his right hand, (and) he drags his feet, he will die.

Flaccid paralysis

When nerve injury or disease prevents the neural stimulus coming from the spinal cord from reaching the muscles that they control, the muscles tend to lose their tone and become limp or flaccid. The most common terms used to describe flaccid paralysis were *ramû* ("to become limp") and *rimūtu* ("limpness").

13.51 DIŠ UB.MEŠ-*š*[*ú ir*]*-mu-ú u* MÚD *i-te-eṣ-ṣi* EGIR-*ta*$_5$ SÌG-*iṣ* GAM (DPS XXII:38 [AOAT 43.255])

**If ⌜his⌝ limbs become ⌜limp⌝ and he excretes blood, he was wounded from behind; he will die.

13.52 DIŠ *šim-ma-tim ù ri-mu-tim* . . . (*BAM* 194 iv 5–6)

**If (you want to cure) numbness and limpness (of the arm) . . .

13.53 DIŠ LÚ *ši-pìr mi-šit-ti šup-šu-ḫi u ri-mu-te* . . . (*AMT* 82/2 iii! 7//*BAM* 138 ii 1–2; *BAM* 138 ii 9–10; *BAM* 398 obv. 1)

**If you want to soothe the effects of a stroke or limpness . . .

Other specialized terms—*saḫāru* ("to turn to one side"), *ṭepû* ("to smooth out"), and *saḫāpu* ("to fall flat")—were used to describe the loss of tone in facial muscles due to trauma. *Saḫāpu* was also used to describe the wasting of facial muscles seen in protein mal-nutrition (see Chapter 7).

13.54 [DIŠ *i-n*] *a* IGI-*šú* SÌG-*iṣ-ma ù* KA-*šú su-ḫur ina* A.[SAG] *i-ṭí-pá-*[*ma is*]*-sà-aḫ-ḫap-ma i-na* KIR$_4$/KA-*šú* UŠ$_{11}$ DU-*ak* ŠU ^{d}EN.ZU BA.[ÚŠ] (*KAR* 211 obv. 15–16)

** [If] he was wounded ⌜on⌝ one side of his face and his mouth is turned (to one side and his skin) smooths out [and] falls flat against (his) ⌜skull⌝, and spittle flows from his nose/mouth, "hand" of Sîn; he will ⌜die⌝.

The *āšipu* also noted if the patient was dragging his feet or allowing them to slap on the ground (see below for additional discussion).

13.55 DIŠ KI.MIN-*ma* GÌR-*šú šá* 15 *i-maš-šar* KA-*šú ṣu-dur mi-šit-ti* MAŠKIM GÍD-*ma* GAM (DPS XV:63 [AOAT 43.154]; DPS XIV A$_2$ iv 3′–4′//C$_2$ iii 30 = *TDP* 142 iv 3′–4′)

**If (it is the first day he is sick) and he drags his left foot (and) his mouth[25] twitches, stroke of a *rābiṣu*; (if) it is prolonged, he will die.

13.56 6,40 *a-wi-lum ši-pa-šu qá-qá-ra-am le-ka* . . . (*BAM* 393 r. 19)

**If a man's feet lick the ground . . .

Spastic paralysis

When injury or disease interrupts the nerves in the spinal cord, there is paralysis of the muscles whose nerves are located below the point of spinal damage. Since the nerves from the spinal cord to the muscles are still intact, they provide a stimulus to the muscles that causes normal or often increased tone (muscle spasm) even though the patient cannot control them. The most commonly used set of terms for spastic paralysis were two words, *šapāku* and *tabāku,* both of which mean literally "to heap up" and which are translated here as "tense"[26] since, when said of flesh, these terms are clearly contrasted with *ramû* which means "limp (flaccid)" (see Chapter 10 with 10.19–10.25).

Tabāku

13.57 DIŠ NA *mi-šit-tú-ma* ŠU-*su u* GÌR-*šú ta-bi-ik* . . . (*AMT* 82/2 iii! 4)

**If a person (has) a stroke and his hand or his foot is tense . . .

13.58 DIŠ NA SA ÚR-*šú ka-la-šu-ma tab-ku* ZI-*a a-tál-lu-ka la i-le-ʾi sa-gal-lum* DIB-*s*[*u*] . . . (*BAM* 130:19–21)

**If all of the muscles of a person's thigh are so tense that he cannot stand up (or) walk about, *sagallu* (see Chapter 11) afflicts ˹him˺ . . .

Šapāku

13.59 [DIŠ GIN$_7$] Ù.SÁ DIB.DIB-*su* UB.NIGIN.NA-*šú iš-šap-pa-ka* GEŠTU^{II}-*šú* GÙ.<DÉ>.MEŠ KA-*šú* DIB-*ma* NU DUG$_4$.DUG$_4$-*ub* ŠU A.LÁ ḪUL (DPS XXVII:21–22 [AOAT 43.298])

**[If something like] a stupor continually afflicts him and his limbs are tense, his ears roar, (and) his mouth is "seized" so that he cannot talk, "hand" of an evil *alû* (coma; see below).

Two other terms, *kasû* and *kamû,* both of which mean "to bind," were also occasionally used to describe spastic paralysis. If the *āšipu* had asked a patient whether his limbs were *šapāku*'d or *tabāku*'d, he would probably have gotten a puzzled look, since, in nonmedical context, these verbs are usually used to describe the heaping up of various commodities for storage. By contrast, the meaning of *kasû* and *kamû* as applied to paralyzed limbs would have been obvious even to ancient Mesopotamians with no medical training. Doctors, whether ancient or modern, have their own professional language that they use when speaking to other doctors whereas other more common terms are used when the doctor is explaining an illness to a patient.

13.60 [DIŠ Š]U^{II}-*šú ka-ma-ma* GÌR^{II}-*šú šad-da* : *šad-na* DINGIR [. . .] (DPS XI A obv. 32//B 31 = *TDP* 92:32//*SpTU* 1.34:31)

**[If] his ˹hands˺ are "bound" (*kamû*) and his feet are pulled taut (var. . . .) [. . .].

13.61 DIŠ NA SAG.DU-*su iṣ-ṣa-na-bat-su šit* x [. . .] MÁŠ.GI$_6$.MEŠ-*šú par-da ina šit-ti-šú ig-d*[*a-na-lu-ut*] *bir-ka-šu ka-si-a ba-ma-as-su šim-ma-*[*tu* . . .] UZ[U]-*šú ru-ṭi-ib-*[*tu*] *im-ta-na-al-lu-šú* LÚ BI *ka-ši-ip* (*AMT* 86/1 ii 3–7)

**If a person's head continually afflicts him, [his] ˹sleep˺ [. . .] his dreams are troubled, he [continually] ˹jerks˺ in his sleep, his knees are "bound" (*kasû*), his chest is numb [. . .] (and) his flesh is continually filled with "dampness," that person is hexed.

13.62 ŠU^{II}-*šú* GÌR^{II}-*šú ka-si-a* (*STT* 403 r. 49 [commentary to DPS III])

**His hands and feet are "bound" (*kasû*).

The *āšipu* also noted whether the paralyzed limb was in a straight or a bent position, as in the following examples.

13.63 DIŠ SAG.DU-*su i-ṭa-mu* GÌR-*šú šá* 150 *ú-kan-na-an-ma* NU LAL Š[U ^{d}. . .] (DPS III C obv. 27 = *TDP* 20:27)[27]

**If his head twists and he bends his right foot and cannot straighten it out, "hand" of [. . .].

13.64 [DIŠ GÌR-*šú*] *šá* 15 *ana šá* 150 NIR-*at* ⌜ŠU⌝ [. . .] (DPS XIV A_2 iv 9′ = TDP 142 iv 9′)[28]

** [If his] left [foot] is stretched out toward his right, "hand" of [. . .].

13.65 ŠU^{II}-*šú* GÌR^{II}-*šú tar-ṣa-šu* = [ŠU^{II}-*šú* GÌR^{II}-*šú*] *šag-ga* (*STT* 403 r. 50 [commentary to DPS III])

**"His hands (and) his feet are stretched out" (means) "[his hands (and) his feet] are stiff."

ABNORMAL MOVEMENTS

The *āšipu* used a number of terms to describe abnormal movements made by his patients. Of these, the most common are a pair of terms, LUḪ/*galātu* and MUD/*parādu*, which are also used to describe forms of nystagmus (see below). Both of the following references are descriptions of seizures. In the first, the seizures are possibly secondary to cysticercosis (see Chapter 3); the second reference describes seizures in infants (see below).

13.66 DIŠ GABA.MEŠ-*šú* KÚ.MEŠ-*šú ma-gal* KÚ-*ma ma-gal* NAG-*ti ik-ta-na-la ma-gal it!-ta-na-al ig-ta-na-lut ù ip-ta-na-ru-ud* LÚ BI *be-en-nu* DIB-*su* LÚ BI *lu ina* KÁ *lu-u ina* TÙR *lu ina* ÍD DIB-*su* (*STT* 89:192–195 [Stol, *Epilepsy* 97])

**If his breasts continually hurt him, he stops eating and drinking a lot (and) he lies down a lot,[29] he continually *galātu*'s and *parādu*'s, *bennu* afflicts that person. It afflicted him either in the door or in the courtyard or in the river.

13.67 DIŠ LÚ.TUR *ig-da-na-al-lut* LÙ.LÙ-*aḫ u* MUD.MUD-*ud* ŠU ^{d}30 *u* ^{d}15 (DPS XL A 47 = *TDP* 222:47)

**If an infant continually *galātu*'s, is restless and *parādu*'s, "hand" of Sîn or of Ištar.

Since LUḪ/*galātu* is used to describe the muscle contractions of tetanus (the first reference below; see Chapter 3) and complex partial seizures (the second reference; see below), it seems to be referring to strong, rapid muscle contractions, that is, "(myoclonic) jerking."

13.68 DIŠ ⌜GÚ⌝-*su i-zur-ma* IGI-*šú gal-ta-át pi-qam* NU *pi-qam* LUḪ-*ut*/MUD-*u*[*d*] SA.DUGUD (DPS X A obv. 11//B obv. 11 = *TDP* 80:11; cf. DPS XXXIII:96 [AOAT 43.357])

**If he twists his neck and his eye jerks (and) he jerks (var. A: shudders) incessantly, *šaššaṭu* (tetanus).

13.69 DIŠ *šá* DIB-*šú šu-te-eq-ru-ub* U$_4$ LÁ-*šú* ŠU^{II}-*šú* GIN$_7$ *šá ku-uṣ-ṣú* DIB-*šú i-ḫe-es-si* GÌR^{II}-*šú* LAL-*aṣ u ma-gal* LUḪ-*ut-ma ina-aḫ* DIB-*su* IGI.BAR-*as* ŠU *ʾe-e-li* (DPS XXVI:43′–44′ [AOAT 43.282])

**If what afflicts him does so in close sequence (and) when it comes over him, he wrings his hands like one whom cold afflicts, he stretches out his feet, he jerks a lot and then is quiet, (and) he gazes at the one who afflicts him, "hand" of the binder.

Cognitive abilities are usually preserved during the jerking movements, but action myoclonias can involve the facial muscles, and even the voice as well as the extremities, making it difficult for the patient to eat or talk as well as walk, as in the following reference.

13.70 DIŠ LÚ ŠÀ.MEŠ-*šú* [*i*] *t-te-ne-en-me-ru*/ *it-te-nen-bi-ṭu* EME-*šú* DIB.DIB-*bat ina ka-ṣa-a-ti ina-al ina* GI$_6$ *i-gal-lu-ut*/MUD-*ud* . . . (*BAM* 361:45–48//*BAM* 386 iv 12′–14′//K 8785:11′–13′)

**If a person's insides are continually colicky/cramped, his tongue is continually "seized," he lies down in the early morning, (and) he jerks/shudders in the night . . .

The "confused" heart of the following reference suggests posthypoxic intention myoclonus, an episode of jerking that can occur as a sequel to a brief cardiorespiratory arrest.

13.71 DIŠ NA *ina* KI.NÁ-*šú* LUḪ.LUḪ-*ut* ŠÀ-*šú e-šu-u ina* KI.NÁ-*šú re-ḫu-su* DU-*ak* NA BI DIB-*ti* ^{d}AMAR.UTU *u* ^{d}EŠ$_4$.DAR UGU-*šú* GÁL-*ši ana* TI-*šú* . . . (*BAM* 205:19′–21′//*STT* 95:16–18//*STT* 280 ii 1–3)

**If a person continually jerks in his bed, his heart(beat) is confused (and) his semen flows in his bed, the anger of Marduk and Ištar is upon that person, to cure him . . .

The fact that MUD/*parādu* is used to describe abnormal movement associated with liver abnormalities (see below) suggests that this term can refer to asterixis, that is, quick arrhythmic movements that occur due to brief interruptions in background tonic contractions. Asterixis is also known as "liver flap" due to the fact that it is commonly observed in liver failure.

13.72 [DIŠ NA] TÙN-*šú* TAG.TAG-*su* [. . .]⸢x⸣-*šú* [NINDA] *u* KAŠ LAL [. . .]x-nam-mu *pi-qam la pi-qam i-par-ru-ud* [ŠÀ-*šú*] ⸢*i*⸣-*sa-bu-u*ʾ ŠÀ-*šú* [. . .] *pit-ru-šú* DÙ-*šú-nu* [. . .]-*šú* NA BI TÙN.GI[G GIG ŠU N]AM.ÉRIM KUR-*su* . . . (*BAM* 87:14–17)

**[If a person]'s liver continually hurts him intensely, [. . .], he loses his appetite for [bread] and beer, [. . .] he *parādu*'s incessantly, [his stomach] churns, (and) his entire abdomen [. . .] him, that person [is sick] with ⸢TÙN.GIG⸣ ("sick liver"); ["hand"] of ⸢curse⸣ has "gotten" him . . .

In other contexts, the *āšipu* may have applied the term to abnormal movements that seemed to him to resemble asterixis. A translation of MUD/*parādu* as "shuddering"[30] is often appropriate, as in the following reference, which refers to a hysterical pseudo ("false") seizure.

13.73 DIŠ *ina ṣa-lu-ti-šú* DIB-*su-ma* DIB-*su* IGI.BAR-*as i-re-eḫ-ḫi-šum-ma* NÍ-*šú i-maš-ši* GIN$_7$ *šá id-ku-šú* MUD-*ud* ZI.ZI-*bé* : U$_4$ *id-de-ku-šú re-ḫi* ŠU LÍL.LÁ.EN.NA *sar-ru ana* MUNUS LÍL.LÁ.EN.NA ZI.ZI-*bé* (DPS XXVI:48′–49′ [AOAT 43.282])

**If it afflicts him in his sleep and he gazes at the one who afflicts him, it flows over him and he forgets himself, he shudders like one whom they have awakened (and) he can still get up (var. when they try to wake him, he is in a stupor), false "hand" of *lilû*. For a woman, a *lilû*; he can get up (afterward).

The *āšipu* distinguished two types of choreic movements (widespread arrythmic movements of a forcible, rapid, restless type) depending on the violence of the movement involved. The affected limbs were either described as "raised up" (*našû*), an expression also used of pelvic thrusting, or "jumping" (*šaḫāṭu*).

13.74 [DIŠ T]ÚG-*su ú-na-kas*$_4$ *u* UB.NÍGIN.NA-*šú na-šá-a* ŠU ^{d}*Šul-pa-è-a* (DPS XXII:45 [AOAT 43.255]; cf. StBoT 36.67 obv. 4′)

**[If] he tears his ⌜garment⌝ and his limbs are raised up, "hand" of Šulpaea.

13.75 U$_4$ GI[G GIG-*m*]*a* GEŠTU-*šu* GÙ-*šu* ŠU *ù* GÌR *šà* 150 ŠÈ 15 *ù šà*! *i-mi-it* ŠÈ 150-*šu i-šà-aḫ-ḫi-iṭ* ŠU *Šu-la-ak ul* TI.LA ÚŠ-*at* (*MDP* 57.11 iv 2′–5′)

**If the ⌜patient⌝ [is sick] ⌜and⌝ his ears ring (and) the right hand and foot jump to the left and the left (hand and foot jump) to his right, "hand" of Šulak. He will not get well; he will die.

The *āšipu* also noted dystonic movements (abnormal posturing resulting from irregular forceful twisting movements). He referred to these twisting movements using a term (*ṭamû*) which literally means "to twine" (i.e., to twist a piece of wool first one way and then another between the fingers), as in the following quote, which appears to describe the abnormal posturing of cerebral malaria (see Chapter 3).

13.76 DIŠ IGI.MEŠ-*šú* NIGIN.ME UB.NÍGIN.NA-*šú i-tar-ru-ra u i-ṭa-ma-a* ŠU ^{d}LUGAL. GÌR.RA *u* ^{d}MES.LAM.TA.È.A : ^{d}LUGAL.BÀN.DA (DPS IX A 64–65 = *TDP* 76:64–65)

**If his face seems continually to be spinning (and) his limbs tremble and twist (*ṭamû*), "hand" of ^{d}LUGAL.GÌR.RA and ^{d}MEŠ.LAM.TA.È.A (var. ^{d}LUGAL.BÀN.DA).

The abnormal posture that results from the twisting movements may be shifting or fixed. The following quote appears to describe a fixed abnormal posture.

13.77 DIŠ SAG.DU-*su i-ṭa-mu* GÌR-*šú šá* 150 *ú-kan-na-an-ma* NU LAL Š[U ^{d}. . .] (DPS III C obv. 27 = *TDP* 20:27)[31]

**If his head twists (*ṭamû*) and he bends his right foot and cannot straighten it out, "hand" of [. . .].

For twisting movements of the trunk and extremities, the *āšipu* also used another term (*šabāṣu*) usually used to describe the posturing of wrestlers (see below under CEREBRAL PALSY). For twisting movements of the neck, there were two further terms (*saḫāru* and *zarû*) that could be used to indicate either a simple turning of the head (*saḫāru*) or a forceful twisting motion (*zarû*), as in the following example, which appears to describe the reflex spasms of tetanus.

> **13.78** [DIŠ NA *šá-á*]*š-šá-ṭa* GIG GÚ-*su i-zu-ur* [IGI^{II}]-*šú* SIG$_7$ ŠUB-*a* [*gal-ta*]-*šú* (*BAM* 129 iv 6′–7′)
>
> **[If a person] is sick with ⸢*šaššaṭu*⸣ (tetanus) (and) he twists (*zarû*) his neck (and) his [eyes] are unevenly colored with yellow [(and) jerk?].

Two other terms were used to describe twitching of the mouth (*ṣadāru*) or face (*ṣapāru*), as in the following quotes, both of which describe strokes.

> **13.79** DIŠ KI.MIN-*ma* GÌR-*šú šá* 15 *i-maš-šar* KA-*šú ṣu-dur mi-šit-ti* MAŠKIM GÍD-*ma* GAM (DPS XV:63 [AOAT 43.154]; cf. DPS XIV A$_2$ iv 3′–4′//C$_2$ iii 30 = *TDP* 142 iv 3′–4′)
>
> **If (it is the first day he is sick) and he drags his left foot (and) his mouth twitches (*ṣadāru*),[32] stroke of a *rābiṣu*; (if) it is prolonged, he will die.
>
> **13.80** DIŠ IGI.MEŠ-*šú ṣap-ru*⸢*ta*⸣-*lam-ma-šú pur-ru-ur* ŠU-*su šá* NÍG.GIG-*ti-šú* ŠUB-*ma* NU ÍL-*ši* GÌR^{II}-*šú i-maš-šar* ŠU *mi-šit-tú* U$_4$.ME-*šú* GÍD.ME NU SI.SÁ (DPS IX A 72–73//B r. 19–20 = *TDP* 78:72–73)
>
> **If his face twitches (*ṣapāru*), his torso is powerless, he lets his right hand drop and is unable to lift (it) (and) he drags his foot, "hand" of a stroke. <Even if> he lives for a long time, he will not straighten up.

Tremors are repetitive muscular spasms. The *āšipu* used four terms to describe trembling patients. One of these (*nâšu*) means literally "to shake" (as of the earth in an earthquake). It was used, inter alia, to describe the movements of the jaws in complex partial seizures (see below).

> **13.81** [DIŠ G]IN$_7$ ŠUB-*ti* ŠUB.ŠUB-*su* IGI^{II}-*šú* MÚD DIRI.MEŠ : IGI^{II}-*šú* BAD-*te u* DUL-*am* ÚNU^{II}-*šú*/[M]E.ZÉ-*šú nu-uš-šá* ŠU^{II}-*šú u* GÌR^{II}-*šú tar-ṣa ina sa-naq a-ši-pi i*ʾ*-a-bat ša* DIB-*šú ina-ṭal* ŠU GIDIM$_7$ *šag-ga-ši* (DPS XXVI:11′–13′ [AOAT 43.279])
>
> **[If] it continually falls upon him ⸢like⸣ a falling spell (and) his eyes are full of blood (var. he opens and closes his eyes), his cheeks/⸢jaws⸣ shake (*nâšu*), his hands and his feet are stretched out, he collapses at the approach of the *āšipu*, (and) he can see the one who afflicts him,[33] "hand" of a murderous ghost.[34]

Of the remaining terms, two (*tarāru* and *ratātu*) were used to describe Parkinson's disease (see below), and probably refer to resting tremors, presumably of differing amplitude. The final term, *ra*ʾ*ābu*, is sometimes contrasted with *tarāru*, as in the following pair of references where dizzy patients were diagnosed as having "hand" of ^{d}LUGAL.GÌR.RA and ^{d}MEŠ.LAM.TA.È.A (possibly cerebral malaria; see Chapter 3) or "hand" of Dapinu in accordance with which type of tremor they exhibited.

> **13.82** DIŠ IGI.MEŠ-*šú* NIGIN.MEŠ SAG.DU-*su* ŠU^{II}-*šú u* GÌR^{II}-*šú i-tar-ru-ra* ŠU ^{d}LUGAL.GÌR.RA *u* ^{d}MEŠ.LAM.TA.È.A / DIŠ IG.MEŠ-*šú* NIGIN.MEŠ ŠU^{II}-*šú u* GÌR^{II}-*šú i-ra*ʾ*-ú-ba* U$_4$.59.KÁM ŠU ^{d}UD.AL.TAR (DPS IX A 57–59//B r. 1–3 = *TDP* 76:57–59)

**If his face seems continually to be spinning (and) his head, his hands, and his feet tremble (*tarāru*), "hand" of ^{d}LUGAL.GÌR.RA and ^{d}MEŠ.LAM.TA.È.A. If his face seems continually to be spinning (and) his hands and his feet tremble (*ra*ʾ*ābu*) (and he has been sick for) fifty-nine days, "hand" of Dapinu.

What this contrast suggests is that the tremor described by *ra*ʾ*ābu* was an intention tremor.[35] Tremors of this sort may be produced by trauma, as in the following reference.

13.83 DIŠ *ina* GÚ-*šú* SÌG-*iṣ-ma* GÌR^{II}-*šú i-ra-*ʾ*-ú-ba* ŠÀ.MEŠ-*šú it-te-nen-bi-ṭu* DIB GIDIM$_7$ (DPS X A obv. 20//B obv. 22 = *TDP* 82:20)

**If he was wounded on his neck and consequently his feet tremble (*ra*ʾ*ābu*) (and) his insides are continually cramped, affliction by a ghost.

The difference between resting and intention tremors is that in the former case the patient trembles continuously unless attempting purposeful activity whereas in the latter case the trembling is discontinuous, occurring only when the patient attempts purposeful activity. Certain infections cause "shaking" chills that are discontinuous (see Chapter 3). It might be expected, then, that if you wished to refer to them as "trembling" chills, you would use the term for intention tremor (*ra*ʾ*ābu*), as in the following example.

13.84 DIŠ U$_4$.1.KÁM DIB-*su* U$_4$.1.KÁM BAR-*šú* U$_4$ LÁ-*šú* LÁ-*šú* UB.MEŠ-*šú* KÚ.MEŠ-*šú* KÚM-*ma i-ra-*ʾ*u-ub* IR ŠUB-*su-ma ina-aḫ u* A *ana* NAG *ma-gal* APIN.MEŠ ŠU ^{d}DÌM.ME DIN (DPS XVI:14–15 [AOAT 43.173])

**If one day it afflicts him and one day it releases him (and) when his confusional state comes over him, his limbs continually hurt him, he is feverish and trembles (*ra*ʾ*ābu*), sweat falls upon him, and then he finds relief and continually asks for a great deal of water to drink, "hand" of Lamaštu; he will get well.

In one passage from the diagnostic/prognostic handbook, the *āšipu* used a series of contrasting references (see Introduction) to explain the difference between Parkinsonian tremors (*tarāru* and *ratātu*) and intention tremors (*ra*ʾ*ābu*), demonstrating once again that he was both an excellent observer and diagnostician.

13.85 DIŠ SAG.DU-*su* ŠU^{II}-*šú u* GÌR^{II}-*šú* 1-*niš i-tar-ru-ra ina* KA-*šú át-mu-šú it-te-ni-ip-r*[*ik-ku* NA BI *lu-*ʾ*-tu*$_4$ *ana ma-al-tak-ti š*] *u-kul*[36] (DPS III C obv. 42 = *TDP* 22:42)

**If his head, his hands, and his feet all tremble (*tarāru*) at once (and) his words hinder each other in his mouth, [that person] ⸢has been fed⸣ [a dirty substance to test (the efficacy of the poison)].[37]

13.86 DIŠ SAG.DU-*su* ŠU^{II}-*šú u* GÌR^{II}-*šú i-ra-*ʾ*-u-ba* KA-*šú ana at-me-e il-la-a* U$_4$[. . .] x / DIŠ SAG.DU-*su* ŠU^{II}-*šú u* GÌR^{II}-*šú* 1-*niš i-ra-*ʾ*-ú-ba* ŠÀ-*šú ana* BURU$_8$ *i-te-ni-il-la-a-ma* ⸢*mim+ma*⸣ [*šá* KÚ ŠÀ-*šú* GUR ŠU ^{d}]20? (DPS III C obv. 43–44 = *TDP* 22:43–44)

**If his head, his hands, and his feet tremble (*ra*ʾ*ābu*), he raises his mouth to the words, [(and) he has been sick for . . .] days, [. . .]. If his head, his hands, and his feet all tremble (*ra*ʾ*ābu*) together (and) his stomach continually rises up to vomit and everything [which he eats, his stomach returns, "hand"] of ⸢Šamaš(?)⸣.

13.87 DIŠ SAG.DU-*su* ŠU^{II}-*šú u* GÌR^{II}-*šú i-rat-tu-ta* KA-*šú ana* DU$_{10}$ *da-an it-te-ni-ip-rik* (coll.) ⌜NA?⌝ [BI *lu-ʾ-a-ti šu-k*] *ul*[38] (DPS III C obv. 45 = *TDP* 22:45)

**If his head, his hands, and his feet tremble (*ratātu*), his mouth is (too) strong for the words (and) they hinder each other, [that] person ⌜has been fed⌝ [dirty substances].

Opisthotonus

This term refers to an arching or bowing of the back caused by severe muscle spasms. If the patient is on his back when the spasm occurs, his pelvis and torso raise up off the bed with his body supported only by his head and heels. Diseases known to have this type of muscle spasm include tetanus (see Chapter 3), strychnine poisoning, and neurological diseases called leukodystrophies (Krabbe's disease and Alexander's disease). The diseases demonstrating this sign are usually serious, and death is a frequent outcome.

13.88 DIŠ KI.MIN-*ma* MURUB$_4$.MEŠ-*šú* ÍL.MEŠ-*šú* GIN$_7$ *i-te-né-ep-pu-šu* NU ZU GAM (DPS XV:48 [AOAT 43.153]; cf. DPS XII D iii 41 = *TDP* 106 iii 41)

**If (it is the first day he is sick) and his pelvic region is continually lifted up (and) he does not realize that he is continually doing (this), he will die.

Cranial Nerve Diseases

There are twelve motor and sensory nerves that leave the brain before the major nerve tracts enter the spinal canal. These cranial nerves ennervate structures in the head and neck. Abnormalities of some of the cranial nerves are described in the references listed below.

SECOND CRANIAL NERVE

Abnormalities of this nerve cause blindness. Partial optic nerve injuries from closed trauma result in blurring of vision, central or paracentral scotomas (blind spots), or sector defects. The text below appears to be referring to visual loss secondary to head trauma, either injury to the second cranial nerve or injury to the occipital portion of the skull where the visual cortex is located. For references to congenital blindness in newborns, see 17.42.

13.89 DIŠ *ina* SAG.DU-*šú* SÌG-*iṣ-ma* IGI^{II}-*šú ur-ru-pa* ŠU ^{d}N[IN].GÍR.SU (DPS III C r. 15 = *TDP* 26:75)

**If he was wounded on his head and, consequently, his eyes are heavily clouded, "hand" of ⌜Ningirsu⌝.

THIRD, FOURTH, AND SIXTH CRANIAL NERVES

These three nerves collectively are responsible for moving the eyeballs. If all three nerves are affected, the eye becomes immobile. The *āšipu* described ocular paralysis with the phrase "the eyes stand (still)." In the second reference below, we believe the cause of paralysis to be Wernicke disease, a thiamine deficiency often seen in severe alcoholism (see Chapter 15).

13.90 DIŠ GIG MURUB$_4$ GIG-*ma* ZI-*bi u* DU$_{10}$.GAM GABA-*su* BAD.BAD-*te* KA-*šú ana* INIM.INIM *da-an* IGI^{II}-*šú* GUB.GUB-*za* GAM (DPS XVII:54–55 [AOAT 43.200])

**If he is sick with an illness of the pelvic region and he gets up and (has to) squat down, he continually bares his chest,[39] his mouth is too strong for the words, (and) his eyes continually stand (still),[40] he will die.

13.91 DIŠ NA KAŠ.SAG NAG-*ma* SAG.DU-*su* DIB.DIB-*su* INIM.MEŠ-*šú im-ta-na-áš-ši ina* DUG$_4$.DUG$_4$-*šú ú-pa-áš-šaṭ ṭè-en-šú la ṣa-bit* NA BI IGI^{II}-*šú* GUB-*za ana* TI-*šú* . . . (*BAM* 575 iii 51–52//*BAM* 59:21–24)

**If a person drinks fine beer and as a result his head continually afflicts him, he continually forgets his words and slurs them when speaking, he is not in full possession of his faculties, and that person's eyes stand still, to cure him . . .

If there is a difference in the nerves affected between the right eye and left eye, the eyes become misaligned or crossed. If both eyes move but they do not maintain their normal alignment, it is called dysconjugate eye movement.[41] This is indicative of brain stem pathology, which often has a poor prognosis. Abnormal eye movements are described in the references below.

13.92 DIŠ SAG.KI-*su* GIN$_7$ *si-ka-a-t*[*i* . . .] IGI^{II}-*šú ip-rik* GAM (DPS IV B r. 34 = *TDP* 44 r. 57)[42]

**If his forehead is [. . .] like brewer's yeast (and) his eyes cross,[43] he will die.

13.93 DIŠ GI$_6$ IGI^{II}-*šú* BAL-*ut-ma* IGI^{II}-*šú ana* ⌜ŠÀ⌝ [. . .] (DPS V G 8 = *TDP* 50 G 8)[44]

**If he rolls his pupils so that his eyes [look] inward [. . .].

The third cranial nerve also controls pupil size and keeps the eyelids open. The *āšipu* described the opening and closing of the eyes with the terms *petû:* "to open" and *katāmu:* "to cover."[45] For dilation and constriction of the pupil, he used the terms *balāṣu:* "to open wide."[46] and *zaqāpu:* "to point forward."[47] He understood that the pupils constrict when a person focuses his eyes, noted the dilation of pupils in infantile seizures, and knew to test for the responsiveness of the pupils in comatose patients.

13.94 DIŠ LÚ *i-na na-ap-lu-sí-šu i-ni-šu za-qá-pa-am ú-qal-la-al-ma la i-le-i* LÚ *šu-ú ṭé-em-šu pu-ur-ru-ur* (Köcher and Oppenheim, *AfO* 18.65 ii 16–17 [physiognomic omens])[48]

**If when a person looks (at something), he is barely able to constrict his eyes, that person's mentation is disconnected.

13.95 DIŠ LÚ.TUR KÚM NU TUKU IGI^{II}-*šú bal-ṣa* ŠU^{II}-*šú u* GÌR^{II}-*šú i-ra-ʾu-ba* ŠU ^{d}30 DIN (DPS XL A 120 = *TDP* 230:120)[49]

**If an infant does not have a fever, his eyes are dilated, (and) his hands and his feet tremble, "hand" of Sîn; he will get well.

13.96 U_4 GIG IGI-*šu bu-ul-lu-ṣú ta-šà-as-sí-šu-ma ul i-še-em-me-ka mi-im-ma šà tu-ka-al-lu-šu ul ú-ma-dì* ŠU *qa-a-a-li* (*MDP* 57.11 iv 15′–18′)[50]

**If the patient's eyes are dilated, you call out to him and he does not hear you, (and) whatever you hold before him he does not recognize, "hand" of the taciturn one.

The following reference describes a "drooping" eye (*kapāṣu*), that is, eyelid paralysis, probably caused by third nerve paralysis. This type of injury may be caused by a lesion such as a tumor or intracerebral bleeding causing the brain to herniate and the patient to die. Muscle weakness such as that seen with myasthenia gravis can also cause a drooping eyelid.

13.97 [*en-šu š*] *a šu-me-e-li i-kap-pa-a*[*ṣ*] *kat-ma-*⌜*at-ma la*⌝*-a*⌜*i-pá!*⌝*-at-ti* BA̤.ÚŠ (StBoT 36.23 r. 9′)[51]

**(If) [his] right [eye] droops (and) it is closed so that he cannot open it, he will die.[52]

FIFTH CRANIAL NERVE

The fifth cranial nerve supplies the sensory nerves of the face and the motor nerves of the jaw (mastication). Interruption of this nerve will cause facial numbness and difficulty chewing. Described below are patients with difficulty chewing, a condition that may have been caused by fifth nerve injury or disease. (Also see the seventh cranial nerve below.)

13.98 DIŠ KA-*šú* DIB.DIB-*ma mim-ma la i-lim* ŠU DINGIR ⌜URU-*šú*⌝[53] [. . .] (DPS VII B obv. 2′ = *TDP* 64:41′)

**If his mouth is continually "seized" so that he cannot eat anything, "hand" of the god of his city [. . .]

Inflammation of this nerve can cause severe facial pain, a condition called trigeminal neuralgia. Ancient physicians recognized and treated the problem, which they attributed to an invisible lion-demon who inhabited the toilet room and who was otherwise responsible for strokes (see below).

13.99 DIŠ NA IGI.MEŠ-*šú* GÚ-*su u* NUNDUN-*su šim-mat* TUKU.MEŠ-*a ù ki-ma* IZI *i-ḫa-am-ma-ṭa-šú* NA BI MAŠKIM *mu-sa-a-ti* DIB-*su ana* DIN-*šú* . . . (*SpTU* 1.46:6–8//*AMT* 60/3 ii 16′–17′)

**If a person's face, his neck, and his lips are continually numb and it burns him like fire, the *rābiṣu* of the lavatory afflicts him; to cure him . . .

SEVENTH CRANIAL NERVE

This nerve supplies the muscles of the face and some of the taste buds of the tongue. In the reference below, smoothing out of the face describes facial paralysis. The text also indicates that the patient is unable to "get his teeth close enough together to be able to eat" and that "his ears roar." This sounds like paralysis of the jaw muscles (fifth nerve; see above) and tinnitus (eighth nerve; see below). This combination of fifth, seventh, and eighth nerve involvement, especially if it is one-sided (unilateral), is compatible with pathology that occurs at the cerebellopontine angle.[54] The usual cause of this pathology is a tumor.

13.100 ŠU.GIDIM.MA GEŠTU^{II}-*šú* GÙ.DÉ.MEŠ *ma-gal iṭ-ṭe-né-pi šin-na-šú ana ma-ka-le-e la ú-qar-ra-ba-ma* (*BRM* 4.32:3–4)

**"Hand" of ghost (is when) his ears roar, (his face) continually smooths out,[55] (and) he cannot get his teeth close enough together to be able to eat.

EIGHTH CRANIAL NERVE

This is a sensory nerve supplying the inner ear where hearing (cochlear) and balance (vestibular) are controlled. Congenital deafness and hearing loss secondary to trauma are discussed in Chapter 17 and below. Injury or disease of the eighth nerve, in addition to deafness, can also cause abnormal balance. Stimulation of the vestibular portion of the eighth nerve can cause dizziness (vertigo). In the final quote below, the patient's vertigo is so severe that he is unable to maintain his balance, and he falls down.

13.101 DIŠ *ina* U[G]U-*šú* SÌG-*ma* GEŠTU^{II}-*šú* NU ŠE.GA-*a* ŠU ^{d}15 *ana* AŠ-*tim* (DPS III A obv. 19//C obv. 10 = *TDP* 18:10; cf. StBoT 36.35 r. 1//StBoT 36.57 r. 8′)

**If he was wounded on his ⌜skull⌝ and, consequently, his ears do not hear, "hand" of Ištar . . .

13.102 DIŠ IGI.MEŠ-*šú* NIGIN.MEŠ ŠU^{II}-*šú u* GÌR^{II}-*šú i-ra-ʾ-ú-ba* U_4.59.KÁM ŠU ^{d}UD.AL.TAR (DPS IX A 59//B r. 3 = *TDP* 76:59)

**If his face seems continually to be spinning (and) his hands and his feet tremble (and he has been sick for) fifty-nine days, "hand" of Dapinu.

13.103 DIŠ NA *ina* LÍL-*šú* KÚM *ana* SAG.DU-*šú ip-pu-uš-ma* SAG.DU-*su* DUGUD-*ma ina* ZI-*šú* SAG.DU-*su ana* IGI-*šú* GÍD.DA-*su ana* DIN-*šú* . . . (*BAM* 3 iii 42–44//*BAM* 480 iv 26–27)

**If during the course of a person's illness, fever/inflammation spreads to his head so that his head (feels like it) is so heavy that it draws him forward[56] when he stands up, to cure him . . .

13.104 DIŠ IGI.MEŠ-*šú* NIGIN.MEŠ *ina* KI.NÁ-*šú* ZI-*ma* ŠUB-*ut* ŠU GIDIM$_7$ (DPS IX A 63//B r. 8 = *TDP* 76:63)[57]

**If his face seems continually to be spinning[58] (and) he gets up from his bed and then falls down (again), "hand" of ghost.

TENTH CRANIAL NERVE

For a possible example of vagus nerve paralysis, see 13.219 (encephalomyelitis).

FIRST, NINTH, ELEVENTH, AND TWELFTH CRANIAL NERVES

These nerves will not be considered here since we have been unable to identify in the references any conditions that seem to be specifically related to these nerves.

Nystagmus

The eyes may have an abnormal movement called nystagmus which can have multiple causes, including dysfunction of the inner ear (vestibular end organ), vestibular nerve, eye, brain stem, and cerebellum and cerebral centers for ocular pursuit. Some drugs such as the antibiotic gentamiacin can cause nystagmus. The movement is rhythmic and involuntary and in some cases may be related to seizure activity. It usually involves both eyes, and the movement may be pendular or jerky. Pendular nystagmus is usually caused by brain stem or cerebellar dysfunction. In pendular nystagmus, the oscillations of the eyes have an equal rate, amplitude, and direction of movement. The *āšipu* appears to have described pendular movement of the eyes using two terms, one of which literally means "to shudder" (*parādu*) and the other "to tremble" (*arāru*).[59] The latter term is possibly describing transient high-frequency, low-amplitude pendular nystagmus.

13.105 [DIŠ MU]RUB$_4$ ⌜*u* ŠÀ⌝-*šú* GIG-*ma* ZI-*bi u* DU$_{10}$.GAM NINDA NU KÚ KAŠ NU NAG IGI^{II}-*šú pár-da* GAM (DPS XII D iv 3–4//E iv 8–9 = *TDP* 106 iv 3–4)

**[If] his ⌜pelvic region⌝ and abdomen are so sick that he gets up and (has to) squat down (again), he does not eat bread, he does not drink beer, (and) his eyes shudder,[60] he will die.

13.106 [DIŠ NA] *it-ta-n*[*a-a*]*d-la-aḫ it-te-nen-biṭ* IGI^{II}-*šú ir-ru-ru* [UZU].MEŠ-*šú i-šam-ma-mu-šú ši-in-na-šu ka-li-ši-na* KÚ.MEŠ-*šú* [NINDA] KÚ KAŠ NAG-*ma i-li-ḫi-ib ana* LÚ BI ZI.KU$_5$.RU.DA *ša* GA.ḪAB DÙ-*su šum-ma* KIN-*šú il-ta-bir* TIL.LA-*ma* TE-*šu-ma* BA.ÚŠ (*BAM* 449 iii 13′–16′)

**[If a person] is continually troubled and cramped, his eyes tremble,[61] his [flesh] goes numb, all of his teeth continually hurt him, (if) he eats [bread] (and) drinks beer, he makes a loud growling noise, ZI.KU$_5$.RU.DA (sorcery) with sour milk has been performed against that person. If his attack persists (and if) he gets well, and then it approaches him (again), he will die.

Jerky nystagmus is generally due to peripheral vestibular dysfunction or an abnormal brain stem neural integrator. The first reference below is probably describing tetanus (see Chapter 3).

13.107 DIŠ GÚ-*su i-zu-ur-ma* IGI-*šú gal-ta-át pi-qam* NU *pi-qam* LUḪ-*ut*/MUD-*ud* SA.DUGUD (DPS X A obv. 11//B obv. 11 = *TDP* 80:11; cf. DPS XXXIII:96 [AOAT 43.357])[62]

**If he twists his neck and his eye jerks[63] (and) he jerks (var. A: shudders) incessantly, *šaššaṭu*.

13.108 [DIŠ . . .]-*su i-na-al* IGI^{II}-*šú gal-ta-ma ina pi-qa la pi-qa i-par-ru-ud*/ *i-ṣar-ru-ut* (*BAM* 131 obv. 9–10//*CT* 23.5–14 iv 18)

**[If] he lies on his [back?], his eyes jerk, and he shudders (var.: breaks wind) incessantly.

Another form of nystagmus is known as periodic alternating nystagmus. In this condition, there is horizontal nystagmus, but it reverses direction every several minutes. This can occur in a congenital form. It is possible that the term *ṭamû*, which means literally "to twine" (i.e., to twist a piece of wool first one way and then another between the fingers) and which was employed by the *āšipu* to describe eye movements in an infant is a reference to periodic alternating nystagmus.[64]

13.109 DIŠ LÚ.TUR IGI^{II}-*šú e-ṭa-ma-a* ŠU ^{d}NIN.GEŠTIN.NA (DPS XL B 72a = *TDP* 226:71a)

**If an infant's eyes oscillate (*ṭamû*), "hand" of Ningeštinanna.

The abnormal eye movements of cerebral malaria (see Chapter 3) are particularly spectacular, including disorders of conjugate gaze, transient ocular bobbing, and both horizontal and vertical nystagmus (jerking eye movements). We believe the following references, which describe the eyes as "spinning (*lamû*)[65] like a spindle whorl," that is, bobbing and "jerking" (*galātu*), to be examples of cerebral malaria.

13.110 DIŠ U$_4$-*ma* UD.DU-*šú* IGI-*šú šá* 150 GIN$_7$ ^{GIŠ}BA[L *i-lam-mi*] IGI-*šu šá* ZAG MÚD DIRI-*at* KA-*šú* [BAD.BAD-*te* EME-*šu*] *ú-na-šak* ^{d}LUGAL.GÌR.RA DIB-*su* [. . .] ÚS.ÚS [. . .] (*STT* 89:109–112 [Stol, *Epilepsy* 92])

**If when it comes over him, his right eye makes (a bobbing motion) like a spindle whorl (when) it [spins] (and) his left eye is full of blood, [he continually opens] his mouth, (and) he bites [his tongue], ^{d}LUGAL.GÌR.RA afflicts him [. . .] continually pursues him [. . .]

13.111 DIŠ U$_4$-*ma* UD.DU-*šú* ŠU-*su šá* 150 IGI-*šú šá* [. . .] GIN$_7$ UR.GI$_7$ *i-šag-gúm* ZÚ.MEŠ-*šú* [. . .] IGI^{II}-*šú gal-ta* ^{d}LUGAL.GÌR.RA DIB-*su ana* TI.LA-*šú qí-ba* NU GAR-*an* (*STT* 89:133–136a [Stol, *Epilepsy* 93])

**If when it comes over him, his right hand (and) his [left] eye [. . .] he growls like a dog, his teeth [. . .] (and) his eyes jerk, ^{d}LUGAL.GÌR.RA afflicts him, the *āšipu* should not make a prognostication as to his recovery.[66]

The direction of the movement is usually horizontal, but vertical nystagmus has been described, especially in patients with brain stem pathology (see below). In the first two references below, we believe that the phrase "his eyes drift downstream" (*neqelpû*) means horizontal and probably pendular nystagmus.[67] A second verb, *ṣabāru* or *ṣapāru*, which literally means "to move back and forth," was used to describe movements of the eyes in connection with grand mal seizures, a condition that is often associated with nystagmus. We believe that this term, translated "to flutter" in the third and fourth references below, refers to rapid horizontal oscillations of the eyes.[68]

13.112 DIŠ IGI^{II}-*šú it-te-neq-lep-pa-a* ŠU ^{d}30 (*STT* 89:207 [Stol, *Epilepsy* 98])

**If his eyes drift downstream, "hand" of Sîn.

13.113 ⸢DIŠ SAG⸣.KI-*su šá* GÙB KÚ-*šú-ma u it-te-néq-lép-pu* ŠU ^{d}30 (*STT* 89:209 [Stol, *Epilepsy* 98])[69]

**If his right temple hurts him and (his eyes) drift downstream, "hand" of Sîn.

13.114 DIŠ IGI-*šú i-ṣa-par* NUNDUN-*šú* DU_8-*á*[*t*] ÚḪ *ina* KA-*šú* DU-*ak* $ŠU^{II}$-*šú* $GÌR^{II}$-*šú* *t*[*a*]-*lam-ma-šú* GIN_7 UDU.NÍTA *ṭa-ab-*[*ḫi*] *i*!-*nap-pa-aṣ* AN.TA.ŠUB.BA DIB-*su* (*STT* 89:141–143 [Stol, *Epilepsy* 94])[70]

**If his eye flutters, his lip(s) come apart, spittle flows from his mouth, his hand, his foot, (and) his buttock thrash around like (those of) a ⌜slaughtered⌝ sheep, AN.TA.ŠUB.BA (seizure) afflicts him.

13.115 DIŠ LÚ *i-ni-šu ki-la-at-tim-ma iṣ-ṣa-pa-ar mu-uḫ-ḫa-šu ma-ḫi-iṣ ki-ma mu-uḫ-ḫi-šu-ma ṭé-em-šu i-ba-aš-ši* (Köcher and Oppenheim, *AfO* 18.65 ii 28–30 [physiognomic omens])[71]

**If both eyes flutter, he was struck on his skull; just as his skull is, so is his mind.

Eye Movements in Seizures

In addition to fluttering (*ṣapāru*; see above), the *āšipu* used two terms to describe movements in the eyes of patients experiencing seizures. One of these, *napalkû*, means "to become wide apart,"[72] which we interpret to mean that the eyes turn upward ("toward the sky") into the sockets so that only the white is visible.

13.116 DIŠ GIG GÚ-*su ana* 150 NIGIN.ME $ŠU^{II}$-*šú u* $GÌR^{II}$-*šú tar-ṣa* IGI^{II}-*šú ana* IGI AN-*e na-pal-ka-a ina* KA-*šú* ÚḪ DU-*ak i-ḫar-ru-ur* NÍ-*šú* NU ZU *ina taq-ti-it* [LÁ-*š*] *ú iḫ-ta-niṭ-ṭa-áš-šú* AN.TA.ŠUB.BA ŠU $^{d}30$[73] (DPS X A obv. 4–6//B obv. 4–6 = *TDP* 80:4–6)

**If the patient continually turns his head to the right, his hands and his feet are stretched out, his eyes are opened wide toward the sky, spittle flows from his mouth, he makes rumbling noises, he does not know who he is at the beginning when ⌜his⌝ [confusional state] comes over him, AN.TA.ŠUB.BA (seizure), "hand" of Sîn.

13.117 [*e-na-a*]-*šu it-ta-na-pal-ka*$_4$-*a* BA.ÚŠ (StBoT 36.23 r. 6′a)[74]

**(If) his [eyes] are continually opened wide, he will die.

The other term, *nabalkutu*: "to roll,"[75] appears to mean eyes rolling to the side (lateral deviation), as suggested by Kinnier Wilson.[76] In the reference below, the head deviates to one side. If our interpretation is correct, one would expect the eyes to deviate to the same side as the head.

13.118 DIŠ GIG GÚ-*su ana* 15 NIGIN.ME $ŠU^{II}$-*šú u* $GÌR^{II}$-*šú am-šá* IGI^{II}-*šú* DUL-*ma* BAL-⌜*ma*⌝ *ina* KA-*šú* ÚḪ DU-*ak i-ḫar-ru-ur* AN.TA.ŠUB.BA (DPS X A obv. 1–2//B obv. 1//DPS IX A 80//B r. 27 = *TDP* 80:1–2//*TDP* 78:80[77]

**If the patient continually turns his head to the left, his hands and his feet are immobilized, he closes and rolls his eyes and spittle flows from his mouth, (and) he makes rumbling noises, AN.TA.ŠUB.BA (seizure).

Parinaud's Syndrome

In the following reference, the patient's pupils are said to have moved downward. This is indicative of paralysis of upward gaze, a sign of midbrain pathology that is frequently fatal. A malignant tumor is a common cause.

13.119 DIŠ U_4.5.KÁM U_4.10.KÁM GIG *dan-na* GIG-*ma uš-tar-di-ma* GI_6 IGI^{II}-*šú uš-ter-di-a* U_4.2.KÁM *ḫu-qu* DIB.DIB-*su ina* U_4.3.KÁM GAM (DPS XVI:53′–54′ [AOAT 43.177])

**If he has been sick with a mighty sickness for five or ten days and the pupils of his eyes persist in (moving) downward[78] (and) *ḫūqu* (gasping respiration; see below) continually afflicts him for two days, he will die on the third day.

Paralysis of Downward Gaze

In the following reference, the patient's pupils are said to have moved upward. This is indicative of paralysis of downward gaze, a rare condition usually caused by occlusion of a midline penetrating artery and bilateral midbrain infarction.

13.120 DIŠ KI.MIN-*ma* GI_6 IGI^{II}-*šú* E_{11}-*a u ḫu-qu* DIB.DIB-*su ana* U_4.3.KÁM GAM (DPS XVI:58′ [AOAT 43.177])

**If (he has been sick for five, ten, or fifteen days) and his pupils (move) upward and *ḫūqu* (gasping respiration; see below) continually afflicts him for three days, he will die.

Trauma to the Head and Spinal Cord

Injury to the nervous system will cause neurologic signs and symptoms, and the war-prone ancient Mesopotamians had many opportunities to sustain these injuries. From the following texts it is apparent that the *āšipu* knew that seizures, loss of sight, loss of hearing, and paralysis could be the result of a head or back injury. The term used by the ancient physician for wound complications was *terdētu*.[79]

TRAUMA TO THE HEAD

SEIZURES The incidence of epilepsy after head injury varies with the severity of the injury to the brain. Seizures occur in 40 percent of patients who sustain penetrating missile wounds, but follow only 10 percent of the blunt injuries characteristic of civilian life. It should not be surprising that Ištar who was, among other things, goddess of war, features prominently among trauma references, including the second text below.

13.121 DIŠ LÚ *i-ni-šu ša ki-la-at-tim-ma iṣ-ṣa-pa-ar mu-uḫ-ḫa-šu ma-ḫi-iṣ ki-ma mu-uḫ-ḫi-šu-ma ṭé-em-šu i-ba-aš-ši* (Köcher and Oppenheim, *AfO* 18.65 ii 28–30 [physiognomic omens])

**If both a person's eyes flutter, he was struck on his skull; just as his skull is, so is his mind.

13.122 DIŠ *ina* SAG.DU-*šú* SÌG-*iṣ-ma u i-ṭa-mu pu-qud-de-e* [d]15 *ana* [d]MAŠ.TAB.BA (DPS III C r. 17//E_2 r. 14 = *TDP* 26:77; cf. StBoT 36.34 obv. 5′)

**If he was wounded on his head and, consequently, he twists, he was entrusted by Ištar to the twin gods.

13.123 DIŠ *ina* SAG.KI-*šú šá* 15/150 SÌG-*iṣ u i-ṭa-mu* [. . .] (DPS IV A obv. 42–43//B obv. 38–39 = *TDP* 36:42–43)

**If he was wounded on his left/right temple and he twists [. . .]

STROKELIKE SYMPTOMS A wound to the left side of the head can mimic a left middle cerebral artery stroke, either by damaging the artery or by direct injury to the left motor cortex, causing right-sided hemiparesis, and in some cases, inability to talk (aphasia). Correspondingly, a wound to the right side of the head can cause left-sided hemiparesis but not aphasia, since the speech center is located on the left side. A wound of this sort was referred to by the *āšipu* as the "wound of a stroke," as in the reference below.

13.124 [*šu-me-el*] *pa-ag-ri-šu ka-la-a-ma* ⌜*ta*⌝*-a*[*b*]*-kà-at*! *da-bá-bá la-a i-le-ʾ-e* [. . . *la-a i-l*] *e-ʾ-e* ŠU [d]*Šu-lak m*[*i*!?*-ḫi-i*]*ṣ me-še-ti ma-ḫi-iṣ* [LÚ]*a-ši-pu a-n*[*a* TI-*šu qí-i-ba l*] *a-a i-ša-kán* (StBoT 36.22 obv. 11–13)[80]

**(If) the entire [right side of] his body is tense[81] (and) he is not able to talk (and) he is [not] ⌜able⌝ to [. . .] "hand" of Šulak (or) he was wounded with the wound of a stroke; the *āšipu* should ⌜not⌝ make a [prognosis as to his recovery].

The texts below specify that the patient was wounded "from in front" (GABA.RI) and "from behind" (EGIR-*tam*), respectively. These statements may indicate on which side of the head the wound was located. Ancient Mesopotamians had the same preponderance of right-handed individuals as we do, and consequently the majority of warriors would have been right-handed. When attacking an enemy face to face (and the term used to describe the direction from which the blow is coming, GABA.RI, is also used to designate a face-to-face rival, a right-handed attacker would be most likely to connect with the left side of the victim's head. Conversely, the same right-handed attacker would be most likely to deal a blow to the right side of the head of a fleeing enemy. In the following references, these assumptions correspond correctly to the side on which the paralysis was observed to have occurred.[82]

13.125 DIŠ ⌜GÙB⌝ LÚ.AD_6-*šú ka-lu-šú-ma tab-kát* GABA.RI SÌG-*iṣ* ŠU [d]*Šu-lak* MAŠKIM *mu-sa-a-ti* MAŠ.MAŠ *ana* DIN-*šú* ME-*a* NU GAR-*an* (DPS XXVII:12–13 [AOAT 43.297]; cf. *AMT* 77/1 i 9–10)

**If the entire right side of his body is tense,[83] he was wounded from in front (or) "hand" of Šulak, the *rābiṣu* of the lavatory; the *āšipu* should not make a prognosis as to his recovery.

13.126 [DIŠ Z]AG LÚ.AD_6-*šú ka-lu-šú-ma tab-kát mi-šit-ti* MAŠKIM EGIR-ta_5 SÌG-*iṣ* (DPS XXVII:10 [AOAT 43.297]; restored from *AMT* 77/1 i 7)

**If the entire left side of his body is tense,[84] stroke of a *rābiṣu* (or) he was wounded from behind.

SKULL FRACTURES If the skin is lacerated over a skull fracture and the underlying meninges are torn, or if the fracture passes through the posterior wall of a nasal sinus, bacteria or air may enter the cranial cavity resulting in meningitis, abscess formation, or pneumocephalus. Alternatively, head trauma that causes bleeding can manifest fever even in the absence of infection.

13.127 DIŠ *ina* SAG.DU-*šú* SÌG-*iṣ-ma* MIR.ŠEŠ ŠUB.ŠUB-⸢*su*⸣ IGI.MEŠ-*šú* SA$_5$ *u* ⸢SIG$_7$ GIN$_7$ DIB⸣-*su* ŠUB-*šú* [U]Š$_4$-*šú* KÚR-*šum-ma i-ṭa-mu* DIB-*it* ^{d}DIM$_{11}$.ME.⸢LAGAB⸣ U$_4$-*me-šú* GÍD.DA.⸢MEŠ-*ma*⸣ GAM (DPS III C r. 22–23 = *TDP* 28:82–83; cf. *KAR* 211 obv. 7–9)

**If he was wounded in the head and, consequently, chills keep falling on him, his face flushes and turns pale (and) when his affliction falls upon him, his ⸢mentation⸣ is altered and he twists, affliction by *aḫḫāzu*.[85] (If) he (is ill) for a long time, he will die.[86]

The reference above with its fatal outcome contrasts sharply with the description below of a relatively benign infected scalp wound.

13.128 DIŠ *ina* SAG.DU-*šú* SÌG-*iṣ-ma* SA SAG.KI-*šú* ŠU [^{II}]-*šú u* [GÌ]R^{II}-*šú* 1-*niš* ZI.MEŠ ⸢SA$_5$⸣ *u* ⸢*i-mim* ŠU DINGIR⸣ TI (DPS III C r. 21 = *TDP* 26:81)[87]

**If he was wounded on his head and, consequently, the blood vessel(s) of his temple, his ⸢hands⸣ and his ⸢feet⸣ all (feel like they) are pulsating together (and) he is reddish and feverish, "hand" of god; he will get well.

CRANIAL NERVE INJURIES Direct facial nerve injury due to a basilar skull fracture may be present immediately or delayed five to seven days secondary to swelling in the facial canal. Petrous fractures, particularly the less common transverse type, are liable to produce this injury.

13.129 [DIŠ *i-n*]*a* IGI-*šú* SÌG-*iṣ-ma ù* KA-*šú su-ḫur* ŠU ^{d}EN.ZU x[. . .] (*KAR* 211 obv. 14)

**[If] he was wounded ⸢on⸣ one side of his face and his mouth is turned (to one side), "hand" of Sîn; [. . .].

13.130 [DIŠ *i-n*]*a* IGI-*šú* SÌG-*iṣ-ma ù* KA-*šú su-ḫur ina* A.[SAG] *i-ṭí-pá-*[*ma is*]-*sà-aḫ-ḫap-ma ina* KA-*šú* UŠ$_{11}$ DU-*ak* ŠU ^{d}EN.ZU BA.[ÚŠ] (*KAR* 211 obv. 15–16)

**[If] he was wounded ⸢on⸣ one side of his face and his mouth is turned (to one side, his skin) smooths out [and] falls flat against (his) ⸢skull⸣ and spittle flows from his mouth, "hand" of Sîn; he will ⸢die⸣.

Injury to the eighth cranial nerve with fractures of the petrous bone causing epidural and/or subdural bleeding may result in loss of hearing, vertigo, and nystagmus immediately after the injury.

13.131 DIŠ *ina* U[G]U-*šú* SÌG-*ma* GEŠTU^{II}-*šú* NU ŠE.GA-*a* ŠU ^{d}15 *ana* AŠ-*tim* (DPS III A obv. 19//C obv. 10 = *TDP* 18:10; cf. StBoT 36.35 r. 1//StBoT 36.57 r. 8′)

**If he was wounded on his ⸢skull⸣ and, consequently, his ears do not hear, "hand" of Ištar . . .

13.132 DIŠ *ina* SAG.DU-*šú* SÌG-*iṣ-ma ḫa-si-si-šú* ⸢*kùd?-du?*⸣[88] *-ta-at* ⸢GEŠTU^{II}? xxxxxxxx ŠU⸣ DINGIR *šag-gaš-šú na-kud* GAM (DPS III C r. 20 = *TDP* 26:80)

**If he was wounded on his head and, consequently, his hearing is low (and) his ears [. . .], "hand" of a murderous god; it is serious; he will die.

13.133 DIŠ IGI.MEŠ-*šú* NIGIN.ME *u su-qat-su* DU$_8$-*át ina* GIG-*šú* ÚŠ (DPS IX A 56 = *TDP* 76:56)

**If his face seems continually to be spinning and his chin was (cut) open, he will die during his illness.

ASSOCIATED GASTROINTESTINAL HEMORRHAGE The majority of patients with severe head injuries develop gastric erosions caused by elevated gastric acidity,[89] but only a few have clinically significant hemorrhages. Gastrointestinal bleeding usually occurs in the first days to one week following the injury. The quotes below describe this trauma complication.

13.134 DIŠ *ina* SAG.DU-*šú* SÌG-*iṣ-ma u* MÚD MUD ŠUB.ŠUB-*a* ŠU ^{d}MAŠ.TAB.BA GAM (DPS III C r. 18 = *TDP* 26:78; cf. StBoT 36.34 obv. 9′)

**If he was wounded on his head and, consequently, he continually produces dark blood, "hand" of the twin gods; he will die.

13.135 DIŠ *ina* SAG.DU-*šú* SÌG-*iṣ-ma u* MÚD *i-ḫa-ḫu* ŠU ^{d}MAŠ.TAB.BA GAM (DPS III C r. 19//E$_2$ r. 16 = *TDP* 26:79)

**If he was wounded on his head and, consequently, he vomits blood, "hand" of the twin gods; he will die.

TRAUMA TO THE SPINAL CORD

CERVICAL SPINE If the spinal cord is completely severed at the neck (cervical) level, it always causes leg paralysis (paraplegia), and depending on the cervical level, either partial or complete paralysis of the arms (quadriplegia).

13.136 DIŠ Á^{II}-*šú tur-ra* NU ZU-*e u* MÚD *i-te-eṣ-ṣi* EGIR-*ta*$_5$ SÌG-*iṣ* GAM (DPS X B r. 3 = *TDP* 86 r. 3)[90]

**If he is unable to turn his arms and he excretes blood, he was wounded from behind; he will die.

13.137 DIŠ UB.MEŠ-*š*[*ú ir*]*-mu-ú u* MÚD *i-te-ez-zi* EGIR-*ta*$_5$ SÌG-*iṣ* GAM (DPS XXII:38 [AOAT 43.255])

**If ⸢his⸣ limbs become ⸢limp⸣ and he excretes blood, he was wounded from behind; he will die.

Incomplete transection of the cord will cause a variable pattern of weakness and paralysis depending on the nerve tracts that have been interrupted. The second quote below lists impotence, a known consequence of cervical injury, while the third reference describes an intestinal problem that is probably ileus (see Chapter 6), and what seems to be either spastic paralysis of the lower extremities or flexion contractures secondary to paralysis.

13.138 DIŠ GÚ-⸢*su*⸣ KÚ-*su-ma* ⸢A⸣.[MEŠ API]N.MEŠ-*iš* ŠU ^{d}15 *ina* GÚ-*šú* SÌG-*iṣ* GAM (DPS X A obv. 8//B obv. 8 = *TDP* 80:8; cf. DPS XV:6 [AOAT 43.150])[91]

**If his neck hurts him (and) he continually ⸢asks⸣ for water, "hand" of Ištar. He was wounded on his neck; he will die.

13.139 DIŠ *ina* GÚ-*šú* SÌG-*iṣ-ma u du-us-su* KAR-*et* ŠU ^{d}15 GAM (DPS X A obv. 18//B obv. 20 = *TDP* 82:18)

**If he was wounded on his neck and his virility is taken away, "hand" of Ištar; he will die.

13.140 DIŠ *ina* GÚ-*šú* SÌG-*ma* ŠÀ.MEŠ-*šú it-te-nen-bi-ṭu u* GÌR^{II}-*šú na-šá-a* DIB GIDIM$_7$ (DPS X A obv. 19//B obv. 21 = *TDP* 82:19)[92]

**If he was wounded on his neck and consequently his insides are continually cramped and his feet are raised up, affliction by a ghost.

13.141 DIŠ *ina* GÚ-*šú* SÌG-*iṣ-ma e-lat* IGI^{II}-*šú* KÚ.ME-*šú* MÚD *ina* KIR$_4$/KA-*šú* ŠUB.ŠUB-*a* ŠU^{II}-*šú u* GÌR^{II}-*šú eṣ-la* NA BI ḪUL DIB-*su* (DPS X A obv. 21//B obv. 23–24 = *TDP* 82:21; cf. *CTN* 4.72 i 15′–19′ [Kinnier Wilson, *Iraq* 19.40–49 (ND 4368)])

**If he was wounded on his neck and consequently the upper part of his eyes continually hurts him, he continually produces blood from his nose/mouth, (and) his hands and his feet are sluggish (var. he lets his hands and feet hang; he cannot move his hands and feet [by himself]),[93] a *gallû* afflicts that person.[94]

SPINAL INJURY IN GENERAL The first quote below is likely to be describing ileus (intestinal paralysis), which is a complication of spinal cord injury (see Chapter 6). The second and third references list seizure of the patient's "nostrils" and "breath." These could be due to a high cervical injury leading to paralysis of the respiratory muscles. In the absence of a mechanical respiratory device, the patient would die quickly from anoxia.

13.142 DIŠ KI.MIN-*ma ina* GÚ.SIG$_4$-*šú* SÌG BAD-*ir-ma* KI.GUB-*su* NU ⸢È⸣-*a* ŠU GIDIM$_7$ *šag-ga-ši* GAM (DPS XV:46 [AOAT 43.152]; cf. DPS XII D iii 35//E iii 38–39 = *TDP* 106 iii 35)[95]

**If (it is the first day he is sick) and he was wounded on his spine and, he is stopped up so that his excrement cannot come out,[96] "hand" of a murderous ghost; he will die.

13.143 DIŠ ^{NA_4}KIŠIB GÚ-*šú* DU$_8$ GAM / DIŠ ^{NA_4}KIŠIB GÚ-*šú* DU$_8$ *na-ḫi-ra-šú* DIB.DIB GAM (DPS X A obv. 22 = *TDP* 82:22; cf. DPS XXI:16 [AOAT 43.247]; StBoT 36.60:7)

**If his vertebra was (cut) open, he will die. If his vertebra was cut open (and) his nostrils are continually "seized,"[97] he will die.

13.144 DIŠ ^{NA_4}KIŠIB GÚ-*šú* DU$_8$ SA.MEŠ-*šú* GAR-*nu u* PA.AN.BI *ina* KIR$_4$-*šú* DIB.DIB GIG BI NU DIN (DPS X A obv. 24//B obv. 27 = *TDP* 82:24; cf. *SpTU* 3.86 obv. 3–4)[98]

**If his vertebra was (cut) open (and) his blood vessels are present but his breath is "seized" in his nose, that patient will not get well.

Headaches

Headache is a very common symptom and is usually benign, although some types (e.g., migraines) can cause considerable discomfort.

13.145 DIŠ NA SAG.KI.DIB.BA TUKU.TUKU-*ši ana* TI-*šú* . . . (*BAM* 158 iv 18; *BAM* 9:21; *BAM* 480 iv 50′//*BAM* 4 iv 2′; *BAM* 482 i 1//*BAM* 11:1; *BAM* 482 iv 2)[99]

*If a person continually has an "affliction of the temples," to cure him . . .[100]

13.146 TUKUM.BI LÚ.Ù SAG.KI DIB-*su* . . . (*AMT* 20/1 i! 21′, 24′, 26′, 28′, 30′, 32′, 34′)

**If a person's temple afflicts him . . .

13.147 DIŠ NA SAG.KI-*šú* KÚ^{II}-*šú* . . . (*BAM* 482 i 64′)

**If a person's temples continually hurt him . . .

13.148 DIŠ LÚ SA SAG.KI-*šú* DIB-*su-ma* KÚ^{II}-*šú* . . . (*BAM* 482 ii 8)

**If the blood vessels of a person's temple afflict him and continually hurt him . . .

13.149 DIŠ ZI (-*ib* SA) SAG.KI *nu-úḫ-ḫi* . . . (*BAM* 482 ii 2//*BAM* 9:61//*BAM* 11:19//Jastrow, *TCPP* r. 13; *BAM* 482 ii 4//*BAM* 9:40; Labat, *RA* 53.10–11 obv. 14)[101]

**If (you want) to calm pulsating[102] of the temples/temporal blood vessels . . .

It would appear from one of the references in the diagnostic/prognostic handbook that a condition often referred to simply by the name of the demon who caused it, the *mukīl rēš lemutti*, was indeed as the literal translation of his name ("holder of the head of evil") implies, a generalized headache.

13.150 DIŠ NA *mu-kil* SAG ḪUL-*tim* DIB-*su* . . . (*BAM* 520 ii 8′)[103]

**If *mukīl rēš lemutti* afflicts a person . . .

13.151 DIŠ SAG.DU-*su* TÉŠ.BI DIB.DIB-*su* ŠU SAG.ḪUL.Ḫ[A.ZA DIN? : ŠU^{d}]⸢15?⸣ (coll.) (DPS III C obv. 38 = *TDP* 22:38)

**If his head continually afflicts him all over, "hand" of ⸢*mukīl*⸣ *rēš lemutti*, [he will get well (var. "hand" of] Ištar).

Modern physicians recognize a number of different types of headache. Similarly, ancient Mesopotamians devised separate treatments for asymmetrical headaches, symmetrical headaches, continuous headaches, and headaches with teary or bloodshot eyes. Headaches that were particularly painful (migraines) and/or particularly persistent (tension headaches) were often blamed on the action of malevolent ghosts.[104]

TENSION HEADACHES

Tension headaches are usually bilateral and viselike in character.

13.152 DIŠ NA SAG.KI.DIB.BA-*ma* SA GÚ-*šú* KÚ.MEŠ-*šú* ŠU.GIDIM.MA . . . (*AMT* 19/1 iv! 27′//*BAM* 482 iv 44′)[105]

**If a person has a headache and his neck muscles continually hurt him, "hand" of ghost . . .

Tension headaches are the only type that exhibit the peculiarity of being absolutely continuous day and night for long periods of time. Although sleep may be possible, whenever the patient awakens, the headache is present.

13.153 DIŠ LÚ GIDIM DIB-*su-ma* SAG.KI.DIB.BA TUKU.TUKU . . . (*BAM* 11:21, 23; *AMT* 102/1 i 8′)

**If a ghost afflicts a man so that he continually has a headache . . .

13.154 DIŠ NA SAG.KI DIB-*su-ma* TA ᵈUTU.È EN ᵈUTU.ŠÚ.A KÚ-*šú* ŠU.GIDIM$_7$.MA *a-ši-pu ki šá i-du-u li-te-ep-pu-uš* . . . (*BAM* 482 iii 7–8)[106]

**If a person's temples afflict him and hurt him from sunrise to sunset, "hand" of ghost; the *āšipu* should do what he knows (how to do) . . .

A common feature of tension headaches is the observation that analgesic remedies have relatively little effect in relieving the pain.

13.155 *šum-ma* SAG.KI.DIB.BA ŠU.GIDIM.MA *ina* SU NA *il-ta-za-az-ma* NU DU$_8$ *ina* IGI *ṣi-in-di* (*nap-šal-ti*) *ù* ÉN NU TAR-*as* . . . SAG.KI.DIB.BA MU.ZI (*AMT* 102/1 i 1–2, 6//*BAM* 483 ii 5′–6′//Jastrow, *TCPP* r. 29–30//*BAM* 9:42; *BAM* 482 iv 51′)

**If headache (and) "hand" of ghost will not let up from a person's body, (and) will not go away in the face of bandages, (salves), and incantations . . . the headache will be removed.

MIGRAINE HEADACHES

Migraine headaches may be asymmetrical with severe pulsating pain. If the migraine is one-sided, blood vessels on the affected side are often dilated, causing the temple on that side to feel warm, as in the last reference below.

13.156 [DIŠ N]A ŠU.GIDIM$_7$.MA DIB-*su-ma* SAG.KI^{II}-*šu i-tar-rak-šú* . . . (*BAM* 227:4′–5′//*AMT* 14/5 r. 3)

**[If] "hand" of ghost afflicts a ⌜person⌝ (so that) his temple throbs . . .

13.157 DIŠ ⌜NA⌝ *ina* DIB-*it* ŠU.GIDIM ZI SAG.KI TUKU.TUKU-[*ši*] *ana* KAR-*šú* . . . (*BAM* 7:1//*BAM* 482 iii 40′//*BAM* 9:1//*BAM* 158 i 1–2//Jastrow, *TCPP* r. 19)

**If a person, as a result of affliction by "hand" of ghost, continually experiences pulsating of the temples, to save him . . .

13.158 DIŠ SAG.KI-*šú šá* 15 ŠED$_7$-*át šá* 150 KÚM-*e-et* ŠU GIDIM$_7$ (DPS IV B obv. 22 = *TDP* 34:22)

**If his left temple (feels like it) is cold and his right one (feels like it) is hot, "hand" of ghost.[107]

Other features of migraine headaches include tearing, bloodshot eyes, nausea, and vomiting.

13.159 DIŠ NA SA SAG.KI 15/150-*šú* ZI-*ma* IGI 15/150-*šú* ÍR *ú-kal* . . . (*BAM* 3 iii 20//*BAM* 35 iv 1′//*AMT* 20/1 ii! 13′; *BAM* 3 iii 24//*BAM* 35 iv 4′//*AMT* 20/1 ii! 15′; *BAM* 6:1–2, 7–8)[108]

**If the blood vessels of a person's left/right temple (feel like they are) pulsating[109] and his left/right eye contains tears . . .

13.160 DIŠ NA SAG.KI 15/150-*šú* DIB-*su-ma* IGI 15/150-*šú* MÚD *ú-kal* . . . (*BAM* 3 iii 28//*BAM* 482 ii 26//*AMT* 20/1 ii! 3′; *BAM* 3 iii 31//*BAM* 482 ii 28//*AMT* 20/1 ii! 5′)[110]

**If a person's left/right temple afflicts him and his left/right eye contains blood . . .

13.161 DIŠ NA SAG.KI^{II}-*šú ṣab-ta-šú-ma* IGI^{II}-*šú* ÍR *ú-kal-la* . . . (*BAM* 482 ii 24//*BAM* 9 obv. 18)[111]

**If a person's temples afflict him and his eyes contain tears . . .

13.162 DIŠ NA SA SAG.KI-*šú* DIB-*su-ma* IGI^{II}-*šú* MÚD *ú-kal-la* . . . (*BAM* 3 iii 15)[112]

**If the blood vessel(s) of a person's temple afflict him and his eyes contain blood . . .

13.163 [DIŠ NA SA SAG.KI-*šú* D]IB-*su-ma* KÚ-*šú ù i-ár-rù* . . . (*BAM* 482 ii 11)

**[If blood vessels of a person's temple] ⌜afflict⌝ him and hurt him and he vomits . . .

FEBRILE HEADACHES

Headaches are also a frequent finding in infectious fevers (see Chapter 3).

13.164 DIŠ SAG.KI^{II}-*šú šá* 15 *u* 150 KÚ.MEŠ-*šú-ma* KÚM-*šú mit-ḫar* ŠU DINGIR-*šú* DIN / DIŠ SAG.KI^{II}-*šú šá* 15 *u* 150 KÚ.MEŠ-*šú-ma* KÚM-*šú* NU *mit-ḫar* ŠU DINGIR URU-*šú* GIG-*su* GÍD.DA-*ma* : [. . .]-*ma* DIN (DPS IV B obv. 32–33//E i 12–13 = *TDP* 36:33–34//*SpTU* 3.88 i 12–13)

**If his left and right temples hurt him and his temperature is normal, "hand" of his god; he will get well. If his left and right temples hurt him and his temperature is not normal, "hand" of the god of his city; his illness may be prolonged (var. [. . .]) but he will get well.

FATAL HEADACHES

Unfortunately, in addition to relatively harmless varieties, headaches may also be a symptom of severe neurological disorders, particularly tumors, abscesses, ruptured cerebral aneurysms, and cranial trauma. The last three references listed below are suggestive of ruptured cerebral aneurysms because of their severity (they are often described as the worst headache possible), but none of these texts provides enough information for a definitive diagnosis.

13.165 DIŠ SAG.KI-*šú* DIB-*su-ma* TA ^{d}UTU.ŠÚ.A EN EN.NUN UD.ZAL.LI *ur-rak* : *ú-šam-šá* GAM (DPS IV B obv. 12 = *TDP* 34:12; cf. *BAM* 482 iv 46′//*AMT* 19/1 iv! 29′)

**If his temple afflicts him and it lasts from sunset until the morning watch (var. it keeps him awake all night), he will die.

13.166 DIŠ *ši-bit* SAG.DU-*šú paṭ-rat* [GAM] / [*ši-bit*] SAG.DU-*šú paṭ-rat* ÚŠ : SAG.DU-*šú* TAG.MEŠ (DPS III A obv. 24//C obv. 15 = *TDP* 20:15 with commentary *STT* 403:22)[113]

**If the seam of his head (feels like it) is open, he will die. (That means) his head continually hurts him intensely.

13.167 DIŠ SAG.KI-*šú* DIB-*su-ma* KI.MIN SA SAG.KI-*šú ma-gal* ZI.MEŠ UGU SAG.DU-*šú* DU$_8$ ŠU GIDIM$_7$ GAM (DPS IV B obv. 8//D 8 = *TDP* 32:8; cf. *BAM* 482 iv 49′//*AMT* 19/1 iv! 32′–33′)

**If his temple afflicts him so that (he continually cries out), his temporal blood vessels (feel like they) are pulsating greatly, (and) the seam of his head (feels like it) is open, "hand" of ghost; he will die.

13.168 DIŠ SAG.KI-*šú* DIB-*su-ma* KI.MIN SA SAG.KI-*šú ma-gal* ZI.MEŠ *u e-li* SAG.DU-*šú ḫa-biš* GAM (DPS IV B obv. 9//D 9 = *TDP* 32:9)

**If his temple afflicts him so that (he continually cries out), his temporal blood vessels (feel like they) are pulsating greatly, (and) the upper part of his head (feels like it) was broken in pieces, he will die.

Seizure Disorders

Seizures occur as part of the symptoms of particular diseases, especially infections, tumors, and trauma. Seizures that recur are called epilepsy. The injured brain commonly reacts by becoming overly excited, a condition that can be visualized in modern times by an electroencephalogram (EEG). This excitement may be manifested by muscle contractions and abnormal sensory perceptions.

The type of changed behavior or neurological abnormality in the person depends upon where the excitement first starts in the brain and whether it spreads throughout the entire brain. If the seizure spreads quite rapidly over the entire brain in an older child or an adult, the seizure may be called grand mal while if the seizure is very brief or remains localized, other types of seizures, including focal seizures, sensory seizures, simple partial seizures, complex partial seizures, or gelastic seizures result. The *āšipu* referred to all of these seizures with the exception of gelastic seizures as "AN.TA.ŠUB.BA."

TECHNICAL TERMS FOR PHASES OF SEIZURES

LUḪ/*galātu* means "to jerk," and was also used to describe the reflex spasms of tetanus (see Chapter 3 with 3.197). When used in connection with a seizure as, for example, in the references below, LUḪ/*galātu* appears to refer to the actual jerking motion of the limbs, in contrast to the beginning of a grand mal seizure when the patient falls to the ground.

13.169 DIŠ NA *ina* KI.NÁ-*šú* LUḪ.LUḪ-*ut* GIN_7 GÙ ÙZ GÙ-*si i-ram-mu-um i-par-ru-ud ma-gal* DUG_4.DUG_4-*ub*/GÙ.GÙ-*si* ŠU[II] *be-en-ni* [d]ÀLAD *šá-né-e* [d]30 *ana* TI-*šú* . . . (BAM 202 r. 5′–7′//*BAM* 311:51′–53′)

**If a person continually *galātus* (LUḪ.LUḪ-*ut*) in his bed, he cries like a goat, he drones, he shudders, (and) he cries out/talks a lot, "hand" of *bennu*, a *šedû* deputized by Sîn; to cure him . . .

13.170 DIŠ NA *ina* KI.NÁ-*šú* LUḪ.LUḪ-*ut* . . . (*BAM* 376 ii 30′//*BAM* 377 iii 4//*BAM* 356 i 21)[114]

**If a person continually *galātus* (LUḪ.LUḪ-*ut*) in his bed . . .

Another word in Akkadian that appears to be related to seizure disorders is *ḫayyattu*. In medicine, *ḫayyattu* and the verb *ḫâṭu* are used to describe the stuporous, comatose state of cholera victims, as well as mental status changes or convulsions due to febrile diseases (see below). Their semantic range also encompasses the confused, disoriented state of mind associated with an epileptic seizure.

13.171 DIŠ LÁ-*šú* LÁ-*šum-ma ina* KA-*šú* ÚḪ DU-*ak* AN.TA.ŠUB.BA (DPS XXVI:15′ [AOAT 43.279])[115]

**If his *ḫayyattu* comes over him and spittle[116] flows from his mouth, AN.TA.ŠUB.BA (seizure).

13.172 DIŠ [L]Á-*šú* LÁ-*šum-ma* ŠU[II]-*šú u* GÌR[II]-*šú ana* GU-*šú ik-tab-ba* AN.TA.ŠUB.BA (DPS XXVI:16′ [AOAT 43.279])

**If his ⌜*ḫayyattu*⌝ comes over him and he bends his hands and his feet toward his neck, AN.TA.ŠUB.BA (seizure).

FEBRILE SEIZURES

Fevers of any cause are capable of triggering seizures, especially in infants and young children. The seizures are often benign and may not recur when the child grows older. The seizures described below are likely to be of this type.

13.173 DIŠ U_4-*mi-šam ana* GIZKIM-*šú* LÁ-*šú u* BAR-*šú* U_4 LÁ-*šú* KÚM-*ma* SA.MEŠ-*šú* KÚ.MEŠ-*šú* IR ŠUB-*su-ma ina-aḫ* LÁ-*ti* UD.DA (DPS XVI:81′–82′ [AOAT 43.179])[117]

**If daily, at the expected time, it comes over him and leaves him (and) when it comes over him, he becomes hot and his muscles continually hurt him (and) sweat comes out on him and then he finds relief, *ḫayyattu* due to *ṣētu* (enteric fever).

13.174 DIŠ NA NAM.ÉRIM DIB-*su-ma* KÚM *u* IR *ma-gal* TUKU.MEŠ U_4.1.KAM DIB-[*su*] U_4.1.KAM BAR-*šú ḫa-a-a-at-ti* KÚM TUKU.MEŠ KÚM *la ḫa-aḫ-ḫaš* DIB-*su-ma ana* KÚM *u ṣir-ḫa* TAR-*si*... (*BAM* 174 r. 29–31)

**If curse afflicts a person so that he has fever and a lot of sweat (and) one day it afflicts [him] (and) one day it releases him (and) he has febrile *ḫayyattu* (and) a lukewarm temperature afflicts him; to keep away fever and burning heat...

SEIZURES IN INFANTS

Seizures in infants may be manifested by a sudden dropping of the head and flexion of the arms.[118] The *āšipu* used the verb ŠUB/ *maqātu*: "to fall" and the related noun ŠUB/ *miqtu*: "falling (spell)" to describe these attacks, which can occur infrequently or hundreds of times a day. These terms were also used to describe the "falling spell" of a grand mal seizure (see below). The seizures in infants may be benign, resolving in childhood, but they can be indicative of a more serious problem. The prognosis tends to be worse as their frequency increases, as noted in the second reference.

13.175 DIŠ LÚ.TUR AN.TA.ŠUB.BA DIB-*su*... (Farber, *Schlaf* 116:1)[119]

**If AN.TA.ŠUB.BA (seizure) afflicts an infant...

13.176 DIŠ LÚ.TUR ŠUB-*tu* ŠUB-*su-ma ib-lu-uṭ* LÍL-*šú ú-ra-ak-ma* BA.ÚŠ (DPS XL A 49 = *TDP* 222:49)

**If *miqtu* falls on an infant and he recovers, (if) his illness is prolonged, he will die.

13.177 DIŠ LÚ.TUR *tu-la-a i-niq-ma mi-iq-tum* ŠUB-*su* ŠU ^{d}[15 : ^{d}30][120] (DPS XL A 60//B 60 = *TDP* 224:60)

**If an infant sucks the breast and then a *miqtu* falls on him, "hand" of [Ištar (var. Sîn)].

13.178 DIŠ LÚ.TUR *ki-ma al-du* U_4.2.KÁM U_4.3.KÁM DU-*ma* GA *la i-maḫ-ḫar mi-iq-tu ki-ma* ŠU.DINGIR.RA ŠUB.ŠUB-*su* ŠU ^{d}15 *ik-ki-im-tum* TAG-*šú* BA.ÚŠ (DPS XL A 26–27 = *TDP* 220:26–27)

**If an infant as soon as he is born (and after) two or three days pass, (his stomach) will not accept the milk and *miqtu* fall on him as in "hand" of god, "hand" of Ištar. The thieving one has touched him; he will die.

Infants having seizures are also described as "jerking," "trembling," and having "confusional states." The first two texts below indicate that the infant recovered, and therefore fit the definition of benign infantile seizures.

13.179 DIŠ LÚ.TUR *ig-da-na-al-lut u* LÙ.LÙ ŠU ^{d}30 AL.TI (DPS XL A 35 = *TDP* 220:35)[121]

**If an infant continually jerks and is restless, "hand" of Sîn; he will get well.

13.180 DIŠ LÚ.TUR KÚM NU TUKU IGI^{II}-*šú bal-ṣa* ŠU^{II}-*šú u* GÌR^{II}-*šú i-ra-ʾu-ba* ŠU ^{d}30 DIN (DPS XL A 120 = *TDP* 230:120)[122]

**If an infant does not have a fever, his eyes are dilated, (and) his hands and his feet tremble, "hand" of Sîn; he will get well.

13.181 DIŠ LÚ.TUR *ig-da-na-al-lut u* LÙ.LÙ-*aḫ ib-ta-nak-ki ip-ta-nar-ru-ud* ŠU^{II}-*šú u* GÌR^{II}-*šú* ÍL.ÍL-*ši* SÌG ^{d}30 *na-ag-mar-ti* TUKU-*ši* (DPS XL A 46//B 46 = *TDP* 222:46)

**If an infant continually jerks and is restless, he continually wails, he continually shudders, (and) he continually raises his hands and his feet, blow of Sîn; it will finish him off.[123]

13.182 KA.INIM.MA LÚ.TUR *le-zu pa-rid* ÍR.MEŠ LUḪ.LUḪ-*ut ḫa-a-a-at-tú* TUKU.MEŠ-*ši* ḪUN.GÁ.KE$_4$ . . . (Farber, *Schlaf* 62:192–193)

**Recitation for the infant continually shuddering, wailing, jerking, and having confusional states, to calm him . . .

Frequent seizures in infants can interfere with nutrition and development, and the following references appear to be describing this problem.

13.183 DIŠ LÚ.TUR ITI.3.KÁM *šu-nu-uq-ma* UZU.ME-*šú im-ta-ṭu-ú* ŠU^{II}-*šú u* GÌR^{II}-*šú it-ta-naq-na-an-na*/[: *im*]*-ta-nag-ga-ga ki-šid* SAḪAR (DPS XL A 4//C 4–5 = *TDP* 216:4)

**If an infant has been suckled for three months and his flesh diminishes (and) his hands and his feet are continually contorted (var. C: are continually ⌜rigid⌝), he was "gotten" by the dust.

13.184 DIŠ LÚ.TUR ITI.3.KÁM *tu-la-a i-niq-ma* ŠU^{II}-*šú u* GÌR^{II}-*šú it-ta-naq-na-an-na* UZU.MEŠ-*šú i-ma-aṭ-ṭu-ú ul-tu* ŠÀ AMA-*šú šu-ul-ḫu kiš-pi ep-šú-šú* (DPS XL A 18–19 = *TDP* 218:18–19)

**If an infant sucks the breast for three months and his hands and his feet are continually contorted (and) his flesh diminishes, sorcerous *šulḫu*[124] has been performed against him from the womb of his mother.

GRAND MAL SEIZURES

Patients with grand mal seizures typically lose all muscle control with violent muscle contractions, loss of consciousness, salivation, and urinary incontinence.[125] They frequently bite their tongues, and injure themselves when they fall.

13.185 DIŠ IGI-*šú i-ṣa*!*-par* NUNDUN-*šú* DU$_8$-*á*[*t*] ÚḪ-*šú*! *ina* KA-*šú* DU-*ak* ŠU^{II}-*šú* GÌR-*šú t*[*a*]*-lam-ma-šú* GIN$_7$ UDU.NITA *ṭa-ab-*[*ḫi*] *i*!*-nap-pa-aṣ* AN.TA.ŠUB.BA DIB-*su* (*STT* 89:141–143 [Stol, *Epilepsy* 94])[126]

**If his eye flutters, his lip(s) come apart, his spittle flows from his mouth, his hand, his foot, (and) his torso thrash around like (those of) a ⌜slaughtered⌝ sheep, AN.TA.ŠUB.BA (seizure) afflicts him.

13.186 DIŠ U$_4$ U$_6$.SÁ *i-re-eḫ-ḫu-šu* U.MEŠ ŠU^{II}-*šú u* GÌR^{II}-*šú i-nap-pa-ṣa* AN.TA.ŠUB.BA *ina ni-du-ti* KI.MIN *ina túb-qí* DIB-*su* (DPS XXVI:69′–70′ [AOAT 43.284])

**If, when a stupor flows over him, his fingers and toes thrash around, AN.TA.ŠUB.BA (seizure). It afflicted him in an abandoned place or in a corner.

Grand mal seizures may be triggered by low blood oxygen as would occur in cardiac arrest (see Chapter 8). Skin pallor ("green")[127] is common prior to or early in a seizure, but as the seizure progresses, the skin usually becomes flushed and even intensely red. Since seizures often occur at night, a patient might appear pallid in the evening prior to and flushed in the morning subsequent to nocturnal seizures.

13.187 [DIŠ ŠUB-*ti* ŠUB-*su-ma ina* U]$_4$.1.KÁM 2-*šú* 3-*šú* DIB-*su u i-ri-iq* GÍD-*ma ina* ŠUB-*ti* TAB.TAB-*šú* (DPS XXVI:6′ [AOAT 43.278]; Arnaud, *Emar* VI/4.694:10′)[128]

**[If a falling spell falls upon him and] it afflicts him/falls on him two or three times a ⌜day⌝ and he turns greenish, (if) it is prolonged, it begins with/grows out of the falling spell.

13.188 [DIŠ ŠUB-*ti* ŠUB-*su-ma*] *ina* U$_4$.1.KÁM 2-*šú* 3-*šú* KÚR/LÁ-*šum-ma*/ŠUB-*su ina šér-ti* SA$_5$ *ina* AN.USAN SIG$_7$ AN.TA.ŠUB.BA (DPS XXVI:5′ [AOAT 43.278]; Arnaud, *Emar* VI/4.694:9′)

**[If a falling spell falls upon him and] (his mentation) alters/(the falling spell) comes over him/falls upon him two or three times a day and in the morning he turns reddish (and) in the evening he turns greenish, AN.TA.ŠUB.BA (seizure).

POSTICTAL STATE

Following a grand mal seizure, patients commonly have weakness or paralysis (Todd's paralysis), and may remain in a confused or stuporous state for minutes or hours. In the following references, this postictal state is referred to by the *āšipu* as a *ḫayyattu* (see above) and attributed to the god Šamaš.

13.189 DIŠ GIG-*su* KU$_4$ *u* È U$_4$ LÁ-*šú* LÁ-*šú* ÍL IGI^{II}-*šú* DUGUD ŠU ^{d}UTU (DPS XVII:34 [AOAT 43.198])

**If his illness enters and leaves (and) when his *ḫayyattu* comes over him, lifting his eyes is difficult, "hand" of Šamaš.[129]

13.190 DIŠ GIG-*su* KU$_4$ *u* È U$_4$ LÁ-*šú* LÁ-*šú* MIN KA-*šú* DIB.DIB-*ma* U$_4$.1.KÁM U$_4$.2.KÁM NU DUG$_4$.DUG$_4$ ŠU 20 (DPS XVII:35–36 [AOAT 43.198])

**If his illness enters and leaves (and) when his *ḫayyattu* comes over him, (lifting his eyes is difficult and) his mouth is "seized" so that he cannot talk for one or two days,[130] "hand" of Šamaš.

In postictal states, muscle pain and tenderness are common, and secondary to the earlier, often violent, muscle contractions.

13.191 DIŠ GIG-*su* KU$_4$ *u* È KI.MIN Á.ÚR.MEŠ-*šú* TÉŠ.BI KÚ.MEŠ-*šú* ŠU ^{d}UTU (DPS XVII:37 [AOAT 43.198])[131]

**If his illness enters and leaves (and when his *ḫayyattu* comes over him), his limbs all hurt him at once, "hand" of Šamaš.

FOCAL SEIZURES

Sometimes the seizure clearly starts on one side of the brain, causing a unilateral reaction in the patient—these are called "focal (Jacksonian) seizures." Often, focal seizures spread to the rest of the brain to become generalized seizures, as in the second reference below.

13.192 DIŠ *ù*ʾ*-a a-i* GÙ.GÙ*-si i-leb-bu* ÚḪ *ina* KA*-šú* DU*-ak u* GÚ*-su ana* 150 *zi-ir* AN.TA.ŠUB.B[A] (DPS XXVI:77′ [AOAT 43.285])

**If he continually cries out: "Ua ai!"[132] he groans, his spittle flows from his mouth and his neck is twisted to the right, ⸢AN.TA.ŠUB.BA⸣ (seizure).

13.193 DIŠ GIG GÚ*-su ana* 15 NIGIN.ME ŠU^{II}*-šú u* GÌR^{II}*-šú am-šá* IGI^{II}*-šú* DUL*-ma* BAL-⸢*ma*⸣ *ina* KA*-šú* ÚḪ DU*-ak i-ḫar-ru-ur* AN.TA.ŠUB.BA (DPS X A obv. 1–2//B obv. 1–2//DPS IX A 80//B r. 27 = *TDP* 80:1–2// *TDP* 78:80)

**If the patient continually turns his head to the left, his hands and his feet are immobilized, he closes and rolls his eyes, and spittle flows from his mouth (and) he makes rumbling noises, AN.TA.ŠUB.BA (seizure).[133]

13.194 DIŠ GIG GÚ*-su ana* 150 NIGIN.ME ŠU^{II}*-šú u* GÌR^{II}*-šú tar-ṣa* IGI^{II}*-šú ana* IGI AN-*e na-pal-ka-a ina* KA*-šú* ÚḪ DU*-ak i-ḫar-ru-ur* NÍ*-šú* NU ZU *ina taq-ti-it* [LÁ*-š*] *ú iḫ-ta-niṭ-ṭa-áš-šú* AN.TA.ŠUB.BA ŠU ^{d}30[134] (DPS X A obv. 4–6//B obv. 4–6 = *TDP* 80:4–6)

**If the patient continually turns his head to the right, his hands and his feet are stretched out, his eyes are opened wide toward the sky, spittle flows from his mouth, he makes rumbling noises, he does not know who he is at the beginning when ⸢his⸣ [confusional state] comes over him, AN.TA.ŠUB.BA (seizure), "hand" of Sîn.[135]

SENSORY SEIZURES

Sometimes a seizure is accompanied by pain somewhere in the body; these are called "sensory seizures."

13.195 *šum*$_4$*-ma* U$_4$*-ma* UD.DU-[*šú*] IGI^{II}*-šú tar-ka i-ḫar-ru-ur* ÚḪ *ina* KA*-šú* DU AN.TA.ŠUB.BA DIB*-su šum*$_4$*-ma* U$_4$ DIB*-šú* ÍR *ina* IGI*-šú* DU*-ak ku-bu-ut-ta i-ṣa-bat a-aḫ-ka la ta-nam-di* (*STT* 89:136b–140 [Stol, *Epilepsy* 93])

**If when it comes over [him], his eyes are dark, he makes rumbling noises, (and) spittle flows from his mouth, AN.TA.ŠUB.BA (seizure) afflicts him. If, when it afflicts him, tears come to his eyes, he is about to enter a difficult (phase); do not be negligent.[136]

13.196 DIŠ ŠUB*-tu* ŠUB*-su-ma* GIN$_7$ GU$_4$ [. . .] *i-ra-mu-um* NUNDUN.MEŠ*-šú* [. . .] AN.TA.ŠUB.BA DIB*-su šum*$_4$*-m*[*a* . . .] ÍR *ár-ḫiš* DU$_8$ *šum*$_4$*-ma* x[. . .] (*STT* 89:148–151 [Stol, *Epilepsy* 94])

**If a falling spell falls upon him and he [. . .] like an ox, he drones, his lips [come apart] [. . .] AN.TA.ŠUB.BA (seizure) afflicts him. If [. . .] the tears will quickly go away; if [. . .]

PETIT MAL SEIZURES

Some seizures are only manifested by brief periods of unresponsiveness, blinking, and blank stares. These are called "absence" or "petit mal" seizures.

13.197 DIŠ DIB-*tu ina* DÙG.GA KÚ NAG *u ḫa-di-*⸢*i*⸣ [DIB-*su-ma* . . .] *ki-ma e-ri-šu-ma* APIN-*iš-ma* NAG [. . .] U_4 DIB-*su um-taš-še-ru* GIN_7 *šá* [. . .] NÍ-*šú* NU ZU AN.TA.ŠUB.BA (*STT* 89:159–162 [Stol, *Epilepsy* 95])

**If the affliction [afflicts him] while he is in a good mood, eating, drinking, and happy [. . .] he asks (for things) just as he was asking (for them before) and drinks [just as he was drinking before?] (but), when his affliction leaves him, like one who [. . .] he himself does not know, AN.TA.ŠUB.BA (seizure).

SIMPLE PARTIAL SEIZURES

Simple partial seizures can occur with motor or sensory signs and symptoms. A simple partial seizure with motor signs consists of contractions of the muscles of one part of the body without loss of consciousness and is caused by epileptiform discharges in the motor cortex on the opposite side. Sensory symptoms (parasthesias and a sensation of dizziness) occur with epileptiform discharges in the opposite sensory cortex. The following sequenced references occur in a part of the diagnostic/prognostic handbook that details types of seizures.[137] Accompanying them is an entry describing hallucinations that may have been included because patients having a simple partial seizure with epileptiform discharges in the temporal and frontal lobes may experience hallucinations.

13.198 DIŠ UB.NÍGIN.NA-*šú i-tar-ru-ra i-ṭa-ma-a u* IGI.MEŠ-*šú* NIGIN.MEŠ-*du* AN.TA.ŠUB.BA *ina ma-šal* U_4-*mi* DUGUD-*su* / DIŠ UB.NÍGIN.NA-*šú i-šam-ma-ma-šú ú-zaq-qa-ta-šú u* IGI.ME-*šú* NIGIN.ME-*du* AN.TA.ŠUB.BA *ina ma-šal* U_4-*mi* DUGUD-*su* (DPS XXVI:71′–72′ [AOAT 43.284])

**If his limbs tremble (and) twist and his face seems continually to spin, AN.TA.ŠUB.BA (seizure) . . . If his limbs go numb (and) sting him and his face seems continually to spin, AN.TA.ŠUB.BA (seizure) . . .

COMPLEX PARTIAL SEIZURES

Complex partial seizures (previously called psychomotor or temporal lobe seizures) are associated with a variety of automatisms, such as lip smacking, hand wringing, or plucking at clothes. Some patients, especially children, may have abdominal complaints associated with these seizures, including nausea, pain, and distention as in the second reference.

13.199 DIŠ *šá* DIB-*šú šu-te-eq-ru-ub* U_4 LÁ-*šú* $ŠU^{II}$-*šú* GIN_7 *šá ku-uṣ-ṣú* DIB-*šú i-ḫe-es-si* $GÌR^{II}$-*šú* LAL-*aṣ u ma-gal* LUḪ-*ut-ma ina-aḫ* DIB-*su* IGI.BAR-*as* ŠU *ʾe-e-li* (DPS XXVI:43′–44′ [AOAT 43.282])

**If what afflicts him does so in close sequence (and) when it comes over him, he wrings his hands like one whom cold afflicts, he stretches out his feet and he jerks a lot and then is quiet, (and) gazes at the one who afflicts him,[138] "hand" of the binder.[139]

13.200 [*ṣi*]-*bit be-en-nim šá ina* MU.7.KÁM Ù.TU IGI *ia-a-az-za* [ŠÀ-*šú*] *i-ta-na-šá-áš ina* ŠUB-*šú* ŠU^{II}-*šú ana* EGIR-*šú* NIGIN-*mi* (K 3628+4009+Sm. 1315 r. 18′–19′)

**⌜Affliction⌝ of *bennu* that is observed in the seventh year (after) birth: he makes senseless noises, [his stomach] is continually upset, (and) during his falling spell he winds his hands behind him.

Some patients may have a warning of an oncoming seizure by an "aura" such as an unusual odor, a feeling that the current experience has happened before, a sudden intense emotional feeling, a sensory illusion, or a specifically formed sensory hallucination. Patients come to recognize these as heralding their seizures.

13.201 ⌜DIŠ⌝ U_4 LÁ-*šú ta-lam-ma-šú* DUGUD-*su u ú-zaq-qat-su* EGIR-*nu* LÁ-*šum-ma* NÍ-*šú i-maš-ši* AN.TA.ŠUB.BA *ina ma-šal* U_4-*mi* DUGUD-*su* (DPS XXVI:26′–27′ [AOAT 43.280])

**If when (a confusional state) comes over him, his torso (feels) heavy and stings him (and) afterward it comes over him and he forgets himself, AN.TA.ŠUB.BA (seizure). (If this happens) in the middle of the day, it will be difficult for him.[140]

13.202 [DIŠ ŠUB-*ti* ŠUB-*su-ma* U_4 ŠUB-*š*] *ú an-nu-ú šu-ú i-qab-bi be-en-nu ṣa-i-du* DIB-*su uš*-[*t*]*e*-⌜*zeb*⌝ (DPS XXVI:4′ [AOAT 43.278]; cf. Arnaud, *Emar* VI/4.694:7′–8′)

** [If a falling spell falls upon him and when it falls upon] ⌜him⌝, he says "This is it," spinning *bennu* afflicts him; he will come through.[141]

13.203 DIŠ KI.MIN U_4 DIB-*šú an-nu-ú šu-ú i-qab-bi* ŠU KI.SIKIL.LÍL.L[Á.EN.NA] (DPS XXVI:39′ [AOAT 43.281])

**If (his affliction always afflicts him in the evening and) when it afflicts him, he says "This is it," "hand" of *ardat* ⌜*lilî*⌝ (see Chapter 19 with 19.55–19.59).

The attribution to a "murderous ghost" in the following references is presumably due to the presence of hallucinations and the fatal outcome (see below under Status Epilepticus).

13.204 [DIŠ G]IN_7 ŠUB-*ti* ŠUB.ŠUB-*su* IGI^{II}-*šú* MÚD DIRI.MEŠ : IGI^{II}-*šú* BAD-*te u* DUL-*am* UNU^{II}-*šú*/[M]E.ZÉ-*šú nu-uš-šá* ŠU^{II}-*šú u* GÌR^{II}-*šú tar-ṣa ina sa-naq a-ši-pi i*ʾ-*a-bat ša* DIB-*šú ina-ṭal* ŠU $GIDIM_7$ *šag-ga-ši* (DPS XXVI:11′–13′ [AOAT 43.279])

** [If] it continually falls upon him ⌜like⌝ a falling spell (and) his eyes are full of blood (var. he opens and closes his eyes), his cheeks/⌜jaws⌝ shake, his hands and his feet are stretched out, he collapses at the approach of the *āšipu* (and) he can see the one who afflicts him,[142] "hand" of a murderous ghost.[143]

13.205 DIŠ *la-am* DIB-*šú ru-qiš* GI[N_7 x] ⌜xxx⌝ ki *it-tap-la-as* GIN_7 *it-tap-la-su da-da-nu-šú* KÚ.MEŠ-*šú ba-mat-s*[*u* . . .] ⌜xx⌝ ŠUB-⌜*ti*⌝ ŠUB.ŠUB-*su* ŠU $GIDIM_7$ *šag-ga-ši* GAM (DPS XXVI:51′–52′ [AOAT 43.283])

**If before it afflicts him, he gazes at something very far off[144] ⌜like⌝ [. . .] (and) when he gazes at it, his neck muscles continually hurt him, ⌜his⌝ chest [. . .], (and) falling spells continually fall upon him, "hand" of a murderous ghost; he will die.

GELASTIC SEIZURES

Gelastic seizures are episodes of laughing unrelated to a situation that would normally trigger laughing, due to abnormal brain wave activity.

13.206 D[IŠ] ⌜GIN$_7$⌝ ŠUB-*šú i-ri-iq-ma ma-gal i-ṣi-iḫ u* GÌR^{II}-*šú it-ta-naq-na-an-na* : ŠU^{II}-*šú u* GÌR^{II}-*šú* ŠU LÍL.LÁ.EN.NA (DPS XXVI:14′ [AOAT 43.279])

**⌜If⌝ when (a falling spell) falls upon him, he turns pale and laughs a lot and his feet (var. his hands and his feet) are continually contorted, "hand" of *lilû*.[145]

STATUS EPILEPTICUS

Seizures occurring one right after another are referred to as "status epilepticus." The severe stress related to this condition can often lead to death unless the process can be stopped.

13.207 [DIŠ ŠUB-*ti* ŠUB-*su-ma ina*] ⌜U$_4$⌝-*mi šu-a-tum* 7-*šú uš-ter-de-ma* DIB-*su uš-te-zeb šum-ma* 8-*šú-nu* ŠUB-*aš-šú ul uš-te-*[*zib*] (DPS XXVI:7′ [AOAT 43.279])

** [If a falling spell falls upon him and] it afflicts him seven times on the same day one after the other, he will come through. If eight of them[146] fall on him, he will not come through.

13.208 DIŠ KI.MIN-*ma i-*[*na* KI.NÁ]-*šú* GIN$_7$ MUŠEN *ù'* GÙ.GÙ-*si u* LUḪ.LUḪ-*ut ana* U$_4$.3.KÁM GAM (DPS XV:90 [AOAT 43.155])

**If (it is the first day he is sick) and like a bird he continually cries out "ua" ⌜in⌝ his [sleep] and he continually jerks, (after he has been sick) for three days, he will die.

13.209 [DIŠ ŠUB]-*ti* ŠUB-*su-ma ina* U$_4$ *šú-a-tum* 7-*šú uš-tir-di-ma i-ḫi-is-su e-nu-ma um-taš-ši-ru-šú i-ṭi-ib* ŠU *šag-ga-ši* GAM (DPS XXVI:9′–10′ [AOAT 43.279])

** [If] a ⌜falling spell⌝ falls on him and, on the same day, (confusional states) come over him seven times one right after the other (and), when (the confusional state) has left him, he feels better,[147] "hand" of a murderous (ghost); he will die.

Narcolepsy-Cataplexy Syndrome

The narcolepsy-cataplexy syndrome is characterized by a tetrad of symptoms: sleep attacks, cataplexy, sleep paralysis, and vivid hypnagogic hallucinations (presleep dreams). The "sleep attacks" appear as clinically normal sleep but are characteristically brief (about fifteen minutes). Patients usually wake refreshed, and there is a refractory period of from one to a few hours before the next attack occurs. Between attacks, the patient is sleepy and inattentive; waking behaviors may become automatic and interrupted by "microsleeps." Nocturnal sleep is usually also disturbed by frequent awakenings. The following reference appears to be describing a "sleep attack."

13.210 DIŠ NA KI.NÁ-*ma šit-ta-šu* UGU-*šú* DÙG.GA ZI-*ma i-ka-šu-uš* GUR-[*ma* KI.NÁ] *ana* TI-*šú* . . . (*AMT* 47/1:1–2)

**If a person goes to sleep and his sleep is pleasing to him (but) when he gets up, he feels exhausted and goes back [to sleep]; to cure him . . .

The following reference, which appears to describe vivid (auditory) hallucinations combined with sleep attacks, may be a description of narcolepsy.

13.211 DIŠ *ik-ki-lu* GÙ.GÙ-*šú* U$_4$ GÙ.GÙ-*šú šú-ú i-ta-nap-pal-šú it-ta-na-as-pak* ZI-*ma i-kàš-šú-uš* ZI-*bé u* DU$_{10}$.GAM GIG-*su uš-te-zeb* MAŠKIM *mur-tap-pi-du* DIB-*su* (DPS XXVI:89′–90′ [AOAT 43.286])[148]

**If a mournful cry continually cries out to him (and) when it cries out to him, he continually answers it, he continually behaves like an animal caught in a trap[149] (and) when he gets up, he feels exhausted (and) he gets up but (has to) squat down, he will come through his illness; a roving *rābiṣu* afflicts him.

The references below may be describing cataplexy (sudden relaxation of muscle tone caused by a generalized motor inhibition) or sleep paralysis (brief episodes of generalized paralysis on wakening). In its most severe form, the cataplectic attack results in total flaccid paralysis and collapse to the floor, as in the first reference. Less severe symptoms may consist of a sagging of the jaw or head, speechlessness, or a feeling of weakening of the knees. The *āšipu* appears to have attributed narcolepsy to the *rābiṣu*-demon and cataplexy to the action of the *gallû*-demon (the ancestor of our "ghoul"). Although 80 percent of patients with narcolepsy also have a history of cataplexy, narcolepsy and cataplexy are best managed by means of two separate classes of drugs, which may explain why the *āšipu* seems to have given them separate diagnoses.

13.212 [DIŠ N]A *ina a-la-ki-šú ana* IGI-*šú* ŠUB-*ma* IGI^{II}-*šú ip-pal-ka-ma tur-ra* ⸢*la i*⸣*-da-a* [Š]U^{II}-*šú* GÌR^{II}-*šú ra-man-šú la ú-na-aš* NA BI ḪUL DIB-*su* GIN$_7$ AN.TA.ŠUB.BA *uš-tar-ri-šú/ir-te-ne-ḫi-šú* (DPS XXVII:16–17 [AOAT 43.298]; *CTN* 4.72 i 3′–5′ [Kinnier Wilson, *Iraq* 19.40–49 (ND 4368)])[150]

**[If] as a ⸢person⸣ is walking,[151] he falls down on his face and he opens his eyes wide and does not know how to turn them (and) he cannot move his hands and feet by himself, a *gallû* afflicts that person. It begins for him/flows over him like AN.TA.ŠUB.BA (seizure).[152]

13.213 [DIŠ NA] GIN$_7$[153] AN.TA.ŠUB.BA *ir-te-ne-eḫ-ḫi-šú* ŠU^{II}-*šú u* GÌR^{II}-*šú* NÍ-*šú la ú-na-aš* NA BI ḪUL DIB-*su* (DPS XXVII:18 [AOAT 43.298]; restored from *CTN* 4.72 i 26′ [Kinnier Wilson, *Iraq* 19.40–49 (ND 4368)]; Nougayrol, *RA* 73.64–65 [AO 7760] iii 7′–9′)

**[If] something like AN.TA.ŠUB.BA (seizure) continually flows over [a person] (and) he cannot move his hands and feet by himself, a *gallû* afflicts that person.

Encephalomyelitis/Encephalopathy

Infections of the brain, spinal cord, or both are called encephalitis, myelitis, or encephalomyelitis, respectively. The cause of these infections is usually a virus: *Herpes simplex, Varicella zoster,* polio virus, or one of many arthropod-borne viruses. Not infrequently, the virus can be an indirect cause of nervous system disease by triggering an immunological process that usually becomes symptomatic after the acute infection has receded. This is referred to as postinfectious encephalopathy.

The general signs and symptoms that are commonly seen in encephalitis include fever, headache, decreased light tolerance (photophobia), and varying levels of depressed cognition. Infections of the spinal cord (myelitis) produce varying degrees of weakness or paralysis in the affected parts of the body. Specific viruses may have a tendency to affect certain parts of the brain or spinal cord, presenting with corresponding neurological abnormalities. However, there is a great degree of variability in affected areas and neurologic findings, making it difficult to determine the causative organism from the clinical presentation. The following two references, both attributed to ghosts, have many of the features of encephalomyelitis or meningoencephalitis (see below), including headache, ringing ears (tinnitus), muscle weakness, low back pain, and light-sensitive eyes (photophobia; see Chapter 9).

13.214 DIŠ NA SAG.KI.DIB.BA TUKU.TUKU-*ši* GEŠTU^{II}-*šú i-šag-gu-ma* IGI^{II}-*šú i-bar-ru-ra* SA.GÚ-*šú* KÚ.MEŠ-*šu* Á^{II}-*šú šim-ma-tum* TUKU.TUKU-*ši* ÉLLAG-*su ú-maḫ-ḫa-as-su* ŠÀ-*šú da-li-iḫ* GÌR^{II}-*šú ri-mu-tú* TUKU.TUKU-*ši* NA BI GIDIM *ri-da-a-ti* ÚS.MEŠ-*šú ana* TI.LA-*šu* . . . (*BAM* 228:23–27//*BAM* 229 obv. 17′–21′//*BAM* 323:89–92)

**If a person continually has headaches, his ears roar, his eyes become dimmed, his neck muscles continually hurt him, his arm(s) are continually numb, his kidney (costophrenic angle) gives him a jabbing pain, his heart is troubled, his feet are continually limp, a pursuing ghost continually follows that person, to cure him . . .

13.215 DIŠ ŠÀ-*šú* MUD.MUD-*ud* SAG ŠÀ-*šú* GU$_4$.UD.MEŠ IGI^{II}-*šú ana e-ṭú-ti* NIR.NIR-*aṣ* ŠU GIDIM$_7$ (DPS XIII B ii 15–16 = *TDP* 118 ii 15–16)

**If his heart flutters, his upper abdomen (epigastrium) pulses rapidly, (and) he stretches out his eyes toward the darkness, "hand" of ghost.

The following three texts display other features of encephalomyelitis, including muscle weakness (paralysis), eyes that "shudder" (probably pendular nystagmus), eyes that "stand still" (ocular paralysis),[154] and a mouth that is "too strong for the words" (presumably spasm or weakness of the muscles involved in speech).

13.216 [DIŠ MURUB$_4$.MEŠ-*šú*] GIG-*ma* ZI-*bi u* DU$_{10}$.GAM *šit-ta-šú* NU *ú-kal* [*u* KA-*šú*] *ana* KA *da-an* GAM [DIŠ MU]RUB$_4$ ⌜*u* ŠÀ⌝-*šú* GIG-*ma* ZI-*bi u* DU$_{10}$.GAM NINDA NU KÚ KAŠ NU NAG IGI^{II}-*šú pár-da* GAM (DPS XII D iv 1–4//E iv 6–9 = *TDP* 106 iv 1–4)

**[If his pelvic region] is so sick that he gets up and (has to) squat down, he does not remember his dreams[155] [and his mouth] is too strong for the words, he will die. [If] his

⌜pelvic region⌝ and abdomen are so sick that he gets up and (has to) squat down, he does not eat bread, he does not drink beer, (and) his eyes "shudder" (exhibit pendular nystagmus), he will die.

13.217 DIŠ GIG MURUB$_4$ GIG-*ma* ZI-*bi u* DU$_{10}$.GAM GABA-*su* BAD.BAD-*te* KA-*šú ana* INIM.INIM *da-an* IGI^{II}-*šú* GUB.GUB-*za* GAM (DPS XVII:54–55 [AOAT 43.200])

**If he is sick with an illness of the pelvic region and he gets up and (has to) squat down, his chest is clear[156] (but) his mouth is too strong for the words (and) his eyes continually stand (still), he will die.

13.218 DIŠ GIG MURUB$_4$ *u* ŠÀ GIG-*ma* ZI-*bi u* DU$_{10}$.GAM *rit-ta-šú paṭ-rat* KA-*šú ana* INIM.INIM *da-an* GAM (DPS XVII:56 [AOAT 43.200])[157]

**If he is sick with an illness of the pelvic region and abdomen and he gets up and (has to) squat down, his hand will open (but) his mouth is too strong for the words, he will die.

The altered breathing described in the following reference ("his breath is 'seized' in his mouth so that he makes his breath go out through his nose") might be due to paralysis of the muscles of respiration and/or the vagus nerve, as happens with polio virus infections.

13.219 DIŠ SAG.DU-*su* KÚM-*im* SA SAG.KI^{II}-*šú* ŠU^{II}-*šú u* GÌR^{II}-*šú* 1-*niš* ZI.MEŠ GÌR^{II}-*šú* EN *kin-ṣi-šú* ŠED$_7$ x[. . .] SAG KIR$_4$-*šú* GI$_6$ 40 U.MEŠ-*šú* SIG$_7$ ŠUB-*ú* ŠÀ IGI^{II}-*šú* SIG$_7$ *u* BABBAR ŠUB PA IGI^{II}-*šú* 2.TA.ÀM DIB.DIB (*ḫe-pí*) x[. . .] *na-pi-is-su ina* KA-*šú* DIB-*ma ina* KIR$_4$-*šú* GARZA *uš-ti-ṣi mu-tim ana* ZI-*šú ú-še-la-a* x x[. . .] (DPS III C obv. 52–54 = *TDP* 24:52–54)

**If his head is hot (and) the blood vessel(s) of his temples, his hands, and his feet all seem to pulsate together, his feet are cold as far as the legs, [. . .], the bulb of his nose is dark, his hands and arms[158] are unevenly colored with yellow, there are yellow and white discolorations in his eyes, both upper and lower eyelids are "seized," [. . .] his breath is "seized" in his mouth so that he makes his breath go out through his nose, it has made death mount to his throat, [. . .][159]

Meningitis

Meningitis is usually an acute bacterial infection of the membranes covering the brain (meninges) plus the exterior surface of the brain. Its signs and symptoms include pain and muscle spasm on bending the neck forward (neck stiffness), fever, focal neurologic abnormalities, and progressive depression of mental activity ending in coma and death. Meningitis must have occurred in ancient Mesopotamia and the following references may be examples.

13.220 DIŠ GEŠTU^{II}-*šú kab-ta-šú* UŠ$_4$-*šu* KÚR.KÚR-*šu u* INIM.INIM-*šu it-te-ni-ip-rik-ku* GAM (DPS VIII 14 = *TDP* 70:14)

**If his ears (feel) heavy, his mentation is continually altered, and his words hinder each other in his mouth, he will die.

13.221 DIŠ LÚ.TUR ITI.1.KÁM ITI.2.KÁM *šu-nu-uq-ma* ŠUB-*tu* ŠUB-*su-ma* ŠU^{II}-*šú u* GÌR^{II}-*šú am-šá* ŠU.DINGIR.RA-*ku* KI-*šú a-lid ina* GÌR-*šú lu* AD-*šú lu* AMA-*šú* ÚŠ (DPS XL A 110 = *TDP* 228/230:110)[160]

**If the infant is breast fed for one or two months and then falling spell(s) fall upon him and his hands and his feet are immobilized, "hand" of god was born with him; either his father or his mother will die at his foot.

13.222 [DIŠ . . .] *niš-mu-šú* DUGUD *ina* LÍL-*šú* GÚ-*su* [ŠUB-*su* . . .] ⌜*šá*⌝ 150 ŠED$_7$ ŠU NAM.ERÍM[161] [GAM] (DPS XIII J5–6 = *TDP* 126 iii 37–38)

**[If. . .] his hearing is difficult, during the course of the illness, his neck falls (i.e., he lets it drop), [his left temple (feels like it) is hot] (and) his right one (feels like it) is cold (i.e., he has a severe headache), "hand" of curse; he will die.

The following reference is unlikely to be describing a patient with bacterial meningitis, since they rarely survive without antibiotic therapy. However, headache, tinnitus, painful neck muscles, back pain, and muscle weakness are also typical of viral meningoencephalitis, which has a much lower fatality rate (see Chapter 17 with 17.151–17.152).

13.223 DIŠ NA SAG.KI.DIB.BA TUKU.TUKU-*ši* GEŠTU^{II}-*šú i-šag-gu-ma* IGI^{II}-*šú i-bar-ru-ra* SA.GÚ-*šú* KÚ.MEŠ-*šu* Á^{II}-*šú šim-ma-tum* TUKU.TUKU-*ši* ÉLLAG-*su ú-maḫ-ḫa-as-su* ŠÀ-*šú da-li-iḫ* GÌR^{II}-*šú ri-mu-tú* TUKU.TUKU-*ši* NA BI GIDIM *ri-da-a-ti* ÚS.MEŠ-*šú ana* TI.LA-*šu* . . . (*BAM* 228:23–27//*BAM* 229 obv. 17′–21′//*BAM* 323:89–92)

**If a person continually has headaches, his ears roar, his eyes become dimmed, his neck muscles continually hurt him, his arm(s) are continually numb, his kidney gives him a jabbing pain, his heart is troubled, his feet are continually limp, a pursuing ghost continually follows that person, to cure him . . .[162]

Space-Occupying Lesions

When a brain tumor, abscess, or any lesion grows inside the brain or spinal canal it will cause neurologic signs and symptoms because of pressure on adjacent nerves. The problem is worsened by the rigid and unyielding nature of the skull and spinal canal. This condition is called a "space-occupying lesion." Many of the findings in the texts attributed to brain tumor and abscess, as seen below, are due to the space-occupying phenomenon.

BRAIN TUMORS

The following text is likely to be a brain tumor because it is slowly progressive, but a fatal outcome is expected. Brain abscesses in ancient Mesopotamia would have had a fatal outcome in most cases, but they would generally have progressed more rapidly than a brain tumor.

13.224 [DIŠ ŠUB-*ti* ŠUB]-*su-ma* MU.1.KÁM ŠUB-*šú-ma ana* GIZKIM-*šú-ma* LÁ-*šú na-kid* AN.TA.ŠUB.BA *ina ma-šal* U$_4$-*mi uš-ta-qar-rab-šú-ma* DUGUD-*su* (DPS XXVI:8′ [AOAT 43.279])

**[If a falling spell falls upon] him and it has been falling upon him for one year and as its sign it comes over him, it is worrisome. If the AN.TA.ŠUB.BA (seizure) comes closely spaced (and) in the middle of the day, it will be difficult for him.

In the following reference, the combination of headache and a cranial nerve sign suggests that the patient might have had a tumor in the brain stem itself or perhaps was deteriorating from increased intracranial pressure brought about by a tumor above the brain stem, which can mimic brain stem signs.

13.225 *šum*$_4$*-ma* SAG.ḪUL.ḪA.ZA GIG-*ma ki-ma* GU$_4$ GÌR IGI.IGI IGI.LÁ GIG BI NU *i-ke-šir* (DPS XXVIII:21 [AOAT 43.310])

**If he is sick with a *mukīl rēš lemutti* (i.e., a mild headache; see above) and just as an ox continually looks at (its own) feet, he looks (at his own feet), that patient will not do well.

BRAIN ABSCESSES

Most brain abscesses in ancient Mesopotamia would have been fatal because surgical drainage would not have been possible, and antibiotic therapy, even if available in some of their medications, was not likely to have been used at the high concentrations achievable in modern pharmaceuticals. In the reference below, the *āšipu* describes a patient with an ear infection with neurologic problems. It seems likely that the ear infection led to a brain abscess, and that the brain abscess was able to drain through the ear to provide a cure.

13.226 [DIŠ DIB DI]B-*su-ma* UZU.MEŠ-*šú* ⌜*ú*⌝*-za!-qat ri-mu-tú* ⌜TUKU⌝-[*š*]*i* [. . .]x-ni *ina* DUG$_4$.DUG$_4$-*šú* ur x GAR-*nu ù ir-te-*[*ḫ*]*a* [*re-ḫ*]*u-ut* ^{d}*Šul-pa-è-a* DIB-*su šum*$_4$*-ma* U$_4$ [D]IB-*šú* [GEŠTU] ZAG-*šú* KÚM TÉŠ.MEŠ-*aš* GIG-*su* DU$_8$ *šum*$_4$*-ma* U$_4$*-ma* DIB-*šú* [GEŠTU] GÙB-*šú* KÚM TÉŠ.MEŠ-*aš* GIG-*šú* GÍD.DA-*ma* (*STT* 89:167–171 [Stol, *Epilepsy* 95])

**[If an affliction] ⌜afflicts⌝ him and his flesh stings(?), he has paralysis [. . .] when he talks [. . .] and it flows over him, ⌜"spawn"⌝ of Šulpaea afflicts him. If when it ⌜afflicts⌝ him, his left [ear] is hot and stinks,[163] his illness will let up. If when it afflicts him, his right [ear] is hot and stinks, his illness may be prolonged (but it will let up).

Strokes

When the arteries that supply the brain develop atherosclerosis, there may be reduced blood supply and eventually complete obstruction. The blockage can be due to fatty plaques in the arteries and associated calcium deposition and/or blood clots. Also the arteries can rupture and bleed into the brain. When any one of these conditions occurs, we call it a stroke. Since any of the arteries in the brain can exhibit these changes, the neurologic findings will depend on which vessel is affected. One of the most common clinical presentations is paralysis of the facial muscles, arm, and leg all on one side of the body (hemiparesis). Since this condition is more common in aging patients, the many texts that describe patients with stroke supports the assumption of relative longevity of individuals in ancient Mesopotamia.

The word for a stroke was *mišittu*,[164] from the Akkadian verb *mašādu*, which has a range of Sumerian equivalents including ŠU.ÙR: "to rub" and RA: "to strike" (usually said of somebody's head with a weapon).[165] What was envisaged was that a demon, usually the *rābiṣu* (see below), had literally rubbed or struck the patient on the affected part, making *mišittu* an almost exact equivalent of the English term *stroke*. The stroke texts are sufficiently detailed that they can be divided by parts of the body affected. There is even a description of a transient ischemic attack (TIA) or a very mild, reversible, stroke.

TIA OR VERY MILD STROKE

When an artery in the brain contracts or goes into spasm, it can cause a transient reduction in blood supply (ischemia) with neurologic abnormalities appropriate for the area of the brain affected. After the artery opens up again, the neurologic function generally returns to normal. This condition commonly is a warning that an irreversible vessel occlusion (blockage) is likely to occur. Also small vessel occlusion can occur with a large surrounding area of inflammation and swelling. With time, the inflammation and swelling will abate, and most of the neurologic changes may disappear. The reference below is likely to be a TIA or stroke involving the middle cerebral artery.

13.227 DIŠ *mi-šit-ti im-šid-su-ma lu* 15 *lu* 150 SÌG-*iṣ* MUD Á-*šú* NU *pa-ṭir* ŠU.SI.MEŠ-*šú* NIR.NIR-*aṣ* ŠU-*su ú-šaq-qá u* NIR-*aṣ* GÌR-*šú i-qan-na-an u* NIR-*aṣ* NINDA *u* KAŠ NU TAR-*us* DIB GIDIM$_7$ *ana* EDIN <U$_4$>.3.KÁM *ni-ši* (DPS XXVII:5–7 [AOAT 43.297]; *AMT* 77/1 i 2–4)

**If he has a stroke and either his left side or his right side is affected (and) his shoulder is not released, (but) he can straighten out his fingers (and) he can lift his hand and stretch it out (and) he can bend his foot and stretch it out again (and) he is not off his food or drink, affliction by a ghost at the steppe; recovery in three (days).

LEFT- OR RIGHT-SIDED STROKE

Occluded arteries on one side of the brain generally cause neurologic loss on the opposite side because the nerve tracts cross in the brain stem. Loss of speech (aphasia) may occur in stroke, but is generally restricted to involvement of the left side of the brain (right-sided paralysis), as in the third reference below.

13.228 DIŠ ZAG-*šú tab-kát mi-šit-ti* MAŠKIM DIN (DPS XXVII:9 [AOAT 43.297]; *AMT* 77/1 i 6; cf. StBoT 36.21 obv. 10b)[166]

**If his left side is tense,[167] stroke of a *rābiṣu*; he will get well.

13.229 DIŠ GÙB-*šú tab-kát* ŠU ^{d}*Šu-lak* (DPS XXVII:11 [AOAT 43.297]; *AMT* 77/1 i 8; cf. StBoT 36.21 obv. 10a)[168]

**If his right side is tense,[169] "hand" of Šulak.

13.230 [*šu-me-el*] *pa-ag-ri-šu ka-la-a-ma* ⸢*ta*⸣-*a*[*b*]-*kà-at*! *da-bá-bá la-a i-le-ʾ-e* [. . . *la-a i-l*] *e-ʾ-e* ŠU ^{d}*Šu-lak m*[*i*!?-*ḫi-i*]*ṣ me-še-ti ma-ḫi-iṣ* ^{LÚ}*a-ši-pu a-n*[*a* TI-*šu qí-i-ba l*]*a-a i-ša-kán* (StBoT 36.22 obv. 11–13)[170]

**[If] the entire [right side of] his body is tense[171] (and) he is not able to talk (and) he is [not] ⌜able⌝ to [. . .], "hand" of Šulak . . . the *āšipu* should ⌜not⌝ make a [prognosis as to his recovery].

STROKE WITH HEADACHE

13.231 DIŠ *m[i-šit-ti im]-šid-su-ma ib-ta-luṭ* SAG.KI-*šú* DIB.DIB-*su u* MUD.MUD-*ud m[u-ki]l* SAG-⌜*šú*⌝ NU *pa-ṭir* (DPS XXVII:2–3 [AOAT 43.297])

**If he has a ⌜stroke⌝ and then gets better (but) his temples continually afflict him and he shudders, the one who ⌜holds⌝ his head has not let go.

13.232 SAG.ḪUL.ḪA.ZA *mi-šit-ti* ŠU^{II} *u* [GÌR^{II}] . . . (BM 76226:8′)

***Mukīl rēš lemutti* (headache; see above) (and) stroke affecting the hands and [feet] . . .

STROKE WITH FOCAL PARALYSIS

Muscular control of various parts of the body is found in particular areas of the motor cortex. Occlusion of an artery supplying the motor cortex will cause weakness or paralysis in the muscles controlled by the area affected.

STROKE WITH FACIAL SYMPTOMS

13.233 DIŠ NA *mi-šit-ti pa-ni i-šu* IGI-*šú i-ṣap-par ur-ra u mu-ša ur-ta-na-at-tú*[172] *la it-ta-na-a-a-al ina* LÀL Ì.NUN.NA IGI.MEŠ-*šú ka-a-a-nam-ma muš-šu-da la i-kal-la* . . . (*AMT* 76/5:11–13+*AMT* 79/4:2–4//*SpTU* 1.46:16–19//*AMT* 35/6:5′–7′)[173]

**If a person has a stroke affecting the face (and) his eye flutters, day and night he is continually wakeful and cannot sleep, (and) he cannot stop <constantly> rubbing his eyes with honey and ghee . . .

13.234 DIŠ NA KA-*šú* NUNDUN-*su ana* ZAG/GÙB *kub-bu-ul-ma da-ba-ba la i-le-[ʾi] da-ba-ab-ta-šú tu-ur-ri* . . . (*BAM* 523 iii 3′–4′, 9′–10′//*BAM* 174 obv. 5′–6′)[174]

**If his mouth (and) his lips are immobilized to the left/right so that he ⌜cannot⌝ talk, in order to restore his speech . . .

13.235 [DIŠ . . . IGI ZA]G-*šú kap-ṣa-at pu-us-su* [. . . NU]NDUN-*su šá* 15 *na-šal-lu-lu* [. . .] (DPS V D i 6–8a = *TDP* 48 E i 6–8a)[175]

**[If his right eye . . .], his ⌜left⌝ [eye(lid)] droops, his forehead [. . .] (and) his left ⌜lip⌝ is slippery [. . .]

In the final reference above, the "slippery" lip is probably due to drooling secondary to the left facial paralysis indicated by the "drooping" left eyelid.

STROKE WITH ARM SYMPTOMS

13.236 [DIŠ] NA *mi-šit-ti a-ḫi* GIG . . . (*AMT* 79/1 iv 21)[176]

**[If] a person is sick with a stroke affecting the arm . . .

13.237 LAL-*ti a-ḫi*... (*BAM* 134 obv. 2′)

**Bandage (for stroke affecting) the arm...

STROKE WITH HIP AND LEG SYMPTOMS

13.238 DIŠ NA *mi-šit-ti* MURUB$_4$ GIG *a-tál-lu-kám* NU ZU MURUB$_4$.MEŠ-*šú ki-iṣ-ra-t*[*i*...]... (*AMT* 79/1 iv 11//*BAM* 136 ii 3′–5′)

**If a person is sick with a stroke affecting the hip (and) he cannot walk (and) his hips and joints [...]...

13.239 DIŠ *ka-bit-ma lu* ŠU-*su lu* GÌR-*šú iq-ta-na-an mi-šit-ti im-šid-su* DIN (DPS XXVII:8 [AOAT 43.297]; *AMT* 77/1 i 5)

**If it is difficult (for him) to bend either his hand or his foot[177] (and) he has had a stroke; he will get well.

13.240 DIŠ NA *mi-šit-tú-ma* ŠU-*su u* GÌR-*šú ta-bi-ik*... (*AMT* 82/2 iii! 4)[178]

**If a person (has) a stroke and his hand or his foot is tense[179]...

STROKE WITH MULTIPLE PARTS OF THE BODY AFFECTED

13.241 [DIŠ NA] *mi-šit-ti pa-ni ma-šid-ma ta-lam-ma-šú i-šam-ma-am-šú* KIN *mi-šit-ti* GIG (DPS XXVII:1 [AOAT 43.297]; DPS XXVI:91′ [AOAT 43.286] (catchline)]; *AMT* 77/1 i 1)[180]

** [If a person] has a stroke affecting the face[181] and his torso goes numb, he is sick with the effect of the stroke.

13.242 DIŠ IGI.MEŠ-*šú ṣap-ru* ⸢*ta*⸣-*lam-ma-šú pur-ru-ur* ŠU-*su šá* NÍG.GIG-*ti-šú* ŠUB-*ma* NU ÍL-*ši* GÌR-*šú i-maš-šar* ŠU *mi-šit-ti* U$_4$.ME-*šú* GÍD.ME NU SI.SÁ (DPS IX A 72–73//B r. 19–20 = *TDP* 78:72–73)[182]

**If his face twitches, his torso is powerless, he lets his right hand drop and is unable to lift (it), (and) he drags his foot, "hand" of a stroke. <Even if> he lives for a long time, he will not straighten up.

13.243 DIŠ KI.MIN-*ma* GÌR-*šú šá* 15 *i-maš-šar* KA-*šú ṣu-dur mi-šit-ti* MAŠKIM GÍD-*ma* GAM (DPS XV:63 [AOAT 43.154]; DPS XIV A$_2$ iv 3′–4′//C$_2$ iii 30 = *TDP* 142 iv 3′–4′)

**If (it is the first day he is sick) and he drags his left foot (and) his mouth[183] twitches,[184] stroke of a *rābiṣu*; (if) it is prolonged, he will die.

Motor System Complexes

Patients can have diseases that prevent them from moving some part of their body voluntarily and normally. Diseases can injure the motor section of the brain, spinal cord, the nerves that control the use of their muscles, or the muscles themselves. Such patients may be partially or fully paralyzed in any muscles, including those of the face. Such diseases can be congenital, such as cerebral palsy, or can begin at any time during life.

The ancient Mesopotamian physicians believed that the diseases that paralyze muscles were due to a demon named Šulpaea.[185] Although in most of the texts, it is hard to be sure exactly what disease is being described, we have made some guesses. The only disease we feel confident in identifying is a text that we believe describes cerebral palsy.

CEREBRAL PALSY

This is a group of persisting, nonprogressive motor disorders caused by fetal anoxia or trauma at birth. Motor development is delayed or abnormal, and the findings include spastic paraplegia, hemiplegia, or quadraplegia. Other signs that may be present include mental retardation, seizures, or ataxia (irregular gait).

13.244 DIŠ LÚ.TUR MU.1.KÁM MU.2.KÁM MU.3.KÁM MU.4.KÁM *šu-ub-bu-uṣ-ma te-ba-a ù ú-zu-uz-za la i-le-ʾ-e* NINDA *a-ka-la la i-le-ʾ-e* KA-*šú ṣu-ub-bu-ut-ma da-ba-ba la i-le-ʾ-e re-ḫu-ut* ᵈ*Šul-pa-è-a* NU SI.SÁ (DPS XL A 21–23 = *TDP* 220:21–23)

**If an infant of one, two, three, (and then) four years writhes in contortion so that he is unable to get up and stand, he is unable to eat bread, (and) his mouth is "seized" so that he is unable to talk, "spawn" of Šulpaea; he will not straighten up.[186]

SPINAL MUSCULAR ATROPHY

The first text below may be a form of spinal muscular atrophy such as Werdnig-Hoffmann disease in small children or amyotrophic lateral sclerosis in adults. The second text describes a patient with severe neck weakness who cannot support his head without it flopping to the right and left. This case also fits into the broad category of spinal muscular atrophy, but a specific diagnosis is not possible. This group of diseases generally has a poor prognosis.

13.245 [DIŠ S]AG.DU-*su* LÚ.ÚŠ-*šú i-na-aš* GÚ-*su ana* 15 *u* 150 ŠUB.ŠUB-*ú* EME-*šú it-te-né-biṭ* EME-*šú it-ta-nak-ṣar*! KA-*šú* ⸢x x⸣ ta Á.ÚR!.MEŠ-*šú tab-ka ina* DU-*šu ú-sa-kar* A.RI.A ᵈ*Šul-pa-è-<a> ana* MAŠ.EN.KAK DIB ḪUL [DUG]UD *uš-ta-mar*!*-raṣ-ma ina la-a* U_4.MEŠ-*šú* (*STT* 89:187–191 [Stol, *Epilepsy* 96–97])

**[If] his ⸢head⸣ (and) his body shake, he continually lets his neck drop to the left or right, his tongue is continually cramped, his tongue is continually in knots,[187] his mouth [. . .] his limbs are tense[188] (and) he blocks (himself) off when he walks,[189] "spawn" of Šulpaea. For a client, (it means) an evil affliction; a ⸢powerful one⸣ will be made ill and (die) before his time.[190]

13.246 DIŠ GÚ-*su* 15 *u* 150 ŠUB.ŠUB-*di* GAM / DIŠ GÚ-*su* 15 *u* 150 ŠUB.ŠUB-*ut* GAM / DIŠ GÚ-*su* TA 15 *ana* 150 *suḫ*₄*-ḫur-ma* ŠUB-*ut* [G]AM (DPS X A obv. 14b–15//B obv. 15–17 = *TDP* 82:14b–15; cf. StBoT 36.62:5)

**If he continually lets his neck drop to the left or right, he will die. If his neck continually falls to the left or right, he will die. If his neck falls when it is turned from left to right, ⸢he will die⸣.

FLOPPY BABY SYNDROME

Modern physicians refer to a group of illnesses in infants and young children as the floppy baby syndrome. This is not a single disease, but a group of diseases involving the central nervous system, peripheral nerves, or muscles and with common characteristics including poor muscle tone (hypotonia) and decreased or absent crying. It is most apparent when the baby cannot hold up its head or when supported under the arms it tends to slip through the examiner's hands. There is a high mortality rate in infants with this syndrome, especially when it occurs early in infancy.

Many diseases fall under this category, including Werdnig-Hoffman disease (see above), Prader-Willi syndrome, and botulism. The references below are part of a series; the first provides the most information and is consistent with this group of diseases.

13.247 [DIŠ A.RI.A ^{d}*Šu*] *l-pa-è-a* KI.BI Ù.TU *ina* GÌR^{II}-*šú* É AD-*šú* ⌜BIR-*aḫ*⌝ [*ana* NU BIR-*aḫ*] *bal-ṭú-us-su ana* ÍD ŠUB-*šu-ma* ḪUL-*šú it-*[*tab-bal* GIZKIM.BI GI] N$_7$ *al-du la ib-ki la is-si la im-t*[*a*]*-ga-*⌜*ag*⌝ [. . .] (DPS XXIX:22–24 [AOAT 43.320]; restored from *KUB* 37.87:7′–9′)[191]

**[If "spawn" of] ⌜Šulpaea⌝ is born with him, the house of his father will be scattered at his feet; [in order for it not to be scattered], you throw him alive into the river and his evil will be ⌜carried away⌝. [Its sign is that, from] the ⌜moment⌝ he is born, he does not wail (or) cry or stiffen up [. . .]

This text is one of only a few examples of euthanasia in ancient Mesopotamia (see below under Huntington's disease). This action was apparently taken because floppy baby syndrome was considered to be a hopeless situation and because of a fear that the rest of the family might somehow be affected ("the house of his father will be scattered at his feet"). Throwing the baby into the river (also the preferred method of disposal of malformed stillbirths) dispatched it to the netherworld from which its spirit (*zaqīqu*) might eventually return for another try at life.

The remaining references in the series (shown below) could also be Werndig-Hoffman disease, since it can occur in late childhood and tends to be less serious the later it develops. Note that the *āšipu* expended as much care on older children with severe neurological problems as he did with adults with epilepsy.

13.248 [DIŠ *ina* MU].⌜3⌝.KÁM ŠUB-*šú* AD-*šú* DINGIR TUKU-*ši* LÚ.TUR BI *ina* MU BI ÚŠ *ana* ZI-*ḫi* . . . (DPS XXIX:25 [AOAT 43.320])

**[If] it falls on him [in] the third[192] [year], his father will obtain a personal god; that infant will die in the same year. To remove it . . .

13.249 DIŠ *ina* MU.7.KÁM <ŠUB-*su*> DINGIR TUKU-*ši ul-tab-bar tás-níq* KUR.[RA GAR-*šú ana* ZI-*ḫi* . . .] (DPS XXIX:29 [AOAT 43.320])

**If it falls on him in the seventh[193] year, he will obtain a personal god; he will live long; dying of old age[194] [was established (by the gods as his fate). To remove it . . .]

13.250 [DIŠ *ina* MU].⌜10⌝.KÁM ŠUB-*su* DINGIR TUKU-*ši ana* ⌜ZI-*ḫi*⌝ . . . (DPS XXIX:30 [AOAT 43.320])

**[If] it falls on him [in] the tenth [year], he will obtain a personal god. To remove it . . .

SPASMODIC TORTICOLLIS

The reference below indicates that the patient's head may be turned to any position but, after it is released by the examiner, it returns consistently to the right or left side. A disease with a chronically rotated head is spasmodic torticollis, a type of dystonia usually caused by a brain lesion in the basal ganglia or brain stem. This can be a very annoying and embarrassing condition, but the prognosis is ultimately determined by the nature of the brain lesion.

13.251 DIŠ GÚ-*su* 15 *u* 150 *ut-ta-nar* GAM (DPS X A obv. 14a//B obv. 14 = *TDP* 82:14a)

**If he continually returns his head to the left or right, he will die.

Dementia

The loss of normal cognitive ability is called dementia, and there are many causes, with Alzheimer's disease being the most common. The following references appear to be clear descriptions of dementia. In the statement that the patient will "die alone like a stranger," it is apparent that the author recognizes the social dissolution that demented patients usually suffer as the disease progresses.

13.252 [DIŠ UŠ$_4$]-*šu* MAN.MAN-*ni* DU$_{11}$.DU$_{11}$-*šú* KÚR.KÚR *mim-mu-ú i-qab-bu-ú i-ma-áš-šú* IM *ku-tal-*[*l*]*i* DIB-*su* 1-*ma* KÚR-*iš* GAM (DPS XXII:49–50 [AOAT 43.255])

**[If] his [mentation] is continually altered, his words are unintelligible, and he forgets whatever he says, a wind from behind afflicts him; he will die alone like a stranger.[195]

13.253 [DIŠ L]Ú *ši-ki-in bi-ti-šu im-ta-na-aš-ši bi-tum šu-ú* [. . .] (Köcher and Oppenheim, *AfO* 18.65 ii 11 [physiognomic omens])[196]

**[If a] ⌜person⌝ continually forgets what his house looks like, that house [will be scattered].

Altered Mental States

Reversible mental status change can be caused by other illnesses. If the primary disease resolves, a return to normal mental functioning may result. Shock (low blood pressure) can result in altered mental function (see Chapter 14). Severe liver disease leads to metabolic abnormalities that affect mentation (hepatic encephalopathy; see Chapter 6). Head trauma (concussion), some infections, and poisons can also alter mental functions (see Chapters 3 and 15).

Autism

Autism is an organic disease of the brain that is manifested in early childhood by the inability of the individual to establish and maintain normal social interactions with other individuals. The texts below may be describing children with this problem.

13.254 BE MUNUS Ù.TU-*ma* AMA-*šú i-zir*... (Šumma Izbu IV 42 [Leichty, *Izbu* 70])

**If a woman gives birth and (the child) rejects its mother...

13.255 BE MUNUS Á.KAM[197] *lu* NITA *lu* MUNUS Ù.TU... (Šumma Izbu I 69 [Leichty, *Izbu* 38])

**If a woman gives birth to an insane (child), either male or female...

Basal Ganglia Disorders

The basal ganglia are located in the center of the brain, and diseases affecting them typically cause unusual involuntary movements of the body. Chorea, Huntington's disease, and Parkinson's disease are disorders of the basal ganglia.

CHOREA

Chorea, a Greek word meaning "to dance," refers to rapid, jerky, and involuntary movements. The arms, legs, and face can be involved. The following references to "hand" of Šulak probably refer to an infectious cause of chorea (encephalitis), since they mention ringing in the ears and a fatal outcome.

13.256 ⸢U$_4$ GIG GIG!-*ma*⸣ GEŠTU-*šu* GÙ-*šu* ŠU *ù* GÌR *šà* 150 ŠÈ 15 *ù šà! i-mi-it* ŠÈ 150-*šu i-šà-aḫ-ḫi-iṭ* ŠU *Šu-la-ak ul* TI.LA ÚŠ-*at* (*MDP* 57.11 v 2′–5′)

**If the patient [is sick] and his ears ring (and) (his) right hand and foot jump to the left and (his) left (hand and foot jump) to his right, "hand" of Šulak. He will not get well; he will die.

13.257 U$_4$ GIG GEŠTU-*šu* <GÙ-*šu*> *ù ší-in-na-šu ne-en-mu-da* MURUB$_4$-*šu ul i-šà-a*[*ḫ-ḫi*]-*ṭá* ŠU ⸢*Šu*⸣-*la-ak* (*MDP* 57.11 v 6′–8′)

**If the patient's ears <ring> and his teeth are gritted (but) his hips do not jump, "hand" of Šulak.

HUNTINGTON'S DISEASE

Some patients manifest a slow, continuous, purposeless movement characterized by the inability to retain their fingers and toes in any one position, which is called athetosis. If this movement is combined with the jerky movement described above, it is called choreoathetosis. When choreoathetosis is combined with mental dysfunction, the condition is likely to be the well-known genetic illness that modern physicians call Huntington's disease.

This condition invariably progresses to advanced dementia and death. Two of the references below (*STT* 89:174–179 and 180–186) appear one after the other in the diagnostic series and therefore probably refer to the same or related medical problems. We believe that Huntington's disease is a likely explanation.

13.258 ⸢DIŠ⸣ TÚG-*su ú-na-kas*$_4$ *u* UB.NÍGIN.NA-*šú i-ṭa-ma-a* ŠU ^{d}*Šul-pa-è-a* [DIŠ T]ÚG-*su ú-na-kas*$_4$ *u* UB.NÍGIN.NA-*šú na-šá-a* ŠU ^{d}*Šul-pa-è-a* (DPS XXII:44–45 [AOAT 43. 255])

**If he tears his garment and his limbs twist, "hand" of Šulpaea. [If] he tears his ⸢garment⸣ and his limbs are raised up, "hand" of Šulpaea.

13.259 DIŠ *ina* DU *ger-ri* DIB-*tu* DIB-*su-ma* U$_4$-*ma* DIB-*šú* ŠU^{II}-*šú* GÌR^{II}-*šú* KI *qaq-qa-*[*r*]*i i-šap-piṣ* IGI^{II}-*šú tar-ka* KIR$_4$.MEŠ-*šú ga-an-ṣa* TÚG-*su i-kal* A.RI.A ^{d}*Šul-pa-è-a ana* GIZKIM-*šú* ZÁḪ É AD-*šú* AD-*šú* AMA-*šú še-re-es-su* ÍL-*ú ana* NU SÁ.SÁ *bal-ṭu-su ina* KI-*ti te-qeb-b*[*e*]*r-*[*š*]*u* ḪUL-*šú* DU$_8$ (*STT* 89:174–179 [Stol, *Epilepsy* 96])

**If an affliction afflicts him while he is going along the road and when it afflicts him he makes his hands and feet writhe in contortion against the earth, his eyes are dark, his nostrils are contracted, (and) he eats his garment, "spawn" of Šulpaea. As its sign, (it portends) destruction of the house of his father. His father and mother will bear his punishment. In order for it not to approach (them) you bury him alive in the earth; its evil will be dispelled.

Mood changes resembling manic-depressive illnesses are common in Huntington's chorea. Patients can have discrete periods of severe depression accompanied by psychomotor retardation and delusions of guilt that may prompt suicide attempts.

13.260 D[IŠ G]IN$_7$ AN.ÚSAN DIB-*tu* DIB-*su-ma* U$_4$-*ma* DIB-*šú ik-kil-lu* GÙ.DÉ-*šú-ma u šu-ú e-*⸢*ta*⸣*-nap-pal* [A]D-*ya* AMA *lu* ŠEŠ.MEŠ-*ya* NIN.MEŠ-*ya* ÚŠ.MEŠ [*ina* N]U ZU!-*e ma-am-ma* GÙ.GÙ-*si ik-ta-na-la* (*ḫe-pí*) EGIR ÍR-*ú i-ṣal-lal-ma* NU ZI-*bé* U$_4$ DIB!-*su um-taš-š*[*e-r*]*u-šu* GIN$_7$ ÍR NU ZU A.RI.A ^{d}*Šul-pa-è-a* NU ZI *ina* GIG-*šú ina* IZI GÍBIL-*šú* (*STT* 89:180–186 [Stol, *Epilepsy* 96])

**⸢If⸣ his affliction afflicts him ⸢in⸣ the evening and when it afflicts him, a mournful cry roars to him and he continually answers it, he continually cries out <without> ceasing: "My ⸢father⸣ (and) mother or my brothers and my sisters will die" [without] recognizing anybody, [he continually wails][198] (and) when he has wailed he goes to sleep and does not get up[199] (and) when his affliction has left him, he does not know what he wailed, "spawn" of Šulpaea; it cannot be removed. In his illness, you burn him with fire.

The preceding two references are further examples of the practice of euthanasia in ancient Mesopotamia. As with floppy baby syndrome, this action was apparently taken because it was considered to be a hopeless situation and because of a fear that the rest of the family might somehow be affected ("[It portends] destruction of the house of his father. His father and mother will bear his punishment").

This approach to a medical problem is in such striking contrast to the often intensive and exhaustive treatment used to cure or ameliorate other medical problems that it demands an explanation. It would appear that the *āšipu* recognized that the disease was passed on to descendants, and was attempting to prevent it by practicing eugenics. The dominant inheritance of the genetic defect in Huntington's disease makes the familial nature of this condition very easy to recognize. This fact plus the devastating consequences of the disease must have been responsible for the *āšipu*'s decision to take such a drastic action.[200]

The choice of killing the patient may be foreign to us but, in view of the grim nature of this incurable condition and the probability that it would be passed on to the next generation, the interests of the family may have been felt to demand the sacrifice of the individual. The fact that the patient in the first case was merely demented and in the second case actually delusional is also reflected in the severity of the reaction. The burial of one victim at least ensured eventual recycling of his spirit; the burning of the second, by contrast, meant that he was gone forever. As the ghost of Enkidu informs Gilgamesh: "'Have you seen him who was set on fire?' 'I did not see him. His smoke went up to heaven (and) his ghost does not dwell in the nether world.'"[201]

The following reference we believe to be another example of Huntington's disease, but in this case it appears to be the Wesphal variant of this condition. This type of Huntington's disease usually begins in childhood with proximal muscle rigidity, mental abnormalities, and seizures. It appears that the *āšipu* used the same approach for a child with this disease as he used for adults, namely, euthanasia of the less severe type (burial).

13.261 DIŠ ^{d}LUGAL.ÙR.RA KI.BI Ù.TU *ina* GÌR^{II}-*šú* É AD-*šú* BIR-*aḫ ana* NU BIR-*aḫ* É AD-*šú* GIN$_7$ ^{d}*Kù-bi tuš-na-al-šu-ma* ḪUL.BI *it-tab-bal* GIZKIM.BI GIN$_7$ ⌜*al-du*⌝ *i-bak-ki i-za-ár ù im-ta-nam-ga-*⌜*ag*⌝ (DPS XXIX:1–3 [AOAT 43.318]; cf. DPS XXVIII:44 [AOAT 43.312])

**If LUGAL.ÙR.RA is born with him, the house of his father will be scattered at his feet, in order that the house of his father not be scattered you lay him to rest as if he were a stillborn child and the evil will be carried away (with him). (LUGAL.ÙR.RA)'s sign is that (the infant), from the moment he is born, wails, twists, and is continually rigid.

PARKINSON'S DISEASE

Patients with Parkinson's disease often have resting movement of the hands, a rigid, masklike face, rigid body, and drooling; when walking they lean forward and move with a mincing, rigid gait. Poor postural reflexes cause falls to be a common problem. This disease tends to occur primarily in the older age groups. We believe that the *āšipu* in the following reference is describing a patient with Parkinson's disease.

13.262 DIŠ SAG.DU-*su i-tar-ru-ur* [G]Ú-*su u* GÚ.MUR$_7$-*šú ka-pí-ip* KA-*šú* N[U].⌜LÁL?⌝[202] [oooooo] ⌜LAL-*e*⌝ (coll.) *ina* KA-*šú* ÚḪ.ME-*šú* DU.MEŠ ŠU^{II}-*šú kìn-ṣa-a-šú u* GÌR^{II}-*šú* 1-*niš i-tar-ru-ra ina* DU-*šú ana* IGI-*šú n*[*a-du-ú* . . . -*m*]*a* ⌜NU⌝.DIN[203] (DPS III C obv. 39–40//D 13–15 = *TDP* 22:39–40)

**If his head trembles, his ⌜neck⌝ and his spine are bent, ⌜he cannot stick out⌝ his tongue (?) or stretch out [. . .], his saliva continually flows from his mouth, his hands, his legs, and his feet all tremble at once, (and) when he walks, he ⌜falls⌝ forward, ⌜(if)⌝ [. . .] he will not get well.[204]

Immediately following this entry in the diagnostic/prognostic series is a sequence of entries that describe patients with similar tremors of the head, hands, and feet but with speech problems of two sorts, difficulties in articulation ("mouth too strong for the words") and abnormal speech patterns ("words hinder each other in the mouth").

13.263 DIŠ SAG.DU-*su* ŠU^{II}-*šú u* GÌR^{II}-*šú i-tar-ru-ra* KA-*šú ana a-ma-ti da-a-an i-na* ⌜KA⌝-[*šú it-te-ne-eṭ-pu* DI]B-*tum* DIB-*su* / DIŠ SAG.DU-*su* ŠU^{II}-*šu u* GÌR^{II}-*šu* 1-*niš i-tar-ru-ra ina* KA-*šú át-mu-šú it-te-ni-ip-r*[*ik-ku* NA BI *lu-ʾ-tu*$_4$ *ana ma-al-tak-ti š*]*u-kul*[205] (DPS III C obv. 41–42 = *TDP* 22:41–42)[206]

**If his head, his hands, and his feet tremble, his mouth is (too) strong for the words (and) [they tumble over one another(?)] in [his] ⌜mouth,⌝ the affliction afflicts him. If his head, his hands, and his feet all tremble at once (and) his words hinder each other in his mouth, [that person] ⌜has been fed⌝ [a dirty substance to test it].[207]

Since Parkinson's disease has recognized speech abnormalities, including short rushes of speech, increased rate of speech, inappropriate silences, and decreased volume, the preceding sequence of references is probably also describing a patient with Parkinson's. It appears from the diagnosis that the *āšipu* suspected that the patient had been poisoned (fed a dirty substance). Although toxic substances are known that can cause Parkinson's disease, they are rare causes of this condition.

Gilles de la Tourette Syndrome

The most unusual feature of this condition is the patient's explosive and uncontrollable verbalization of obscene words and phrases. Coupled with this are jerking and gyrating movements of the head, pelvis, or arms. These unfortunate individuals often are socially ostracized because of their bizarre but neurologically driven behavior. In most cases, the disease is genetically acquired but can rarely be secondary to another disease.

The texts below list the major features of Tourette's syndrome, both jerking movements and "frightful," presumably obscene, and antisocial speech. Since this syndrome usually begins in the first two decades of life, it is not surprising that the *āšipu* attributed this problem to a malevolent class of demons (*lilû, lilītu, ardat lilî*) that specialized in attacking adolescent victims (see Chapter 12). The rule for this class of demons was to victimize persons of the opposite sex. Consequently, the *āšipu* could distinguish between syndromes that afflicted both boys and girls (*lilû* or *lilītu*) and syndromes that primarily afflicted boys (*ardat lilî*). It was presumably for this reason that this syndrome, which affects boys four times more frequently than girls, was attributed to the *ardat lilî*.

13.264 DIŠ ŠÀ ŠÀ GÙ.GÙ-*si* MURUB$_4$.ME-*šú* ÍL.ME IGI.LÁ-*šú* LÁ-*šú* U$_4$ LÁ-*šú* LÁ-*šú par-di-iš* DUG$_4$.DUG$_4$-*ub* ŠU [KI.SIKIL.LÍL.LÁ] (DPS XIII G$_2$ 18 = *TDP* 124 iii 25)

**If he continually cries out: "My insides, my insides!" he continually raises his pelvic region,[208] his confusional state(s)[209] come over him (and) when they come over him, he continually talks in a frightful manner, "hand" of [*ardat lilî*].

13.265 DIŠ GIG-*su* KU_4 *u* È KI.MIN *par-diš* DUG_4.DUG_4-*ub* ŠU KI.SIKIL.LÍL.LÁ (DPS XVII:40 [AOAT 43.199])

**If his illness enters and leaves (and when his confusional state comes over him), he continually talks in a frightful manner, "hand" of *ardat lilî.*

Peripheral Neuropathy

The long nerves running through the arms and especially the legs are subject to damage by diseases such as diabetes and by chemicals and poisons. When this damage occurs, the patient may experience pain, numbness, itching, and paralysis in varying combinations. It is likely that this common condition was also seen in ancient Mesopotamia. Some of the quotes that follow probably represent neuropathies.

13.266 [DIŠ NA GÌR^{II}-*šú i-š*]*am-ma-ma-šú a-tal-la-kám la i-l*[*e-ʾ-i*] . . . (*BAM* 119:4′)[210]

**[If a person's feet] ⌜go numb⌝ (and) he ⌜cannot⌝ walk . . .

13.267 DIŠ NA GÌR^{II}-*šú šim-ma-tú* TUKU-*a* KÚ.MEŠ-*šú* SA GÌR^{II}-*šú sa-ag-gu-ma* GÌR^{II}-*šú* BAL.BAL.MEŠ-*šu* . . . (*BAM* 122 obv. 8–10//*AMT* 70/7 ii 7′–8′)[211]

**If a person's feet are numb (and) hurt him, the muscles of his feet are stiff, and his feet shift constantly under him . . .[212]

13.268 DIŠ ŠU^{II}-*šú it-te-nen-ṣi-la-šú u it-ta-naq-na-an-na* ŠU ^{d}*D*[*il-bat* . . .] (DPS XI A obv. 18//B 17 = TDP 90:18//*SpTU* 1.34:17, cf. StBoT 36.35 obv. 13′//StBoT 36.57 r. 2′)

**If his hands are continually sluggish and are continually contorted, "hand" of ⌜Dilbat (Ištar)⌝ [. . .].

13.269 DIŠ NA GÌR^{II}-*šú it-te-nen-ṣi-la u it-ta-naq-na-an-na* ŠU ^{d}[. . .] x ana kur me ru (DPS XIV A_2 iv 13′–14′//G iv 3′–4′ = *TDP* 142 iv 13′–14′)

**If a person's feet are continually sluggish and continually contorted, "hand" of [. . .].

13.270 DIŠ NA GÌR^{II} *u* Š[U^{II} *qu-u*]*n-nu-na-ma la i-tar*[*-ra-aṣ*] . . . (*AMT* 68/1 obv. 14)

**If a person's feet and ⌜hands⌝ are ⌜contorted⌝ so that he cannot ⌜stretch them out⌝ . . .

As the patient's condition worsens, sensory loss moves centripetally in a graded fashion with a distribution that mimics the location of a glove or stocking. Patients experience difficulty walking on their heels during examination and their feet may slap the ground while walking. Later, the knee jerk reflex disappears and foot drop becomes more apparent. Foot drop may occur as part of a generalized neuropathy, but it may also be an isolated problem when the deep peroneal nerve is injured. This condition is colorfully described in the second reference below. Patients with foot drop cannot raise their feet up (dorsiflex) to avoid tripping so they must lift their legs high to achieve clearance for their toes. Even then their toes may scrape the ground. In this maneuver the patient's foot appears to be "licking the ground."

The *āšipu* would not have referred to these sensory deficits as "stockings" or "gloves," since these had yet to be invented. Instead, he drew on an analogy still current today, if in a different form, that of putting a letter into an envelope. In ancient Mesopotamia, letters were written on clay tablets that were enclosed in clay envelopes. When a distal extremity was numb, it was said to be covered by an envelope.

13.271 [DIŠ NA GÌR.MEŠ *i*]*t-ta-na-aq-na-na-šú šá-pu-la-šú* BAL.BAL-*šú* NA BI *a-ri-im* [. . .] *ana* TI-*šú* . . . (*AMT* 70/3 i 3–4)[213]

**[If a person's feet] ⸢continually⸣ become contorted (and) his inguinal regions shift constantly under him,[214] that person is "enveloped" [. . .] to cure him . . .

13.272 6,40 *a-wi-lum ši-pa-šu qá-qá-ra-am le-ka* . . . (*BAM* 393 r. 19)

**If a man's feet lick the ground . . .

Coma

Coma is a neurological condition where the patient cannot be aroused by vigorous visual, auditory, or painful stimuli. Coma may be graded in the following manner: the higher the grade the more serious the patient's condition.

Stage I — The patient can be roused for brief periods. This is referred to as a stupor.
Stage II — The patient cannot be roused, even with painful stimuli although she or he may moan and make semi-purposeful avoidance movements.
Stage III —Painful stimuli fail to produce a response or they lead to decerebrate posturing (extension and pronation of arms).
Stage IV — The patient is no longer breathing, and his or her muscles are flaccid; the patient is brain dead. Stage IV can be indicated by bilateral fixed, dilated pupils, which usually indicate irreversible brain stem damage if they last longer than five minutes.

Ancient Mesopotamian doctors had a test to distinguish between the first two stages and the second two stages (see DPS XVI:63′–64′ [AOAT 43.177–178] in the Neurological Testing section [13.286] below). Stage I was attributed to the baneful influence of an evil *alû*,[215] as in the following references.

13.273 [DIŠ GIN$_7$] Ù.SÁ DIB.DIB-*su* UB.NIGIN.NA-*šú iš-šap-pa-ka* GEŠTU^{II}-*šú* GÙ.<DÉ>.MEŠ KA-*šú* DIB-*ma* NU DUG$_4$.DUG$_4$-*ub* ŠU A.LÁ ḪUL (DPS XXVII:21–22 [AOAT 43.298])

** [If something like] a stupor continually afflicts him and his limbs are tense,[216] his ears roar, (and) his mouth is "seized" so that he cannot talk, "hand" of an evil *alû*.

13.274 DIŠ GIN$_7$ Ù.SÁ DIB.DIB-*su* U$_4$ DIB-*šu* GEŠTU^{II}-*šú* GÙ.DÉ.MEŠ KA-*šú* DIB-*ma* NU DUG$_4$.DUG$_4$-⸢*ub*⸣ ŠU A.LÁ ḪUL (DPS XXVII:23 [AOAT 43.298–299])

**If something like a stupor continually afflicts him and, when it afflicts him, his ears roar (and) his mouth is "seized" so that he cannot talk, "hand" of an evil *alû*.

13.275 (A.LÁ.ḪUL) *šá ki-ma i-ga-ri i-qup-pu-ma* UGU LÚ [*i*]*b-ba-tu at-ta*$_5$ . . . (A.LÁ.ḪUL) *šá pa-a la i-šu-ú at-ta* . . . (A.LÁ.ḪUL) *la še-mu-ú at-ta* (A.LÁ.ḪUL) *šá ina ma-a-a-al mu-ši* LÚ *ina šit-ti i-re-eḫ-ḫu-ú at-ta* . . . (A.LÁ.ḪUL) *e-kim šit-ti šá* LÚ *ana ta-ba-li iz-*[*za-az-zu at-ta*] . . . (*CT* 16.27:5, 9, 13, 19, 21)[217]

**You are the evil *alû*-demon who buckled like a wall and fell on the person . . . you are the evil *alû*-demon who has no mouth . . . you are the evil *alû*-demon who does not hear . . . you are the evil *alû*-demon who flows over[218] a person in his sleep on his night bed . . . you are the evil *alû*-demon who deprives a person of his sleep and stands (beside him) to carry him off . . .

Stages II–III were considered to have a dismal prognosis.[219]

13.276 DIŠ KI.MIN IGI^{II}-*šú ú-zaq-qap* SÌG-*su ina* SAG-*šú* GUB-*az* ÚŠ (DPS XXVI:80′ [AOAT 43.285])

**If (he continuously goes through the motions of getting into and out of his clothing and) he makes (the pupils of) his eyes constrict, the one who strikes him stands at his head; he will die.

13.277 DIŠ *i-ta-nar-ra-ar* IGI^{II}-*šú ú-zaq-qap* SÌG-*su ina* SAG-*šú* GUB-*ma* GAM (DPS XXVI:81′ [AOAT 43.285])[220]

**If he trembles (and) makes (the pupils of) his eyes constrict, the one who strikes him stands at his head and consequently he will die.

In addition to observing the comatose patient's movements and the responsiveness of his pupils, the *āšipu* also noted several of the distinctive respiratory patterns that accompany comas. Rapid, deep (Kussmaul) breathing usually implies metabolic acidosis but may also occur with pontomesencephalic lesions.

13.278 DIŠ ZI-*šú* GU$_4$.UD.ME *u* ŠÀ.MEŠ-*šú it-te-nen-bi-ṭu* GAM / DIŠ ZI-*šú* GU$_4$.UD.ME *u* SA.MEŠ-*šú šap-ku* GAM / DIŠ ZI-*šú i-tar-rak-ma qit-ru-bat* [G]AM (DPS X A obv. 30–31//B obv. 34–36 = *TDP* 84:30–31)

**If his breath becomes rapid[221] and his insides are continually cramped, he will die. If his breath becomes rapid[222] and his muscles are tense,[223] he will die. If his breath throbs and comes closely spaced, ⌜he will die⌝.

Gasps, held in inspiration, reflect bilateral lower brain stem damage and are well known as the terminal respiratory pattern of severe brain damage. The *āšipu* referred to this breathing pattern by the onomatopoeic expression *ḫūqu*.[224]

13.279 DIŠ U$_4$.5.KÁM U$_4$.10.KÁM GIG *dan-na* GIG-*ma uš-tar-di-ma* GI$_6$ IGI^{II}-*šú uš-ter-di-a* U$_4$.2.KÁM *ḫu-qu* DIB.DIB-*su ina* U$_4$.3.KÁM GAM (DPS XVI:53′–54′ [AOAT 43.177])

**If he has been sick with a mighty sickness for five or ten days and the pupils of his eyes persist in (moving) downward (and) *ḫūqu* continually afflicts him for two days, he will die on the third day.

13.280 DIŠ KI.MIN-*ma* GI$_6$ IGI^{II}-*šú* E$_{11}$-*a u ḫu-qu* DIB.DIB-*su ana* U$_4$.3.KÁM GAM (DPS XVI:58′ [AOAT 43.177])[225]

**If (he has been sick for five, ten, or fifteen days) and the pupils of his eyes (move) upward and *ḫūqu* continually afflicts him for three days, he will die.

Neurologic Testing

The ancient Mesopotamian physician tried to separate one disease from another not only by careful observation of signs and symptoms, but by performing specific clinical tests. Five of the tests involved the nervous system, and modern physicians use these same tests today.

MORO REFLEX TEST

The neurologic status of an infant can be evaluated by placing it on its back on a table with its head supported. When the physician withdraws support, suddenly allowing the head to fall backward, the infant quickly flexes its extremities and then extends its arms wide open. Absence of this response in an infant, which modern physicians call the Moro reflex, is a bad prognostic indicator. From the following reference it is clear that the ancient Mesopotamian physician knew and used this test, but, of course, without its modern name.[226]

13.281 DIŠ LÚ.TUR *ki-ša-da-nu-uš-šú tuš-qa-lal-šu-ma la i-gal-lut u i-di-šú la i-tar-ra-aṣ ki-šid* SAḪAR (DPS XL A 3//C 3 = *TDP* 216:3)

**If you suspend an infant by his neck and he does not jerk and does not stretch out his arms, he was "gotten" by the dust.

EXTREMITY REFLEX TEST

Today physicians test the sensorimotor pathway through the spinal cord (deep tendon reflex) by tapping a tendon with a hard object. Typically this is done by striking the knee just below the knee cap, but similar tests can be performed at other sites such as the ankle and elbow. A normal response is for the leg to kick forward immediately after the knee is struck. If this fails to occur it indicates a neurologic abnormality. We believe that the following reference demonstrates that the *āšipu* used this test and understood its significance.

13.282 DIŠ U$_4$*-ma* UD.DU*-šú* GIN$_7$ TU.K[UR$_4$^{MUŠEN} *i-dam-mu-um*] IGI^{II}*-šú it-ta-na-aš-d*[*a*]*-da* [. . .] *ina ṭur-ri* KA*-šú* D[U*-m*]*a* ŠÀ-[*šú* . . .] A ŠUB U$_4$*-ma* UD.DU*-šú* [S]A SAG.K[I*-šú* ZI.MEŠ ŠÀ.MEŠ*-šú*][227] *na-šu-u ina* KIN TUR Z⸢A⸣BAR SÌG*-m*[*a* . . .] *ár-ḫiš* LUḪ*-ut* GIG*-su* DU$_8$[*-ár* . . . *šúm-ma*] *ina* IGI SÌG*-ka* NU LUḪ*-ut* GIG-[*su* . . .] (*STT* 89:152, 158 [Stol, *Epilepsy* 95])

**If when it comes over him, [he moans] like a ⸢dove⸣, his eyes (feel) like they are continually pulled forward, [. . .] comes out of the "band" of his mouth,[228] his insides [. . . his eyes(?)] water(?),[229] (and if) when it comes over him the blood [vessels] of [his] ⸢temple⸣ [(feel like they) are pulsating (and) his insides] are puffed up, you strike with a small copper object ⌜and⌝ [. . .], he immediately jerks,[230] his illness will relent . . . [If (however)] he does not jerk despite your striking, [his] illness [. . .].

TESTS FOR PARALYSIS

The *āšipu* actively evaluated patients for evidence of weakness or paralysis by performing some of the observations or maneuvers listed below.

13.283 DIŠ GÚ-*su* 15 *u* 150 *ut-ta-nar* GAM / DIŠ GÚ-*su* 15 *u* 150 ŠUB.ŠUB-*di* GAM (DPS X A obv. 14//B obv. 14–15 = *TDP* 82:14)

**If he continually returns his head to the left or right, he will die. If he continually lets his neck drop to the left or right, he will die.

13.284 DIŠ GÚ-*su* 15 *u* 150 ŠUB.ŠUB-*ut* GAM / DIŠ GÚ-*su* TA 15 *ana* 150 *suḫ*$_4$-*ḫur-ma* ŠUB-*ut* [G]AM (DPS X A obv. 15//B obv. 16–17 = *TDP* 82:15; cf. StBoT 36.62:5)

**If his neck continually falls to the left or right, he will die. If his neck falls when it is turned from left to right, ⌜he will die⌝.

13.285 DIŠ *mi-šit-ti im-šid-su-ma lu* 15 *lu* 150 SÌG-*iṣ* MUD Á-*šú* NU *pa-ṭir* ŠU.SI.MEŠ-*šú* NIR.NIR-*aṣ* ŠU-*su ú-šaq-qá u* NIR-*aṣ* GÌR-*šú i-qan-na-an u* NIR-*aṣ* [NIN]DA *u* KAŠ NU TAR-*us* DIB GIDIM$_7$ *ana* EDIN <U$_4$>.3.KÁM *ni-ši* (DPS XXVII:5–7 [AOAT 43.297]; *AMT* 77/1 i 2–4)

**If he has a stroke and either his left side or his right side is affected (and) his shoulder is not released, (but) he can straighten out his fingers (and) he can lift his hand and stretch it out (and) he can bend his foot and stretch it out again[231] (and) he is not off his ⌜food⌝ or drink, affliction by a ghost at the steppe; recovery in three (days).

COMA EVALUATION TESTS

Modern physicians often test for the presence of coma by applying a strong auditory or pain stimulus to an apparently unresponsive patient. Shouting, shaking, nasal tickle with a cotton wisp, and deep pressure on the knuckles or bony prominences are preferred forms of noxious stimulus. The ancient physician used a variation on this approach by splashing water in the patient's face, as shown in the following text (see Coma above). The second and third quotes use an auditory stimulus.

13.286 DIŠ U$_4$.6.KÁM LÍL-*ma ina* U$_4$.7.KÁM NU PA.AN-*uš* A *ana* IGI.MEŠ-*šú i-sal-la-ú-ma šum*$_4$-*ma* IGI^{II}-*šú* NU BAD GAM *šum*$_4$-*ma* IGI^{II}-*šú* BAD *u* DUL-*tam ana* A *šá is-lu-ḫu-šú* ÍR DIN (DPS XVI:63′–64′ [AOAT 43.177–178])[232]

**If he has been sick for six days and he does not get a respite[233] on the seventh, they throw water on his face and if he does not open his eyes, he will die. If he opens and closes his eyes at the water that they throw over him (and) wails, he will get well.

13.287 U$_4$ GIG IGI-*šu bu-ul-lu-ṣú ta-šà-as-si-šu-ma ul i-še-em-me-ka mi-im-ma šà tu-ka-al-lu-šu ul ú-ma-dì* ŠU *qa-a-a-li* (*MDP* 57.11 v 15′–18′)

**If the patient's eyes are dilated, you call out to him and he does not hear you, (and) whatever you hold before him he does not recognize,[234] "hand" of the taciturn one.

13.288 *a-lu-ú zu-um-ri i-te-di-iq ṣu-ba-ti ki-ma šu-uš-kal-li ú-kàt-ti-man-ni šit-tú bal-ṣa-a-ma ul i-na-aṭ-ṭal i-na-a-a pi-ta-a-ma ul i-šim-ma-a uz-na-a-a kal pag-ri-ia i-ta-ḫaz ri-mu-tú* . . . [*iš*]*-du-ud mu-tu i-te-rim pa-ni-ia* [*i-ḫa*]*-*⌜*sa*⌝*-sa-ni-ma ša-ʾi-i ul ap-pal* (Lambert, *BWL* 42:71–75, 81–82)

**My body has donned an *alû*-demon as one would a garment; he covered me with sleep[235] as with a net. My eyes are dilated and do not see; my ears are open but do not hear. Paralysis has gripped my whole body . . . Death has ⌜drawn⌝ (the curtain); it has covered my face. He ⌜listens⌝ to me, but I do not answer the one who questions me.

Another consciousness test used by the *āšipu* sought to determine whether the patient was able to follow simple instructions.

13.289 DIŠ *ana* KA-*šú* A.MEŠ ŠUB-*ma* A.MEŠ *ina* [K]A-*šú ú-kal* [DIN] (DPS III A obv. 4//B 4)

**If you pour water into his mouth and he can hold the water in his ⌜mouth⌝, [he will live].

MEMORY TESTING

A patient's mental clarity can be tested by a physician asking the patient to recall past events or facts. In the quote that follows, the *āšipu* has performed this test on his patient.

13.290 ⌜DIŠ⌝ U$_4$ LÁ-*šú* UB.NÍGIN.NA-*šú i-šam-ma-ma-šú i-re-eḫ-ḫi-šum-ma* NÍ-*šú i-maš-ši* U$_4$ *ir-te-ḫu-šú* IGI^{II}-*šú* SAR-*ṭa* IGI.MEŠ-*šú* SA$_5$: *suḫ$_4$-ḫu-ru* SA.MEŠ-*šú* ZI.MEŠ *u i-leb-bu ap-pat* U.MEŠ ŠU^{II}-*šú u* GÌR^{II}-*šú ka-ṣa-a* GIG BI MAŠ.MAŠ *ú-šad-bab-šú-ma ša ú-šad-ba-bu-šú i-qab-bi* U$_4$ *un-deš-ši-ru-šú šá id-bu-bu* NU ZU ŠU LÍL.LÁ.EN.NA *la-ʾ-bi* (DPS XXVI:22′–25′ [AOAT 43.280])

**If when (a confusional state) comes over him, his limbs go numb, as it flows over him he forgets himself, when it has flowed over him, his eyes (look) "(wind) blasted,"[236] his face flushes (var. he turns away), his blood vessels (feel like they) are pulsating and he groans, the tips of his fingers and toes are cold (and) the *āšipu* makes that patient say (something) and (the patient) says what (the *āšipu*) has him say (but) when (the confusional state) has left him, (the patient) does not know what he said, infectious "hand" of *lilû*.

Summary

A strong indication of the importance of precise description of observations was the complexity of the vocabulary used. The technical terminology devised by the *āšipu* to describe pain, loss of sensation and movement, and abnormal movement is especially extensive and complex, and more clinical tests were associated with neurologic disorders than with any other discipline of ancient Mesopotamian medicine. The wealth of unique neurologic signs and symptoms permitted ancient Mesopotamian physicians to separate and characterize neurologic diseases with particular success. Most impressive are the descriptions of brain trauma, including damage to the cranial nerves and all of the major categories of seizure disorders and strokes.

CHAPTER 14

Trauma and Shock

If he was crushed in his mouth and continually
produces black blood [. . .]

—DPS VII B obv. 8′ = *TDP* 64:47′

Trauma

*Āšipu*s were provided with ample opportunities to observe trauma victims. The armies of Assyrian kings contemporary with the bulk of the surviving medical texts were protected by shields, helmets, and flexible suits of armor made from iron scales sewn onto a cloth backing. Wars were unavoidably frequent, at times virtually annual events, as during the reign of Sargon II. Swords were made of iron hardened by heating and quenching in cold water and coated with bronze to maintain a consistently sharp edge. Attacking soldiers were greeted with showers of sling-stones and iron-tipped arrows, shot from composite bows. Below are some examples of common injuries. Trauma resulting in neurological abnormalities is discussed in Chapter 13, trauma to the ears in Chapter 9, and infected abdominal wounds in Chapter 3.

MINOR, TREATABLE WOUNDS

The extensive use of sandals by ancient Mesopotamians made feet particularly liable to injuries to the heel, as in the second and third references below, to which the *āšipu* applied medicinal bandages. For information on treatable wound and soft tissue infections, see Chapter 3.

14.1 DIŠ NA NUNDUN.MEŠ-*šú* *ku*-[*bu-ra*] . . . DIŠ KI.MIN NUNDUN-*su* *ḫe-pa-at* . . . (*BAM* 543 i 51′, 55′)

**If a person's lips are ⌜thickened⌝ . . . If (a person's lips are thickened and) his lip is broken . . .

14.2 DIŠ NA *a-si-da-šú pur-ru-ur*. . . (*AMT* 75/1+ iv 17)

**If a person's heels were bored into . . .

14.3 DIŠ NA *a-si-da-šú lu-ut-ta-a* . . . (*AMT* 75/1+ iv 19)

**If a person's heels were split . . .

SEVERE FACIAL AND HEAD INJURY

14.4 DIŠ SA SAG.KI-*šú* [. . .]x *zi-iz* DIŠ KÚM-*im* SILIM-*ma* DIN / DIŠ SA SAG.KI-*šú zi-iz u* GI_6 GIG-*su* DUGUD GABA.RI SÌG-*iṣ* (DPS IV E ii 17–18 = *SpTU* 3.88 ii 17–18)[1]

**If a blood vessel of his temple [. . .] was cut through (divided), if he is (merely) feverish, he is safe and will get well. If a blood vessel of his temple was cut through and is dark, his illness will get worse; he was wounded on the front side.

14.5 DIŠ IGI^{II}-*šú pa-ʾ-a-ṣa-ma* IM.G[Ú DIRI . . .] (DPS V A 8′ = *TDP* 46 B 8)[2]

**If his eyes were smashed and, as a consequence, [are full] of ⌜sediment⌝ [. . .].

14.6 DIŠ $GEŠTU^{II}$-*šú* DU_8.DU_8-*ra* GAM (DPS VIII 7b = *TDP* 68:7b)[3]

**If (both) his ears were (broken) open, he will die.

14.7 [DIŠ KIR_4-*šú* . . .] / DIŠ KIR_4-*šú ur-ru-ub* GAM (DPS VI A obv. 5 = *TDP* 54:5)[4]

**If his nose is [. . .] If his nose was knocked in all over, he will die.

14.8 DIŠ EME-*šú* GI_6-*at ina* KA-*šú* S[ÌG-*iṣ* . . .] (DPS VII A obv. 23 = *TDP* 62:23)[5]

**If his tongue is black, he was ⌜wounded⌝ on his mouth [. . .].

14.9 DIŠ *ina* KA-*šú i-ḫaš-šal u* MÚD GI_6 ŠUB.ŠUB-*a* [. . .] (DPS VII B obv. 8′ = *TDP* 64:47′)

**If he was crushed in his mouth and continually produces black blood [. . .]

14.10 DIŠ EME-*šú ina* ZÚ.MEŠ-*šú na-šik* UGU ⌜SÌG⌝-[*iṣ* . . .] (DPS VII A obv. 17 = *TDP* 62:17)

**If his tongue was bitten with his teeth, the top of the head was hit [. . .]

The last reference above describes one of the two ways that an individual can bite his tongue during a hostile interchange. If a person's tongue happens to be extended out beyond his teeth when he receives a downward blow to the top of his head or an upward blow to his chin, he will in most cases bite his tongue. The *āšipu* clearly understood the nature of this injury. See Chapter 13 for other descriptions of head wounds.

FATAL NECK WOUND

14.11 DIŠ *ina gir-ri-šú* SÌG-*iṣ* ŠU ^{d}MAŠ.T[AB.BA GAM] (DPS X A obv. 54b = *TDP* 86:54b)

**If he was wounded on his throat, "hand" of the ⌜twin gods⌝; [he will die].

Neck wounds could have caused death by bleeding, airway obstruction, or spinal cord injury with death from respiratory paralysis.

FATAL CHEST/ABDOMINAL WOUNDS

14.12 DIŠ KI.MIN-*ma* ŠÀ ŠÀ GÙ.GÙ-*si u* SÍG-*su ú-ban-qam ina ban-ti-šú* SÌG-*iṣ* GAM (DPS XV:38′ [AOAT 43.152]; cf. DPS XIII G_2 r. 16 = *TDP* 124 iii 23)

**If (it is the first day he is sick) and he cries: "My insides, my insides!" and he tears his hair, he was wounded on his chest (thorax); he will die.

The chest wound in the reference above possibly caused death by bleeding or pneumothorax (air entering the chest around the lungs and preventing the lungs from expanding). The air could enter the chest either through a chest wall wound or from a punctured lung.

The reference below appears to be a penetrating wound of the abdomen and chest resulting in a tear in the diaphragm. This wound would have interrupted normal breathing mechanisms and almost certainly have involved severe bleeding and injury to the liver or spleen.

14.13 [DIŠ. . .]x BÀD ŠÀ-*šú ana* ḪAR-*šú is-niq* [GAM] (DPS XIII J 8 = *TDP* 126 iii 40)

**[If he keeps crying out: "My insides, my insides"] (and) the wall of his abdomen approaches his lung, [he will die].[6]

FATAL LEG WOUNDS

Leg wounds may lead to a fatal outcome primarily from blood loss if a major vessel is damaged or from severe wound infections. In the former case, the patient might suffer from hemorrhagic shock and in the latter from septic shock (see below). In the following references, blood loss would be the more likely cause of shock since the day of the injury would have been too recent for a serious infection to develop.

14.14 DIŠ KI.MIN-*ma ina* ḪÁŠ.<GAL>-*šú šá* 15 SÌG-*iṣ* UŠ$_4$-*šú* NU DIB [*ina* NU ZU *ú-rap-pad* GAM] (DPS XV:57 [AOAT 43.154]; cf. DPS XIV A_2 i 15//C_2 i 5+C i 19 = *TDP* 132 i 66)

**If (it is the first day he is sick) and he was wounded on his left inguinal region,[7] he is not in full possession of his faculties [(and) he wanders about[8] without knowing (where he is), he will die].[9]

14.15 DIŠ KI.MIN-*ma ina* ḪÁŠ.GAL-*šú šá* 150 SÌG-*iṣ* GIN$_7$ GÙ.GÙ N[U ZU GAM] (DPS XV:58 [AOAT 43.154]; cf. DPS XIV A$_2$ i 16//C$_2$ i 6+C i 20 = *TDP* 132 i 67)

**If (it is the first day he is sick) and he was wounded on his right inguinal region (and) he does ⌜not⌝ [know] that he is continually crying out, [he will die].[10]

14.16 DIŠ KI.MIN-*ma ina kur-ri-šú šá* 15 SÌG-*iṣ-ma* NÍ-*šú ma-ši* ŠU ^{d}ŠUL.PA.È.A GAM (DPS XV:49 [AOAT 43.153]; cf. DPS XII D iv 23//E iv 30 = *TDP* 108 iv 23)

**If (it is the first day he is sick) and he was wounded on his left groin (femoral crease)[11] and consequently he forgets himself, "hand" of Šulpaea; he will die.

14.17 DIŠ *ina kin-ṣi-šú šá* 15 [SÌG-*i*]*ṣ u ina* KA-*šú* MÚD BURU$_8$ [GÍD-*ma*? GAM] / DIŠ *ina kin-ṣi-šú šá* 150 SÌG-*iṣ u ina* KA-*šú* MÚD MUD [ŠUB-*di* GAM] (DPS XIV C iii 27–28+C$_2$ iii 26b–27//F 15–16; cf. DPS XV:59–60 [AOAT 43.154])

**If he was ⌜wounded⌝ on his left leg (and) he vomits blood from his mouth, [(if) it is prolonged(?), he will die]. If he was wounded on his right leg and he [produces] dark blood from his mouth, [he will die].

Nerve damage, as noted in the reference below by the patient's inability to raise his foot, would not by itself lead to death (unless it prevented him from fleeing the enemy).

14.18 DIŠ KI.MIN-*ma ina kur-ri-šú šá* 150 SÌG-*iṣ-ma* GÌR-*šú* NU ZI-*aḫ ina* ^{d}UTU È <SÌG-*iṣ*> ŠU ^{d}15 GAM (DPS XV:50 [AOAT 43.153]; cf. DPS XII D iv 24–25//E iv 31–32 = *TDP* 108 iv 24–25)

**If (it is the first day he is sick) and he was wounded on his right groin (femoral crease)[12] and consequently he cannot uproot his foot (from the ground) (and) he <was wounded> at sunrise, "hand" of Ištar; he will die.

Constipation and abdominal cramps mentioned in the following references suggest peritonitis (see Chapter 3), which in turn suggests that the wound extended from the thigh into the pelvis or that a second wound penetrated the abdomen.

14.19 DIŠ KI.MIN-*ma ina* ÚR-*šú šá* 15 SÌG-*iṣ u e-sil* GAM (DPS XV:54 [AOAT 43.153]; cf. DPS XIV A iii 6//C$_2$ iii 1 = *TDP* 140 iii 40′)

**If (it is the first day he is sick) and he was wounded on his left crotch/thigh and he is constipated, he will die.

14.20 DIŠ KI.MIN-*ma ina* ÚR-*šú šá* 150 SÌG-*iṣ* ŠÀ.MEŠ-*šú eb-ṭú* SAG.KI-*šú ḫe-sa-át* [GAM] (DPS XV:55 [AOAT 43.153]; cf. DPS XIV A iii 7 = *TDP* 140 iii 41′)

**If (it is the first day he is sick) and he was wounded on his right crotch/thigh, his stomach is cramped (and) he has a viselike headache,[13] [he will die].

BLEEDING, EXTERNAL AND INTERNAL

The ancient Mesopotamian physician would have readily recognized the potentially serious consequence of visible bleeding as a cause of shock (see below) and ultimately death.

14.21 DIŠ GIG GAR-*šú* GIN_7 KUD-*is* UDU.NÍTA MÚD *ṣar-ḫa ú-*[*š*]*e-ṣi* GI.DÙ.A gul lu su *ana* TI-*šú* x e xx [. . .] (DPS XXXIII:33 [AOAT 43.355])

**If the nature of the wound is that it produces hot blood like a sheep with its throat cut [. . .], to cure him [. . .].

The presence of internal bleeding would have been difficult for the *āšipu* to determine. Without modern screening procedures only bleeding that could make its way to the outside through some opening or under the skin would be noted. The two references below are examples of trauma-induced internal bleeding that came to the attention of the ancient physician.

14.22 DIŠ NA *ina* DÚR-*šú* MÚD *ú-tab-ba-ka* GIN_7 MUNUS ^{GIŠ}TUKUL *ma-ḫi-iṣ ana* TI-*šú* . . . (*BAM* 152 iii 8–9//*BAM* 99:27)

**If a person pours blood from his anus like a woman, he was wounded with a weapon, to cure him . . .

14.23 DIŠ NA *ina* GÌŠ-*šu* MÚD *ú-tab-ba-ka* GIN_7 MUNUS ^{GIŠ}TUKUL *ma-ḫi-iṣ ana* TI-*šú* . . . (*BAM* 159 i 9–10//*BAM* 396 iv 3//*BAM* 182 obv. 6′)

**If a person pours blood from his penis like a (menstruating) woman, he was wounded with a weapon, to cure him . . .

Shock

The term *shock* is usually used when blood pressure drops to the point that tissue circulation is inadequate for normal function, although it is also used to describe the mental changes that occur due to the stress of war. Although the cause of the shock in the following references is unspecified, the collapse of the blood vessels[14] and the anticipated death of the patient demonstrate its presence.

14.24 DIŠ SAG.KI-*šú šal-mat* DIN / DIŠ SAG.KI-*šú* ŠUB-*ut* GAM (DPS IV A obv. 5//B obv. 5 = *TDP* 32:5)[15]

**If his temple is normal, he will get well; if (the blood vessels of) his temple have collapsed, he will die.

14.25 DIŠ SAG.KI-*šú* ŠUB-*ut-ma* IGI^{II}-*šú a-ši-a*/ÍR-*a*[16] GAM (DPS IV A obv. 6+A_2 obv. 1//B obv. 6//D 6 = *TDP* 32:6)[17]

**If (the blood vessels of) his temple have collapsed and his eyes are "confused"/shed tears, he will die.

The following references have been separated into the type of shock that they appear to describe. However, it is impossible in all cases to be certain that they are properly categorized. Some patients may be experiencing both hemorrhagic shock and post-traumatic stress syndrome.

HEMORRHAGIC SHOCK

Rapid blood loss (hemorrhage) is one cause of shock. Often the first noticeable change is altered mental function, including confusion and disorientation, with the patient eventually lapsing into coma. If uncorrected, this condition will end in death. In the following references, the first patient died as a result of a wound to the abdomen; the second was literally stabbed in the back (perhaps trying to flee the field of battle). The last two seem to have been run through with the shaft of a spear or arrow passing through the back with the point emerging through the rib cage.

14.26 DIŠ KI.MIN-*ma* ŠU-*su ina* LI.DUR-*šú* GAR-*at-ma* ŠU^{II}-*šú u* GÌR^{II}-*šú ka-ṣa-a ina* NU ⌜ZU-*e*⌝ [DUG$_4$.DUG$_4$-*ub*] ZI-*bi u* TÚŠ-*ab ina* LI.DUR-*šú* SÌG-*iṣ* ŠU ^{d}*Dil-bat* [GAM] (DPS XV:13–14 [AOAT 43.151]; cf. DPS XI A obv. 9//B 8 = *TDP* 90:9//*SpTU* 1.34:8)

**If (it is the first day he is sick) and his hand is placed on his navel and his hands and his feet are cold,[18] he talks without knowing (what he is saying and) he gets up and sits down (again), he was wounded on his navel. "Hand" of Dilbat (Ištar); [he will die].

14.27 DIŠ KI.MIN-*ma ina* ÉLLAG-*šú šá* 150 SÌG-*iṣ* UŠ$_4$-*šú* NU DIB *u* MÚD BURU$_8$ ŠU ^{d}7.BI GAM (DPS XV:40 [AOAT 43.152]; cf. DPS XII D iii 22 = *TDP* 104 iii 22)

**If (it is the first day he is sick) and he was wounded on his right kidney, he is not in full possession of his faculties, and he vomits blood, "hand" of the Sibitti; he will die.

14.28 DIŠ KI.MIN-*ma* TI-*šú šá* 15 GI$_6$ KA-*šú* ḪÁD.MEŠ *u it-ta-nag-ra-ár* ŠU ^{d}*Da-mu ina* ÉLLAG-*šú* SÌG-*iṣ* GAM (DPS XV:42 [AOAT 43.152])

**If (it is the first day he is sick) and his left rib is dark, his mouth is continually dry, and he rolls over and over, "hand" of Damu. He was wounded on his kidney; he will die.

14.29 DIŠ KI.MIN-*ma* TI-*šú šá* 150 GI$_6$ MÚD BURU$_8$ *u* ZI.IR.MEŠ *ina* U$_4$ BI SÌG-*iṣ* GAM (DPS XV:43 [AOAT 43.152])

**If (it is the first day he is sick) and his right rib is dark, he vomits blood, and (his insides) are continually upset (and) he was wounded that same day, he will die.

The texts below graphically describe massive bleeding from a head wound and the expected outcome, death.

14.30 [DIŠ SA SAG.KI^{II}-*š*] *ú ip-te-ru-nim* [. . .] GAM (DPS IV A$_2$ r. 9//G r. 8 = *TDP* 40 r. 9//*LKU* 94 r. 8; cf. Labat, *Syria* 33.125 r. 10)

** [If the blood vessel(s)] of ⌜his⌝ [temples] vomit forth [. . .], he will die.

14.31 [DIŠ SA SAG.KI^{II}]-*šú* ⌜MÚD⌝ *il-<te>-qú-m*[*a* . . .] GAM (DPS IV A$_2$ r. 11//G r. 10 = *TDP* 40 r.11//*LKU* 94 r.10; cf. Labat, *Syria* 33.125 r. 12)

** [If the blood vessel(s) of] his [temples] water the ground with blood [. . .], he will die.

Often used in descriptions of shock is the Akkadian term *rapādu*, which means literally "to wander about" and which is used almost exclusively to describe fatal syndromes associated with disorientation, trauma, and fever. In the following references, the first patient died as a result of a wound to the chest and the second was stabbed in the back.

14.32 DIŠ KI.MIN-*ma ina* GABA-*šú* SÌG-*ma* MÚD *ú-tab-ba-ka u ú-rap-pad* ŠU ^{d}U.GUR GABA.RI⌜SÌG⌝-*iṣ* GAM (DPS XV:32 [AOAT 43.152]; cf. DPS XII A 4 = *TDP* 100 i 4)[19]

**If (it is the first day he is sick) and he was wounded on his breast and, as a consequence, he continually pours out blood and wanders about, "hand" of Nergal; he was wounded on the front side; he will die.

14.33 DIŠ KI.MIN-*ma ina* ÉLLAG-*šú šá* 15 SÌG-*iṣ* UŠ$_4$-*šú* NU DIB *ina* NU ZU *ú-rap-pad* ŠU ^{d}MAŠ.TAB.⌜BA⌝ GA[M] (DPS XV:39 [AOAT 43.152]; cf. DPS XII D iii 21//E iii 22 = *TDP* 104 iii 21)[20]

**If (it is the first day he is sick) and he was wounded on his left kidney, he is not in full possession of his faculties, (and) he wanders about without knowing (where he is), "hand" of the twin gods; he will die.[21]

POST-TRAUMATIC STRESS SYNDROME

Severe mental and/or physical (traumatic) stress may produce psychological changes that can be confused with some of the early mental changes associated with low blood pressure. However, this illness will not cause the death of a patient. Modern physicians call this the post-traumatic stress syndrome. The quotes below may be describing this syndrome.

14.34 DIŠ GIG [INIM-*šú*] KÚR.KÚR-*ir ana* U$_4$.3.[KÁM . . .] KA-*šú* [. . .] *u ra-pa-du su-ud-dur-šú ana* U$_4$.3.K[ÁM . . .] (DPS VII B r. 3–4 = *TDP* 64:59′–60′)

**If his words are unintelligible for three days [. . .] his mouth [. . .] and he experiences wandering about for three days in a row [. . .].

14.35 *ra-pa-du su-ud-dur-*[*šú*] = [*šá-n*]*e-e ṭè-e-me sa-dir-šú* (*SpTU* 1.32 r. 8–9 [commentary to DPS VII B r. 3–4 = *TDP* 64:59′–60′])

**"He experiences wandering about (for three) consecutive (days)" means "he experiences ⌜alteration⌝ of mentation (for three) consecutive (days)."

14.36 DIŠ INIM-*šú* KÚR.KÚR[-*ir*] *u a-šu-uš-tum* ⌜ŠUB⌝.ŠUB-*su ana* U$_4$.DUG$_4$.GA-⌜*šú ana*⌝ U$_4$.3.K[ÁM . . .] (DPS VII B r. 8 = *TDP* 66:64′)[22]

**If his words are unintelligible and depression keeps falling on him at regular intervals (and he has been sick) for three days [. . .].

SEPTIC SHOCK

In some forms of severe infection, another serious complication develops that is variously called septic shock, sepsis syndrome, or systemic inflammatory response syndrome. This condition usually causes low blood pressure, but by mechanisms other than blood loss. As with hemorrhagic shock, there are usually early changes in mental status similar to those described above, and without treatment, the patient usually dies.

14.37 DIŠ KI.MIN-*ma* U.MEŠ ŠU^{II}-*šú ina* [KA-*šú ú-man-zaq* KÚM] ⌜ÚḪ⌝ ŠÀ-*šú na-pi-iḫ u ú-rap-pad ina* GÚ-*šú* SÌG-*iṣ* ⌜ŠU⌝ ^{d}⌜*Ba*⌝-*ú* GAM (DPS XV:26 [AOAT 43.151]; cf. DPS XI A r. 36 = *TDP* 96 r. 36)[23]

**If (it is the first day he is sick) and he sucks his fingers in his mouth, he burns with fever,[24] his abdomen is bloated, and he wanders about, he was wounded on his neck. "Hand" of Bau; he will die.

14.38 DIŠ KI.MIN-*ma ri-bit-su šá* 15 *nap-ḫat-ma* GI_6-*át ina* NU ZU *ú-rap-pad* ŠU [d]IŠKUR *ina* $AN.BAR_7$ SÌG-*iṣ* GAM (DPS XV:52 [AOAT 43.153]; cf. DPS XIV A iii 10–11//C_2 iii 3//I 6–7 = *TDP* 140 iii 44′–45′)[25]

**If (it is the first day he is sick) and the left side of his abdomen is swollen and dark (and) he wanders about without knowing (where he is), "hand" of Adad. <If> he was wounded at noon; he will die.

14.39 LU.UL.LU.PA.AP.ḪA.AL.LA ([*m*]*u-ut-ta-al-li-kam*) [D]I.A N[U.U]N.ZA.A (*i-na la i-du-ú*) BA.NI.IB.DI.IB.BI LU.BI ŠU.SI.IQ.QA BA.AN.ŠE GI.RI.SI.IQ.QA BA.AN.ŠE SA.AD.NI.IM IM.ŠU.UB ZA.AG.ŠE (*a-ḫa-a-šu*) IM.G[U].G[U.R]A (*ku-us-sà*) A.GI.GA. I.I (Falkenstein, *ZA* 45.12–41:14–19)[26]

**That person was afflicted with going about without knowing (where he was going). That person's wounded hand was made cold; his wounded foot was made cold. Wandering about in a daze[27] fell upon (him). His arms were bent/bound; he complained bitterly.

In some cases of septic shock, because of a combination of low blood pressure and increased blood coagulability, the patient's hands or feet may become gangrenous. We believe that the dark hands mentioned in the quote below are due to gangrene. A further complication of septic shock is increased bleeding. This occurs when the increased coagulability runs its course, consuming all the available clotting proteins and platelets. This may result in bleeding into the tissues, potentially contributing to the "dark" appearance of the hands and feet.

14.40 DIŠ $ŠU^{II}$-*šú* GI_6.MEŠ-*ma* AD_6-*šú* KÚM-*im* [. . .] (DPS XI A obv. 15//B 14 = *TDP* 90:15//*SpTU* 1.34:14)

**If his hands are dark and his body is feverish [. . .]

In the texts below, the *āšipu* refers to the "bellies" of the fingers and toes and to the "breasts" of the hands and feet as being "dark." The clinical outcome in all cases is death. We believe the "bellies" to be the pads or tips of the digits.[28] Since the tips of the fingers and toes are usually the first areas to show signs of gangrene due to their peripheral location, it is probable that these are cases of septic shock.

14.41 DIŠ KI.MIN-*ma kar-ši* U.MEŠ $ŠU^{II}$-*šú* GI_6.MEŠ *u i-ṭa-me* ŠU.GÍDIM.⌜MA⌝ GAM (DPS XV:29 [AOAT 43.152])[29]

**If (it is the first day he is sick) and the "bellies" of his fingers are dark and he twists, "hand" of ghost; he will die.

14.42 DIŠ *kar-ši* U.MEŠ $GÌR^{II}$-*šú* GI_6.MEŠ *i-ṭa-mu* GAM (DPS XIV A iv 14//K 8 = *TDP* 144 iv 49′; cf. DPS XV:66 [AOAT 43.154])

**If the "bellies" of his toes are dark (and) he twists, he will die.

The texts that mention the "dark breasts" of the hands and feet are less clear. These "breasts" may be the prominent padded areas of the palms and soles near the base of the fingers and toes,[30] areas that would also be highly susceptible to gangrene.

> **14.43** DIŠ KI.MIN-*ma* GABA.MEŠ *šá* ŠU^{II}-*šú* GI$_6$.MEŠ ŠU DINGIR⸢URU⸣-*šú* GAM (DPS XV:28 [AOAT 43.152])
>
> **If (it is the first day he is sick) and the "breasts" of his hands are dark, "hand" of the god of his city; he will die.
>
> **14.44** DIŠ GABA.MEŠ *šá* GÌR^{II}-*šú* GI$_6$.MEŠ ŠU ^{d}15 GÍD-*ma* GAM (DPS XIV A iv 16//K 10 = *TDP* 144 iv 51′; cf. DPS XV:65 [AOAT 43.154])
>
> **If the "breasts" of his feet are dark, "hand" of Ištar; (if) it is prolonged, he will die.

Whether it is caused by blood loss or sepsis, shock eventually results in a significant decrease in blood pressure. This will ultimately lead to a drop in body temperature. In the quotes below, the *āšipu* appears to be evaluating core (central) body temperature using the ear canal and mouth. Low temperatures in these areas are indicative of shock and a poor prognosis. (See Chapter 20 for more details on core body temperature and its prognostic significance.)

> **14.45** [DIŠ ŠÀ]-*š*[*ú*] KÚM *r*[*uq-q*]*í* GEŠTU^{II}-*šú* ŠED$_7$.MEŠ *ḫaṭ-ṭu* ŠED$_7$.MEŠ *ina* KA-*šú* DU.MEŠ GÍD-*ma* GAM (DPS XIII B i 52′–53′//F 11//G$_2$ 2 = *TDP* 116 i 56′–57′)
>
> **[If] ⸢his⸣ [abdomen] is hot (and) his ear ⸢canals⸣[31] are cold (and) the scepter of the cold goes to his mouth, (if) it is prolonged, he will die.
>
> **14.46** [DIŠ ŠÀ-*šú*] KÚM.MEŠ *ruq-qí* GEŠTU^{II}-*šú* KÚM.MEŠ *ḫaṭ-ṭu* KÚM.MEŠ *ina* KA-*šú* DU.MEŠ *ni-ši* (DPS XIII B i 54′–55′//F 12//G$_2$ 3 = *TDP* 116 i 58′–59′)
>
> **[If his abdomen] is continually hot (and) his ear canals are hot (and) the scepter of the heat goes to his mouth, (there will be a) recovery.

Summary

Although this chapter lists only a small number of traumatic wounds and their consequences, the total number of trauma references is quite large. They competed with infections in commanding the attention of the ancient Mesopotamian physician. Although the lack of modern surgical skills and blood replacement technology would have prevented the *āšipu* from significantly affecting the outcome in many cases, he did not bleed his patients or put them on a starvation diet, as recommended by other ancient medical traditions. Those wounded patients who could be helped, the *āšipu* attended closely, and he bandaged their wounds with care. There is nothing to suggest that wounds were stitched or held together in any way except by bandages. Although he was of limited help in this situation, it is quite likely that this experience served to educate the *āšipu* about human anatomy, helping him to understand and deal with other medical problems.

CHAPTER 15

Poisons

That person has been fed (something) in bread,
been given (something) to drink in beer,
been rubbed (with something) in oil.

—*BAM* 232 i 20′

A poison is any substance which, when relatively small amounts are ingested, inhaled, or absorbed, will cause illness or death. Ancient cultures must have first learned of such harmful substances in their efforts to find edible plants. Poisonous plants would have been quickly identified and knowledge of them entered into the shared information of the culture.[1] Knowledge of poisonous animals and minerals would also have been important.

Poisons can have medicinal and social uses. Some substances that may cause illness and death in larger doses may have therapeutic roles in lower doses. Poisons may be used for revenge, to gain social advantage, or to commit suicide. The list of poisonous substances is very long; this chapter will discuss only those that may have been responsible for illnesses described in ancient Mesopotamian texts.

Parasympathetic Nerve Poisons

The parasympathetic nervous system has many roles in controlling day-to-day bodily functions such as heart rate, breathing, and intestinal movement. There are two major classes of plant toxins with opposing effects on this system: belladonna drugs (atropine and scopolamine) and muscarinic drugs. Belladonna drugs inhibit parasympathetic nerves, whereas muscarinic drugs stimulate them.

Plants containing belladonna drugs are widely distributed in nature, especially the Solanaceae plants (deadly nightshade, jimson weed, and henbane). Both atropine and scopolamine have significant central nervous system effects. Atropine causes restlessness, irritability, disorientation, hallucinations, and delirium, while scopolamine leads to drowsiness, amnesia, fatigue, and dreamless sleep. These drugs otherwise have similar physiologic actions including cutaneous (skin) flushing and decreased sweating, dry nose and mouth causing difficulty swallowing, rapid heart rate with intermittent slowing, decreased intestinal and bladder contraction, and fever. These same physiologic actions can make this class of drugs useful as therapeutic agents when used in small doses to counteract excessive parasympathetic activity.

Certain mushrooms such as *Amanita muscaria* produce muscarinic drugs while others including *Amanita phalloides* produce other toxins that can cause fatality due to gastrointestinal, liver, and kidney damage. Muscarinic drugs cause increased salivation and lacrimation (tearing), headache, visual disturbance, nausea and vomiting, diarrhea, abdominal colic, bronchospasm, slow heart rate, low blood pressure, and shock. *Amanita muscaria* has other toxins including atropine-like compounds that can cause irritability, restlessness, unsteady gait (ataxia), hallucinations, delirium, drowsiness, and sedation.

Mesopotamian physicians were well versed in the uses of plants in both their toxic and therapeutic functions. From some of the references listed below, it is quite evident that the toxins were ingested, but the physicians were also aware that the toxins in some cases could be absorbed transdermally since there is reference to substances in oil rubbed on the patient's skin that caused illness. Although the poisoning may in some cases have been accidental or due to suicide attempts, clearly the physicians were aware that it was often related to attempted murder.

BELLADONNA DRUGS

There are three references listed below that have many similar signs and symptoms as well as being attributed to the combined effects of pursuing ghosts and the Babylonian god Marduk (otherwise responsible for angina). Included in the complaints are dry mouth, mental status changes (confusion, disorientation, forgetfulness, and hallucinations), pains in back, neck, breast, and shoulders, nausea and vomiting, and fever. This illness is likely to be due to belladonna drugs. It is evident that ancient physicians believed that the poisoning could be intentional. Since belladonna drugs, used in conjunction with ergotamine, are an appropriate treatment for some of the ailments attributed to ghosts (such as migraine headaches), it is possible that some of the poisonings arose accidentally through attempted self-medication.

15.1 DIŠ NA MURUB$_4$ UGU-*šú* ⌜SAG⌝.KI.MEŠ-*šú* TAG.TAG-*s*[*u*] GEŠTU^{II}-*šú i-šag-gu-ma liq pi-šú i-ta-na-b*[*al*] *šim-ma-tú ri-mu-tú* TUKU.TUKU-*ši* GABA.MEŠ-*šú* KÚ.MEŠ-⌜*šú*⌝ ZI-*šú ik-ta-nàr-rù* SÍG UGU-*šú* GUB.GUB-*az ḫur-ba-šú* ŠUB.ŠUB-*su mi-na-tu-šú i-šam-ma-ma-šú ḫu-uṣ* GAZ ŠÀ-*bi* TUKU.TUKU-*ši a-šu-uš-tum* ŠUB.ŠUB-*su bi-bil* ŠÀ-*bi* TUKU-⌜*ma*⌝ NU KÚ ⌜*la*⌝ *ina-aḫ* [*ur-r*]*a u* [GI$_6$ *i*]-*ár-ru* LÚ BI GID[IM *mu*]*r-tap-pi-du* DIB-*su ù lu-ba-ṭù* ⌜ŠU^{II}⌝ ^{d}AMAR.UT[U] *ana* KAR-*šú* . . . (*LKA* 88 obv. 1–9//*LKA* 87 obv. 1′–10′; cf. *AMT* 54/2 r. 2′)

**If the middle of a person's scalp (and) his temples continually hurt ⌜him⌝ intensely, his ears roar, his palate keeps getting ⌜dry⌝, he continually has numbness and paralysis, his breasts keep hurting him, he is continually short of breath, the hair of his scalp constantly (feels like it) is standing on end, chills keep attacking him, his limbs go numb, he continually has a crushing sensation in the chest, depression continually falls on him, he has an appetite but then cannot eat, without relief he ⸢vomits⸣ ⸢day⸣ and [night], a roving ghost afflicts that person and/or *lubāṭu*, "hand" of ⸢Marduk⸣; to save him . . .[2]

15.2 [. . .] IGI^{II}-*šú i*-[*ṣa-nun-du* . . . *kin-ṣa-šú*] GÌR^{II}-*šú i-kaṣ*-[*ṣa-ṣa-šú* . . .] su *ana* ZI-*e u* GUB-⸢*zi*⸣ [*u* DUG$_4$.DUG$_4$ *mu-uq* . . .] *za-mar* SA$_5$ *za-mar* SI[G$_7$ KI ŠÀ-*šú* DUG$_4$.DUG$_4$ ŠÀ-*ba-š*]*ú nu-ul-la-a-te i-ta-ma* [*ṭè-en-šú il-ta-na-ni*]-*šú qí-bit* KA-*šú im-ta-na-áš-ši* [*um-mu mun-ga li-ʾ-ba*] *u ta-dir-ta* TUKU [MÁŠ.GI$_6$.MEŠ-*šú ma*]-*ʾ-da* ^{LÚ}ÚŠ.MEŠ IGI.IGI-*mar* [KI ÚŠ.ÚŠ DUG$_4$.D]UG$_4$-*ub* ŠÀ-*šú šá-pil ik-ka-šú ku-ri* [MÁŠ.GI$_6$.MEŠ *ša im-ma-r*]*u la ú-kal* ŠÀ-*šú i-aʾ-šam-ma* [*la i-ár-ru in*]*a* KI.NÁ-*šú ip-ta-nar-ru-ud* [. . .]x *ḫur-ba-šu* TUKU.TUKU-*ši* ZI.GA *i-ḫé-rid* [. . .]x-*su ḫu-uṣ* GAZ ŠÀ TUKU.TU [K]U-*ši* [*ina* É *ṣal*]-*tu ina* SILA *pu-uḫ-pu-uḫ-ḫu-ú* GAR-*šú* [*ni-ip-q*]*u-šú qer-buʾ-ú-a i-qab-bi a-a i-šá-si* [NINDA *u*] KAŠ LAL *ana* MUNUS DU-*ka* LAL *ana* MUNUS ŠÀ-*šú* NU ÍL-*šú* [K]A-*šú* BAD.BAD-*te im-ta-nag-gag uš-ta-na-aḫ* [ ]x-*na-aḫ-ḫi a-ḫu-lap-ya i-qab-bi* [DUG$_4$-*š*]*ú* LÙ.LÙ-*aḫ* NA BI *ina* NINDA *šu-kul ina* KAŠ NAG *ina* Ì ŠÉŠ [NU.MEŠ-*šú*] KI LÚ.ÚŠ *šu-nu-lu ana* GIDIM *ri-da-a-te paq-du* [. . .] ^{d}AMAR.UTU GUR-*ma* GIDIM *ri-da-a-te* ÚS.MEŠ-*šú* [*ana* TI.LA]-*šú u mu-ru-uṣ* DÙ.A.BI BÚR . . . (*BAM* 232 i 1′–23′)[3]

**[If . . .] his eyes [(feel like they) are spinning . . . his shins (and)] his feet give him a ⸢gnawing pain⸣ [. . . he is slow] to rise and to stand [and to speak . . .] he is now flushed and now pale, [he talks to himself, his heart] ponders untruths, [his mentation continually alters], he continually forgets what he has said, he has [fever, *mungu* (stiffness), *liʾbu* (fever) and] apprehensiveness, [his dreams] are ⸢numerous⸣, he continually sees dead persons [(and) continually] ⸢talks⸣ [with dead persons], his heart is down, his breath is short, he cannot remember [the dreams that he] ⸢saw⸣, his stomach is nauseous but then [he does not vomit], he continually shudders ⸢in⸣ his bed [. . .] he continually has chills [. . .] he continually has a crushing sensation in his heart, he experiences ⸢quarrels⸣ [in the house] and disturbances in the street, he has closely spaced [fits of] ⸢choking⸣, he says "oh" (and) cries: "ah!" his appetite for [bread] and beer is diminished, his (desire for) going to a woman is diminished, at (the sight of) a woman, he cannot get an erection,[4] he continually opens his ⸢mouth⸣, he is continually rigid, he is continually dejected [. . .] he says "have mercy on me!" (and) [his words] are troubled, that person has been fed (something) in bread, been given (something) to drink in beer, been rubbed (with something) in oil; [his figurines] have been laid (in the ground) with a corpse (and) entrusted to a pursuing ghost; [. . .] have been turned to Marduk so that pursuing ghosts continually pursue him; [to cure] him and to loosen every sort of illness . . .

KIŠPU

The term *kišpu* means "sorcery." In many references in which it is used, the signs and symptoms develop quite suddenly. This may have suggested to the *āšipu* the possibility that the illness resulted from a deliberate act by a sorcerer. The *kišpu* texts do not appear to represent a single disease, but the entities they describe seem to fall into a number of separate categories.

One group of texts describe signs and symptoms that appear to be quite similar to muscarinic poisoning such as increased salivation, heart "fluttering," depression, insomnia, "jerking," vomiting, and abdominal bloating. It seems likely that in these cases the patient was exposed to some plant derivative, most likely a mushroom. Some of the quotes speak of *kišpu* as a food or a drink that could be ingested, further supporting the idea that the food or drink could have been poisoned.[5]

15.3 DIŠ NA ÚḪ *ina* KA-*šú* NU TAR-*as* NA BI *ka-šip ana* TI-*šú* . . . (*AMT* 31/4:14, 16)[6]

**If the saliva in a person's mouth never stops, that person is *kišpu*'d, to cure him . . .

15.4 [DIŠ L]Ú TÙN.ŠÀ DIB.DIB-*su bir-ka-šú i-ta-na-na-ḫa* x x *šú* ⸢*ù*⸣ *ša-sal-la-šu* KÚ.KÚ-*šú ú-man-ga-ag in-né-eṣ-ṣil* [*i*]*l-la-ta-šú* ZAG *u* GÙB *il-la-ka* KÚM ŠÀ-*šu* TUKU-*ši* ŠÀ-*šu pi-qa la pi-qa* MUD-*ut* LÚ BI *ka-šip a-na* TI-*šu* . . . (*BAM* 397:33–37)[7]

**If his liver continually afflicts him, his knees continually become tired, his [. . .] and his back continually hurt him, he is stiff and sluggish, his spittle flows left and right, he has internal fever, (and) his heart flutters incessantly, that person is *kišpu*'d, to cure him . . .

15.5 DIŠ NA SAG.DU-*su iṣ-ṣa-na-bat-su šit* x [. . .] MAŠ.GI$_6$.MEŠ-*šú par-da ina šit-ti-šú ig-d*[*a-na-lu-ut*] *bir-ka-šu ka-si-a ba-ma-as-su šim-ma-*[*tu* . . .] UZ[U]-*šú ru-ṭi-ib-*[*tu*] *im-ta-na-al-lu-šú* LÚ BI *ka-ši-ip* . . . (*AMT* 86/1 ii 3–7)

**If a person's head continually afflicts him, [his] ⸢sleep⸣ [. . .] his dreams are troubled, he [continually] ⸢jerks⸣[8] in his sleep, his knees are "bound," his chest is ⸢numb⸣, [. . .] (and) his flesh is continually filled with ⸢dampness⸣, that person is *kišpu*'d . . .

A second group of *kišpu* references includes complaints of chest pain, fever, phlegm, and "sick lungs." These texts are compatible with pneumonia, and are discussed in Chapter 3 with 3.82–3.85. A third category (see below) lists gastrointestinal complaints involving mucus coming from the gastrointestinal tract.

15.6 DIŠ SAG ŠÀ-*šú ru-púl-ta* TUKU.MEŠ-*ši* SAG ŠÀ-*šú ú-ṣa-rap-šú ur-ra u* GI$_6$ *la i-ṣal-lal* NINDA *u* A LAL UZU^{II}-*šú tab-ku* NA BI *kiš-pi* KÚ *u* NAG *a-na šup-šu-ri* . . . (*AMT* 48/2:1-3)

**If his upper abdomen (epigastrium) continually has mucus, his upper abdomen (epigastrium) burns him hotly, he cannot sleep day or night, he loses his appetite for bread and water, (and) his flesh is tense,[9] that person has eaten or drunk *kišpu*, to dispel it . . .

15.7 DIŠ NA SAG ŠÀ-*šú ru-púl-ta* TUKU-*ši* SAG ŠÀ-*bi-šú ú-ṣar-rap-šú* NINDA *u* A/KAŠ LAL UZU.MEŠ-*šú tab-ku* NA BI UŠ$_{11}$.ZU KÚ *u* NAG *ana šup-šu-ri-šú* . . . (*BAM* 190: 22–24//*STT* 102:7–9//*BAM* 193 ii 2′–5′//K 8469:1–3 [Abusch, *Mesop. Witchcr.* 81])

**If a person's upper abdomen continually has mucus, his upper abdomen burns him hotly, he loses his appetite for bread and water/beer, (and) his flesh is tense,[10] that person has eaten or drunk *kišpu*, to make it release him . . .

15.8 [DIŠ NA SAG] ŠÀ-*šú ik-ta-na-su-šú* ŠÀ-*šú i-ḫa-áš* GABA.MEŠ-*šú ir-*<*ta*>*-na-*[*mu*]*-ú* DIB-*it* ŠÀ TUKU.MEŠ-*ši* SAG ŠÀ-*šú* ÚḪ TUKU.MEŠ-*ši* NA BI ⸢*ka-šip*⸣ [*ana e-t*]*e-ri-šú* . . . (*BAM* 90:9′–11′//*BAM* 434 iii 10–13)

**[If a person]'s ⌜upper abdomen⌝ continually gnaws at him, his stomach heaves, both sides of his chest are ⌜relaxed⌝, he continually has affliction of the stomach, (and) his upper abdomen continually contains mucus, that person is *kišpu*'d, ⌜to save⌝ him . . .

One possible explanation for these three references might be an allergy or hypersensitivity reaction; however, the information provided in these texts is too scanty to allow a single diagnosis. Allergic reactions often develop quite suddenly following inhalation, ingestion, or skin exposure to allergens, which might have suggested to the *āšipu* the possibility of a deliberate act of sorcery. We suspect that the "tense flesh" mentioned in some of the texts represents edematous or inflamed skin due to an allergic reaction. Some allergens, including moldy hay and grain, pigeon droppings, wheat weevils, moldy barley, and wood dust, all of which would have been present in ancient Mesopotamia, can also result in a form of respiratory allergy (which may be the source of mucus). It is puzzling, however, that none of the references describes wheezing or shortness of breath, complaints that are very common in respiratory allergies.

The remaining category of *kišpu* references is a grab bag of miscellaneous ailments of uncertain etiology including possible cases of ergot poisoning discussed below.

Ergot

The fungal genus *Claviceps* parasitizes grasses including edible grains such as rye and wheat. A possible reference to ergot is to be found in an Old Babylonian recitation.

15.9 *er-ṣe-tum ú-li-id lu-ḫa-ma lu-ḫu-mu-ú ú-li-id i-ši-na i-ši-nu-um ú-li-id šu-bu-ul-tam šu-bu-ul-tum ú-li-id me-er-ḫa* (Landsberger, *JNES* 14.15:1–8)

**The earth bore the dirt, the dirt bore the stalk, the stalk bore the ear of grain, the ear of grain bore the *merḫu*.

The recitation goes on to state that the *merḫu* subsequently entered the eye of the patient from which it is to be removed in the course of treatment. This passage clearly has nothing to do with ergotism as such, but it is possible (as B. Landsberger suggests)[11] that *merḫu* is a sty and that the purplish cockspur-shaped ergot was described by Akkadian speakers as the "sty" on an ear of grain. It is, of course, equally possible that what produced this grain "sty" was some other fungus infecting wheat or barley.

Claviceps produces ergot, which can be a poison or a medicine and has been known by Chinese physicians since the Han dynasty. Ergot may be used to cause uterine contractions or to treat migraine headaches. When used in toxic doses, ergot can cause chest pressure and pain, heaviness and pain of the extremities, local or generalized convulsions, nausea and vomiting, and confusion and hallucinations. In another form of the disease, called ergot gangrene, a prominent feature is pain in the extremities with limbs turning black, numbness, and eventual autoamputation due to inadequate blood supply. The quote listed below has many features consistent with ergot poisoning, including chest (heart) pain, focal convulsions, numbness and pain in the extremities, and gastrointestinal disturbance. The spittle that is mentioned could be secondary to seizure activity.

It should be noted that the extracts used for medicine are specifically derived from the ergot of rye, a plant that was probably not grown in ancient Mesopotamia. *Claviceps* does parasitize other grasses besides rye, and cases of ergotism from wheat grown in Mesopotamia were likely to have occurred. Epidemic ergotism, however, has historically been confined to areas such as France, where the poor subsisted on cheap rye bread. In addition to ergotism, it is possible that the reference below is due to a case of complex poisoning containing mixtures of cardiotoxic and convulsion-inducing plants other than ergot. It is probable that the poisons (as is certainly the case with North African mixtures containing *Atractylis gummifera*) would have had additional agents to inhibit vomiting in order to allow the poisons to work.[12]

15.10 DIŠ NA *ḫu-uṣ-ṣa* GAZ ŠÀ TUKU.TUKU-*ši* [. . .] EME-*šú it-te-nen-biṭ* EME-*šú ú-na-a*[*š-šak*] GEŠTU^{II}-*šú* GÙ.GÙ-*a* ŠU^{II}-*šú i-šam-ma-ma-šú* [. . .] *i-kaṣ-ṣa-ṣa-šú* SAG ŠÀ-*šú it-ta-n*[*a-áš-qàr*] *ana* MUNUS DU LAL *ḫur-ba-šú* ŠUB.ŠUB-*su* [. . .] ÚḪ *ina* KA-*šú it-ta-na-ad-d*[*i*. . .] NA BI *ina* NINDA *šu-kul ina* KAŠ NAG *ina* Ì Š[ÉŠ] . . . (*BAM* 445:10–16)

**If a person continually has a crushing sensation in his heart [. . .] his tongue[13] is continually cramped, he ⌜bites⌝ his tongue, his ears continually ring, his hands go numb, [his knees (and) his shins] give him a gnawing pain, his upper abdomen (epigastrium) continually ⌜protrudes⌝, his sexual appetite is diminished, chills keep falling on him, [. . .], he continually lets spittle fall from his mouth, [. . .], that person has been fed (something) in bread, been given (something) to drink in beer, been ⌜rubbed⌝ (with something) in oil . . .

There is an article by Biggs[14] which argues that "there may have been frequent bouts—probably even epidemics—of ergotism or other mycotoxicoses in ancient Mesopotamia." His evidence is drawn largely from letters and nonmedical omens. It includes references in letters to multiple deaths of children in a single household and to mysterious deaths among fattened cattle. Other references, drawn from the apodoses (prediction sections) of omens, mention spontaneous abortion due to infections (*liʾbu*). Biggs also cites references in medical texts to jaundice and the plague in the Assyrian army at Sennacherib's siege of Jerusalem (2 Kings 18:13–19:37).

We find these arguments tenuous. In the absence of rye cultivation, deaths from ergotism would have been sporadic events, not epidemics. Jaundice is not a sign of ergotism, and *liʾbu* was a term usually used to describe a type of fever (see Chapter 3).

15.11 *li-ʾ-bu ina* KUR *ú-la-ʾ-ib* MUNUS.PEŠ$_4$.MEŠ *šá* ŠÀ-*ši-na* NU SILIM.MEŠ (Rochberg-Halton, AfO Beih. 22.243:4)

**Infection (*li-ʾ-bu*) will infect (*ú-la-ʾ-ib*) people in the land; pregnant women will not bring their fetuses to term.

Infectious diseases, especially typhoid, typhus, brucellosis, and listeria, are common causes of febrile abortions, and seem a more likely explanation for a generalized failure to carry children to term than ergot-induced abortion. More interesting are the cases of mysterious deaths among cattle being stall-fattened for use in sacrifice and in particular a Mari letter cited by Biggs as a possible example of the gangrenous form of ergotism.

15.12 1 GUD *i-gi-[se-e] é-kál-lim ši-ra-am im-la-a-ma ik-k[a-b]i-it-ma i-na ú-zu-uz-zi-im ša-ap-la-nu-um še-pí-šu da-mu-um iṣ-ba-at-ma ú-zu-[u]z-za-a[m] ú-ul i-li-i ù a-<na>* ŠÀ.GAL-*šu i-na* x x nu *uš-ta-na-at-bu-šu* GUD *šu-ú a-la-k[am] a-na Ma-ri*^{KI} *ú-ul i-li-i* (*ARM*[*T*] 2.82:29–35).

**One ox, a ⌜palace offering⌝, has fleshed out and gotten heavy, but when he (tries to) stand up, blood afflicts the lower part of his feet so that he cannot stand and he has to be forced to get up to eat . . . He cannot go to Mari.

This condition is certainly not gangrenous ergotism, since gangrene means the absence of circulation to the extremities, not bleeding. However, it may have been a case of what is known to veterinarians as "sweet clover disease." This disease is characterized by the development of a gradually increasing prolongation in the time required for the blood to coagulate. It is usually fatal, death resulting from hemorrhage either in the tissues of the body or from surgical or accidental wounds.[15]

Sweet clover is mentioned in Arab herbals, and four varieties grow currently in Iraq: *Melilotus officinalis, M. alba, M. indica,* and *M. messanensis.*[16] Fresh or properly cured sweet clover is harmless, and a valuable feed crop. It is the spoiled, moldy, or damaged fodder that is dangerous to cattle, a fact that suggests that whoever was stall feeding the ox for sacrifice was cutting a few corners (and risking more literally than usual the wrath of the gods).

Although only moldy sweet clover is dangerous, the cause of the problem is a constituent of the plant itself, dicoumarol (which is the source of its distinctive aroma and taste familiar to connoisseurs of Swiss Chapziger cheese). Warfarin, a synthetic compound that mimics the action of dicoumarol, is used clinically to prevent abnormal (excessive) clotting within blood vessels (thrombosis) in certain high-risk clinical situations.[17]

Alcohol

Alcohol (ethanol)[18] is another toxin that, when taken in large enough quantities, can cause acute intoxication, and if consumed over a long enough period of time, can cause a number of chronic illnesses. Acute alcoholic intoxication is sufficiently well known that its description is unnecessary. This self-inflicted disease must have been very common due to the widespread use of beer and wine as beverages. The latter was mostly imported and would have been used largely by the wealthy, but the former was made locally in enormous quantities. Like modern Belgian beers, many brews were flavored. Being very full-bodied and more than slightly sweet, it was almost as much a food as a drink, and a very popular supplement to the diet of the poor. The widespread use of alcoholic beverages might have been due not only to the central nervous system effects but the antibacterial action of alcohol that would have made it safer to drink than river water.

The two quotes below describe the early and late effects of an alcoholic binge and the ancient physicians' efforts to treat it.

15.13 DIŠ NA KAŠ.SAG NAG-*ma* SUḪUŠ.MEŠ-*šú pa-al-qa di-ig-la ma-a-ṭi ana* TI-*šú* . . . (*BAM* 575 iii 49)[19]

**If a person drinks fine beer and then he is unsteady on his foundations (and) his eyesight is diminished, to cure him . . .

15.14 DIŠ INIM-*šú* KÚR.[KÚR-*i*]*r u* KAŠ APIN.MEŠ-*iš ana* U_4.10.[KÁM . . .] / DIŠ INIM-*šú* K[ÚR.KÚR-*i*]*r u* GIŠGEŠTIN APIN.MEŠ-*iš ana* U_4.DUG_4.GA-[*šu ana* U_4.10. KÁM . . .] (DPS VII B r. 13–14 = *TDP* 66:69′–70′)[20]

**If his words are ⸢unintelligible⸣ and he continually asks for beer (and he has been sick) for ten days [. . .]. If his words are ⸢unintelligible⸣ and he continually asks for wine at regular intervals (and he has been sick) [for ten days . . .]

It appears from the text below that the ancient Mesopotamians had a method for increasing the intoxicating effects of alcohol with an additive. It would be interesting to know whether this additive was used to reduce the cost of getting drunk, as a harmless party prank, or to gain control over another individual for some nefarious purpose.[21] Another possible use was to alleviate the pain of medical procedures such as the insertion of a tube into the urethra, is suggested by Geller and Cohen.[22]

15.15 DIŠ NA *a-na šu-uk-ku-ri* KU.KU GIŠTÚG *ina* TÚG.GADA *t*[*a*]*-ra-kás ina* GEŠTIN ŠUB-*di* NAG-*ma i-šak-kir* (*BAM* 260:1–3)[23]

**If (you want) to make a person drunk, you tie up powdered *taskarinnu* in a linen cloth. You steep it in wine. If he drinks it, he will get drunk.

The *āšipu* seems to have attributed the effects of prolonged and excessive drinking (alcoholism) to affliction by a ghost. These denizens of the waterless steppe were otherwise blamed for dehydration and dehydrating illnesses such as cholera (see Chapter 3). References to "hand" of ghost appear to describe alcoholic ketoacidosis as well as respiratory distress, a common complication of ketoacidosis. It may be the dehydrating aspects of ethanol poisoning that suggested affliction by a ghost as the cause of many of the effects of alcoholic binge drinking. The presence of severe headache, abdominal pain, and hallucinations, all of which were independently attributed to ghosts, would have helped confirm the correctness of the *āšipu*'s analysis. For more details, see 19.295–19.303 with discussion.

Drinking alcohol on an empty stomach can also induce hypoglycemia, producing sweating, tremor, tachycardia, anxiety, and hunger. A complex of anxiety, sweating, and hunger would appear to be described in the following references.

15.16 DIŠ ZI.IR ŠUB.ŠUB-*su mim-ma šá im-ma-ru ú-ṣal-la* UB.NIGIN.NA-*šú* KÚM *u* IR *u_4-mi-šam-ma* TUKU-*ši a-zu-za-a bi-bil* ŠÀ *ma-dam-ma* TUKU.MEŠ EN *ú-bal-lu-niš-šú* ŠÀ *i-ḫa-ḫu* U_4 *ú-ba-lu-niš-šú* IGI.BAR-*ma la i-lem* ŠU GIDIM_7 *šá ina* A SÌG-[*iṣ*] (DPS XXVII:29–31 [AOAT 43.299–300])

**If worry continually afflicts him (and) he makes supplication to whatever he sees, his limbs are hot and he sweats every day, he has a big appetite at unpredictable times, (and) until they bring him what he wants, he vomits, (but) when they bring it to him he looks at it and doesn't eat it, the "hand" of a ghost who was struck in the water.

15.17 DIŠ *ina* U_4.GURUM.MA DIB-*su* DIB.DIB-⸢*su*⸣ U_4 DIB-*šú* KÚM NU *ma-dam-ma u* IR.ME[Š] SAG.KI-*šú* IGI^{II}-*šú i-se-ʾa u* ŠÀ-*šú* KÚ-*šú* ŠU GIDIM_7 (DPS XXVI:50′ [AOAT 43.282])

**If his affliction always afflicts him in the late afternoon (and) when it afflicts him, his temperature does not seem very great but sweat presses down on his temples[24] (and) his eyes, and his abdomen hurts him, "hand" of ghost.[25]

A more serious consequence of excessive alcohol intake is delirium tremens (DTs), which the following reference appears to describe.

15.18 DIŠ *tu-gu-un-šú ú-zaq-qat-su* GEŠTU^{II}-*šú* GÙ.DÉ.MEŠ SÍG SU-*šú* GUB.GUB-*az kal* LÚ.AD$_6$-*šú* GIN$_7$ *kal-ma-tum i-ba-šú-ú i-nam-muš u* ŠU-*su ub-bal-ma la i-ba-áš-šú* : *la ig-gi-ig* ŠU GIDIM$_7$ UD.DA LÚ GIN$_7$ ^{GIŠ}NÍG.GIDRU *šá* ^{d}30 GÌR^{II}-*šú* ŠU GIDIM$_7$ (DPS XXVII:32–34 [AOAT 43.300])

**If (the skin under) his headband stings him, his ears roar, the hair of his body continually seems to stand on end, his whole body crawls as if there were lice but when he brings his hand up, there is nothing to scratch, "hand" of ghost *ṣētu* (dehydration);[26] (if) the person (bends and stretches out) his feet as in the scepter of Sîn, "hand" of ghost.

The "scepter of Sîn" in the reference above is also mentioned in connection with ghosts in the following, very similar references. One of these is drawn from the diagnostic series and the other appears in a therapeutic text, with accompanying treatment.

15.19 DIŠ ^{GIŠ}NÍG.GIDRU *šá* ^{d}30 GAR-*su-ma* GÌR-*šú i-kap-pap u i-tar-ra-aṣ i-ram-mu-um u* ÚḪ *ina* KA-*šú* DU-*ak* ŠU GIDIM$_7$ *mur-tap-pi-du ina* EDIN DIB-*su* (DPS XXVII:35–36 [AOAT 43.300])

**If the scepter of Sîn has been placed on him so that he bends and stretches out his foot, he drones and saliva flows from his mouth, "hand" of a ghost roving in the steppe afflicts him.

15.20 [DIŠ GIG] LÚ GIN$_7$ ^{GIŠ}GIDRU *ša* ^{d}EN.ZU GAR-*šum-ma* G[ÌR]-*šú i-kap-pap u i-tar-ra-aṣ i-ra-am-mu-um u* ⸢*ru-ʾu-tú*⸣ [*ina*] ⸢KA-*šú*⸣ DU-*ak* GIDIM *mur-tap-pi-du ina* EDIN DIB-*su* . . . (*BAM* 385 i 15′–17′//*BAM* 471 ii 21′–22′)

**[If] the person's [illness] sets upon him like the scepter of Sîn so that he bends his ⸢foot⸣ and then stretches (it) out, (and if) he drones and saliva flows [from] his mouth, a ghost roving in the steppe afflicts him . . .

What appears to be described in the above texts are seizures of the grand mal type.[27] Seizure disorders may occur within twenty-four hours after the cessation of drinking. Interesting in view of the association of the "scepter of Sîn" with both delirium tremens and grand mal seizures is the fact that approximately one-third of the patients with alcohol-induced seizure disorders progress to develop delirium tremens.

Alcohol may cause some long-term complications such as numbness of the extremities (polyneuropathy) and cirrhosis with secondary bleeding esophageal varices (dilated varicose veins in the esophagus). The references below may describe conditions that had chronic alcohol addiction as the underlying cause.

15.21 ŠU.GIDIM.MA *šim-mat* ŠU^{II} *u* GÌR^{II} . . . (*UET* 4.150:10)

**"Hand" of ghost (and) numbness of hands and feet . . .

15.22 DIŠ ZI SAG.KI TUKU-*ši-ma* ŠU^{II}-*šú u* GÌR^{II}-*šú i-šam-ma-ma-šú* ŠU GÍDIM (DPS IV A r. 6+A_4 r. 5//B r. 18//E iv 2 = *TDP* 42 r. 39//*SpTU* 3.88 iv 2)[28]

**If he experiences pulsating temporal (arteries) and his hands and feet go numb, "hand" of ghost.

15.23 DIŠ SAG.KI-*šú* DIB-*su-ma* GÙ.GÙ-*si* MÚD *ina* KIR_4/KA-*šú* DU-*ku* ŠU $GIDIM_7$ (DPS IV B obv. 7//D 7 = *TDP* 32:7)[29]

**If his temple afflicts him so that he continually cries out (and) blood flows from his nose/mouth, "hand" of ghost.

The neurological disease called Wernicke-Korsakoff syndrome is caused by thiamine deficiency brought on by chronic alcoholism. Its findings include confusion, amnesia, paralysis of the muscles for eye movement (ophthalmoplegia), staggering gait (ataxia), and abnormal eye movements (nystagmus). Kinnier Wilson[30] has cited the following reference as an example of this condition, and we concur.

15.24 DIŠ NA KAŠ.SAG NAG-*ma* SAG.DU-*su* DIB.DIB-*su* INIM.MEŠ-*šú im-ta-na-áš-ši ina* DUG_4.DUG_4-*šú ú-pa-áš-šaṭ ṭè-en-šú la ṣa-bit* NA BI IGI^{II}-*šú* GUB-*za ana* TI-*šú* . . . (*BAM* 575 iii 51–52//*BAM* 59:21–24)[31]

**If a person drinks beer and as a result his head continually afflicts him, he continually forgets his words and slurs them when speaking, he is not in full possession of his faculties, and that person's eyes stand still, to cure him . . .

The following reference to a "family ghost" describes unsteady stance ("contorted feet") and gait ("shifting inguinal regions") which could be due to ethanol poisoning, especially in view of the presence of headache and unpleasant sensations ("stinging flesh").

15.25 [DIŠ NA IGI.ME]Š-*šú* NIGIN.MEŠ UZU-*šú i-zaq-qat-uš*[32] [. . . ÍR.MEŠ-*š*]*ú* DU.DU-*ka-ma la ina-ṭal* [. . .]x *u-ku-u-ku-šú šá-pu-la-šú* BAL.BAL-*šú* [. . .] GÌR^{II}-*šú iq-qa-an-na-an* SAG.DU-[*su*] DIB.DIB-*su* [. . .] x GIDIM IM.RI.A-*šú* DIB.DIB-[*su ana* TI-*šú*] . . . (*AMT* 54/3 r. 5′–9′)

**[If a person's] ⌜face⌝ continually seems to spin, his flesh stings him, ⌜his⌝ [tears] flow so (copiously) that he cannot see, [. . .] his pelvis (inguinal regions) shifts constantly under him, [. . .] his feet become contorted, [his] head constantly afflicts him, [. . .] his family ghost is continually afflicting [him; to cure him] . . .

River Toxins

There is an interesting group of twelve references that identify illnesses associated with exposure to river water. Six texts mention patients being in the water for bathing or some other purpose. The remaining six texts indicate that the patient had drunk water from a hoisting device used to move river water onto irrigated garden plots. The illnesses that followed exposure developed very quickly, in some cases even before the patient got out of the water.

15.26 DIŠ NA ŠUB-*ta ina* A ÍL-*ši* GIG-*su lu ana a-ḫ*[*i* . . .] *ip-pu-uš* IM DIRI *u i-ra-aq ana* TI-*šú* . . . (*AMT* 87/6:3–4//*AMT* 1/5:3′–4′)

**If a falling spell comes upon a person in the water and his illness spreads either to one side [or . . .], he fills up with "wind" and empties out, to cure him . . .

Most of the references describe neurological abnormalities including seizures (see text above), vertigo (spinning), paralysis (immobilization), twisting (abnormal posturing), and altered mentation. The final reference below mentions an abnormality of the diaphragm. This abnormality was probably a paralysis of the diaphragm recognized by failure of the abdominal wall to move with respiration.

15.27 DIŠ A.MEŠ *ina* TU_5-*šú* TA ÍD *ina* E_{11}-*šú* ⸢NIGIN-*ma*⸣ ŠUB-⸢*ut*⸣ [MA]ŠKIM ÍD SÌG-[*s*]*u*[33] (DPS XXVII:24 [AOAT 43.299]; Ni. 470:9–10 [Kraus, *ZA* 77.197])

**If when he is bathing, when he comes up from the river, he (feels like he) is spinning and falls down, the ⸢*rābiṣu*⸣ of the river struck ⸢him⸣.

15.28 DIŠ TA A.MEŠ *ina* E_{11}-*šú* LÚ.AD_6-*šú iḫ-mi-šu-ma* NIGIN-*ma* ⸢ŠUB-*ut* MAŠKIM⸣ ÍD SÌG-[*s*]*u* (DPS XXVII:25 [AOAT 43.299]; Ni. 470:11 [Kraus, *ZA* 77.197])[34]

**If when he comes up from the water, his body is paralyzed[35] and he (feels like he) is spinning and falls down, the *rābiṣu* of the river struck ⸢him⸣.

15.29 DIŠ *ina* GIG-*šú i-ṣa-ád* A ^{GIŠ}BAL ÍD NAG (DPS XVII:21 [AOAT 43.196])

**If during his illness he (feels like he) is spinning, he drank water from a hoisting device of the river.

15.30 DIŠ *ina* GIG-*šú i-ṭa-mu* A ^{GIŠ}BAL ÍD NAG (DPS XVII:22 [AOAT 43.196])[36]

**If during his illness he twists, he drank water from a hoisting device of the river.

15.31 DIŠ SAG ŠÀ-*šú* KÚM *ú*!-*kal* UŠ_4-*šú* KÚR.KÚR-*šú* A ^{GIŠ}BAL ÍD NAG *ana* ⸢MÁ.ÚR.RA TAG-*ma*⸣[37] GAM (DPS XIII B i 29′ = *TDP* 114 i 33′)[38]

**If his upper abdomen (epigastrium) holds fever (and) his mentation is altered, he drank water from a hoisting device of the river. (If) it affects (his) diaphragm, he will die.

Other symptoms and signs were seen including fever, bloating, and skin lesions (*bubuʾtu*: blisters).

15.32 DIŠ TA A *ina* E_{11}-*šú* ŠÀ.MEŠ-*šú nap-ḫu* A ^{GIŠ}BAL ÍD NAG (DPS XVII:64 [AOAT 43.201])

**If when he comes up from the water, his insides are bloated, he drank water from a hoisting device of the river.

15.33 D[IŠ N]A ŠUB-*ta ina* A ÍL-*ši* UZU.MEŠ-*šú ut-tap-pa-ḫ*[*u* . . . U_4.BÚ.B]Ú.UL *ina* U_4.BÚ.BÚ.UL *ina* SU-*šú* E_{11}-*a* [. . .] (*BAM* 568:1–2)

**⸢If⸣ a falling spell comes upon a ⸢person⸣ in the water, his flesh is made to swell [. . .] (and) *bubuʾtu* (blisters) ride on top of *bubuʾtu* in his body [. . .]

The very rapid development of the disease following river water exposure makes an infectious etiology quite unlikely. Neurotoxin exposure, however, is compatible with the rapid onset of neurological problems. There are a number of aquatic microorganisms and animals that harbor neurotoxins, which could be the cause of this disease. Toxic dinoflagellates including *Gonyaulax catenella* and *Ptychodiscus brevis* can multiply to large numbers in coastal waters and because of their pigmentation are called a red tide. They are ingested by shellfish and mussels, and consequently the toxin becomes concentrated. Eating the shellfish or mussels can cause gastrointestinal complaints, paralysis, ataxia, and death from respiratory paralysis.

A dinoflagellate, *Pfiesteria piscicida*, recently has been recognized to cause neurological problems, especially memory loss in fishermen working in rivers on Maryland's eastern shore.[39] Additional complaints include abdominal cramps, diarrhea, and rash.

Another neurotoxin-producing water organism that often occurs in nutrient-rich fresh waters is the blue-green algae, *Anabaena flos-aqua*. It produces anatoxin A(s), which is a water-soluble organophosphorus cholinesterase inhibitor. Ingestion of very small amounts of this material can cause seizures, salivation, vomiting, tremors, slow heart rate, paralysis of the respiratory muscles, and death.[40] Brain cholinesterase remains normal, but blood, muscle, and lung cholinesterases are inhibited.

Neurotoxins can also be delivered by the bites of marine animals including sea snakes, scorpion fish, stonefish, sea urchins, and stingrays. It is impossible to know if one or more of the above organisms were responsible for this disease, especially since there is no information about the water conditions. Some of the above will not live in fresh water, but may require either brackish or salt water, as is found in the lower reaches of the southern Mesopotamian marshlands. Stinging fish are mentioned in lexical texts[41] and, since the verb used to describe the sting (*zaqātu*) refers specifically to scorpions, it seems likely that scorpion fish were present. There was no mention of eating seafood before the attack, nor was there any statement about an animal bite, but we cannot exclude either of these possibilities. We believe, however, that it is highly likely that a neurotoxin producing organism was the cause. The *āšipu* attributed this condition to a river *rābiṣu* (river demon), but he understood the association between the river and the disease. This permitted him to advise others on how to prevent this problem.

Snakes and Scorpions

Toxins from the bites of snakes and scorpions were known, and treatments were available. The success of the treatments is unknown.

15.34 DIŠ NA MUŠ *iš-šuk-šú* . . . (*BAM* 42:63//*AMT* 92/7:6′; *BAM* 42:64, 65)[42]

**If a snake bit a person . . .

15.35 Ú SÌG-*iṣ* MIR . . . (*CT* 14.23 [K 9283]:12–13//*STT* 92 i 12–13)

**Plant for the bite of a *šibbu*-snake . . .

15.36 6,40 *a-wi-lum zu-qì-qì-pu-um i-iz-qú-*[*ut*] . . . (*BAM* 393 obv. 19)[43]

**If a scorpion ⸢stung⸣ a man . . .

15.37 Ú GAZ GÍR.TAB . . . (*CT* 14.23 [K 9283]:14–16//*STT* 92 i 14–16)[44]

**Plant to "crush" a scorpion (sting) . . .

15.38 DIŠ NA *šim-mat* GÍR.TAB GIG . . . (*AMT* 91/1 r. 4)[45]

**If a person is sick with numbness due to a scorpion (sting) . . .

15.39 DIŠ U.MEŠ ŠU^{II}-*šú šá* 15 ZÉ DIRI-*ma* KÚ.MEŠ-*šú* [. . .] (DPS XI A r. 41 = *TDP* 98 r.41)[46]

**If the fingers of his hands, the ones on the left are full of venom[47] and continually hurt him [. . .]

Summary

The physicians of ancient Mesopotamia understood that exposure to certain substances added to food or drink, or oil applied to the skin could lead to serious illness. It is not clear to what extent they considered the symptoms to be produced by a spirit or demon, but there was clearly enough experience with some poisonous materials and their "uses" to realize that other humans were the primary cause of the problem.

CHAPTER 16

Mental Illness

If a person is well, but his behavior is sick.

—BM 64174:9//*BAM* 326 ii 7′

There is a sufficient record in many cultures, regions of the world, and times for us to conclude that mental illness is a problem common to human society. The peoples of ancient Mesopotamia must have shared this problem, and the medical texts discussed in this chapter show that the *āšipu* had a clear idea of what was normal and what was "sick" behavior. However, since virtually all of the signs and symptoms of psychiatric disease can be produced by organic brain disease or metabolic abnormalities, it is difficult to read a single text and know with certainty whether it is an organic or purely psychiatric problem. There is also a risk in applying modern Western standards of normality, which are embedded in our own cultural norms and expectations, to ancient texts.[1] Even in the modern era, mental illnesses in different cultures have clinical presentations that do not always fit standard definitions of specific diseases and, where cultural differences are particularly great, there is always a danger of serious misinterpretation. For this reason, we have tried to base our diagnoses on findings that were considered by the ancient Mesopotamians to be abnormal, and to be especially cautious in assigning possible modern equivalents.

Signs and Symptoms of Mental Illness

Ancient Mesopotamian physicians recognized many abnormal behavioral patterns and emotional responses. In many cases they failed to provide sufficient information for us to reach a diagnosis understandable in modern terms. However, the extent of their observations bears testimony to their concerns about mental illness.

GNASHING TEETH (BRUXISM)

It is generally recognized that certain people when under stress will gnash or grind their teeth either during sleep or when awake. The first of the references that follow indicates that the *āšipu* was aware that worry and bruxism were related. See Chapter 18 for additional discussion.

16.1 [DIŠ LÚ] *i-na ṣa-la-li-šu ši-*[*i*]*n-*[*ni-šu*] *i-ka-ṣa-aṣ* [*i-na*]*-an-zi-iq* (Köcher and Oppenheim, *AfO* 18.64 i 41–42 [physiognomic omens])

**[If a person] gnashes his ⌜teeth⌝ in his sleep, [he is] worried.

16.2 NA$_4$.MEŠ DIŠ NA ZÚ.MEŠ-*šú i-ka-ṣa-ṣa* . . . (*BAM* 372 iii 5′)[2]

**Stones for cases where a person gnashes his teeth . . .

16.3 KA.INIM.MA DIŠ NA ZÚ.MEŠ-*šú i-kaṣ-ṣa-aṣ* . . . (*BAM* 30:8′)

**Recitation (for cases where) a person gnashes his teeth . . .

16.4 DIŠ NA *ina i-tu-li-šú* ZÚ.MEŠ-*šú i-kaṣ-ṣa-as* . . . (*BAM* 30:47′–48′//*BAM* 157 obv. 6′)[3]

**If a person when he lies down to sleep gnashes his teeth . . .[4]

STRESS HEADACHE

Headaches can occur during periods of mental stress, and the texts below seem compatible with this association. For the personal god and goddess of the patient as causers of stress, see 19.35–19.38, with discussion.

16.5 DIŠ *ina* SAG.DU-*š*[*ú*]/SAG.KI-*šú* DIB-*su* DIB DINGIR-*t*[*i*] (DPS XIX/XX:100′ [AOAT 43.232])

**If it afflicts him in his head/temple(s), divine anger.

16.6 DIŠ SAG.KI^{II}-*šú šá* 15 *u* 150 KÚ.MEŠ-*šú-ma* KÚM-*šú mit-ḫar* ŠU DINGIR-*šú* DIN (DPS IV B obv. 32//E i 12 = *TDP* 36:33//*SpTU* 3.88 i 12)[5]

**If his left and right temples continually hurt him and his temperature is normal, "hand" of his god; he will get well.

NIGHTMARES

The goddess Ištar was responsible for nightmares in small children (see Chapter 17). In adults as well as in children, disturbing dreams are a frequent consequence of mental stress.

16.7 NA$_4$.MEŠ MÁŠ.GI$_6$.MEŠ ḪUL.MEŠ SIG$_5$ . . . (*BAM* 376 i 30′; cf. *SpTU* 4.129 ii 6)[6]

**Stones to make bad dreams good . . .

16.8 *šá mal-di* ${}^{\text{GIŠ}}$NÁ.MU *it-ti-iq ú-pal-liḫ-an-ni ú-šag-ra-*[*ra-an-ni*] *šu-na-a-tú pàr-da-a-tú ú-kal-lam-an-ni* . . . (*SpTU* 3.82 iv 12–13//Ebeling, *ArOr* 21.403:1–2)

**(The demon) who crosses the edge of my bed, frightens me makes me roll over and over, shows me troubled dreams . . .

16.9 DIŠ N[A M]ÁŠ.GI$_6$ *par-d*[*a* IGI-*mar* . . .] BÚR-*ri-šú* . . . (*STT* 107:12′–13′)

**If a ⌜person⌝ [sees] a ⌜troubled dream⌝ [. . .], to dispel it . . .

16.10 NA$_4$ MÁŠ.GI$_6$.MEŠ *par-da-te* . . . (*BAM* 377 iii 18)

**Stones for troubled dreams . . .

One particular sort of bad dream that receives special mention in the texts is having visions of "dead persons." Generally ghosts are believed to bother people in dreams because they have needs that are not being attended to or because their victim did them some wrong while they were alive.

16.11 DIŠ NA GID[IM DIB-*s*]*u-*⌜*ma*⌝ *ina* KI.NÁ-*šú* ÚŠ.MEŠ IGI.MEŠ . . . (*CT* 23.15–22+ iv 5 [Scurlock, *MMTGI* no. 54])

**If a ⌜ghost⌝ [afflicts] a person so that he continually sees dead persons (when he is) in his sleep . . .

16.12 DIŠ NA *ina* MÁŠ.GI$_6$-*šú* ÚŠ.MEŠ IGI.MEŠ . . . (*SpTU* 4.134:7; *CT* 23.15–22+ iv 13 [Scurlock, *MMTGI* no. 25]; *SpTU* 4.135 iii 9)

**If a person continually sees dead persons in his dreams . . .

INSOMNIA

Ancient Mesopotamians lost sleep because of stress and worry just like modern humans.

16.13 *i-na ni-zi-iq-ti-ka mu-ši-a-tim ú-ul a-ṣa-la-al* (*TCL* 18.152:33 [Oppenheim, *Letters* no. 18])

**I cannot sleep at night because of worry about you.

SLEEP TALKING

Talking aloud while asleep is considered to be a sign of stress. This is not mentioned in the preserved diagnostic texts but does appear in physiognomic omens, where it was used for predictions of the future. The last reference below indicates that there was a treatment, now unfortunately lost.

16.14 [DIŠ LÚ] *i-na ṣa-la-li-šu iṣ-ṣí-iḫ* . . . (Köcher and Oppenheim, *AfO* 18.64 i 39, 43)

**[If a person] laughs/⌜cries⌝ in his sleep . . .

16.15 DIŠ LÚ *i-na ṣa-la-li-šu i-da-ab-bu-ub* . . . (Köcher and Oppenheim, *AfO* 18.64 ii 1)

**If a person talks in his sleep . . .

16.16 DIŠ NA *ina* KI.NÁ-*šú* GÙ.GÙ-*si iṣ-ṣe-né-eḫ* . . . (*BAM* 30:54′)

**If a person continually cries out (or) continually laughs in his sleep . . .

STRESS ANGINA

Patients who are under mental stress have physiological changes that might include increased heart rate and blood pressure. With a normal heart, the physiological changes are usually well tolerated, but with decreased coronary artery blood flow, the stress could produce heart pain (angina) because of the increased demand on the heart. The text below identifies two well-known triggers of angina, namely, eating and mental stress. (See Chapter 8.)

16.17 DIŠ NA *ina ma-ka-li-šú* ŠÀ-*šú* GAZ.MEŠ-*šú ina* É *ṣal-te ina* SILA *pu-úḫ-pu-ḫu-u* GAR-*šú šá* NA BI *ki-mil-ti* ^{d}MES/ ^{d}AMAR.UTU UGU-*šú* GÁL-*ši* (DIB-*ti* ^{d}AMAR.UTU) *ana* BÚR-*ri*. . . (*STT* 95 i 7–8//*BAM* 317 r. 27–28//*AMT* 40/2:4′–6′)

**If when a person eats, his heart continually crushes him (and) in the house quarrel and in the street disturbance are inflicted upon him, the anger of Marduk is upon that person, to loosen (the anger of Marduk) . . .

ANXIETY

Severe mental and emotional stress may cause anxiety, which is manifested by a variety of signs and symptoms including sleeplessness, loss of appetite, nightmares, depression, fearfulness, and muscle tenseness. This condition seems to have been attributed by the *āšipu* to the patient's being abandoned by his personal god and goddess. Below are references that describe an anxious patient.

16.18 DIŠ NA GAZ ŠÀ-*bi* TUKU.MEŠ-*ši ur-ra u* GI$_6$ *pu-luḫ-tú* TUKU-*ši* DINGIR-*šú* KI-*šú ze-ni* DINGIR-*šú* KI-*šú ana* SILIM-*me*. . . (*BAM* 316 iii 13′–14′//*BAM* 317 r. 16–17//*STT* 95 iv 145//*BAM* 447:4′)

**If a person continually has crushing of the heart (and) day and night he has fearfulness/shuddering, his god is angry with him; in order to make his god at peace with him . . .

16.19 DIŠ *ina ši-mi-tan lu* LÚ.TI *lu* LÚ.ÚŠ *lu* ⌜*mu-da-šú lu*⌝[7] *la m*[*u-da-šú*] *lu mam-ma lu mim-ma* IGI-*ma* LUḪ-*uṭ i-tu-ram-ma* GIN$_7$ *šá* Ì.ḪAB *tu* [. . .] KA-*šú* DIB-*ma šá i-ta-a-šú ṣal-lu šá-sa-a* NU ZU-*e* ŠU GIDIM$_7$: ŠU [. . .] (DPS XVII:83–85 [AOAT 43.203])[8]

**If in the evening, he sees either a living person or a dead person or someone known to him or someone not ⌜known to him⌝ or anybody or anything and becomes afraid; he turns around but, like one who has [been hexed with?] rancid oil, his mouth is seized so that he is unable to cry out to one who ⌜sleeps⌝ next to him, "hand" of ghost or "hand" of [. . .].

16.20 DIŠ NA *mi-iḫ-ru ma-ḫi-ir-ma ki-i im-ḫu-ru-šu ul i*!-[*di*] . . . GAZ ŠÀ-*bi* TUKU.TUKU-[*ši*] DUG$_4$.GA NU ŠE.GA *sa-su-u la ap-pa-lu i-zi-im-tú* KA UN.MEŠ.ḪI.A [. . .] *i-na* KI.NÁ-*šú* MUD.MUD-*ud ri-mu-tu* TUKU-*ši a-du bi-nu-te-šú ana* DINGIR *u* LU[GAL] ŠÀ-*bi-šú ma-li mi-na-tu-šú* DUB.DUB-*ak pi-qa la pi-qa i-pár-ru-ud ur-ra u* GI$_6$ *la* NÁ-*lal* MÁŠ.GI$_6$.MEŠ *pár-da-a-ti* IGI.DU$_8$.A.MEŠ *ri-mu-tu* TUKU.TUKU NINDA *u* KAŠ *muṭ-ṭu a-mat i-qab-bu-ú i-maš-ši* LÚ BI *šib-sat* DINGIR *u* ^{d}EŠ$_4$.DAR UGU-*šú* TUKU-*ši* DINGIR-*šú u* ^{d}EŠ$_4$.DAR-*šú* KI-*šú ze-nu-ú ana* NA BI ŠU.NAM.RIM.MA ŠU.DINGIR.RA ŠU NAM.LÚ.U$_{19}$.LU GIG *ḫi-*

im-ma-te GIG *ár-ni* AD *u* AMA ŠEŠ *u* NIN IM.RI.A IM.RI.A IM.RI.A DIB-*šú a-na* DU_8- «*ri*»-*ri-ma a-di-ra-te-šú a-na la ka-šá-d*[*i*] . . . (*BAM* 234:1, 4–12 [Ritter and Kinnier Wilson, *AnSt* 30.23–40])

**If something untoward has happened to a person and he ⌜does not know⌝ how it happened to him . . . (he is experiencing financial losses and animals and people in his household are dying) he continually has a crushing sensation in his chest,[9] speaking and not being heard,[10] calling out and not being answered, (and) [not attaining] commonly desired things;[11] he continually shudders in his bed, he has limpness as regards his shape (i.e., he looks like a wet dishrag), he is continually enraged against god and ⌜king⌝, his limbs are continually tense,[12] he incessantly shudders, he cannot sleep day or night, he continually sees troubled dreams, he continually has limpness,[13] his appetite for bread and beer is diminished, (and) he forgets whatever he says, the anger of god and goddess are upon him (and) his god and goddess are angry with him. In order to loosen "hand" of curse (anorexia; see 19.307 with discussion); "hand" of god (ill-defined or stress-related illnesses; see 19.35–38, 19.347–363, with discussion),[14] or "hand" of mankind-sorcery[15] or being sick with an illness involving (hysterical) paralysis[16] or the sins of his father or mother, brother or sister or most distant relations that afflict him and for his worries not to "get" that person . . .

ANXIETY AND SEIZURES

The following reference combines apparent seizure activity with behavior that seems anxious, depressed, even paranoid. The patient is having difficulty getting along with others; he has bad dreams, and is in a fearful state. "His understanding(?) is continually altered; he continually forgets what he has (just) said" and he "frightens (even) himself." In addition, he is losing weight; he is very irritable, has little interest in sex, and has no energy to do anything. He also "ponders untruths," that is, he suspects others wrongly of harboring malice against him (see below under PARANOIA). If it was not simply a coincidence that the person for whom this ritual was designed was having emotional problems and seizures at the same time, it is possible that he had suffered a concussion or, alternatively, was in withdrawal from alcohol. Both conditions can produce spontaneously remitting seizures and serious emotional problems, particularly anxiety.

16.21 DIŠ NA AN.TA.ŠUB.BA LUGAL.ÙR.RA ŠU.DINGIR.RA ŠU ^{d}INNIN [ŠU.GIDIM.MA] ⌜ŠU⌝ NAM.ÉRIM ŠU NAM.LÚ.U_{19}.LU UGU-*šú* GÁL-*ši* A.LÁ ḪUL ŠÚ.ŠÚ-*šú i-qab-bi-ma* NU ŠE.GA-*šú* ŠU.SI ḪUL-*tim* EGIR-*šú* LAL-*at* DINGIR *ù* ^{d}$EŠ_4$.DAR KI-*šu ze-nu-ú* MÁŠ.GI_6.MEŠ *pár-da-te* ḪUL.MEŠ NU ŠE.GA.MEŠ IGI.IGI-*mar pu-ul-ḫu* GAR-*šú ana* IGI DINGIR *u* ^{d}$EŠ_4$.DAR *ug-gat* ŠÀ-*bi* TUKU.TUKU-*ši nu-ul-la-te* ŠÀ-*šú i-tam-mu* NÍ-*šú šup-luḫ ina* KA UN.MEŠ-*šú zi-i-ru* GAR-*šú* DINGIR LUGAL IDIM *u* NUN *da-ṣu-šu i-qab-bu-šu-ma la i-nam-di-nu-šú ka-la* UZU.MEŠ-*šú šim-ma-tú* TUKU.MEŠ-*ú* IGI.MEŠ-*šú* SA_5 SIG_7 *u* GI_6 SU-*šú* KÚR.KÚR-*ir* INIM.MEŠ-*šu im-ta-na-aš-ši* MUNUS ŠÀ-*šú la ir-ri-su a-na* KUR-*ád* ÁŠ ŠÀ-*šú la* ÍL-*šu a-na gi-mir* TI.LA DÙ.A.BI *ana* NA NU TE-*e* . . . (*KAR* 26 obv. 1–10 and parallels [Mayer, *OrNS* 68.145–163])

**(This ritual is to be performed) if various sorts of seizures (see Chapter 19 with 19.60–19.79), "hand" of curse (wasting; see p. 506), and "hand" of mankind-sorcery are upon a person. An evil *alû*-demon overwhelms him (if taken literally, this would put him in a coma [see Chapter 13, with 13.273–275]; walking about "like a zombie" is presumably what is meant). (If) he says (something), people do not agree with him; people say bad things about him behind his back. God and goddess are angry with him; he continually sees troubled dreams that are bad and ill-omened. He is in a fearful state; he is continually enraged against god and goddess; his heart ponders untruths. He frightens (even) himself; his people say hateful things about him. God, king, magnate, and prince oppress him; they promise him (things) and then will not give (them) to him. All of his flesh is continually numb. His face flushes, turns pale, and darkens.[17] His understanding(?) is continually altered; he continually forgets his words. His woman does not want him (anymore); he cannot get up the energy to accomplish what he wants. In order for this not to approach the person for absolutely his entire life . . .[18]

ANOREXIA

Mental stress may cause opposite responses to food. Some patients increase food intake to alleviate stress, others lose their appetite and eat less. In the quote below, the patient has lost his appetite (anorexia). The attribution of this problem to a "murderous" ghost indicates that the patient was expected to die. Incinerated ghosts typically made their victims scream, or conversely, go completely silent due to a linguistic pun between the verb *qalû*: "to burn" and a near homophone *qâlu*: "to be silent."

16.22 DIŠ UB.NÍGIN.NA-*šú* GIN$_7$ *šá bal-ṭi ne-ḫa-ma i-qá-al u mim-ma la i-lem* ŠU GIDIM$_7$ *šag-ga-ši šá-niš* ⸢ŠU GIDIM$_7$ *qa-li-i*⸣ (DPS XXVI:76′ [AOAT 43.285])

**If his limbs are as still as those of a healthy person (but) he is silent (*i-qá-al*) and does not take any food, "hand" of a murderous ghost (var. "hand" of the ghost of someone burned to death [*qa-li-i*])

LOVE-SICKNESS

A specific form of stress is "love-sickness." It is caused by the uncertainty that the love is reciprocal, and the confusion of the "patient" about what he or she should do to attract the beloved individual. This stress causes behavioral abnormality and psychosomatic complaints (see below). The descriptions of love-sickness that follow are quite recognizable and understandable in spite of the thousands of years that have transpired since their writing.

16.23 DIŠ *iš-ta-na-ʾ-i* KA ŠUB.ŠUB-*su* KI ŠÀ-*šú* DUG$_4$.DUG$_4$-*ub ṣu-uḫ la pak-ki iṣ-ṣe-né-eḫ* GIG *ra-mi* GIG *ana* NITA *u* MUNUS 1-*ma* (DPS XXII:6–7 [AOAT 43.251])

**If he continually flutters about, he is continually insolent, he continually talks with himself, (and) he continually laughs for no reason, he is sick with love-sickness; it is the same for a man and a woman.

16.24 DIŠ NÍG.ZI.IR ŠUB.ŠUB-*su* ZI.MEŠ-*šú* LÚGUD.MEŠ[19] NINDA KÚ A/KAŠ NAG-*ma* UGU-*šú* NU DU-*ak ʾù-a* ŠÀ-*bi i-qab-bi u uš-tan-na-aḫ* GIG *ra-mi* GIG *ana* NITA *u* MUNUS 1-*ma* (DPS XXII:8–9 [AOAT 43.251–252])[20]

**If depression continually falls upon him, his breath is continually short, he eats bread (and) drinks water/beer but it does not agree with him, he says "Ua my heart!" and he is dejected, he is sick with love-sickness; it is the same for a man and a woman.

PSYCHOSOMATIC ILLNESS

As indicated above, mental stress may have physiological effects on the heart and blood pressure, but other tissues and organs may also be affected. Increased blood flow or flushing may occur, the respiratory rate can increase, and intestinal movement (peristalsis) may increase. Abdominal cramping and diarrhea are common. The patient may interpret these symptoms to be organic disease when in fact they are secondary to mental stress.[21] In the second reference, the sensation of laryngeal constriction describes a lump in his throat, another common symptom of mental stress. However, the quote could also be describing a physical disease causing difficulty swallowing (dysphagia).[22]

16.25 DIŠ NA ŠÀ-*bi* ŠÀ-*bi i-qab-bi*/GÙ.GÙ-*si* ŠÀ-*šú* NU KÚ-*šú* NINDA NU KÚ A/KAŠ NU NAG *i-dam-mu-um* NA BI DIB-*ti* DINGIR-*šú u* ^{d}EŠ$_{4}$.DAR-*šú* UGU-*šú* GÁL-*ši*... (*BAM* 316 iv 3–4//*STT* 95 ii 70–72//*KAR* 92 r. 4–6)

**If a person says/cries out: "My insides, my insides!" (but) his stomach does not hurt him, he cannot eat bread (and) he cannot drink water/beer (and) he moans, the anger of his god or goddess is upon that person . . .

16.26 DIŠ GÚ.MUR-*su ḫa-niq* NÍG.GIG DINGIR-*šú* KÚ : *uš-te-zeb* (DPS X A obv. 28//B obv. 32 = *TDP* 84:28)

**If his larynx is constricted, he ate something offensive to his god (var. he will get through).

In the three references below, the *āšipu* appears to have concluded that the patient's problems were in response to guilt. The first text describes flushing and stress headache probably brought on by an act of theft. The second and third patients have insomnia (and mysterious pains) due to incest. The phrase "the son of her god has approached her sexually" indicates that she has had sexual relations with her brother.

16.27 DIŠ ⸢TA⸣ [SAG.DU]-*šú* EN MURUB$_{4}$-*šú* KÚM TA MURUB$_{4}$-*šú* EN ⸢GÌR⸣^{II}-*šú* ⸢ŠED$_{7}$⸣ SAG.KI-*su* ⸢SÌG⸣.SÌG-*su* [. . .]x *ina* SAG *šá* ^{GIŠ}⸢MÁ⸣ *iš-riq* DINGIR *ka-a-ri* DIB-*su* ⸢BÚR⸣-*ma* DIN (DPS III A r. 3′–4′//C r. 26–27 = *TDP* 28:86–87)

**If he is hot from his [head] to his hip region (and) cold from his hip region to his feet (and) his temple continually gives him a jabbing pain [. . .], he stole something[23] from the prow of a boat and the god of the quay afflicts him; (if) it lets up, he will get well.

16.28 DIŠ MU[NUS *ina bal-ṭ*]*ú-ti-šá ú-šam-šá u ina* GIG-*šá ú-šam-šá* DUMU DINGIR-*šú* TE-*ši* (DPS XXXVII A obv. 20 = *TDP* 214:20)

**If a ⸢woman⸣ is kept up all night [when] she is ⸢healthy⸣ and when she is sick, the son of her god has approached her (sexually).

16.29 DIŠ MU[NUS . . .]x *lu* ŠU^{II}-*šá lu* GÌR^{II}-*šá ú-ṣa-⌜bi-ta⌝-ši* DUMU DINGIR-*šú* TE-*ši* : DIŠ KI.NÁ-*šá* ŠUB.ŠUB-*ši* É-*sà* ⌜BIR⌝ (DPS XXXVII A obv. 21 = *TDP* 214:21)

**If a ⌜woman⌝ [is kept up all night(?)] (and) either her hands or her feet continually afflict her, the son of her god has approached her (sexually). If the bed continually throws her off, her household will be scattered.

MOURNFUL OR WORRIED EXPRESSION

16.30 DIŠ IGI.MEŠ-*šú ad-ru* DIN (DPS IX A 41//B obv. 40 = *TDP* 74:41)

**If a person's face is mournful/worried, he will get well.

16.31 NA$_4$.MEŠ DIŠ NA *gi-na-a a-dir* . . . (*BAM* 372 ii 17//*BAM* 373 ii 5)

**Stones for cases where a person is continually mournful/worried . . .

16.32 NA$_4$.MEŠ DIŠ NA *gi-na-a a-dir* Ḫ[UL ŠÀ TUKU.TUKI-*ši*] KI NÍ-*šú i-ta-mu uš-tan-na-aḫ uš-tád-dar šib-sat* DINGIR *u* [^{d}15] UGU-*šú* GÁL.MEŠ . . . (*SpTU* 3.85 ii 2–4)

**Stones for cases where a person is continually mournful/worried, [he is continually] ⌜sorrowful⌝, he talks to himself, he is continually exhausted and unhappy, god and [goddess] are angry at him . . .

16.33 DIŠ NA *gi-na-a šu-dur ur-ra u mu-ši ina-an-ziq* . . . MÁŠ.GI$_6$.MEŠ-*šú* ḪUL.MEŠ *ina* MÁŠ.GI$_6$-*šú* ÚŠ.MEŠ IGI.MEŠ GAZ ŠÀ-*bi* TUKU-*šú* MÁŠ.GI$_6$ IGI NU DIB-*át ina* MÁŠ.GI$_6$-*šú* GIN$_7$ *šá* KI MUNUS *uš-ta-ḫu*! *u* A.RI.A-*šú i-ṣar-ru-ru šib-sat* DINGIR *u* ^{d}15 UGU-*šú* GÁL-*ši* . . . (*SpTU* 2.22 i 16, 19–21)[24]

**If a person is continually made sad/worried, he is upset day and night . . . (he is having serious financial losses; people slander him, lie to him, and talk about him behind his back), his dreams are bad, in his dream he continually sees dead persons, he has a crushing sensation in his heart, he cannot remember the dream that he sees, (and) during his dream, his semen flows like one who has congress with a woman, god and goddess are angry with him . . .

ALTERED MENTATION

This term indicates any change in the usual patterns of an individual's behavior.

16.34 DIŠ UŠ$_4$-*šú* MAN.MAN-*šu uz-zi* DINGIR (DPS XXII:47b [AOAT 43.255])[25]

**If his mentation is continually altered, anger of a god.

16.35 [DIŠ U]Š$_4$-*šú šá-ni-šu-ma* UŠ$_4$-*šú* NU DIB ŠU GIDIM *mur-tap-pi-du* GAM (DPS XXII:47a [AOAT 43.255])

** [If] his ⌜mentation⌝ is altered so that he is not in full possession of his faculties, "hand" of a roving ghost; he will die.

16.36 DIŠ UŠ$_4$-[*šú* KÚR-*ir* IN]IM.MEŠ-*šú it-te-né-ep-rek-ka-a* GIDIM *mu-šam-šu-ú* DIB-*su* [:] KI.SIKIL.LÍL.LÁ *šum$_4$-ma* LÚ.LÍL.LÁ (DPS XXII:51–52 [AOAT 43.255])

**If [his] mentation [is altered] (and) his ⸢words⸣ hinder each other (in his mouth), a ghost who wanders about at night[26] afflicts him ([var.] *ardat lilî* or *lilû*).

16.37 DIŠ UŠ$_4$-*šú* KÚR-⸢*ir*⸣ [. . .] x *maš-u-tú* INIM.MEŠ-*šú it-te-né-ep-rek-ka-a* GIDIM$_7$ *mut-tag-gi-šú* DIB-*su* [. . .].MEŠ-*ma* DIN KI.MIN ŠU LÚ.LÍL.LÁ (DPS XXII:53–54 [AOAT 43.256])

**If his mentation is altered, [. . .] forgetfulness(?) (and) his words hinder each other in his mouth, a roaming ghost afflicts him. If [. . .] he will get well. Alternatively, "hand" of *lilû*.

16.38 DIŠ UŠ$_4$-*šú* KÚR.KÚR-*šú* ŠU ^{d}UTU AZAG KÚ (DPS XXII:55a [AOAT 43.256])

**If his mentation continually alters, "hand" of Šamaš; he has transgressed a taboo.

MUMBLING AND USING UNINTELLIGIBLE WORDS

In addition to psychiatric diseases, this problem could be caused by organic brain disease and abnormalities of the tongue or larynx.

16.39 DIŠ EME-*šú ik-ka-ṣir-ma* KA *la ip-te*[27] [. . .] NIN.DINGIR DINGIR-*šú iš-šiq* AZAG [DINGIR-*šú* KÚ] (DPS VII A obv. 19–20 = *TDP* 62:19–20)[28]

**If his tongue is tied in knots and he cannot open (his) mouth [. . .], he has kissed the *ēntu*-priestess of his god;[29] [he has done] something offensive [to his god].

16.40 [DIŠ UŠ$_4$]-*šú* MAN.MAN-*šu u* EME-*šú ir-ta-nap-pu-ud* GAM (DPS XXII:48 [AOAT 43.255])

**[If] his [mentation] is continually altered and his tongue continually roves about, he will die.

16.41 DIŠ KA-*šú* [KÚR.KÚR-*i*]*r u* ⸢*i-ram*⸣-*mu-um*[30] *ana* [U$_4$.10.KÁM . . .] (DPS VII B r. 15 = *TDP* 66:71′)

**If his words are ⸢unintelligible⸣ and he drones for [ten days . . .]

16.42 DIŠ AL.ZU.BI NAM.BA.ZU.BI *u* INIM-*šú* KÚR.KÚR-*ir* GAM (DPS XXII:56 [AOAT 43.256])

**If he does not recognize one who is known to him[31] and his words are continually unintelligible, he will die.

EXCESSIVE TALKING (LOGORRHEA)

This condition may be a response to stress as well as to more severe psychiatric problems such as the manic phase of bipolar disorder (see below).

16.43 DIŠ NA DIMMA.KÚR.RA DIB-*su-*[*m*]*a ṭè-en-šú iš-t*[*a-nu*] *a-ma-tu-šú* KÚR.KÚR-*ra ṭé-em-šú* ŠUB.ŠUB-*su u ma-gal* DUG$_4$.DUG$_4$-*ub a-na ṭè-me-šú tur-r*[*i*]-*šú* . . . (*BAM* 202 obv. 1–3//*STT* 286 ii 14–16)

**If derangement seizes a person [so] that his mentation ⸢alters⸣, his words are unintelligible, his thinking continually fails him, and he continually talks a lot, to restore his mind to him . . .

16.44 DIŠ *pa-rid-ma it-te-né-et-bi ma-gal* DUG$_4$.DUG$_4$-*ub u i*[*g-d*]*a*-⸢*na*⸣-*al-lu-u*[*t*] *ana* MUNUS LÍL.L[Á].EN.NA *ana* NITA SAL.LÍL.LÁ.EN.NA ZI.ZI-*bé* (DPS XXVI:82′–83′ [AOAT 43.285])

**If he shudders and he can get up (afterward), he talks a lot, and he continually ⸢jerks⸣, for a woman, a *lilû*, for a man, a *lilītu*; he can get up (afterward).

16.45 DIŠ *ina* GIG-*šú* DUG$_4$.DUG$_4$-*ub* GIDIM *ár-da-na-an* ÚŠ DIB-*su* DIN (DPS XVII:17 [AOAT 43.196])

**If, during his illness, he talks continually, a ghost, the "double" of a dead person has seized him (but) he will get well.

MUTISM

At the opposite extreme, patients may speak less or cease speaking completely. Severely frightened patients may respond to this stress by becoming mute (see above), and patients with catatonic schizophrenia also may have this problem. Of course, abnormalities of the larynx and tongue can cause the same finding.

16.46 DIŠ UB.NÍGIN.NA-*šú* GIN$_7$ *šá bal-ṭi ne-ḫa* KA-*šú* DIB-*ma* NU DUG$_4$.DUG$_4$-*ub* ŠU GIDIM$_7$ *šag-ga-ši* : ŠU GIDIM$_7$ *qa-li-i* (DPS XXVI:75′ [AOAT 43.285])

**If his limbs are as still as those of a healthy person (but) his mouth is "seized" so that he cannot talk, "hand" of a murderous ghost (var.: "hand" of the ghost of someone burned to death).

16.47 DIŠ UB.NÍGIN.NA-*šú* GIN$_7$ *šá bal-ṭi ne-ḫa-ma i-qá-al u mim-ma la i-lem* ŠU GIDIM$_7$ *šag-ga-ši šá-niš* ⸢ŠU GIDIM$_7$ *qa-li-i*⸣ (DPS XXVI:76′ [AOAT 43.285])

**If his limbs are as still as those of a healthy person (but) he is silent and does not take any food, "hand" of a murderous ghost (var.: "hand" of the ghost of someone burned to death).[32]

CONFUSION

The *āšipu* described some patients as wandering about in a daze, staring off into space, and staring at body parts.

WANDERING ABOUT IN A DAZE

16.48 DIŠ GIG [KA-*šú*] KÚR.KÚR-*ir ana* U$_4$.3.[KÁM . . .] KA-*šú* [. . .] *u ra-pa-du su-ud-dur ana* U$_4$.3.K[ÁM . . .] (DPS VII B r. 3–4 = *TDP* 64:59′–60′)

**If his words are unintelligible for three days [. . .] his mouth [. . .] and he experiences wandering about for three days in a row [. . .]

16.49 *ra-pa-du su-ud-dur-*[*šú*] = [*šá-n*]*e-e ṭè-e-me sa-dir-šú* (*SpTU* 1.32 r. 8–9 [commentary to DPS VII B r. 3–4 = *TDP* 64:59′–60′])

**"He experiences wandering about (for three) consecutive (days)" means "he experiences ⌜alteration⌝ of mentation (for three) consecutive (days)."[33]

16.50 DIŠ *ú-rap-pad ú-ma-aq it-ta-na-an-di* : ŠUB.ŠUB-*ut* GAM (DPS XXII:57 [AOAT 43.256])

**If he wanders about, he does things slowly,[34] (and) he is continually thrown down (var. falls down), he will die.

STARING OFF INTO SPACE

16.51 DIŠ *ina ṣal-lu-ti-šú* DIB-*su-ma* DIB-*su* IGI.BAR-*as i-re-eḫ-ḫi-šum-ma* NÍ-*šú i-maš-ši* GIN$_7$ *šá id-ku-šú* MUD-*ud* ZI.ZI-*bé* : U$_4$ *id-de-ku-šú re-ḫi* ŠU LÍL.LÁ.EN.NA *sar-ru ana* MUNUS LÍL.LÁ.EN.NA ZI.ZI-*bé* (DPS XXVI:48′–49′ [AOAT 43.282])

**If it afflicts him in his sleep and he gazes at the one who afflicts him, it flows over him and he forgets himself, he shudders like one whom they have awakened (and) he can get up (var. when they try to wake him, he is groggy), false "hand" of *lilû*. For a woman, a *lilû*; he can get up (afterward).

16.52 [DIŠ] LÚ *i-na na-ap-lu-sí-šu a-wi-lam la ú-te-ed-di* LÚ *šú-ú a-na qá-ti mu-tim pa-qí-id* (Köcher and Oppenheim, *AfO* 18.65 ii 12–13 [physiognomic omens])

** [If] a person does not recognize (another) person while gazing at him, that person has been entrusted into the hands of death.

16.53 DIŠ LÚ *i-na na-ap-lu-sí-šu i-ni-šu za-qá-pa-am ú-qal-la-al-ma la i-le-i* LÚ *šu-ú ṭé-em-šu pu-ur-ru-ur* (Köcher and Oppenheim, *AfO* 18.65 ii 16–17 [physiognomic omens])

**If when a person looks, his eyes are barely able to constrict[35] so that he can't (actually look), that person's mentation is weak.

STARING AT BODY PARTS

16.54 [DIŠ ŠU^{II}-*šú* I]GI.BAR.MEŠ BAL.BAL Z[I]-*bi u* DU$_{10}$.GAM *ina* SAG [GI$_6$ TAG-*it* ...] (DPS XI A obv. 38 = *TDP* 92:38)[36]

** [If] he continually ⌜gazes⌝ at [his hands], he has changes of mood, he ⌜gets up⌝ and (has to) squat down, (and) [he is particularly affected] at the beginning of [the night ...]

16.55 DIŠ SA SAG.KI^{II}-*šú* ŠU^{II}-*šú u* GÌR^{II}-*šú šá* 15 *u* 150 *it-ta-na-aš-gag-gu u* BAL.MEŠ / DIŠ ⌜*e-sa*⌝ *ú-šaq-qa-ma* LÚ.AD$_6$-*šú* IGI.BAR.MEŠ ŠU ^{d}UTU MU DAM LÚ (DPS IV A$_2$ r. 31–32//B r. 11–12 = *TDP* 42 r. 31–32)

**If the blood vessels of his temples,[37] his hands, or his feet, the ones on the left or right <"go" but the ones on the right or left are present and the muscles of the feet> on the left or right side continually become stiff and continually shift under (him), (his feet) have a viselike pain(?) (but) he can lift (them) and he continually gazes at his body, "hand" of Šamaš on account of a man's wife.

INAPPROPRIATE USE OF CLOTHING

This includes repetitive dressing and undressing, refusing to wear clothes, and tearing off clothes.

16.56 DIŠ *i-te-ner-ru-ub* TÚG-*su* ŠUB.ŠUB-*di iš-ta-na-su ma-gal* DU [G$_4$.DUG$_4$-*ub*] NINDA *u* KAŠ NU GUR-*ma* KÚ *u la i-ṣal-lal* ŠU ^{d}15 GAR ⸢TI⸣ (DPS XXVI:78′–79′ [AOAT 43.285])

**If he keeps beginning to get into and taking off his garments, he continually cries out(!), he continually ⸢talks⸣ a lot, bread and beer do not come back up on him so that he can eat but he cannot sleep, "hand" of Ištar is laid (on him); he will get well.[38]

16.57 [DIŠ TÚ]G-*su* ŠUB.ŠUB-*di u i-te-ner-ru-ub* ŠU ^{d}MAŠ.TAB.BA GAM (DPS XXII:46 [AOAT 43.255])

**[If] he keeps taking off and beginning to get into his ⸢garments⸣, "hand" of the twin gods; he will die.

16.58 DIŠ MUNUS GIG-*ma* DIB-*sa ina* AN.ÚSAN DIB.DIB-*si u* TÚG-*sa* ŠUB.ŠUB-*di* DIB-*it* LÍL.LÁ.EN.NA (DPS XXXVII A obv. 13 = *TDP* 214:13)

**If a woman is sick and her affliction always afflicts her in the evening and she continually takes her clothes off, it is an affliction of *lilû*.

16.59 [DIŠ] ŠU^{II}-*šú ana* KA-*šú ú-ḫab-bat* TÚG-*su it-ta-na-as-suk u* UŠ$_4$-*šú* NU [DIB *lu-ʾ-a-tú šu-kul* GAM] (DPS XI A obv. 28//B 27 = *TDP* 92:28//*SpTU* 1.34:27; cf. DPS XV:16 [AOAT 43.151])

**[If] he moves his hands across his mouth,[39] he continually throws off his garment, (and) he is not in full [possession] of his faculties, [he has been made to eat dirty substances;[40] he will die].

ABNORMAL HANDLING OF BODY PARTS

Patients may repetitively rub, suck, hit, or bite their own or another's hands, feet, or other body parts. This behavior in its more extreme form may cause self-mutilation, and is described below.

16.60 [DIŠ ŠU^{II}-*šú*] LÚ.AD$_6$-*šú ma-gal* TAG.MEŠ GIN$_7$ TAG.MEŠ NU ZU [GAM] (DPS XI A obv. 30//B 29 = *TDP* 92:30//*SpTU* 1.34:29)[41]

**[If his hands] continually rub his body a lot (and) he does not realize that they are continually rubbing (it), [he will die].

16.61 DIŠ ŠU^{II}-*šú ina* KA-*šú* GAR-*na-ma ta-tab-bal-ma ana* KA-*šú ú-tar* [GAM] (DPS XI A obv. 26//B 25 = *TDP* 92:26//*SpTU* 1.34:25)[42]

**If his hands are placed in his mouth and (if) you take (them) out, he returns (them) to his mouth, [he will die].[43]

16.62 DIŠ KI.MIN-*ma* ŠU^{II}-*šú ana* KA-*šú ú-ḫab-bat* TÚG-*su it-ta-na-as-suk lu-ʾ-a-tú šu-*[*kul* GAM] (DPS XV:16 [AOAT 43.151]; cf. DPS XI A obv. 28//B 27 = *TDP* 92:28//*SpTU* 1.34:27)

**If (it is the first day he is sick) and he moves his hands across his mouth[44] (and) continually throws off his garment, he has been made [to eat] dirty substances;[45] [he will die].

16.63 DIŠ IGI.MEŠ-*šú* SÌG.SÌG-*aṣ u* GÙ.DÉ.DÉ.ME-*si* GIDIM *qá-li-i* DIB-*su* (DPS IX A 76//B r. 23 = *TDP* 78:76)

**If he continually strikes his face and screams, the ghost of someone burned to death afflicts him.

16.64 DIŠ EME-*šú ú-na-aš-šak* [. . .] (DPS VII A obv. 16 = *TDP* 62:16)

**If he bites his tongue [. . .]

The *āšipu* used three special terms to convey the exact manner in which the patient rubbed his body: *ḫanāṣu*: "to rub (something against something else)"; *kapāru*: "to wipe off"; and *kâru*: "to rub (raw)."

16.65 ⌜DIŠ GÚ⌝-*su i-tar-rak* SAG.DU-*su* ŠUB.ŠUB-*ut* ŠU^{II}-*šú u* GÌR^{II}-*šú it-ta-na-aš-gag-gu u ana qaq-qa-ru ú-ḫa-an-na-aṣ* KI.SIKIL.LÍL.LÁ DIB-*su* (DPS X A obv. 12–13//B obv. 12–13 = *TDP* 80:12–13)

**If his neck throbs, his head continually falls (i.e., he lets it drop), his hands and feet continually become stiff, and he rubs (them) on the ground, *ardat lilî* afflicts him.

16.66 DIŠ U$_4$ LÁ-*šú* SAG.KI^{II}-*šú* KÚ.MEŠ-*šú* ŠÀ-*šú* GAZ.MEŠ-*šú* EGIR-*nu* ŠU^{II}-*šú u* GÌR^{II}-*šú ú-kap-p*[*ár*] BAL.BAL-*ut* ÚḪ NU TUKU : *it-ta-nag-ra-ár* ŠUB-*tu* : *ḫa-mi-tum* ŠU ^{d}15 ZI-*bé* (DPS XXVI:28′–29′ [AOAT 43.280])

**If when (confusional states) come over him, his temples continually hurt him, he continually has a crushing sensation in his heart (and) afterward he wipes off his hands and his feet, he rolls over and over (but) he does not have any spittle (var. he rolls over and over), falling spell (var. paralysis) of "hand" of Ištar; he can get up (afterward).

16.67 DIŠ NA ŠÀ-*šú ik-ta-na-ar* . . . (*BAM* 574 ii 41)

**If he continually rubs his abdomen raw . . .

HALLUCINATIONS

When sensations are perceived by a patient in the absence of the stimulus that normally causes the sensation, it is called a hallucination. This abnormal sensation can be visual, auditory, tactile, or for that matter any of the sensations that we normally perceive including smell and taste. Auditory and visual hallucinations are most common, and they usually indicate a more severe mental illness or organic brain disease.

TACTILE

16.68 DIŠ *tu-gu-un-šú ú-zaq-qat-su* GEŠTU^{II}-*šú* GÙ.DÉ.MEŠ SÍG SU-*šú* GUB.GUB-⌜*az*⌝-*kal* LÚ.AD$_6$-*šú* GIN$_7$ *kal-ma-tum i-ba-šú-ú i-nam-muš u* ŠU-*su ub-bal-ma la i-ba-áš-šú* : *la ig-gi-ig* ŠU GIDIM$_7$ UD.DA LÚ GIN$_7$ ^{GIŠ}GIDRU *šá* ^{d}30 GÌR^{II}-*šú* ŠU GIDIM$_7$ (DPS XXVII:32–34 [AOAT 43.300])

**If (the skin under) his headband stings him, his ears roar, the hair of his body continually (feels like) it is standing on end, his whole body crawls as if there were lice but when he brings his hand up, there is nothing to scratch, "hand" of ghost *ṣētu* (dehydration); (if) the person (bends and stretches out) his feet as in the scepter of Sîn, "hand" of ghost.

VISUAL

16.69 DIŠ UB.NÍGIN.NA-*šú* GIN$_7$ *šá bal-ṭi ne-ḫa* IGI^{II}-*šú* BAD.MEŠ-*ma* U$_4$ DIB-*su ina-ṭal* KI-*šú* DUG$_4$.DUG$_4$-*ub u* NÍ-*šú ut-ta-na-kar* ŠU LÍL.LÁ.EN.NA DUMU *šip-ri šá* DINGIR-*šú* (DPS XXVI:73′–74′ [AOAT 43.284])

**If his limbs are as still as those of a healthy person, (and) he continually opens his eyes and, when he sees the one who afflicts him, he talks with him[46] and continually changes himself, "hand" of *lilû*, messenger of his god.[47]

16.70 DIŠ *mi-šit-ti im-šid-su-ma* SAG.KI-*šú* DIB.DIB-*su mu-kil* SAG-*šú ina-ṭal* : SAG.ḪUL.ḪA.ZA IGI GAM (DPS XXVII:4 [AOAT 43.297])

**If he has a stroke and his temples continually afflict him (and) he can see the one who holds his head, he will die.

AUDITORY[48]

16.71 DIŠ *ik-kil-lu* GÙ.GÙ-*šú u šu-ú i-ta-nap-pal-šú* U$_4$ GÙ.GÙ-*šú at-ta$_5$ man-nu* DUG$_4$.GA *mu-ut-til-lu*^{MUŠEN} TAG-*ma* KI-*šú* KEŠDA *ina* SAG-*šú* GUB-*az* GAM (DPS XXVI:86′–87′ [AOAT 43.285–286])

**If a mournful cry continually cries out to him and he continually answers it (and) when it cries out to him, he says: "Who are you?" a *muttillu*-bird has touched him and is bound with him (and) stands at his head; he will die.

16.72 DIŠ *ik-kil-lu* GÙ.GÙ-*šú u šu-ú i-ta-nap-pal-šú* ZI-*bé u* DU$_{10}$.GAM-*is* MAŠKIM *ḫar-ba-ti* DIB-*su* DIŠ *ik-kil-lu* GÙ.GÙ-*šú* U$_4$ GÙ.GÙ *šú-ú i-ta-nap-pal-šú it-ta-na-as-pak* ZI-*ma i-káš-šú-uš* ZI-*bé u* DU$_{10}$.GAM GIG-*su uš-te-zeb* MAŠKIM *mur-tap-pi-du* DIB-*su* (DPS XXVI: 88′–90′ [AOAT 43.286])

**If a mournful cry continually cries out to him and he continually answers it (and) he gets up and (has to) kneel down, the *rābiṣu* of the wastes afflicts him. If a mournful cry continually cries out to him (and) when it cries out, he continually answers it, he continually behaves like an animal caught in a trap[49] (and) when he gets up, he feels exhausted, he gets up and (has to) kneel down, he will come through his illness; a roving *rābiṣu* afflicts him.

INAPPROPRIATE EMOTIONS

16.73 DIŠ *iš-ta-na-ʾ-i* KA ŠUB.ŠUB-*su* KI ŠÀ-*šú* DUG$_4$.DUG$_4$-*ub ṣu-uḫ la pak-ki iṣ-ṣe-né-eḫ* GIG *ra-mi* GIG *ana* NITA *u* MUNUS 1-*ma* (DPS XXII:6–7 [AOAT 43.251])

**If he continually flutters about, he is continually insolent, he continually talks with himself, (and) he continually laughs for no reason, he is sick with love-sickness; it is the same for a man and a woman.

16.74 DIŠ *iṣ-ṣe-né-eḫ* ŠU ^{d}SAG.ḪUL.ḪA.ZA GAM : ŠU ^{d}*Iš-tar* (DPS XXII:62 [AOAT 43.256])

**If he continually laughs, "hand" of *mukīl rēš lemutti*; he will die (var. "hand" of Ištar).

16.75 DIŠ *ḫa-di u pa-rid* ŠU SAG.ḪUL.ḪA.ZA GAM : ŠU ^{d}*Iš-tar* (DPS XXII:63 [AOAT 43.256])[50]

**If he rejoices and is terrified, "hand" of *mukīl rēš lemutti*; he will die (var. "hand" of Ištar).

ANTISOCIAL BEHAVIOR

16.76 ŠU.DINGIR.RA : DINGIR.MEŠ *i-nam-zar šil-lat i-qab-bi šá im-mar i-maḫ-ḫaṣ* (*BRM* 4.32:2)

**"Hand" of god (is when) he curses the gods, speaks blasphemy, (and) strikes whatever he sees.

SELF-MUTILATION

The range of harm that a patient may inflict on himself or herself is great, from something as minor as fingernail chewing, to damage to structures such as hands, fingers, and eyes that can severely reduce their function. This phenomenon can be triggered by mental stress, but the more extreme forms are usually seen in psychotic individuals. Patients with an inherited metabolic disease, Lesch-Nyhan syndrome, characteristically manifest self-mutilation (see Chapter 7).

16.77 [DIŠ NA *ma-a*] *m-ma* IGI-*ma* TÚG-*su it-ta-na-as-suk ú-rap-pad* IGI^{II}-*šú ú-ma-ḫa-aṣ* NA BI ḪUL DIB-*su* (DPS XXVII:19 [AOAT 43.298])

**[If a person] sees ⌜somebody⌝ and continually throws off his garment, he wanders about (and) strikes his eyes, a *gallû* afflicts that person.

16.78 DIŠ KI.MIN-*ma* ÚR-*šú ú-maḫ-ḫaṣ* ŠU^{II}-*šú ú-na-aš-šak* Á^{II}-*šú ana ku-tal-li-šú* GUR ŠU ^{d}MAŠ.T[AB.BA GAM] (DPS XV:56 [AOAT 43.154]; cf. DPS XIV A iii 1–2 = *TDP* 140 iii 35′–36′)

**If (it is the first day he is sick) and he strikes his crotch, chews on his hands,[51] (and) they have to put his arms behind him (to restrain him), "hand" of the ⌜twin gods⌝; [he will die].

16.79 DIŠ Á^{II}-*šú ú-na-aš-šak ina šag-gaš-ti* LÚ *ú-šaḫ-niq-ma ár-da-na-an* ÚŠ DIB-*su* (DPS X B r. 6 = *TDP* 88 r. 6)[52]

**If he chews on his arms, he had a person strangled to death and the "double" of the dead person afflicts him.

ADDICTION

It appears that alcohol was the primary form of substance abuse in ancient Mesopotamia. Beer was readily available at all levels of society, and wine was also known and used.

Marijuana (cannabis) may or may not have been used as a recreational drug but it was probably used as a medicine, and was called *azallû*. The medical diseases caused by alcohol addiction are discussed in Chapter 15. Available references do not indicate how the ancient physician or society dealt with addicted individuals.

16.80 DIŠ NA KAŠ.SAG NAG-*ma* SUḪUŠ.MEŠ-*šú pa-al-qa di-ig-la ma-a-ṭi ana* TI-*šú* . . . (*BAM* 575 iii 49)

**If a person drinks fine beer and then he is unsteady on his foundations (and) his eyesight is diminished, to cure him . . .

16.81 DIŠ NA KAŠ.SAG NAG-*ma* SAG.DU-*su* DIB.DIB-*su* INIM.MEŠ-*šú im-ta-na-áš-ši ina* DUG$_4$.DUG$_4$-*šú ú-pa-áš-šaṭ ṭè-en-šú la ṣa-bit* LÚ BI IGI^{II}-*šú* GUB-*za ana* TI-*šú* . . . (*BAM* 575 iii 51–52//*BAM* 59:21–24)

**If a person drinks fine beer and as a result his head continually afflicts him, he continually forgets his words and slurs them when speaking, he is not in full possession of his faculties, and that person's eyes stand still, to cure him . . .

16.82 DIŠ INIM-*šú* K[ÚR.KÚR-*i*]*r u* ⸢^{GIŠ}GEŠTIN⸣ APIN.MEŠ-*iš ana* U$_4$.DUG$_4$.GA-[*šu ana* U$_4$.10.KÁM . . .] (DPS VII B r. 14 = *TDP* 66:70′)[53]

**If his words are ⸢unintelligible⸣ and he continually asks for wine at regular intervals (and he has been sick) [for ten days . . .]

MOOD DISORDERS

An individual's mood represents his or her internal emotional state or affect in response to external conditions. When mood does not properly reflect the external factors, it can be due to a pathological mood disorder that is manifested by inappropriate depression or mania. Modern physicians define patients that vacillate between depression and mania as having bipolar disorder. More common are patients who alternate between periods of clinical depression and normal emotional response (unipolar depression). Patients with mania demonstrate expansiveness, flight of ideas, decreased sleep, heightened self-esteem, and grandiose ideas. Depressed patients have loss of interest and energy, loss of appetite, and thoughts of suicide. Symptoms compatible with manic and depressed states were described in ancient Mesopotamian texts.

DEPRESSED

16.83 NA$_4$.MEŠ DIŠ NA *gi-na-a a-dir* Ḫ[UL ŠÀ TUKU.TUKI-*ši*] KI NÍ-*šú i-ta-mu uš-tan-na-aḫ uš-tád-dar šib-sat* DINGIR *u* [^{d}15] UGU-*šú* GÁL.MEŠ . . . (*SpTU* 3.85 ii 2–4)[54]

**Stones for cases where a person is continually worried, [he is continually] ⸢sorrowful⸣, he talks to himself, he is continually exhausted and unhappy, god and [goddess] are angry at him . . .

16.84 DIŠ NA *ḫu-uṣ-ṣa* GAZ ŠÀ-*bi u* SAG.PA.KIL TUKU.MEŠ-*ši nu-ul-la-ti* ŠÀ-*šú i-ta-mu* . . . (*BAM* 316 iii 23′–24′; *KAR* 92 obv. 1–2)

**If a person continually has a crushing sensation in his chest and depression (and) his heart ponders untruths . . .

16.85 DIŠ INIM-*šú* KÚR.KÚR-[*ir*] *u a-šu-uš-tum* ⸢ŠUB⸣.ŠUB-*su ana* U$_4$.DUG$_4$.GA-⸢*šú ana*⸣ U$_4$.3.K[ÁM . . .] / DIŠ INIM-*šú* KÚR.KÚR-[*i*] *r u* ÍR.MEŠ [*ana*] U$_4$.DUG$_4$.GA-*šú ana* U$_4$.3.[KÁM . . .] (DPS VII B r. 8–9 = *TDP* 66:64′–65′)

**If his words are unintelligible and depression keeps falling on him at regular intervals (and he has been sick) for three days, [. . .] If a person's words are unintelligible and he continually weeps at regular intervals (and he has been sick) for three days, [. . .]

16.86 Ú SAG.PA.KIL . . . (*BAM* 1 i 59)[55]

**Plant for depression . . .

MANIC

16.87 DIŠ NA DIMMA.KÚR.RA DIB-*su-*[*m*]*a ṭè-en-šú iš-t*[*a-nu*] *a-ma-tu-šú* KÚR.KÚR-*ra ṭé-em-šú* ŠUB.ŠUB-*su u ma-gal* DUG$_4$.DUG$_4$-*ub a-na ṭè-me-šú tur-r*[*i*]-*šú* . . . (*BAM* 202 obv. 1-3//*STT* 286 ii 14–16)

**If derangement seizes a person [so] that his mentation ⸢alters⸣, his words are unintelligible, his thinking continually fails him, and he continually talks a lot, to restore his mind to him . . .

16.88 DIŠ *i-te-ner-ru-ub* TÚG-*su* ŠUB.ŠUB-*di iš-ta-na-su ma-gal* DU[G$_4$.DUG$_4$-*ub*] NINDA *u* KAŠ NU GUR-*ma* KÚ *u la i-ṣal-lal* ŠU ^{d}15 GAR ⸢TI⸣ (DPS XXVI:78′–79′ [AOAT 43.285])

**If he keeps beginning to put on and throwing off his garments, he continually cries out(!), he ⸢talks⸣ a lot, bread and beer do not come back up on him so that he can eat but he cannot sleep, "hand" of Ištar is laid (on him); he will get well.

PSYCHOTIC STATES

In modern times, schizophrenia is a relatively common problem, affecting about one percent of the population. It usually begins before the age of twenty-five, and it persists throughout life. Its clinical presentation can be quite varied, but common aspects are a marked social withdrawal and absence of goal-directed behavior. Auditory or visual hallucinations are often present. Schizophrenics frequently have peculiar behavior, abnormal affect, unusual speech, bizarre ideas, and strange perceptual experiences. They may be talkative or mute, and may have reduced emotions or overactivity with extreme rage, happiness, or anxiety.

The texts below have some features that are compatible with schizophrenia including auditory or visual hallucinations, bizarre ideas, and personality changes, but there is insufficient information to meet the modern criteria for this disease. The first reference might also be describing a person with depressive psychosis.

16.89 D[IŠ G]IN$_7$ AN.ÚSAN DIB-*tu* DIB-*su-ma* U$_4$-*ma* DIB-*šú ik-kil-lu* GÙ.DÉ-*šú-ma u šu-ú e-t*[*a*]-*nap-pal* [A]D-*ya* AMA *lu* ŠEŠ.MEŠ-*ya* NIN.MEŠ-*ya* ÚŠ.MEŠ [*ina* N]U ZU!-*e ma-am-ma* GÙ.GÙ-*si ik-ta-na-la* (*ḫé-pí*) EGIR ÍR-*ú i-ṣal-lal-ma* NU ZI-*bé* U$_4$ DIB-*su um-taš-š*[*e-r*]*u-šu* GIN$_7$ ÍR NU ZU A.RI.A ^{d}*Šul-pa-è-*<*a*> NU ZI (*STT* 89:180–186)

**⸢If⸣ his affliction afflicts him in the evening and when it afflicts him, a mournful cry roars to him and he continually answers it, he continually cries out <without> ceasing: "My ⸢father⸣ (and) mother or my brothers and my sisters will die" [without] recognizing anybody, [he continually wails][56] (and) when he has wailed he goes to sleep and does not get up[57] (and) when his affliction has left him, he does not know what he wailed, intractable "spawn" of Šulpaea.

16.90 DIŠ UB.NÍGIN.NA-*šú* GIN$_7$ *šá bal-ṭi ne-ḫa* IGI^{II}-*šú* BAD.MEŠ-*ma* U$_4$ DIB-*su ina-ṭal* KI-*šú* DUG$_4$.DUG$_4$-*ub u* NÍ-*šú ut-ta-na-kar* ŠU LÍL.LÁ.EN.NA DUMU *šip-ri šá* DINGIR-*šú* (DPS XXVI:73′–74′ [AOAT 43.284])

**If his limbs are as still as those of a healthy person, (and) he continually opens his eyes and, when he sees the one who afflicts him, he talks with him and continually changes himself, "hand" of *lilû*, messenger of his god.

DISSOCIATIVE STATE

Patients who manifest a sudden transient alteration in the normally integrated functions of consciousness, motor behavior, and identity are said to have a dissociative state. Varieties of this condition include multiple personality disorder, psychogenic amnesia, psychogenic fugue, and depersonalization disorder.

The references which follow indicate that the patient had a change of self or confusion of self, suggesting a dissociative state. The second text also describes signs and symptoms compatible with an infectious disease. The stress of a systemic disease may help to trigger a dissociative state, which presumably is the case here.

16.91 DIŠ LÚ *i-na na-ap-lu-sí-šu i-na-šu it-ta-na-za-az-za di-li-iḫ ra-ma-ni-šu na-di-i-šu* (Köcher and Oppenheim, *AfO* 18.65 ii 18–19 [physiognomic omens])

**If a person's eyes continually stand still while he is looking, a confusion of self has come down over him.

16.92 DIŠ U$_4$ DIB-*šú* ŠÀ-*bi* ŠÀ-*bi* GÙ.GÙ-*si* IGI^{II}-*šú* BAD-*te u* DUL-*am* KÚM *li-ʾ-ba i-šu* SAG KIR$_4$-*šú ú-lap-pat ap-pat* ŠU.SI.MEŠ ŠU^{II}-*šú u* GÌR^{II}-*šú ka-ṣa-a* GIG DIB-*šú ina-ṭal* KI-*šú* DUG$_4$.DUG$_4$-*ub u* NÍ-*šú ut-ta-na-kar* ŠU LÍL.LÁ.EN.NA *la-ʾ-bi* (DPS XXVI:66′–68′ [AOAT 43.284])

**If when it afflicts him, he continually cries out: "My insides, my insides!" he opens and shuts his eyes, he has *liʾbu* fever (see Chapter 3), he rubs the bulb of his nose, the tips of his fingers and toes are cold, he can see the illness that afflicts him, he talks with it and continually changes him self, infectious "hand" of *lilû*.

PARANOIA

Paranoia is a delusional disorder that lacks symptoms of major mood disorder and the bizarre quality of delusions seen in schizophrenia. As a delusion, it does not have an identifiable basis in reality. Patients often seem suspicious, eccentric, or hostile. They may believe that they are being followed, poisoned, or harmed in some physical or social manner. The delusion may involve feelings of jealousy or persecution.

The quotes below appear to be from patients with paranoid delusions. The last reference is both the most interesting and the most uncertain. One has the feeling that the adversities listed are not real. However, if they are, then paranoia would not be an appropriate diagnosis.[58]

16.93 DIŠ NA *nu-ul-la-ti* ŠÀ-*šú i-ta-mu at-mu-šú i-šá-an-ni za-mar ṣa-lil za-mar e-er u* UŠ$_4$-*šú* NU DIB-*al* DIB-*ti* DINGIR-*šú* UGU-*šú* GÁL-*ši* . . . (*BAM* 316 vi 4′–6′//*STT* 95 ii 84–86)

**If a person's heart ponders untruths, he repeats his words, he is now sleeping, now awake, and he cannot make up his mind (to do anything), the anger of his god is upon him . . .

16.94 DIŠ NA ŠÀ-*šú nu-ul-la-ti i-ta-mu* . . . (*BAM* 316 iii 20′//*BAM* 317 r. 31)

**If a person's heart ponders untruths . . .

16.95 DIŠ NA *gi-na-a šu-dur ur-ra u* GI$_6$ *ina-ziq* ZI.GA *sa-dir-šú iš-di-iḫ-šú* KUD-*is kar-ṣi-šú* KÚ.MEŠ *da-bi-ib* KI-*šú kit-te* NU DUG$_4$.DUG$_4$-*ub* ŠU.SI ḪUL-*tim* EGIR-*šú* LAL-*ṣi ina* É.GAL GUB-*zu la maḫ-ra-šú* MÁŠ.GI$_6$.MEŠ-*šú par-da ina* MÁŠ.GI$_6$-*šú* ÚŠ.MEŠ IGI.IGI-*mar* GAZ ŠÀ GAR-*šú šib-sat* DINGIR *u* ^{d}EŠ$_4$.DAR UGU-*šú* GÁL-*a* DINGIR-*šú u* ^{d}EŠ$_4$.DAR-*šú* KI-*šú ze-nu-u* (*kiš-pi ep-šú-šú* KI DINGIR *u* ^{d}EŠ$_4$.DAR *šu-zu-ur* ÁŠ.MEŠ-*šú dal-ḫa* DINGIR MAN IDIM NUN *šu-zu-qú-šú*) KI ^{LÚ}ḪAL *u da-gi-li*/LÚ.DINGIR.RA *u* ENSI *di-in-šú* EN 7-*šú* NU SI.SÁ *qá-bu-u* NU *še-mu-ú* GAR-*nu-šú* . . . (*BAM* 316 ii 5′–13′//BM 64174: 1–6//*STT* 95:130–137; cf. *BAM* 315 iii 1–8; BM 64174:15–16)

**If a person is continually made sad, he is upset day and night, he is having serious financial losses and making no profit, people slander him, the person who talks with him does not tell him the truth, people say bad things about him behind his back; they will not see him in the palace where he stands, his dreams are troubled, in his dream he continually sees dead persons, a crushing sensation in his chest is established for him . . . (god and goddess are angry with him, sorcery has been performed against him, he has been cursed before god and goddess), his desires are confused, god, king, patron, and prince cause him grief, he cannot get an answer to his problems out of diviner or seer (var. ecstatic or dream interpreter) even after seven (attempts), nobody listens to him . . .

Summary

Ancient Mesopotamian physicians recognized and documented abnormal behaviors and actions, and these abnormalities were often recognized as mentally based. They showed the same concern and attention to these problems as they did to physical illnesses. It is not always clear, however, where they drew the line between mental and physical conditions. Even modern physicians wrestle with this issue. Many illnesses previously categorized as mental problems have later been found to have a physical basis.

CHAPTER 17

Pediatrics

If a mother gives birth to a powerless (child).

—Šumma Izbu I 56

The birth process and the early years of life are subject to many risks of morbidity and mortality in the current era, and those risks were even greater in ancient Mesopotamia. Inherited diseases often become evident early in life, and the immature immune system of children places them at greater risk for infectious diseases. The *āšipu* reserved a tablet of the diagnostic/prognostic series exclusively for diseases of infants and small children (^{LÚ}TUR/*šerru*). A section of the omen series Šumma Izbu also discussed malformations in newborns and their ominous significance. This chapter will cover only those conditions that are unique to childhood diseases; those that have signs, symptoms, and outcomes similar to adult diseases will be included in the relevant sections of other chapters.

Birth

DIFFICULT BIRTHS

17.1 BE MUNUS Ù.TU-*ma uš-tap-ši-iq* . . . (Šumma Izbu IV 45 [Leichty, *Izbu* 70])

**If a woman is too narrow to give birth . . .

Difficult births are caused by many factors, some of which have been discussed in the obstetrics and gynecology chapter (Chapter 12). Some problems specifically relating to the fetus are covered in this chapter.

STILLBIRTHS: THE KŪBU-DEMON

The Kūbu-demon[1] was a ghoulish nuisance whose malevolence was particularly directed at newborn babies (see Chapter 19 with 19.335–19.342) for the simple reason that Kūbu was the demonic manifestation of stillborn children, as may be seen from the following references.[2]

17.2 **Kūbu who was not buried in a grave . . .[3]

17.3 **Like Kūbu, never able to suck his mother's milk . . .[4]

17.4 **The Kūbu of *nadītu, qadištu, kulmašītu,* and *ištarītu* of Anu (holy women whose duties included supervising childbirth); the little ones who do not know their own names (and) who never saw the sun . . .[5]

"Seeing the light of the sun" is a typical metaphor for live birth.[6] Kūbu is presumably described as "not buried in a grave" because, as in early twentieth-century C.E. Iraq,[7] stillbirths were not buried in the cemetery with the adults, but under the threshold of the house or by the door of the mother's room. Like the *lilû* family of demons (see Chapter 12), Kūbu's personality profile falls into a pattern whereby the victim of demonic attack is confronted by the unattractive possessor of unfulfilled desires.[8]

PREMATURE DELIVERIES

Premature deliveries are described in medical and omen texts with the terse "she will not bring her fetus to term," reflecting the fact that this is a problem that is associated with very real fetal risk.

17.5 DIŠ TU *ip-ta-na-ar-ru ul ú-šal-lam* (DPS XXXVI A 81 = *TDP* 208:81)

**If a pregnant woman continually vomits, she will not bring (her fetus) to term.

17.6 *li-ʾ-bu ina* KUR *ú-la-ʾ-ib* MUNUS.PEŠ$_4$.MEŠ *šá* ŠÀ-*ši-na* NU SILIM.MEŠ (Rochberg-Halton, *AfO* Beih. 22.243:4)

**Infections will infect people in the land; pregnant women will not bring their fetuses to term.

With regard to the second quote above, many infections appear capable of inducing premature delivery, but cholera and brucellosis are well documented as having this effect.

POST MATURE DELIVERIES

The *āšipu* considered a normal pregnancy to last 10 months rather than 9 months as in the modern era. This is due to the practice of reckoning time using lunar months, measured from new moon to new moon and lasting for an average of 28 days. In both eras, the usual gestation period was 40 weeks. In the text below, periods of 11 and 12 lunar months are marked as abnormal. Since this is an omen text, there is little to suggest the medical significance of this abnormality. Delayed deliveries, however, carry some risk to the fetus, since fetal wasting and other signs of placental insufficiency may be present.

17.7 [BE] MUNUS *lu* ITI.11.KAM *lu* 12.KAM *ú-bi-il-ma* Ù.TU-*ma* [...] (Šumma Izbu IV 46 [Leichty, *Izbu* 70])

**[If] a woman carries (the child) for eleven or twelve months and gives birth and [...]

FOOTLING BIRTHS

The position of the fetus when it passes through the birth canal has a very significant effect on the degree of difficulty in delivering the fetus. Normally the fetus exits head first. When the fetus comes out feet first the delivery is more difficult, and injury to the fetus (especially the brain) is more likely. The examples below mention this problem in twin births.[9]

17.8 BE MUNUS 2 NITA.MEŠ *še-pa-nu-šu-nu* Ù.TU ... (Šumma Izbu I 85 [Leichty, *Izbu* 39])

**If a woman gives birth to two boys feet first...

17.9 BE MUNUS 2 MUNUS.MEŠ *še-pa-nu-ši-na* Ù.TU ... (Šumma Izbu I 103 [Leichty, *Izbu* 42])

**If a woman gives birth to two girls feet first...

MULTIPLE FETUSES

The joy that can be associated with pregnancy and procreation should increase when the pregnant woman carries more than one fetus. Unfortunately, however, this is tempered by the realization that both the mother and the fetus are at greater risk of illness and death, and the risk increases as the number of fetuses increases. Much of the risk to the fetus is due to premature delivery and low birth weight. The texts that follow are omen texts that utilize the number, sex, and survival of the fetuses for predicting the future.

TWINS (MAŠ.TAB.BA/*MAŠTÛ*)

17.10 BE MUNUS 2 NITA.MEŠ Ù.TU ... (Šumma Izbu I 83 [Leichty, *Izbu* 39])[10]

**If a woman gives birth to two boys...

17.11 BE MUNUS 2 Ù.TU-*ma* 1 NITA 1 MUNUS ... (Šumma Izbu I 86 [Leichty, *Izbu* 39])[11]

**If a woman gives birth to two (children) and one is a boy, one a girl...

17.12 BE MUNUS 2 MUNUS.MEŠ Ù.TU ... (Šumma Izbu I 100 [Leichty, *Izbu* 42])[12]

**If a woman gives birth to two girls...

Pangas[13] points out that the following reference reflects a recognition that certain women have a special predisposition to multiple pregnancies.[14]

17.13 BE MUNUS MAŠ.TAB.BA *uš-ta-aš-ni-ma* Ù.TU . . . (Šumma Izbu I 90 [Leichty, *Izbu* 40])

**If a woman gives birth to a second set of twins . . .

TRIPLETS (*TAKŠÛ*)[15]

17.14 BE MUNUS 3 MUNUS.MEŠ *šu-ta-ḫa-a-ti* Ù.TU . . . (Šumma Izbu I 101 [Leichty, *Izbu* 42])[16]

**If a woman gives birth to three identical girls . . .

17.15 BE MUNUS 3 NITA.MEŠ Ù.TU . . . (Šumma Izbu I 104 [Leichty, *Izbu* 42])

**If a woman gives birth to three boys . . .

17.16 BE MUNUS 3 Ù.TU-*ma* 2 MUNUS.MEŠ 1 NITA . . . (Šumma Izbu I 109 [Leichty, *Izbu* 42])[17]

**If a woman gives birth to three (children) and two are girls, one a boy . . .

QUADRUPLETS

17.17 BE MUNUS 4 NITA.MEŠ Ù.TU . . . (Šumma Izbu I 105, 116 [Leichty, *Izbu* 42,43])[18]

**If a woman gives birth to four boys . . .

17.18 BE MUNUS 4 Ù.TU-*ma* 2 NITA.MEŠ 2 MUNUS.MEŠ . . . (Šumma Izbu I 119 [Leichty, *Izbu* 43])

**If a woman gives birth to four (children) and two are boys, two girls . . .

QUINTUPLETS

17.19 BE MUNUS 5 NITA.MEŠ Ù.[TU] . . . (Šumma Izbu I 106 [Leichty, *Izbu* 42])[19]

**If a woman ⌜gives birth⌝ to five boys . . .

17.20 BE MUNUS 5 Ù.TU-*ma* 3 NITA.MEŠ 2 MUNUS.MEŠ . . . (Šumma Izbu I 125 [Leichty, *Izbu* 44])[20]

**If a woman gives birth to five (children) and three are boys, two girls . . .

In the texts below that mention quadruplets, some references state that the infants live and others that they die. It is curious that, in the texts where the infants die, the omens are more favorable than in those where they live. We believe that this is due to the tendency in ancient Mesopotamian omen texts for more typical events to be regarded as favorable and uncommon events as unfavorable. If this interpretation is correct, then they must have witnessed quadruple pregnancies and learned that the infants usually died.

17.21 BE MUNUS 4 NITA.MEŠ/MUNUS.MEŠ Ù.TU-*ma* TI.MEŠ . . . (Šumma Izbu I 117, 121 [Leichty, *Izbu* 43])

**If a woman gives birth to four boys/girls and they live . . .

17.22 BE MUNUS 4 NITA.MEŠ/MUNUS.MEŠ Ù.TU-*ma* ÚŠ.MEŠ . . . (Šumma Izbu I 118, 122 [Leichty, *Izbu* 43])

**If a woman gives birth to four boys/girls and they die . . .

Since omens were believed to be the language of the gods by means of which mankind was given fair warning of impending difficulties, there was an obvious interest in filling out apparent gaps in the record by speculating as to the potential meaning of ominous events that had not actually occurred. The listing of multiple fetuses as high as nine suggests that the following references are to such theoretical possibilities rather than to observed events.

17.23 BE MUNUS 5 *ú-lu* 6 NITA.MEŠ/MUNUS.MEŠ Ù.TU . . . (Šumma Izbu I 127–128 [Leichty, *Izbu* 44])[21]

**If a woman gives birth to five or six boys/girls . . .

17.24 BE MUNUS 6 Ù.TU . . . (Šumma Izbu I 129 [Leichty, *Izbu* 44])

**If a woman gives birth to six (children) . . .

17.25 BE MUNUS 7 Ù.TU . . . (Šumma Izbu I 130 [Leichty, *Izbu* 44])

**If a woman gives birth to seven (children) . . .

17.26 BE MUNUS 8 *ú-lu* 9 Ù.TU . . . (Šumma Izbu I 131 [Leichty, *Izbu* 44])

**If a woman gives birth to eight or nine (children) . . .

HYDATIDIFORM MOLE

This intrauterine mass may be delivered like a fetus, but it is only a portion of the fertilized ovum with no recognizable organs or human morphology. It consists of many small cystic structures that resemble bunches of grapes or fish roe. The following text clearly describes this anomaly.

17.27 BE MUNUS *bi-nu-ut* KU_6 Ù.TU . . . (Šumma Izbu I 22 [Leichty, *Izbu* 33])

**If a woman gives birth to (what looks like) fish roe . . .

OTHER ABNORMAL FETAL TISSUES

There are other abnormal structures that can form from the fertilized ovum that fail to develop a recognizable fetal configuration, and have no chance for survival outside the uterus. When this occurred in ancient Mesopotamia, it must have been an awesome and frightening event. The last reference below describes a recognized fetal anomaly caused by abnormal twin development.

17.28 BE MUNUS *mu-ut-ta-at* NAM.LÚ.U_{18}.LU Ù.TU . . . (Šumma Izbu I 76 [Leichty, *Izbu* 38])

**If a woman gives birth to a half human (child) . . .

17.29 BE MUNUS *bi-ni-it* NITA/MUNUS Ù.TU . . . (Šumma Izbu I 58–59 [Leichty, *Izbu* 37])

**If a woman gives birth to a male/female creature . . .

17.30 BE MUNUS *iz-ba-am* Ù.TU*-ma ina* ŠÀ*-šú iz-bu* MAN*-ma* GAR . . . (Šumma Izbu I 48 [Leichty, *Izbu* 35])[22]

**If a woman gives birth to a malformed fetus and there is another malformed fetus inside it . . .

Ancient texts describe a wide variety of material delivered from a woman's uterus, including "(what looks like) a head",[23] a hand,[24] a foot,[25] the likeness of a tortoise,[26] a gecko,[27] a goat horn,[28] matted hair,[29] clay,[30] and a membrane of flesh full of blood.[31]

Birth Defects

Congenital abnormalities are relatively common in the current era.[32] In live births one to five percent have some type of genetic or acquired abnormality, and the incidence is even higher in stillbirths. Data collected in the United States from 1970 to 1987 by the Centers for Disease Control identify the types and frequency of abnormalities. They are expressed below as prevalence per 10,000 live and stillbirths.[33]

Cardiovascular 35.9
Musculoskeletal 30.3
Central Nervous System 19.0
Orofacial (includes cleft lip and palate) 14.3
Gastrointestinal (includes intestinal atresia and imperforate anus) 5.2
Eye 1.9
Respiratory 1.7
Genitourinary 1.6

The references from ancient Mesopotamia mention all of the above categories except cardiovascular and respiratory abnormalities.[34] There are only equivocal references to these latter birth defects, which would have been difficult to identify without modern diagnostic technologies.

Most of the information on congenital abnormalities in ancient Mesopotamia comes from an omen series known as Šumma Izbu ("If a malformed fetus"), which contains much valuable information but is less reliable than either the diagnostic/prognostic handbook or the therapeutic texts. The diviner (*barû*), for whose use Šumma Izbu was intended, seems to have wanted to be prepared to state the prognostic significance of any malformed fetus that might conceivably be shown to him. Many (perhaps most)[35] of the references in Šumma Izbu are quite consistent with common birth defects. However, some seem to represent logical (if improbable) extensions of observed anomalies (such as conjoined twins with sirenomelia; see below), and a few are almost certainly legendary (see Tall Tales below).

SKIN

Many congenital skin abnormalities are apparent at birth. Below are references to skin lesions noted at birth, some of which are likely to be lesions commonly seen today. Other congenital and acquired skin lesions are described in Chapter 10.[36] In the following references, the verb translated "disfigured" *(nakāru)* literally means "to change for the worse." It is not clear whether this is meant to convey the presence of one or only a few spots or, alternatively, a diffuse and abnormal coloration of the skin.

RED SKIN

17.31 [BE MUNUS] Ù.TU-*ma* MIN-*ma* SA_5 *na-kìr*... (Šumma Izbu IV 15 [Leichty, *Izbu* 67])

**[If a woman] gives birth and (from the beginning the newborn) is disfigured with red ...

If *nakāru* refers to spots, the text above is likely to be describing port-wine hemangiomas or cavernous hemangiomas. Port-wine hemangiomas are flat areas of skin that are red to purple in color. They are often on the individual's face, and can be highly unsightly. These lesions persist throughout life. Cavernous hemangiomas are red elevated lesions that often disappear toward the end of childhood.

Alternatively, if *nakāru* means a diffusely red child, this could be due to one of a number of infections that can produce rashes in newborns. These include herpes simplex, enteroviruses, and bacterial sepsis.

WHITE SKIN

17.32 [BE MUNUS] Ù.TU-*ma* MIN-*ma* BABBAR *na-kìr*... (Šumma Izbu IV 14 [Leichty, *Izbu* 67])

**[If a woman] gives birth and (from the beginning) it is disfigured with white ...

If *nakāru* refers to spots, white spots (leukoderma) can be caused by both congenital defects and a variety of acquired conditions. The white color is due to the absence of melanin pigmentation. On the other hand if *nakāru* means a diffusely white or pale child, then the cause is likely to be anemia.

BLACK (DARK) SKIN

17.33 [BE MUNUS] Ù.TU-*ma* MIN-*ma* GI_6 KÚR... (Šumma Izbu IV 13 [Leichty, *Izbu* 67])

**[If a woman] gives birth and (from the beginning) it is disfigured with black...

If *nakāru* refers to a single black spot, this is most likely to be describing a congenital nevus that can be of any size. Conversely, if diffuse coloration of the skin was intended, the cause is less certain. It is unlikely that a naturally dark-skinned child would be described in this manner. It seems more reasonable that Cadelli[37] is correct in suggesting that cyanosis due to congenital heart disease is causing the dark skin color.

ALBINO There are inherited defects in the production of melanin, the substance that gives skin pigmentation. It is likely that the following quote is describing such a case. Another possible explanation would be severe anemia in a fair-skinned infant, although that condition may have been described as "disfigured with white" (see above).

17.34 [BE MUNUS] Ù.TU-*ma* MIN-*ma* GIN_7 ^{NA_4}GIŠ.NU_{11}.GAL BABBAR . . . (Šumma Izbu IV 12 [Leichty, *Izbu* 67])

**[If a woman] gives birth and (from the beginning the child) is as white as alabaster . . .

In albinism, the absence of pigment affects not only the skin, but also the iris whose pigmentation is lost, resulting in a red-colored iris. A red iris is mentioned alongside a "shining" (blue), a "dark red" (brown), or a "yellow" (green) iris in physiognomic omens.[38]

NEUROFIBROMATOSIS (VON RECKLINGHAUSEN'S DISEASE) Patients with neurofibromatosis may have a variety of flat, pigmented, and at times elevated and grossly distorted masses. The references below are possibly examples of this disease, although the skin lesions at birth may be minimal only to grow larger throughout life. Other skin lesions such as nevuses and warts caused by the papilloma virus could also be responsible for these abnormalities.[39]

17.35 BE MUNUS *šu-la-nam* Ù.TU . . . (Šumma Izbu I 64 [Leichty, *Izbu* 37])

**If a woman gives birth to a warty (child) . . .

17.36 BE MUNUS Ù.TU-*ma* MIN-*ma ep-qá ma-li* . . . (Šumma Izbu IV 4 [Leichty, *Izbu* 66])

**If a woman gives birth and (from the beginning the child) is full of *epqu* (patches of thickened skin) . . .

17.37 BE MUNUS Ù.TU-*ma* MIN-*ma a-bu-sa-at* UZU *ma-šid* . . . (Šumma Izbu IV 16 [Leichty, *Izbu* 67])

**If a woman gives birth and (from the beginning the child) has a lump in the form of a forelock of flesh . . .

17.38 BE MUNUS Ù.TU-*ma* MIN-*ma ṭup-pa šá* UZU *ma-šid* . . . (Šumma Izbu IV 17 [Leichty, *Izbu* 68])[40]

**If a woman gives birth and (from the beginning the child) has a lump in the form of a "tablet" of flesh . . .

17.39 [BE MUNUS] Ù.TU-*ma* MIN-*ma ma-aš-tam šá* UZU *ma-ši-id* . . . (Šumma Izbu IV 19 [Leichty, *Izbu* 68])[41]

**[If a woman] gives birth and (from the beginning the child) has a lump in the form of a staff of flesh . . .

Patients with neurofibromatosis often have neurologic problems in addition to the skin lesions. Nerve trunk tumors form to cause pain and impaired sensory and motor function. Tumors also may grow within the spinal cord and brain to cause focal neurologic abnormalities, mental deficiency, and seizures, as in the following reference.

17.40 BE MUNUS Ù.TU-*ma ina* UGU SAG.DU-*šú* UZU GIN$_7$ *ku-ub-ši* GAR-*ma* SUḪUŠ-*su ḫa-niq u im-ta-na-qut* IGI-*šú šá* 15 *ub-bu-ṭa-at* ŠU-*su u* GÌR-*šú šá* 15 *a-ka-at u* ZÚ.MEŠ-*šú* È.MEŠ . . . (Šumma Izbu II 19 [Leichty, *Izbu* 47])

**If a woman gives birth and there is a piece of flesh set on top of (the child)'s head like a turban and its base is constricted and (the child) continually falls down, his left eye is blind,[42] his left hand and foot are weak and his teeth have erupted . . .[43]

GRAY HAIR

Graying of hair in childhood is associated with many diseases including ataxia telangiectasia, cri du chat syndrome, hyperthyroidism, progeria, and Werner's disease. Some infants have white patches of hair from birth, such as patients with Waardenburg's disease. There is no way to know what underlying disease has caused the graying in the following patient.

17.41 BE MUNUS Ù.TU-*ma ul-la-nu-um-ma* SAG.DU-*su ši-pa-a-ti* DIRI . . . (Šumma Izbu IV 1 [Leichty, *Izbu* 66])[44]

**If a woman gives birth and from the beginning (the child)'s head is full of gray hair . . .

EYES[45]

CONGENITAL BLINDNESS

17.42 BE MUNUS IGI.NU.TUKU Ù.TU . . . (Šumma Izbu I 60 [Leichty, *Izbu* 37])[46]

**If a woman gives birth to a blind (child) . . .

CYCLOPIA An uncommon but awesome anomaly is the birth of a child with a single eye centrally placed on the forehead. This is associated with severe brain defects, and most fetuses with this defect are stillborn. This fetal anomaly was probably the source of the Cyclops in Greek legend including the one encountered by Odysseus in Homer's *Odyssey*. The quotes below are examples of this anomaly from ancient Mesopotamian sources.

17.43 BE MUNUS Ù.TU-*ma* IGI-*šú* 1-*at-ma u* GAL . . . (Šumma Izbu II 49 [Leichty, *Izbu* 50])

**If a woman gives birth and (the child) has only one eye and it is large . . .

17.44 BE MUNUS Ù.TU-*ma* IGI-*šú* 1-*at-ma ina* SAG.KI-*šú* GAR-*at* . . . (Šumma Izbu II 50 [Leichty, *Izbu* 50])[47]

**If a woman gives birth and (the child) has only one eye and it is placed on its forehead . . .

MICROPHTHALMIA Some infants are born with abnormally small eyes.[48]

17.45 BE *iz-bu* IGI.MEŠ-*šú ṣa-aḫ-ra-a* . . . (Šumma Izbu X 36 [Leichty, *Izbu* 124])

**If a malformed fetus's eyes are (too) small . . .

OTHER EYE MALFORMATIONS

17.46 BE MUNUS Ù.TU-*ma* IGI 15-*šú* GAL IGI 150-*šú* TUR . . . (Šumma Izbu II 46 [Leichty, *Izbu* 50])

**If a woman gives birth and (the child)'s left eye is big (and) its right eye is small . . .

17.47 [BE MUNUS Ù.TU]-*ma* IGI 15-*šú* NU GÁL . . . (Šumma Izbu II 47 [Leichty, *Izbu* 50])

**[If a woman gives birth] and (the child) does not have a left eye . . .

17.48 BE MUNUS Ù.TU-*ma* IGI.MEŠ-*šú* NU GÁL.MEŠ . . . (Šumma Izbu II 48 [Leichty, *Izbu* 50])[49]

**If a woman gives birth and (the child) does not have eyes . . .

17.49 [BE MUNUS] Ù.TU-*ma* 2 IGI.MEŠ-*šú ina* SAG.KI-*šú* GAR.MEŠ . . . (Šumma Izbu II 52 [Leichty, *Izbu* 50])[50]

**[If a woman] gives birth and (the child)'s two eyes are placed on its forehead . . .

17.50 BE MUNUS Ù.TU-*ma* IGI^{II}-*šú* GIN_7 SIG_4 BÀD . . . (Šumma Izbu II 65 [Leichty, *Izbu* 52])[51]

**If a woman gives birth and (the child)'s eyes are like the bricks of a wall (i.e., two bumps) . . .

EARS

CONGENITAL DEAFNESS

17.51 BE MUNUS GEŠTU.LAL Ù.TU . . . (Šumma Izbu I 63 [Leichty, *Izbu* 37])[52]

**If a woman gives birth to a deaf (child) . . .

CONGENITAL MALFORMATION Ear abnormalities that are apparent at birth include hypoplastic ears (small ears: microtia) that are in abnormal (ectopic) locations, and large external ears (jug-ears). These anomalies are described in the following references.

Microtia

17.52 BE MUNUS Ù.TU-*ma* GEŠTU 15/150-*šú* TUR . . . (Šumma Izbu III 5–6 [Leichty, *Izbu* 54])

**If a woman gives birth and (the child)'s left/right ear is (abnormally) small . . .

17.53 BE MUNUS Ù.TU-*ma* $GEŠTU^{II}$-*šú* TUR.MEŠ . . . (Šumma Izbu III 7 [Leichty, *Izbu* 54])

**If a woman gives birth and (the child)'s ears are (abnormally) small . . .

Ectopic locations

17.54 BE MUNUS Ù.TU-*ma* GEŠTU 15/150-*šú ina* TE-*šú ṭe₄-ḫa-a-at* . . . (Šumma Izbu III 11–12 [Leichty, *Izbu* 54])[53]

**If a woman gives birth and (the child)'s left/right ear is near its cheek . . .

Jug-ears

17.55 BE MUNUS Ù.TU-*ma* GEŠTU UR.MAḪ GAR . . . (Šumma Izbu III 1 [Leichty, *Izbu* 53])

**If a woman gives birth and (the child) has the ear of a lion . . .

Other ear abnormalities

17.56 BE MUNUS Ù.TU-*ma* GEŠTU 15/150-*šú* NU GÁL . . . BE MUNUS Ù.TU-*ma* GEŠTU^{II}-*šú* NU GÁL.MEŠ . . . (Šumma Izbu III 2–4 [Leichty, *Izbu* 53])[54]

**If a woman gives birth and (the child) does not have a left/right ear . . . If a woman gives birth and (the child) does not have ears . . .

17.57 BE MUNUS Ù.TU-*ma* 2 GEŠTU.MEŠ-*šú ina* ZAG/GÙB GAR.MEŠ-*ma šá* GÙB/ZAG NU GÁL . . . (Šumma Izbu III 18–19 [Leichty, *Izbu* 55])

**If a woman gives birth and (the child) has two ears on the left/right but none on the right/left . . .

17.58 BE MUNUS Ù.TU-*ma* GEŠTU 15/150-*šú uq-qá-at* . . . (Šumma Izbu III 14–15 [Leichty, *Izbu* 54–55])[55]

**If a woman gives birth and (the child)'s left/right ear is withered . . .

17.59 BE MUNUS Ù.TU-*ma* MIN-*ma* GEŠTU-*šú šá* 15/150 BA.RA.BÙRU-*at* . . . BE MUNUS Ù.TU-*ma* MIN-*ma* GEŠTU^{II}-*šú ki-lat-tan* BA.RA.BÙRU.MEŠ . . . (Šumma Izbu IV 36–38 [Leichty, *Izbu* 69–70])

**If a woman gives birth and (from the beginning the child)'s left/right ear is imperforate (no opening) . . . If a woman gives birth and (from the beginning) both ears are imperforate . . .

NOSE

CONGENITAL MALFORMATION

17.60 BE MUNUS Ù.TU-*ma* KIR₄ *u na-ḫi-ri* NU GÁL . . . (Šumma Izbu III 29 [Leichty, *Izbu* 56])[56]

**If a woman gives birth and (the child) does not have a nose or nostrils . . .

17.61 BE MUNUS Ù.TU-*ma na-ḫi-ir* 15/150-*šú* NU GÁL . . . (Šumma Izbu III 30-31 [Leichty, *Izbu* 29])[57]

**If a woman gives birth and (the child) does not have a left/right nostril . . .

17.62 DIŠ LÚ.TUR KIR$_4$-[*šú ki-ma i-ṭi-im ṣa-li-im*] . . . (Šumma Izbu IV 64′ [Leichty, *Izbu* 72])[58]

**If the infant'[s] nose [is as black as pitch] . . .

The last reference above is probably describing a pigmented congenital nevus located on the nose.

MOUTH AND LIPS

HARE-LIP (CLEFT LIP AND PALATE)[59]

17.63 DIŠ TU I[GI]^{II}-*šá* BAL.BAL.MEŠ *ar-na-ab-ba* ÍL *šà*-ŠÀ-*šà* GAM (DPS XXXVI A 89 = *TDP* 208:89)

**If a pregnant woman continually rolls her ⌜eyes⌝ (and) she carries a hare, her fetus will die.

In the reference above, the statement that the pregnant woman "carries a hare" probably means that the child has a hare-lip deformity.[60] Without surgery, children with hare-lip deformity often die because of a defect in their palates that leads to ear infections and aspiration pneumonia. The rolling of the eyes probably describes some sort of seizure activity (see Chapter 13). There is a two- to threefold higher incidence of fetal malformations, including cleft lip and palate, in offspring of epileptic women.

17.64 DIŠ SAG KIR$_4$-*šú maš-du bi-bi-en* KIR$_4$-*šú* NUNDUN.ME-*šú* BAR-*ma su*[*q-ti-šú* . . .] (Böck, *Morphoskopie* 250:6)

**If the head of his nose is flattened, his nasal septum[61] (and) his lip are divided in two (and) [his] ⌜chin⌝ [. . .]

The preceding reference is drawn from the physiognomic omens, which means that the child with a hare-lip must have survived to adulthood, an indication of a minor deformity in the lip and either a small or no palatal defect. The nose is somewhat deformed, possibly secondary to the nasal septal defect.

OTHER CONGENITAL MALFORMATIONS

17.65 BE MUNUS Ù.TU-*ma pi-a* NU TUKU . . . (Šumma Izbu III 37 [Leichty, *Izbu* 57])[62]

**If a woman gives birth and (the child) does not have a mouth . . .

17.66 BE MUNUS Ù.TU-*ma* NUNDUN-*su* AN.TA KI.TA U$_5$ . . . (Šumma Izbu III 40 [Leichty, *Izbu* 58])

**If a woman gives birth and (the child)'s upper lip rides the lower one . . .

17.67 BE MUNUS Ù.TU-*ma* NUNDUN-*su* KI.TA AN.TA U$_5$ . . . (Šumma Izbu III 41 [Leichty, *Izbu* 58])

**If a woman gives birth and (the child)'s lower lip rides the upper one . . .

JAW AND CHIN

CONGENITAL MALFORMATION

17.68 BE MUNUS Ù.TU-*ma la-ḫu-šú* KI.TA NU GÁL.MEŠ . . . (Šumma Izbu III 34 [Leichty, *Izbu* 57])[63]

**If a woman gives birth and (the child) has no lower jaw . . .

17.69 BE MUNUS Ù.TU-*ma* ZAG.GA-*šu ku-ra-a* . . . (Šumma Izbu III 36 [Leichty, *Izbu* 57])[64]

**If a woman gives birth and (the child)'s chin is (too) short . . .

Although a small (hypoplastic) jaw may occur as an isolated defect, it may also be part of the Pierre Robin syndrome. This condition also includes a cleft palate and a retracted tongue (glossoptosis).

SPINAL CORD DEFECT

When the vertebral bodies in the developing fetus fail to fuse, the resulting condition is called spina bifida.[65] This abnormality commonly causes malfunction of the nerves that are located below the defect. Secondary infection is a common problem. In the reference below, the defect is at the cervical (neck) level, giving this patient a very poor prognosis.

17.70 DIŠ LÚ.TUR *šap-pu ul-ti* GÚ-*šú* EN GÚ.MURGU-*šú kàs-lu-šu* DU_8.MEŠ BA.ÚŠ (DPS XL A 41//B 41 = *TDP* 222:41)

**If the transverse processes[66] of a bent-over[67] infant's neck including his spine are open, he will die.

OMPHALOCELE

This is an abdominal wall defect that may permit the intestines to herniate into the umbilical cord of the newborn. In this abnormality, the intestines bulge through the abdominal wall defect, and can be easily seen through a clear covering membrane. The reference below clearly describes this condition.

17.71 BE MUNUS Ù.TU-*ma ir-ru-šú ina* LI.DUR-*šú a-ṣú-ú u* UZU *ku-ut-tu-mu* . . . (Šumma Izbu III 67 [Leichty, *Izbu* 61])[68]

**If a woman gives birth and (the child)'s intestines protrude from its navel and are covered with flesh . . .[69]

CONJOINED ("SIAMESE") TWINS

When the fertilized egg of a woman divides completely, it forms two identical structures that may develop into identical twins. If the embryo starts to divide, but fails to divide completely, two humans fused at some portion of their bodies is the result. The fusion may result in shared nonduplicated organs, and limb and head malformations. These congenital anomalies are described in some detail in ancient Mesopotamian omen literature.[70]

ONE CHILD WITH TWO HEADS

17.72 BE MUNUS Ù.TU-*ma* 2 SAG.DU.MEŠ-*šú* . . . (Šumma Izbu II 20 [Leichty, *Izbu* 47])

**If a woman gives birth and (the child) has two heads . . .

17.73 [BE MUNUS Ù.TU]-*ma* 2 IGI.MEŠ-*šú* . . . (Šumma Izbu II 64 [Leichty, *Izbu* 52])[71]

**[If a woman gives birth] and (the child) has two faces . . .[72]

ONE CHILD WITH TWO HEADS AND TWO SETS OF EXTREMITIES

17.74 [BE MUNUS Ù.TU-*ma* 2] SAG.DU.MEŠ-*šú* 2 KA-*šú* 4 IGI.MEŠ-*šú u* 4 ŠU.MEŠ-*šú* 4 GÌR.MEŠ-*šú* . . . (Šumma Izbu II 25 [Leichty, *Izbu* 48])[73]

**[If a woman gives birth and (the child) has two] heads, two mouths, four eyes, and four hands, (and) four feet . . .

JOINED TWINS

17.75 BE MUNUS 2 NITA.MEŠ/MUNUS.MEŠ Ù.TU-*ma* ŠÀ-*šu-nu*/ŠÀ-*ši-na* 1-*ma* . . . (Šumma Izbu I 84, 102 [Leichty, *Izbu* 39, 42])

**If a woman gives birth to two boys/girls and they have only one abdomen . . .

17.76 [BE MUNUS Ù.TU-*ma* 2 SAG.DU.MEŠ-*šú*] 2 KA-*šú* 2 GÚ.MURGU-*šú* 4 ŠU.MEŠ-*šú* 4 GÌR.MEŠ-*šú* 4 GU.DU.MEŠ-*šú* . . . (Šumma Izbu II 27 [Leichty, *Izbu* 48])[74]

**[If a woman gives birth and (the child) has two heads], two mouths, two spines, four hands, four feet, (and) four buttocks . . .

17.77 [BE MUNUS Ù.TU-*ma* 2 SAG.DU.MEŠ-*šú*] 2 KA-*šú* 2 GÌŠ.MEŠ-*šú* 4 ŠU.MEŠ-*šú* 4 GÌR.MEŠ-*šú* 4 GU.DU.MEŠ-*šú* . . . (Šumma Izbu II 29 [Leichty, *Izbu* 49])

**[If a woman gives birth and (the child) has two heads], two mouths, two penises, four hands, four feet, (and) four buttocks . . .

JOINED TRIPLETS

17.78 BE MUNUS 3 MUNUS.MEŠ Ù.TU-*ma* ŠÀ-*ši-na* 1-*ma* . . . (Šumma Izbu I 115 [Leichty, *Izbu* 43])

**If a woman gives birth to three girls and they have only one abdomen . . .

17.79 BE MUNUS 3 Ù.TU-*ma i-lik-šú-nu* 1-*ma* . . . (Šumma Izbu I 112 [Leichty, *Izbu* 43])

**If a woman gives birth to three (children) and they have only one waist . . .

TWINS JOINED AT THE WAIST

17.80 [BE MUNUS Ù.TU-*ma* 2 SAG.DU].MEŠ-*šú* 2 KA-*šú* 4 ŠU.MEŠ-*šu* 4 GÌR.MEŠ-*šú* *ina* $MURUB_4$-*šú-nu* 1-*ma* . . . (Šumma Izbu II 31 [Leichty, *Izbu* 49])

**[If a woman gives birth and (the child) has two heads], two mouths, four hands, (and) four feet but there is only one waist . . .

TWINS JOINED AT THE RIBS

17.81 [BE MUNUS Ù.TU-*ma* 2 SAG].DU.MEŠ-*šú* 2 GÚ.MEŠ-*šú* 2 GÚ.MURGU-*šú* 2 GABA.MEŠ-*šú* 4 ŠU.MEŠ-*šu* 4 GÌR.MEŠ-*šú* [*ina* TI]-*šú-nu* DIB.DIB . . . (Šumma Izbu II 32 [Leichty, *Izbu* 49])[75]

**[If a woman gives birth and (the child) has two] ⌜heads⌝, two necks, two spines, two breasts, four hands, four feet, (and) they are joined [at] their [rib(s)] . . .

17.82 BE MUNUS MAŠ.TAB.BA Ù.TU-*ma ina* TI-*šú-nu* DIB.DIB-*tum* . . . (Šumma Izbu I 91 [Leichty, *Izbu* 40])

**If a woman gives birth to twins and they are joined at their rib(s) . . .

17.83 BE MUNUS MAŠ.TAB.BA Ù.TU-*ma ina* TI-*šú-nu* DIB.DIB-*ma šá* 15/150 ŠU-*su šá* 15/150 NU GÁL . . . (Šumma Izbu I 92–93 [Leichty, *Izbu* 40])

**If a woman gives birth to twins and they are joined at their rib(s) and the one on the left/right does not have a left/right hand . . .

17.84 BE MUNUS MAŠ.TAB.BA Ù.TU-*ma* MIN-*ma šá* 15/150 ŠU.MEŠ-*šú-nu* NU GÁL.MEŠ . . . (Šumma Izbu I 94–95 [Leichty, *Izbu* 41])

**If a woman gives birth to twins and (they are joined at their ribs) and they do not have hands on the left/right (side) . . .

17.85 BE MUNUS MAŠ.TAB.BA Ù.TU-*ma* MIN-*ma šá* 15/GÙB GÌR-*šú šá* 15/GÙB NU GÁL . . . (Šumma Izbu I 96–97 [Leichty, *Izbu* 41])

**If a woman gives birth to twins and (they are joined at their ribs) and the one on the left/right does not have a left/right foot . . .

17.86 BE MUNUS MAŠ.TAB.BA Ù.TU-*ma* MIN-*ma šá* 15/150 GÌR.MEŠ-*šú-nu* NU GÁL.MEŠ . . . (Šumma Izbu I 98–99 [Leichty, *Izbu* 41])

**If a woman gives birth to twins and (they are joined at their ribs) and they do not have feet on the left/right (side) . . .

TWINS JOINED AT THE BACK

17.87 BE MUNUS 2 Ù.TU-*ma ina* GÚ.MURGU-*šú-nu in-nem-du-ma pa-nu-šú-nu a-ḫe-e* GAR . . . (Šumma Izbu I 88 [Leichty, *Izbu* 40])

**If a woman gives birth to two (children) and they come together at their spine so that their faces are turned towards the outside . . .

17.88 [BE MUNUS Ù.TU-*ma* 2] SAG.DU.MEŠ-*šú* 2 GÚ.MEŠ-*šú* 2 GABA.MEŠ-*šú* 4 ŠU.MEŠ-[*šú*. . .] DIB.[DIB] . . . (Šumma Izbu II 33 [Leichty, *Izbu* 49])[76]

**[If a woman gives birth and (the child) has two] heads, two necks, two breasts, four hands [. . .] (and) they are joined . . .

TWINS CROSSED OVER

17.89 BE MUNUS 2 Ù.TU-*ma* GIN_7 GU_4.DUMU.^{d}UTU *ti-iṣ-bu-ti*. . . (Šumma Izbu I 87 [Leichty, *Izbu* 40]; cf. Šumma Izbu I 10 [Leichty, *Izbu* 33])

**If a woman gives birth to two (children) and they are joined grasping one another like the Bullgod, son of Šamaš . . .

TWINS FACE TO FACE AND JOINED IN TWO PLACES

17.90 BE MUNUS Ù.TU-*ma* 2 SAG.DU.MEŠ-*šú* ŠEŠ *ana* IGI ŠEŠ KA-*šú-nu* 1!-*ma* 4 IGI.MEŠ-*šú-nu* 2 GÚ.MURGU-*šú-nu* 4 GEŠTU.MEŠ-*šú-nu* 2 GABA.MEŠ-*šú-nu* 4 ŠU-*šú-nu* 4 GÌR.MEŠ-*šú-nu* [$MURUB_4$-*šú-nu*] GIŠ.KUN-*šú-nu* 1-*ma* . . . (Šumma Izbu II 21 [Leichty, *Izbu* 48])

**If a woman gives birth and (the child) has two heads, one facing the other but only one mouth, four eyes, two spines, four ears, two breasts, four hand(s), four feet, but only one [waist] and hip . . .

TWINS WITH ONE HEAD

17.91 [BE MUNUS Ù.TU]-*ma* 2 IGI.MEŠ-*šú* 4 ŠU.MEŠ-*šú* 4 GÌR.MEŠ-*šú* . . . (Šumma Izbu II 66 [Leichty, *Izbu* 52])[77]

**[If a woman gives birth] and (the child) has two eyes, four hands, (and) four feet . . .

Probably falling into the category of omens produced by artificially filling out the record rather than by direct observation are the following extremely unlikely, if not impossible, examples of conjoined twins.

17.92 [BE MUNUS Ù.TU-*ma* 2 SAG.DU.MEŠ-*šú*] 2 KA-*šú* 2 EME.MEŠ-*šú* 4 IGI.MEŠ-*šú* 4 GÚ.MURGU-*šú* 4 ŠU.MEŠ-*šú* 4 GÌR.MEŠ-*šú* . . . (Šumma Izbu II 30 [Leichty, *Izbu* 49])

**[If a woman gives birth and (the child) has two heads], two mouths, two tongues, four eyes, four spines, four hands, four feet . . .

17.93 BE MUNUS Ù.TU-*ma* GÌR-*šú* 1-*at u* MIN 2 *pag-ru-šu* . . . (Šumma Izbu III 93 [Leichty, *Izbu* 63])

**If a woman gives birth and (the child) has only one foot and (it is weak and the child) has two bodies . . .

17.94 BE MUNUS Ù.TU-*ma* 4 GÌR.MEŠ-*šú* GÌŠ *u* GAL_4.LA GAR . . . (Šumma Izbu III 98 [Leichty, *Izbu* 64])

**If a woman gives birth and (the child) has four feet, a penis, and a vulva . . .

The last reference above seems to be describing a type of conjoined twin that has two sets of genitalia, one male and the other female. This does not seem possible since incompletely separated twins are always of the same sex. Since, however, conjoined fetuses with two vulvae, or two penises would have been seen on occasion by the diviner, he must have wanted to be prepared for the occurrence of conjoined fetuses with both types of genitalia.

EXTREMITY MALFORMATIONS

FINGERS Extra fingers and toes are relatively common malformations, and were seen by the *āšipu*. Modern physicians surgically remove the extra digits, but the ancient physicians would probably have avoided surgery in all but life-threatening conditions, because of the high risk of wound infection.

17.95 BE MUNUS Ù.TU-*ma* 6 ŠU.SI.MEŠ-*šú šá* 15/150 . . . (Šumma Izbu III 54–55 [Leichty, *Izbu* 59])

**If a woman gives birth and (the child) has six fingers on the left/right (hand) . . .

17.96 BE MUNUS Ù.TU-*ma* 6.TA.ÀM ŠU.SI.ME ŠU^{II}-*šú šá* 15 *u* 150 . . . (Šumma Izbu III 56 [Leichty, *Izbu* 59])

**If a woman gives birth and (the child) has six fingers each on the left and right hands . . .

17.97 [BE MUNUS Ù.TU-*ma* 6.TA].ÀM ŠU.⸢SI.ME GÌR^{II}-*šú šá* 15 *u* 150⸣ . . . (Šumma Izbu III 57 [Leichty, *Izbu* 59])[78]

** [If a woman gives birth and (the child) has six toes] ⸢each⸣ on the left and right feet . . .

17.98 [BE MUNUS Ù.TU]-⸢*ma* 6.TA.ÀM ŠU.SI⸣.[ME ŠU^{II}-*šú šá* 15 *u* 150 *u* GÌR^{II}-*šú šá* 15 *u* 150] . . . (Šumma Izbu III 60 [Leichty, *Izbu* 60])

** [If a woman gives birth] and (the child) has six digits each [on the left and right hands and left and right feet] . . .

CLUB FOOT (EQUINOVARUS DEFORMITY) In this congenital anomaly, the foot is flexed downward (plantar flexed), and the forefoot curves inward (Varus). We believe that the following references are describing this anomaly.

17.99 BE MUNUS Ù.TU-*ma* GÌR 15/150-*šu* GIN$_7$ GÌR BAL.GI^{KU}6 . . . (Šumma Izbu III 87–88 [Leichty, *Izbu* 63])[79]

**If a woman gives birth and (the child)'s left/right foot is like the foot of a tortoise . . .

17.100 BE MUNUS Ù.TU-*ma* ⸢*kab*⸣-[*bar-tum*] NIGIN-*ma* GÚ.DU-*su* IGI . . . (Šumma Izbu II 17 [Leichty, *Izbu* 47])

**If a woman gives birth and the ⸢side of (the child)'s foot(?)⸣ is turned and faces its buttocks . . .

SIRENOMELIA When the lower extremities develop, they may fail to separate into two structures. The resulting condition is called sirenomelia. Pangas[80] suggests that the following reference is describing this abnormality.

17.101 BE MUNUS Ù.TU-*ma* GÌR-*šú* 1-*at-ma ù ma-ka-a-at* . . . (Šumma Izbu III 92 [Leichty, *Izbu* 63])[81]

**If a woman gives birth and (the child) has only one foot and it is weak . . .

PARTIAL OR TOTAL ABSENCE OF LIMBS (PHOCOMELIA) This is an uncommon congenital abnormality in which the arm, forearm, or hand as well as the thigh or foot may be missing or small (hypoplastic). In the recent past the use of thalidomide during pregnancy caused a marked increase in the occurrence of this condition. Congenital varicella infection is also a known cause of this defect (see below). It was known to occur in ancient Mesopotamia, as may be seen from the following references.

Arm, forearm, or hand

17.102 BE MUNUS Ù.TU-*ma* ZAG-*šú*/GÙB-*šú ku-rat* . . . (Šumma Izbu III 43–44 [Leichty, *Izbu* 58])[82]

**If a woman gives birth and (the child)'s left/right (arm) is (too) short . . .

17.103 BE MUNUS Ù.TU-*ma* Á-*šú iš-ti-a-at* . . . (Šumma Izbu III 46 [Leichty, *Izbu* 58])[83]

**If a woman gives birth and (the child) has only one forearm . . .

17.104 BE MUNUS Ù.TU-*ma* [Á.MEŠ-*šu u*] $ŠU^{II}$-*šú* NU GÁL.MEŠ . . . (Šumma Izbu II 13 [Leichty, *Izbu* 47])[84]

**If a woman gives birth and (the child) does not have [forearms and] hands . . .

17.105 BE MUNUS Ù.TU-*ma* ŠU-*su šá* 15/150 NU GÁL . . . BE MUNUS Ù.TU-*ma* ŠU.MEŠ-*šu* NU GÁL.MEŠ . . . (Šumma Izbu III 48–50 [Leichty, *Izbu* 59])[85]

**If a woman gives birth and (the child) does not have a left/right hand . . . If a woman gives birth and (the child) does not have hands . . .

17.106 BE MUNUS Ù.TU-*ma* ŠU.SI.MEŠ-*šú šá* 15/150 NU GÁL.MEŠ . . . (Šumma Izbu III 51–52 [Leichty, *Izbu* 59])[86]

**If a woman gives birth and (the child) does not have fingers on the left/right . . .

Thigh or foot

17.107 BE MUNUS Ù.TU-*ma* ÚR 15/150-*šu* NU GÁL . . . (Šumma Izbu III 77–78 [Leichty, *Izbu* 62])[87]

**If a woman gives birth and (the child) does not have a left/right thigh . . .

17.108 BE MUNUS Ù.TU-*ma* GÌR 15/150-*šú* NU GÁL . . . (Šumma Izbu III 80–81 [Leichty, *Izbu* 62])[88]

**If a woman gives birth and (the child) does not have a left/right foot . . .

17.109 BE MUNUS Ù.TU-*ma* GÌR 15/150-*šú ša-bu-lat* . . . (Šumma Izbu III 85–86 [Leichty, *Izbu* 63])[89]

**If a woman gives birth and (the child)'s left/right foot is withered . . .

17.110 BE MUNUS Ù.TU-*ma* 6 *qar-ši* ŠU.SI.MEŠ GÌR-*šú šá* 15/150 . . . (Šumma Izbu III 61–62 [Leichty, *Izbu* 60])[90]

**If a woman gives birth and (the child) has six stumps of toes on his left/right foot . . .

17.111 BE MUNUS Ù.TU-*ma a-si-id* 15/150-*šú* NU GÁL . . . (Šumma Izbu III 99–100 [Leichty, *Izbu* 64])

**If a woman gives birth and (the child) does not have a left/right heel . . .

DWARFISM

There are many causes of abnormally small body size, or dwarfism. One of the most common types is achondroplasia. One of its major characteristics is a relatively normal-sized torso and markedly shortened extremities. The following quote is probably describing an achondroplastic dwarf.[91]

17.112 BE MUNUS LÚ.BA.AN.ZA Ù.TU . . . (Šumma Izbu I 54–55 [Leichty, *Izbu* 36])[92]

**If a woman gives birth to a male/female (child with) short (limbs) . . .

ABSENCE OF SEX ORGANS

There are many causes of sex organ abnormalities. In males, the urethral opening may not be at the tip of the penis but lower on the shaft (hypospadia). In this condition, the penis may be malformed or rudimentary. Also associated with hypospadia may be a downward bowing of the penis (chordee). Undescended testes, where the structures remain in the abdominal cavity leaving the scrotum empty, is a common problem. There are also congenital hormonal abnormalities that can affect sex organ size and configuration. Congenital adrenal hyperplasia is a group of enzyme abnormalities that may cause increased production of male sex hormone. When this occurs in females, the clitoris enlarges and may look like a penis.

In the following references, the absence of testes is probably due to undescended testes. The remaining references may actually be describing atrophied, aplastic, or malformed sex organs, since these are not rare conditions, whereas complete absence is quite unusual. For additional abnormalities, see Hermaphroditism below.

17.113 BE MUNUS Ù.TU-*ma* GÌŠ-*šú* NU GÁL . . . (Šumma Izbu III 68 [Leichty, *Izbu* 61])[93]

**If a woman gives birth and (the child) does not have a penis . . .

17.114 BE MUNUS Ù.TU-*ma* GÌŠ-*šú u* ŠIR.MEŠ-*šú* NU GÁL.MEŠ . . . (Šumma Izbu III 69 [Leichty, *Izbu* 61])

**If a woman gives birth and (the child) does not have a penis or testicles . . .

17.115 BE MUNUS Ù.TU-*ma* ŠIR.ME-*šú* NU GÁL.MEŠ . . . (Šumma Izbu III 72 [Leichty, *Izbu* 61])

**If a woman gives birth and (the child) does not have testicles . . .

17.116 BE MUNUS Ù.TU-*ma* GAL_4.LA NU TUKU . . . (Šumma Izbu III 73 [Leichty, *Izbu* 61])[94]

**If a woman gives birth and (the child) does not have a vulva . . .

HERMAPHRODITISM

Congenital anomalies include fetuses with both male and female gonadal tissue. When this occurs the infant may have both male and female sexual organs. In pseudohermaphroditism, which is more common, the patient has male and female genitalia, but the gonads are of only one sex. The reference below describes these phenomena. The second text mentions a spirit, Lamassu, which was thought to possess both a penis and a vulva. This implies that the infant had the same genital anatomy as the spirit.

17.117 BE MUNUS Ù.TU-*ma* GÌŠ *u* GAL_4.LA GAR . . . (Šumma Izbu III 70 [Leichty, *Izbu* 61])

**If a woman gives birth and (the child) has a penis and a vulva . . .[95]

17.118 BE MUNUS Ù.TU-*ma* ᵈLAMMA *u bu-nu* NAM.LÚ.U_{18}.LU GAR . . . (Šumma Izbu II 67 [Leichty, *Izbu* 52])

**If a woman gives birth and (the child) is a *lamassu* with a human face (comm. It has a penis and a vulva) . . .

IMPERFORATE ANUS

A fetus can survive to delivery if the anal opening fails to develop, but it cannot survive long after delivery without surgical intervention. The ancient Mesopotamian text below describes such a case, but it is unclear whether the *āšipu* would have attempted to surgically relieve this problem.

17.119 BE MUNUS Ù.TU-*ma* GU.DU-*su pe-ḫa-a-at* . . . (Šumma Izbu III 75 [Leichty, *Izbu* 62])[96]

**If a woman gives birth and (the child)'s anus is closed . . .

INTESTINAL ATRESIA

The intestinal opening may be blocked at birth. This can occur at any level, but most commonly in the ileum. In modern times, this condition can be surgically corrected, but failure to do this will certainly lead to death. Infants with this problem in ancient Mesopotamia would have died because surgery of this type would have been impossible. In the reference below, the term *blocked off* indicates a complete and permanent blockage (as opposed to simple constipation, which was referred to by the term *esēlu*; see Chapter 6 with 6.67). A grim prognosis is suggested by the fact that Damu was a youth who died before his time. Since there were no tests available to the *āšipu* that could have diagnosed this disease before death, it is likely that an autopsy was performed to identify the problem.

17.120 DIŠ LÚ.TUR ŠÀ.MEŠ-*šú suk-ku-ru* ŠU ᵈ*Da-mu* (DPS XL B 73a = *TDP* 226:72a; cf. DPS XIII B ii 44 = *TDP* 120 ii 44)

**If an infant's insides are blocked off, "hand" of Damu.

Brain Diseases

BRAIN INJURY

Brain damage can result from intrauterine infection or trauma that occurs during delivery. Also, there are genetic and congenital metabolic diseases that can result in brain damage or malfunction. Diseases such as cerebral palsy can result from injury to the motor portions of the brain, spinal cord, or the nerves that control the use of muscles. Such patients may be partially or fully paralyzed in any muscles, including the face. For more on cerebral palsy, see Chapter 13.

17.121 BE MUNUS *a-ka-a-am* Ù.TU . . . (Šumma Izbu I 56 [Leichty, *Izbu* 36])[97]

**If a woman gives birth to a powerless (child) . . .

17.122 BE MUNUS *ku-ub-bu-lam* Ù.TU . . . (Šumma Izbu I 62 [Leichty, *Izbu* 37])

**If a woman gives birth to an immobilized (child) . . .

17.123 BE MUNUS *ṣu-un-du-ru* Ù.TU . . . (Šumma Izbu I 72 [Leichty, *Izbu* 38])

**If a woman gives birth to a twitching (child) . . .

MENTAL RETARDATION

The references listed below identify mental deficiency occurring at birth. The causes of this problem are not possible to determine with the amount of information available, but it seems likely that Down syndrome would have been commonly seen.

17.124 BE MUNUS LÚ.LIL Ù.TU . . . (Šumma Izbu I 52 [Leichty, *Izbu* 36])[98]

**If a woman gives birth to a fool . . .

17.125 BE MUNUS SAL.LIL Ù.TU . . . (Šumma Izbu I 53 [Leichty, *Izbu* 36])

**If a woman gives birth to a female fool . . .

SEIZURES IN INFANTS

In Chapter 13, in a section on seizure disorders, there is a discussion of seizures in infants that range from frequent and life-threatening to infrequent, benign, and transient.

AUTISM

This is considered to be an organic brain defect, but it is manifested by an inability of the individual to establish social relationships with others. The problem becomes apparent in early childhood when the child fails to respond socially to other children or adults.

17.126 BE MUNUS Ù.TU-*ma* AMA-*šú i-zir*... (Šumma Izbu IV 42 [Leichty, *Izbu* 70])

**If a woman gives birth and (the child) rejects its mother...

17.127 BE MUNUS Á.KAM[99] *lu* NITA *lu* MUNUS Ù.TU ... (Šumma Izbu I 69 [Leichty, *Izbu* 38])

**If a woman gives birth to an insane (child), either male or female...

SECKELS SYNDROME

The texts below describe newborns with abnormal heads that resemble those of birds. Although no other characteristics are listed, it seems quite possible that they are patients with Seckels syndrome. Besides having "bird-shaped" heads, they typically have small heads (microcephaly), mental retardation, an underdeveloped (hypoplastic) face with a prominent nose, and low-set, malformed ears.

17.128 BE MUNUS MUŠEN Ù.TU ... (Šumma Izbu I 23 [Leichty, *Izbu* 34])

**If a woman gives birth to (what looks like) a bird...

17.129 BE MUNUS Ù.TU-*ma* SAG.DU MUŠEN GAR ... (Šumma Izbu II 8 [Leichty, *Izbu* 46])[100]

**If a woman gives birth and (the child) has the head of a bird...

17.130 BE MUNUS Ù.TU-*ma* KIR_4 MUŠEN GAR... (Šumma Izbu III 24 [Leichty, *Izbu* 56])[101]

**If a woman gives birth and (the child) has the nose of a bird...

Normal Variants

The following are some conditions that are considered unusual, but are not diseases or abnormalities.[102] However, because they are unusual they were thought to have some significance in predicting the future. In the first three texts below a child is born with some teeth already erupted. The first omen would probably have required cancellation through the performance of an apotropaic ritual to avert bad omens (NAM.BÚR.BI), since it is the queen's child who is involved. To judge from the preserved examples, the precocious presence of teeth signaled rapaciousness, as reflected in the overthrow of the father by the son, the using up of stored royal resources, and famine in the land (due to overpopulation or excessive taxation).[103]

17.131 BE SAL.LUGAL Ù.TU-*ma ul-la-nu-um-ma* ZÚ.MEŠ-*šú a-ṣa-a*... (Šumma Izbu IV 50 [Leichty, *Izbu* 71])[104]

**If the queen gives birth and from the beginning (the child)'s teeth have emerged . . .

17.132 BE MUNUS Ù.TU-*ma* MIN-*ma* 1-*at* ZÚ-*šú a-ṣa-at* . . . (Šumma Izbu IV 27 [Leichty, *Izbu* 69])

**If a woman gives birth and (from the beginning) one of (the child)'s teeth has emerged . . .

17.133 BE MUNUS Ù.TU-*ma* MIN-*ma* 2 ZÚ.MEŠ-*šú* È.MEŠ . . . (Šumma Izbu IV 28 [Leichty, *Izbu* 69])[105]

**If a woman gives birth and (from the beginning) two of (the child)'s teeth have emerged . . .

Newborns with hair present at birth were also described.

17.134 BE MUNUS Ù.TU-*ma* MIN-*ma pi-ir-tum* TUKU . . . (Šumma Izbu IV 34 [Leichty, *Izbu* 69])

**If a woman gives birth and (from the beginning the child) has a full head of hair . . .

17.135 [BE MUN]US Ù.TU-*ma* MIN-*ma ab-bu-ut-ta* GAR . . . (Šumma Izbu IV 22 [Leichty, *Izbu* 68])

**[If] a ⌜woman⌝ gives birth and (from the beginning the child) has a lock of hair on its head[106] . . .

17.136 [BE MUN]US Ù.TU-*ma* MIN-*ma ke-zi-ir* . . . (Šumma Izbu IV 23 [Leichty, *Izbu* 68])

**[If] a ⌜woman⌝ gives birth and (from the beginning the child) has curls . . .

Tall Tales

The second-millennium kings of Mari took a particular interest in malformed fetuses; one letter records a case that occurred among some rather ordinary folks' flocks but which was brought to the governor for inspection, after which it was sent on to the king for his personal examination.[107] The wisdom of insisting on actual evidence as opposed to accepting reports of anomalies at face value may readily be seen by the presence in the omen series of a number of highly implausible, if not physically impossible, examples, some of which find ready parallels in the folklore of other cultures.

17.137 BE MUNUS Ù.TU-*ma* MIN-*ma* SU$_6$.MEŠ-*šú* È.MEŠ . . . (Šumma Izbu IV 32 [Leichty, *Izbu* 69])[108]

**If a woman gives birth and (from the beginning the child) has grown his beard . . .

17.138 BE MUNUS Ù.TU-*ma* MIN-*ma* KA-*šú* BAD-*ma id-bu-ub* . . . (Šumma Izbu IV 35 [Leichty, *Izbu* 69])

**If a woman gives birth and (from the beginning the child) opens its mouth and talks . . .

17.139 BE MUNUS Ù.TU-*ma* 1/2 KUŠ *la-an-šú* SU_6 *za-kin i-da-ab-bu-ub* GIN.GIN *u* ZÚ.MEŠ-*šú* È.MEŠ *ti-ig-ri-ilu* MU-*šú*... (Šumma Izbu I 82 [Leichty, *Izbu* 39])[109]

**If a woman gives birth and (the child) is half a cubit tall, he is bearded, he can talk and walk, and his teeth have erupted, it is called a *tigrilu*...

17.140 BE MUNUS Ù.TU-*ma* GÌR-*šú* 1-*at-ma it-ti* LI.DUR-*šú rak-sat-ma qá-qá-ra* NU *i-kaš-[šad]*... (Šumma Izbu III 96 [Leichty, *Izbu* 64])[110]

**If a woman gives birth and (the child) has only one foot and it is attached to its navel and does not ⌜reach⌝ the ground...

Acquired Diseases of Infants and Small Children[111]

It is generally accepted that the term that we are translating "infant" (LÚ.TUR) refers to children who are still nursing.[112] In ancient Mesopotamia, children were generally wet-nursed for two to three years, with supplements for the older children of a ready-to-hand baby food, ripe dates.[113]

A special category of recitation was designed to hush the cries of cranky babies.

17.141 *ṣe-eḫ-ru-um wa-ši-ib bi-it ek-[le-tim] lu ta-ta-ṣa-am ta-ta-ma-ar n[u-ur*ᵈUTU-*ši] a-mi-in ta-ba-ki a-mi-in tu-g[a-li-it?] ul-li-ki-a a-mi-in la ta-ab-[ki] i-lí bi-tim te-ed-ki ku-sa-ri-[k] u-u[m] i-gi-il-tim ma-nu-um id-ki-a-ni ma-nu-um ú-ga-li-ta-ni ṣe-eḫ-ru-um id-ki-ka ṣe-eḫ-ru-um ú-ga-li-it-ka ki-ma ša-tu-ù ka-ra-ni-im ki-ma ma-ar sà-bi-tim li-im-qù-ta-šum ši-tum* (W. Farber, *Schlaf* 34:1–11)

**Infant who dwelt in the house of ⌜darkness⌝ (the womb), you have come out; you have seen the ⌜light⌝ [of day]. Why do you cry? Why do you ⌜startle⌝ (people)? Why did you not ⌜cry⌝ when you were there? You roused the household god, startled the *kusarikku* ("bison"). (They say:) "Who roused me?! Who startled me?!" The infant roused you; the infant startled you. May sleep fall upon him like one who drinks wine, like the gazelle's young.

Affluent families hired wet (*mušēniqtu*) and dry (*tarîtu*) nurses to care for their children.[114] Wet-nursing was a respectable and profitable if somewhat hazardous occupation. On the one hand, contracts indicate that the nurse could expect up to three years of food, oil, wool, and clothing[115] and on the other there was the danger of being caught trying to handle too many charges at once.

17.142 *šum-ma a-wi-lum* DUMU-*šu a-na mu-še-ni-iq-tim id-di-in-ma* DUMU *šu-ú i-na qá-at mu-še-ni-iq-tim im-tu-ut mu-še-ni-iq-tum ba-lum a-bi-šu ù um-mi-šu* DUMU *ša-ni-a-am-ma ir-ta-ka-ás ú-ka-an-nu-ši-ma*... UBUR-*šá i-na-a-ki-su* (Laws of Ḫammurapi § 194)

**If a person turns his child over to a wet nurse and that child dies in the hands of the wet nurse, if they convict the wet nurse of having made a contract for another child without (the consent) of its (the first child's) father and mother... they cut off her breast.

NURSING PROBLEMS

Infants may fail to nurse adequately for a variety of reasons, causing them to lose weight. In the first reference below, the wet nurse was said to have weak breasts, suggesting inadequate milk production. However, it also mentions a bitter taste in the milk. Since many of the substances that enter the woman's circulation can also enter the breast milk, it is quite possible that the wet nurse was taking in some food or medicine that entered the milk and altered its taste.

17.143 DIŠ LÚ.TUR *ina te-ni-qí-šú* UZU.MEŠ *i-šaḫ-ḫu-ḫu u mu-še-niq-ta-šú* UBUR SIG-*at* UBUR ÍL-*šum-ma* NU KÚ UBUR *šú-ú mur-ra i-šú ana* UBUR *eš-ši tu-na-kar-šú-ma* TI (DPS XL A 36–37 = *TDP* 220–222:36–37)

**If an infant's flesh wastes away while he is nursing and his wet nurse's breast is weak (and if) you raise the breast to him he will not eat, that breast has a bitter taste. (If) you move him to a new breast, he will get well.

The following reference mentions an infant with *ašû* or *samānu* who improves with a new wet nurse and a recitation. *Ašû* is a nonspecific term meaning a generalized rash (see Chapter 10). If the child developed this rash in reaction to something in the breast milk, switching wet nurses might indeed be helpful.

17.144 DIŠ LÚ.TUR *a-šu-ú u sa-ma-ni* DIB-*su ana tu-la-a eš-šá tu-na-kar-šu-ma u* ÉN ŠUB.ŠUB-*šum-ma* TI (DPS XL A 38/B 38 = *TDP* 222:38)[116]

**If *ašû* or *samānu* afflicts an infant, you move him to a new breast and also continually say a recitation over him and he will get well.

Samānu means soft tissue infection (see Chapter 3), and it seems unlikely that a new wet nurse would resolve this problem unless it was the nurse and not the infant who had the infection. There is a Sumerian recitation for *samānu* which, to judge from context, may be the very one that the *āšipu* would have recited over the infant. This recitation indicates that *samānu* ("the red dragon") prevented the *qadištu* and *kulmašītu* (holy women whose duties included overseeing wet nursing) from performing their functions and could result in the infant's never being weaned and never growing up to be an adolescent boy or girl able to have children of his or her own.

17.145 DUMU.GA.KE$_4$ NINDA.GURU$_5$.NA BA.NI.RÁ.A.GIN$_7$ KI.SIKIL.LE DU$_8$.ITI.ITI.A.NA BA.NI.RÁ.A.GIN$_7$ GURUŠ.E ZAG.MAŠ.MAŠ.A.NA BA.NI.RÁ.A.GIN$_7$ NU.GIG.E NAM.NU.GIG.GA.NA BA.NI.R[A].A.RÁ.A.GIN$_7$ NU.BAR.E NAM.NU.BAR.RA.NA BA.NI.RÁ.A.GIN$_7$ (Nougayrol, *ArOr* 17/2.213–214:11–15; cf. Finkel, *Fs. Borger* 73–76)

**When the suckling is denied his baby food, the adolescent girl her menses, the adolescent boy his virility; when *qadištu* is prevented from performing her functions as *qadištu*, the *kulmašītu* from performing her functions as *kulmašītu*.[117]

The description suggests a wet nurse with breast cellulitis (mastitis). *Streptococcus pyogenes* can cause mastitis, and may also produce a serious and even fatal infection in a nursing infant. Switching wet nurses would certainly have been recommended, with or without the accompanying recitation.

FAILURE TO THRIVE

Modern physicians use the term *failure to thrive* when an infant nurses but does not grow. There are many causes of this problem. The quote below mentions an infant who is nursing but losing weight and who "pours it out." The expression "pour out" is usually used of voluminous watery diarrhea from the anus. Infectious enteritis with diarrhea could be the explanation, but an obstructive congenital gastrointestinal defect with vomiting could also explain it. There are many other causes for failure to thrive, including milk allergy, malabsorption, lactase deficiency, and many chronic or recurrent infections.

17.146 DIŠ LÚ.TUR *la-ʾ-ḫu ki-ma al-du ṣir-ti i-ni-qu ina* ŠÀ-*šú la i-bi-ma i-tab-bak ù* UZU.MEŠ-*šú im-ta-ṭu-ú ki-ši-id e-pi-ru* (DPS XL A 1–2//C 1–2 = *TDP* 216:1–2)

**If an infant as soon as he is born sucks the teat (but) does not get fat from it but pours (it) out and his flesh diminishes, he was "gotten" by the dust.[118]

TEETHING

Most parents and physicians are acquainted with teething problems. The child is cranky and drooling, may have a low-grade temperature, and is reluctant to eat. This problem can last for weeks with parents losing sleep and a very unhappy baby. Fortunately the prognosis is excellent. The four references that follow indicate that the *āšipu* understood this problem.[119]

17.147 DIŠ LÚ.TUR SAG.DU-*su* KÚM *ú-kal pa-gar-šú* KÚM *la ḫa-aḫ-ḫa-aš* IR *la i-ši* ŠU^{II}-*šú u* GÌR^{II}-*šú* ŠA *em-ma il-la-tu-šú* DU-*ka u ú-šar-ra-aḫ ma-la* KÚ *ina* ŠÀ-*šú la ina-aḫ-ma i-tab-ba-ka* LÚ.TUR.BI ZÚ.MEŠ-*šú* È.MEŠ-*ni* U_4.15.KÁM : U_4.20.KÁM *dan-nat* IGI-*ma* DIN! (DPS XL A 10–12 = *TDP* 218:10–12)

**If the infant's head holds fever (and) his body (holds) a lukewarm temperature (and) he does not sweat (but) his hands and feet are hot, his saliva flows and he drools,[120] whatever he eats does not rest easy in his stomach and he then pours (it) out, that infant's teeth are coming out. He will suffer for fifteen or twenty days and then get well.[121]

17.148 DIŠ LÚ.TUR *pa-gar-šú* KÚM *la ḫa-ḫaš* SAG.DU-*su* KÚM TUKU UBUR KÚ-*ma ma-gal ú-sar-ra-aḫ* ZÚ.ME-*šú* È.ME-*ni* U_4.14.KÁM : U_4.20.KÁM SAL.KALAG.GA IGI-*ma* DIN (DPS XL A 115 = *TDP* 230:115)

**If an infant's body (has) a lukewarm temperature (and) his head has fever, he eats (from) the breast and then drools a lot, his teeth are coming out. He will suffer for fourteen or twenty days and then get well.

17.149 DIŠ LÚ.TUR KÚM NU TUKU SAG.DU-*su* KÚM ZÚ.MEŠ-*šú* È.MEŠ-*ni* U_4.21.KÁM SAL.KALAG.GA IGI-*ma* DIN (DPS XL A 116 = *TDP* 230:116)

**If the infant does not have a fever (but) his head is feverish, his teeth are coming out. He will suffer for twenty-one days and then get well.

17.150 *ṣa-ra-ḫu ša* SAG.DU-*su* Á^{II}.MEŠ-*šú* GÌR^{II}.MEŠ-*šú i-ṣar-ḫu-u-ni* TA* *pa-an* ZÚ.MEŠ-*šú* ZÚ.MEŠ-*šú a-na ú-ṣe-e* TA* *pa-ni šu-ú it-ta-aṣ-raḫ bé-ta-nu-uš-šu ú-sa-pi-il* (*ABL* 586 [*SAA* 10.302]:11-r. 7)[122]

**The burning (fever) that burns his head, his arms, (and) his feet is due to his teeth. His teeth are trying to come out, and it is for this reason that he has been burned (with fever). It has gone down inside him.[123]

OPEN FONTANELLES

The skull bones of a newborn infant are not yet fused into a single structure to protect the brain as is the case in adults. This allows the brain to continue to grow in size during early childhood. The skull of the infant has six fontanelles, which are at the junctions of the calvarial bones. Since these areas plus portions of the sutures between the calvarial bones are not yet shielded by bone, they can reflect pressures within the skull. When the fluid around the brain has increased pressure due to meningitis or congenital hydrocephalus, the fontanelles further separate and bulge. The fontanelles can bulge during crying, but this reverts promptly to normal when crying stops.

The texts that follow indicate an awareness by the *āšipu* that fontanelle size has significance. No other symptoms (such as fever) are given, however, which makes it difficult to decide between meningitis and hydrocephalus as the cause for the "forehead getting wider."[124] Congenital hydrocephalus without modern therapy is often progressive but occasionally remits spontaneously. Children with bacterial meningitis usually die without antibiotic therapy; children with viral meningitis, on the other hand, not infrequently recover without therapy. This means that bulging fontanelles were not likely to be reversible in bacterial meningitis, but might be with viral meningitis. A hint that it was indeed two forms of meningitis that were being differentiated is the mention in the first reference that the child was expected to get well if the illness remitted after seven or eight days. The most common causes of viral (aseptic) meningitis in infants and young children are the enteroviruses. The prognosis with enteroviral meningitis is good and most patients are well within a week.

17.151 DIŠ LÚ.TUR *ši-bit* SAG.DU-*šú paṭ-rat-ma mu-uḫ-ḫa-šu i-rap-pu-uš u* NU *i-ṣa-lal* U$_4$.7.KÁM U$_4$.8.KÁM GIG-*ma* DIN/BA.ÚŠ (DPS XL A 44//B 44 = *TDP* 222:44)

**If the seam of the infant's head is open and his forehead is getting wider and he cannot sleep, (if) he is sick for (only) seven or eight days, he will get well (var. B: he will die).

17.152 DIŠ LÚ.TUR *ši-bit* SAG.DU-*šú paṭ-rat-ma mu-uḫ-ḫa-šu i-rap-pu-uš* BA.ÚŠ (DPS XL A 45//B 45 = *TDP* 222:45)

**If the seam of the infant's head is open and his forehead is getting wider, he will die.

ANKYLOBLEPHARON

In the following reference, the infant's eyes are described as being closed like those of a puppy. This could be explained by a neurologic condition preventing the lid muscles from opening the eyes or, as Fincke suggests,[125] by fusion of the eyelids (ankyloblepharon). As she notes, the eyes of puppies normally remain fused for the first two weeks of life.

17.153 BE *iz-bu* IGI.MEŠ-*šú ki-i šá* UR.TUR *la-ki-i kát-ma* . . . (Šumma Izbu X 38′ [Leichty, *Izbu* 125])

**If the malformed birth's eyes are closed like those of a young puppy . . .

OPHTHALMIA NEONATORUM

As suggested by Fincke,[126] the text below appears to be describing ophthalmia neonatorum.[127] This is a superficial eye infection that is acquired by the newborn from the mother's birth canal during delivery. In the absence of antibiotic treatment, it will produce scarring, membrane formation, and blindness. The most common organism causing this condition currently is the gonococcus, but other organisms might also be involved.

17.154 BE *iz-bu* IGI.MEŠ-*šú ši-ši-tam ár-ma* . . . (Šumma Izbu X 26′ [Leichty, *Izbu* 123])

**If the malformed birth's eyes are enveloped by a membrane . . .

CONGENITAL CHICKENPOX (*VARICELLA ZOSTER* VIRUS)

Mothers who develop chickenpox (*Varicella zoster* virus; VZV) during pregnancy may transmit the infection to their fetuses. Infection in early pregnancy can cause a variety of congenital defects including microcephaly, mental retardation, and eye, skeletal (see Phocomelia above), kidney, and gastrointestinal abnormalities. In mid-pregnancy, the fetus may develop local dermal scars (pockmarks). Transmission of the virus late in pregnancy will not produce congenital defects, but it can cause severe illness and death, as well as extensive vesicles that are often hemorrhagic. Liver, lung, brain, kidney, and heart injury may occur. We believe that the references that follow are describing the scars and vesicles that may be seen in congenital varicella.

17.155 [BE MUNUS] Ù.TU-*ma* MIN-*ma ši-li* DIRI . . . (Šumma Izbu IV 21 [Leichty, *Izbu* 28])

**[If a woman] gives birth and from the beginning it is full of pockmarks (*šīlu*) . . .

17.156 [BE MUNUS Ù].TU-*ma* MIN-*ma bu-bu-ʾ-tum ma-li* . . . (Šumma Izbu IV 7 [Leichty, *Izbu* 66])

**[If a woman] ⸢gives birth⸣ and from the beginning it is full of *bubuʾtu* (vesicles; see Chapter 10) . . .

BUʾŠĀNU

Buʾšānu appears to have been a syndrome involving the mouth and pharynx that included *Herpes simplex* virus infection, Vincent's angina, and diphtheria (see Chapter 3). The *buʾšānu* references with infants are somewhat vague, but not incompatible with one or more of these diseases. The second text below states that the infant's cry is stifled, suggesting laryngeal (vocal cord) involvement. Laryngeal diphtheria would be one possible cause.

17.157 DIŠ LÚ.TUR ŠÀ.MEŠ-*šú eb-ṭú u* KA-*šú ka-bit bu-ʾ-šá-nu* DIB-*su* / DIŠ LÚ.TUR *il-la-tu-šú* DU.MEŠ-*ka bu-ʾ-šá-nu* DIB-*su* / DIŠ LÚ.TUR *il-la-tu-šú* MÚD *ú-kal-la bu–ʾ-šá-nu* DIB-*su* / DIŠ LÚ.TUR UGU-*šú* GABA-*su u šá-šal-la-šú* KÚM.MEŠ *bu-ʾ-šá-nu* DIB-*su* / DIŠ LÚ.TUR KÚM *la ḫa-aḫ-ḫaš u* ŠÀ.MEŠ *eb-ṭú bu-ʾ-šá-nu* DIB-*su* (DPS XL A 97–101 = *TDP* 228:97–101; cf. DPS XXXIII:88–91 [AOAT 43.357])

**If an infant's insides are cramped and his mouth (feels) heavy, *buʾšānu* afflicts him. If an infant's spittle continually flows, *buʾšānu* afflicts him. If an infant's spittle contains blood, *buʾšānu* afflicts him. If an infant's head, his breast, and his upper back are feverish, *buʾšānu* afflicts him. If an infant has a lukewarm temperature and his insides are cramped, *buʾšānu* afflicts him.

17.158 DIŠ LÚ.TUR *ik-kil-la-šú e-sír ú-pa-ṭi* NU *i-šu* BI.LU *ṣab-tu-šú* (DPS XL A 114 = *TDP* 230:114)

**If an infant's cry is stifled (but) he does not have nasal discharge, *buʾšānu* afflicts him.

For infantile kala-azar, see 19.319–19.334. For infantile leptospirosis, see 19.335–19.342. For congenital syphilis, see 4.23–4.24.

CHOKING

Inability to breathe because of upper airway obstruction must have been a problem well known even to early humans. In the quote below the infant's pharynx is constricted, leading to anoxia and collapse. We have no information with which to determine the cause but, in childhood, aspiration of a foreign body that blocks the airway is a common cause. Infections that lead to airway obstruction such as diphtheria and hemophilus epiglottitis are discussed in Chapter 3.

17.159 DIŠ LÚ.TUR GÚ.MUR-*su ḫa-niq šá-niš* GUB-*ma ina šu-ba-as-su im-qut* . . . (BM 62376:1–2)

**If an infant's pharynx is constricted and moreover he stands up and then falls down on his seat . . .

A drawing of a LÍL sign on the above tablet suggests that the cause of the problem was a *lilû*-demon. This class of demon, which is discussed in Chapter 12, usually victimized adolescents. However, since the demon in question was recruited from the ghosts of young men who died before being able to have children, it was also known to pester infants as in the following reference.

17.160 DIŠ *a-na* LÚ.TUR LÚ.LÍL.LÁ NU TE-*e* . . . (Farber, *Schlaf* 126:1)

**If (you want) *lilû* not to approach an infant . . .

INFANT COLIC

Many infants have this benign but distressing problem. They have bouts of fussing, crying, fist clenching, and leg flexing, and evidence of abdominal pain. Excessive belching and flatus are common. The cause of the problem is unknown, but the children grow out of it without any residual problems. The following references, which appear in sequence in the diagnostic/prognostic handbook, are likely to be examples of colic.

17.161 DIŠ LÚ.TUR ŠÀ.MEŠ-*šú it-te-nin-mi-ru* IGI^{II}-*šú* DUGUD-*šú* ŠU DINGIR DIN / DIŠ LÚ.TUR ŠÀ.MEŠ-*šú* MÚ.MÚ-*ḫu u ib-ta-nak-ki* ŠU DINGIR DIN / DIŠ LÚ.TUR ŠÀ.MEŠ-*šú* MÚ.MEŠ-*ḫu* ŠU DINGIR DIN / DIŠ LÚ.TUR ŠÀ.MEŠ-*šú it-te-nin-bi-ṭu* ŠU DINGIR DIN (DPS XL A 63–66//B 64–67 = *TDP* 224:63–226:66)

**If an infant's insides are continually colicky (and) his eyes (feel) heavy, "hand" of god; he will get well. If an infant's insides are continually bloated and he continually wails, "hand" of god; he will get well.[128] If an infant's insides are continually bloated, "hand" of god; he will get well. If an infant's insides are continually cramped, "hand" of god; he will get well.

GREEN STOOLS

The text below is prognostic in nature, and indicates that the infant is likely to die. Other than the prognosis, the only information provided is that the infant is crying at the breast (instead of nursing), and that its stools (intestines) contain bile.

17.162 DIŠ LÚ.TUR *ina* UBUR AMA-*šú* ÍR.MEŠ *ir-ru-šú* ZÉ *ú-kal-lu* BA.ÚŠ (DPS XL A 102 = *TDP* 228:102)

**If an infant continually wails at the breast of his mother (and) his intestines contain bile, he will die.

The presence of bile in the intestines was undoubtedly determined by green colored stools. What is very interesting is that modern pediatricians make the same association of bile-colored stools and reduced food intake. Food and its byproducts, when mixed with bile, cause the loss of bile's green color. Infants that do not or cannot eat are certainly at risk of death, and this was especially true when intravenous fluids and nutrition were not available.

PERITONITIS

Serious injury to the infant's abdomen and subsequent infection can also result in abdominal pain and distention and eating problems.

17.163 DIŠ LÚ.TUR UBUR ÍL-*šum-ma* NU KÚ ŠÀ.MEŠ-*šú še-eb-r*[*u*] (DPS XL B 74 = *TDP* 226:73)[129]

**If you raise the breast to an infant and he will not eat, his insides ⸢have been seriously injured⸣.[130]

In contrast to infant colic, peritonitis would have been fatal. The *āšipu* seems to have used a water test to determine the diagnosis. As with a similar test for adults,[131] the point seems to have been that an abdomen distended and rigid from peritoneal infection would not have an indentation that could hold water.

17.164 DIŠ LÚ.TUR *it-ta-na-as-la-ʾ-ma* A.MEŠ *ana* UGU ŠÀ-*šú* DUB-*ak-ma* ŠÀ-*šú la ú-šel-la-a* ŠÀ-*šú še-bir* (DPS XL A 13 = *TDP* 218:13)

**If an infant is continually ill and (if) you pour water onto his abdomen, it does not pool[132] in his abdomen, his abdomen has been seriously injured.[133]

BED WETTING (ENURESIS)

Bed wetting (enuresis) is a problem of childhood. Emotional disturbances can delay the child's ability to achieve this control. This topic has been covered in Chapter 5.

NIGHTMARES

This phenomenon is so common in children that it is hard to consider it an abnormality. However, it is more frequent and disturbing when the child is under excessive stress.

17.165 DIŠ LÚ.TUR *ina* KI.NÁ-*šú ina* NU ZU-*ú is-si-ma* ŠU ^{d}*Iš-tar* (DPS XL A 112 = *TDP* 230:112; cf. K 3628+4009 obv. 6′)

**If a young child screams in his bed without knowing (it), "hand" of Ištar.

17.166 DIŠ LÚ.TUR *ina* KI.NÁ-*šú is-si-ma mim-ma šá i-mu-ru i-qab-bi* ŠU ^{d}15 *ik-ri-bu* DIB.ME-*šú* (DPS XL A 113 = *TDP* 230:113; cf. K 3628+4009 obv. 7′)

**If a young child screams in his bed and says whatever he sees, "hand" of Ištar; (unfulfilled) vows afflict him.

FISTED THUMB

The text below provides some interesting clues that suggest a diagnosis. The infant's thumb that "turns inward" appears to be describing an important pediatric neurologic sign called "fisting" or "fisted" thumb. This means that the infant makes a fist with his or her fingers wrapped around the thumb. A "fisted" thumb is a typical sign of a child with cerebral hypotonia, a large group of different diseases that are characterized by severe neurologic damage and reduced muscle tone. These patients are so severely involved that survival even in modern times is unlikely, with death resulting from poor nutrition and wasting. The significance of the infants' laughing is not clear.[134]

17.167 DIŠ LÚ.TUR ŠU.SI-*šú* GAL-*tum* <*ana*> ŠÀ-*šú*/ŠÀ ŠU^{II}-*šú tur-rat u ma-diš iṣ-ṣe-né-eḫ* UZU.MEŠ-*šú mur-ṣa i-šu-ú šiḫ-ḫat* UZU TUKU-*ši ina* ŠÀ-*bi* ÚŠ (DPS XL A 62//B 62–63 = *TDP* 224:62)

**If an infant's thumb is turned inward (var. B: toward his hands)[135] and he laughs a great deal, his flesh has a sick (look and) he has wasting away of the flesh, he will die of it.

SHORT INTESTINES

Infants may be born with intestines that are shorter than normal. If the bowel length is too short, the child will have inadequate absorption of nutrients, and is likely to die. The reference above describes this condition, which must have been diagnosed after death by an autopsy.

17.168 BE MUNUS Ù.TU-*ma ir-ru-šú i-ṣu* . . . (Šumma Izbu III 66 [Leichty, *Izbu* 61])

**If a woman gives birth and (the child)'s intestines are (too) few . . .

Summary

The *āšipu* appears to have been as concerned with the care of infants and children as he was with adults. He understood common, benign childhood problems such as teething and colic, as well as serious and life-threatening infections. Congenital anomalies were also described. The omen texts (Šumma Izbu) provide a richer source of information on congenital abnormalities; however, this material appears less reliable than the medical texts.

CHAPTER 18

Dental and Oral Diseases

(If) a tooth worm eats (a person's tooth) . . .

—*STT* 279:14

Many of the conditions that manifest oral signs or symptoms are complex and often systemic diseases. In these cases, the references and associated discussions are included in other chapters, but are cross-referenced here. Toothache, however, is a focal problem which can reach a level of intensity that totally absorbs the patient's mind and demands attention. The quotes below make it clear that ancient Mesopotamians had their share of toothaches.

Teeth and Gums

In ancient Mesopotamia there were no dentists or health care workers devoted exclusively to dental care. Certainly drilling and filling teeth would not have been possible. It is probable that, as in the Middle East today, people chewed on branches of the "toothbrush tree" (*Salvadora persica*) to freshen the breath and keep their teeth "shining" (see below). The *āšipu* also had a plant with which he could clean patient's teeth.

18.1 ^{Ú}*mar-gu-ṣu* Ú ZÚ.ZÚ *ka-pa-ri* NU *pa-tan* ZÚ.MEŠ-*šú ta-kap-par* (*BAM* 1 i 15//*CT* 14.23 [K 259]:16; cf. *CTN* 4.194:10).

***Marguṣu*, plant to wipe the teeth clean. You wipe his teeth clean (in the morning) before he has eaten.

There is no direct evidence that rotten, abscessed, or loose teeth were pulled[1] by the *āšipu* or *asû*, but there is a reference (18.15 below) that suggest that pulling of teeth occurred. The *āšipu* did observe and describe abnormalities of teeth and the surrounding gums.

PAIN

Dental pain was listed in some texts, but in general the cause of the pain is not clear. Dental caries (cavities) leading to a dental apical abscess were probably a common cause.[2]

18.2 DIŠ NA ZÚ-*šú* KÚ [. . .] (*BAM* 538 i 28)

**If a person's tooth hurts [. . .]

18.3 DIŠ ZÚ-*šú* KÚ-*š*[*ú*] *u* ÚḪ-*su* ŠUB-*di* [. . .] (DPS VI A r. 4//B_1 r. 1+B_2 r. 5 = *TDP* 60 r. 35′)

**If his tooth hurts ⌜him⌝ and he lets his spittle fall, [. . .].

18.4 DIŠ NA ZÚ.MEŠ-*šú i-saḫ-ḫa-la-šú ana* TI-*šú* . . . (*BAM* 26:1–2)

**If a person's teeth give him a piercing pain, to cure him . . .

18.5 DIŠ NA ZÚ.MEŠ-*šú* GIG . . . (*BAM* 538 i 1, iv 50′; *BAM* 543 iv 60b)[3]

**If a person's teeth are sore . . .

LOOSE TEETH

Teeth loosen mainly by three mechanisms: (1) the primary (milk) teeth of children normally loosen as the second teeth begin to erupt; (2) periodontitis is a chronic infection of the gums and the tissues surrounding the tooth socket; as the infection progresses, the bone in the tooth socket resorbs, and eventually the tooth loosens and falls out;[4] (3) trauma can loosen or remove teeth. Loose or weak teeth are described in the references below which are likely to be due to periodontitis. Red and bleeding gums are mentioned, common signs of this condition. There is no mention of trauma, and it seems unlikely that the physicans were describing the loss of primary teeth.

18.6 DIŠ NA *gi-mir* ZÚ.MEŠ-*šú i-na-áš u ri-šu-tú* TUKU-*ši* . . . (*BAM* 159 v 10–11//*BAM* 543 i 1; *BAM* 538 iv 50′)[5]

**If all of a person's teeth move and (the gums) have redness . . .

18.7 DIŠ NA ZÚ.MEŠ-*šú nu-uš-šá-ma* MÚD *i-ḫi-il-la ana* TI-*šú* . . . (*STT* 279:1//*BAM* 543 i 17)

**If a person's teeth move and ooze blood, to cure him . . .

18.8 DIŠ NA ZÚ.MEŠ-*šú en-šá lu* MÚD *i-ḫi-il-la* [. . .] MÚD *i-ḫa-al ana* TI-*šú* . . . (*BAM* 543 i 13–14)

**If a person's teeth are wobbly or ooze blood [. . .] oozes blood, to cure him . . .

18.9 Ú ZÚ.MEŠ *un-nu-šá-ti* . . . (*BAM* 1 i 11; *CT* 14.23 [K 259]:12–15; *CTN* 4.194:9)[6]

**Plant for wobbly teeth . . .

18.10 ZU.LÚM.MA NU KÚ ZÚ.MEŠ-*šú i-nu-uš-ša* (Labat, *Hémérologies* 124:41–42, 170:38; ND 5545:22 [Hulin, *Iraq* 21.46–53])

**He should not eat dates (or) his teeth will become wobbly.

There is a less common cause of loose teeth and bleeding gums, namely, scurvy.[7] Scurvy is due to vitamin C deficiency; it used to be common among sailors on long voyages and may also have occurred in ancient Mesopotamia (see Chapter 7 with 17.19–17.20).

CARIES

Bacteria can attach to the dental surface and multiply, especially if the individual eats a lot of sweet, sugared food. The sugar permits the bacteria to multiply and form plaque on the tooth surface. The acids produced by the bacteria will eventually erode the tooth and can cause the tooth to rot away.

The references below use the word *tultu.* Lexical texts equate this term on one hand with the Sumerograms ZÚ.MUŠ ("tooth snake") or MUR.DÚR.RA (a type of worm) and on the other with the Sumerogram TÚL ("well" or "excavation in the form of a truncated pyramid"). The *āšipu,* presented with a badly decayed tooth with only a rim of tooth structure intact and a deep, rotted center, seems to have observed that the cavity becomes larger as it deepens, like the excavations made by human ditch diggers, and to have concluded from this that the hole in question was produced by an invisible worm eating away at the tooth.

18.11 MIN (DIŠ NA ZÚ-*šú*) *tul-tú* KÚ . . . (*STT* 279:14)

**(If) a tooth worm eats (a person's tooth) . . .

18.12 6,40 *a-wi-lum ši-in-na-šu tu-ul-tum* . . . (*BAM* 393 obv. 8, r. 9)

**If a man's tooth has a tooth worm . . .

18.13 Ú *tul-te* . . . (*BAM* 1 i 7; *CT* 14.23 [K 259]:7)

**Plant for the tooth worm . . .

18.14 *i-na mu-úḫ-ḫi ši-in-ni ša tu-⌜ul-tim ta-ša-ak-ka-an⌝* (*YOS* 11.29:22)[8]

**You put it on the tooth that has a tooth worm.

There is a picturesque recitation that explains how the "tooth worm" developed its rather peculiar diet. Particularly interesting is the statement that, besides sucking the blood of the tooth, the "tooth worm" was feeding on the food particles left in the mouth after eating. The reference to "driving in a peg" and "getting hold of the foot" is somewhat obscure but might have been preliminary to extraction of the rotten tooth.[9]

18.15 *ul-tu* ^{d}*A-nu-um* [*ib-nu-ú* AN-*ú*] AN-*ú ib-nu-ú* [*er-ṣe-tam*] *er-ṣe-tum ib-nu-ú* ÍD.MEŠ ÍD.MEŠ *ib-na-a a-tap-pa-ti a-tap-pa-ti ib-na-a ru-šum-ta ru-šum-ta ib-nu-ú tu-ul-tu il-lik tu-ul-tu ana* IGI ^{d}UTU *i-bak-ki ana* IGI ^{d}*É-a il-la-ka di-ma-ta-ta mi-na-a ta-at-ta-an-na a-na a-ka-li-ia mi-na-a ta-at-ta-an-na a-na mun-zu-qí-ia at-tan-nak-ki* ^{GIŠ}PÈŠ *ba-ši-il-ta ar-ma-na-a* ^{GIŠ}ḪAŠḪUR *ana-ku am-mi-na-an-na-a* ^{GIŠ}PÈŠ *ba-ši-il-ta ù ar-ma-na-a* ^{GIŠ}ḪAŠḪUR *šu-uk-na-an-ni-ma ina bi-rit ši-in-ni ù la-áš-ḫi šu-ši-ba-an-ni ša ši-in-ni-ma lu-uz-zu-qa da-mi-šu ù ša la-áš-ḫi-«ši»-im lu-uk-su-u*[*s*] *ku-sa-se-e-šu sik-ka-ta ri-te-ma* GÌR *ṣa-ba-at aš-šum an-na-a taq-bi-i tu-ul-tu lim-ḫa-aṣ-ki* ^{d}*É-a i-na dan-na-ti ri-it-ti-šu* / KA.INIM.MA ZÚ.GIG.GA.KÁM . . . (*CT* 17.50:1–24//*AMT* 23/6:1′–6′//*BAM* 538 iv 31′–37′)

**When (the sky-god) Anu [created the heavens], the heavens created [the earth]. The earth created the rivers, the rivers created the branch canals. The branch canals created the dampness, the dampness created the tooth worm. The tooth worm came, crying, before Šamaš (god of justice); before Ea (god of wisdom) his tears flowed. "What will you give for me to eat? What will you give for me to suck?" "I will give you the ripe fig (and) the apricot." "What would I want with the ripe fig or the apricot? Put me among the teeth and set me in the jaw so that I may suck the blood of the tooth and chew up the chewed up (food particles collected) in the jaw." Drive in a peg and so get hold of the foot (of the tooth). Because you said (all this), O tooth worm, may Ea strike you with his mighty hand. — Recitation for "sick tooth" . . .

The text below appears to connect the tooth worm (dental cavities) to *buʾšānu*. In fact, there is a close association between tooth decay, poor dental hygiene, and Vincent's angina, one of the forms of *buʾšānu* (see Chapter 3).

18.16 ÉN ^{d}*A-nu-ma* ^{d}*A-nu* ^{d}*A-nu pu-ḫur* AN-*e* ^{d}*A-nu pu-ḫur* KI-*ti* KI-*tum ib-ta-ni t*[*ul-tum*] *tul-tum ib-ta-ni bu-ʾ-šá-nu šá bu-ʾ-šá-ni* KAL-*an* DIB-*su* GIN_7 UR.MAḪ *nap-šá-tú i-*[. . .] *ki-ma* UR.BAR.RA *iṣ-ṣa-bat lu-ʾ-a iṣ-bat ap-pu nu-ru-ub ap-*[*pi iṣ-bat*] UZU.ḪAR *ina bi-rit* ZÚ.MEŠ *na-da-at* ^{GIŠ}GU.ZA-*šú* (*BAM* 538 ii 52′–55′)

**Only Anu is Anu. Anu is the entire heavens; Anu is the entire earth. The earth created the ⌜tooth worm⌝; the tooth worm created *buʾšānu*. Mighty is the affliction of *buʾšānu*. It [. . .] the breath like a lion; it seized the throat like a wolf. It seized the nose, the mucus from the ⌜nose⌝; [it seized] the lungs. It set up its throne among the teeth.[10]

TOOTH LOSS

The quotes below describe teeth falling out. This problem is most likely due to periodontitis, as described above. Teeth with caries rot away and eventually disappear, but without a simultaneous periodontitis they are not likely to fall out.

18.17 MIN (DIŠ NA ZÚ-*šú*) *na-da-at* . . . (*STT* 279:12)

**(If a person's tooth) is falling out . . .

18.18 Ú ZÚ ŠUB-*te* . . . (*BAM* 1 i 8, 9, 10; *CT* 14.23 [K 259]:8–10)

**Plant for a tooth falling out . . .

TOOTH COLOR

Teeth were described as yellow, dark, and shining. The yellow color could be due to dental plaque and poor dental hygiene. Pangas[11] suggests another possible explanation for yellow teeth, namely, fluorosis due to excess fluoride in drinking water. Studies of skeletal remains from ancient Bahrain show that this condition was common there.[12] Tetracycline has been found in the bones of pre-antibiotic skeletons throughout the Near East. Since the fungus that produces tetracycline is present in the soil, it has been postulated that bread and beer made from grain grown in tetracycline-rich soil came to contain this antibiotic.[13] Tetracycline is known to adhere to both bone and teeth, and could also have caused the yellow teeth described below. Dark or black teeth can develop when the tooth has lost its nerve supply secondary to trauma or decay. Finally, the reference to shining teeth that predict recovery may constitute a good prognosis because the patient is well enough to maintain good dental hygiene.

18.19 DIŠ NA ZÚ.MEŠ-*šú* SIG_7 ŠUB-*a* KIR_4/KA-*šú* [. . .] (*BAM* 543 i 26)

**If a person's teeth are colored with yellow, his nose/mouth [. . .]

18.20 DIŠ ZÚ.MEŠ-*šú tar-k*[*a*] GIG-*su* GÍD.DA (DPS VI A r. 7a//B_1 r. 3+B_2 r. 8 = *TDP* 60 r. 38′a)[14]

**If his teeth are dark, his illness will be prolonged.

18.21 DIŠ ZÚ.MEŠ-*šú nam-*[*ra*] DIN DPS VI A r. 5a = *TDP* 60 r. 36′a)[15]

**If his teeth ⌜shine⌝, he will get well.

TEETH GRINDING (BRUXISM)

Teeth grinding is a common sign of emotional tension and disturbance. It can occur when the individual is awake or asleep. The first reference below demonstrates that the *āšipu* understood the role of emotional disturbance in causing the problem.

18.22 [DIŠ LÚ] *i-na ṣa-la-li-šu ši-*[*i*] *n-*[*ni-šu*] *i-ka-ṣa-aṣ* [*i-na*] *-an-zi-iq* (Köcher and Oppenheim, *AfO* 18.64 i 41–42 [physiognomic omens])

** [If a person] grinds his ⌜teeth⌝ in his sleep, [he is] worried.

18.23 NA_4.MEŠ DIŠ NA ZÚ.MEŠ-*šú i-ka-ṣa-ṣa* . . . (*BAM* 372 iii 5′)[16]

**Stones for cases where a person gnashes his teeth . . .

18.24 KA.INIM.MA DIŠ NA ZÚ.MEŠ-*šú i-kaṣ-ṣa-aṣ* . . . (*BAM* 30:8′)

**Recitation (for cases where) a person gnashes his teeth . . .

18.25 DIŠ [N]A [*ina*] K[I.NÁ]-*šú* ZÚ.MEŠ-*šú* GÙRUŠ-*aṣ* . . . (*BAM* 311:87′)

**If a ⌜man⌝ [in] his ⌜bed⌝ gnashes his teeth . . .

18.26 DIŠ NA *ina i-tu-li-šú* ZÚ.MEŠ-*šú i-gaṣ-ṣa-aṣ* . . . (*BAM* 30:47′–48′//*BAM* 157 obv. 6′)

**If a person when he lies down to sleep gnashes his teeth . . .

Bruxism can be so severe that it becomes audible, and can be a source of annoyance to others. It can also occur during seizures and other conditions that cause muscle spasms such as tetanus.[17]

18.27 DIŠ ZÚ.MEŠ-*šú* ZÚ.GUZ $ŠU^{II}$-*šú u* $GÌR^{II}$-*šú ú-n*[*a-aš* ŠU] $^{d}30$ GAM (DPS VI A r. 12//B_1 r. 9+B_2 r. 13 = *TDP* 60 r. 43′; cf. StBoT 36.40 obv. 7′)

**If he gnashes his teeth (and) he ⌜moves⌝ his hands and feet (spasmodically), ["hand"] of Sîn; he will die.

Lips

SWOLLEN LIPS

One common cause of swollen lips is an allergic reaction. Another less likely explanation is angioneurotic edema, a rare inherited abnormality of the complement immune system. For further discussion, see Chapter 8 with 8.91. Trauma can also cause swollen lips, as is described below.

18.28 DIŠ NA NUNDUN.MEŠ-*šú ku-*[*bu-ra*] . . . DIŠ KI.MIN NUNDUN-*su ḫe-pa-at* . . . (*BAM* 543 i 51′, 55′)

**If a person's lips are ⌜thickened⌝ . . . If (a person's lips are thickened and) his lip was broken . . .

GLAZED LIPS

The two texts below describe patients who are very sick and ultimately die. Although not enough information is available to establish the primary disease with confidence, liver disease (see Chapter 6) is a possibility. Part of the clinical description is the observation that the patient's lips have a glaze. The cause of the glaze may be dried saliva or vomitus that a very weak or unconscious patient cannot wipe off.

Another less likely explanation is that the glaze is uremic frost. Patients with advanced renal failure may deposit urea on their skin, especially the face. The urea looks like a fine white powder on the surface of the skin.

18.29 DIŠ IGI.MEŠ-*šú* IM.GÁ.LI ŠUB-*ú* NUNDUN.MEŠ-*šú ši-ši-tú* DIRI.MEŠ IGI^{II}-*šú* SIG$_7$ ŠUB.ŠUB-*a u* IGI-*šú šá* 15 *i-ṣa-par* GAM (DPS IX A 29//B obv. 27–28 = *TDP* 74:29)

**If his face is unevenly colored with *kalû*-clay (light) yellow, his lips are full of glaze,[18] his eyes are continually colored with yellow, (and) his left eye flutters, he will die.

18.30 DIŠ IGI.MEŠ-*šú* BABBAR *u* SIG$_7$ ŠUB.ŠUB-*ú* KA-*šú* NUNDUN.ME-*šú ši-ši-tu* IGI-*šú šá* 150 *i-ṣap-par* GAM (DPS IX A 8–9 = *TDP* 72:8–9)

**If his face is unevenly colored with white and yellow, his mouth (and) his lips (have) a glaze, and his right eye flutters, he will die.

Tongue

PAIN

A painful tongue was described, but not enough information is available in the first reference to identify the cause. The pain in the second reference would seem from context to be due to trauma. If the patient cannot return his tongue to his mouth, it must be extremely swollen.

18.31 DIŠ NA EME-*šú* GIG . . . (*SpTU* 2.50:25)

**If a person's tongue is sore . . .

18.32 DIŠ EME-*šú* GI_6-*at ina* KA-*šú* S[ÌG-*iṣ* . . .] / DIŠ EME-*šú la ú-tar-ra ina* [. . .] / DIŠ EME-*šú* KÚ-*šú u* ÚḪ-*s*[*u* ŠUB . . .] (DPS VII A obv. 23–25 = *TDP* 62:23–25)

**If his tongue is black, he was ⌜wounded⌝ on his mouth [. . .]. If he cannot return his tongue to [his mouth . . .]. If his tongue hurts him and [he lets] his spittle [fall] [. . .]

ENLARGED TONGUE (MACROGLOSSIA)

Enlargement of the tongue can be caused by a number of diseases, including cancer and amyloidosis, a disease where an abnormal protein, amyloid, infiltrates and swells the tissues. The text below describes a patient with tongue enlargement,[19] but with insufficient information to determine the etiology.

18.33 DIŠ NA EME-*šú eb-ṭe-et-ma* KA-*šú* DIRI-*at* . . . (*SpTU* 1.46:1//*BAM* 543 i 49′; *SpTU* 1.44:84)

**If a person's tongue is cramped (enlarged) so that it fills his mouth . . .

ENLARGED TONGUE WITH MENTAL RETARDATION The text below refers to a patient with a tongue "hanging out" and some type of mental disorder, possibly mental retardation. Modern pediatricians recognize at least four conditions that have large tongues (macroglossia) and mental retardation, namely, Down syndrome, cretinism (childhood hypothyroidism due to iodine deficiency), Hurler's syndrome, and gangliosidosis. Certainly, patients with Down syndrome and cretinism frequently allow their tongues to hang out. It is likely that patients with enlarged tongues due to other causes also let their tongues hang out, but the evidence to support this is less solid. Down syndrome must have occurred in ancient Mesopotamia, and cretinism, since it is common in modern Iraq, was probably seen as well. Hurler's syndrome and gangliosidosis are rare genetic diseases.

18.34 DIŠ EME-*šú i-tál-lal u* $UŠ_4$-*šú* NU DIB [. . .] (DPS VII A 22 = *TDP* 62:22)

**If his tongue hangs out and he is not in full possession of his faculties [. . .].

TONGUE THAT HANGS OUT The following reference immediately precedes the text that we have been discussing and was presumably meant to contrast with it (see Introduction). This text also refers to a patient's tongue "hanging out" but in this case it is only a temporary condition, caused by shortness of breath (panting). When the fever resolves, the tongue will presumably no longer hang out.

18.35 DIŠ EME-*šú i-tal-lal* GIG-*su* TAK_4-*šum-ma* [. . .] (DPS VII A obv. 21 = *TDP* 62:21)

**If his tongue hangs out, his illness is leaving him [. . .].

SHRIVELING

We suggest dehydration as the cause of the shriveled tongue in the first reference, especially given the upper abdominal complaints. See Chapter 3 for a discussion of infectious diarrhea and dehydration.

18.36 [DIŠ SA] G ŠÀ-*šú* DIB.DIB-*su u* EME-*šú ḫe-em-ret ana* KI GIG GAM (DPS XIII B i 8′ = *TDP* 110:12′)

**[If] his ⌜upper abdomen (epigastrium)⌝ continually afflicts him and his tongue is shriveled, he is at an acute stage[20] of the illness; he will die.

18.37 DIŠ KI.MIN-*ma* SAG ŠÀ-*šú* GI$_6$-*ma* EME-*šú ḫe-em-ret ana* GIZKIM GIG GAM (DPS XV:33 [AOAT 43.152]; cf. DPS XIII A 2)

**If (it is the first day he is sick) and his upper abdomen (epigastrium) is dark and his tongue is shriveled, he is at an acute stage[21] of the illness, he will die.

TONGUE COLOR

The references below list tongue colors of red, white, black or dark, and yellow.

WHITE

18.38 DIŠ SAG.KI-*su* BABBAR EME BABBAR GIG-*su* GÍD.DA-*ma* DIN (DPS IV B r. 23 = *TDP* 44 r.46)

**If his forehead is white (and) the tongue is white, his illness may be prolonged (but) he will get well.

The white tongue might have this color because of severe anemia. A superficial fungal infection (*Candida albicans*; monilia) can coat the tongue, giving it a white appearance. This infection usually occurs in patients with severe immune or metabolic abnormalities.

RED The red tongue is probably the result of normal levels of red blood cells and blood oxygen, and therefore should be associated with a good prognosis.

18.39 DIŠ GIG EME-*šú* SA$_5$-*át* DIN (*SpTU* 1.32 r. 14)

**If the patient's tongue is red, he will get well.

18.40 DIŠ IGI.MEŠ-*šú šal-mu* EME-*šú* SA$_5$ GIG-*su* GÍD-*ma* DIN-*uṭ* (DPS IX A 40//B obv. 39 = *TDP* 74:40)

**If his face is healthy (and) his tongue is red, his illness may be prolonged (but) he will get well.

YELLOW

18.41 DIŠ IGI.MEŠ-*šú* KÚR.KÚR-*ru* EME-*šú* SIG$_7$: SU-*šú* SIG$_7$ TÙN.GIG *ana* U$_4$.3.KÁM GAM (DPS IX A 31 = *TDP* 74:31)

**If his face continually alters (and) his tongue is yellow (var. his body is yellow), TÙN.GIG ("sick liver"); (if he has been sick) for three days, he will die.

The yellow tongue represents the jaundice that affects all parts of the body with circulating blood vessels.

BLACK/DARK The text below mentions a black tongue and a mouth wound. The black color in this case probably represents bleeding into the tissues of the tongue secondary to the trauma. The blood as it degrades in the tissues takes on a brown or black color.

18.42 DIŠ EME-*šú* GI$_6$-*at ina* KA-*šú* S[ÌG-*iṣ* . . .] (DPS VII A obv. 23 = *TDP* 62:23)

**If his tongue is black, he was ⸢wounded⸣ in his mouth [. . .]

Mouth

LUDWIG'S ANGINA

Infections of the mouth, especially abscessed teeth, can lead to infection of the floor of the mouth. With swelling in this area, the tongue is pushed upward and backward and there is swelling below the jaw. Pain, redness, and heat are present, and the patient has difficulty speaking, eating, and eventually breathing. Death from airway obstruction and/or overwhelming infection would be common without antibiotics and modern surgery to maintain an open airway. The text below is almost certainly an example of this condition.

18.43 DIŠ LÚ ⸢KA-*šú*⸣ MAŠKIM DIB-*it-ma*[22] KA.DIB.BI.DA TUKU.MEŠ-*ši* [EM]E?-*šú e-bíṭ na-piš* KA-*šú* DUGUD-*it* ÚḪ.MEŠ-*šú* DU.MEŠ-*ma la* TAR.MEŠ [Z]Ú.MEŠ-*šú* SIG.MEŠ-*šú ù da-mu i-ḫi-la* . . . (*BAM* 533:1–3//*BAM* 28 obv. 1–3)

**If a *rābiṣu* seizes a person's mouth so that he continually has inability to talk, his ⸢tongue⸣ is cramped, his breathing is difficult, his saliva flows and will not stop, his ⸢teeth⸣ are weak and ooze blood . . .

PAIN

In the texts below, there is mention of mouth soreness, but no signs or symptoms are available to identify the cause. Infections caused by bacteria, viruses, and occasionally fungi are the most common causes of mouth pain. References that describe these illnesses can be found in the infectious diseases chapter (Chapter 3 with, e.g., 3.64–3.70).

18.44 DIŠ [K]A-*šú* KÚ-*šú u* ÚḪ-*su* ŠUB-*di* x [. . .] (DPS VII B obv. 5′ = *TDP* 64:44′)[23]

**If his ⸢mouth⸣[24] hurts him and he lets his spittle fall . . .

18.45 ⸢*šum-ma* LÚ *pí-šu*⸣ *ḫa-mi-iṭ* . . . (*YOS* 11.28:1)

**If a person's mouth burns . . .

RED/BLACK MOUTH

In the text below, a red mouth gives a good prognosis, while a black mouth predicts the death of the patient. It seems likely that the color reflects the level of oxygenation of the patient's blood. If the patient is breathing and absorbing oxygen, the tissues of the mouth will be red, but failure to absorb adequate oxygen levels will cause the mouth to appear "black" (dark blue/cyanotic). In patients with heavy skin pigmentation, the color of tissue in the mouth would be an important site to evaluate color changes as determined by oxygenation.

18.46 DIŠ KA-*šú* SA_5 DIN : DIŠ KA-[*šú*...] / DIŠ KA-*šú* GI_6 GAM / DIŠ KA-*šú* [...] DPS VII A obv. 27–28 = *TDP* 62:27–28)

**If his mouth is red, he will get well. If [his] mouth is [...]. If his mouth is black, he will die. If his mouth is [...]

BUʾŠĀNU

The term *buʾšānu* appears to refer to at least three different infections involving the mouth and pharynx: diphtheria, *Herpes simplex* type 1, and Vincent's angina. Cases of infectious mononucleosis and scurvy may also have been included. A discussion of *buʾšānu* is found in Chapter 3.

DROOLING

Drooling commonly occurs in patients, especially children, with severe mouth or pharyngeal pain on swallowing, making the patient reluctant to swallow saliva. Below is a quote of a patient with *bubuʾtu* (water blisters) in the mouth, probably caused by *Herpes simplex* type 1 (HSV1), a very painful condition.

18.47 DIŠ KA-*šú* U_4.BU.BU.UL DIRI *u il-la-tu-šú* [DU-*ka*...] (DPS VII B obv. 4′ = *TDP* 64:43′; cf. DPS XXXIII:87 [AOAT 43.357])

**If a person's mouth is full of *bubuʾtu* and his saliva [flows, *buʾšānu*].

Patients undergoing a grand mal seizure are also likely to drool (see Chapter 13).

SEIZED MOUTH (STUTTERING)

The text below refers to a "seized" mouth that causes a problem with saying a particular word, *annu* (yes). Stuttering is a common problem in speech development that may be triggered by certain words or sounds.

18.48 DIŠ [K]A-*šú* DIB.DIB-*ma an-na ma-gal la ip-pal-lum ana* DINGIR x [...] (DPS VII B obv. 3′ = *TDP* 64:42′)

**If his ⸢mouth⸣ is continually "seized" so that he cannot frequently answer: *annu* (yes), [he has...] to a god.

Summary

Although many of the problems localized to the teeth and mouth are not life-threatening, they can interfere with eating and speech, and cause the patient much distress. The *āšipu* must have been called upon to diagnose and treat these conditions. The tooth worm was a creative device to explain how a solid tooth could be invaded and destroyed. The success of the *āšipu* in treating this and other oral conditions is as yet unclear, but there are numerous texts that document his treatment efforts.

CHAPTER 19

Ancient Etiologies: The Naming of Disease Patterns

This chapter will explore the approaches used by ancient Mesopotamian physicians to identify and name syndromes or patterns of disease (ancient etiologies). Although ancient Mesopotamian medicine was remarkable for its foundation in prior observations, the *āšipu* was still an intellectual. He was expected to be well versed in the scribal arts, Sumerian, classics of literature, and a wide variety of "magical" rituals in addition to the forty tablets of the diagnostic/prognostic handbook and innumerable therapeutic texts. Moreover, like intellectuals everywhere, it was not possible for him to approach a medical problem without bringing to it a bit of preconceived theory. This is particularly noticeable in his determination to see significance in right/left variations in signs or symptoms (see Introduction). The *āšipu* was also predisposed to explain illness in terms of the influence ("hands") of the various gods/goddesses, ghosts, demons/demonesses, and demonic forces such as curses and sorcery that populated his spirit world.

In part, this was simply his way of dealing with broad categories of disease such as mental illness, neurologic conditions, arthritis, skin diseases, heart and circulatory problems, illness due to trauma, and fevers. Ancient Mesopotamian religion was polytheistic, with many gods/goddesses already present and the possibility, by divination, of establishing new gods/goddesses at will. Thus, his religion provided the *āšipu* with a relatively flexible system for the assignment of diseases to causal agents.

If the *āšipu* so desired, there were methods of divination that could have been used to assign his patients' medical problems to "hands" of gods/goddesses or demons/demonesses in a perfectly arbitrary fashion. What is interesting, therefore, is the apparent reluctance of the *āšipu* to allow his theories to run roughshod over observed realities. He seems not infrequently to have been unhappy with the attribution of specific problems to *any* of the spirits or demonic forces known to him.[1] In some of these cases where known gods/goddesses or demons/demonesses were not invoked as causal agents, associations were made with anatomic areas. If diagnosis by this method did not seem appropriate, a set or several sets of connected symptoms might be given a name that referred to some characteristic of the disease (see below under Specially Named Syndromes). Some of these specially named syndromes evolved, over time, into demonic forces in their own right (see below under Named Syndromes That Evolved into Demons).

As a rule, syndromes identified by the *āšipu* as "sick *x* or *y* body part" or by a syndrome name are much easier for the modern observer to puzzle out than those attributed to "hands" of ancient Mesopotamian gods/goddesses or demons/demonesses. However, with some syndromes attributed to divine or demonic "hands," we may not be able to identify every individual reference, but the organizing principle that inspired grouping all of the attested references under one diagnosis is still relatively clear (see below under Clearly Organized Syndromes Attributed to Divine or Demonic "Hands"). An interesting example is a set of diagnoses that seems collectively to have been the ancient equivalent of our category of "unknown etiology" (see below under Ill-defined Syndromes of the Sort Gods/Goddesses Might Cause and Mystery Syndromes).

At least in part, "hands" are more difficult to pin down to a single disease or set of related syndromes. As an intellectual, the *āšipu* will have been inclined to try to make things uncomplicated and with the fewest number of causal agents possible. Also, at least in theory, there should have been a tendency for independent-minded gods and demons to cause a variety of different problems. Even so, with some of the better-attested gods/goddesses and demons/demonesses, reasons logical, exegetical, or theological can still be found to explain why at least some of the syndromes were attributed to that particular god/goddess or demon/demoness (see below under Syndromes Assigned in Accordance with Known Predilections of Specific Gods/Goddesses or Demons/Demonesses).

Part of the difficulty in puzzling out the godly and demonic "hands" is that there are many gods/goddesses or demons/demonesses that have only one or two associated references or who are given as causal agents for syndromes that we have been unable to identify (see below under Problem Syndromes Due to Insufficient Information). It is always possible that our inability to identify syndromes attributed to divine or demonic "hands" is simply due to the fact that the attribution was determined by divination. However, there are enough gods/goddesses where the attributions seem to make sense in modern terms or where reasons can readily be generated for the attribution of specific syndromes to particular divinities to suggest that we should give the ancients the benefit of the doubt and to suppose that if we knew as much about these divinities as the *āšipu*, we would better understand why particular gods/goddesses and demons/demonesses were assigned specific diseases.

Gods/Goddesses of Mental Illnesses

A number of ancient Mesopotamian gods/goddesses and demons/demonesses were given responsibility for causing various forms of what the *āšipu* was first to call "alteration of mentation." Given our own association of madness with the moon ("lunatic"), we might have expected the moon-god, Sîn, to be a major producer of mental symptoms. In fact, in the hot and dry climate of ancient Mesopotamia, an association of bizarre behavior with "having been out in the sun too long" seemed more obvious to the *āšipu*.

ŠAMAŠ

19.1 DIŠ UŠ$_4$-*šú* KÚR.KÚR-*ir-šú* ŠU ^{d}UTU AZAG KÚ (DPS XXII:55a [AOAT 43.256])

**If his mentation continually alters, "hand" of Šamaš; he has violated a taboo.

Šamaš was not only god of the sun but also of justice. As such, he seemed an appropriate deity to punish misbehavior. The type of "alteration of mentation" he caused is spelled out in other references. The specific reason given for the god's anger was the failure of the patient to pay his tithes, which were used to make low-interest loans to the needy.

19.2 DIŠ *ina* GABA-*šú* A *i-sal-lu ù* KA-*šú* KIR$_4$.ŠU.GÁL ŠU ^{d}UTU MU KÙ.BABBAR ZAG.GAR.RA (DPS XII A 5 = *TDP* 100 i 5)

**If he sprinkles water on his breast and makes gestures of supplication, "hand" of Šamaš on account of silver for a tithe.

19.3 DIŠ KÙŠ.MEŠ-*šú ana* SU-*šú* NU TE-*ḫi* ŠU 20 MU KÙ.BABBAR ZAG.GAR.RA (DPS X B r. 15 = *TDP* 88 r. 15)[2]

**If he does not bring his forearms close to his body, "hand" of Šamaš on account of silver for a tithe.

19.4 DIŠ *ki-ṣir* KÙŠ.MEŠ-*šú ana* SAG-*šú* GAR.GAR-*an* ÚḪ.ME-*šú i-s[al-l]u* GIG *na-kam-ti* ŠU.ZAG.GAR.RA DIN (DPS X B r. 18 = *TDP* 88 r. 18)

**If he continually places his elbows on his head (and) he ⌜sprays⌝ his spit, he (has) a sickness of excess(?),[3] "hand" of a tithe; he will get well.

Other forms of aberrant behavior were laid at the door of Šamaš's twin sister, the goddess Ištar.

IŠTAR

Ištar is usually known as a goddess of "love and war." What connects these diverse activities is her true function, which was as a goddess of liminality.[4] Ancient Mesopotamians conceived of the cultural world (including kingship, and male and female roles in society) as governed by a set of defining regulations, or "*me*s." Humans and gods alike were bound by the "*me*s," which were controlled by the goddess Ištar. This was because Ištar was the goddess of boundaries. What makes kings, kings and commoners, commoners and what makes men, men and women, women are the boundaries that define the differences between them. Like the Roman god Janus, who gave his name to our month January, which ends the old year and begins the new, Ištar was the household guardian of the doorpost, the part of the house that marks the transition between the inside and the outside.[5]

However, according to a basic principle of ancient religion, the goddess of boundaries was also the goddess of the transgression of boundaries. At her festivals, men dressed as women and children as old people, in the spirit of carnival, to honor the goddess. Like Hermes, the Greek god associated with boundaries, she acted as psychopomp, sending young men to their deaths on the field of battle (see below 19.150–19.164), and steering the boat that brought human souls up from the netherworld to be born.

She also governed age transitions. Songs about her love for Dumuzi and her reluctance to leave her girlhood haunts were sung at weddings to ease the transition from virgin girl to adult woman, a transition also marked by the menstrual cramping that generated one of her subsyndromes (see under Syndromes Assigned in Accordance with Known Predilections of Specific Gods/Goddesses or Demons/Demonesses). Those who offended the goddess could experience another, less pleasant transition, that from sanity to madness.

19.5 DIŠ SAG.DU-*su* DIB.DIB-*su* GÚ-*su* TAG.TAG-*su* GABA-*su* KÚ.MEŠ-*šú*! ŠÀ-*šú* GAZ.MEŠ-*šú i*[*t-ta-na-ad-là*] *ḫ*[6] K[Ú] *u* N[A]G NU GUR-*ma* KÚ *u* NAG ^{d}15 MU É *er-bet-tim* ÚS.ME-*šú šá-niš ana* MUNUS MU *a-rin u sa-ma-li* [*ana* KI.SIKIL.BÀN.D]A[7] MU *ki-gul-lim áš-tam-mi* (DPS III C obv. 32–33 = *TDP* 20/22:32–33)

**If his head continually afflicts him, his neck continually hurts him intensely, his breast continually hurts him, his heart continually gives him a crushing sensation (and) [is continually troubled], (but) he eats and drinks and it does not return (to his mouth) so that he can eat and drink, Ištar continually pursues him because (he built) a house at the crossroads.[8] For a woman, it is because of well and cup; [for an adolescent girl], it is because of place of mourning(?)[9] and tavern.

If the male victim did indeed build himself a house at a crossroads, he was certainly asking for trouble. Crossroads have in virtually every culture and every time period in history come to be associated with the netherworld. Possibly what was meant was a house with four entrances lined up so as to form a cross; this would effectively have placed the center of the house at a crossroads, thus inadvertently signaling a desire for members of the household to die. The reason for Ištar's anger at the woman and adolescent girl was probably the violation of age taboos. It was most likely the job of girls, not of women, to gad about the well collecting water and of women, not girls, to carry out funerary rites. Unmarried girls in ancient Mesopotamia would certainly have had no business frequenting taverns, which often doubled as places of prostitution (also patronized by the goddess Ištar).

It was the fact that the patient described in the quote above was not vomiting that suggested to the *āšipu* that nothing was seriously wrong with him, but that his problem was Ištar attacking him as also in the following quote, which describes a manic patient (see Chapter 16).

19.6 DIŠ *i-te-ner-ru-ub* TÚG-*su* ŠUB.ŠUB-*di iš-ta-na-su ma-gal* DU[G_4.DUG_4-*ub*] NINDA *u* KAŠ NU GUR-*ma* KÚ *u la i-ṣal-lal* ŠU ^{d}15 GAR ⌜TI⌝ (DPS XXVI:78′–79′ [AOAT 43.285])

**If he keeps beginning to put on and throwing off his garments, he continually cries out(!), he ⌜talks⌝ a lot, bread and beer do not come back up on him so that he can eat but he cannot sleep, "hand" of Ištar has been laid (on him); he will get well.

In addition to mania, Ištar also caused depression and mood swings.

19.7 DIŠ *iṣ-ṣe-né-iḫ* . . . ŠU ᵈ15 (DPS XXII:62 [AOAT 43.256])

**If he continually laughs . . . "hand" of Ištar.

19.8 [. . .] *a-šu-uš-tú* ŠUB.ŠUB-*su* ŠU ᵈINNIN ᵈx[. . .] (*BAM* 584 ii 23′)

**[If . . .] (and) depression continually falls upon him, "hand" of Ištar and [. . .]

19.9 DIŠ *ḫa-di u pa-rid* . . . ŠU ᵈ15 (DPS XXII:63 [AOAT 43.256])

**If he rejoices and is terrified . . . "hand" of Ištar.

Not surprisingly, Ištar afflicted small children with nightmares (see Chapter 17) and plagued adults with visions of ghosts.

19.10 DIŠ LÚ.TUR *ina* KI.NÁ-*šú ina* NU ZU-*ú is-si-ma* ŠU ᵈ*Iš-tar* / DIŠ LÚ.TUR *ina* KI.NÁ-*šú is-si-ma mim-ma šá i-mu-ru i-qab-bi* ŠU ᵈ15 *ik-ri-bu* DIB.ME-*šú* (DPS XL A 112–113 = *TDP* 230:112–113; cf. K 3628+4009 obv. 6′–7′)

**If an infant screams in his bed without realizing (it), "hand" of Ištar. If an infant screams in its bed and says whatever it sees, "hand" of Ištar; (unfulfilled) vows afflict him.

19.11 DIŠ NA ÚŠ.MEŠ IGI.MEŠ ŠU ᵈINNIN *a-na* ÚŠ.MEŠ TAR-*si* . . . (*KAR* 234 obv. 27//*SpTU* 4.134:1)

**If a person continually sees dead persons, "hand" of Ištar; to keep the dead persons away . . .

In the first reference to "hand" of Ištar quoted above (19.5), the patient was afflicted with mysterious pains in the head, neck, and breast and was experiencing chest pain. Ištar also caused headaches alone and chest pain alone, both presumably psychosomatic.

19.12 DIŠ SAG.DU-*su* DIB.DIB-*su u* KÚM NU TUKU ŠU ⸢ᵈ⸣15 (DPS III C obv. 35 = *TDP* 22:35)

**If his head continually afflicts him and he does not have a fever, "hand" of Ištar.

19.13 ŠU ᵈINNIN.NA: *ḫu-uṣ-ṣi* GAZ ŠÀ TUKU.TUKU-*ši ši-nun*(?) DUG_4.MEŠ-*šú im-ta-na-aš-ši* (*BRM* 4.32:2–3)[10]

**"Hand" of Ištar (is when) he continually has a crushing sensation in the chest (and) continually forgets the . . . of his words.

Both of these symptoms (headache and chest pain) might be combined in another problem caused by Ištar, patients having what looked like seizures but which were not. What alerted the *āšipu* to the fact that these were not seizures (AN.TA.ŠUB.BA; see Chapter 13) but pseudo-seizures[11] were the headache and chest pain, the rubbing and rolling, the absence of spittle, and the "crying out." These findings, inconsistent with true seizures, are described in the references below. Also, the patient in both cases was able to "get up (afterward)," that is, there was no postictal state.

19.14 DIŠ U_4 LÁ-*šú* SAG.KI^{II}-*šú* KÚ.MEŠ-*šú* ŠÀ-*šú* GAZ.MEŠ-*šú* EGIR-*nu* ŠU^{II}-*šú u* GÌR^{II}-*šú ú-kap-p*[*ár*] BAL.BAL-*ut* ÚḪ NU TUKU : *it-ta-nag-ra-ár* ŠUB-*tu* : *ḫa-mi-tum* ŠU ^{d}15 ZI-*bé* (DPS XXVI:28′–29′ [AOAT 43.280])

**If when (confusional states) come over him, his temples continually hurt him, he continually has a crushing sensation in his heart (and) afterward he ⌜rubs⌝ his hands and his feet, he rolls over and over (but) he does not have any spittle (var. he rolls over and over), falling spell (var. paralysis)[12] of "hand" of Ištar; he can get up (afterward).[13]

19.15 DIŠ ITI.1.KÁM ITI.2.KÁM *ina* GI_6 ŠUB-*su u* GÙ-*si pi-rit-ti*[14] ŠU ^{d}15 ZI-*bé* (DPS XVI:80′ [AOAT 43.179])[15]

**If (what looks like a falling spell) falls upon him in the night for one or two months and he cries out, it is shuddering of "hand" of Ištar; he can get up (afterward).

These seizures fall into a category known to us as "hysteria."[16] It should, therefore, come as no surprise that Ištar was responsible for "hysterical" behavior in pregnant women (see Chapter 12), although similar behavior in adolescents of both sexes was laid at the door of the *lilû* class of demons (see below).

19.16 DIŠ MUNUS *ina* GIG-*šá* ŠÀ-*bi ku-ri i-qab-bi* ŠU ^{d}15 AL.TI (DPS XXXVII A obv. 17 = *TDP* 214:17)

**If a woman during her illness says: "My womb is (too) short," "hand" of Ištar; she will get well.

Fortunately, in stark contrast to trauma and some of the other conditions caused by the goddess Ištar, her psychiatric problems seem to have fallen into the category of treatable illnesses. When prognoses are mentioned, they are good.

19.17 DIŠ KI.MIN *ana* ŠU ^{d}INNIN GUR-*šú* KI.MIN (DPS XXVIII:34 [AOAT 43.311])

**If (he is ill with a prolonged illness and) it turns into "hand" of Ištar for him, (if you treat him, he will get well).

LILÛ, LILĪTU, AND *ARDAT LILÎ*

Lilû, lilītu, and *ardat lilî* were a class of demons who were believed to be recruited from among young persons who died just before or just after marriage. These demons tended to victimize persons of the opposite sex but of the same age as themselves.[17] For example, the adolescent female *ardat lilî* was responsible for Gilles de la Tourette syndrome, a disorder that primarily affects boys in the first two decades of life (see Chapter 13). Among the psychiatric symptoms that they caused were what would now be classed as "hysteria" in teenagers. For more details, see Chapter 12 with 12.71–12.76.

19.18 DIŠ MUNUS GIG-*ma* DIB-*sa ina* AN.ÚSAN DIB.DIB-*si u* TÚG-*sa* ŠUB.ŠUB-*di* DIB-*it* LÍL.LÁ.EN.NA (DPS XXXVII A obv. 13 = *TDP* 214:13)[18]

**If a woman is ill and her affliction always afflicts her in the evening and she continually takes her clothes off, it is an affliction of *lilû*.

Individuals presenting with seizure-like symptoms that are in fact hysterical "pseudo-seizures" are even today difficult to distinguish from genuine epileptics. Hysterical seizures are characterized by nonphysiologic events such as a twitching of all four extremities without loss of consciousness or by careful attention to avoid injury by moving away from a wall or bed edge while having convulsions. Hysterical seizures may also have frankly sexual overtones, with pelvic thrusting or genital manipulation.

These sorts of "pseudo-seizures" seem to have been referred to by the *āšipu* as "(lying) hand" of *lilû* or *lilītu*, as in the references below. What made it possible for the *āšipu* to be sure that this was a "lying," that is, false or pretended, seizure was the absence of a postictal state as ascertained by seeing whether the patient could get up afterward (see above under IŠTAR with 19.14–19.15).

19.19 DIŠ *ina ṣal-lu-ti-šú* DIB-*su-ma* DIB-*su* IGI.BAR-*as i-re-eḫ-ḫe-šum-ma* NÍ-*šú i-maš-ši* GIN_7 *šá id-ku-šú* MUD-*ud* ZI.ZI-*bé* : U_4 *id-de-ku-šú re-ḫi* ŠU LÍL.LÁ.EN.NA *sar-ru ana* MUNUS LÍL.LÁ.EN.NA ZI.ZI-*bé* (DPS XXVI:48′–49′ [AOAT 43.282])

**If it afflicts him in his sleep and he gazes at the one who afflicts him, it flows over him and he forgets himself, he shudders like one whom they have awakened (and) he can still get up,[19] "lying hand" of *lilû*.[20] For a woman, *lilû*; she can get up (afterward).[21]

19.20 DIŠ *pa-rid-ma it-te-né-et-bi ma-gal* DUG_4.DUG_4-*ub u i*[*g-d*] *a-*⌜*na*⌝*-al-lu-u*[*t*] *ana* MUNUS LÍL.L[Á].EN.NA *ana* NITA SAL.LÍL.LÁ.EN.NA ZI.ZI-*bé* (DPS XXVI:82′–83′ [AOAT 43.285])

**If he shudders and he can get up (afterward), he talks a lot and he continually ⌜jerks⌝, for a woman, *lilû*, for a man, *lilītu*; he can get up (afterward).[22]

Also attributed to this class of demon was an atypical seizure accompanied by profuse nosebleed (epistaxis), an oddity that is also described in the miracle stories associated with the shrines of a number of medieval European saints.

19.21 DIŠ U_4 LÁ-*šú* $ŠU^{II}$-*šú* IGI.BAR-*as* BABBAR IGI^{II}-*šú* BAL-*ut u* MÚD *ina* KIR_4-*šú* DU-*ku ana* MUNUS LÍL.LÁ.EN.NA *ana* NITA SAL.LÍL.LÁ.EN.NA (DPS XXVI:30′ [AOAT 43.280–281])

**If when (a confusional state) comes over him, he gazes at his hands, he rolls the whites of his eyes, and blood flows from his nose, for a woman, *lilû*; for a man, *lilītu*.[23]

Apart from "hysteria," the *lilû* class of demons caused a form of insanity characterized by slurred speech, dissociative states, and visual hallucinations, as in the following references. The reason for the attribution of this disorder to the *lilû* was probably that the majority of patients developed characteristic symptoms in adolescence or early adulthood. This pattern of onset is characteristic of some mental disorders as, for example, schizophrenia.

19.22 DIŠ $UŠ_4$-[*šú* KÚR-*ir* IN]IM.MEŠ-*šú it-te-né-ep-rek-ka-a* GIDIM *mu-šam-šu-ú* DIB-*su* [:] KI.SIKIL.LÍL.LÁ *šum*$_4$-*ma* LÚ.LÍL.LÁ (DPS XXII:51–52 [AOAT 43.255])[24]

**If [his] mentation [is altered] (and) his ⌜words⌝ hinder each other in his mouth . . . *ardat lilî* or *lilû*.

19.23 DIŠ UB.NÍGIN.NA-*šú* GIN$_7$ *šá bal-ṭi ne-ḫa* IGI^{II}-*šú* BAD.MEŠ-*ma* U$_4$ DIB-*su ina-ṭal* KI-*šú* DUG$_4$.DUG$_4$-*ub u* NÍ-*šú ut-ta-na-kar* ŠU LÍL.LÁ.EN.NA DUMU *šip-ri šá* DINGIR-*šú* (DPS XXVI:73′–74′ [AOAT 43.284])

**If his limbs are as still as those of a healthy person, (and) he continually opens his eyes and, when he sees the one who afflicts him, he talks with him and continually changes himself, "hand" of *lilû*, messenger of his god.

Also laid at the door of the *lilû* class of demons were similarly described mental status changes accompanying "infectious" fevers of the *liʾbu* type, as described in the following references. As we know from other contexts, *liʾbu*-fevers can be accompanied by a macular rash (see Chapter 3). That this is true of the type of *liʾbu* associated with *lilû* may be seen from the commentary to the first quote below which explains "infectious" (*laʾbu*) as referring to "what the *lilû* left behind" (i.e., the characteristic "infectious" lesions).[25] Note also the lexical equation of *laʾbu* with KI.TAG.GA,[26] which literally means "the place that was touched." It seems likely, therefore, that fever and a macular rash were part of this syndrome in addition to severe abdominal discomfort (cries of "oh my insides"). Fever, a macular rash, and gastritis are consistent with syphilis, as are the mental status changes noted. In the modern era, however, the former are part of secondary syphilis and the latter of tertiary neurosyphilis. Since neurosyphilis only appears many years after secondary syphilis resolves, it seems unlikely that this is a description of syphilis as we know it.

19.24 DIŠ U$_4$ DIB-*šú* ŠÀ-*bi* ŠÀ-*bi* GÙ.GÙ-*si* IGI^{II}-*šú* BAD-*te u* DUL-*am* KÚM *li-ʾ-ba i-šu* SAG KIR$_4$-*šú ú-lap-pat ap-pat* ŠU.SI.MEŠ ŠU^{II}-*šú u* GÌR^{II}-*šú ka-ṣa-a* GIG DIB-*šú ina-ṭal* KI-*šú* DUG$_4$.DUG$_4$-*ub u* NÍ-*šú ut-ta-na-kar* ŠU LÍL.LÁ.EN.NA *la-ʾ-bi* (DPS XXVI:66′–68′ [AOAT 43.284])

**If when it afflicts him, he continually cries out: "My insides, my insides!" he opens and shuts his eyes, he has *liʾbu*-fever (KÚM *li-ʾ-ba*), he rubs the bulb of his nose, the tips of his fingers and toes are cold, he can see the illness that afflicts him, he talks with it and continually changes him self, infectious "hand" of *lilû*.

19.25 DIŠ U$_4$ DIB-*šú* ŠÀ-*bi* ŠÀ-*bi* GÙ.GÙ-*si* IGI^{II}-*šú* BAD-*te u* DUL-*am* KÚM *li-ʾ-ba i-šu* SAG KIR$_4$-*šú ú-lap-pat ap-pat* ŠU.SI.MEŠ ŠU^{II}-*šú u* GÌR^{II}-*šú* ŠED$_7$-*a* GIG *šú-a-tu tu-šad-bab-šú-ma la ip-pal* ŠU LÍL.LÁ.EN.NA (DPS XXVI:64′–65′ [AOAT 43.284])

**If when it afflicts him, he continually cries out: "My insides, my insides!" he opens and shuts his eyes, he has *liʾbu*-fever (KÚM *li-ʾ-ba*), he rubs the bulb of his nose, the tips of his fingers and toes are cold, (and if) you try to make that patient talk, he does not answer, "hand" of *lilû*.[27]

GALLÛ

The name of this demon, our ghoul, is usually written in the diagnostic series with the otherwise unusual Sumerogram ḪUL.[28] Although ḪUL literally means "evil," an epithet frequently used for ghosts, *gallû*, and other demons, the significance of the choice of ideogram may lie in a philological word game. One way in which the *āšipu* teased more meaning out of written words was to deconstruct them. We have already seen one example in Chapter 2, where the name for the demon Šulak was explained by breaking it down into its constituent syllables, ŠU, LA, and KU and then "translating" the results as ŠU = "hand," LA = "not," and KÙ = "clean." More extreme examples of ancient deconstructionism are also attested, whereby individual cuneiform signs were broken down into two or more separate signs and then similarly "translated." A very clear example of this process appears in the commentary *SpTU* 1.49:35–36. One way of writing "ghost" is with the GIDIM$_2$ sign which, if split into two signs, consists of a BAR and a U.[29] BAR appears in lexical lists with the meaning "to open" and U (read BÙR) as "ear." GIDIM$_2$ was correspondingly "translated" by the *āšipu* as "the one who opens the ears."

Applying the same methodology to the sign used to designate the *gallû*-demon, ḪUL, we split it into its two constituent signs, a ŠI and an UR. "Translating" these two signs as if they were pseudo-Sumerian yields IGI TÉŠ, or "the eye comes to shame." Curiously, the only obvious link that connects the various ills that are blamed on the *gallû*-demon is the fact that, in each separate syndrome, an eye symptom is prominently mentioned. There is pain in the upper part of the eyes in the *gallû* trauma reference (see 19.176), and ocular paralysis in the references to a *gallû*-induced bleeding syndrome (see 19.177) and in the cataplexy references to *gallû* (see Chapter 13 with 13.212). In no other syndrome attributed to the *gallû*-demon, however, do the eyes come quite so literally "to shame" as in the following psychiatric reference.

19.26 [DIŠ NA *ma-a*] *m-ma* IGI-*ma* TÚG-*su it-ta-na-as-suk ú-rap-pad* IGI^{II}-*šú ú-ma-ḫa-aṣ* NA BI ḪUL DIB-*su* (DPS XXVII:19 [AOAT 43.298])

**[If a person] sees ⸢somebody⸣ and continually throws off his garment, he wanders about (and) strikes his eyes, a *gallû* afflicts that person.

GHOST

Self-destructive behavior that did not particularly focus on the eyes was laid at the door of another netherworld denizen, the ghost. Those who lived a full life and died in the bosom of their families were the contented recipients of food offerings made on a regular basis by grieving relatives. Those who died by violence, however, had scores to settle with the living.

19.27 DIŠ IGI.MEŠ-*šú* SÌG.SÌG-*aṣ u* GÙ.DÉ.DÉ.ME-*si* GIDIM *qá-li-i* DIB-*su* (DPS IX A 76//B r. 23 = *TDP* 78:76)

**If he continually strikes his face and screams, the ghost of someone burned to death afflicts him.

19.28 DIŠ Á^{II}-*šú ú-na-aš-šak ina šag-gaš-ti* LÚ *ú-šaḫ-niq-ma ár-da-na-an* ÚŠ DIB-*su* (DPS X B r. 6 = *TDP* 88 r. 6)[30]

**If he chews on his arms, he had a person strangled to death and the "double" of the dead person afflicts him.

The preceding references to self-abuse suggest something between a very guilty conscience and physical possession by the avenging ghost. The victim of ghost affliction seems either to have talked more than he should (as in the first two examples below) or not at all (as in the last reference). The suspicion that it was specifically an incinerated ghost that produced the patient's mutism is probably due to a linguistic pun between the verb *qalû*: "to burn" and a near homophone *qâlu*: "to be silent."

19.29 DIŠ *ina* GIG-*šú* DUG$_4$.DUG$_4$-*ub* GIDIM *ár-da-na-an* ÚŠ DIB-*su* DIN (DPS XVII:17 [AOAT 43.196])

**If during his illness, he continually talks, a ghost, the "double" of a dead person afflicts him; he will get well.

19.30 DIŠ ŠÀ ŠÀ GÙ.GÙ *it-bi-ma il-su-um* GIDIM *ár-da-na-an*[31] ÚŠ [DIB-*su*] (DPS XIII G$_2$ r. 19 = *TDP* 124 iii 26)

**If he keeps crying out: "My insides, my insides" and he gets up and runs, a ghost, the "double" of a dead person [afflicts him].

19.31 DIŠ UB.NÍGIN.NA-*šú* GIN$_7$ *šá bal-ṭi ne-ḫa* KA-*šú* DIB-*ma* NU DUG$_4$.DUG$_4$-*ub* ŠU GIDIM$_7$ *šag-ga-ši* : ŠU GIDIM$_7$ *qa-li-i* (DPS XXVI:75′ [AOAT 43.285])[32]

**If his limbs are as still as those of a healthy person (but) his mouth is "seized" so that he cannot talk, "hand" of a murderous ghost (var. "hand" of the ghost of someone burned to death).

Assyrian kings drafted their citizens in rotation (one year for military service, one year for public works, one year at home), which means that, in periods when wars were frequent, a significant portion of the male population was subjected to the stress of battle in one campaign season out of every three. Although ancient warfare was considerably less terrifying than the modern version, it is likely that a portion of these draftees experienced battle fatigue (post-traumatic stress syndrome; see Chapter 14). Some of the psychological signs and symptoms attributed by ancient Mesopotamians to ghosts are compatible with this stress disorder. It is not difficult to imagine why the *āšipu* would have supposed such patients to be haunted by the ghosts of those whom they had killed or whose violent deaths (say by incineration via fire arrows) they had personally witnessed. Note in particular the association of ghost-induced mutism with vivid nightmares in the following reference.

19.32 DIŠ *ina ši-mi-tan lu* LÚ.TI *lu* LÚ.ÚŠ *lu* ⸢*mu-da-šú lu*⸣[33] *la m*[*u-da-šú*] *lu mam-ma lu mim-ma* IGI-*ma* LUḪ-*ut i-tu-ram-ma* GIN$_7$ *šá* Ì.ḪAB *tu* [. . .] KA-*šú* DIB-*ma šá i-ta-a-šú ṣal-lu šá-sa-a* NU ZU-*e* ŠU GIDIM$_7$: ŠU [. . .] (DPS XVII:83–85 [AOAT 43.203])[34]

**If in the evening, he sees either a living person or a dead person or someone known to him or someone not ⸢known to him⸣ or anybody or anything and becomes afraid; he turns around but, like one who has [been hexed with?] rancid oil, his mouth is seized so that he is unable to cry out to one who sleeps next to him, "hand" of ghost (var. hand of [. . .])

"Roving" or "roaming" ghosts were also blamed for alteration of mentation (as in our "wandering mind"). Given the association of ghosts with various forms of alcoholism (see Chapter 15), it is possible that these are references to slurring of speech and loss of cognitive functions produced by ethanol poisoning.

19.33 [DIŠ U]Š$_4$-*šú šá-ni-šu-ma* UŠ$_4$-*šú* NU DIB ŠU GIDIM *mur-tap-pi-du* GAM (DPS XXII:47a [AOAT 43.255])

**[If] his ⌜mentation⌝ is altered so that he is not in full possession of his faculties, "hand" of a roving ghost; he will die.

19.34 DIŠ UŠ$_4$-*šú* KÚR-⌜*ir*⌝ [. . .] x *maš-u-tú* INIM.MEŠ-*šú it-te-né-ep-rek-ka-a* GIDIM$_7$ *mut-tag-gi-šú* DIB-*su* [. . .].MEŠ-*ma* DIN (DPS XXII:53–54 [AOAT 43.256])[35]

**If his mentation is altered, [. . .] (and) forgetfulness(?) (and) his words hinder each other in his mouth, a roaming ghost afflicts him. (If) [. . .], he will get well.

PERSONAL GOD OR GODDESS

Every ancient Mesopotamian had his own personal god or goddess, a sort of guardian angel. When this god or goddess became angry, the result was what we call stress. In some people, this resulted in mysterious aches and pains.

19.35 DIŠ SAG.KI^{II}-*šú šá* 15 *u* 150 KÚ.MEŠ-*šú-ma* KÚM-*šú mit-ḫar* ŠU DINGIR-*šú* DIN (DPS IV B obv. 32//E i 12 = *TDP* 36:33//*SpTU* 3.88 i 12)[36]

**If his left and right temples continually hurt him and his temperature is normal, "hand" of his god; he will get well.

19.36 DIŠ NA ŠÀ-*bi* ŠÀ-*bi i-qab-bi*/GÙ.GÙ-*si* ŠÀ-*šú* NU KÚ-*šú* NINDA NU KÚ A/KAŠ NU NAG *i-dam-mu-um* NA BI DIB-*ti* DINGIR-*šú u* ^{d}*Eš$_4$-dar-šú* UGU-*šú* GÁL-*ši*. . . (*BAM* 316 iv 3–4//*STT* 95 ii 70–72//*KAR* 92 r. 4–6)[37]

**If a person says/cries out: "My insides, my insides!" (but) his stomach does not hurt him, he cannot eat bread (and) he cannot drink water/beer (and) he moans, the anger of his god or goddess is upon that person . . .

In others, an angry personal god or goddess could lead to a complete nervous breakdown.

19.37 DIŠ NA *nu-ul-la-ti* ŠÀ-*šú i-ta-mu at-mu-šú i-šá-an-ni za-mar ṣa-lil za-mar e-er u* UŠ$_4$-*šú* NU DIB-*al* DIB-*ti* DINGIR-*šú* UGU-*šú* GÁL-*ši* (*BAM* 316 vi 4′–6′//*STT* 95 ii 84–86)

**If a person's heart ponders untruths, he repeats his words, he is now sleeping, now awake, and he cannot make up his mind (to do anything), the anger of his god is upon him.

Other gods/goddesses besides the personal god or goddess of the patient could also become angry with the patient, the resulting "alteration of mentation"[38] in this case being, rather curiously, completely irreligious and antisocial behavior.

19.38 ŠU.DINGIR.RA : DINGIR.MEŠ *i-nam-zar šil-lat i-qab-bi šá im-mar i-maḫ-ḫaṣ* (*BRM* 4.32:2)

**"Hand" of a god (is when) he curses the gods, speaks blasphemy, (and) strikes whatever he sees.

Gods/Goddesses of Neurologic Conditions

In dividing up neurologic syndromes, the *āšipu* made good use of the presence of numerous potential causal agents. For example, Ningirsu was responsible for injuries to the second cranial nerve and ghosts for abnormalities of the fifth, seventh, and eighth cranial nerves. Trauma to the fifth cranial nerve was blamed on Sîn; the *rābiṣu* of the lavatory claimed responsibility for inflammation of the trigeminal nerve producing trigeminal neuralgia. Traumatic injury to the eighth cranial nerve was caused by Ištar, but sensory hearing loss and dizziness produced by disease in the same nerve came under the purview of ghosts (see Chapter 13 with 13.89–13.104).

Various forms of nystagmus were similarly divided, with ocular bobbing and disorders of conjugate gaze going to Lugalgirra, horizontal pendular nystagmus to Sîn, and nystagmus in infants to Ningeštinanna. For more details on all of these associations and their possible explanations, see Chapter 13 with 13.105–13.115.

^{d}LUGAL.ÙR.RA VERSUS ^{d}LUGAL.GÌR.RA

These two divinities with very similar names provide an interesting study in comparisons and contrasts. Ostensibly, they are easily confused[39] since both produced neurologic symptoms involving the eyes and both could also produce a severely ill patient cradling his head in his hands.

19.39 DIŠ U_4 UD.DU-*šú* IGI-*šú šá* 15/150 GIN_7 ^{GIŠ}BAL *i-lam-*[*mi*] IGI-*šú šá* 150/ZAG MÚD DIRI-*at* KA-*šú* BAD.BAD-*te* EME-[*šú*] *ú-na-šak* ^{d}LUGAL.GÌR.RA DIB-*su* (*STT* 89:103–105a, 109–111)

**If when it ⌜comes⌝ over him, his left/right eye (makes bobbing movements similar to what) a spindle (does) when it spins (and) his right/left eye is full of blood, he continually opens his mouth (and) he bites [his] tongue, ^{d}LUGAL.GÌR.RA afflicts him.

19.40 ^{d}LUGAL.ÙR.RA : IGI^{II} 15-*šú u* 150-*šú i-kap-pi-iṣ* (*BRM* 4.32:2)

**^{d}LUGAL.ÙR.RA (is when) he lets his left and his right eye droop.

19.41 DIŠ ŠU^{II}-*šú ina* SAG.DU-*šú* GAR-*na-ma la ur-ra-da-ni* ŠU ^{d}LUGAL.GÌR.RA *u* ^{d}MES.L[AM.TA.È.A . . .] (DPS XI A obv. 24//B 23 = *TDP* 90:24//*SpTU* 1.34:23)

**If his hands are placed on his head and he does not bring them down, "hand" of ^{d}LUGAL.GÌR.RA and ⌜^{d}MES.LAM.TA.È.A⌝; [. . .]

19.42 DIŠ MUNUS GIG-*ma ú-ru-úḫ-šá bé-e-er ana* U_4.2.KÁM *ana* U_4.3.KÁM BA.ÚŠ / DIŠ MUNUS GIG-*ma* ŠU^{II}-*šá ina* SAG.DU-*šá* GAR-*na-ma la ur-ra-da-ni* ŠU EN ÙR KI.MIN MAŠKIM ÙR SÌG-*aṣ* ÚŠ (DPS XXXVII A obv. 10–11 = *TDP* 214:10–11)

**If a woman is ill and her head hair is fine (lit. select) (and) she has been sick for two or three days, she will die. If a woman is ill and her hands are placed on her head and she does not bring them down,[40] "hand" of the lord of the roof (^{d}LUGAL.ÙR.RA).[41] Alternatively, the *rābiṣu* of the roof[42] has struck her; she will die.

Subtle differences, however, reveal an important distinction. The eye movements described in connection with ^{d}LUGAL.GÌR.RA and his twin ^{d}MES.LAM.TA.È.A are consistent with cerebral malaria (see Chapter 3), whereas the drooping eyes of ^{d}LUGAL.ÙR.RA suggest myasthenia gravis. That cerebral malaria should produce a severely ill patient (with head cradled in the hands) comes as no surprise. More interesting is the fact that the other severely ill patient is expected to be a woman and that the alternative diagnosis to ^{d}LUGAL.ÙR.RA is a *rābiṣu* of the roof. Among other ills, the *rābiṣu* was responsible for thyrotoxicosis, a potentially fatal condition that is more common in women than in men (see Chapter 7), as is myasthenia gravis. About 5 percent of patients have both myasthenia gravis and thyrotoxicosis, usually simultaneously.

GHOST

On a more mundane level, the *āšipu* distinguished between generalized headaches, attributed to the *mukīl rēš lemutti*, and more protracted or painful frontal headaches, which he attributed to the baneful influence of ghosts. Also attributed to ghosts were particularly severe headaches resulting in fatality. Ghosts were notorious for causing pain, and particularly the type that "divides the right side from the left side of the body." Since migraine headaches are often unilateral, it is not surprising that ghosts were blamed for this condition (see Chapter 13 with 13.156–13.158).

Another factor in the attribution is possibly the fact that migraine sufferers not infrequently report that the headache seems to start from the ear on the affected side. Ghosts were assumed to be at work in many other syndromes involving the ears. A final connection was ophthalmologic migraine, which can cause a patient to see dazzling zigzag lines; flashes in the eyes was also a condition caused by ghosts. For more details, see Chapters 9 and 13.

Headaches, neckaches, and dizziness, all of which were separately caused by ghosts, were not surprisingly also attributed to ghosts when they occurred together, as in the following references.

19.43 DIŠ SAG.KI-*šú* DIB-*su-ma* IGI.ME-*šú* NIGIN-*du* ZI-*bi u* ŠUB-*ut* ŠU $GIDIM_7$ (DPS IV B obv. 18 = *TDP* 34:18)[43]

**If his temple afflicts him and his face continually seems to spin (and) he gets up but then falls down, "hand" of ghost.

19.44 [DIŠ NA *ina* DIB] ŠU $GIDIM_7$ GÚ-*su* KÚ-*šú* IGI.MEŠ-*šú* NIGIN.MEŠ-*du* (*BAM* 312:9)

**[If, as a result of affliction] by "hand" of ghost, a [person]'s neck hurts him, (and) his face seems continually to spin.

RĀBIṢU OF THE RIVER

The *āšipu* recognized a number of illnesses that he associated with exposure to river water. Most of the references describe neurologic abnormalities including seizures, vertigo (spinning), paralysis (immobilization), twisting (abnormal posturing), and altered mentation, and are probably due to the ingestion or absorption of neurotoxins. He further subdivided this class of illness into two syndromes. One was attributed to the fact that the patient "drank water from a hoisting device of the river." The other was diagnosed as *rābiṣu* of the river, or "ghost of one who died in the water," the understanding being that those who drowned lurked about the river like demons, eager to cause the deaths of other swimmers. In the second reference below, the comment "it will be difficult for him in the middle of the day" is usually appended to seizure disorders. For more details, see Chapter 15 with 15.26–15.33.

19.45 DIŠ TA A.MEŠ *ina* E_{11}-*šú* LÚ.AD_6-*šú iḫ-mi-šu-ma* NIGIN-*ma* ŠUB-*ut* ⸢MAŠKIM⸣ ÍD SÌG-[*i*]*ṣ* (DPS XXVII:25 [AOAT 43.299]; cf. Ni. 470:11 [Kraus, *ZA* 77.197])[44]

**If (after bathing) when he comes up from the (river) water, his body is paralyzed and he (feels like he) is spinning and falls down, the *rābiṣu* of the river has struck ⸢him⸣.

19.46 DIŠ *šá* DIB DIB.DIB-*su* U_4 DIB-*šú* $ŠU^{II}$-*šú u* IGI.ME-*šú ú-maš-šad* $GIDIM_7$ *šá ina* A ÚŠ DIB-*su ina ma-šal* U_4-*mi* DUGUD-*su* : MAŠKIM ÍD SÌG-*s*[*u*] (DPS XXVI:42′ [AOAT 43.282])[45]

**If that which afflicts continually afflicts him (and) when it afflicts him, he massages his hands and face, the ghost (of one) who died in water afflicts him. It will be difficult for him in the middle of the day. Alternatively, the *rābiṣu* of the river has struck ⸢him⸣.

SÎN AND IŠTAR IN INFANTS

SEIZURES In addition to a fever with neurologic findings (see 19.259–19.265), Sîn, the moon-god, was also one of the causes of seizures in infants. For more details, see Chapter 13. Some of the moon-god's infantile seizures were fatal and some were not.

19.47 DIŠ LÚ.TUR *ig-da-na-al-lut u* LÙ.LÙ ŠU ^{d}30 AL.TI (DPS XL A 35 = *TDP* 220:35)

**If an infant continually jerks and is restless, "hand" of Sîn; he will get well.

19.48 DIŠ LÚ.TUR *ig-da-na-al-lut u* LÙ.LÙ-*aḫ ib-ta-nak-ki ip-ta-nar-ru-ud* $ŠU^{II}$-*šú u* $GÌR^{II}$-*šú* ÍL.ÍL-*ši* SÌG ^{d}30 *na-ag-mar-ti* TUKU-*ši* (DPS XL A 46//B 46 = *TDP* 222:46)

**If an infant continually jerks and is restless, he continually wails, he continually shudders, he continually raises his hands and his feet, blow of Sîn; it will finish him off.[46]

Note in the preceding references the presence of signs and symptoms ("jerking" and "restless" in particular) similar to those of the moon-god's neurologic fever in adults (see 19.259–19.265). It may be this similarity that attracted the diagnosis. However, Sîn's fever was "the same for adults and children," whereas the syndrome caused by this god involving infants exclusively was not invariably accompanied by a fever, as is indicated in the following references.

19.49 DIŠ LÚ.TUR KÚM NU TUKU IGI^{II}-*šú bal-ṣa* $ŠU^{II}$-*šú u* $GÌR^{II}$-*šú i-ra-ʾu-ba* ŠU ^{d}30 DIN / DIŠ LÚ.TUR KÚM NU TUKU *u i-ra-ʾ-ub* ŠU ^{d}30 / DIŠ LÚ.TUR KÚM NU TUKU *ra-ʾ-i-ba* DIB.DIB-*su* ŠU ^{d}30 (DPS XL A 120–122 = *TDP* 230:120–122)

**If an infant does not have a fever, his eyes are dilated, (and) his hands and his feet tremble, "hand" of Sîn; he will get well. If an infant does not have a fever and he trembles, "hand" of Sîn. If an infant does not have a fever (but) trembling continually afflicts him, "hand" of Sîn.

Besides Sîn, the goddess Ištar was also involved in causing infantile seizures.[47] Her seizures were often difficult to distinguish from those of the moon god, even for the *āšipu*. In the following references, the clinical findings, which include seizures, swollen hands and feet, and constricted pupils, might have been caused by congenital syphilis (see Chapter 4).

19.50 DIŠ LÚ.TUR *ig-da-na-al-lut* LÙ.LÙ*-aḫ u* MUD.MUD*-ud* ŠU ^{d}30 *u* ^{d}15 (DPS XL A 47 = *TDP* 222:47)[48]

**If an infant continually jerks, is restless, and shudders, "hand" of Sîn or Ištar.

19.51 DIŠ LÚ.TUR ŠU^{II}*-šú u* GÌR^{II}*-šú it-ta-na-an-pa-ḫa* IGI^{II}*-šú uz-za-na-qap* ^{GIŠ}GIDRU ^{d}30 *u* ^{d}15 (DPS XL A 56 = *TDP* 224:56)

**If an infant's hands and feet are continually swollen (and) he continually constricts[49] (the pupils of) his eyes, scepter of Sîn or Ištar.

"ABDOMINAL EPILEPSY" In the references below, the infants display a variety of gastrointestinal symptoms including vomiting, diarrhea, and intestinal colic (cramping, pain, and bloating). In addition, the infants have jerking, restlessness, shuddering, rigidity, and sluggishness.

19.52 DIŠ LÚ.TUR *i-šá-as-si i-gal-lut* LÙ.LÙ*-aḫ ib-ta-nak-ki u* MUD.MUD*-ud ṣir-tú ma-la* NAG *ut-ta-nar-ra* ŠU ^{d}30 *u* ^{d}15 (DPS XL A 55 = *TDP* 224:55)

**If an infant screams, jerks, is restless, continually wails, and continually shudders (and) as much as he drinks from the breast (his insides) continually return, "hand" of Sîn or Ištar.

Such problems were assigned to the two gods that usually caused infantile seizures; Sîn was usually blamed where vomiting and diarrhea were prominent and Ištar when apparent seizures were accompanied by colic.

19.53 DIŠ LÚ.TUR *ma-la* KÚ *i-ḫa-ḫu* KI.MIN *iṣ-ṣa-na-aḫ* ŠU^{II}*-šú u* GÌR^{II}*-šú it-te-ṣi-la-šú qí-bit* KA *ana* ^{d}30 TUKU*-ši* (DPS XL A 48 = *TDP* 222:48)[50]

**If an infant vomits as much as he eats; alternatively, (if) he has diarrhea (and) his hands and his feet become sluggish, there is an (unfulfilled) promise to Sîn.

19.54 DIŠ LÚ.TUR KÚM NU TUKU ŠÀ.MEŠ*-šú eb-ṭu u i-bak-ki ṣi-bit* DUMU.MUNUS ^{d}*A-nim* / DIŠ LÚ.TUR *i-bak-ki u im-ta-nag-ga-ag* DUMU.MUNUS ^{d}*A-nim* DIB*-su* / DIŠ LÚ.TUR U$_4$*-ma u mu-šu i-bak-ki* DUMU.MUNUS ^{d}*A-nim* DIB*-su* (DPS XL A 106–108 = *TDP* 228:106–108)[51]

**If an infant does not have a fever (but) his insides are cramped and he wails, affliction by the daughter of Anu.[52] If an infant wails and is continually rigid, the daughter of Anu afflicts him. If an infant wails day and night, the daughter of Anu afflicts him.

We suspect that, in making these assignments, the *āšipu* was making the same mistake that modern physicians have made in the recent past. The jerking, shuddering, and posturing of infants with gastrointestinal problems can mimic seizures. Modern physicians therefore had a category of seizures called abdominal epilepsy until further investigation demonstrated that it was not true epilepsy.

LILÛ, LILĪTU, AND *ARDAT LILÎ*

We have already met this class of demons who were believed to be recruited from among young persons who died just before or just after marriage and to victimize persons of the opposite sex but of the same age as themselves. In addition to the psychiatric symptoms and "hysterical" seizures that he attributed to their influence, the *āšipu* seems also to have blamed them for real seizures in adolescents. What is distinctive about this group of references is that the descriptions specifically mention auras and laughing (gelastic) seizures but not the "thrashing about like a slaughtered sheep" of grand mal seizures (AN.TA.ŠUB.BA).

19.55 DIŠ KI.MIN U$_4$ DIB-*šú an-nu-ú šu-ú i-qab-bi* ŠU KI.SIKIL.LÍL.L[Á.EN.NA] (DPS XXVI:39′ [AOAT 43.281])

**If (his affliction always afflicts him in the evening and) when it afflicts him, he says "This is it," "hand" of *ardat lilî*.[53]

19.56 D[IŠ] ⌜GIN$_7$⌝ ŠUB-*šú i-ri-iq-ma ma-gal i-ṣi-iḫ u* GÌR^{II}-*šú it-ta-naq-na-an-na* : ŠU^{II}-*šú u* GÌR^{II}-*šú* ŠU LÍL.LÁ.EN.NA (DPS XXVI:14′ [AOAT 43.279])

**⌜If⌝ when (a falling spell) falls upon him, he turns pale and laughs a lot and his feet (var. his hands and his feet) are continually contorted, "hand" of *lilû*.

Also interesting to note is the fact that the flushing associated with *lilû*-seizures was not generalized as it was with AN.TA.ŠUB.BA-seizures. In the third reference below, "letting the hips drop" refers to the absence of pelvic thrusting, a sign that the *āšipu* associated with the hysterical seizures produced by the same family of demons (see above with 19.18–20).

19.57 [DIŠ ŠUB-*ti* ŠUB-*su-ma*] *ina* U$_4$.1.KÁM 2-*šú* 3-*šú* KÚR/LÁ-*šum-ma*/ŠUB-*su ina šér-ti* SA$_5$ *ina* AN.USAN SIG$_7$ AN.TA.ŠUB.BA (DPS XXVI:5′ [AOAT 43.278]; Arnaud, *Emar* VI/4.694:9′)

**[If a falling spell falls upon him and] (his mentation) alters/(the falling spell) comes over him/falls on him two or three times a day and in the morning he flushes (and) in the evening he turns pale, AN.TA.ŠUB.BA (seizure).

19.58 [DIŠ ŠUB-*ti* ŠUB-*su-ma* U$_4$ ŠUB-*šú*] ⌜IGI.MEŠ⌝-[*šú*] SA$_5$ SIG$_7$ [ŠU] KI.SIKIL.LÍL.[LÁ.EN.NA] (DPS XXVI:3′ [AOAT 43.278])[54]

**[If a falling spell falls upon him and when it falls upon him, his] face flushes and turns pale, ["hand"] of *ardat lilî*.[55]

19.59 DIŠ *ina* EN.NUN.MURUB$_4$.BA *šá* DIB DIB.DIB-*su* U$_4$ DIB-*šú* ŠU^{II}-*šú u* GÌR^{II}-*šú ka-ṣa-a ma-gal ú-te-te-eṭ-ṭe* KA-*šú* BAD.BAD-*te* IGI.MEŠ-*šú* SA$_5$ *u* SIG$_7$ MURUB$_4$.ME-*šú*

ŠUB.ŠUB-*di* ŠU KI.SIKIL.LÍL.LÁ.EN.NA GÍD-*ma* GAM : *ana* MUNUS LÍL.LÁ.EN.NA *ana* NITA SAL.LÍL.LÁ.EN.NA (DPS XXVI:45′–47′ [AOAT 43.282])

**If that which afflicts continually afflicts him during the middle watch of the night (and) when it afflicts him his hands and his feet are cold, he continually becomes darkened (i.e., passes out),[56] he continually opens his mouth,[57] his face flushes and turns pale, (and) he continually lets his hips drop, "hand" of *ardat lilî*. If it is prolonged, he will die (var. for a woman, a *lilû*; for a man, a *lilītu*).

What this suggests is that adolescents, and young men in particular (hence the diagnoses of *ardat lilî*), were observed by the *āšipu* to have a higher proportion of focal seizures than adults. If so, the probable cause was the service of young men in ancient armies. Even today, in adolescents and young adults, cranial trauma is a major cause of focal epilepsy, whereas generalized tonic-clonic seizures are often associated with drug or alcohol withdrawal, a syndrome apparently described by the *āšipu* as "scepter" of Sîn and attributed to ghosts (see Chapter 15 with 15.19–15.20).

SEIZURE DISORDERS

In accordance with similar principles of subdivision, seizures were described as AN.TA.ŠUB.BA but the postictal state was laid at the door of the sun-god Šamaš, and what we call status epilepticus (continual or rapidly recurring seizures) was the sign of the involvement of a ghost. What appears to be the narcolepsy-cataplexy syndrome was also separately defined, narcolepsy being caused by the *rābiṣu* and cataplexy by the *gallû*-demon. For more details on these syndromes, see Chapter 13 with 13.210–13.213.

In one series of references in the neurological section of the diagnostic and prognostic series, the *āšipu* seems to have attempted to account for observed variations in seizure disorders in terms of the influence of various gods/goddesses. The author of this section also used "hands" of gods/goddesses to designate the phases of the disorder being described. The terminology is nowhere defined, but taken for granted or meant to be explained orally. Moreover, the use of "hands" seems often to be idiosyncratic. For these reasons, it is particularly difficult to puzzle out what was meant, as may be seen from the following reference.

19.60 DIŠ AN.TA.ŠUB.BA *ana* ŠU.GIDIM.MA GUR-*šú* SAG.ḪUL.ḪA.ZA TUKU.TUKU-*ši* ŠU [d]15 ŠU MAŠKIM *ana* KAR-*šú* . . . (DPS XXVIII:4–6 [AOAT 43.308])

**If AN.TA.ŠUB.BA turns into "hand" of ghost (and) he continually has a *mukīl rēš lemutti* (and) "hand" of Ištar, "hand" of a *rābiṣu*; to save him . . .[58]

In the reference above, AN.TA.ŠUB.BA refers to a seizure or seizure-like disorder, and the diagnosis of "hand" of *rābiṣu* to what may be narcolepsy (see Chapter 13). We believe that narcolepsy was separately described by the *āšipu* as follows.

19.61 DIŠ *ik-kil-lu* GÙ.GÙ-*šú* U_4 GÙ.GÙ-*šú šu-ú i-ta-nap-pal-šú it-ta-na-as-pak* ZI-*ma i-káš-šú-uš* ZI-*bé u* DU_{10}.GAM GIG-*su uš-te-zeb* MAŠKIM *mur-tap-pi-du* DIB-*su* (DPS XXVI:89′–90′ [AOAT 43.286])[59]

**If a mournful cry continually cries out to him (and) when it cries out to him, he continually answers it, he continually behaves like an animal caught in a trap[60] (and) when he gets up, he feels exhausted (and) he gets up but (has to) squat down, he will come through his illness; a roaming *rābiṣu* afflicts him.

Collating this reference with the preceding one allows us to know what was meant by "hand" of ghost, *mukīl rēš lemutti*, and "hand" of Ištar in this context. The first symptom described in the text above is: "If a mournful cry continually cries out to him (and) when it cries out to him, he continually answers it." This should correspond to the first "hand" of DPS XXVIII:4–6 (AOAT 43.308), which is "hand" of ghost. The attribution of a "mournful cry" to a ghost makes a certain amount of sense, since ghosts were known to pester people by crying in their houses. Supporting this attribution is a second reference from this same section of the diagnostic and prognostic series that describes a patient with some form of "spawn" of Šulpaea developing "hand" of ghost.

19.62 DIŠ ^{d}LUGAL.ÙR.RA *ana* ŠU ^{d}INNIN GUR-*šú* A.RI.A ^{d}*Šul-pa-è-a ana* ŠU.GIDIM. MA GUR-*šú* NU *i-ke-šir* (DPS XXVIII:20 [AOAT 43.310])

*If . . . "spawn" of Šulpaea turns into "hand" of ghost, he will not do well.

As it happens, "(if) a mournful cry roars to him and he continually answers it" is specifically mentioned in connection with "spawn" of Šulpaea in *STT* 89:180–186, which appears to describe the mood changes associated with Huntington's chorea (see Chapter 13), a disease for which the prognosis would indeed have been very poor.

The second symptom described in DPS XXVI:89′–90′ (AOAT 43.286), cited above, is: "He continually behaves like an animal caught in a trap." This should correspond to the second causal agent of DPS XXVIII:4–6 (AOAT 43.308), which is *mukīl rēš lemutti*. *Mukīl rēš lemutti* usually refers to a benign headache, but in this context, it seems to refer to wild swings in emotion and terror such as might be experienced by an animal caught in a trap. The following sequence of references to fatal cases of *mukīl rēš lemutti* seems to describe this syndrome.

19.63 DIŠ *iṣ-ṣe-né-eḫ* ŠU ^{d}SAG.ḪUL.ḪA.ZA GAM . . . / DIŠ *ḫa-di u pa-rid* ŠU SAG.ḪUL.ḪA.ZA GAM . . . / DIŠ *ud-daḫ-ḫa-as* GAM : ŠU SAG.ḪUL.ḪA.ZA (DPS XXII:62–64a [AOAT 43.256])

**If he continually laughs, "hand" of *mukīl rēš lemutti*; he will die . . .[61] If he rejoices and is terrified, "hand" of *mukīl rēš lemutti*; he will die . . . If he feels harassed, he will die (var. "hand" of *mukīl rēš lemutti*).

The third symptom described in DPS XXVI:89′–90′ (AOAT 43.286) is: "When he gets up, he feels exhausted (and) he gets up but (has to) squat down." This should correspond to the third "hand" of DPS XXVIII:4–5 (AOAT 43.308), which is "hand" of Ištar. This, too, seems plausible, since the goddess is invoked when symptoms of lassitude or prostration are mentioned, with or without other accompanying symptoms, as in the following reference.

19.64 DIŠ KI.MIN-*ma* ŠU-*su ina* LI.DUR-*šú* GAR-*at-ma* ŠU^{II}-*šú u* GÌR^{II}-*šú ka-ṣa-a ina* NU ⌜ZU-*e*⌝ [DUG$_{4}$.DUG$_{4}$-*ub*] ZI-*bi u* TUŠ-*ab ina* LI.DUR-*šú* SÌG-*iṣ* ŠU ^{d}*Dil-bat* [GAM] (DPS XV:13–14 [AOAT 43.151]; cf. DPS XI A obv. 9//B 8 = *TDP* 90:9//*SpTU* 1.34:8)[62]

**If (it is the first day he is sick) and his hand is placed on his navel and his hands and his feet are cold, [he talks] without knowing (what he is saying and) he gets up and sits down (again), he was wounded on his navel; "hand" of Dilbat (Ištar); [he will die].

If we may assume that all examples in the same section use the same "code,"[63] the presence of these "translations" gives us a head start at puzzling out some of the remaining references. If "hand" of ghost in these contexts refers to auditory (or visual) hallucinations, then the following would appear to be a reference to a seizure preceded by an aura. The diagnosis "hand" of city god and the positive prognosis suggests that the *āšipu* recognized this as a normal variant, and had no firm idea as to which god/goddess might have caused it.

19.65 DIŠ *šum*$_4$*-ma* ŠU.GIDIM.MA *ana* AN.TA.ŠUB.BA GUR-*šú* LÚ BI ŠU DINGIR URU-*šú* GIG *ina* ŠU DINGIR URU-*šú* KAR-*šú* . . . (DPS XXVIII:1–2 [AOAT 43.307])

**If "hand" of ghost turns into AN.TA.ŠUB.BA, that person is sick with "hand" of his city god; in order to save him from "hand" of his city god . . .[64]

A complication arises with the use of ^{d}LUGAL.ÙR.RA and "spawn" of Šulpaea in the following reference, also given a favorable prognosis and attributed to the city (or personal) god.

19.66 DIŠ ^{d}LUGAL.ÙR.RA A.RI.A ^{d}*Šul-pa-è-a ana* AN.TA.ŠUB.BA GUR-*šú* ŠU DINGIR-*šú*/DINGIR URU-*šú ana* KAR-*šú* . . . (DPS XXVIII:19 [AOAT 43.310])

**If ^{d}LUGAL.ÙR.RA (or) "spawn" of Šulpaea turns into AN.TA.ŠUB.BA, "hand" of his god (var. his city god); to save him . . .

Patients with cerebral palsy (a category included under "spawn" of Šulpaea; see Chapter 13 with 13.244) can develop seizures (AN.TA.ŠUB.BA), which may be what is being referred to by "spawn" of Šulpaea "turning into" AN.TA.ŠUB.BA. But what about ^{d}LUGAL.ÙR.RA "turning into" AN.TA.ŠUB.BA? In addition to being responsible for myasthenia gravis (see above), ^{d}LUGAL.ÙR.RA not infrequently appears listed alongside other types of seizure activity.

19.67 *lu* AN.TA.ŠUB.BA [*l*]*u* ^{d}LUGAL.ÙR.RA *lu* ^{d}LUGAL.AMAŠ.PA.È . . . (*BBR* 45:5–6)

**Either AN.TA.ŠUB.BA ⌜or⌝ ^{d}LUGAL.ÙR.RA or ^{d}LUGAL.AMAŠ.PA.È . . .

An obvious suggestion is that, in these contexts, ^{d}LUGAL.ÙR.RA refers to focal seizures.[65] Simple or complex partial seizures can indeed progress to ("turn into") generalized seizures either immediately or after an interval of a few minutes.

Another normal variant of uncertain etiology, according to the *āšipu*, was a patient who had experienced a seizure finding himself in a state of exhaustion ("hand" of Ištar) afterward, as in the following reference.

19.68 DIŠ AN.TA.ŠUB.BA *ana* ŠU ^{d}INNIN GUR-*šú* ŠU NAM.ÉRIM ŠU DINGIR URU-*šú* KI.MIN ŠU ^{d}INNIN URU-*šú ana* KAR-*šú* . . . (DPS XXVIII:7–8 [AOAT 43.308])

**If AN.TA.ŠUB.BA turns into "hand" of Ištar, "hand" of curse, "hand" of the god of his city. Alternatively, "hand" of the goddess of his city; to save him . . .

Headache and drowsiness are common sequelae of grand mal seizures, and the individual may not return to normal functioning for days afterward. Patients with focal seizures (^{d}LUGAL.ÙR.RA) were not expected to be similarly exhausted ("hand" of Ištar) unless there was also progression to a generalized seizure (AN.TA.ŠUB.BA). When this happened, it was due to the influence ("hand") of the goddess who caused the exhaustion, namely, Ištar.

19.69 DIŠ ^{d}LUGAL.ÙR.RA *ana* AN.TA.ŠUB.BA GUR-*šú ana* ŠU ^{d}INNIN GUR-*šú* ŠU ^{d}15 *ana* KAR-*šú* . . . (DPS XXVIII:17 [AOAT 43.309–310])

**If ^{d}LUGAL.ÙR.RA turns into AN.TA.ŠUB.BA (and then) turns into "hand" of Ištar, "hand" of Ištar; to save him . . .

Patients who were exhausted by focal seizures were presumably having a whole series of them in a row, which may account for the following bad prognosis.

19.70 DIŠ ^{d}LUGAL.ÙR.RA *ana* ŠU ^{d}INNIN GUR-*šú* A.RI.A ^{d}*Šul-pa-è-a ana* ŠU. GIDIM.MA GUR-*šú* NU *i-ke-šír* (DPS XXVIII:20 [AOAT 43.310])

**If ^{d}LUGAL.ÙR.RA turns into "hand" of Ištar . . . , he will not do well.

When the prostration *preceded* the seizure, the *āšipu* had reason to suspect that some other factors were at work. The choice of Sîn, Šamaš, and Ištar as problem-causers might suggest that the prostration in question was produced by a febrile illness (see 19.266–19.268).

19.71 DIŠ ŠU ^{d}INNIN *ana* AN.TA.ŠUB.BA GUR-*šú* ŠU ^{d}30 : ŠU ^{d}15 *ana* KAR-*šú* . . . (DPS XXVIII:11 [AOAT 43.309])

**If "hand" of Ištar turns into AN.TA.ŠUB.BA, "hand" of Sîn (var. "hand" of Ištar); to save him . . .

19.72 DIŠ ŠU ^{d}INNIN *ana* ^{d}LUGAL.ÙR.RA GUR-*šú* ŠU ^{d}UTU *ana* KAR-*šú* . . . (DPS XXVIII:14 [AOAT 43.309])

**If "hand" of Ištar turns into ^{d}LUGAL.ÙR.RA, "hand" of Šamaš; to save him . . .

In a subsequent section of the diagnostic and prognostic series, the *āšipu* included a discussion of the prognostic (and ominous) implications of the first appearance of seizures of different types in a patient at various ages: at birth, three years, seven years, ten years, twenty years, thirty years, and fifty years (roughly corresponding to our categories of infant, young child, child, adolescent, young adult, and older adult). For ^{d}LUGAL.ÙR.RA (focal seizures; see above), he was most concerned with patients who were seven or younger and thirty or older.

19.73 DIŠ *ina* MU.3.<KÁM> ŠUB-*su uš-ta-sak*(*a*)*-pá-ma* ÚŠ *a-na* NU ÚŠ-*šu* . . . / DIŠ *ina* MU.7.KÁM ŠUB-*su ina* MU BI ÚŠ *a-na* NU ÚŠ-*šu* . . . (DPS XXIX:4, 6 [AOAT 43.318])

**If it falls on him in the third year, it will knock him flat(?) and he will die; in order for him not to die . . . If it falls on him in the seventh year, he will die that same year;[66] in order for him not to die . . .

19.74 DIŠ *ina* MU.10.KÁM ŠUB-*su ul-tab-bar tas-níq* KUR.RA GAR-*šú ana* ZI-*ḫi* . . . [DIŠ *ina* MU].20.KÁM ŠUB-*su* NÍG.TUKU NÍG.GA DAGAL.ME *ana* ZI-*ḫi* . . . (DPS XXIX:8, 15 [AOAT 43.319])[67]

**If it falls on him in the tenth year, he will live long; dying of old age[68] is established for him; to remove it . . . [If] it falls on him [in] the twentieth [year], he will become rich (and) his possessions will be numerous; to remove it . . .

Many seizures in children under the age of five occur in connection with febrile infections, whereas focal seizures in young adults are most commonly due to trauma. Many patients with post-traumatic seizures (up to 75 percent) either spontaneously recover or have medically controllable seizures.

19.75 ⌜DIŠ⌝ *ina* MU.30.KÁM ŠUB-*su ina* GÌR^II^-*šú* É AD-*šú* BIR-*aḫ ana* ZI-*aḫ* . . . [DIŠ *ina* M]U.5[0?.KÁM ŠU]B-*su ina* GÌR^II^-*šú* É AD-*šú* BIR-*aḫ* NU [*i-ke-šir*?] (DPS XXIX:18, 20 [AOAT 43.319–320])

**If it falls on him in the thirtieth year, the house of his father will be scattered at his feet;[69] to remove it . . . [If] it ⌜falls⌝ on him [in] the ⌜fiftieth (?)[70] year⌝, the house of his father will be scattered at his feet; [he will] not [do well(?)].

Brain tumors become more common causes of seizures in individuals between the ages of thirty and fifty, particularly in patients who first develop focal seizures at that age. After fifty, cerebrovascular disease emerges as the most common cause of focal or generalized seizures.

The *āšipu* also attached significance to the occurrence of seizures under particular circumstances. For example, a person experiencing a seizure on a journey might lay this at the door of the god to whom one typically prayed when setting out on a journey, namely, the sun-god Šamaš, as in the following reference.

19.76 DIŠ *ina a-lak gi-ru* ŠUB-*su* KAR ^d^UTU . . . (BM 56605:44 [AOAT 43.119]; cf. DPS XXIX:63′ [AOAT 43.322])

**If (a falling spell) falls on him while he is going on a journey, quay[71] of Šamaš . . .

The stay-at-home, by contrast, might suspect the influence of "the lordly" Marduk in seizures experienced in the process of going about in what the ancient Mesopotamians referred to as "lordly" fashion, that is, not having to answer to anyone else for what you do.

19.77 DIŠ *ina ṭú-ub a-la-ki-šú* ŠUB-*su lu* ŠU ^d^AMAR.UTU *lu* Š[U . . .] (DPS XXIX:67′ [AOAT 43.322]; cf. BM 56605:26 [AOAT 43.118])

**If it falls on him while he is going about wherever he pleases, either "hand" of Marduk or ⌜"hand"⌝ of [. . .]

Similarly, the god of the city got you when you went outside the walls to take a swim in the river, and the moon-god, Sîn, during the night.

19.78 DIŠ *ina* ⸢ÍD *ṭe₄*⸣*-bi-šú* ŠUB-*su* ŠU DINGIR URU-*šú* . . . (DPS XXIX:65′ [AOAT 43.322]; cf. BM 56605:12 [AOAT 43.118])

**If it falls on him while he is going down to the river (to swim), "hand" of the god of his city . . .

19.79 DIŠ *ina mu-ši* ŠUB-*su* KAR ᵈ30 *ana* ZI.BI . . . (BM 56605:24 [AOAT 43.118])

**If it falls on him in the night, quay of Sîn; to remove it . . .

STROKES

Severe strokes were the work of the *rābiṣu,* whereas ghosts produced very mild, reversible, strokes. Strokes were further differentiated into those affecting the right and left sides of the body by the simple expedient of dividing off Šulak, the *rābiṣu* specifically associated with the lavatory, from an unnamed colleague. For more details, see pp. 327–329.

ŠULAK

In many cases, the *āšipu*'s concern with handedness was of no modern clinical relevance. In this case, however, he was justified. Strokes that cause right-sided hemiparesis may also leave the patient unable to talk, since the speech center is located on the left side of the brain, as is the motor cortex that controls the muscles on the right side of the body. As the *āšipu* put it, it was specifically Šulak, causer of "tenseness" in the right side of the body, who "seized the patient's mouth."[72]

19.80 [*šu-me-el*] *pa-ag-ri-šu ka-la-a-ma* ⸢*ta*⸣*-a*[*b*]*-kà-at*! *da-bá-bá la-a i-le-ʾ-e* [. . . *la-a i-l*] *e-ʾ-e* ŠU ᵈ*Šu-la-ak m*[*i*!?*-ḫi-i*]*ṣ me-še-ti ma-ḫi-iṣ* ᴸᵁ́*a-ši-pu a-n*[*a ba-la-ṭi-šu qí-i-ba l*] *a-a i-ša-kán* (StBoT 36.22 obv. 11–13)[73]

**(If) the entire [right side of] his body is tense (and) he is not able to talk (and) he is [not] ⸢able⸣ to [. . .] "hand" of Šulak (or) he was wounded with the wound of a stroke; the *āšipu* should ⸢not⸣ make a [prognosis as to his recovery].

19.81 KA.⸢INIM⸣.MA *šum-ma* MAŠKIM KA LÚ *uṣ-ṣab-*[*bit*] // MAŠKIM KA LÚ *uṣ-ṣab-b*[*it*] . . . A PÚ *šá* E-*ú* : *ina* ŠÀ-*šá* MAŠKIM *mu-sa-a-*[*tú*] ᵈ*Šu-lak* : *lu-ú* ᵈ*Šu-lak šá mu-sa-a-*[*tú*] (*SpTU* 1.46:27[74] with its commentary *SpTU* 1.47 obv. 13–15)

**"Recitation for cases where a *rābiṣu* ⸢seizes⸣ a person's mouth." (The commentary goes on to analyze this text as follows) "a *rābiṣu* seizes a person's mouth" . . . when it says (you are to use) well water (for this), it is because the *rābiṣu* of the ⸢lavatory⸣ is Šulak. It is truly Šulak of the ⸢lavatory⸣ (who causes this).

It was presumably the accompanying numbness of the face and lips that attracted the diagnosis of Šulak to trigeminal neuralgia (see above). Possibly, the disturbances of speech that are associated with Sydenham's chorea are what caused chorea of infectious origin also to be blamed on Šulak. For more details, see Chapter 13 with 13.256–13.257.

RĀBIṢU'S FOOTSTEPS

Sydenham's chorea is a delayed manifestation of rheumatic fever, and *rābiṣus* were otherwise held responsible for irregularities in heartbeat (see 19.115–19.120) including rapid heart beat (tachycardia), which can be a manifestation of rheumatic carditis. In view of these connections between Sydenham's chorea and rapid heart rate (tachycardia) and the *rābiṣu* it is possible that the following references, which are attributed to the patient's having trod in the footsteps of a *rābiṣu*, and which describe a complex of fever and arthritis, are due to rheumatic fever.[75] In the first reference below, the left temple's "seeming to shake" and the right temple's being hot seems to be the *āšipu*'s way of saying that both temples were hot and "shaking" at the same time. What was exactly meant by "shaking" is unclear, but a possible suggestion is that this was the patient's perception of what the *āšipu* called a "jumping" (i.e., very rapid) pulse.

19.82 DIŠ SAG.KI-*šú šá* 15 *i-rad-ma šá* 150 KÚM KI.ÚS SAG.TUKU KI.ÚS-*us* DIN (DPS IV B obv. 23 = *TDP* 34:23)

**If his left temple (seems to) shake[76] and the right one is hot, he has trod in the footsteps of a *rābiṣu*;[77] he will get well.

19.83 DIŠ GÌR^{II}-*šú it-t*[*a-n*] *a-aš-gag-ga ina* KI.ÚS MAŠKIM GUB-*iz* DIN (DPS XIV A$_2$ iv 15′//G iv 5′ = *TDP* 142 iv 15′)

**If his feet ⸢continually⸣ become stiff, he stood in the footsteps of a *rābiṣu*; he will get well.

19.84 DIŠ NA GÌR^{II}-*šú* GIG-*ma te-ba-a u ú-zu-za la i-*[*le-ʾ-i*] *ù* ŠU^{II}-*šú* GÌR^{II}-*šú i-ra-ʾu-ba* NA BI *man-za-az* MAŠKIM x [. . .] *ana* GÌR^{II}-*šú bul-lu-ṭi* . . . (*AMT* 69/2:2–4//*BAM* 152 iv 1–3; *AMT* 70/7 i 9′)

**If a person's feet are so sore that he ⸢can⸣ not get up and stand and his hands and feet tremble, that person [trod? on] the emplacement of a *rābiṣu*, to cure his feet . . .

ŠULPAEA

If chorea and paralysis due to strokes were the product of Šulak, choreoathetosis and paralysis due to degenerative diseases of the brain or spinal cord were the specialties of an obscure god known as Šulpaea. The syndromes that he produced include what appear to be Huntington's disease, cerebral palsy, and Werdnig-Hoffmann disease in small children or amyotrophic lateral sclerosis in adults. For more details, see Chapter 13 with 13.244–13.247, 13.258–13.260. Šulpaea was also implicated in a type of brain abscess.

19.85 [DIŠ DIB DI]B-*su-ma* UZU.MEŠ-*šú* ⸢*ú*⸣-*za*!-*qat ri-mu-tú* T[UKU-*š*]*i* [. . .]x-ni *ina* DUG$_4$.DUG$_4$-*šú* ur x GAR-*nu ù ir-te-*[*ḫ*] *a* [*re-ḫ*] *u-ut* ^{d}*Šul-pa-è-a* DIB-*su šum$_4$-ma* U$_4$ [D]IB-*šú* [GEŠTU Z]AG-*šú* KÚM TÉŠ.MEŠ-*aš* GIG-*su* DU$_8$ *šum$_4$-ma* U$_4$-*ma* DIB-*šú* [GEŠTU] GÙB-*šú* KÚM TÉŠ.MEŠ-*aš* GIG-*šú* GÍD.DA-*ma* (*STT* 89:167–171)

**[If an affliction] ⸢afflicts⸣ him and his flesh stings(?), he ⸢has⸣ paralysis [. . .] when he talks [. . .] and it flows over him, ⸢"spawn"⸣ of Šulpaea afflicts him. If when it ⸢afflicts⸣ him, his ⌜left⌝ [ear] is hot and stinks,[78] his illness will let up. If when it afflicts him, his right [ear] is hot and stinks, his illness may be prolonged (but it will let up).

In the preceding quote, the "hot" and "stinking" suggests a middle ear or mastoid infection as the source of the abscess. The specific mention of paralysis is suggestive of a cerebral abscess. For more details, see Chapter 13 with 13.226.

DAPINU

Šulpaea, designated by the epithet *Dapinu* ("the ferocious"), was associated with the planet Jupiter (normally Marduk) for two months of the year.[79] It was, with the exception of the first reference below, this form of the god that was held responsible for producing the perception on the part of the patient of loss of a sector of the visual field in one eye.

19.86 DIŠ SAG.KI-*šú šá* 150 KÚ-*šú u* IGI-*šú šá* 150 GISSU DÙ ŠU [d]*Šul-pa-è-a* BÚR-*ma* DIN (DPS IV B obv. 28//E i 8 = *TDP* 36:28//*SpTU* 3.88 i 8)

**If his right temple hurts him and his right eye makes a shadow, "hand" of Šulpaea. (If) it goes away, he will get well.

Although it is not apparent in the reference above, this one-sided vision loss could take several days to develop, as in the following reference.

19.87 DIŠ U_4.2.KÁM GIG-*ma* SAG.KI-*šú šá* 15 KÚ-*šú* IGI-*šú šá* 15 GISSU DÙ ŠU [d]UD.AL.TAR BÚR-*ma* DIN (DPS XVI:21–22 [AOAT 43.174])

**If he has been sick for two days and his left/right temple hurts him and his left/right eye makes a shadow, "hand" of Dapinu. (If) it goes away, he will get well.

It is difficult given such limited signs and symptoms to attempt a diagnosis. However, a possibility would be some form of retrobulbar optic neuropathy, which can produce severe loss of vision over the course of a few days. There is often pain on movement of the eye or on pressure on the globe. After a few days or weeks, the other eye may become similarly involved with loss of central vision but with some preservation of peripheral vision. In a high percentage of patients, no cause can be found, and after days or weeks there may be a spontaneous recovery of vision.

In addition to vision problems, Dapinu also produced symptoms more to be expected of a by-form of Šulpaea.

19.88 DIŠ IGI.MEŠ-*šú* NIGIN.MEŠ ŠU[II]-*šú u* GÌR[II]-*šú i-ra-ʾ-ú-ba* U_4.59.KÁM ŠU [d]UD.AL.TAR (DPS IX A 59//B r. 3 = *TDP* 76:59)

**If his face seems continually to be spinning (and) his hands and his feet tremble (and he has been sick for) fifty-nine days, "hand" of Dapinu.

The term used to describe "trembling" (*raʾābu*) may specifically indicate an intention tremor (see Chapter 13 with 13.82). As to what might have connected transient vision loss with a several months-long attack of "spinning" dizziness and "trembling" extremities in the mind of the *āšipu*, 40 percent of patients with multiple sclerosis experience an episode of optic neuritis either as their first difficulty or at some point in the course of their disease. Conversely, 15 to 40 percent of patients with retrobulbar optic neuropathy will develop other signs and symptoms consistent with multiple sclerosis within ten to fifteen years, and even more will do so if the patients are observed for longer periods.

Gods/Goddesses of Pain

A fairly clear example of the use of various gods/goddesses and demons/demonesses to differentiate individual syndromes within a disease class is in the treatment of arthritic pain. In addition to describing joints with stiffness, pain, swelling, sluggishness, and "shrinking," the *āšipu* distinguished between arthritis in old and exceptionally young patients and assigned symptoms consistent with arthritis to DÚR.GIG (see Chapter 6), the *rābiṣu*-demon (see 19.83–19.84), "semen made to lie with a corpse" (see Chapter 11 with 11.54–11.56), and the "hand"s of Šamaš and Ištar. Ištar probably caused gonococcal arthritis (see Chapter 11 with 11.49–11.53) and Šamaš perhaps psoriatic arthritis (see Chapter 11 with 11.42–11.48). The *āšipu* also separately discussed lower back pain, of which he recognized two grades. This seems to have been attributed to ghosts, presumably because it tends to be one-sided (see above, p. 441). For more details, see Chapter 11 with 11.61.

Gods/Goddesses of Skin Disease

Skin conditions with "hand" diagnoses are the hardest to justify in terms of signs and symptoms, suggesting a more than usually arbitrary assignment of causal agents. Some of the divinities involved were constellations or heavenly bodies, and it is possible that there was some formula whereby the "divine writing" in the heavens (i.e., the stars) was mapped onto the skin surface.

PABILSAG

Associated with the city of Isin, Pabilsag was also the constellation we call Sagittarius. He produced what is either a mixed sexually transmitted disease (STD) involving *Herpes simplex* type 2 (HSV2) and chancroid or a painful suppurating ulcer surrounded by redness (see Chapter 4 with 4.32).

19.89 DIŠ GIG MIN *ul-la-nu-ma ḫa-ri-is* ŠÀ-*ba-šu* KAK.MEŠ DIRI KAK.MEŠ-*šú* BAD KÚ[M] *u* DU-*ak lam-ṣa-at ḫi-la-a-ti* NÍTA MU.NI IM *iš-biṭ-su-ma si-ḫi-*[*ip-ti*] ^{d}PA.BIL.SAG DUG$_4$.GA GAR-*an ana* ZI-*šú* . . . (*BAM* 580 iii 15′–17′)

**If a sore (comes out on a person's body), it has been itching for a long time, the inside of it is full of *sikkatu* (peg-shaped lesions), it encloses its *sikkatu*, it is hot and it flows, it is called a male suppurating *lamṣātu*-ulcer. (If) "wind" has blasted him, ⌜overwhelming⌝ by Pabilsag. You may make a (favorable) prognosis; to remove it . . .

TWIN GODS

The "twin gods" gave us the name of our constellation Gemini. They produced what is either a mixed STD involving HSV2 and syphilis or a painless suppurating ulcer surrounded by redness (see Chapter 4 with 4.25).

19.90 DIŠ GIG MIN *ul* KÚ-*šú* IGI UZU.MEŠ-*šú-ma* GAR-*in* MÚD-*šú-ma* MÚD.[BABBAR] *šur-du-ma* DU-*ak lam-ṣa-at ḫi-la-a-te* MUNUS MU.NI IM *iš-*[*biṭ-su-ma*] *si-ḫi-ip-ti* ^{d}MAŠ.TAB.BA *qí-ba* GAR-*an ana* ZI-*šú* . . . (*BAM* 580 iii 20′–22′)

**If a sore (comes out on a person's body), it does not hurt him, it is placed only on the surface of his flesh, (and) its blood (and) pus flows freely, it is called a female suppurating *lamṣātu*-ulcer. (If) "wind" has ⌜blasted him,⌝ overwhelming by the twin gods. You may make a (favorable) prognosis. To remove it . . .

EA

This god of the sweet waters was a patron of the healing arts, but also presided over the lowest of the ancient Mesopotamian heavens, the "path of Ea" through which the stars passed each night. He was responsible for clustered (as opposed to solitary) lesions (*ummedu*; see Chapter 10). Was the reference perhaps to clusters of stars?

19.91 *um-me-di* [Š]U ^{d}*É-*[*a*] (DPS XXXIII:109 [AOAT 43.358])

** *Ummedu* (are caused by) ⌜"hand"⌝ of ⌜Ea⌝.

IŠTAR

Ištar was also the planet Venus; what sore she produced is unfortunately lost in a lacuna.

19.92 *a-na si-ḫi-ip-ti* ^{d}EŠ$_{4}$.DAR [. . .] *ana* IGI GIG Ì.NUN.NA ŠÉŠ [. . .] (*BAM* 582 ii 5′–6′)

**For overwhelming by Ištar [. . .] you rub ghee on the sore and [. . .]

SÎN

Sîn, the moon-god, was dreaded for his tendency to inflict those who angered him with lesions that were or resembled those of Hansen's disease (*saḫaršubbû*; see Chapter 3).[80] In this enterprise, Sîn was assisted by other members of his family (his son Šamaš[81] and his daughter Ištar).[82] Since the *epqu*-lesions of *saḫaršubbû* came in a variety of colors (see Chapter 10), it is possible that the division of labor was the same as for generalized *bubu'tu* lesions (see below), namely, that "white" lesions went to Šamaš, "black" or "dark" to Ištar, and "red" to Sîn. That this was indeed the case would seem to be indicated by the following reference.

19.93 KI.MIN SAḪAR.ŠUB.BA SIG$_{7}$ SA$_{5}$ ŠU ^{d}30 *ana* ZI-*šú* . . . (Tsukimoto, *Priests and Officials* 199–200:60)

**(If the patient has) yellow and red *saḫaršubbû*, "hand" of Sîn, to remove it . . .

When all possible colors were present, the *āšipu* used what appears to have been his "god only knows" category, "hand" of god (see below under Ill-defined Syndromes of the Sort Gods/Goddesses Might Cause).

19.94 KI.MIN SAḪAR.ŠUB.BA SA_5 BABBAR GI_6 ŠU DINGIR LÚ *ana* ZI-*šú* . . . (Tsukimoto, *Priests and Officials* 199–200:61, 70)

**(If the patient has) red, white, and black *saḫaršubbû*, "hand" of the person's god, to remove it . . .

This division of labor may also explain the attribution of what appear to be descriptions of congenital syphilis either to "hand" of god or to Sîn and Ištar. In this case, Sîn and Ištar would indicate the presence of a rash that consists of reddish lesions (Sîn) and gray plaques (Ištar). "Hand" of god would indicate the additional presence of another color, yellow, possibly due to faded subcutaneous petechiae or ecchymoses (see Chapter 6 with 6.123–6.125).

19.95 DIŠ LÚ.TUR $ŠU^{II}$-*šú u* $GÌR^{II}$-*šú it-ta-na-an-pa-ḫa* IGI^{II}-*šú uz-za-na-qap* ^{GIŠ}GIDRU ^{d}30 *u* ^{d}15 (DPS XL A 56 = *TDP* 224:56)

**If an infant's hand and feet are continually swollen (and) he continually constricts[83] (the pupils of) his eyes, scepter of Sîn and/or Ištar.

19.96 DIŠ LÚ.TUR UZU.MEŠ-*šú* SIG_7 ŠUB-*ú* ŠÀ.MEŠ-*šú eb-ṭu* $ŠU^{II}$-*šú* GÌR-*šú nap-ḫa li-ʾ-ba ma-gal* TUKU *ḫa-še-e* GIG ŠU DINGIR TI (DPS XL A 29 = *TDP* 220:29)

**If an infant's flesh is unevenly colored with yellow, his insides are cramped, his hands (and) feet are swollen, he has lots of *liʾbu* (see Chapter 3), and the lungs are sick, "hand" of god; he will get well.

NINGAL

Ningal, Sîn's wife, was considered responsible for guinea worm infestations.

19.97 DIŠ GIG *ina* SU NA È GIN_7 *i-ba-ri* È *lu* IGI UZU-*šú-ma pa?-še-er u na-kis ni-lu-gu*$_4$ MU.NI ŠU ^{d}NIN.GAL *qí-ba* GAR-*an ana* ZI-*šú* . . . (*BAM* 417 obv. 14–15)

**If a sore comes out on a person's body (and) it comes out like an *ibaru*-lesion or it comes through(?) his skin and is cut off, its name is *nilugu*;[84] "hand" of Ningal. You may make a (favorable) prognosis; to remove it . . .

OTHER DIVINITIES

Other divinities to whom skin lesions were attributed had little if anything to do with stars. Ningeštinanna was the sister of Ištar's lover Dumuzi and scribe to Ereškigal, queen of the nether world. She has one reference[85] that is unfortunately too fragmentary to allow a great deal to be said about it. Nergal was the husband of Ereškigal and king of the netherworld. It was probably his close association with pestilence that caused his name to be written ^{d}Ù/U_4.BU.BU.UL: "god of *bubuʾtu* (vesicles)" in several god lists.[86] The reference is presumably to fever blisters. For some unknown reason, Adad, god of thunderstorms, joined Marduk, head of the Babylonian pantheon, in causing serious cases of acne.[87]

We are on somewhat firmer ground with the skin conditions and their godly causers, which appear on the skin tablet (Tablet XXXIII) of the diagnostic series. These include Gula,[88] Ninurta, Marduk, and Šamaš.[89]

GULA

As goddess of health, Gula was a lady not to be crossed. According to Middle Babylonian curse formulae, those who broke oaths sworn by the gods had to fear the possibility that Gula might inflict upon them a "persistent sore."[90]

19.98 *ṣi-i-tu*$_4$ ŠU ^{d}*Gu-la* . . . *ṣar-ri-šu* ŠU ^{d}*Gu-la* (DPS XXXIII:104–105 [AOAT 43.357])

**Growths (are caused by) "hand" of Gula . . . proliferating (sores are caused by) "hand" of Gula.

NINURTA

19.99 *ša-*[*da*]*-nu* ŠU ^{d}NIN.[IB] *ta-kal-tu*$_4$ ŠU ^{d}NIN.IB *aḫ-ḫ*[*a-z*]*u* ŠU ^{d}[NIN.IB] (DPS XXXIII:106–107 [AOAT 43.358])

**⸢*šadānu*⸣ (is caused by) "hand" of ⸢Ninurta⸣. (Sick) liver[91] (is caused by) "hand" of Ninurta; ⸢*aḫḫāzu*⸣-jaundice (is caused by) "hand" of [Ninurta].

For the association of the god Ninurta with the liver, see below, 19.365–19.367. As the *āšipu* knew, some forms of liver disease were accompanied by "tense flesh," that is, skin lesions (see Chapter 6 with 6.123–6.125) or jaundice, which accounts for the inclusion of this entry in a discussion of skin conditions. The context in which Ninurta was associated with *šadānu* was as causer of plague or plaguelike illness, as shown below.[92] For more details, see Chapter 3.

19.100 DIŠ GIG GAR-*šú ki-ma* NA$_4$ *da-an qer-bi-nu-um-ma* GAL *qer-bi-nu-um-ma* DU-*ak* ÍL-*šú* ⸢ZI!⸣-*a* [*u*] DU.ME[Š GUB-*za*] *la i-le-eʾ-e šá-da-nu* MU.NI TAG ^{d}AMAR.UTU *u* [^{d}NIN.IB] (DPS XXXIII:31 [AOAT 43.354–355] restored from *BAM* 409 obv. 33′–36′)

**If the nature of his sore is that it is hard as a rock, as it grows down inside, it continually goes down inside (and) he is not able to lift (his foot),[93] to get up, to walk (or) to stand, its name is *šadānu*; "touch" of Marduk and [Ninurta].

MARDUK

As we know from other references, the god Marduk commonly caused chest pain (see 19.111).

19.101 *di-ik-šú* ŠU ^{d}AMAR.UTU (DPS XXXIII:108 [AOAT 43.358])

**Needling pain (is caused by) "hand" of Marduk.

What justified the inclusion of this entry on the tablet of the diagnostic series dealing with skin conditions was presumably the occasional association of Marduk's chest pain with skin lesions. Two such lesions are attested for this god: *ziqtu* (whitehead; see Chapter 10 with 10.108–10.109) and yellow *ramīṭu*-lesions.

19.102 DIŠ IGI.MEŠ-*šú* ḪÁD.A SIG$_7$.MEŠ DIRI.MEŠ ŠU ^{d}BAD DIN (DPS IX A 45//C 13 = *TDP* 74:45)

**If his face is full of yellow *ramīṭu*-lesions, "hand" of Bel ("the lord"; i.e., Marduk); he will get well.

Ramīṭu-lesions were plaquelike and, depending on which etymology you favor, either caused by overexposure to sunlight or pale in color or both (for more details, see Chapter 10 with 10.161–10.170). Pale yellow plaques occurring in quantity on the face sounds like a reasonable description of what we call xanthelasma. These lesions, a sign of plasma lipid abnormalities, may indeed accompany heart problems (specifically myocardial infarctions). Hypercholesterolemia, a familial genetic disorder, is characterized by elevation (up to eight times normal) in the amount of LDL cholesterol in the bloodstream, and is a major risk factor for coronary artery disease.

ŠAMAŠ

"Scratchies" (*ekketu*; see Chapter 10) and *girgiššu* (perhaps erysipelas attributed to the god of the sun due to the reddening of the face; see Chapter 10) may have been due to irritation and/or infection of the skin, in the latter case by group A streptococci.

19.103 *gir-giš-šum* ŠU ^{d}UTU . . . *ek-ke-tum* ŠU ^{d}UTU (DPS XXXIII:110–111 [AOAT 43.358])

***girgiššu* (is caused by) "hand" of Šamaš . . . *ekketu* (is caused by) "hand" of Šamaš.

When group A streptococci enter the body via scratching or mosquito bites, glomerulonephritis can result. It is, therefore, interesting to note that Šamaš was also held responsible for "swelling." The edema of glomerulonephritis tends to appear initially in areas of low tissue pressure, such as around the eyes, but may subsequently lead to ascites and circulatory congestion.

19.104 DIŠ IGI.MEŠ-*šú* ŠÀ.MEŠ-*šú* ⸢ŠU⸣^{II}-*šú u* GÌR^{II}-*šú* MÚ.ME *nap-paḫ-tú* GIG ŠU ^{d}20 (DPS IX A 68//B r. 14 = *TDP* 78:68)

**If his face, his insides, his hands, and his feet are continually swollen, he is ill with swelling; "hand" of Šamaš.[94]

In their fullest form (and in slightly different order), the following references to Šamaš and other members of his family (his father Sîn and his sister Ištar) appear elsewhere in the diagnostic series.[95] The last of these references, at least, appears to refer to the characteristic lesions of *Herpes simplex* type 1 (HSV1). For more details, see Chapter 10 with 10.82–10.84.

19.105 Ù.BU.BU.U[L] BABBAR ŠU ^{d}UTU TI-*uṭ* [Ù.BU.BU.UL GI$_6$] ŠU ^{d}*Iš-tar* TAG-*it* NAM.TAR NU DIN-*uṭ* Ù.BU.B[U.U]L [S]A$_5$ ŠU ^{d}30 KI.MIN (DPS XXXIII:113–114 [AOAT 43.358])

**White ⸢*bubu'tu*⸣ : "hand" of Šamaš; he will get well. [Black *bubu'tu*] : "hand" of Ištar; "touch" of (his) personal death demon; he will not get well. ⸢Red *bubu'tu*⸣ : "hand" of Sîn; (he will get well).

Also distributed among Šamaš and his family on grounds of the color of the lesion and the color of the surrounding skin were the vesicles of sexually transmitted *Herpes simplex* type 2 (HSV2) (see Chapter 10 with 10.85–10.87).

19.106 [DIŠ T]A SAG.DU-*šú* EN [GÌR^{II}-*š*] *ú* U$_4$.BU.BU.UL BABBAR/GI$_6$ DIRI *u* SU-*šú* GI$_6$/SA$_5$ KI.MIN ŠU ^{d}UTU (DPS III A r. 11′–12′//C r. 34–35 = *TDP* 28:94–95)[96]

** [If] ⌜from⌝ his head to [his feet], he is full of white/dark *bubuʾtu* and his skin/body is dark/red, (he was "gotten" in bed with a woman), "hand" of Šamaš.

Possibly to be connected with the preceding reference are the two other examples of affliction by Šamaš that follow.

19.107 DIŠ NA GÌŠ SÌG.SÌG-*šú i-te-e[b]-bi* KI A-*šú* MURUB$_4$.MEŠ-*šú* KÚ.MEŠ-*šú šá* NA BI ⌜xx⌝ *ki-mil-ti* ^{d}UTU UGU-*šú* GÁL-*ši* . . . (*STT* 95 i 42–43)

**If a person's penis continually gives him a jabbing pain, he gets up (to urinate and) with his water his pelvic region hurts him, that person [. . .]; the anger of Šamaš is upon him . . .

19.108 DIŠ *ina mu-šar-ri-šú* MÚD SUR ŠU ^{d}UTU MU KI.NU.GI GAM (DPS XIV A ii 37//C ii 12//F 3 = *TDP* 134 ii 37)

**If blood drips from his penis, "hand" of Šamaš on account of sexual intercourse with a woman;[97] he will die.

HSV2 urethritis can produce pain and small amounts of bleeding ("drips"). That the second reference suspects that "intercourse with a woman" was the source of the patient's problem is suggestive, although kidney stones can produce the same symptoms. Since stones are usually diagnosed as such, however, it is possible that the *āšipu* meant "hand" of Šamaš to refer to pain and bleeding where no stone was present.

Gods/Goddesses of Heart Problems

PERSONAL GOD OR GODDESS

As we already noted, every ancient Mesopotamian had his own personal god and goddess, a sort of guardian angel. When these personal guardians became angry, their charges became stressed and/or experienced chest pain.

19.109 DIŠ NA ŠÀ-*šú* GAZ.MEŠ-*šú pi-qam* NU *pi-qam i-pár-ru-ud* NA BI DIB-*ti* DINGIR *u* ^{d}*Eš$_4$-dar* UGU-*šú* GÁL-*ši* DINGIR-*šú* KI-*šú ze-ni ana* BÚR . . . (*BAM* 316 iii 8′–10′)[98]

**If a person's heart continually crushes him (and) shudders incessantly, the anger of god or goddess is upon him, his god is angry with him, to loosen (it) . . .

19.110 DIŠ NA *gi-na-a šu-dur ur-ra u mu-ši ina-an-ziq* . . . MÁŠ.GI$_6$.MEŠ-*šú* ḪUL.MEŠ *ina* MÁŠ.GI$_6$-*šú* ÚŠ.MEŠ IGI.MEŠ GAZ ŠÀ-*bi* TUKU-*šú* MÁŠ.GI$_6$ IGI NU DIB-*át ina* MÁŠ.GI$_6$-*šú* GIN$_7$ *šá* KI MUNUS *uš-ta-ḫu*!-*u* A.RI.A-*šú i-ṣar-ru-ru šib-sat* DINGIR *u* ^{d}15 UGU-*šú* GÁL-*ši* . . . (*SpTU* 2.22 i 16, 19–21)[99]

**If a person is continually made sad, he is upset day and night . . . (he is having serious financial losses; people slander him, lie to him, and talk about him behind his back), his dreams are bad, in his dream he continually sees dead persons, he has a crushing sensation in his heart, he cannot remember the dream that he sees, (and) during his dream, his semen flows like one who has congress with a woman, the anger of god or goddess is upon him . . .

MARDUK

In causing chest pain, the personal god and goddess were joined by the god Marduk. As we know from the Creation Epic, Marduk became king of the gods by virtue of his defeat of the monstress Tiamat from whose corpse he created the universe. Given the commonplace associations of the heart with courage,[100] it seems plausible that Marduk was associated with chest pain because he epitomized divine heroism and bravery.

19.111 DIŠ NA *ina ma-ka-li-šú* ŠÀ-*šú* GAZ.MEŠ-*šú ina* É *ṣal-te ina* SILA *pu-úḫ-pu-ḫu-u* GAR-*šú šá* NA BI *ki-mil-ti* [d]AMAR.UTU UGU-*šú* GÁL-*ši* DIB-*ti* [d]AMAR.UTU *ana* BÚR-*ri* . . . (*BAM* 317 r. 27–28//*AMT* 40/2:4′–6′//*STT* 95 i 7–8)[101]

**If when a person eats, his heart continually crushes him (and) in the house quarrel and in the street disturbance are inflicted upon him, the anger of Marduk is upon that person, to loosen the anger of Marduk . . .

In addition to causing chest pain all by himself, Marduk might be joined with other deities in cases where heart symptoms were prominent but where the problem did not originate with the heart. For example, Marduk joined with pursuing ghosts to cause poisoning by belladonna drugs (see Chapter 15). In addition, he joined with Ištar to produce the symptoms of what could be disseminated gonococcal infection (see 8.1).

19.112 DIŠ NA *ina* KI.NÁ-*šú* LUḪ.LUḪ-*ut* ŠÀ-*šú e-šu-u ina* KI.NÁ-*šú re-ḫu-su* DU-*ak* NA BI DIB-*ti* [d]AMAR.UTU *u* [d]EŠ$_4$.DAR UGU-*šú* GÁL-*ši ana* TI-*šú* . . . (*BAM* 205: 19′–21′//*STT* 95:16–18//*STT* 280 ii 1–3)

**If a person continually jerks in his bed, his heart (beat) is confused, (and) his semen flows in his bed, the anger of Marduk and Ištar is upon that person, to cure him . . .

19.113 DIŠ *ina* SAG ŠÀ-*šú* [*di-ik-šú* GAR-*su-ma ur*]-*qá* ŠUB-*a* ŠU [d]AMAR.UTU : ŠU [d]15 GAM (DPS XIII B i 42′//F 4 = *TDP* 114 i 46′)

**If [a needling pain is firmly established] in his upper abdomen (epigastrium) (and) he is unevenly colored with ⸢yellow spots⸣, "hand" of Marduk (var. "hand" of Ištar); he will die.

The reason for Marduk's association with Ninurta in causing plague is less clear, but may have to do with the pericarditis that can be associated with it. Also potentially relevant is the development by some patients of disseminated intervascular coagulopathy and bleeding. Marduk caused bleeding in the context of hemorrhagic fever (see Chapter 3 with 3.237–3.238).

19.114 DIŠ GIG GAR-*šú ki-ma* NA_4 *da-an qer-bi-nu-um-ma* GAL *qer-bi-nu-um-ma* DU-*ak* ÍL-*šú* ⌜ZI!⌝-*a* [*u*] DU.ME[Š GUB-*za*] *la i-le-e*ᵓ*-e šá-da-nu* MU.NI TAG ᵈAMAR.UTU *u* [ᵈNIN.IB] (DPS XXXIII:31 [AOAT 43.354–355] restored from *BAM* 409 obv. 33′–36′)

**If the nature of his sore is that it is hard as a rock, as it grows down inside, it continually goes down inside, (and) he is not able to lift (his foot),[102] to get up, to walk, (or) to stand, its name is *šadānu*; "touch" of Marduk and [Ninurta].

BLOW OF A *RĀBIṢU*

This demon was normally blamed for severe strokes (see 13.228). The following reference, however, appears to describe a case of thyrotoxicosis. In patients over forty, cardiovascular and myopathic symptoms dominate the clinical picture. In addition to velvety skin, silky hair, excessive sweating, and heat intolerance, patients experience rapid heart beat ("pulsating temporal blood vessels"), systolic murmurs, and, at times, overt heart failure ("protruding upper abdomen" due to ascites). For more details on thyrotoxicosis, see Chapter 7.

19.115 DIŠ *ú-ru-uḫ* SAG.KI-*šú šá* 15 *bé-e-er* SA.MEŠ-*šú šá* 150 ZI.MEŠ DIB-*it* ŠÀ TUKU *u* SAG ŠÀ-*šú i-ru-ur* SÌG-*iṣ* MAŠK[I]M GAM (DPS IV B r. 20//E iv 4 = *TDP* 44 r. 41–42//*SpTU* 3.88 iv 4)

**If the hair of his left temple is fine (lit. "select"), his blood vessels, the ones on the right (feel like they) are pulsating (i.e., the fine head hair and pulsating temporal blood vessels appeared simultaneously), he has affliction of the abdomen and his upper abdomen (epigastrium) rumbles, blow of a *rābiṣu*; he will die.

It may have been the rapid heart rate ("pulsating temporal blood vessels"), which is one of the prominent findings of thyrotoxicosis, that attracted the diagnosis of "blow of a *rābiṣu*" to this disease. We believe this because rapid heart beat (tachycardia) when appearing by itself was also diagnosed as "blow of a *rābiṣu*." Sometimes, the *āšipu* could actually feel the vessels pulsating rapidly; often, however, he recognized this condition from the fact that his patient's rapidly beating heart produced a pulse that was too weak to detect. As explained in Chapter 8, the term "*go*" in the following reference describes a weak or absent pulse.

19.116 [DIŠ SA SA]G.KI^{II}-*šú* ⌜*šá*⌝ 15 *u* 150 *ina* DU-*ki im-taḫ-ru* SÌG-*iṣ* [MA]ŠKIM SÌG-*iṣ* ^{LÚ}MAŠ.MAŠ DÙ-*uš* ⌜DIN⌝ [: GAM] (DPS IV A_2 r. 20–21+A_5 r. 4–5//B r. 2 = *TDP* 40 r. 20–21; cf. Labat, *Syria* 33.125 r. 13)[103]

**[If the blood vessel(s) of] his ⌜temples⌝, the ones on the left and the ones on the right,"go" to an equal extent, he was struck with the blow of a ⌜*rābiṣu*⌝. You may do his medical treatment; he will get well [or die].

The *āšipu* was aware that rapid heart rate (tachycardia) was not necessarily fatal, and looked for accompanying symptoms to aid in his prognoses.[104] In some cases, the rapid heart beat (tachycardia) was accompanied by upper or generalized abdominal pain or "changes of mood." The pain and emotional distress might have been due to cardiac angina or myocardial infarction. The patient sometimes survived, but usually died.

19.117 [DIŠ SA S]AG.KI^{II}-*šú šá* 15 *u* 150 1-*niš* DU.MEŠ SAG ŠÀ-*šú* DIB.DIB-*su* SÌG-*iṣ* MAŠKIM SÌG-*iṣ* [MAŠ].MAŠ-*su* DÙ-*ma* DIN (DPS IV A_2 r. 26–27+A_5 r. 10–11//B r. 7 = *TDP* 40 r. 26–27; cf. Ni. 470:5–6 [Kraus, *ZA* 77.197])

**[If the blood vessel(s)] of his ⌜temples⌝, the ones on the left and the ones on the right "go" at the same time (and) his upper abdomen (epigastrium) continually afflicts him, he was struck with the blow of a *rābiṣu*. (If) you do his ⌜medical treatment⌝ (right away), he will get well.

19.118 [DIŠ SA S]AG.KI^{II}-*šú šá* 15 *u* 150 1-*niš* DU.ME-*ma u šu-ú* BAL.BAL SÌG-*iṣ* MAŠKIM GAM (DPS IV A_2 r. 28+A_5 r. 12//B r. 8 = *TDP* 42 r. 28; cf. Ni. 470:7 [Kraus, *ZA* 77.197])

**[If the blood vessel(s)] of his ⌜temples⌝, the ones on the left and the ones on the right "go" at the same time and he has changes of mood, blow of a *rābiṣu*; he will die.

Other grave signs for a victim of a blow by a *rābiṣu* were peripheral cyanosis ("black hands") and syncope (loss of consciousness).

19.119 DIŠ SA SAG.KI-*šú te-bu-ú* [SÌG-*iṣ* MAŠKIM . . .] / DIŠ ŠU^{II}-*šú ṣa-al-ma ù* [LÚ.AD$_6$-*šú ma-ši* SÌG-*iṣ* MAŠKIM . . .] (Ni. 470:1–2 [Kraus, *ZA* 77.197])[105]

**If his temporal blood vessel(s) (feel like they) are pulsating, [blow of a *rābiṣu* . . .]. If his hands are black and [he loses consciousness, blow of a *rābiṣu* . . .]

19.120 [DIŠ DIB-*su* DIB].DIB-*su ir-te-né-eḫ-ḫi-šú u iš-ta-na-da-as-su* MÁ[ŠK]IM KI-*šú* KEŠDA *ina* SAG-*šú* GUB-*az* GAM (DPS XIX/XX:117′ [AOAT 43.233])

**[If his affliction continually] afflicts him, flows over him, and pulls him taut, a ⌜*rābiṣu*⌝ is bound with him, (and) stands at his head; he will die.

There could be many causes of the symptoms described above, but sinus node dysfunction causing atrial fibrillation is probably included among them. This is very interesting in view of the fact that the *rābiṣu* was also blamed for severe strokes. Atrial fibrillation commonly leads to blood clots in the heart that may break off, travel to the brain, and result in stroke.

Cerebral embolism is the most common cause of ischemic stroke, and the heart can be the source of the embolus. When this occurs, it lodges in the middle cerebral artery 80 percent of the time. The *āšipu*, therefore, may have associated the abnormal cardiac rhythm of atrial fibrillation with the development of stroke.

"HAND" OF MANKIND

What may be a description of myocardial infarction (the reference below; see 8.11) was attributed by the *āšipu* to "hand" of mankind, a form of *kišpu*-sorcery.[106] The point of the diagnosis was that the demonic force ("hand") causing the affliction was allegedly unleashed upon the victim by a fellow human being.

19.121 DIŠ NA IGI.MEŠ-*šú* NIGIN-*du*.ME GÌR^{II}.MEŠ-*šú* DUB.DUB-*ka ḫu-uṣ-ṣa* GAZ [ŠÀ] *pi-rit-tum* TUKU.TUKU-*ši* ŠU.NAM.LÚ.U$_{18}$.LU UGU-*šú* GÁL-*ši* (*BAM* 317 r. 24–25)

**If a person's face seems continually to be spinning, his feet are continually tense, he continually has a crushing sensation in his heart and fluttering, "hand" of mankind is upon him.

As the following reference explains, the form of sorcery known as "hand" of mankind could be performed by laying figurines that the sorcerer had manufactured to his victim's specifications in a grave with a corpse with the nefarious intent of turning him into one.

19.122 DIŠ *ri-mu-tu* ŠUB.ŠUB-*su* SAG ŠÀ-*šú* DIB.DIB-*su ma-gal in-né-sil* GIG-*su* ŠU. NAM.LÚ.U$_{18}$.LU NU.MEŠ-*šú šu-nu-lu* MAŠ.MAŠ *ana* DIN-*šú* ME-*a* NU GAR-*an* (DPS XXII:2–3 [AOAT 43.250–251])

**If limpness[107] continually falls upon him, his upper abdomen (epigastrium) continually afflicts him, (and) he is very sluggish, his illness is "hand" of mankind. His figurines have been made to lie (with a corpse); the *āšipu* should not make a prognosis as to his recovery.

LAYING FIGURINES WITH A CORPSE

"Laying figurines with a corpse" is separately mentioned as a diagnosis, usually in connection with symptoms compatible with congestive heart failure (see Chapter 8), as in the following reference.

19.123 [DIŠ NA *a-ka-li*]-*šú muṭ-ṭu ana da-ba-bi* ŠÀ-*šú š*[*a-pil ḫu-u*]*ṣ* GAZ ŠÀ TUKU. MEŠ-*ši mi-na-ti-šú it-*[*ta-na-áš-pa-ka* EME-*šú*] *it-te-nen-bi-iṭ* NUNDUN.MEŠ-*šú ú-na-áš-šak* GEŠTU^{II}-*šú* G[Ù.GÙ-*a*] ŠU^{II}-*šú i-šam-ma-ma-šú bir-ka-šú kim-ṣa-šú i-kas-s*[*a-sa-šú*] SAG ŠÀ-*šú it-ta-na-áš-qàr ana* MUNUS DU-*ka mu*[*ṭ-ṭu*] *ana* MUNUS ŠÀ-*šú* NU ÍL-*šú ḫur-ba-šu* ŠUB.ŠUB-[*su*] *i-kab-bir i-ba-aḫ-ḫu* ÚḪ *ana* KA-*šú it-ta-na-*[*at-la-ak*] *ik-ka-šú* LÚGUD. DA.MEŠ KI.NÁ NU ÍL *pi-qa la pi-qa ú-ta-ṣal* NA BI *ka-*[*šip*] NU.MEŠ-*šu* DÙ-*ma ina* ÚR LÚ.ÚŠ *šu-nu-*[*lu*] . . . (*BAM* 438 obv. 5–14)[108]

**[If a person]'s [appetite] is diminished, his heart is [too low] for (him) to speak, he continually has a crushing sensation in his heart, his limbs are continually [tense, his tongue] is continually cramped, he bites his lips, his ears [continually] ⌜ring⌝, his hands go numb, his knees (and) his shins give him a gnawing pain, his upper abdomen (epigastrium) continually protrudes, his desire to go to a woman ⌜is diminished⌝, (and) he cannot get an erection for a woman, chills keep falling on [him], he is now fat (and now) thin, spittle continually ⌜comes⌝ to his mouth, his breath is continually short, he cannot stand the bed (and) he is incessantly sluggish, that person is ⌜*kišpu*'d⌝; figurines of him were manufactured and made to ⌜lie⌝ in the lap of a corpse . . .

Where heart symptoms were involved, the *āšipu* was not always sure whether the patient had merely been hexed from a safe distance by "laying figurines in the ground with a corpse"[109] or whether the effects had been created by poisoning him, more properly described as "fed (something) in bread, been given (something) to drink in beer, been rubbed (with something) in oil."[110] Since diet can indeed have significant effect on heart problems, the *āšipu* was not entirely wrong in suspecting the patient's food and beer as potential contributing factors.

Gods/Goddesses of Circulatory Problems

GOD OF HIS CITY

Since each ancient Mesopotamian city had its own set of gods and goddesses, this vaguely described divinity could literally be any member of the ancient Mesopotamian pantheon. In view of this fact, it is probable that this diagnosis, like the similar "hand of his god" or "hand" of god, was meant to indicate uncertainty on the part of the *āšipu* as to which god or goddess was actually responsible (see under Ill-defined Syndromes of the Sort Gods/Goddesses Might Cause). Nonetheless, as with *kišpu*, the other ancient Mesopotamian catch-all category, it is sometimes possible to guess what was being described for the individual syndromes.

The following quote, which describes an apparently absent pulse on one side of the body, could be an example of atherosclerosis with one side having greater obstruction than the other. For more details, see Chapter 8.

19.124 DIŠ SA SAG.KI^{II}-*šú* ŠU^{II}-*šú u* GÌR^{II}-*šú* <*šá* 150> DU-*ku-ma šá* 15 GAR-*nu* ŠU DINGIR URU-*šú* : ŠU ^{d}UTU (DPS IV A_2 r. 30//B r. 10 = *TDP* 42 r. 30)[111]

**If the blood vessel(s) of his temples, his hands, or his feet, <the ones on the right> "go" and the ones on the left are present, "hand" of the god of his city (var: "hand" of Šamaš).

The potential involvement of the god Šamaš (in the variant) is explained by the immediately following entry in the diagnostic/prognostic handbook, which is apparently somewhat abbreviated but which seems to describe weakness and pain in the affected limb when the patient attempts to walk (exercise-induced claudication due to atherosclerosis). Both weakness of the sort described and pain in the leg and foot were otherwise caused by the god Šamaš (see Chapter 11 with 11.43, 11.46, and below, 19.272).

19.125 DIŠ SA SAG.KI^{II}-*šú* ŠU^{II}-*šú u* GÌR^{II}-*šú šá* 15 *u* 150 *it-ta-na-aš-gag-gu u* BAL.MEŠ ⌜*e?-sa*⌝ *ú-šaq-qa-ma* AD$_6$-*šú* IGI.BAR.MEŠ ŠU ^{d}UTU MU DAM LÚ (DPS IV A_2 r. 31–32//B r. 11–12 = *TDP* 42 r. 31–32)

**If the blood vessels of his temples,[112] his hands, or his feet, the ones on the left or right <"go" but the ones on the right or left are present and the muscles of the feet> on the left or right side continually become stiff and continually shift under (him), (his feet) have a viselike pain(?) (but) he can lift (them) and he continually gazes at his body, "hand" of Šamaš on account of a man's wife.

In addition to the apparent loss of pulse on one side of the body, the city god was responsible for one type of gangrene. In some cases of shock, because of a combination of low blood pressure and increased blood coagulability, the patient's hands or feet may become gangrenous. For more details, see Chapter 14.

The *āšipu* distinguished three different types of gangrene, which he attributed to the goddess Ištar, a ghost, and the "god of his city." Since the city god was apparently associated with circulation problems, it is possible that his (the city god's) gangrene was due to acute arterial occlusion, producing a sudden interruption of the blood supply. The patient first feels pain, then numbness and loss of sensation, followed within six hours by ischemic muscular contracture associated with subcutaneous hemorrhage and focal areas of gangrene. In the first quote below, "immobilization of the hands (or) feet" could possibly refer to muscular contracture. The comment that he is able to speak calmly may have been intended to distinguish this from similar signs and symptoms accompanying encephalitis or meningitis ("hand" of Šamaš; see 19.271). The second quote would, then, refer to focal gangrene.

19.126 DIŠ KI.MIN-*ma* ŠU^{II}-*šú u* GÌR^{II}-*šú* ⌜*am*⌝-*šá* ⌜DUG$_4$⌝ [*ne*]-⌜*e-ḫe*⌝-*e* DUG$_4$.GA DINGIR URU-*šú* SÌG-*su* [GAM] (DPS XV:20 [AOAT 43.151])

**If (it is the first day he is sick) and (either or both of) his hands or feet are immobilized (and) he speaks ⌜calmly(?)⌝; the god of his city has stricken him; [he will die].

19.127 DIŠ KI.MIN-*ma* GABA.MEŠ *šá* ŠU^{II}-*šú* GI$_6$.MEŠ ŠU DINGIR URU-*šú* GAM (DPS XV:28 [AOAT 43.152])

**If (it is the first day he is sick) and the "breasts" of his hands are dark, "hand" of the god of his city; he will die.

IŠTAR

Ostensibly, the difference between Ištar's gangrene and that of the city god was whether the hands or feet were affected. However, it seems likely that the real distinction lies elsewhere. Ištar was a goddess of war, blamed for many types and consequences of trauma, including hemorrhagic shock, as described in the second reference below. It seems likely, then, that her gangrene victims (described in the first quote below) were suffering from shock secondary to trauma.

19.128 DIŠ GABA.MEŠ *šá* GÌR^{II}-*šú* GI$_6$.MEŠ ŠU ^{d}15 GÍD-*ma* GAM (DPS XIV A iv 16//K 10 = *TDP* 144 iv 51′; cf. DPS XV:65 [AOAT 43.154])

**If the "breasts" of his feet are dark, "hand" of Ištar; (if) it is prolonged, he will die.

19.129 DIŠ KI.MIN-*ma* ŠU-*su ina* LI.DUR-*šú* GAR-*at-ma* ŠU^{II}-*šú u* GÌR^{II}-*šú ka-ṣa-a ina* NU ⌜ZU-*e*⌝ [DUG$_4$.DUG$_4$-*ub*] ZI-*bi u* TÚŠ-*ab ina* LI.DUR-*šú* SÌG-*iṣ* ŠU ^{d}*Dil-bat* [GAM] (DPS XV:13–14 [AOAT 43.151]; cf. DPS XI A obv. 9//B 8 = *TDP* 90:9//*SpTU* 1.34:8)

**If (it is the first day he is sick) and his hand is placed on his navel and his hands and his feet are cold, he talks without knowing (what he is saying and) he gets up and sits down (again), he was wounded on his navel. "Hand" of Dilbat (Ištar); [he will die].

GHOST

Gangrene attributed to ghosts was accompanied by pain or bruxism ("gnashing of teeth") and posturing ("twisting").

19.130 DIŠ ZÚ.MEŠ-*šú* ZÚ.GUZ ŠU^{II}-*šú u* GÌR^{II}-*šú* GI$_6$ D[IB] ⌜GU⌝$_4$ GAM (DPS VI A r. 11//B$_1$ r. 8+B$_2$ r. 12 = *TDP* 60 r. 42′)

**If he gnashes his teeth (and) his hands or his feet are dark, ⌜affliction⌝ by a ghost; he will die.[113]

19.131 DIŠ KI.MIN-*ma kar-ši* U.MEŠ ŠU^{II}-*šú* GI$_{6}$.MEŠ *u i-ṭa-me* ŠU.GÍDIM.⌜MA⌝ GAM (DPS XV:29 [AOAT 43.152])[114]

**If (it is the first day he is sick) and the undersides of the fingers of his hands are dark and he twists, "hand" of ghost; he will die.

Gods/Goddesses of Illness Due to Trauma

Wounds are described in the diagnostic handbook with the formula: "If a person was struck on such and such a body part." Uses of the word *struck* in nonmedical texts include "hitting" with a club or stick, "stabbing" with a sword, "shooting" with an arrow, and "striking" with a bare hand.[115] Many of these "strikings" of the body were attributed to the influence of godly or demonic "hands," the variability of wound locations and their sequelae being explained by the influence of different spirits. Which spirit was chosen for which particular wound often looks suspiciously like it was determined by divination, but there are patterns in the material that suggest that the assignments are not always as arbitrary as they appear. For example, wounds for that gods of the netherworld such as Nergal and Ereškigal were responsible were invariably fatal (see below).

Also noticeable is a pattern of assigning wounds to divinities who cause other problems affecting the same parts of the body and/or displaying the same symptoms as the wound complications, a pattern that can facilitate the restoration of broken ends of lines, as in the following pair of references to "hand" of god (see below).

19.132 DIŠ *ina* SAG.DU-*šú* SÌG-*iṣ-ma* SA SAG.KI-*šú* ŠU[^{II}]-*šú u* [GÌ]R^{II}-*šú* 1-*niš* ZI.MEŠ ⌜SA$_{5}$⌝ *u* ⌜*i-mim* ŠU DINGIR⌝ TI (DPS III C r. 21 = *TDP* 26:81)

**If he was wounded on his head and, consequently, the blood vessel(s) of his temple, his ⌜hands⌝ and his ⌜feet⌝ all (feel like they) are pulsating together, (and) he is flushed and feverish, "hand" of god; he will get well.

19.133 DIŠ SAG.DU-*su* KÚM-*im* SA SAG.KI^{II}-*šú* ŠU^{II}-*šú u* GÌR^{II}-*šú* 1-*niš* ZI.MEŠ SA$_{5}$ *u i-mim* ŠU [DINGIR DIN] (DPS III C obv. 55 = *TDP* 24:55)

**If his head is feverish (and) the blood vessel(s) of his temples, his hands, and his feet all (feel like they) are pulsating together (and) he is flushed and feverish, "hand" of [god; he will get well].

Although not all trauma references can be matched with a corresponding nontrauma reference with the same diagnosis, this occurs frequently enough to suggest that many (if not most) of the trauma references were assigned on the basis of this principle. For example, the most obvious reason that the twin gods were blamed for trauma to the arms is that, in a nontrauma context, they caused cold arms, as is shown by the following references.

19.134 DIŠ Á^{II}-*šú ik-ta-na-ṣa-a* ŠU ^{d}MAŠ.TAB.BA (DPS X B r. 7 = *TDP* 88 r. 7)

**If his arms are continually cold, "hand" of the twin gods.

19.135 DIŠ *ina* Á-*šú* SÌG-*iṣ* ŠU ^{d}MAŠ.TAB.BA (DPS X B r. 11 = *TDP* 88 r. 11)

**If he was wounded on his arm, "hand" of the twin gods.

Moreover, in a nontrauma context, the twin gods caused fever with upset stomach and, as gods of trauma, trauma to the abdomen producing upset stomach, as in the following references. It is to be noted that the prognosis given in the texts is based on observation, not on any presumed predilection of the causal agent. A "twin god" fever with upset stomach was not a problem; a "twin god" abdominal wound with a similarly upset stomach was.

19.136 DIŠ SAG.DU-*su* ^{LÚ}AD$_{6}$-*šú* KÚM ÚḪ *u i-ta-na-šu-*<*uš*> ŠU ^{d}MAŠ.TAB.BA DIN *šum*$_{4}$-*ma* ⌜*ina* DÚR⌝-[*šú* MÚD SUR . . .] (DPS III C r. 7//E$_{1}$ 8+E$_{2}$ 4 = *TDP* 26:67)

**If his head and body burn with fever and (his stomach) is continually upset, "hand" of the twin gods; he will get well. If [blood drips] from [his] anus [. . .]

19.137 DIŠ *ina* ŠÀ-*šú* SÌG-*ma u* ZI.IR.MEŠ ŠU ^{d}MAŠ.TAB.BA GAM (DPS XIII B ii 19b = *TDP* 118 ii 19b; cf. DPS XV:36 [AOAT 43.152])

**If he was wounded on his abdomen and, consequently, (it) is continually upset, "hand" of the twin gods; he will die.

Similarly, the god Ninurta, despite his associations with warfare, caused only one type of trauma.

19.138 DIŠ IGI.MEŠ-*šú u* IGI^{II}-*šú* MÚ.MEŠ KI.A IGI^{II}-*šú* SA$_{5}$ IM KIR$_{4}$-*šú* KÚM : *ṣa-bit* ⌜KÀŠ⌝.MEŠ-*šú ta-ba-ka* NU ZU-*e* GABA.RI SÌG-*iṣ* ŠU ^{d}MAŠ (DPS IX A 69–70//B r. 15–16 = *TDP* 78:69–70)

**If his face and his eyes are swollen, the rims of his eyes are red, the breath of nose is hot (var. seized), (and) he is not able to pour out his urine, he was wounded on the front side; "hand" of Ninurta.

The most obvious reason for the attribution of this particular wound complication to Ninurta is that the body swelling and anuria described were also seen as part of a separate, nontraumatic syndrome that fell under the charge of Ninurta). For other examples of this principle at work see below under Trauma caused by Gods/Goddesses of Fever or Gods/Goddesses of Neurological Conditions.

Trauma Caused By Gods/Goddesses of Warfare

ADAD

Twenty texts are available that mention Adad or "hand" of Adad, all of them in the diagnostic series.[116] Analysis of these references indicates a heavy emphasis (seventeen out of twenty) on problems involving the head, neck, and abdomen. There were two references to the extremities, one back (kidney) problem, and no chest findings.

19.139 DIŠ *ina* SAG ŠÀ-*šú* SÌG-*iṣ* ŠU ^{d}IŠKUR : *pu-qud-de-e* ^{d}UTU *ana* ^{d}MAŠ.TAB.BA (DPS XIII B i 32′//D 6 = *TDP* 114 i 36′)[117]

**If he was wounded on his upper abdomen (epigastrium), "hand" of Adad (var. he was entrusted by Šamaš to the twin gods).

19.140 DIŠ *ina ri-biti-šú* SÌG-*iṣ-ma ina* KA-*šú* MÚD MUD ŠUB.ŠUB-*a* ŠU ^{d}IŠKUR GAM (DPS XIV A iii 17 = *TDP* 140 iii 51′)[118]

**If he was wounded on the side of his abdomen and, consequently, he continually produces black blood from his mouth, "hand" of Adad; he will die.

19.141 DIŠ *ina* ÉLLAG-*šú* SÌG-*iṣ* ŠU ^{d}IŠKUR : ŠU ^{d}*Kù-bi* (DPS XII D iii 19 = *TDP* 104 iii 19)

**If he was wounded on his kidney, "hand" of Adad . . .

The types of medical findings were quite varied with only a few examples of each, including pain, redness, swelling, darkness, and mental confusion. Where a prognosis was mentioned, it was usually poor (seven out of eight).[119] Wounds, however, were quite frequent (thirteen out of twenty). Adad was a storm-god, associated with thunderstorms, hail, and floods, but he was also associated with warfare. A Neo-Assyrian stela from Arslan Tash shows him astride a bull wielding thunderbolts in martial pose. His standard was carried into battle by the forward divisions of the Neo-Assyrian army. This facet of his activities clearly fits well with the medical syndrome that bears his name. It appears that the Adad syndrome was predominately restricted to wounds (probably war wounds) involving the head, neck, and abdomen. The name of Adad was invoked especially when the wound was left-sided, perhaps because the Adad division was on that side of the Neo-Assyrian army.

19.142 DIŠ *ina* SAG.DU-*šú šá* 15 SÌG-*iṣ* ŠU ^{d}IŠKUR (DPS III C r. 13 = *TDP* 26:73)

**If he was wounded on his head to the left, "hand" of Adad.

19.143 DIŠ *ina*[120] EME-*šú* SÌG-*iṣ* ŠU ^{d}IŠKUR [. . .] (DPS VII A obv. 26 = *TDP* 62:26)[121]

**If he was wounded on his tongue, "hand" of Adad; [. . .]

19.144 DIŠ KI.MIN-*ma ri-bit-su šá* 15 *nap-ḫat-ma* GI$_{6}$-*át ina* NU ZU *ú-rap-pad* ŠU ^{d}IŠKUR *ina* AN.BAR$_{7}$ SÌG-*iṣ* GAM (DPS XV:52 [AOAT 43.153]; cf. DPS XIV A iii 10–11//C$_{2}$ iii 3//I 6–7 = *TDP* 140 iii 44′–45′)

**If (it is the first day he is sick) and the left side of his abdomen is swollen and dark (and) he wanders about without knowing (where he is), "hand" of Adad. <If> he was wounded at noon, he will die.

19.145 DIŠ KI.MIN-*ma* ŠU^{II}-*šú u* GÌR^{II}-*šú* [. . .] DUG$_{4}$-*šú ú-rap-pad ina* AN.BAR$_{7}$ SÌG-*iṣ* ŠU ^{d}⸢10⸣[122] [GAM] (DPS XV:21 [AOAT 43.151])

**If (it is the first day he is sick) and his hands and his feet [. . .], his speech wanders about,[123] (and) he was wounded at noon, "hand" of Adad; [he will die].

Although the condition could have a fatal outcome, wound complications were seldom listed, probably because death (when it occurred) was usually rapid.

19.146 DIŠ *ina* ŠÀ-*šú* SÌG-*iṣ* U$_{4}$.9.KÁM ŠU ^{d}MAŠ.TAB.BA DIŠ 2-*i* ŠU ^{d}IŠKUR / DIŠ *šal-šú* ŠU ^{d}*É-a* DIŠ 4 ŠU DINGIR.MAḪ DIŠ 5 ŠU ^{d}*Papsukkal* (DPS XIII B ii 17–18 = *TDP* 118 ii 17–18)

**If he was wounded on his abdomen (and has been sick for) nine days, "hand" of the twin gods. If (it is) the second (day), "hand" of Adad. If the third, "hand" of Ea. If the fourth, "hand" of Dingirmaḫ. If the fifth, "hand" of Papsukkal.

19.147 DIŠ KI.MIN-*ma i-*[*siḫ-ti* KI.MA]Ḫ-*šú i-si-iḫ* SÌG-*iṣ* ^{d}DIM$_{11}$.ME GAM : SÌG-*iṣ* ^{d}IŠKUR DUMU ^{d}*A-nim* GA[M] (DPS XV:91 [AOAT 43.155])

**If (it is the first day he is sick) and he makes the ⸢assignments⸣ for his ⸢tomb⸣ . . . wound of Adad, son of Anu; he will die.

Other gods such as Ištar, Ningirsu, the twin gods, Nergal, Ningizzida, and the Sibitti were considered responsible for wound complications. Note, for example, the following references, in which Adad causes an uncomplicated wound to the neck and Ištar the same neck wound but with loss of virility.

19.148 DIŠ *ina* GÚ-*šú* SÌG-*iṣ* ŠU ^{d}IŠKUR (DPS X A obv. 16//B obv. 18 = *TDP* 82:16)

**If he was wounded on his neck, "hand" of Adad.

19.149 DIŠ *ina* GÚ-*šú* SÌG-*iṣ-ma u du-us-su* KAR-*et* ŠU ^{d}15 GAM (DPS X A obv. 18//B obv. 20 = *TDP* 82:18)

**If he was wounded on his neck and his virility is taken away, "hand" of Ištar; he will die.

IŠTAR

Of this dread goddess it was said that "her play was battle." It is hardly surprising, then, that eighteen of the ninety-one texts bearing her name are references to trauma. Many of the wounds were on the head, neck, back, and arms, but wounds of the abdomen, pelvis, and lower extremities were also listed. The complaints related to these injuries were those that would be expected, namely, pain, neurologic abnormalities, infection, blood loss, and mental confusion probably caused by a combination of brain injury and shock. Prognosis, when stated, was usually bad.

19.150 DIŠ KI.MIN-⸢*ma*⸣ ⸢GÚ-*su*⸣ [K]Ú-*šú*-[*ma* A APIN.MEŠ] ŠU ^{d}15 *ina* GÚ-*šú* SÌG-*iṣ* GAM (DPS XV:6 [AOAT 43.150]; cf. DPS X A obv. 8//B obv. 8 = *TDP* 80:8)

**If (it is the first day he is sick) and his neck ⸢hurts him⸣ [and he continually asks for water, "hand"] of Ištar. He was wounded on his neck; he will die.

19.151 DIŠ KI.MIN-*ma* ŠU-*su ina* LI.DUR-*šú* GAR-*at-ma* ŠU^{II}-*šú u* GÌR^{II}-*šú ka-ṣa-a ina* NU ⸢ZU-*e*⸣ [DUG$_4$.DUG$_4$-*ub*] ZI-*bi u* TÚŠ-*ab ina* LI.DUR-*šú* SÌG-*iṣ* ŠU ^{d}*Dil-bat* [GAM] (DPS XV:13–14 [AOAT 43.151]; cf. DPS XI A obv. 9//B 8 = *TDP* 90:9//*SpTU* 1.34:8)

**If (it is the first day he is sick) and his hand is placed on his navel and his hands and his feet are cold, [he talks] without knowing (what he is saying and) he gets up and sits down (again), he was wounded on his navel; "hand" of Dilbat (Ištar); [he will die].

19.152 DIŠ ŠÀ.MEŠ-*šú nap-ḫu-ma* SA.MEŠ ŠÀ-*šú šu-ud-du-du* ŠU ^{d}15 NU ⸢DIN⸣ (DPS XIII B ii 46//G$_2$ 37+G$_1$ 20 = *TDP* 120 ii 46)

**If his insides are bloated and the muscles of his abdomen are pulled taut, "hand" of Ištar; he will not get well.

Ištar was also, not surprisingly, responsible for one of the forms of gangrene. For details, see 19.128 and Chapter 14 with 14.44. The name of Ištar was invoked especially when the wound was right-sided, perhaps because the Ištar division was on that side of the Neo-Assyrian army. Note that the third reference below pairs with one of the trauma references of Adad, who was on the left side of the army (see above).

19.153 DIŠ KI.MIN-*ma ina kur-ri-šú šá* 150 SÌG-*iṣ-ma* GÌR-*šú* NU ZI-*aḫ ina* dUTU È <SÌG-*iṣ*> ŠU d15 GAM (DPS XV:50 [AOAT 43.153]; cf. DPS XII D iv 24–25//E iv 31–32 = *TDP* 108 iv 24–25)

**If (it is the first day he is sick) and he was wounded on his right groin area (femoral crease) and consequently, he cannot uproot his foot (from the ground) (and) he <was wounded> at sunrise, "hand" of Ištar; he will die.

19.154 DIŠ KI.MIN-*ma ina* GÌR-*šú šá* 150 SÌG-*iṣ* ŠU d15 GÍD-[*ma* GAM] (DPS XV:62 [AOAT 43.154]; cf. DPS XIV C_2 iv 5b)

**If (it is the first day he is sick) and he was wounded on his right foot, "hand" of Ištar. [(If)] (his illness) is prolonged, [he will die].

19.155 DIŠ KI.MIN-*ma re-bit-su šá* 150 *nap-ḫat-ma* GI_6-*át ina* NU ZU *ú-rap-pad* ŠU d*Dil-bat ina šat ur-ri* SÌG-[*i*]*ṣ* GAM (DPS XV:53 [AOAT 43.153]; cf. DPS XIV A iii 12–13//C_2 iii 4//I 8–9 = *TDP* 140 iii 46′–47′)

**If (it is the first day he is sick) and the right side of his abdomen is swollen and dark (and) he wanders about without knowing (where he is), "hand" of Dilbat (Ištar). <If> he was wounded in the morning, he will die.

Whereas Adad seems to have caused simple wounds to the head and neck (see above), Ištar's head and neck wounds were sure to result in complications. In particular, she caused injuries to the eighth cranial nerve as well as parasthesias and seizures.

19.156 DIŠ *ina* U[G]U-*šú* SÌG-*ma* GEŠTUII-*šú* NU ŠE.GA-*a* ŠU d15 *ana* AŠ-*tim* (DPS III A obv. 19//C obv. 10 = *TDP* 18:10; cf. StBoT 36.35 r. 1//StBoT 36.57 r. 8′)

**If he was wounded on his skull and consequently his ears do not hear, "hand" of Ištar for a gift (which she wants).[124]

19.157 DIŠ *ina* SAG.DU-*šú* SÌG-*iṣ-ma* Á.ÚR.MEŠ-*šú* 1-*niš* KÚ.ME-*šú* ŠU d15 *ana* BÚR *ú-qàt-ti*[125] *ni-ši* (DPS III C r. 16//E_1 r. 17+E_2 r. 13 = *TDP* 26:76; cf. StBoT 36.35 obv. 16′–17′//StBoT 36.57 r. 6′–7′)[126]

**If he was wounded on his head and, consequently, his limbs all hurt him at once, "hand" of Ištar. (If) it completely goes away, (there will be a) recovery.

19.158 DIŠ *ina* SAG.DU-*šú* SÌG-*iṣ-ma u i-ṭa-mu pu-qud-de-e* d15 *ana* dMAŠ.TAB.BA (DPS III C r. 17//E_2 r. 14 = *TDP* 26:77; cf. StBoT 36.34 obv. 5′)[127]

**If he was wounded on his head and consequently he twists, he was entrusted by Ištar to the twin gods.

In addition, Ištar caused serious abdominal wounds accompanied by the vomiting of blood. This is probably related to the attribution to her of abdominal pain and bleeding (see 19.373).

19.159 DIŠ *ina* SAG ŠÀ-*šú* SÌG-*iṣ* ŠU^{II}-*šú u* GÌR^{II}-*šú am-šá* ŠU ^{d}DUMU.MUNUS ^{d}*A-nim* (DPS XIII B i 33′//D 7 = *TDP* 114 i 37′)

**If he was wounded on his upper abdomen (epigastrium) (and) his hands and his feet are immobilized, "hand" of (Ištar), daughter of Anu.

19.160 DIŠ Á^{II}-*šú tur-ra* NU ZU-*e u* MÚD BURU$_{8}$ ŠU ^{d}15 GÍD-*ma* GAM (DPS X B r. 4 = *TDP* 86 r. 4)

**If he is unable to turn his arms and he vomits blood, "hand" of Ištar. (If) it is prolonged, he will die.

Probably the most obvious attribution to Ištar, in view of her role as goddess of lust and venereal diseases, was spinal or abdominal trauma resulting in a loss of virility.

19.161 DIŠ *ina em-ši-šú* SÌG-*iṣ-ma u du-u*[*s-su* KAR-*et* ŠU ^{d}15 . . .] (DPS XIII D r. 4 = *TDP* 126 iv 13′)

**If he was wounded on his lower abdominal (hypogastric) region and [his] ⸢virility⸣ [is taken away, "hand" of Ištar . . .]

19.162 [DIŠ MIN-*ma*] ÍL ŠÀ-*šú ṣa-bit* ŠU ^{d}15 *ana* KI G[IG! GAM] (DPS XIII J 9 = *TDP* 126 iii 41)

**[If he keeps crying out: "My insides, my insides"][128] (and) he is impotent, "hand" of Ištar, he is at an acute stage of the ⸢illness⸣;[129] [he will die].

Also noticeable in the Ištar trauma references is a predilection for wounds affecting bones and joints.

19.163 [DIŠ *ina*] ⸢TUGUL⸣-*šú u* GU.DU-*šú* SÌG-*iṣ* ŠU ^{d}15 / [DIŠ *ina* TU]GUL-*šú u kin-ṣi-šú* SÌG-*iṣ* ŠU ^{d}15 (DPS XIV A$_{2}$ i 10–11 = *TDP* 132 i 61–62)

**[If] he was wounded [on] his hip socket and his buttock, "hand" of Ištar. [If] he was wounded [on] his ⸢hip socket⸣ and his leg, "hand" of Ištar.

19.164 DIŠ *ina* GÌR-*šú* MURUB$_{4}$.MEŠ-*šú* Á.MEŠ-*šú u* GÚ-*šú* SÌG-*iṣ* U$_{4}$.41.KÁM ŠU ^{d}15 (DPS XIV A iv 4–5//C$_{2}$ iv 9 = *TDP* 144 iv 39′–40′)[130]

**If he was wounded on his foot, his hips, his arms, (and) his neck, (and he has been sick for) forty-one days, "hand" of Ištar.

NINGIRSU AND BAU

Ningirsu and Bau were a married couple and the chief divinities of the neighboring cities of Lagash and Girsu. This Sumerian city-state in southern Mesopotamia is probably best known today from the inscriptions of a city ruler or ensi named Gudea who memorialized his rebuilding of Ningirsu's temple with a series of very elegant basalt statuettes that now grace many of the world's museums. Ningirsu was also syncretized with Ninurta, another god of warfare. Both husband and wife were responsible for neurologic trauma, differing from Ištar (see above) in the exact nature of the injury. Bau was to blame for cranial trauma resulting in strokelike paralysis of the extremities (in contrast to the seizures caused by Ištar). Bau also caused death from infected neck wounds.

19.165 DIŠ GÌR-*šu šá* 150 *i-maš-šar* SÌG-*iṣ* ᵈ*Ba-ú* SÌG-*iṣ* GAM (DPS XIV A_2 iv 5′//C_2 iii 31 = *TDP* 142 iv 5′; cf. DPS XV:64a [AOAT 43.154])

**If he drags his right foot, he was wounded with a wound of Bau; he will die.

19.166 DIŠ KI.MIN-*ma* U.MEŠ ŠU^{II}-*šú ina* [KA-*šú ú-man-zaq* KÚM] ⌜ÚḪ⌝ ŠÀ-*šú na-pi-iḫ u ú-rap-pad ina* GÚ-*šú* SÌG-*iṣ* ŠU ᵈ*Ba-ú* GAM (DPS XV:26 [AOAT 43.151]; cf. DPS XI A r. 36 = *TDP* 96 r. 36)[131]

**If (it is the first day he is sick) and he sucks his fingers in his mouth, he burns with fever,[132] his abdomen is bloated, and he wanders about, he was wounded on his neck; "hand" of Bau; he will die.

Bau's husband, Ningirsu, caused injuries to the second cranial nerve with loss of vision in contrast to Ištar's eighth cranial nerve injuries causing loss of hearing. This particular assignment is probably related to the fact that "clouding" of the eyes also appears in the only other known reference to Ningirsu.

19.167 DIŠ *ina* SAG.DU-*šú* SÌG-*iṣ-ma* IGI^{II}-*šú ur-ru-pa* ŠU ᵈ*N*[*in*]-*gír-su* (DPS III C r. 15 = *TDP* 26:75)

**If he was wounded on his head and, consequently, his eyes are heavily clouded, "hand" of ⌜Ningirsu⌝.

19.168 [DIŠ . . .] *u* IGI^{II}-*šú ur-ru-pa* U_4.12.KÁM ŠU ᵈ*Nin-gír*-[*su*] (DPS XIX/XX:15′ [AOAT 43.227])

**[If . . .] and his eyes are heavily clouded (and) it is the twelfth day (he has been sick), "hand" of ⌜Ningirsu⌝.

Trauma Caused by Ghosts, Demons, and Gods/Goddesses of the Netherworld

GHOSTS

Since these spirits of the dead were conceived of as walking skeletons, one might have expected them to be responsible for trauma involving the skeletal parts of the anatomy. The following references describe cranial trauma, trauma to the chest, and complications of vertebral trauma.

19.169 DIŠ *ina* SAG.KI-*šú šá* 15 SÌG-*iṣ* ŠU GIDIM ŠU DINGIR DIN (DPS IV E i 18b = *SpTU* 3.88 i 18b)

**If he was wounded on his left temple, "hand" of ghost . . . he will get well.

19.170 [DIŠ *ip-ru-ma* ZA]G *u* GÙB SÌG-*iṣ* ŠU *šag-ga-š*[*i* GAM] (DPS XXIII:4 [AOAT 43.272])

**[If he vomits(?) and] he was wounded on the ⌜left⌝ or right side, "hand" of a murderous (ghost); [he will die].

19.171 DIŠ *ina* GÚ-*šú* SÌG-*iṣ-ma* GÌR^{II}-*šú i-ra-ʾ-ú-ba* ŠÀ.MEŠ-*šú it-te-nen-bi-ṭu* DIB GIDIM$_7$ (DPS X A obv. 20//B obv. 22 = *TDP* 82:20)[133]

**If he was wounded on his neck and, as a consequence, his feet tremble, (and) his insides are continually cramped, affliction by a ghost.

19.172 DIŠ KI.MIN-*ma ina* GÚ.MURGU-*šú* SÌG BAD-*ir-ma* KI.GUB-*su* NU ⌜È⌝-*a* ŠU GIDIM$_7$ *šag-ga-ši* GAM (DPS XV:46 [AOAT 43.152]; cf. DPS XII D iii 35//E iii 38–39 = *TDP* 106 iii 35)

**If (it is the first day he is sick) and he was wounded on his spine and he is stopped up so that his excrement cannot come out,[134] "hand" of a murderous ghost; he will die.

NERGAL AND EREŠKIGAL

Ereškigal was the queen of the netherworld and wife of Nergal. Both caused fatal trauma, but of different types. Ereškigal seems to have been responsible for multiple injuries involving the ribs.

19.173 DIŠ *ina* SAG ŠÀ-*šú* SAG.KI-*šú u* TI-*šú* SÌG-*iṣ* ŠU ^{d}*Ereš-ki-gal* GAM (DPS XIII B i 35′//D 9 = *TDP* 114 i 39′)[135]

**If he was wounded on his upper abdomen (epigastrium), his temple and one of his ribs, "hand" of Ereškigal; he will die.

Nergal's speciality was wounds to the chest or abdomen that produced profuse amounts of blood. Given his associations with the netherworld, and the fact that plague was sometimes described as Nergal or other gods of pestilence "eating"[136] the plague victims, it is not unlikely that he was imagined as being literally thirsty for human blood.

19.174 DIŠ KI.MIN-*ma ina* GABA-*šú* SÌG-*ma* MÚD *ú-tab-ba-ka u ú-rap-pad* ŠU ^{d}U.GUR GABA.RI ⌜SÌG⌝-*iṣ* GAM (DPS XV:32 [AOAT 43.152]; cf. DPS XII A 4 = *TDP* 100 i 4)

**If (it is the first day he is sick) and he was wounded on his breast and, as a consequence, he continually pours out blood and wanders about, "hand" of Nergal; he was wounded on the front side; he will die.

19.175 DIŠ *ina* ŠÀ-*šú u ri-bit* 150-*šú* SÌG-*iṣ-ma u* MÚD *i-ḫa-ḫu* U$_4$.31.KÁM ŠU $^{d⌜}$U.GUR⌝ GAM (DPS XIII B ii 21 = *TDP* 118 ii 21)[137]

**If he was wounded on his abdomen or on the right side of his abdomen and he vomits blood (and he has been sick) for thirty-one days, "hand" of Nergal; he will die.

GALLÛ

The *gallû* was the distant ancestor, via Arabic, of our "ghoul," and probably also inherently rather bloodthirsty. His trauma resulted in bleeding combined with symptoms relating to the eyes (see 19.26). In contrast to either the Sibitti (see 19.178) who caused hemorrhagic shock from wounds to the back and Nergal (see 19.174) who made victims bleed to death from wounds to the chest and abdomen, the *gallû*'s bleeding seems to have largely taken place inside the body of the patient.

19.176 DIŠ *ina* GÚ-*šú* SÌG-*iṣ-ma e-lat* IGI^{II}-*šú* KÚ.ME-*šú* MÚD *ina* KIR$_4$KA-*šú* ŠUB.ŠUB-*a* ŠU^{II}-*šú u* GÌR^{II}-*šú eṣ-la* NA BI ḪUL DIB-*su* (DPS X A obv. 21//B obv. 23–24 = *TDP* 82:21; cf. *CTN* 4.72 i 15′–19′)

**If he was wounded on his neck and consequently the upper part of his eyes continually hurts him, he continually produces blood from his nose/mouth, (and) his hands and his feet are sluggish (var. he lets his hands and feet hang; he cannot move his hands and feet [by himself])[138] a *gallû* afflicts that person.

Other references to this demon mention uncontrollable internal bleeding but not trauma. It may be that the prior trauma was not mentioned, because it was considered to be obvious.

19.177 DIŠ NA *si-mat* IGI.ME-*šú* KÚR.KÚR-*ir* IGI^{II}-*šú it-ta-nap-ra-ra* ⌜NUNDUN⌝-*šú su-qat-su ú-*⌜*lap*⌝*-pat* (*u*) MÚD *ina* KIR$_4$KA-*šú* DU-*ka* NU *par-su*/ *la*⌜*i*⌝*-kal-lu-ú* NA BI ḪUL DIB-*su* (DPS XXVII:14–15 [AOAT 43.298]; cf. *CTN* 4.72 i 10′–12′)[139]

**If a person's facial appearance changes (for the worse), his eyes are continually disconnected from one another,[140] he rubs his lips and chin and blood does not stop flowing/they cannot stop the blood (which) flows from his nose/mouth, a *gallû* afflicts that person.

A number of the subsidiary symptoms described in these references could be related secondarily to the bleeding. For example, the "sluggish" hands and feet could have resulted from bleeding into the joints. The pain in the upper part of the eyes and the statement that the eyes were "disconnected" from one another could possibly be a reference to neurologic problems due to bleeding into and around the brain.

Trauma Caused by Gods/Goddesses of Fever or Gods/Goddesses of Neurologic Conditions

Another category of Gods/Goddesses of Illness Due to Trauma seems to have been gods/goddesses who actually specialized in causing fevers or neurological syndromes. To judge from the trauma assigned to them, they appear to have been invoked to explain cases where either the wound location or the wound complications, or both, could somehow be related to the fever or neurological condition that they independently caused. For example, two of the sets of gods (the Sibitti and the "twin gods") whose fevers involved extensive bleeding were invoked to account for aspects of bleeding in trauma.

TRAUMA CAUSED BY GODS OF FEVER

SIBITTI This was a group of seven gods who were identified with a cluster of seven stars known to us as the Pleiades. Like Nergal, they seem to have had a predilection for blood, causing one of the two varieties of viral hemorrhagic fever recognized by the *āšipu* (see 19.234). Severe bleeding from the chest was Nergal's preserve; what the Sibitti caused was hemorrhagic shock from injuries to the back.

19.178 DIŠ KI.MIN-*ma ina* ÉLLAG-*šú šá* 150 SÌG-*iṣ* $UŠ_4$-*šú* NU DIB *u* MÚD $BURU_8$ ŠU ^{d}7.BI GAM (DPS XV:40 [AOAT 43.152]; cf. DPS XII D iii 22 = *TDP* 104 iii 22)

**If (it is the first day he is sick) and he was wounded on his right kidney (costophrenic angle), he is not in full possession of his faculties and he vomits blood, "hand" of the Sibitti; he will die.

TWIN GODS "Twin gods" is an abbreviated way of referring to the twin gods ^{d}LU-GAL.GÌR.RA and MES.LAM.TA.È.A. These divinities were by-forms of Nergal as god of pestilence, and were responsible for various aspects of bleeding in febrile patients (see 19.236). They were also associated with the kidneys (see 19.368). For these reasons, they joined with the Sibitti in causing hemorrhagic shock from injuries to the back.

19.179 DIŠ *ina* ÉLLAG-*šú šá* 15 SÌG-*ma* $UŠ_4$-*šú* NU DIB *ina* NU ZU *ú-ra*[*p*]-*pad* ŠU ^{d}MAŠ.TAB.BA GAM (DPS XII D iii 21//E iii 22 = *TDP* 104 iii 21; cf. DPS XV:39 [AOAT 43.152])

**If he was wounded on his left kidney, he is not in full possession of his faculties, (and) he wanders about without knowing (where he is), "hand" of the twin gods; he will die.

Another specialty of the twin gods was to cause vomiting of blood. This vomiting might be from cranial trauma (see Chapter 13 with 13.134–13.135) or abdominal wounds, as in the following references.

19.180 DIŠ *ina* SAG.DU-*šú* SÌG-*iṣ-ma u* MÚD MUD ŠUB.ŠUB-*a* ŠU ^{d}MAŠ.TAB.BA GAM / DIŠ *ina* SAG.DU-*šú* SÌG-*iṣ-ma u* MÚD *i-ḫa-ḫu* ŠU ^{d}MAŠ.TAB.BA GAM (DPS III C r. 18–19//E_2 r. 15–16 = *TDP* 26:78–79; cf. StBoT 36.34 obv. 9′)

**If he was wounded on his head and he continually produces dark blood, "hand" of the twin gods; he will die. If he was wounded on his head and vomits blood, "hand" of the twin gods; he will die.

19.181 DIŠ *ina* ŠÀ-*šú* SÌG-*ma u* MÚD MUD ŠUB.ŠUB-*a* DIB-*it* ^{d}MAŠ.TAB.BA GAM (DPS XIII B ii 20 = *TDP* 118 ii 20)

**If he was wounded on his abdomen and, consequently, he continually produces dark blood, affliction by the twin gods; he will die.

Throat wounds were known to produce vomiting of blood (see Chapter 8 with 8.92). It may be for this reason that the twin gods were implicated in throat wounds.

19.182 DIŠ *ina gir-ri-šú* SÌG-*iṣ* ŠU ^{d}MAŠ.T[AB.BA GAM] (DPS X A obv. 54b = *TDP* 86:54b)

**If he was wounded on his throat, "hand" of the ⌜twin gods⌝; [he will die].

In the following reference, the formula "Šamaš entrusted (the patient) to the twin gods" may indicate that the patient vomited blood after the appearance of other symptoms appropriate to the entrusting god, such as a feverish upper abdomen with profuse sweating (i.e., Šamaš-type symptoms; see 19.255–19.256, 19.258). Adad, the god to whom the variant attributes this trauma, was otherwise known to cause vomiting of blood subsequent to abdominal wounds.[141]

19.183 DIŠ *ina* SAG ŠÀ-*šú* SÌG-*iṣ* ŠU ^{d}IŠKUR : *pu-qud-de-e* ^{d}UTU *ana* ^{d}MAŠ.TAB.BA (DPS XIII B i 32′//D 6 = *TDP* 114 i 36′)

**If he was wounded on his upper abdomen (epigastrium), "hand" of Adad; (var.) he was entrusted by Šamaš to the twin gods.

In the following references, the formula "Ištar entrusted (the patient) to the twin gods" would seem to indicate a complicated head wound of the sort expected of Ištar accompanied by mental status changes and abnormal posturing ("twisting") such as are characteristic of the twin gods' fever (see 19.238).

19.184 DIŠ KI.MIN-*ma* [*i-na* SAG.DU-*šú* SÌG-*iṣ-ma*] LÁ!-*sú na-kud* GAM : *pú-qud-de-e* ^{d}15 *ana* ^{d}MAŠ.TAB.BA GAM (DPS XV:92 [AOAT 43.155])

**If (it is the first day he is sick) and [he was wounded on his head(?) and] (a confusional state) comes over him; it is worrisome; he will die (var. he was entrusted by Ištar to the twin gods).

19.185 DIŠ *ina* SAG.DU-*šú* SÌG-*iṣ-ma u i-ṭa-mu pu-qud-de-e* ^{d}15 *ana* ^{d}MAŠ.TAB.BA (DPS III C r. 17//E_2 r. 14 = *TDP* 26:77; cf. StBoT 36.34 obv. 5′)

**If he was wounded on his head and consequently he twists, he was entrusted by Ištar to the twin gods.

The twin gods' fever could also produce shock resulting in vascular collapse and cold extremities (see 19.237). It may be that this aspect of the twin gods is being invoked in the following references to foot wounds. By itself, a wound in the foot should not have produced fatality. When, however, such a wound became seriously infected (as it might have been very liable to do since many ancient Mesopotamians wore no or minimal foot coverings) the patient would have been at grave risk. In the following sequence of references, the gods Ištar and Šamaš were held responsible for the initial injury to the foot but, when the wound failed to heal and the patient began to cry with pain, the initial problem-causers were said to have turned him over to the twin gods.

19.186 [DIŠ *ina* GÌR-*š*] *u šá* 15 SÌG-*iṣ* ŠU ^{d}UTU *ana* [U_4.3.KÁM GAM] / DIŠ *ina* GÌR^{II}-*šu šá* 150 SÌG-*iṣ* ŠU ^{d}15 GÍD-*ma* GAM / [DIŠ *ina* GÌR-*š*] *u šá* 15 SÌG-*iṣ u* GÙ.[GÙ]-*si pu-qud-de-e* ^{d}UTU *ina* ŠU ^{d}MAŠ.TAB.BA / DIŠ *ina* G[ÌR-*š*] *u šá* 150 SÌG-*iṣ u* GÙ.[GÙ]-*si* *pu-qud-de-e* ^{d}15 *ana* ^{d}MAŠ.TAB.BA (DPS XIV C_2 iv 5a–b; cf. DPS XV:61–62 [AOAT 43.154]; DPS XIV C_2 iv 6; DPS XIV A iv 1–2//C_2 iv 7 = *TDP* 144 iv 36′–37′)[142]

**[If] he was wounded [on] ⸢his⸣ left [foot], "hand" of Šamaš. <If> (he has been sick) for [three days, he will die]. If he was wounded on his right foot, "hand" of Ištar. (If) (his illness) is prolonged, he will die. [If] he was wounded [on] ⸢his⸣ left [foot] and he [continually] cries out, he was entrusted by Šamaš to the twin gods. If he was wounded on ⸢his⸣ right ⸢foot⸣ and he [continually] cries out, he was entrusted by Ištar to the twin gods.

AḪḪĀZU This demon was responsible for biphasic fevers presenting with jaundice (see 3.30–3.31). Louse-borne relapsing fever produces high temperatures accompanied by some alteration in mental status. Meningismus (irritation of the meninges without direct infection) also occurs in 40 percent of patients. It was probably this sort of behavior that attracted to *aḫḫāzu* the attribution of skull fractures accompanied by fever, mental status changes, and abnormal posturing ("twisting"; see 13.76–13.77) as described in the following reference.

19.187 DIŠ *ina* SAG.DU-*šú* SÌG-*iṣ-ma* MIR.ŠEŠ ŠUB.ŠUB-⸢*su*⸣ IGI.MEŠ-*šú* SA_5 *u* ⸢SIG_7 GIN_7 DIB⸣-*su* ŠUB-*šú* [U]$Š_4$-*šú* KÚR-*šum-ma i-ṭa-mu* DIB-*it* $^{d}DIM_{11}$.ME.⸢LAGAB⸣ U_4-*me-šú* GÍD.DA.⸢MEŠ-*ma*⸣ GAM (DPS III C r. 22–23 = *TDP* 28:82–83; cf. *KAR* 211 obv. 7–9)

**If he was wounded in the head and, consequently, chills keep falling on him, his face flushes and turns pale, (and) when his affliction falls upon him, his ⸢mentation⸣ is altered and he twists, affliction by *aḫḫāzu*.[143] (If) he (is ill) for a long time, he will die.[144]

KŪBU It is suggested below[145] that Kūbu was essentially a demon of infant diseases whose specialty was leptospirosis. If so, it is conceivable that the frontal headache and severe aching in the muscles of the thigh and lumbar regions caused by leptospirosis was what suggested Kūbu to the *āšipu* as a possible cause of wounding to the temple and kidney.

19.188 DIŠ *ina* SAG.KI-*šú* SÌG-*iṣ* ŠU ^{d}*Kù-bi* (DPS IV B obv. 35a//E i 16 = *TDP* 36:37//*SpTU* 3.88 i 16)

**If he was wounded on his temple, "hand" of Kūbu.

19.189 DIŠ *ina* ÉLLAG-*šú* SÌG-*iṣ* ŠU ^{d}IŠKUR : ŠU ^{d}*Kù-bi* (DPS XII D iii 19 = *TDP* 104 iii 19)

**If he was wounded on his kidney . . . "hand" of Kūbu.

ŠAMAŠ Headache and lower back pain caused by Šamaš's fever may similarly have drawn the attribution of the following trauma references.

19.190 DIŠ *ina* SAG.DU-*šú šá* 150 SÌG-*iṣ* ŠU ^{d}UTU AL.GAM (DPS III C r. 14 = *TDP* 26:74)

**If he was wounded on his head to the right, "hand" of Šamaš; he will die.

19.191 DIŠ *ina* ÉLLAG-*šú šá* 15 SÌG-*iṣ ana* U_4.14.KÁM ŠU ^{d}UTU (DPS XII D iii 20//E iii 21//G_2 iii 17 = *TDP* 104 iii 20)

**If he was wounded on his left kidney (and he is sick) for fourteen days,[146] "hand" of Šamaš.

Since Šamaš did not otherwise cause abdominal wounds, it is probable that it was the feverish abdomen and sweating of the wounded patient in the first reference below that suggested Šamaš as the cause. Note the similarity between the wording of this reference to Šamaš's trauma and the second reference below, which appears just before it in the diagnostic series and which describes Šamaš's fever.

19.192 DIŠ ŠÀ-*šú* KÚM IR ŠUB.ŠUB-*su lu* ŠU ^{d}UTU *lu* ^{d}*Šu-*⸢*lak* GABA⸣.RI SÌG-*iṣ* (DPS XIII B ii 10 = *TDP* 118 ii 10)

**If his abdomen is hot (and) sweat continually falls upon him, "hand" of Šamaš or "hand" of Šulak; he was wounded on the front side.

19.193 DIŠ ŠÀ-*šú* KÚM-*ma* IR GIN$_7$ *lu-ba-ṭi* ŠUB.ŠUB-*su u* ŠED$_7$ U$_4$.31.KÁM ŠU ^{d}20 (DPS XIII B ii 9 = *TDP* 118 ii 9)

**If his abdomen is hot, sweat keeps falling upon him as in *lubāṭu* (excessive sweating; see Chapter 10), and he has been cold (for) thirty-one days, "hand" of Šamaš.

The final reference to trauma caused by the god Šamaš may relate to his role in causing a type of arthritis (see Chapter 11 with 11.42–11.48). This reference is paired with another, already quoted above,[147] which may have been drawn to Ištar in consideration of her role as causer of arthritis.

19.194 DIŠ KI.MIN-*ma ina* GÌR-*šú šá* 15 SÌG-*iṣ* ŠU ^{d}UTU *ana* U$_4$.3.[KÁM GAM] (DPS XV:61 [AOAT 43.154]; cf. DPS XIV C$_2$ iv 5a)

**If (it is the first day he is sick) and he was wounded on his left foot, "hand" of Šamaš. <If> (he has been sick) for three days, [he will die].

TRAUMA CAUSED BY GODS/GODDESSES OF NEUROLOGIC CONDITIONS

ŠULAK The clearest example of gods/goddesses of neurology causing trauma related to their neurologic symptoms is the class of demons known as the *rābiṣu*. Šulak, the *rābiṣu* of the lavatory, and an unnamed colleague were responsible for strokes, and caused trauma to the head that produced strokelike symptoms. For more details, see 13.124–126, 13.228–230.

19.195 DIŠ ⸢GÙB⸣ ^{LÚ}AD$_6$-*šú ka-lu-šú-ma tab-kát* GABA.RI SÌG-*iṣ* ŠU ^{d}*Šu-lak* MAŠKIM *mu-sa-a-ti* MAŠ.MAŠ *ana* DIN-*šú* ME-*a* NU GAR-*an* (DPS XXVII:12–13 [AOAT 43.297]; cf. *AMT* 77/1 i 9–10)

**If the entire right side of his body is tense, he was wounded from in front; "hand" of Šulak, the *rābiṣu* of the lavatory; the *āšipu* should not make a prognosis as to his recovery.

19.196 [DIŠ Z]AG ^{LÚ}AD$_6$-*šú ka-lu-šú-ma tab-kát mi-šit-ti* MAŠKIM EGIR-*ta*$_5$ SÌG-*iṣ* (DPS XXVII:10 [AOAT 43.297]; cf. *AMT* 77/1 i 7)

**[If] the entire ⌜left⌝ side of his body is tense, stroke of a *rābiṣu* (or) he was wounded from behind.

The remaining trauma references may have been attributed to Šulak because the signs and symptoms were similar to those associated with an infectious neurologic syndrome that he produced (see Chapter 13 with 13.256–13.257).[148]

ŠULPAEA There is only a single reference to this god as a cause of trauma. The reason for the attribution is not completely clear but may relate to the fact that most of his neurologic syndromes (see 13.258–13.260) involved malfunctioning of the limbs and that some included mental status changes.

19.197 DIŠ KI.MIN-*ma ina kur-ri-šú šá* 15 SÌG-*iṣ-ma* NÍ-*šú ma-ši* ŠU ᵈ*Šul-pa-è-a* GAM (DPS XV:49 [AOAT 43.153]; cf. DPS XII D iv 23//E iv 30 = *TDP* 108 iv 23)

**If (it is the first day he is sick) and he was wounded on his left groin (femoral crease) and, consequently, he forgets himself, "hand" of Šulpaea; he will die.

SÎN Sîn was god of the moon and the father of Ištar and Šamaš, whom he joined in causing both types of *Herpes simplex* virus infections (HSV1 and HSV2; see 10.82–10.87). The presence of vesicles on the genitals in sexually transmitted HSV2 is possibly what drew Sîn as the causal agent for trauma to the testicles.[149] Injury to the coccyx is a bit more difficult to explain but may be due to the numbness and tingling of buttock or perineal areas which sometimes occurs with HSV2 infections.

19.198 DIŠ KI.MIN-*ma ina* GIŠ.KUN-*šú* SÌG-*iṣ* : *ina* ŠIR-*šú* ŠU ᵈ30 GÍD-*ma* GAM (DPS XV:41 [AOAT 43.152])

**If (it is the first day he is sick) and he was wounded on his coccyx[150] (or) on his testicle,[151] "hand" of Sîn. (If) it is prolonged, he will die.

In addition, Sîn shared with his daughter Ištar the role of causer of cranial nerve trauma. Whereas she produced injuries to the eighth cranial nerve, he specialized in injuries to the facial nerves (see Chapter 13 with 13.129–13.131).

19.199 [DIŠ *i-n*] *a* IGI-*šú* SÌG-*iṣ-ma ù* KA-*šú su-ḫur ina* A.[SAG] *i-ṭí-pá-*[*ma is*]*-sà-aḫ-ḫap-ma ina* KA-*šú* $UŠ_{11}$ DU-*ak* ŠU ᵈEN.ZU BA.[ÚŠ] (*KAR* 211 obv. 15–16)[152]

**[If] he was wounded ⌜on⌝ one side of his face and his mouth is turned (to one side and his skin) smooths out [and] falls flat against (his) ⌜skull⌝ and spittle flows from his mouth, "hand" of Sîn; he will ⌜die⌝.

This may be due to the fact that reactivation of HSV1 infections can cause idiopathic facial paralysis (Bell's palsy) or cranial polyneuritis. Also possibly related to the HSV infections that Sîn and family caused is an infectious neurologic syndrome involving fever and seizures that is described in 19.259–19.265. The remaining trauma references for Sîn share some of the symptoms that are described in connection with this syndrome.

19.200 DIŠ *ina* SAG.KI-*šú šá* 150/ZAG SÌG-*iṣ u* IGI[I][I-*šú* ÉR ŠU [d]EN.ZU] : DIŠ *ina* SAG.KI-*šú šá* 150 SÌG-*iṣ u* IGI[II]-*šú* DIRI.MEŠ-*ḫa* [ŠU [d]EN.ZU] (DPS IV A obv. 40–41//B obv. 36b–37 = *TDP* 36:40–41; cf. *KAR* 211 obv. 21–22)

**If he was wounded on his left/right temple and [his] eyes [shed tears, "hand" of Sîn]. If he was wounded on his right temple and his eyes are "soaked" ["hand" of Sîn].[153]

19.201 DIŠ KI.MIN-*ma* ⌜Á⌝-*šú šá* 150 GI_6-*át i-ṭa-mu* [SÌG-*i*] *ṣ* [d]30 *u uš-te-zeb* [: GAM] (DPS XV:10 [AOAT 43.151]; cf. DPS X B r. 1 = *TDP* 86 r. 1)

**If (it is the first day he is sick) and his right arm is dark (and) he twists, ⌜blow⌝ of Sîn but he will get through [(var. he will die)].

The blow to the temple described in the first reference above could produce a lengthwise fracture in the petrous bone that could, in turn, as pointed out by Fincke,[154] damage the facial nerves resulting in an inability to fully close the eye. Conjunctival irritation, inflammation, and tearing can be a consequence of an eye that cannot close properly. The fact that Sîn is otherwise associated with injuries to the facial nerves (see above) strengthens the possibility that the patient's "soaked" and "tearing" eyes in these trauma references were the result of a petrous bone fracture.

Other Gods/Goddesses of Trauma

The remaining cases of trauma were divided up among minor and sometimes quite obscure divinities or assigned to what appears to have been the *āšipu*'s residual category, "hand" of god (see below).

DAMU AND NINGIŠZIDA

Damu was a god of healing associated, like the goddess Gula, with the city of Isin. He caused intestinal narrowing (atresia; see 17.120) and penetrating wounds. He was either the son of or else identical with Ningišzida who, not surprisingly, caused ileus from abdominal wounds.[155] Both were gods who, according to tradition, themselves died, that is, they were banished to the netherworld.

19.202 DIŠ KI.MIN-*ma* TI-*šú šá* 15 GI_6 KA-*šú* ḪÁD.MEŠ *u it-ta-nag-ra-ár* ŠU [d]*Da-mu ina* ÉLLAG-*šú* SÌG-*iṣ* GAM (DPS XV:42 [AOAT 43.152])

**If (it is the first day he is sick) and his left rib is dark, his mouth is continually dry, and he rolls over and over, "hand" of Damu. He was wounded on his kidney; he will die.

19.203 DIŠ *ina ri-biti-šú* SÌG-*iṣ-ma* DÚR-*šú* BAD.BAD-*ir* ŠU [d]*Nin-giš-zi-da* (DPS XIV A iii 18 = *TDP* 140 iii 52′)[156]

**If he was wounded on the side of his abdomen and consequently his anus is continually stopped up, "hand" of Ningišzida.

PAPSUKKAL

This divinity was vizier/messenger for the gods and in particular the god Anu. He caused skull wounds and was part of the queue of abdominal wound causers that began with Adad and ended with the twin gods (19.146). A blow to the skull was probably attributed to Papsukkal because his master, Anu, had a special relationship with that part of the head (see 19.369–19.372).

19.204 DIŠ *ina* U[G]U-*šú* SÌG-*iṣ* ŠU ^{d}*Papsukkal* KI.MIN ŠU ^{d}[. . .] (DPS III A obv. 18//C obv. 9 = *TDP* 18:9)

**If he was wounded on the ⌜top of his head⌝, "hand" of Papsukkal or "hand" of [. . .]

19.205 DIŠ *ina* SUḪUŠ KIR$_4$-*šú* SÌG-*iṣ ana* U$_4$.15 ŠU ^{d}*Papsukkal* (DPS VI A obv. 31b//C i 18 = *TDP* 56:31)

**If he was wounded on the base of his nose, (if he has been sick) for fifteen days, "hand" of Papsukkal.

To judge from the arrangement of entries in the third tablet of the diagnostic series,[157] the following fragmentary references to gastrointestinal symptoms as complications of head wounds (see Chapter 13 with 13.134–13.135) may also have originally been attributed to Papsukkal. If so, this might account for Papsukkal's association with trauma to the abdomen (see 19.146).

19.206 DIŠ *ina* U[G]U-*šú* SÌG-*ma kìn-ṣa-a-šú* DÚB.MEŠ *u* ŠÀ-*šú* DIB.DIB-*su* DIB-*it* [. . .] / DIŠ *ina* U[G]U-*šú* SÌG-*ma* ŠÀ.MEŠ-*šú* MÚ.MÚ-*ḫu* DIB-*iṭ* [. . .] (DPS III A obv. 20–21//C obv. 11–12 = *TDP* 18:11–12)

**If he was wounded on the top of his head and consequently his legs tremble and his stomach continually afflicts him, affliction by [. . .]. If he was wounded on the top of his head and consequently his insides are continually bloated, affliction by [. . .]

"HAND" OF GOD

The references to trauma attributed to "hand" of god or "hand" of the (personal) god of the patient can generally be related to one of the nontrauma syndromes with similar attribution. For example, "hand" of his (personal) god was blamed for mysterious aches and pains in the chest and upper body (see 19.109–19.110) and (paired with "god of his city") for wounding to the upper back, as in the following reference.

19.207 DIŠ KI.MIN-*ma ina šá-šal-li-šú šá* 15/150 SÌG-*iṣ u ú-rap-pad* ŠU DINGIR-*šú ina ša-at ur-ra*/<EN.NUN> MURUB$_4$-*ti* SÌG-*iṣ* GAM (DPS XV:44–45 [AOAT 43.152]; cf. DPS XII D iii 23–24//E 24–27 = *TDP* 104 iii 23–24)

**If (it is the first day he is sick) and he was wounded on his left/right upper back and he wanders about, "hand" of the god of his city/"hand" of his god. <If> he was wounded in the dawn watch/middle watch, he will die.

Other wound references seem to have been attributed by parallelism with the headaches and other aches and pains induced by personal god stress (see 19.35–19.36). In the first two quotes below, the references to baked goods and scatter offerings explain the reason for the personal god's anger.

19.208 U_4 GIG GABA-*su* DU_8-*at* NU *el-lu is-su* É[Š] *e-pu-ti* DINGIR-*šu iṭ-ḫi* (*MDP* 57.11 iv 15′–16′)

**If the patient's breast was (cut) open, his arm approached the baked goods of his god when he was in an unclean state.

19.209 DIŠ GIG GABA-*su* KÚ-*šú* ŠU DINGIR-*šú ana si-riq ga*[*b-b*]*i* [. . .] (DPS XII A 1 = *TDP* 100 i 1)

**If the patient's breast hurts him, "hand" of his god for scatter offerings of all [sorts . . .]

19.210 DIŠ *ina* SAG.KI-*šú šá* 150 SÌG-*iṣ* ŠU DINGIR-*šú* : DIŠ *ina* SAG.KI-*šú šá* 15 SÌG-*iṣ* ŠU GIDIM ŠU DINGIR DIN (DPS IV B obv. 36a//E i 18 = *TDP* 36:39//*SpTU* 3.88 i 17–18)

**If he was wounded on his right temple, "hand" of his god. If he was wounded on his left temple . . . "hand" of god; he will get well.

19.211 DIŠ SAG.KI^{II}-*šú šá* 15 *u* 150 KÚ.MEŠ-*šú-ma* KÚM-*šú mit-ḫar* ŠU DINGIR-*šú* DIN (DPS IV B obv. 32//E i 12 = *TDP* 36:33//*SpTU* 3.88 i 12)[158]

**If his left and right temples continually hurt him and his temperature is normal, "hand" of his god; he will get well.

Similarly, headache and deafness produced by a god in a nontrauma patient seems to have attracted the attribution to a "murderous god" to head wounds with diminished hearing.

19.212 DIŠ SAG.KI *ḫe-si-ma* GEŠTU^{II}-*šú* NU ŠE.GA-*a* ŠU DINGIR-*šú* UGU-*šú um-mu-da* GAM (DPS IV B obv. 4 = *TDP* 32:4)

**If he has a viselike headache[159] and his ears do not hear, the "hand" of his god has been imposed on him; he will die.

19.213 DIŠ *ina* SAG.DU-*šú* SÌG-*iṣ-ma ḫa-si-si-šú* ⌜*kùd*?-*du*?[160]⌝-*ta-at* ⌜GEŠTU^{II}? xxxxxxxx ŠU⌝ DINGIR *šag-gaš-šú na-kud* GAM (DPS III C r. 20 = *TDP* 26:80)

**If he was wounded on his head and, consequently, his hearing is low (and) his ears [. . .], "hand" of a murderous god; it is serious; he will die.

The final set of references[161] seems linked to the role of unspecified gods in producing nonspecific fever. In other words, both the trauma (the first reference below) and the fever (the second reference below) affected the bulb of the nose.

19.214 DIŠ *ina* SAG KIR_4-*šú* SÌG-*iṣ* ŠU DINGIR-*šú* (DPS VI A obv. 31a//C i 17 = *TDP* 56:31a)

**If he was wounded on the bulb of his nose, "hand" of his god.

19.215 DIŠ SAG KIR_4-*šú na-ru-ub* KÚM-*im u* $ŠED_7$ ŠU DINGIR-*šú* DIN (DPS VI A obv. 22 = *TDP* 56:22)

**If the bulb of his nose is soft (and) he is hot and then cold, "hand" of his god; he will get well.

Gods/Goddesses of Fever

The presence of multiple potential disease-causers provided the *āšipu* with ample opportunity to create and subdivide categories of infectious diseases that produced fever. As is discussed in the infectious diseases chapter (Chapter 3), he distinguished biphasic from continuous fevers and subdivided these two fever patterns into two further categories, those with and those without jaundice.

LIʾBU-FEVERS

Liʾbu was an intermittent fever, accompanied by a flat (macular) or raised (papular) rash. Patients with *liʾbu*-fever but without jaundice might be further diagnosed as having *ṣibit šadî.*

ṢIBIT ŠADÎ

19.216 DIŠ SAG.DU-*su* KÚM-*im* SAG KIR_4-*šú* ŠU^{II}-*šú u* GÌR^{II}-*šú* $ŠED_7$ DIḪ KUR DIB-*su* KI.MIN *kiš-pi* DIB.MEŠ[-*šú* . . .] (DPS III C obv. 51 = *TDP* 24:51)

**If his head is hot (and) the tip of his nose, his hands, and his feet are cold, *liʾbu* (*ṣibit*) *šadî* afflicts him . . .

19.217 DIŠ NA TA GÌR^{II}.MEŠ-*šú a-di* MAŠ.SÌLA.MEŠ-*šú i-tar-rak* NA BI *li-i-bu šá-di-i* DIB-*su* (K 2581 obv. 20′–21′//*AMT* 53/7+K 6732:1)

**If from his feet to his shoulders it throbs, *liʾbu* (*ṣibit*) *šadî* afflicts that person.

Ṣibit šadî means literally "affliction of/by the mountain." This could theoretically mean a disease that originated in the mountains to the east of Mesopotamia (KUR/*šadû* also means "east"). Alternatively, the reference is not to a real geographic location but to the netherworld mountain[162] whose lord, Nergal, was a god of pestilence. The two following quotes describe a fever course that is classically seen in malaria and typhoid, although it may occur with many infections. For more details, see Chapter 3 with 3.10–3.11.

19.218 DIŠ U_4.2.KÁM ŠUB-*šú-ma ina* U_4.3.KÁM DIB-*su* U_4-*ma* DIB-*šú im-ta-na-ag-ga-gu* EGIR *im-ta-na-gag-ga ra-ʾ-i-ba* TUKU-*ši* UB.MEŠ-*šú* KÚ.MEŠ-*šú* ŠU^{II}-*šú u* GÌR^{II}-*šú* $ŠED_7$-*a* EGIR-*nu* KÚM 1-*niš i-rak-kab-šú* : *i-re-eḫ-ḫi-šú u* IR ŠUB-*su-ma ina-aḫ* DIB KUR-*i* DIB-*su* (DPS XVI:25–27 [AOAT 43.174–175])

**If it falls upon him for two days and then afflicts him on the third day and when it afflicts him, he continually becomes rigid and after he continually becomes rigid, he has a trembling, his limbs continually hurt him, his hands and his feet are cold (and) afterward fever rides (var. flows) over him everywhere at once and sweat falls upon him and then he finds relief, *ṣibit šadî* afflicts him.

19.219 [DIŠ NA *li-ʾ*] *-bu ṣi-bit* KUR-*i* DIB-*su-ma* [*ú-maš-šir*] *-šu-ma ina* U$_4$.3.KÁM DIB-*su ir-te-dá-aš-šu um-ma ṣa-ar-ḫa li-ʾ-ba dá-an-na ù zu-ʾ-ta-am ma-ʾ-tam* TUKU.MEŠ-*ši si-li-ʾ-ta-šu ú-ta-ar-ri-ik-ma it-ta-dim-šu* . . . (Meier, *ZA* 45.208 v 15–21)

**[If] ⌜*liʾbu*⌝ *ṣibit šadî* afflicts [a person] and then [it releases] him and then, on the third day, it afflicts him (and) pursues him, he continually has burning fever, severe *liʾbu*, and lots of sweat, his illness has been prolonged and has knocked him down . . .

Irregular or inverted fever patterns (two days in a row of paroxysms and a third day of rest) were also noted.

19.220 DIŠ U$_4$.2.KÁM DIB-*su-*⌜*ma*⌝ *ina* U$_4$.3.KÁM *i-re-eḫ-ḫi-šú* DIB-*it* KUR-*i* : GAM (DPS XVI:28 [AOAT 43.175])

**If it afflicts him for two days and flows over him on the third day, *ṣibit šadî* (var. he will die).

A final reference to *ṣibit šadî* has a rather picturesque way of describing febrile illnesses that never quite seem to go away.

19.221 *pa-na i-šu ar-ka-tam ú-ul i-šu* . . . KA.INIM.MA *ṣi-bi-it* KUR.RA (BM 64526:2, 5; cf. 10)

**It has a face; it does not have a back . . . recitation for *ṣibit šadî*.

FATHER'S GOD Another syndrome defined by the *āšipu* that included *liʾbu*-fever but with extensive gastrointestinal involvement and dehydration was *ṣētu* (enteric fever; see Chapter 3 with 3.121–3.156). Aspects of *ṣētu* that particularly affected the head seem to have been attributed to "hand" of his father's god.

19.222 DIŠ U$_4$.1.KÁM GIG-*ma* SAG.DU-*su* KÚ-*šú* UD.DA TAB.BA ŠU DINGIR AD.A.NI DIN GAM (DPS XVI:1 [AOAT 43.171–172]; cf. DPS XV:93 [AOAT 43.155]; catch-line)[163]

**If it is the first day he is sick and his head hurts him, he burns with *ṣētu*, "hand" of his father's god; he will get well or die.

LAMAŠTU *Liʾbu* fever, which could be accompanied by jaundice, was likely to be diagnosed as "hand" of the demoness Lamaštu.[164] Although recitations and rituals designed to placate her can be very folkloric and picturesque, she may actually have originated as a name for this type of fever (see below under Named Syndromes That Evolved into Demons).

19.223 DIŠ IGI.MEŠ-*šú* SIG$_7$.MEŠ ^{d}DIM$_{11}$.ME DIB-*su* (DPS IX A 11 = *TDP* 72:11)

**If his face is yellow, Lamaštu afflicts him.[165]

19.224 DIŠ LÚ.TUR *um-ma li-ʾ-ba ú-kal u ik-ta-na-aṣ-ṣa ṣi-bit* ^{d}DIM$_{11}$.ME : ŠU DUMU.MUNUS ^{d}*A-nim* (DPS XL A 51 = *TDP* 224:51)

**If *liʾbu*-fever grips an infant and he is continually cold, affliction by Lamaštu (var. "hand" of the daughter of Anu).[166]

19.225 DIŠ U_4.1.KÁM DIB-*su* U_4.1.KÁM BAR-*šú* U_4 LÁ-*šú* LÁ-*šú* UB.MEŠ-*šú* KÚ.MEŠ-*šú* KÚM-*ma i-ra-ʾu-ub* IR ŠUB-*su-ma ina-aḫ u* A *ana* NAG *ma-gal* APIN.MEŠ ŠU ᵈDIM_{11}.ME[167] DIN (DPS XVI:14–15 [AOAT 43.173])[168]

**If one day it afflicts him and one day it releases him (and) when his confusional state comes over him, his limbs continually hurt him, he is feverish and trembles, sweat falls upon him, and then he finds relief and continually asks for a great deal of water to drink, "hand" of Lamaštu; he will get well.

Lamaštu's fever produced severe headache, abdominal discomfort[169] and bloating, and mental status changes. Most of the descriptions would fit either typhus or typhoid. For more details, see Chapter 3 with 3.20, 3.25–3.26.

19.226 DIŠ MUNUS *eʾ-re-et-ma u* IM *ud-du-pat* DIM_8.ME DIB . . . (*BAM* 240:28′)

**If a woman is colicky and is puffed up with wind, Lamaštu afflicts (her) . . .

19.227 DIŠ SAG.DU-*su* DIB.DIB-*su u* KÚM TÉŠ.BI UNU-*su*[170] GIG-*su* TAK_4-*šum*$_4$-*ma* NÍG.NIGIN TUKU *šu*[*m-ma* KI] ⸢LAL⸣[171] -*šú* LAL-*šú* $UŠ_4$-*šú* KÚR-*šum-ma ina* NU ZU-*ú ú-rap-pad* GIN_7 DIB-*it* $GIDIM_7$ ᵈDIM_{11}.ME ⸢DIB⸣-[*su uš*]-*te-zib*[172] (DPS III C obv. 36–37 = *TDP* 22:36–37)

**If his head continually afflicts him[173] and fever (has) its seat[174] equally all over (and) when his illness leaves him, he has dizziness (and) ⸢if⸣, [when] his confusional state comes over him, his mentation is altered so that he wanders about without knowing (where he is) as in affliction by a ghost, Lamaštu afflicts [him]. ⸢He will come through.⸣

An interesting feature of Lamaštu's fever was that it was recognizably the same in infants as it was in adults. This is made explicit in the first reference below, but note also the similarity in the descriptions of the fever in the remaining references to infant and older child or adult versions.

19.228 DIŠ LÚ.TUR GIN_7 DIB-*it* ᵈDIM_9.ME *u*$_4$-*mi-šam-ma* DIB.DIB-*su* ŠU ᵈDIM_9.ME (DPS XL A 58//B 57 = *TDP* 224:58)

**If something continually afflicts an infant daily like affliction by Lamaštu, "hand" of Lamaštu.

19.229 DIŠ LÚ.TUR ŠÀ-*šú i-mim* $ŠED_7$ *u* A.MEŠ *ana* NAG-*e ma-gal i-te-ner-reš-ma i-šat-ti* ŠU ᵈDIM_9.ME (DPS XL A 53 = *TDP* 224:53)[175]

**If an infant's abdomen gets hot (and) gets cold and he asks for a lot of water to drink and drinks it, "hand" of Lamaštu.

19.230 DIŠ ŠÀ-*šú* KÚM-*im u* $ŠED_7$ A UL_4-*gal* APIN-*ma* NAG ŠU ᵈDIM_{10}.ME (DPS XIII B ii 11 = *TDP* 118 ii 11)

**If his abdomen gets hot and gets cold (and) he asks for a lot of water and drinks it, "hand" of Lamaštu.

19.231 DIŠ ŠÀ-*šú* KÚM-*im u* $ŠED_7$ A *ana* TU_5 UL_4-*gal* APIN.MEŠ ŠU ᵈDIM_{10}.ME DIN (DPS XIII B ii 12 = *TDP* 118 ii 12)[176]

**If his abdomen gets hot and gets cold (and) he continually asks for a lot of water to bathe in, "hand" of Lamaštu; he will get well.

In favor of typhoid as the specific fever caused by Lamaštu[177] is the fact that this demoness had a fearsome reputation as a baby snatcher who produced abortions in pregnant women and deaths in young children. Curiously, she did not do these things out of malice or ill will but because she was a frustrated mother who inadvertently killed in her overeagerness to nurture, as is described in the following recitation.

19.232 **The daughter of Anu daily counts the pregnant women; she goes around ⌜after⌝ those (about to) give birth. She counts up their [months]; she marks the days (of their confinement) onto the wall. For the lying-in women giving birth (this) is (her) incantation: "Bring me your sons so that I can give them suck; let me put the breast into the mouth of your daughters" (*LKU* 33:18–22).

One of the few striking differences between typhus and typhoid is that in typhus the prognosis is actually more favorable for younger patients. In children under ten years, the disease is usually mild and fatalities are uncommon. Mortality rates rise with age, reaching over 60 percent in untreated patients over fifty. Typhoid, by contrast, is dangerous to persons at both extremes of age. Moreover, in pregnant women, typhoid fever produces abortions or premature labor in 60 to 80 percent of cases.[178]

BIPHASIC FEVERS

LABAṢU Labaṣu, although apparently a demoness whose name is written with a variant of the Sumerogram for Lamaštu, has no personality profile and is also probably simply a demon of disease, specifically biphasic fevers without jaundice such as rat bite-fever. For more details, see Chapter 3 with 3.35.

The *āšipu* separately described what appears to be leptospirosis and which he attributed to "hand" of Kūbu. For more details, see 19.335–19.342. The term used to describe biphasic fevers with jaundice, *aḫḫāzu*, is also used to describe a type of jaundice (see pp. 138–139).

OTHER FEVERS WITH JAUNDICE

RĀBIṢU One further type of fever with jaundice was distinguished by the *āšipu*. It would appear from the description to be hepatitis A (see Chapter 6 with 6.127). For some obscure reason, and in spite of numerous differences between hepatitis A and the kinds of symptoms more normally caused by this demon (as, for example, 13.211), this type of fever with jaundice was blamed on a *rābiṣu*.[179]

19.233 DIŠ *ina taš-rit* GIG-*šú* KÚM ÚḪ NINDA KAŠ GURUN *ma-da* KÚ *ina* ŠÀ-*šú* NU ḪUN DUB-*ka* U-*šú* LAL-*aṣ* IGI^II^-*šú* BAD.BAD-*te ana* ⌜AKKIL⌝ *i-qal* NÍ-*šú ú-dam-ma-aq* ZI.IR.MEŠ *u* IGI.MEŠ-*šú i-ta-nar-ri-qu* MAŠKIM SÌG-*su* TA TAG-*ma* KI-*šú* [K]EŠDA *ina*

NINDA *ik-ka-lu* KÚ *ina* A NAG-*ú* NAG NA BI *ana* U_4.5.KÁM : *ana* U_4.7.KÁM DIN (DPS XVII:10–13 [AOAT 43.195–196])

**If at the beginning of his illness he burns with fever, he eats a lot of bread, beer, and fruit (but) it does not rest easy in his stomach (and) he pours it out, he can stretch out his finger, he continually opens his eyes, at a mournful cry, he is silent, he treats himself well, (his stomach) is continually upset, and his face continually turns yellow, a *rābiṣu* has struck him (and) after it touched him, it was ⌜bound⌝ with him (or) he ate it with the bread he ate (or) drank it with the water he drank; (if he is sick) for five (var. seven) days, he will get well.

That the *āšipu* was not completely ignorant of the true source of this infection is shown by the comment "he ate it with the bread he ate (or) drank it with the water he drank."

FEVERS WITH BLEEDING

SIBITTI The Sibitti were a group of seven gods associated with a constellation containing seven stars which is currently known as the Pleiades. They were responsible for one of two types of viral hemorrhagic fever recognized by the *āšipu*, as well as for hemorrhagic shock (see 19.178).

19.234 DIŠ *ina* GIG-*šú* IGI[II]-*šú* NU ÍL-*ši ina* IGI[II]-*šú* KIR_4-*šú* KA-*šú* GEŠTU[II]-*šú u* GÌŠ-*šú* MÚD TÉŠ.BI È.ME-*a* ŠU 7-*bi* . . . (DPS XVII:25–26 [AOAT 43.197])

**If during his illness, he does not raise his eyes (and) blood comes out of his eyes, his nose, his mouth, his ears, and his penis all at the same time, "hand" of the Sibitti . . .

MARDUK What distinguished the variety of hemorrhagic fever caused by Marduk were symptoms indicating something wrong with the heart: fluttering and/or needling pain,[180] as in the following example. For more details, see Chapter 3 with 3.237–3.238.

19.235 DIŠ GABA-*su* DU_8.MEŠ-*át* SAG.KI-*šú* ŠUB-*ut* MÚD *ina* KA/KIR_4-*šú pi-qam la p*[*i-qam*] ⌜DU⌝-*k*[*a*] ŠÀ-*šú pi-qam la pi-qam* MUD-*ud* ŠU [d]AMAR.UTU *a-dir-ma* BA.ÚŠ (DPS XII A 2–3 = *TDP* 100 i 2–3)[181]

**If his chest is clear,[182] (the blood vessels of) his temple have collapsed, blood incessantly flows from his mouth/nose, (and) his heart incessantly shudders, "hand" of Marduk; he will be worried and die.

The god Marduk was also given partial responsibility (with Ninurta) for plague (*šadānu*; see Chapter 3 with 3.226), which has a marked hemorrhagic tendency. The connection of Marduk with plague is possibly due to the involvement of the spleen, which was associated with Marduk's planet (Jupiter) in popular tradition.[183]

TWIN GODS Joining with the Sibitti in causing bleeding in connection with fever as well as hemorrhagic shock from injuries to the back (see 19.179) were the "twin gods" [d]LU-

GAL.GÌR.RA and ^{d}MES.LAM.TA.È.A, also the constellation Gemini. Whereas the Sibitti's bleeding developed quickly, the victim of the twin gods' fever or fevers did not begin to bleed until well into the course of the illness.

Bleeding could be so severe as to mimic viral hemorrhagic fevers, producing vascular collapse ("cold arms") and mental status changes including abnormal posturing, as is described in the following references. A likely cause of this bleeding would have been the consumption of clotting factors and the blood clotting cells (platelets, thrombocytes), a condition referred to as disseminated intravascular coagulopathy.

> **19.236** DIŠ *ina* GIG-*šú* IGI^{II}-*šú* NU ÍL-*ši ina* IGI^{II}-*šú* KIR$_4$-*šú* KA-*šú* GEŠTU^{II}-*šú u* GÌŠ-*šú* MÚD TÉŠ.BI È.ME-*a* . . . U$_4$.31.KÁM ŠU ^{d}MAŠ.TAB.BA (DPS XVII:25–26 [AOAT 43.197])
>
> **If during his illness, he does not raise his eyes (and) blood comes out of his eyes, his nose, his mouth, his ears, and his penis all at the same time . . . (and he has been sick for) thirty-one days, "hand" of the twin gods.
>
> **19.237** DIŠ Á^{II}-*šú ik-ta-na-ṣa-a* ŠU ^{d}MAŠ.TAB.BA (DPS X B r. 7 = *TDP* 88 r. 7)
>
> **If his arms are continually cold, "hand" of the twin gods.
>
> **19.238** DIŠ KI.MIN-*ma* ÚR-*šú ú-maḫ-ḫaṣ* ŠU^{II}-*šú ú-na-aš-šak* Á^{II}-*šú ana ku-tal-li-šú* GUR ŠU ^{d}MAŠ.T[AB.BA GAM] (DPS XV:56 [AOAT 43.154]; cf. DPS XIV A iii 1–2 = *TDP* 140 iii 35′–36′)[184]
>
> **If (it is the first day he is sick) and he strikes his crotch, chews on his hands, (and) they have to put his arms behind him, "hand" of the ⌜twin gods⌝; [he will die].

Victims of the twin gods had a high fever that could be accompanied by convulsions. The stomach was also upset, but as long as severe vomiting did not develop, the patient could survive.

> **19.239** [DIŠ GIG IGI.M]EŠ-*šú* IR *ú-kal u* DUL.DUL-*tam* ŠU ^{d}MAŠ.TAB.BA [MAŠ]. ⌜MAŠ-*su*⌝ DÙ-*uš u* ŠU.GUR.GUR-*šu-ma* DIN (DPS IX A 1–2//B obv. 1–2 = *TDP* 70:1–2)
>
> **[If a patient]'s [face] holds sweat and he veils himself (i.e., withdraws from social intercourse), "hand" of the twin gods. (If) you do his ⌜treatment⌝ and you continually wipe him off, he will get well.
>
> **19.240** DIŠ SAG.DU-*su* AD$_6$-*šú* KÚM ÚḪ *u i-ta-na-šu-<uš>* ŠU ^{d}MAŠ.TAB.BA DIN *šum$_4$-ma* ⌜*ina* DÚR⌝-[*šú* MÚD SUR . . .] (DPS III C r. 7//E$_1$ 8+E$_2$ 4 = *TDP* 26:67)
>
> **If his head and body burn with fever and (his stomach) is continually upset, "hand" of the twin gods; he will get well. If [blood drips] from [his] anus [. . .]
>
> **19.241** DIŠ SAG.DU-*su* KÚM NAR *ina* KÚM-*šú*?[185] LUḪ.ME ŠU ^{d}MIN DIN *šum$_4$-ma ina* DÚR-*šú* ZÉ SUR *u* ZÉ/MÚD *i-ta-n*[*a-ḫu* . . .] (DPS III C r. 8//E$_1$ 9+E$_2$ 5 = *TDP* 26:68)
>
> **If his head burns (?)[186] with fever (and) during the course of his? fever, he continually jerks, "hand" of the twin gods; he will get well. If bile drips from his anus and he continually ⌜vomits (?)⌝ bile/blood[187] [. . .]

FEVERS WITH JOINT PAIN (ARTHRALGIA) AND RASH

EA Ea was the god of sweet water and, working as a team with his son Asaluḫi, a major patron of the *āšipu* and his craft. Apart from appearing on day 3 in the abdominal wound sequence quoted in 19.146, he was responsible for a high fever with much sweat accompanied by arthritis-like symptoms including severe ("hand" of ghost) pain and stiffness in the joints and lower back pain (*maškādu*).

19.242 DIŠ *ma-gal* GÙ.GÙ-*si* KÚM.KÚM-[*i*]*m* ŠU.GIDIM.MA *šá-<né>-e* ^{d}*É-a* (DPS XXII:59 [AOAT 43.256])

**If he cries out a lot (and) is continually feverish, "hand" of ghost, deputy of Ea.

19.243 DIŠ MIN-*ma* IR *la-ba-ṣi ma-at-tú* TUKU.TUKU-*ši u ḫur-ba-šu* ŠUB.ŠUB-*su* ŠU ^{d}*aš-ṭi* ^{d}ÀLAD *šá-né-e* ^{d}*É-a* DIŠ *ina* ŠU ^{d}*aš-ṭi* KAR-*šú* . . . (*CTN* 4.72 vi 14′–16′)

**If . . . he continually has much sweat (as in) Labaṣu and chills keep falling upon him, "hand" of "stiff," a *šedû*-demon deputized by Ea. If (you want) to save him from "hand" of "stiff" . . .[188]

19.244 *ana* SA.GIG A.RÁ *šá-nim* ^{d}IDIM [S]IG$_5$ . . . (*STT* 93:42′)

(The plant) is good for *maškādu*, a *šedû* deputized by Ea . . .

The attribution of these symptoms to the deputy of Ea rather than to the god himself suggests that the fever and arthralgia were expected to be followed in due course by some other manifestation of the illness, perhaps a rash consisting of the clustered lesions (*ummedu*) otherwise attributed to the god's "hand" (see 19.91).

19.245 [. . .] *ina* ÚNU-*šú* È [ŠU] ^{d}*É*-[*a*] (DPS XXXIII:81 [AOAT 43.357])

**[If . . .] erupt on the middle of the cheek, ["hand"] of ⌜*Ea*⌝.

19.246 *um-me-di* [Š]U ^{d}*É*-[*a*] (DPS XXXIII:109 [AOAT 43.358])

***Ummedu* (are caused by) ⌜"hand"⌝ of ⌜Ea⌝

Various possibilities suggest themselves for Ea's fever, including German measles, hepatitis B, and viral fevers of the type represented by modern Chikungunya, a mosquito-carried disease that is still prevalent in Africa and India. Cikungunya, like a number of other arbovirus infections, is associated with a fever over 100°F, arthritis, backache, and a maculopapular eruption that may appear at any point during the febrile course.

BENIGN SÎN FAMILY FEVERS WITHOUT NEUROLOGIC SYMPTOMS

A further group of fevers is represented by the family of Sîn, Šamaš, and Ištar. Ghosts also were closely associated with this family for a variety of reasons, including the fact that Šamaš was a patron of uncared-for ghosts, that Sîn was involved in necromancy, and that Ištar made people see dead persons in their dreams. Curiously, many of the possibilities for specific diseases that might have been blamed on this family of causal agents are viral (including herpetic infections and venereally transmitted hepatitis B; see Chapter 4 with 4.18, 4.34). Fevers caused by this family divide roughly into two categories: those with and those without neurologic symptoms (other than headache and bone or joint pain).

GHOST This spirit of the dead caused a benign fever accompanied by painful, swollen eyes as is described in a sequence of references in the diagnostic series. Probably to be connected with these references are a number of therapeutic texts in which "hand" of ghost, deputy of Ištar is blamed for a similar complex of headache and swollen or stinging eyes.[189] The "deputy of Ištar" probably indicates that the illness left the patient exhausted (see 19.64). A variety of illnesses, including influenza, could be responsible for the described symptoms. For more details, see Chapter 9 with 9.52–9.56.

19.247 DIŠ SAG.KI-*šú* DIB-*su-ma* SA IGI^{II}-*šú* KÚ.MEŠ ŠU GIDIM$_7$ / DIŠ SAG.KI-*šú* DIB-*su-ma* KÚM ŠED$_7$ *u* IGI^{II}-*šú* *nu-up-pu-ḫa* ŠU GIDIM$_7$ (DPS IV B obv. 16–17 = *TDP* 34:16–17; cf. *BAM* 482 iii 5)

**If his temple afflicts him and his eye muscles continually hurt, "hand" of ghost. If his temple afflicts him and he gets hot (and then) cold and his eyes are swollen,[190] "hand" of ghost.

One or more upper respiratory illnesses would seem appropriate to the preceding references since ghosts were otherwise blamed for ear infections (see Chapter 9 with 9.106, 9.112) and pharyngitis (see below).

19.248 DIŠ *gir-ra-a-šú* ŠUB.MEŠ-*ma* KÚ.ME-*šú* ŠU GIDIM$_7$ (DPS X A obv. 54a//D 14 = *TDP* 86:54a)

**If both sides of his throat continually (look) terrible and continually hurt him, "hand" of ghost.[191]

The quote below describes a chronic illness with headache and feverishness, rhinorrhea and a stiff and edematous ("distended") bullneck. There are a number of infections that could cause this type of pharyngeal and neck involvement.

19.249 DIŠ NA GÚ *ú-ḫa-ma-šú u* ⌜SA⌝ (coll.) GÚ-*šú* ⌜*aš-ṭa ṣu-mur*⌝ (coll.) SAG.DU-*su* DIB.DIB-*su pi-qam la pi-qam na-ḫi-ra-šú ṣab-ta em-ma ši-ḫat* UZU.MEŠ TUKU.TUKU-*ši* NA BI ŠU.[GID]IM DIB-*su ana* TI-*šú* . . . (Labat, *RSO* 32.112 v 6′–9′)

**If a person's neck is paralyzed and his neck muscle(s) are stiff (and) distended, he continually has headaches, again and again his nostrils are "seized" (and) hot, (and) he continually has wasting away of the flesh, "hand" of ⌜ghost⌝ afflicts that person, to cure him . . .

ŠAMAŠ AND IŠTAR These twin children of the moon-god Sîn seem to have caused a benign fever or perhaps a pair of fevers, differentiated by duration and characterized by a frontal headache, nausea, and a very high temperature. The temples "going at the same time"[192] in the second quote below is probably a reference to a pulse sufficiently rapid that the *āšipu* is having difficulty in finding it on either side. Since, in other contexts, both Šamaš and Ištar were responsible for arthritis, it may have been understood that the pair of fevers caused by these divinities were also characterized by severe pain in the limbs or joints. A number of modern fevers of viral origin would fit these descriptions (frontal headache, temperatures in excess of 100°F, and muscle pain [myalgias] or joint pain [arthralgias]).

19.250 [DIŠ SU-*šú* KÚ]M ÚḪ TUKU-*ma* ŠU^{II}-*šú u* GÌR^{II}-*šú*-[*ma*] *mar-ṣa it-te-nin-ṣi-la-šú* [. . .]-*a-šú* KÚ.MEŠ-*šú* GÌR^{II}-*šú* x.[M]EŠ ŠU 15 : ŠU ^{d}*Kù-bi* (DPS XVIII:5–6 [AOAT 43.218])

**[If his body] burns with ⸢fever⸣, his hands and his feet are sore and sluggish, his [legs?] continually hurt him (and) his feet [. . .], "hand" of Ištar . . .

19.251 U$_4$ GIG *um-ma-šu ṣa-ru-uḫ zu-ʾ-ta ki me-e ra-mi-ik* ŠU ^{d}UTU ŠU *ik-ri-bi-šu* (*MDP* 57.11 iii 4)

**If the patient burns with fever (and) is bathed in sweat like water, "hand" of Šamaš, "hand" of his vow.

19.252 DIŠ SAG.KI^{II}-*šú* 1-*niš* DU.MEŠ *u* IR-*su it-ta-nag-ra-ár ú-gaš* ŠU ^{d}15 : ŠU ^{d}UTU (DPS IV A obv. 65//E ii 10 = *TDP* 38:65//*SpTU* 3.88 ii 10)[193]

**If (the blood vessels of) his temples "go" at the same time and his sweat rolls down (and) he vomits, "hand" of Ištar (var. "hand" of Šamaš).

19.253 DIŠ SAG.KI-*šú šá* 15 KÚ-*šú* ŠU ^{d}UTU DIN / DIŠ SAG.KI-*šú šá* 150 KÚ-*šú* ŠU ^{d}15 DIN (DPS IV B obv. 25–26//E i 5–6 = *TDP* 34:25–26//*SpTU* 3.88 i 5–6; cf. *SpTU* 1.30 obv. 11–12)

**If his left temple hurts him, "hand" of Šamaš; he will get well. If his right temple hurts him, "hand" of Ištar; he will get well.

19.254 DIŠ SAG.DU-*su* DIB.DIB-*su u* KÚM ŠUB.ŠUB-*su* ŠU [^{d}]⸢15⸣ (DPS III C obv. 34 = *TDP* 22:34)

**If his head continually afflicts him and fever continually falls upon him, "hand" of Ištar.

19.255 DIŠ SA GÌR^{II}-*šú* ZI.MEŠ-*ú* IGI^{II}-*šú ana* ÍL DUGUD SAG.DU-*su u* SAG ŠÀ-*šú e-em* ŠU ⸢20?⸣ [: AL].TI (DPS XIV A iv 26–27//C$_2$ iv 21//L 5–6 = *TDP* 146 iv 61′–62′)

**If the blood vessel(s) of his feet (feel like they are) pulsating, it is difficult for him to raise his eyes, (and) his head and his epigastrium are hot, "hand" of Šamaš(?) (var. he will get well).

19.256 DIŠ ŠÀ-*šú* KÚM IR GIN$_7$ *lu-ba-ṭi* ŠUB.ŠUB-*su u* ZI.IR.MEŠ ŠU 20 MAŠ.MAŠ-*su* DÙ-*uš u* ŠU.⸢ÚR?⸣-*šú-ma* DIN (DPS XIII B ii 5–6 = *TDP* 116 ii 5–6)[194]

**If his abdomen is hot, sweat keeps falling upon him as in *lubāṭu*, and (his stomach) is continually upset, "hand" of Šamaš. (If) you do his treatment and you continually wipe him off, he will get well.

The major discernible difference between the two fevers seems to have been their respective duration. A duration of approximately five days ("hand" of Ištar) would fit many viral fevers. Some have relapses or second attacks occurring two to twelve weeks after the first which, if counted all together might give you the thirty days of Šamaš's fever. The "shaking" temples in the first quote below is probably a reference to a bounding pulse.

19.257 DIŠ SAG.KI^{II}-*šú ki-lat-tan* 1-*niš i-rad-da-šú* : DU.MEŠ *u* IR-*su it-ta-nag-ra-ár* U_4.5. KÁM ŠU ^{d}15/[15] *u* 20 (DPS IV A obv. 66–67+A_2 obv. 1–2//E ii 11 = *TDP* 38:66–67// *SpTU* 3.88 ii 11)

**If both temples seem to shake (var. "go") at the same time and his sweat rolls down (and) it is the fifth day, "hand" of Ištar (var. A: Ištar and Šamaš).

19.258 DIŠ ŠÀ-*šú* KÚM-*ma* IR GIN_7 *lu-ba-ṭi* ŠUB.ŠUB-*su u* $ŠED_7$ U_4.31.KÁM ŠU 20 (DPS XIII B ii 9 = *TDP* 118 ii 9)

**If his abdomen is hot, sweat keeps falling upon him as in *lubāṭu*, and he has been cold (for) thirty-one days, "hand" of Šamaš.

SÎN FAMILY FEVERS WITH PROMINENT NEUROLOGIC SYMPTOMS

A number of ancient Mesopotamian gods/goddesses had "deputies" of whose signs and symptoms we have descriptions. The moon-god Sîn's deputy was known as *bennu*, and may have been responsible for cysticercosis, an illness with signs and symptoms of meningoencephalitis produced by infestation with pork tapeworm larvae. For more details, see Chapter 3 with 3.267–3.274. With a little help from his children Šamaš and Ištar, Sîn also caused afebrile infantile seizures (see 19.47–19.51), cranial nerve trauma, and herpetic infections. In addition, Sîn, Šamaš, and Ištar and ghosts were also blamed for febrile illnesses with neurologic abnormalities. Since these gods/goddesses were family members or related hangers on, it is probably safe to assume that the *āšipu* would have used them for different but related syndromes that he could separate along clinical lines.

SÎN This god of the moon produced a febrile syndrome involving prominent neurologic symptoms that is described in two noncanonical diagnostic tablets. The first of these gives the symptoms of the moon-god's fever, as shown in the reference below. It is probable from this description that the *āšipu* included in his diagnosis of "hand" of Sîn forms of viral encephalitis characterized primarily by fever, prostration, tremors, and nystagmus.

19.259 [DIŠ G]IG SU-*šú i-mim* $ŠED_7$ DIB-*su* KÚR.KÚR ŠU ^{d}30 / [DIŠ] IGI^{II}-*šú ma-aḫ-ḫa* ŠU ^{d}30 / [DIŠ N]A IGI^{II}-*šú it-te-neq-lep-pa-a* ŠU ^{d}30 / [DIŠ N]A IGI-*šú šá* GÙB *kab-ṣa-at u i-sa-šú nu-uš* ŠU ^{d}30 / [DIŠ N]A SAG.KI-*šú šá* 150 KÚ-*šú-ma u it-te-nék-lep-pu* ŠU ^{d}30 [. . .] / [DIŠ LUḪ.LU]Ḫ-*ut* LÙ.LÙ ŠU ^{d}30 . . . [DIŠ . . . KÚM *u* I]R NU TUKU ŠU 30 AL.TI *šá-niš ana* GAL *u* TUR ŠU-*ma* (*STT* 89:205–210, 212 [Stol, *Epilepsy* 98])

**[If] the ⸢patient's⸣ body is hot (and then) cold (and) his affliction keeps changing (for the worse), "hand" of Sîn. [If] his eyes are "soaked," "hand" of Sîn. [If] a ⸢person's⸣ eyes drift downstream (horizontal nystagmus; see Chapter 13), "hand" of Sîn. [If] a ⸢person's⸣ right eye droops and his jaws shake, "hand" of Sîn.[195] [If] a ⸢person's⸣ right temple hurts him and <his eyes> drift downstream, "hand" of Sîn [. . .] [If he continually] ⌜jerks⌝ and is restless, "hand" of Sîn . . . [If he has been sick for only one or two(?) days (and) he is hot but] he does not have ⌜sweat⌝, "hand" of Sîn; he will get well. Moreover, it is the same for adults and infants.[196]

The second diagnostic text describes Sîn's neurologic fever in very similar terms.

19.260 DIŠ KÚM-*im* ŠED$_7$ A.[M]EŠ *ana ra-ma-ki*⌜*-i*⌝*-[te-ner-ri-iš] li-pit* ᵈEN.ZU [. . .] / DIŠ *ina šèr-tim* KÚM-*im ina* AN.ÚSAN ŠED$_7$ *i-r[a-ʾ-ub]* IGI^{II}-*šú im-ta-na-aḫ-ḫa-aḫ* ŠU^{II}-*šú u* GÌR^{II}-*šú ú-n[a]-aš* (*KAR* 211 obv. 10–13)

**If he is hot (and then) cold (and) he [continually asks] for water to bathe in, "touch" of Sîn [. . .][197] If in the morning he is hot (and) in the evening he is cold and ⌜trembles⌝, his eyes are continually "soaked" (and) his hands and his feet ⌜shake⌝, <"hand" of Sîn>.

Many of the same signs and symptoms are also attributed to "hand" of Sîn in scattered references in the diagnostic series. These references fall into two distinct groups. The first describes the moon-god's fever with its noticeably elevated temperatures in the morning and accompanying tremors.

19.261 DIŠ *ina šèr-ti* KÚM-*im ina le-lá-a-ti* ŠED$_7$ *u i-ra-ʾ-ub* ŠU ᵈ30 / DIŠ *ina šèr-ti* KÚM-*em ina le-lá-a-ti* ŠED$_7$ *ina* ⌜GI$_6$⌝ *ma-šil ùʾ* DUG$_4$.GA ŠEŠ-*šú ma-a-a-ta-nu* KI-*šú* KEŠDA / DIŠ *ina šèr-ti* KÚM-*im ina le-lá-a-ti* ŠED$_7$ ŠU ᵈ30 / DIŠ *ina šèr-ti* KÚM-*ma* ŠU^{II}-*šú u* GÌR^{II}-*šú i-ra-ʾ-ú-ba* ŠU ᵈ30 (DPS XVII:90–94 [AOAT 43.204])[198]

**If in the morning he is hot (and) in the evening he is cold and trembles, "hand" of Sîn.[199] If in the morning he is hot, in the evening he is cold, (and) in the middle of the night he says, "Ua!" his dying brother is bound with him (i.e., one child has infected another). If in the morning he is hot (and) in the evening he is cold, "hand" of Sîn. If in the morning he is hot and his hands and his feet tremble, "hand" of Sîn.

Two apparently contrasting quotes would seem to indicate that the shorter the duration of the fever, the better the patient's chance of survival.

19.262 DIŠ U$_4$.5.KÁM U$_4$.10.KÁM GIG-*ma* KÚM *u* IR NU TUKU ŠU ᵈ30 GAM (DPS XVI:56′ [AOAT 43.177])[200]

**If he has been sick for five or ten days and he is hot but he does not have sweat, "hand" of Sîn; he will die.

19.263 [DIŠ . . . KÚM *u* I]R NU TUKU ŠU 30 AL.TI (*STT* 89:212; DPS XIX/XX:11′ [AOAT 43.227])

**[If he has been sick for only one or two(?) days (and) he is hot but] he does not have ⌜sweat⌝, "hand" of Sîn; he will get well.

The neurologic symptoms of the moon-god's fever appear for the most part to have been listed separately in the diagnostic series but are also described in terms similar to those found in the noncanonical diagnostic texts, with headache,[201] "shaking" hands and feet,[202] mental status changes,[203] and "eyes drifting downstream,"[204] that is, horizontal nystagmus (see Chapter 13 with 13.112–13.113). Further clues as to the nature of Sîn's neurologic fever are provided by the sequence of references, also diagnosed as "hand" of Sîn, which follow the description of the moon-god's fever in the second noncanonical diagnostic text (*KAR* 211:14–22). Most are examples of trauma to the cranial nerves producing signs of the sort that would not be out of place in Sîn's fever. Two nontrauma references falling in the middle of the sequence are, however, of great interest.

19.264 [DIŠ ŠU]B-*tu* ŠUB-*su-ma i-sal-li-iḫ* [*i-ra-*ʾ]*-ub u i-ni-šú* [. . . :] DIRI x [Š]U ^{d}EN.ZU (*KAR* 211 obv. 17–18)

**[If a] ⌜falling⌝ spell falls on him and he shakes (and) ⌜trembles⌝ and his eyes [. . .] (var. are "soaked"), ⌜"hand"⌝ of Sîn.

19.265 [DIŠ TA] SAG.DU-*šú* EN GÌR^{II}-*šú* Ù.BU.BU.UL GAR-*ma* ⌜SU⌝-*šú* [BABBAR/GI$_{6}$] KI MUNUS *ina* NÁ *ka-*[*š*] *id* ŠU ^{d}[EN.ZU] (*KAR* 211 obv. 19–20)

**[If from] his head to his feet, there are *bubuʾtu*-vesicles and his skin/body is [white/black], he was "gotten" in bed with a woman; "hand" of [Sîn].

What this suggests is that Sîn's neurologic fever was connected in the mind of the *āšipu* with the sexually transmitted vesicles of *Herpes simplex* virus type 2 (HSV2), which he attributed to Sîn acting in concert with his children Šamaš and Ištar (for details, see Chapter 4). We know from other sources that Sîn was also deemed responsible for the characteristic facial vesicles of HSV1 (see Chapter 4 with 4.16). Both HSV1 and HSV2 cause encephalitis in adults, but HSV2 rarely produces fatalities, whereas HSV1 has a high fatality rate.

HSV encephalitis is still the most common identified cause of encephalitis in the United States and a direct connection could potentially have been made between HSV2 encephalitis and the venereal disease in adult patients whose fever was accompanied by radicular pain, since this pain is often temporally associated with eruptions of genital herpes. Also, as we noted above, the *āšipu* recognized infantile cases of "hand" of Sîn. Infants with HSV2 encephalitis are typically born to infected adults, which might have made it easier for the ancient physician to make a connection between the two.

The clinical hallmark of HSV encephalitis is the acute onset of fever and the presence of focal neurological symptoms. For what it is worth, when the "falling spells" produced by "hand" of Sîn are described, they are specifically described as focal seizures, as in the following example. For more details on focal seizures, see Chapter 13 with 13.194.

19.266 DIŠ GIG GÚ-*su ana* 150 NIGIN.ME ŠU^{II}-*šú u* GÌR^{II}-*šú tar-ṣa* IGI^{II}-*šú ana* IGI AN-*e na-pal-ka-a ina* KA-*šú* ÚḪ DU-*ak i-ḫar-ru-ur* NÍ-*šú* NU ZU *ina taq-ti-it* [LÁ-*š*] *ú iḫ-ta-niṭ-ṭa-áš-šú* AN.TA.ŠUB.BA ŠU ^{d}30[205] (DPS X A obv. 4–6//B obv. 4–6 = *TDP* 80:4–6)[206]

**If the patient continually turns his head to the right, his hands and his feet are stretched out, his eyes are opened wide toward the sky, spittle flows from his mouth, he makes rumbling noises, he does not know who he is at the beginning when ⌜his⌝ [confusional state] comes over him, AN.TA.ŠUB.BA (seizure), "hand" of Sîn.

The "not knowing who he is," which was supposed to precede the seizure in the quote above, presumably indicates that the patient was conscious but completely disoriented before he went into convulsions. This is reminiscent of the following references drawn from the "turns into" section of the diagnostic series subsection on neurology, which we discussed above with 19.71–19.72.

> **19.267** DIŠ ŠU ^{d}INNIN *ana* AN.TA.ŠUB.BA GUR-*šú* ŠU ^{d}30 : ŠU ^{d}15 *ana* KAR-*šú* . . . (DPS XXVIII:11 [AOAT 43.309])
>
> **If "hand" of Ištar turns into AN.TA.ŠUB.BA (seizure), "hand" of Sîn (var. "hand" of Ištar); to save him . . .
>
> **19.268** DIŠ ŠU ^{d}INNIN *ana* ^{d}LUGAL.ÙR.RA GUR-*šú* ŠU ^{d}UTU *ana* KAR-*šú* . . . (DPS XXVIII:14 [AOAT 43.309])
>
> **If "hand" of Ištar turns into ^{d}LUGAL.ÙR.RA, "hand" of Šamaš; to save him . . .

In this sequence, "hand" of Ištar appears to refer to extreme lethargy or drowsiness, indicating that the patient was prostrate before the seizures developed. In this case, the *āšipu* appears, as he did with the skin lesions of *Herpes simplex* type 2 (HSV2), to have taken advantage of the presence of other members of the family ("hand" of Ištar and "hand" of Šamaš) to account for minor variations.

^{d}LUGAL.ÙR.RA, which appears in the second quote above, generally refers to the patient allowing his eyes to droop.

> **19.269** ^{d}LUGAL.ÙR.RA : IGI^{II} 15-*šú u* 150-*šú i-kap-pi-iṣ* (*BRM* 4.32:2)
>
> **^{d}LUGAL.ÙR.RA (is when) he lets his left and his right eye droop.

In the specific context of 19.268, what is presumably meant by ^{d}LUGAL.ÙR.RA is the prominent appearance of neurologic symptoms relating to the eyes. The seizures of herpes encephalitis can take the form of generalized, focal motor, temporal lobe, or myoclonic phenomena. Involvement of larger or deeper portions of the cerebrum is, however, signaled by the appearance of hemiparesis, conjugate deviation of the eyes, or aphasia. If our guess is correct, the *āšipu* who compiled the neurological section of the diagnostic series noted the variation and adjusted his diagnoses accordingly, using "hand" of Šamaš for cases exhibiting aphasia, conjugate deviation of the eyes, or hemiparesis.

SÎN AND ŠAMAŠ We suggested above that occasionally survivable fevers accompanied by prostration, tremors, and nystagmus would have tended to be diagnosed as "hand" of Sîn. Some cases, however, appear to have been attributed instead to Sîn's son Šamaš or to both gods working in concert.

> **19.270** DIŠ SAG.KI^{II}-*šú* GEŠTU^{II}-*šú* KÚM *la ḫa-aḫ-ḫaš* [. . .] DU$_8$ DIB-*it* SAG.DU TUKU.TUKU-*ši lu* ŠU ^{d}30 *l*[*u*] ^{d}20/[ŠU] 30 *u* 20 (DPS IV A obv. 56–57//E ii 2//G obv. 9–10 = *TDP* 38:56–57//*SpTU* 3.88 ii 2//*LKU* 94:9–10)[207]
>
> **If his temples (and) his ears are lukewarm, [. . .] is uncongested (and) he continually has "affliction of the head," either "hand" of Sîn ⸢or⸣ Šamaš (var. ["hand"] of Sîn and Šamaš).

We presume that the intent of the *āšipu* was to distinguish forms of encephalitis or meningitis characterized by paralysis, conjugate deviation of the eyes, or aphasia. The association of "hand" of Šamaš with conjugate deviation of the eyes (^{d}LUGAL.ÙR.RA) has already been mentioned above. We also know that Šamaš was blamed in nonfebrile contexts for paralysis with aphasia (the postictal state; see Chapter 13 with 13.189–13.191), which would strengthen the possibility that fevers with similar signs and symptoms would have been attributed to Šamaš. The following references describe a sudden onset problem blamed on "hand" of Šamaš. The victim was left helpless and disoriented, with paralysis of the extremities, and the prognosis was grim, suggestive of some form of encephalitis or meningitis.

19.271 DIŠ KI.MIN-*ma* ŠU^{II}-*šú am-šá-ma* LAL NU ZU-*e u* UŠ$_4$-*šú* NU DIB ŠU 20 [GAM] (DPS XV:18 [AOAT 43.151]; cf. DPS XI A obv. 20//B 19 = *TDP* 90:20//*SpTU* 1.34:19)[208]

**If (it is the first day he is sick) and his hands are immobilized so that he is unable to stretch (them) out and he is not in full possession of his faculties, "hand" of Šamaš; [he will die].

Patients who have had *Herpes simplex* type 2 (HSV2) meningitis are often left with weakness of the lower extremities that can persist for many months. In view of the apparent association of Šamaš with HSV infections, it is possible that in the reference below the second sentence was meant to refer to postmeningitis weakness in the legs (causing the inguinal regions to appear to shift under the patient when he attempted to stand). Normally when this weakness appeared, the *āšipu* as is indicated in the first sentence below was well aware that it was likely to get progressively worse. If, however, it seemed instead to improve, then the "shifting" was due to the fever of the god Šamaš which the patient had experienced, and a full recovery could be expected.

19.272 [DIŠ *šá-p*] *u-la-šu* BAL.BAL-*ut* GIG-*su* MAN-*ni* / [DIŠ *šá*] *-pu-la-šu* BAL.BAL-*ut u* UŠ$_4$ LÍL-*šú* KÚR-*šú* ŠU ^{d}UTU DIN (DPS XIV A$_2$ i 12–13//C$_2$ i 3–4+C i 17–18 = *TDP* 132 i 63–64)

**[If] his ⌜inguinal regions⌝ shift constantly under him, his illness will change (for the worse). [If] his ⌜inguinal regions⌝ shift constantly under (him) but the nature of his disease alters, "hand" of Šamaš; he will get well.

GHOST In addition to "hand" of Sîn and "hand" of Šamaš, the *āšipu* recognized a further category of fevers with neurologic symptoms which included "roaring in the ears." As with other examples of distorted sensory perception, this category was attributed to a ghost.

A sequence of references in the diagnostic series describes what appears to be a neurologic illness that includes roaring in the ears plus fever. Curiously, as seems to have been the case with other fevers with neurologic symptoms, the fever itself is mentioned last, almost as an afterthought.

19.273 DIŠ DIB-*su ina* AN.USAN DIB.DIB-*su* DIB GIDIM$_7$ / DIŠ DIB-*su ina* AN.USAN DIB.DIB-*su* SAG.ŠÀ-*šú* MÚ.MEŠ-*aḫ* GÌR^{II}-*šú* ÍL-*a* DIB GIDIM$_7$ / DIŠ DIB-*su ina* AN.USAN DIB.DIB-*su* ŠÀ.MEŠ-*šú* MÚ.MEŠ-*ḫu* EN EN.NUN.MURUB$_4$.BA *id-lip* DIB GIDIM$_7$ / DIŠ DIB-*su ina* AN.USAN DIB.DIB-*su* IGI^{II}-*šú ur-ru-pa* GEŠTU^{II}-*šú* GÙ.DÉ.MEŠ DIB GIDIM$_7$ / DIŠ DIB-*su ina* AN.USAN DIB.DIB-*su* GEŠTU^{II}-*šú* GÙ.DÉ.MEŠ DIB GIDIM$_7$ / DIŠ DIB-*su ina* AN.USAN DIB.DIB-*su* GEŠTU^{II}-*šú i-šam-ma-*

ma-šú DIB GIDIM$_7$ / DIŠ DIB-*su ina* AN.USAN DIB.DIB-*su* SAG.KI-*šú* KÚ-*šú* DIB GID[IM$_7$] / DIŠ KI.MIN U$_4$ DIB-*šú* KÚM TA EN.NUN.AN.USAN EN EN.NUN. MURUB$_4$.BA *id-da-lip-šú* DIB GID[IM$_7$] (DPS XXVI:31′–38′ [AOAT 43.281])

**If his affliction always afflicts him in the evening, . . .[209] his upper abdomen (epigastrium) is continually bloated, his feet are raised up,[210] . . . his eyes are heavily clouded, his ears roar, . . . his ears go numb . . . his temples continually hurt him, . . . (and) when it afflicts him, fever keeps him awake from the evening watch until the middle watch of the night, affliction by a ⌜ghost⌝.[211]

It may be the ghost's role in producing this neurologic fever that inspired the attribution to ghosts of the following trauma references.

19.274 DIŠ *ina* GÚ-*šú* SÌG-*ma* ŠÀ.MEŠ-*šú it-te-nen-bi-ṭu u* GÌR^{II}-*šú na-ša-a* DIB GIDIM / DIŠ *ina* GÚ-*šú* SÌG-*iṣ-ma* GÌR^{II}-*šú i-ra-ʾ-ú-ba* ŠÀ.MEŠ-*šú it-te-nen-bi-ṭu* DIB GIDIM$_7$ (DPS X A obv. 19–20//B obv. 21–22 = *TDP* 82:19–20)

**If he was wounded on his neck and, as a consequence, his insides are continually cramped and his feet are raised up, affliction by a ghost. If he was wounded on his neck and, as a consequence, his feet tremble (and) his insides are continually cramped, affliction by a ghost.

In a pair of examples, one drawn from the diagnostic series[212] and the other from a therapeutic text with treatment quoted below, ghosts seem to have caused a combination of fever and very closely spaced seizures. The attribution of these references to the ghost is probably due to his association with status epilepticus (see Chapter 13 with 13.209).

19.275 DIŠ NA GIDIM DIB-*su-ma i-mi-im i-ka-aṣ-ṣa* [*ma-d*] *a-a-at ḫa-a-a-at-ta-šú qer-bet* U$_4$ *u* GI$_6$ *la i-na-a-aḫ* GÙ-*šú* GIN$_7$ GÙ ANŠE/ÙZ *it-ta-*ŠUB-*di* ŠU GIDIM *a-ḫi-i ina ḫar-ba-ti* DIB-*su ana* TI-*šú* . . . GIDIM *šá* DI[B-*šú* TAR-*as*] (*BAM* 471 ii 26′–28′, 31′//*BAM* 385 i 23′–26′//*BAM* 323:65–67)

**If a ghost afflicts a person and, as a result, he gets hot and then cold, his confusional states are ⌜numerous⌝? and close together, he gets no rest day or night (and he continually emits) his cry like the cry of a donkey/goat, ("hand" of) a strange ghost has seized him in the wasteland, to cure him . . . The ghost that ⌜afflicts⌝ [him will be kept away].[213]

In short, fevers that prominently featured roaring in the ears or closely spaced seizures were assigned by the *āšipu*, for that reason, to "hand" of ghost. In addition, a number of scattered references mention roaring in the ears alongside other neurologic symptoms. Two of the references attributed to ghosts have many of the features of encephalomyelitis or meningoencephalitis, including headache, ringing ears (tinnitus), muscle weakness, low back pain, and light-sensitive eyes (photophobia). For more details, see Chapters 9 with 9.15 and 13 with 13.214–13.215. Photophobia is a symptom of migraine, which ghosts also caused.

Other ghost references combine roaring or ringing in the ears with pulsating headache, dizziness, and tenseness or stinging pains in the limbs.

19.276 DIŠ NA SAG.DU-*su* GÍR.GÍR-*su* SAG.DU-*su i-šag-gum* GEŠTU^{II}-*šú* GÙ.GÙ-*a* ŠU.SI.MEŠ-*šú ú-zaq-qa-ta-šú* NA BI DIB-*it* GIDIM/GIDIM DIB-*su*/ŠU.GIDIM.MA *ana* TI-*šú* . . . (*BAM* 9:51–52//*AMT* 14/5:1//*BAM* 481 obv. 13′–15′//*BAM* 493 i 2′–3′)[214]

**"If a person's head continually stings him, his head (seems to) roar, his ears ring, (and) his finger(s) sting him, that person (is afflicted with) affliction by a ghost (var. a ghost afflicts him/"hand" of ghost), to cure him . . .

The "shaking" temples in the second reference below probably refers to the patient's perception of a bounding pulse.

19.277 [DIŠ N]A SAG.KI-*šú šá* ZAG *u* GÙB *ki-ma* DIB-*bat* GIDIM ZI-*ma uz-na-šú i-ša-sa-ma* [IGI^{II}-*šú*] ÍR DIRI-*a*. . . (*AMT* 14/5:6–7)

**[If a] ⌜person's⌝ left or right temple seems to pulsate as in affliction by a ghost, his ears ring and [his eyes] are full of tears . . .

19.278 DIŠ IGI.MEŠ-*šú* NIGIN.MEŠ GEŠTU^{II}-*šú* GÙ.DÉ.MEŠ UB.NÍGIN.NA-*šú* DUB.DUB-*ka* ŠU GIDIM$_7$ / DIŠ IGI.MEŠ-*šú* NIGIN.MEŠ GEŠTU^{II}-*šú i-šag-gu-ma* SAG.KI^{II}-*šú ú-maḫ-ḫa-ṣa-šú u i-rad-da-šú* ŠU GIDIM$_7$ (DPS IX A 60–61//B r. 4–5 = *TDP* 76:60–61)

**If his face seems continually to spin, his ears roar, (and) his limbs get tense, "hand" of ghost. If his face seems continually to spin, his ears roar, (and) his temples give him jabbing pains and seem to shake, "hand" of ghost.

It is probable that fatal neurologic fevers displaying other characteristic signs and symptoms of ghost affliction would also have been attributed to "hand" of ghost. These signs and symptoms should have included some combination of severe headache, neckache, and partial paralysis of the third, fourth, fifth, sixth, seventh, or eighth cranial nerve as described in the following references.

19.279 [DIŠ . . .]⌜II⌝-*šú* ŠED$_7$-*ma* IGI^{II}-*šú it-te-né-ep-rek-ka-a* [. . . GIDIM *mu-ša*] *m-šu-u* DIB-*su* (DPS XVIII:17–18 [AOAT 43.218–219])

**[If] his [. . .] are cold and his eyes are continually crossed [. . . a ghost who wanders about at] ⌜night⌝[215] afflicts him.

19.280 ŠU.GIDIM.MA GEŠTU^{II}.MEŠ-*šú* GÙ.DÉ.MEŠ *ma-gal iṭ-ṭe-né-pi šin-na-šú ana ma-ka-le-e la ú-qàr-ra-ba-ma* (BRM 4.32:3–4 [Campbell Thompson, *JRAS* 1924.452])

**"Hand" of ghost (is when) his ears roar, (his face) continually smooths out,[216] (and) he cannot get his teeth close enough together to be able to eat.

The obvious semantic association between the roving of uncared-for ghosts and patients' wandering minds seems also to have invited the attribution to ghosts[217] of mental status changes, as is described in the following references.

19.281 [DIŠ U]Š$_4$-*šu šá-ni-šu-ma* UŠ$_4$-*šú* NU DIB ŠU GIDIM *mur-tap-pi-du* GAM . . . [DIŠ UŠ$_4$]-*šú* MAN.MAN-*šu u* EME-*šú ir-ta-nap-pu-ud* GAM (DPS XXII:47a, 48 [AOAT 43.255])

**[If] his ⌜mentation⌝ is altered so that he is not in full possession of his faculties, "hand" of a roving ghost; he will die . . . [If] his [mentation] is continually altered and his tongue roves about, he will die.

19.282 DIŠ UŠ$_4$-[*šu* KÚR-*ir* IN]IM.MEŠ-*šú it-te-né-ep-rek-ka-a* GIDIM *mu-šam-šu-ú* DIB-*su* [:] KI.SIKIL.LÍL.LÁ *šum*$_4$*-ma* LÚ.LÍL.LÁ (DPS XXII:51–52 [AOAT 43.255)[218]

**If [his] mentation [is altered] (and) his ⌜words⌝ hinder each other in his mouth, a ghost who wanders about at night afflicts him . . .

Some of the syndromes potentially included under this rubric of fevers with neurologic signs and symptoms featuring some combination of severe headache, neckache, dizziness, mental status changes, seizures, altered sensory perception involving the eighth cranial nerve, partial paralysis of facial cranial nerves, and tenseness or stinging pains in the limbs are forms of meningitis or encephalitis or brain abscess. A further connection between such problems and the ghost as causal agent may be the fact that ghosts were otherwise closely associated with ear infections and mastoiditis. For more details, see Chapter 9. Partial paralysis of the third, fourth, and sixth nerves as well as other cranial nerves are particularly frequent with pneumococcal meningitis, and acute otitis media and mastoiditis are underlying causes in about one-fourth of patients. Pneumococcal meningitis is also more common in patients suffering from alcoholism, another syndrome attributed to ghosts (see 19.297). These overlaps could easily have suggested a ghost to the *āšipu* as a cause of this and other neurologic fevers with similar signs and symptoms.

IŠTAR The final member of the Sîn family, the goddess Ištar, also produced neurologic symptoms. Although none of the references with neurologic symptoms clearly mentions fever,[219] the skin lesions described (see below) are strongly suggestive of an infectious process.

Primarily, Ištar caused prostration (see 19.64). The "letting drop" in these references presumably means that the *āšipu* has lifted the patient's head or hand above the bed and then let go to test whether the patient is able to hold it up unaided.

19.283 DIŠ ZÚ.[ME]Š-*šú* ZÚ.GUZ SAG.DU-*su* ŠUB.ŠU[B-*di*] ŠU ^{d}15 (DPS VI A r. 13//B$_1$ r. 10+B$_2$ r. 14 = *TDP* 60 r. 44′)

**If he gnashes his teeth (and) ⌜continually⌝ lets his head drop, "hand" of Ištar.

19.284 DIŠ ZÚ.⌜MEŠ⌝-*šú* ZÚ.GUZ ŠU-*su* ŠUB.Š[UB-*d*] *i* ŠU ^{d}15 (DPS VI A r. 14//B$_1$ r. 11+B$_2$ r. 15 = *TDP* 60 r. 45′; cf. StBoT 36.35 obv. 14′//StBoT 36.57 r. 3′–4′)

**If he gnashes his teeth (and) ⌜continually⌝ lets his hand drop, "hand" of Ištar.

19.285 DIŠ ZÚ.[MEŠ]-*šú* ZÚ.GUZ *u* G[ÌR]-*su* ŠUB.ŠUB-*di* GA[M KI.MIN] ŠU ^{d}15 MU TAG-*te* (DPS VI A r. 15//B$_1$ r. 12+B$_2$ r. 16 = *TDP* 60 r. 46′)

**If he gnashes his teeth (and) continually lets his ⌜foot⌝ drop, he will die. [Alternatively], "hand" of Ištar on account of touching the cheek.[220]

In addition, Ištar could be responsible for seizures ("shuddering"), severe pain ("gnashing of teeth"), and hearing loss, as is described in the following references.

19.286 DIŠ ⌜ZÚ⌝.[MEŠ-*šú*] *ig-ta-na*[*-aṣ*]*-ṣa-aṣ* IGI.[MEŠ-*šú*] ŠED$_7$.MEŠ GIG.[BI DIB.D]IB-*su* ŠU ^{d}15 BI GAR-*šú* (DPS VI A r. 16//B$_1$ r. 13+B$_2$ r. 17 = *TDP* 60 r. 47′)

**If he continually ⌜gnashes⌝ [his] teeth, his face is continually cold, (and) [his] illness [continually] afflicts him, the "hand" of Ištar has been laid on him.

19.287 DIŠ GEŠTU^{II}-*šú i-šag-gu-mu u* UGU-*šú i-šam-ma-am-ma-šu* ŠU ^{d}15 (DPS VIII 13 = *TDP* 70:13)

**If his ears roar and his skull goes numb, "hand" of Ištar.

19.288 DIŠ ZI.ḪA.ZA SAG.ÚS DIB.DIB-*su u* MUD-*ud* ŠU ^{d}15 [GAM] (DPS X A obv. 37 = *TDP* 84:37)

**If persistent "grabbing" of the throat continually afflicts him and he continually shudders, "hand" of Ištar; [he will die].

It may be this association of Ištar with severe prostration, pain, hearing loss, and seizures that led to the attribution to her of some of the trauma references (see 19.150–19.164). As to what could have differentiated Ištar's neurologic fevers from what would appear to be very similar neurologic fevers blamed on ghosts by the *āšipu*, the most obvious difference is that ghosts are never attested in connection with skin lesions of any kind, whereas a by-form of the goddess (the scorpion-shaped Išḫara) could cause lesions on the upper abdomen and subcutaneous bleeding (ecchymosis) on the fingers ("uneven yellow color"; see Chapter 6 with 6.123), as is described in the following quotes.

19.289 DIŠ U.MEŠ-*šú* SIG$_7$ ŠUB-*a* ŠU ^{d}*Iš-ḫa-ra* NU DIN (DPS XI A r. 48a = *TDP* 98 r. 48a)

**If his fingers are unevenly colored with yellow, "hand" of Išḫara; he will not get well.

19.290 [. . .] *ina* SAG ŠÀ-*šú* È ⌜IGI⌝.[ME]Š-*šú* KÚR.KÚR-*ru* ŠU ^{d}*Iš-ḫ*[*a-ra*] (DPS XXXIII:83 [AOAT 43.357])[221]

**[If . . .] erupt on his upper abdomen (epigastrium) (and) his face continually changes (for the worse), "hand" of ⌜Išḫara⌝.

Meningococcal meningitis is more likely than other forms of meningitis to produce a petechial or purpuric skin eruption (such a rash accompanies approximately half of the cases). If this illness had been seen by the *āšipu*, he would have had good reason to blame it on this man-hungry goddess of war. This organism usually causes an overwhelming infection, prostration, shock, and usually death. This disease pattern is consistent with the signs and symptoms associated with Ištar. Meningococcal meningitis also has a military connection. It tends to occur more commonly during war when soldiers are crowded together, permitting ready transmission of the bacteria. The nonvisual aspects of Strachan's syndrome (see Chapter 7 with 7.17–7.18), which also occurs more commonly in wartime, were attributed to Ištar of Arbela, presumably for this same reason. Naturally, other forms of meningitis or encephalitis with similar signs and symptoms would have been included under the diagnosis of "hand" of Ištar.

MISCELLANEOUS FEVERS WITH NEUROLOGIC SYMPTOMS

A remaining category of fevers that were sufficiently similar to one another to be almost indistinguishable was classed by the *āšipu* under the rubric of "hand" of (personal/city) god. Included in this category of nonspecific fevers were also forms of encephalitis or meningitis that were sufficiently nondescript as to prevent their attribution to any of the Sîn family of neurological fevers. For details on fevers without associated neurologic symptoms, see 19.360–19.363.

19.291 DIŠ *i-leb-bu* KÚM U_5-*šú* : DIŠ GÙ.GÙ-*si* ŠU MU DINGIR-*šú* GAM (DPS XXII:58 [AOAT 43.256])

**If he groans (and) fever rides him (var. If he continually cries out), "hand" of an oath (sworn by) his god; he will die.

19.292 DIŠ SAG.KI *ḫe-si-ma* GEŠTU.MEŠ-*šú* NU ŠE.GA-*a* ŠU DINGIR-*šú* UGU-*šú um-mu-da* GAM (DPS IV B obv. 4 = *TDP* 32:4)[222]

**If he has a viselike headache[223] and his ears do not hear, the "hand" of his god has been imposed on him; he will die.

19.293 DIŠ *gir-ra-a-šú ma-aq-ta* GÌR^{II}-*šú na-šá-a ú-šam-šá* ŠU DINGIR URU-*šú*/DINGIR-*šú ana* ÚŠ GAR-*šú* (DPS X A obv. 53/D 13 = *TDP* 86:53)[224]

**If both sides of his throat (look) terrible, his feet are raised up,[225] (and) it keeps him awake all night, the "hand" of the god of his city (var. A: "hand" of his god) has been placed on him for death.

19.294 DIŠ KI.MIN-*ma i-*[*na* KI.NÁ-*šú* G]Ù.GÙ-*si u de-ki-šu la ip-pal* ŠU DINGIR-*šú* GAM (DPS XV:89 [AOAT 43.155])[226]

**If (it is the first day he is sick) and he continually cries out ⌜in⌝ [his sleep] and does not answer the one trying to wake him, "hand" of his god; he will die.

Gods/Goddesses of Wet and Dry

As we saw in Chapter 3 with 3.165–3.168, the *āšipu* seems to have made a distinction not made by modern physicians, between forms of enteric fever with dehydration (*ṣētu*) and forms without (*di'u*). The wet/dry distinction was also invoked to distinguish between two major classes of plant toxins with opposing effects on the parasympathetic nervous system, belladonna drugs (atropine and scopolamine) and muscarinic drugs. Belladonna drugs cause cutaneous (skin) flushing and decreased sweating, dry nose and mouth causing difficulty swallowing, rapid heart rate with intermittent slowing, decreased intestinal and bladder contraction, and fever. Muscarinic drugs cause increased salivation and lacrimation (tearing), headache, visual disturbance, nausea and vomiting, diarrhea, abdominal colic, bronchospasm, slow heart rate, low blood pressure, and shock. Belladonna drug poisoning was blamed by the *āšipu* on the combined action of Marduk and ghosts and muscarinic mushroom poisoning on sorcery (*kišpu*). For more details, see Chapter 15 with 15.1–15.5.

This association of *kišpu* with wetness (increased salivation) and of ghosts with dryness (dry nose and mouth) is a consistent pattern that seems to have suggested the attribution of many of the syndromes associated with these two causal agents.

GHOST

As denizens of the waterless steppe, it is not terribly surprising to see ghosts being blamed for dehydration, and particularly the ghosts of those who had died of thirst or who, in their desperation for water, had drowned while trying to drink directly from the river. The provision of water by libation was an important component of funerary offerings provided by ancient Mesopotamian families for the ancestral dead.

19.295 [DIŠ NA Š]À(!).MEŠ-*šú it-te-⸢nem⸣-mi-ru liq* KA-*šú i-ta-nab-b*[*al*] [Á^{II}.MEŠ]-*šú šim-ma-tú* TUKU.MEŠ-*a i-ge-eš-šú az-zu-za-a bi-bil* ŠÀ TUKU.MEŠ [IGI.DU]$_8$-*ma* UGU-*šú* NU DÙG.GA MUNUS ŠÀ-*šú ḫa-šiḫ-ma* MUNUS IGI.DU$_8$-*ma* ŠÀ-*šú* NU ÍL-*šú* [ŠÀ-*šú a*]-*na da-ba-bi ša-pil* NA BI ŠU.GIDIM.MA ÚS-*šú ana* TI-*šú* . . . (*AMT* 76/1:4–7)[227]

**[If a person's] ⸢insides⸣ are continually colicky, his palate continually ⸢dries up⸣, his [arms] are continually numb, he belches, he has plenty of appetite (for food), but when [he sees it], it does not please him; he wants a woman, but when he sees a woman, he cannot get an erection;[228] [his heart] is (too) depressed (for him) to speak—"hand" of ghost is pursuing that person; to cure him . . .

Cholera, which causes rapid dehydration creating a shrunken body with a skeletal look, would have been a particularly strong candidate for a problem caused by a ghost. We believe the following ghost reference is describing cholera. For more details, see Chapter 3 with 3.101–3.112.

19.296 [D]IŠ U$_4$ LÁ-*šú* UB.NÍGIN.NA-*šú i-šaḫ-ḫu-ḫa* ŠÀ-*šú* DIB.DIB-*su* ŠÀ.MEŠ-*šú* SI.SÁ.MEŠ-*šú* ŠU GIDIM$_7$ / DIŠ U[$_4$] LÁ-*šú* UB.NÍGIN.NA-*šú i-šam-ma-ma-šú* IGI.MEŠ-*šú* NIGIN.MEŠ-*du* ŠÀ-*šú i-šaḫ-ḫu-uḫ u mim-ma šá ana* KA-*šú* GAR-*ár ina* U$_4$-*me-šú ma-ti-ma ina* DÚR-*šú* ŠUB-*šú* ŠU GIDIM$_7$ *šá ina šag-gaš-ti* GAM (DPS XXVI:19′–21′ [AOAT 43.279–280])[229]

**⸢If⸣ when (a confusional state) comes over him, his limbs waste away (and) his abdomen continually afflicts him (and) his bowels are continually loose, "hand" of ghost. If when (a confusional state) comes over him, his limbs go numb, his face seems continually to spin, his abdomen wastes away and whatever he puts to his mouth is always excreted from his anus on the very same day, "hand" of a ghost who died through murder.

Ghosts were also held responsible for a complex of gastrointestinal complaints that included bloating, abdominal or upper abdominal pain, and vomiting, leading, presumably, to dehydration.

19.297 DIŠ SAG ŠÀ-*šú e-bi-iṭ ša-šal-la-šú* KÚ.MEŠ-*šú* ŠU GIDIM$_7$ (DPS XIII B i 12′ = *TDP* 112 i 16′)[230]

**If his upper abdomen (epigastrium) is cramped (and) his back continually hurts him, "hand" of ghost.

19.298 DIŠ SAG ŠÀ-*šú* MÚ.MEŠ DIB GIDIM$_7$ (DPS XIII B i 14′ = *TDP* 112 i 18′; cf. StBoT 36.41 r. 8′–9′)[231]

**If his upper abdomen (epigastrium) is continually bloated, affliction by a ghost.

19.299 [DIŠ NA GIDIM] DIB-*su-ma i-ḫa-rù* NINDA.MEŠ *u* KAŠ.MEŠ [LAL?] *ana* TI-*šú* ... (*BAM* 221 ii 2′–3′//*AMT* 81/7:5)[232]

**[If a ghost] afflicts [a person] so that he vomits (and) [he loses his appetite(?)] for bread and beer, to cure him . . .

Interestingly, the medicines used to treat the first quote below (and similar references) are in every instance identical with those used in potions for hallucinations (seeing ghosts). In view of this fact, as well as the severe headache that is mentioned in many of the examples, some of these references to gastrointestinal complaints may be due to alcoholic ketoacidosis, which is frequently associated with severe vomiting, dehydration, abdominal pain, and, in 75 percent of cases, with pancreatitis (also a cause of severe abdominal pain). The hallucinations of delirium tremens (DTs) were likely to have occurred in many patients with alcoholic ketoacidosis.

19.300 [DIŠ NA GIDIM D]IB-*su-ma* ŠÀ-*šú* KÚ.MEŠ-*šú* . . . (*BAM* 165 i 16′)[233]

** [If a ghost] ⸢afflicts⸣ [a person] and as a result his insides continually hurt him . . .

19.301 DIŠ NA SAG.KI.DIB.BA-*ma* ŠÀ ŠÀ-*bi* GÙ.GÙ-*si* ŠU.GIDIM.MA *šá-ne-e* ^{d}*Iš-tar* ÚŠ (*BAM* 482 iv 47′//*AMT* 19/1 iv! 30′)[234]

**If a person has a headache and he keeps crying out: "My insides, my insides," "hand" of ghost, deputy of Ištar; he will die.

19.302 DIŠ SAG.KI-*šú* DIB-*su-ma* KI.MIN *ma-gal* i_{16}-*à-ru u* KI.NÁ NU ÍL ŠU GIDIM$_7$ GAM (DPS IV B obv. 11 = *TDP* 32:11)[235]

**If his temple afflicts him and (he keeps crying out: "my insides, my insides"), he vomits a lot and cannot stand the bed, "hand" of ghost; he will die.

Although other conditions could be responsible for the signs and symptoms described, it is interesting to note that respiratory distress, a common complication of ketoacidosis, was also blamed on thirsty ghosts, as in the reference quoted below.

19.303 DIŠ NA *ina* DIB-*it* ŠU.GIDIM.MA IGI.MEŠ NIGIN-*du ù* ZI.MEŠ-⸢*šú ik-ta-nar-ru*⸣ ZI.MEŠ-*šú* GIN$_7$ *šá* A.MEŠ *ṣa-mu-ú i-ta-na-šá-áš* GIDIM *mur*!-*tap-pi*!-*du ina* EDIN DIB-*su ana* ZI-*šú* . . . (*BAM* 216:55′–57′//Scheil, *RA* 14.88 ii 6′–9′//Labat, *RSO* 32.112 v 1′–3′)[236]

**If, as a result of affliction by "hand" of ghost, a person('s) face seems to spin and he is also continually short of breath (and) his breaths come in spasms as if he were thirsting for water, a roving (!) ghost has seized him in the steppe; to remove it . . .

It may be that the dehydrating aspects of ethanol poisoning suggested affliction by a ghost as the cause of many of the effects of alcoholic binge drinking. The presence of severe headache, abdominal pain, and hallucinations, all of which were independently attributed to ghosts, would have helped confirm the correctness of the *āšipu*'s analysis. Other aspects of alcoholism that appear to have been blamed on ghosts include delirium tremens, seizures on withdrawal, polyneuropathy, and cirrhosis with secondary bleeding esophageal varices. For more details, see Chapter 15 with 15.16–15.25.

KIŠPU

As we saw above, *kišpu* ("sorcery") was blamed for muscarinic mushroom poisoning. This was part of a more general pattern of assigning to "sorcery" syndromes in which hypersalivation or the production of phlegm was prominently involved.

> **19.304** DIŠ NA *ina* DUG$_4$.DUG$_4$-*šú el-la-tú-šú* DU-*ka* ÚḪ-*su ina* IGI *a-wi-lim i-šal-lu* DUG$_4$.MEŠ-*šú im-ta-na*[-*áš*]-*šú* KA-*šú iḫ-ta-na-aṭ-ṭaš-šu zi-qí* KA-*šú te-bu-u* NA BI *nu-ul-la-a-ti šu-kul*... (*BAM* 161 ii 16′–21′//*BAM* 436 vi 12′–15′//*BAM* 282:2′)
>
> **If, when a person speaks, his saliva flows,[237] he sprays his spit on (the other) person, he continually ⸢forgets⸣ his words, he continually stutters and burps, that person has been fed deceitful things...
>
> **19.305** [DIŠ NA] GÌR^{II}-*šú i-ra-ʾu-ba* KA-*šú ru-pu-uš-tú* [DIRI UŠ$_{11}$ KÚ] NAG ŠÉŠ ALAM ZI.K[U$_5$.RU.DA *ep-šu-šu* UŠ$_{11}$] *pa-ṭa-ri-im*-⸢*ma* ZI⸣.[KU$_5$.RU.DA BÚR.RU.DA.KÁM]... (*BAM* 452:10′–12′)
>
> **[If a person]'s feet tremble (and) his mouth [is full of] phlegm, [there was *kišpu* in something he ate], drank, or rubbed on; a figurine of ⸢ZI.KU$_5$.RU.DA⸣ [was made of him]; to loosen [the *kišpu*] and [dissolve] the ⸢ZI.KU$_5$.RU.DA⸣...

This attribution was probably due to the fact that one very common way of hexing somebody was to make use of the sorcerer's infected spittle or phlegm as a contaminating agent. Apart from the poisoning and mystery references, there is another group of *kišpu* references that include complaints of chest pain, fever, phlegm, and "sick lungs." These texts are compatible with pneumonia, and are discussed in Chapter 3 with 3.82–3.85. What links the pneumonia caused by *kišpu* to cases of poisoning and/or hypersalivation is the production of phlegm by the patient, which is taken as a sign that he or she, like the victim of poisoning, has been brought into contact with sorcerous phlegm.

A further category of *kišpu* references list vaguely described gastrointestinal complaints involving mucus coming from the gastrointestinal tract. For more details, see Chapter 15 with 15.6–15.8. In addition to the excess production of saliva or phlegm, the victim of sorcery might be expected to display what appeared to the physician to be an uncontrollable flow of another phlegmlike substance, namely, semen.[238] The *āšipu*'s explanation for the appearance of urethritis combined with arthritis and skin lesions (what we call reactive arthritis) was, as might be expected, also a form of sorcery, specifically the laying of a person's semen with a corpse. For details, see Chapter 11 with 11.54–11.56.

Specially Named Syndromes

A surprisingly high percentage of the illnesses recognized by the *āšipu* were not believed by him to have either a divine or demonic cause. It is unclear why no demon or deity came forth to claim these diseases but, in some of these cases, associations were made instead with anatomic areas. Examples of this method of describing illnesses include IGI.GIG ("sick eye"; see Chapter 9), ḪAR.MEŠ.GIG ("sick lungs"; see Chapter 3), TÙN.GIG ("sick liver"; see Chapter 6), ZÉ.GIG ("sick gall bladder"; see Chapter 6), and ZÚ.GIG ("sick tooth"; see Chapter 18). Perhaps the most interesting example of this type of diagnosis is DÚR.GIG, "sick peroneal (pelvic) area." Ancient physicians tended to use this diagnosis for patients with diseases where urethral or rectal excretion was impeded, and where these problems tended to be relatively chronic and afebrile. For more details, see Chapter 6 with 6.176–6.187.

In other cases, the *āšipu* did not attribute diseases to either ghosts, gods/goddesses or demons, or regions of the body. Instead, names were used that related to some characteristic of the disease. Clear examples of this process are *buʾšānu, muruṣ kabbarti,* and "touched in the steppe."

BUʾŠĀNU

Ancient physicians distinguished three types of *buʾšānu* (BI.LU in Sumerian), a category of mouth and throat problems. We believe that these three types of *buʾšānu* refer to at least three separate diseases: diphtheria, oral infection with *Herpes simplex* virus type 1 (HSV1), and anaerobic infection of the gingiva and throat (Vincent's angina, or trench mouth). In addition, cases of the viral infection, infectious mononucleosis, which can mimic diphtheria, and scurvy (see Chapter 7)[239] may also have been included in this category. What all have in common is that the patient exhibits a noticeably foul odor (*buʾšānu* literally means "stinking") and have lesions or exudates that are grayish in contradistinction to the bright red ("skinned") appearance of streptococcal throat infections. For more details, see Chapter 3 with 3.61–3.70.

MURUṢ KABBARTI

Muruṣ kabbarti, lit. "sickness of thickening," appears to be the same condition that modern physicians call mycetoma or Madura foot. This is a chronic fungal or actinomyotic infection that primarily involves the feet of people living in tropical or subtropical regions who work in the soil without shoes, conditions that must have existed in ancient Mesopotamia. As the disease progresses, the foot and ankle become swollen, the skin becomes thickened, the joint loses mobility, muscles are damaged, and multiple sinus tracts drain pus containing granules that are small colonies of the organisms that are causing the infection. For more on this condition, see Chapter 3 with 3.241–3.253.

"TOUCHED IN THE STEPPE"

We have found in the ancient Mesopotamian medical literature sixteen references that include the phrase "touched in the steppe." Twelve of these describe changes in the hair of the patient's head. These references also indicate that the hair changes were associated with a very poor prognosis (worrisome) or a fatal outcome. Another quote that suggests a fatal outcome does not mention hair changes but describes changes in the patient's face that clearly indicate a wasted or cadaveric appearance. These findings are all highly compatible with protein malnutrition, or kwashiorkor. In addition, there are three "touched in the steppe" quotes that do not seem to fit this diagnosis, but which may refer to cases of diabetes, since untreated diabetes commonly causes severe wasting that can mimic protein malnutrition. For more details, see Chapter 7 with 7.1–7.10.

Buʾšānu, *muruṣ kabbarti*, and "touched in the steppe" are some of the more striking examples of ancient specially named syndromes. For others, see especially Chapter 10 (ancient Mesopotamian terms for skin lesions) but also note *aganutillû* (Chapter 8), A.GA.ZI/*tugānu* (Chapter 6), *amurriqānu* (Chapter 6), AN.TA.ŠUB.BA (Chapter 13), *ašû* (Chapter 3), *bennu* (Chapter 3), *diʾu* (Chapter 3), *ḫarasu* (Chapter 3), *maškādu* (Chapter 11), *meḫru* (Chapter 3), *mišittu* (Chapter 13), *muruṣ nâki* ("sickness of sexual intercourse"; see Chapter 4), *muruṣ râmi* ("love-sickness"; see Chapter 16), *mūṣu* (Chapter 4), *naḫšātu* (Chapter 12), *pašittu* (Chapter 6), *sagallu* (Chapter 11), *saḫaršubbû* (Chapter 3), *samānu* (Chapter 3), *sinlurma* (Chapter 9), *ṣētu* (Chapter 3), *šadānu* (Chapter 3), *šaššaṭu* (Chapter 3), and *šibiṭ šāri* ("wind blasting"; see Chapter 4).

Named Syndromes That Evolved into Demons

The most obvious example of names evolving into demons is the term *aḫḫāzu*, for which see above under GODS/GODDESSES OF FEVER. Another possible example, also discussed there, is the demoness Lamaštu. She is known to us as a "baby-snatching demon," a rejected daughter of the sky-god Anu, who literally hurled her from heaven. She was also a frustrated mother who killed human children in her attempts to suckle them with her poisonous milk. It has been suggested[240] that this colorful and apparently folkloric personality was actually derived from the symptoms that she produced in her victims, namely, "fever," for which the Akkadian word *ummu* resembles the Akkadian word for "mother" (also *ummu*) and "bile" for which the Akkadian word *martu* resembles the Akkadian word for daughter (*mārtu*). Lamaštu, therefore, may originally have been the name of a fever with jaundice which, due to a fearsome reputation as a baby-killer, was eventually transformed into a demon.

A third candidate for a demon that evolved from an original medical syndrome is *alû*, a demon whose name is written with the Sumerogram: A.LÁ. Since the verb LÁ is frequently used in medical texts to describe a confusional state "coming over" a patient, it is not surprising that A.LÁ (lit. "that which comes over (you)")[241] caused stage I coma, as described in the following reference.

19.306 DIŠ GIN$_7$ Ù.SÁ DIB.DIB-*su* U$_4$ DIB-*šú* GEŠTU^{II}-*šú* GÙ.DÉ.MEŠ KA-*šú* DIB-*ma* NU DUG$_4$.DUG$_4$-⌈*ub*⌉ ŠU A.LÁ ḪUL (DPS XXVII:23 [AOAT 43.298–299])

**If something like a stupor continually afflicts him and, when it afflicts him, his ears roar (and) his mouth is "seized" so that he cannot talk, "hand" of an evil *alû*.

Mišittu (strokes) seem also to have been in the process of demonization, as is reflected in occasional references to "hand" of *mišittu*.[242] For more details, see Chapter 13. A final example of observed symptoms generating a custom-designed demonic cause is the "tooth worm," discussed in Chapter 18 with 18.11–18.16.

Clearly Organized Syndromes Attributed to Divine or Demonic "Hands"

Ancient Mesopotamian curses are a good example of a set of syndromes where the organizing principle that inspired grouping the attested references under one diagnosis is relatively clear.

CURSE

Thirty-eight reasonably well-preserved medical texts contain the diagnosis "curse" or "hand" of curse. The strongest impression conveyed by our review of these texts is that the conditions described tended to be chronic processes.[243] When the signs and symptoms suggested to us a diagnosis, the diseases were inherently chronic: leprosy (3.214), mycetoma (3.252), and nontropical sprue (7.21).

Signs and symptoms that are by their nature chronic, such as wasting, were often listed in references containing a "curse" attribution, as in the following reference.

19.307 [DIŠ SA.MEŠ ŠÀ].MEŠ-*šú šá* 15 *u* 150 *ana pi-rik* ŠÀ-*šú šu-ud-*[*du-du*] NAM.ERÍM DIB-[*su*] (DPS XIII J14–15 = *TDP* 126 iii 46)

**[If the muscles] of his [abdomen], those of the left and right sides, are ⌜drawn taut⌝ across his abdomen,[244] a curse afflicts [him].

The affected regions of the body and organ systems primarily included the chest and lungs, the abdomen and gastrointestinal tract, and the joints. The nervous system, both central and peripheral, and the urinary tract were largely unrepresented in the references (only three examples). There were twelve texts that mentioned fever, and there were other signs typically associated with infections such as cough and sputum production.

19.308 DIŠ NA NAM.ÉRIM DIB-*su-ma* KÚM *u* IR *ma-gal* TUKU.MEŠ U_4.1.KAM DIB-[*su*] U_4.1.KAM BAR-*šú ḫa-a-a-at-ti* KÚM TUKU.MEŠ KÚM *la ḫa-aḫ-ḫaš* DIB-*su-ma ana* KÚM *u ṣir-ḫa* TAR-*si*. . . (*BAM* 174 r. 29–31)

**If curse afflicts a person so that he has fever and a lot of sweat (and) for one day it afflicts [him] (and) for one day it releases him (and) he has a febrile confusional state (and) a lukewarm temperature afflicts him, to keep away fever and burning heat . . .

19.309 DIŠ ŠÀ-*šú* KÚM-*ma* NINDA KÚ-*ma* KAŠ NAG-*ma ú-gan-na-aḫ* SAG ŠÀ-*šú u* MAŠ.SÌLA.MEŠ-*šú* KÚ.MEŠ-*šú ú-sa-al ú-na-ḫaṭ u* ÚḪ-*su i-šal-lu* NA BI ⌜NAM.ÉRIM⌝ *u* NAM.TAG.GA DIB-*su* (DPS XXII:29–30 [AOAT 43.254])[245]

**If his stomach feels hot, he eats bread and drinks beer, and then *guḫḫu*-coughs (brassy; see Chapter 8 with 8.67–8.69), his upper abdomen (epigastrium) and his shoulders continually hurt him, he *su'ālu*-coughs (barking; see Chapter 8 with 8.65–8.66), he breathes deeply[246] and he sprays his saliva, curse or wrongdoing afflicts that person.

We conclude, therefore, that infections were an important part of this disease subset. We believe that some of the references were describing bacterial pneumonia (see Chapter 3 with 3.77–3.78), a condition that is usually thought of as acute in the current antibiotic era. However, in the absence of effective antibiotic therapy, it is likely that some of the cases would have been subacute or chronic processes. Since "curse" seems to be applied at least in part to chronic febrile conditions with wasting and multiorgan system involvement, it is quite possible that tuberculosis, the pulmonary variety of which has a clinical presentation that can be similar to bacterial pneunomia, was also included in this syndrome.

Gastrointestinal tuberculosis, once a common complication of extensive pulmonary tuberculosis, and which produced bleeding and other symptoms resembling gastrointestinal cancer or atypical ulcerative colitis, may be represented by references that compare "curse" or "hand" of curse with DÚR.GIG. The latter is another ancient Mesopotamian syndrome that may have included gastrointestinal cancer and/or ulcerative colitis but did not typically produce fever or affect the lungs (see Chapter 6 with 6.176–6.187).

19.310 DIŠ NA DÚR.GIG GIG-*ma* ḪAR.MEŠ [. . .] KÚM ŠUB.ŠUB-*su* NAM.RIM [. . .] (*BAM* 96 ii 20–21)

**If a person is (apparently) sick with DÚR.GIG but his lungs [. . .], and fever continually falls upon him, (he has) a curse [. . .]

19.311 DIŠ NA *kin-ṣa-*⸢*a*⸣-[*šú* KÚ.MEŠ-*šú* . . .]-zi *e-ṣil ši-ḫat* UZU TUKU-*ši* MÚD DUB.MEŠ NA BI DÚR.GIG ŠU ^{d}NAM.ÉRIM *ana* TI-*šú* . . . (*BAM* 95:19–20//*AMT* 53/9:5′–6′)[247]

**If a ⸢person's⸣ legs [hurt him . . .], he is sluggish, he has wasting away of the flesh and pours out blood, that person (has) DÚR.GIG (or) "hand" of curse, to cure him . . .

Alternatively, some or all of these references may simply represent the more chronic forms of DÚR.GIG. Renal tuberculosis can result in urethral narrowing (stricture). However references[248] that place "curse" alongside other urinary tract problems may simply indicate a recurrent urinary tract infection. Similarly, although tuberculous peritonitis is often mistaken for hepatic cirrhosis, the following references to "hand" of curse are probably due to cirrhosis with chronic jaundice accompanied by wasting, leading ultimately to liver failure.

19.312 DIŠ *ina* DUG_4.DUG_4-*šú il-la-tu-šú* DU.MEŠ *aḫ-ḫa-zu* IGI.MEŠ-*šú* DIRI.MEŠ $ŠÀ^{II}$-*šú i-šá-ru-šú* ŠU *ma-mit* GAM (DPS XXII:16 [AOAT 43.253]; cf. Labat, *Syria* 33.121–126 obv. 6)[249]

**If a person's spittle flows when he speaks, *aḫḫāzu*-jaundice fills his face,[250] (and) his bowels are loose, "hand" of curse; he will die.

19.313 DIŠ [D]IRI.MEŠ-*pú* ŠÀ.MEŠ-*šú* MÚ.MEŠ-*ḫu* $PIŠ_{10}$ IGI^{II}-*šú* MÚ.MEŠ-*ḫu* MURGU $GÌR^{II}$-*šú* MÚ.MEŠ *u* MÚD *ina* KIR_4-*šú šá* GÙB DU-*ku* ŠU NAM.ÉRIM.MA GAM (DPS XXII:19–20 [AOAT 43.253])

**If (his eyes) drift downstream, his insides are bloated, the rims of his eyes are swollen, the soles of his feet are swollen, and blood flows from his right nostril, "hand" of curse; he will die.[251]

The text below has a number of findings suggestive of a neurologic disease including hearing difficulty, inability to hold one's head up, and severe headache. Meningitis is one possible explanation, but since "hand" of curse is mentioned, the disease would appear to be one that is chronic with wasting. Although meningitis is more commonly an acute condition, there are some forms that may have a subacute or chronic course. Patients with tuberculous meningitis may follow an acute course; however, a small but significant subset of cases can be chronic. A severe headache, as described in the text below, would be more common with the chronic form of meningitis. A fatal outcome would also be expected.

19.314 [DIŠ . . .] *niš-mu-šú* DUGUD *ina* LÍL-*šú* GÚ-*su* [ŠUB-*su* . . .] ⸢*šá*⸣ 150 ŠED$_7$ NAM.ERÍM[252] [GAM] (DPS XIII J 5–6 = *TDP* 126 iii 37–38)

**[If he keeps crying out: "My insides, my insides"][253] (and) his ⸢hearing⸣ is difficult, during the course of his illness, his neck ["falls" (i.e., he lets it drop), his left temple (feels like it) is hot], (and) his right one (feels like it) is cold (i.e., he has a severe headache), "hand" of curse; [he will die].

Besides leprosy, mycetoma, nontropical sprue, and pneumonia or tuberculosis, other chronic infectious and noninfectious diseases would almost certainly have been included under the rubric "curse" or "hand of curse." Conditions such as *kis libbi* (indigestion; see Chapter 6 with 6.84–6.87) and diseases such as *ṣētu* (enteric fever; see Chapter 3 with 3.121–3.156), when they ran a prolonged course, were sometimes said to evolve into "curse."[254]

19.315 *ki-is* ŠÀ-*bi ir-ta-n*[*a-aš-ši*] *ma-aš-qí-it ki-is* ŠÀ-*bi ki á*[*š-ta-qu-ú-ši*] *iš-ta-na-at-ti* ^{Ú}GUR$_5$!.U[Š]! *ù* ^{GIŠ}GEŠTIN SUR.RA *ba-ti-iq be-lí li-še-bi-lam lu-uš-ta-aq-qí-ma a-na* ŠU.NAM.<ER>ÍM.MA *la i-tar-ši* (*PBS* 1/2.72:21–26, apud Parpola, AOAT 5/2.496)[255]

**She keeps ⸢having⸣ *kis libbi* (indigestion). Since I [gave her] a potion for *kis libbi* [to drink] she has continually been drinking (it). *Šarmadu* and drawn wine are in short supply; let my lord send (some) to me. I want to give it (to her) to drink so that it does not turn into "hand" of curse for her.

There are a group of "hand" of curse references that contain findings suggestive of sickle cell crisis. Although sickle cell disease is most common in Africa, it does occur in the Middle East in modern times, and probably occurred in ancient Mesopotamia. It is characterized by severe pain almost anywhere in the body secondary to infarction from aggregated sickle red blood cells. Painful, spontaneous penile erection (priapism) often occurs in men. Patients with sickle cell disease follow a chronic wasting course.

19.316 DIŠ *su-ḫar* GÌR^{II}-*šú* ŠED$_7$ KI.A IGI^{II}-*šú nu-up-pu-ḫa* GÌŠ-*šú aš-ṭa-at* LI.DUR-*su* DU$_8$-*át* ŠU NAM.ÉRIM.MA *ú-zab-bal-ma* GAM (DPS XIV A iv 17–18 = *TDP* 144 iv 52′–53′)

**If the soles of his feet are cold, the rims of his eyes are swollen, his penis is stiff and hard, (and) his navel is supple, "hand" of curse; (if) he lingers, he will die.[256]

19.317 DIŠ NA IGI^{II}-*šú* [. . .] x [. . .] ŠÀ-*šú* x x [. . .] *it-te-*[. . .] *bur-ka-šú tab*?!*-ka* a ga? zi x [. . .] ⌜*u*⌝ *it-ta-*⌜*na*⌝*-an-*⌜*ga*⌝*-ag* GABA.MEŠ-*šú* TAG.GA[-*šú*] *u* SAG.MEŠ-*šú e-te-nen-nu u* IM *ina* ŠÀ-*šú i-le-eb-bu ni-ḫi-is* ^{GIŠ}GIGIR NU ÍL NA BI ^{d}NAM.ÉRIM DIB-⌜*su*⌝ *ana* TI-*šú* . . . (*BAM* 49:1′-6′//*BAM* 50 obv. 1–7)

**If a person's eyes [. . .], his stomach [. . .], his knees are tense(?) [. . .] and is continually stiff, his breasts hurt [him] intensely, he keeps changing the (side of his) head (he sleeps on), "wind" groans in his stomach, (and) he is unable to bear being jostled in a chariot,[257] "hand" of curse afflicts that person, to cure him . . .

19.318 DIŠ NA SAG ŠÀ-*šú* KÚM TUKU.MEŠ-*ši* ŠÀ-*šú* GIG NINDA *u* A.MEŠ ŠÀ-*šú* NU IGI-*šú* GABA.MEŠ-*šú ir-te-nem-mu-u* ŠÀ-*šú ina pi-qi ana* ḪAL-*e* DÙ.DÙ-*uš* NU *i-par*$_5$*-ru* IM *ina* ŠÀ-*šú i-sa-na-ḫur i-le-eb-bu* ŠÀ.MEŠ-*šú eb-ṭú* NA BI ^{d}ŠU.NAM.ÉRIM DIB-*su ana* TI-*šú* . . . (*BAM* 49:9–14′//*BAM* 50 obv. 11–15//*BAM* 51:1′–3′)[258]

**If a person's upper abdomen (epigastrium) continually has fever, his stomach is sick, his stomach will not accept bread and water, both sides of his chest are continually relaxed, his stomach suddenly makes as if to vomit but he cannot throw up, the "wind" in his stomach continually roils (and) groans (and) his insides are cramped, "hand" of curse afflicts that person, to cure him . . .

Gods/Goddesses of Infants' Diseases

Also falling into the category of "hands" which more or less make sense in modern terms are two of the gods/goddesses who caused diseases in infants, namely, Gula and Kūbu.

GULA

There are twenty-six medical references that mention the goddess Gula. She was a patroness of healing and of the city of Isin, whose doctors were renowned for their skill. Her temples were associated with burials of dogs (her characteristic animal) and with ex-votos[259] showing patients clutching the body parts that had been (or it was hoped would be) healed by her intercession.

Nineteen of the references specify "infants," a term which, due to lengthy nursing periods, could include children as old as four years. Other characteristics were fever, weight loss, and skin color changes (yellow, white, and black). The process also appears to have been chronic in nature, with abdominal protrusion. Also included in this condition were problems involving the mouth, larynx, and skin.

Assuming, as seems likely, that at the very least the symptoms that appear in sequence in the diagnostic series (DPS XL A 75//B 76 = *TDP* 226:75 through DPS XL A 96 = *TDP* 228:96) were intended to represent a single syndrome,[260] the most probable major disease responsible for these signs and symptoms is visceral leishmaniasis, or kala-azar. This is caused by the parasite, *Leischmania donovani*, which is transmitted by the bite of the sandfly *Phlebotomus papatasii* (see Chapter 10 with 10.110). Visceral leishmaniasis occurs in many parts of the world, but in the Middle East it is usually a disease of young children, causing fever, jaundice, and weight loss. Since it invades and enlarges the liver and spleen, the children have a curious combination of emaciated extremities and a distended ("fat") abdomen. Kala-azar is a Hindi word meaning "black sickness," and it refers to a dark gray skin color seen in many patients. Other characteristics are anemia and frequent secondary infections due to the chronic and debilitating nature of this disease. Without treatment, the prognosis is very poor.

Many of the signs of visceral leishmaniasis are included in the sequenced Gula references. The syndrome that she caused is a characteristically chronic process, persisting for as long as five years.

19.319 DIŠ LÚ.TUR *it-ta-na-as-ḫur it-ta-na-as-la-*ʾ ŠU [^{d}*Gu-la*] (DPS XL A 82 = *TDP* 226:82)

**If an infant is repeatedly[261] (and) continually sick, "hand" of [Gula].[262]

Patients can have a petechial rash (the uneven yellow color),[263] and anemia could be the cause of the pallor ("turns white"). With more advanced disease, a dark gray (black) color may develop. At this stage, the prognosis is very poor.

19.320 [DIŠ] LÚ.TUR UZU.MEŠ-*šú* SIG_7 ŠUB-*ú* ŠU ^{d}*Gu-la* (DPS XL A 76//B 77a = *TDP* 226:76)[264]

** [If] an infant's flesh is unevenly colored with yellow, "hand" of Gula.[265]

19.321 DIŠ IGI.MEŠ-*šú* GI_6.MEŠ *u* BABBAR.MEŠ GAM (DPS IX A 17 = *TDP* 72:17)[266]

**If his face turns black and turns white, he will die.

19.322 DIŠ LÚ.TUR BABBAR *u* GI_6 ŠU ^{d}*Gu-*[*la*] (DPS XL A 87 = *TDP* 226:87)

**If an infant turns white and turns black, "hand" of ⸢Gula⸣.

Fever, weight loss, and abdominal protuberance are also consistent with visceral leishmaniasis.

19.323 DIŠ LÚ.TUR SAG ŠÀ-*šú za-qir* ŠU ⸢^{d}⸣*Gu-la* (DPS XL A 78//B 78 = *TDP* 226:78)

**If an infant's upper abdomen (epigastrium) protrudes, "hand" of Gula.[267]

19.324 DIŠ LÚ.TUR KÚM TUKU *u* UZU.MEŠ-*šú i-maṭ-ṭu-ú* ŠU ^{d}*Gu-la* (DPS XL A 89 = *TDP* 226:89)[268]

**If an infant has a fever and his flesh diminishes, "hand" of Gula.

The following reference may be attempting to describe the curious appearance of a child with emaciated extremities and a "fat" abdomen due to an enlarged liver and spleen.

19.325 DIŠ LÚ.TUR UZU.ME-*šú za-mar i-šaḫ-ḫu-ḫu za-mar i-šal-li-mu* ŠU ^{d}*G*[*u-la*] (DPS XL A 85 = *TDP* 226:85)

**If an infant's flesh wastes away in some places and gets more healthy (-looking—a.k.a. fat) in others, "hand" of ⸢Gula⸣.

19.326 DIŠ LÚ.TUR *i-ba-aḫ-ḫi ù i-kab-bir* ŠU ^{d}*Gu-la* (DPS XL A 88 = *TDP* 226:88)

**If an infant gets thin and gets fat, "hand" of Gula.

Other references suggest the presence of complications such as dysentery (see 3.117–3.119),[269] a common problem in visceral leishmaniasis.

19.327 DIŠ LÚ.TUR KÚM TUKU *u* ŠÀ.MEŠ-*šú eb-ṭu* ŠU [^{d}*Gu-la*] (DPS XL A 79 = *TDP* 226:79)

**If an infant has a fever and his insides are cramped,[270] "hand" of [Gula].

A number of Gula texts that are not part of the Gula sequence mention pain and a yoke around the neck, abdomen, or pelvis. The association of "hand" of Gula with *samānu* (cellulitis; see 3.172–3.182) and *ašû* (see 10.89–10.101)[271] suggests that the yoke was reddish and a macular (flat), papular (raised), or vesicular (blistered) eruption. This description is compatible with shingles, a skin infection caused by *Varicella zoster* (chickenpox) virus that lies dormant in the dermal nerves. When it reactivates, it causes local skin infection. It characteristically resembles chickenpox lesions (included by the *āšipu* under *ašû*; see Chapter 10) except that it is in a bandlike distribution affecting only one-half of the body. Reduction in immunity is known to be responsible for this condition, and it would be a likely complication of visceral leischmaniasis.

19.328 DIŠ ⸢ÚR⸣.KUN-*šú* KÚ-*šú* ŠU ^{d}*Gu-la* DIŠ *ni-ri* ÍL-*ma* NIGIN-*šú* (DPS XII D iv 16//G_2 iv 14 = *TDP* 108 iv 16)

**If his coccyx hurts him, "hand" of Gula. If a yoke-shaped lesion rises and curves round, ("hand" of Gula).

19.329 [DIŠ] ŠÀ-*šú* DIB-[*su-ma ú-a* D]UG$_4$.GA ŠU ^{d}ME.ME DIŠ *ni-ri ina* GÚ-*šú* GAR-*ma* NIGIN (DPS XIII B i 51′//F 10//G_2 1 = *TDP* 116 i 55′)

**[If] his abdomen afflicts [him so that] he ⸢says⸣ ["wah!"], "hand" of Gula. If a yoke-shaped lesion is established on his neck and curves round, ("hand" of Gula).

There is also a reference in the sequence that mentions *buʾšānu* as part of the Gula syndrome. By itself, *buʾšānu* appears to have been a syndrome that included *Herpes simplex* virus infection, Vincent's angina, and diphtheria (see Chapter 3). When mentioned in connection with other symptoms of "hand" of Gula, such as jaundice and discoloration of the skin, *Herpes simplex* virus infection and diphtheria[272] could be complicating secondary infections brought on in part by the reduced immunity seen in kala-azar.

19.330 DIŠ LÚ.TUR ŠÀ.MEŠ-*šú eb-ṭú u* SU-*šú* SIG$_7$ *bu-ʾ-šá-nu* DIB-*su* ŠU ^{d}*Gu-la* (DPS XL A 96 = *TDP* 228:96)

**If an infant's insides are cramped, his body is yellow, (and) *buʾšānu* afflicts him, "hand" of Gula.

19.331 DIŠ LÚ.TUR UZU.MEŠ-*šú ur-qá it-ta-du-ú* KÚM *la ú-kal* SAG.KI^{II}-*šú ma-aq-ta*$_5$ *ap-pi-šu ma-gal i-si-ir ú-pa-ṭi la i-šu* [BI.LU][273] *ṣab-tu-šú* (DPS XL A 5//B 5–6 = *TDP* 218:5)

**If an infant's flesh is unevenly colored with yellow, he does not "hold" fever, (the blood vessels of) his temples have collapsed, (and) he rubs his nose in a downward direction a lot (but) does not have snot, [*buʾšānu*] afflicts him.

19.332 DIŠ LÚ.TUR UZU.MEŠ-*šú* GI$_6$.MEŠ : ŠUB-*tu u ap-pa-šú us-sà-na-ar di-im-tum ina* IGI^{II}-*šú* DU-*ak* BI.LU (*ḫi-pi*) [. . .] (DPS XL A 61//B 61 = *TDP* 224:61)

**If an infant's flesh is dark (var. looks terrible) and he continually rubs his nose in a downward direction (and) tears flow from his eyes, *bu'šānu* [afflicts him . . .]

Such superinfection might account for the laryngeal constriction and choking in the following sequenced "hand" of Gula references.

19.333 DIŠ LÚ.TUR *ur-us-su ḫa-niq* ŠU ^{d}*Gu-la* (DPS XL A 91 = *TDP* 228:91)

**If an infant's larynx is constricted, "hand" of Gula.[274]

19.334 DIŠ LÚ.TUR *ú-nap-paq* UBUR NU NAG *u* SU-*šú* SIG$_7$ ŠU ^{d}*Gu-la* (DPS XL A 93 = *TDP* 228:93)[275]

**If an infant chokes (and) will not drink from the breast and his body is yellow, "hand" of Gula.[276]

Finally, it must be admitted that other conditions could have mimicked visceral leishmaniasis and been included within the syndrome of "hand" of Gula. It is even possible that *Leishmania donovani* did not exist in ancient Mesopotamia, and that some other pathogen was capable of producing similar signs and symptoms.

KŪBU

Eighteen texts were found that referred to Kūbu or "hand" of Kūbu. Since Kūbu was the demonic personification of stillborn children (see Chapter 17 with 17.2–17.4), and since such ghosts might be supposed to be jealous of siblings who were successfully born, it seems likely that the bulk of these references, trauma aside (see 19.188–19.189), are to one or more childhood illnesses.[277] In fact, four texts specifically mention infants, while another three indicate that the patient was wailing and/or refused to drink milk, behaviors more associated with children than adults. Fever was prominently mentioned.

19.335 DIŠ SAG.KI^{II}-*šú* KÚM-*ma* GEŠTU^{II}-*šú* ŠED$_7$.MEŠ *lu* ŠU DINGIR-*šú lu* ŠU ^{d}*Kù-bi* (DPS IV A obv. 64//E ii 9 = *TDP* 38:64//*SpTU* 3.88 ii 9)

**If his temples are hot and his ears are cold, either "hand" of his god or "hand" of Kūbu.

There are four references that mention fever, and another four with related complaints, namely, two with cold sensations and two with "shaking" chills (see below). We began by examining the four sequenced references that specify infants as patients.

19.336 DIŠ LÚ.TUR *mit-ḫar-riš em-ma u* SAG ŠÀ-*šú za-qir* ŠU ^{d}*Kù-bi* / DIŠ LÚ.TUR SA.MEŠ ŠÀ-*šú* SA$_5$ *u* SIG$_7$ ŠUB-*ú* ŠU ^{d}*Kù-bi* / DIŠ LÚ.TUR ŠÀ.MEŠ-*šú eb-ṭú-ma* SIG$_7$ ŠUB-*ú* ŠU ^{d}*Kù-bi* / DIŠ LÚ.TUR *ik-ta-na-aṣ-ṣa u* ZÚ.MEŠ-*šú i-gaṣ-ṣa-aṣ* GIG-*su ir-ri-ik ṣi-bit* ^{d}*Kù-bi* (DPS XL A 31–34 = *TDP* 220:31–34)

**If an infant is equally hot (all over) and his upper abdomen (epigastrium) protrudes, "hand" of Kūbu.[278] If the muscles of an infant's abdomen are unevenly colored with red and yellow, "hand" of Kūbu.[279] If an infant's insides are cramped and he is unevenly colored with yellow, "hand" of Kūbu. If an infant is continually cold and he gnashes his teeth, his illness will be prolonged; affliction by Kūbu.

The infants with Kūbu were suffering from fever with a red rash. The uneven yellow color could be due to jaundice appearing where the rash was not prominent. Alternatively, the red and yellow could be referring to subcutaneous bleeding (ecchymoses) in different stages of evolution (see Chapter 6 with 6.123). The protruding upper abdomen could be due to an enlarged liver, and the teeth gnashing to abdominal pain. "Prolonged" probably indicates a febrile disease lasting more than five to seven days.

These symptoms are consistent with leptospirosis. This is a bacterial infection acquired from the contaminated urine of wild and domesticated animals. It can range in severity from asymptomatic to a severe and occasionally fatal infection with hemorrhagic manifestations and kidney failure. It is typically a biphasic illness with muscle pain, headache, abdominal pain, vomiting, fever, and conjunctivitis (red eye) in the first phase. In the second phase, fever may return along with rash, liver and kidney involvement, hemorrhage, and meningitis.

The remaining references are also potentially consistent with leptospirosis, although none with the possible exception of the following reference to abdominal symptoms makes a particularly strong case.

19.337 [DI]Š ŠÀ.MEŠ-*šú* MÚ.MÚ-*ḫu* ŠU ᵈ*Kù-bi*: [. . .] / [DI]Š ŠÀ.MEŠ-*šú* MIN *u* ÍR.MEŠ ŠU ᵈ*Kù-bi*: ⌜ŠU⌝ [. . .] / [DI]Š ŠÀ.MEŠ-*šú* MIN *u* IGI^{II}-*šú* DUGUD-*šú* ŠU ᵈ*Kù-bi*: ŠU ᵈ[. . .] (DPS XIII I 7–9 = *TDP* 122 iii 7–9)[280]

**⌜If⌝ his insides are continually bloated, "hand" of Kūbu (var. [. . .]). ⌜If⌝ his insides (are continually bloated) and he continually wails, "hand" of Kūbu (var. "hand" of [. . .]). ⌜If⌝ his insides (are continually bloated) and his eyes bother him, "hand" of Kūbu (var. "hand" of [. . .]).

Children with leptospirosis frequently have acalculous cholecystitis (i.e., gallbladder inflammation in the absence of stones). This often produces abdominal distention and hypoactive bowel sounds, which may account for the specific references to "bloating (with air)" in the quote above.

What is particularly suggestive is the "bothersome" (lit. "heavy") eyes. This eye symptom is usually associated with fever, as in the following quote. A possible suggestion is that this is a reference to conjunctival suffusion as perceived by the patient. Conjunctival suffusion, if this is what is being described, is a common physical sign of leptospirosis.

19.338 DIŠ SAG ŠÀ-*šú* KÚM-*ma* SA SAG.KI^{II}-*šú* ŠU^{II}-*šú* *u* GÌR^{II}-*šú* ZI.ME IGI^{II}-*šú* DUGUD-*šú* (DPS XIII B i 27′ = *TDP* 112 i 31′)[281]

**If his upper abdomen (epigastrium) is hot and the blood vessels of his temples, his hands, and his feet continually (feel like they) are pulsating, (and) his eyes bother him.

Another set of references to symptoms produced by Kūbu mentions a viselike headache with fever and cramping (which is common) or diarrhea (which occasionally occurs) in leptospirosis.

19.339 DIŠ SAG.KI *ḫe-si-ma* KÚM-*im* : ŠED$_7$ ⸢ŠU⸣ ᵈ*Kù-bi* / DIŠ SAG.KI *ḫe-si-ma* ŠÀ.MEŠ-*šú* AL.DU ŠU ᵈ*Kù-bi* / DIŠ SAG.KI *ḫe-si-ma* ŠÀ.MEŠ-*šú it-te-nin-bi-ṭu* ŠU ᵈ*Kù-bi* (DPS IV B obv. 1–3//DPS III A r. 30 = *TDP* 32:1–2)

**If he has a viselike headache[282] and he is hot (var. cold), "hand" of Kūbu. If he has a viselike headache and his bowels are loose,[283] "hand" of Kūbu. If he has a viselike headache and his insides are continually cramped, "hand" of Kūbu.

A further set of references mentions wailing, loss of appetite (anorexia), and "shaking" (lit. "quaking" as in earthquakes), possibly a reference to the recurrent chills and high spiking temperatures of the first phase of the disease. Alternatively, it may be describing meningitis-induced seizures.

19.340 DIŠ *ina ši-mi-tan* ÍR.MEŠ *u* GA NU NAG ŠU ⸢ᵈ*Kù*⸣-[*bi*] / DIŠ *ina* IGI NÁ-*šú ú-na-*ʾ*-aš* ŠU ᵈ*Kù*-⸢*bi*⸣ / DIŠ ÍR.MEŠ *u ú-na-*ʾ*-aš* ŠU ᵈ*Kù-bi* (DPS XVII:87–89 [AOAT 43.203])

**If in the evening he continually wails and will not drink milk, "hand" of ⸢Kūbu⸣. If before he goes to bed he shakes, "hand" of Kūbu. If he continually wails and shakes, "hand" of Kūbu.

Also suggestive of the first phase of leptospirosis is the severe muscle pain (myalgia) mentioned in the following reference.

19.341 [DIŠ SU-*šú* KÚ]M ÚḪ TUKU-*ma* ŠU^{II}-*šú u* GÌR^{II}-*šú*-[*ma*] *mar-ṣa it-te-nen-ṣi-la-šú* [. . .]-*a-šú* KÚ.MEŠ-*šú* GÌR^{II}-*šú* x.[M]EŠ ŠU 15 : ŠU ᵈ*Kù-bi* (DPS XVIII:5–6 [AOAT 43.218])

** [If his body] burns with ⸢fever⸣, his hands and his feet are sore and sluggish, his [legs?] continually hurt him, (and) his feet [. . .] . . . "hand" of Kūbu.

Finally, there is a set of references that may be describing the signs and symptoms of the second phase of leptospirosis. These include "jerking" and "roaring" (?) in the ears, perhaps produced by meningitis, "affliction" of the abdomen, "puffing up (with liquid)" and "thickening," which suggest the liver and kidney involvement of leptospirosis.

19.342 [U$_4$ GIG *ig-da-n*] *a-al-lu-ut il-ta-*[*na-as-si*? ŠU ᵈ*Ku*] -*bi* U$_4$ GIG GEŠTU.MEŠ-*šu* [*i-šà-ag-gu-ma*? ŠU ᵈ*K*] *u-bi* [U$_4$ GIG (SAG) Š]À-*šú it-ta-na-aṣ-*[*ba-at-su* ŠU ᵈ*Ku-b*] *i* U$_4$ GIG TA *ši-pi* [. . .] *it-ta-aš-šu* ŠU ᵈ*Ku-bi* [U$_4$ GIG . . .] *kab-ba-ru* ŠU ᵈ*Ku-bi* [U$_4$ GIG . . .] *it-ta-na-aṣ-ba-ta* [. . .]-*ṣa ù ik-*[. . . ŠU ᵈ*Ku-b*] *i* [U$_4$ GIG . . . *i-ta-na*] -*na-ḫa* [. . .] (*MDP* 57.11 ii 10–20)

** [If the patient ⸢continually jerks⸣ (and) ⸢continually⸣ [cries out, "hand"] of ⸢Kūbu⸣. If the patient's ears [roar?, "hand"] of ⸢Kūbu⸣. [If the patient]'s upper abdomen (epigastrium)/abdomen is continually ⸢afflicted⸣, ["hand"] of ⸢Kūbu⸣. If the patient's [. . .] from the feet [to the . . .] are puffed up, "hand" of Kūbu. [If the patient's . . .] are thickened, "hand" of Kūbu. [If the patient's . . .] is continually afflicted (and) he [. . .] and [. . . "hand"] of ⸢Kūbu⸣. [If the patient's . . .] ⸢are continually tired⸣ [. . .]

AZU

Azu is attested outside of medical texts only in personal names.[284] The fact that he is called Azu (as in the healing specialist from whom the *asû* and *āšipu* were descended; see Introduction) would seem to indicate that, like Gula, he was a god of medicine. He was associated with a five-day illness producing headache, chills, and pain inside the ear. These symptoms are suggestive of an ear infection. Ear infections are most common in children between the ages of two and ten.

19.343 DIŠ SAG.KI^{II}-*šú* KÚ.MEŠ-*šú u* ŠED$_7$.MEŠ ŠU ^{d}A.ZU / DIŠ SAG.KI^{II}-*šú* MURUB$_4$.MEŠ-*šú*/GEŠTU^{II}-*šú* KÚ.MEŠ-*šú u* ŠED$_7$.MEŠ U$_4$.5.KÁM ŠU ^{d}A.ZU (DPS IV A obv. 62–63//E ii 7–8 = *TDP* 38:62–63//*SpTU* 3.88 ii 7–8)

**If his temples continually hurt him and he continually has chills, "hand" of Azu. If his temples (and) the middle parts (of his ears)[285] continually hurt him and he continually has chills (and) it is the fifth day (he has been sick), "hand" of Azu.

DINGIR.MAḪ, BELIT-ILI, AND NUSKU

A few final examples appear also to belong to the category of gods of childhood or infant diseases, but there are too few references to be absolutely sure of this. DINGIR.MAḪ was a "birth goddess" who caused abdominal problems in infants, which probably explains her appearance in the sequence of abdominal trauma (see 19.146).

19.344 DIŠ LÚ.TUR *i-mi-iš-ti* ŠÀ-*bi i-šu* KA-*šú* BAD.BAD-*te ma-la* KÚ *ut-ta-nar-ru* ŠU DINGIR.MAḪ : ŠU DINGIR TI (DPS XL A 50//B 49 = *TDP* 222:50)

**If an infant has intestinal colic, he continually opens his mouth, and as much as he eats (his insides) continually return, "hand" of Dingirmaḫ . . . he will get well.

Belit-ili's name means "mistress of the gods." Those who offended her had good reason for considerable embarrassment; she caused eneuresis.

19.345 DIŠ NA *ina* KI.NÁ-*šú* KÀŠ *iš-tin* ŠU ^{d}NIN.M[AḪ]/^{d}*Be-lit*-DINGIR.MEŠ (*STT* 238:1; cf. *BAM* 115 obv. 14′)

**If a person urinates in his bed, "hand" of Belit-ili.

Since bed-wetting is usually a problem of childhood, and since Belit-ili was a "birth goddess," this attribution makes a certain amount of sense, but we cannot be absolutely sure that this was all that Belit-ili did. The same may be said for Nusku, the god of lamps. He caused fever in infants that could be detected by placing a hand on the top of the head, a not inappropriate choice for causal agent if you can imagine the head of a feverish child being lit like a lamp.

19.346 DIŠ LÚ.TUR UGU-*šú* KÚM.KÚM-*im* ŠU ^{d}*Nusku* (DPS XL A 117 = *TDP* 230:117)[286]

**If the top of an infant's head is continually feverish, "hand" of Nusku.

Ill-Defined Syndromes of the Sort Gods/Goddesses Might Cause

A number of ills are attributed to the personal god or goddess of the victim or the god worshiped in his city[287] or quite simply to "hand" of god. For only two of these references is the reason behind their attribution obvious. Both are fatal abdominal complaints attributed to goddesses, and one is of venereal origin. Such problems, in view of the propensities of the goddess Ištar (whose name came to mean "*the* goddess"), would seem naturally to fall to female divinities.[288]

19.347 DIŠ SAG ŠÀ-*šú* ÍL ḪÁŠ-*su da-an* ŠED$_7$ *u* KÚM-*im* ŠU *il-ti* NU DIN (DPS XIII B i 28′ = *TDP* 112 i 32′)

**If his upper abdomen (epigastrium) is puffed up and his lower abdomen (hypogastrium) is hard (and) he is cold and then hot, "hand" of a goddess; he will not get well.

19.348 [DIŠ GÌŠ-*šú u* SAG ŠÀ-*šú* KÚM Ú]Ḫ *ú-kal* TÙN ŠÀ-*šú* KÚ-*šú u* ŠÀ-*šú ma-ḫu* Á^{II}-*šú* GÌR^{II}-*šú* ŠÀ-*šú* KÚM NA BI GIG *na-a-ki* GIG ŠU DINGIR-*šú* : ^{d}15-*šú* (DPS XIV A ii 34–36//C ii 10–11 = *TDP* 134 ii 34–36)[289]

**[If his penis and his upper abdomen (epigastrium)] hold ⌜burning⌝ [fever], his liver[290] hurts him and his stomach goes crazy (and) his arms, his feet, (and) his stomach are hot, that person is sick with a disease of intercourse; "hand" of his god (var. his goddess).

Two further references, which have the personal and city gods acting in concert, describe symptoms that are sufficiently dramatic to make it possible to hazard a diagnosis.

19.349 DIŠ U$_4$.2.KÁM GIG-*ma* SAG.KI-*šú šá* 15 *u* 150 KÚ.MEŠ-*šú* IGI^{II}-*šú šá* 15 *u* 150 GISSU *ib-na-a* NA BI DINGIR-*šú u* DINGIR URU-*šú iz-zur* BÚR-*ma* DIN (DPS XVI:23–24 [AOAT 43.174])

**If he has been sick for two days and his left and right temple continually hurt him and his left and right eye make a shadow, he cursed his god and the god of his city. (If) it goes away, he will get well.

19.350 DIŠ SAG.KI-*šú šá* 15 *u* 150 KÚ.MEŠ-*šú* IGI^{II}-*šú šá* 15 *u* 150 GISSU DÙ-*a* LÚ BI DINGIR-*šú u* DINGIR URU-*šú iz-zur ik-ri-ba ana* DINGIR-*šú iq-bi* BÚR-*ma* DIN (DPS IV B obv. 29//E i 9 = *TDP* 36:29–30//*SpTU* 3.88 i 9)[291]

**If his left and right temple hurt him and his left and right eye make a shadow, he cursed his god and the god of his city; he made a vow to his god. (If) it goes away, he will get well.

The *āšipu* distinguished at least two conditions involving a "shadow" made by the patient's eye. What was involved was probably the perception on the part of the patient of a sector of vision loss in one or both eyes. For more details, see Chapter 9. Of these conditions, one was attributed to Dapinu (see 19.86–19.87) and one to the patient's having cursed his god and the god of his city.

Simultaneous impairment of vision in the two eyes with central scotomas occurring over a period of days or weeks is usually due to a toxic or nutritional disorder. Nutritional optic neuropathy was a common occurrence during the Second World War and Korean War, due to a lack of B vitamins in the diet of many prisoners. Conditions in besieged cities in ancient Mesopotamia would probably have been equally grim. Indeed, this syndrome was observed in the besieged population of Madrid during the Spanish Civil War. If the victim of this condition was caught inside a city under siege, he would have had good reason to curse his luck (as we would say) or (as the *āšipu* might say) to curse his personal god and the god of his city.

Strengthening the possibility that the above references were due to nutritional optic neuropathy is the separate description of a condition that strikingly resembles what American prisoners of war called "burning feet" (peripheral neuropathy). This peripheral nerve disorder, characterized by distorted sensory perception (parasthesias), painful hyperesthesias of the feet, loss of superficial and deep sensation, and ataxia, was experienced by the prisoners in combination with the optic neuropathy described above. These two together, with other attendant symptoms, form what is known as Strachan's syndrome (see Chapter 7 with 7.17–7.18).

That the description of peripheral neuropathy is separate from the eye disease and not said to be the "hand" of god and city god and not explicitly blamed on those causal agents is to be expected. For better or worse, ancient ophthalmology seems to have been a subspecialty with its own subseries of therapeutic treatments, and eye problems tend therefore to be discussed in isolation.

19.351 DIŠ LÚ GÌR^{II}-*šú šim-ma-tú ú-kal-la* KÚM.MA TUKU-*a ù a-na a-tál-lu-ku* DUGUD-*šú* . . . (*BAM* 122 obv. 16–17; cf. *BAM* 406 r. 2′)

**If numbness grips a person's feet, they are feverish and it is difficult for him to walk . . .

19.352 DIŠ NA GÌR^{II}-*šú* KÚM TUKU-*a* DUGUD-*šú na-šá-a a-tál-lu-ka la i-le-ʾi ana* TI-*šú* . . . (*AMT* 69/7 ii 8–9; cf. *CTN* 4.117:10)[292]

**If a person's feet are feverish (and) it is difficult for him to lift (them or) to walk, to cure him . . .

For the rest of the references to personal or city gods or "hand" of god, the symptoms quoted are varied, and would not for the most part have been terribly helpful in arriving at a firm diagnosis. They include *birdu*-nodules on the face,[293] iritis,[294] choking,[295] slow pulse,[296] arthritic necks, feet, legs, and hips,[297] difficulty eating,[298] mild hematuria (blood in the urine),[299] and the loss of facial hair, as described in the following reference.

19.353 DIŠ NA SÍG TE.MEŠ-*šú ma-gal i-šaḫ-ḫu-uḫ* NA BI DINGIR-*šú* ^{d}EŠ$_{4}$.DAR-*šú* KI-*šú ze-nu-u* . . . (*BAM* 480 iii 48)

**If the hair on a person's cheeks falls out a lot, his god and goddess are angry with that person . . .

On the surface of it, the obvious suggestion is that "hand" of god was for the ancient physician something akin to what his modern counterpart would call "god only knows," in this case, perhaps better "gods, goddesses, and guardian angels only know (what it is)." Approximately one-third of the nontrauma references are to what we would call stress-related illnesses (see 19.35–19.38). A handful appear to describe normal variations of seizures (see 19.65–19.66, 19.68).[300] Two references[301] involve cases where the characteristic color of lesions produced by three different divinities appeared simultaneously in a single patient (see 19.94). Another one-third of the references to "hand" of god and the like are to vaguely described illnesses of infants.[302] One of these descriptions is compatible with congenital syphilis (see 4.23), several more appear to describe infant colic (see 17.161) or possibly meningitis (see 13.221). The remainder of the infant references mention gastrointestinal problems or flushing and sweating.

19.354 DIŠ LÚ.TUR *i-mi-iš-ti* ŠÀ-*bi i-šu* KA-*šú* BAD.BAD-*te ma-la* KÚ *ut-ta-nar-ra* ŠU DINGIR.MAḪ : ŠU DINGIR TI (DPS XL A 50//B 49 = *TDP* 222:50)

**If an infant has intestinal colic, he continually opens his mouth and as much as he eats (his insides) continually return . . . "hand" of god; he will get well.

19.355 DIŠ LÚ.TUR UGU [K]IR$_4$-*šú* IR DU-*ak* SA$_5$ *u* SIG$_7$ ŠU DINGIR DIN (DPS XL B 68 = *TDP* 226:67)

**If sweat flows over an infant's nose (and) he flushes and turns pale, "hand" of god; he will get well.

19.356 DIŠ LÚ.TUR ⌜*pa-ru*⌝-*ta ma-li* ŠU DINGIR DIN / DIŠ LÚ.TUR *pa-ru-ta sa-li-iḫ u liq* KA-*šú* ⌜*i-ta!-nab-bal*⌝-*šú* ŠU DINGIR [DIN] / DIŠ LÚ.TUR ⌜*pa-ru*⌝-*ta sa-li-iḫ* ŠU D[INGIR DIN] (DPS XL B 69–71 = *TDP* 226:68–70)

**If an infant is full of vomiting, "hand" of god; he will get well. If an infant is sick with vomiting and his palate continually dries up, "hand" of god; [he will get well]. If an infant is sick with vomiting, "hand" [of god; he will get well].

Probably to be connected with these references are a series of infants whose ill-defined problems were attributed to an "unfulfilled vow," that is, the parents made a promise of offerings to some god or goddess in return for some requested benefit. They got what they asked for but then failed to pay what they had promised and their child became ill as a result.

19.357 DIŠ LÚ.TUR *ina* UBUR AMA-*šú* LÙ.LÙ-*aḫ* LÍL.LÍL-*a*' KI.MIN *i-bak-ki u* KÚM DIB.DIB-*su ik-ri-bu* DIB.ME-*šú* (DPS XL A 20 = *TDP* 220:20)

**If an infant is continually restless at the breast of his mother (and) is continually sick; alternatively, (if) he wails and fever continually afflicts him, (unfulfilled) vows afflict him.

19.358 DIŠ LÚ.TUR *ina* UBUR AMA-*šú* LÙ.LÙ-*aḫ ik-ri-bu ṣab-tu-šu* / DIŠ LÚ.TUR UBUR ÍL-*šum-ma* NAG-*ma ú-šar-ra-aḫ ik-ri-bu* DIB.MEŠ-*šu* / DIŠ LÚ.TUR UBUR ÍL-*šum-ma* NU KÚ *u* ŠÀ.MEŠ-*šú nap-ḫu ik-ri-bu ṣab-tu-šu* (DPS XL A 103–105 = *TDP* 228:103–105)

**If an infant is continually disturbed at the breast of his mother, (unfulfilled) vows afflict him. If (when) you raise the breast to an infant, he drinks and then drools, unfulfilled vows afflict him. If (when) you raise the breast to an infant, he will not eat and his insides are bloated, (unfulfilled) vows afflict him.

19.359 DIŠ LÚ.TUR *i-lab-bu-ma* UBUR ÍL-*šum-ma* NU KÚ *ik-ri-bu* DIB-*šu* (DPS XL A 109 = *TDP* 228:109)

**If an infant groans and (if) you raise the breast to him he will not eat, (unfulfilled) vows afflict him.

Many of the remaining references to "hand" of god and the like describe nonspecific fevers, usually mentioning elevated temperatures detected in various parts of the body.[303]

19.360 DIŠ SAG.DU-*su* KÚM *ḫa-ḫaš* SA.ME SAG.KI^{II}-*šú* ZI.MEŠ KÚM-*im u* ŠED$_7$ ŠU DINGIR-*š*[*u*] (coll.) (DPS III C obv. 50 = *TDP* 24:50)

**If his head (has) a very hot temperature, the blood vessels of his temples seem to pulsate, (and) he is hot and then cold, "hand" of ⌜his⌝ god.

19.361 DIŠ SAG.DU-*su* KÚM-*im* SA SAG.KI^{II}-*šú* ŠU^{II}-*šú u* GÌR^{II}-*šú* 1-*niš* ZI.MEŠ SA$_5$ *u i-mim* ŠU [DINGIR DIN] (DPS III C obv. 55 = *TDP* 24:55)

**If his head is hot (and) the blood vessel(s) of his temples, his hands, and his feet all seem to pulsate together (and) he is flushed and feverish, "hand" of [god; he will get well].

19.362 DIŠ SAG ŠÀ-*šú* DIG-*ub i-mim u* ŠED$_7$ ^{GIŠ}GIDRU *šá* DINGIR-*šú ana* GAL *u* TUR 1-*ma* (DPS XIII B i 25′ = *TDP* 112 i 29′)[304]

**If his upper abdomen (epigastrium) is soft (and) he is hot and then cold, scepter of his god. It is the same for adults and children.

In addition to elevated temperatures, the references describe symptoms that often occur with fevers such as headache,[305] trembling hands,[306] abdominal bloating,[307] vomiting,[308] diarrhea,[309] and muscle pain (myalgia).[310]

19.363 DIŠ SAG ŠÀ-*šú* DIB.DIB-*su* ŠÀ.MEŠ-*šú* KÙŠ.ME-*šú kin-ṣa-a-šú u* GÌR^{II}-*šú* KÚ.MEŠ-*šú* ŠU DINGIR-*šú ni-ši* (DPS XIII B i 11′ = *TDP* 112 i 15′)

**If his upper abdomen (epigastrium) continually afflicts him (and) his insides, his upper arms, his legs, and his feet continually hurt him, "hand" of his god; (there will be) recovery.

A final group of "hand" of god or "hand" of his (personal/city) god references appear to describe fevers with neurologic symptoms that the *āšipu* was unsure how to place (see under 19.291–19.294).

Mystery Syndromes

Another set of categories used by the *āšipu* was "cutting of the breath" (ZI.KU$_5$.RU.DA)[311] or other forms of sorcery (*kišpu*). Ancient Mesopotamian physicians apparently used this set of diagnoses to designate syndromes that had specific signs and symptoms but seemed bizarre and mysterious (see below).

In some cases, we believe that we know what the *āšipu* was trying to describe. Both Graves' disease (hyperthyroidism) and Addison's disease (adrenal insufficiency) seem to have been blamed on the machinations of sorcerers. The former was specifically brought about by "cutting of the breath" using wax and tallow figurines. The thought was presumably that sorcery was causing the patient to "melt away" like wax, a description that reflects the weight loss of patients with this disease (for more details, see Chapter 7 with 7.24). Another disease blamed on "cutting of the breath" with figurines, this time devoted to Gilgameš in his capacity as judge of the netherworld, was rabies (see 2.34). Figurines laid in the ground with a corpse were invoked to explain congestive heart failure or cardiotoxic poisons (see 8.28, 15.2), and figurines devoted to the queen of the netherworld, Ereškigal, for Ménière's syndrome (see 9.117), as in the following reference.

19.364 *šum*$_4$*-ma* NA IGI.MEŠ-*šú* NIGIN.DU-*šú* GEŠTU.MEŠ-*šú i-šag-gu-ma* UZU.MEŠ-*šú šim-ma-ta* TUKU.TUKU-*ú* ŠÀ-*šú it-ta-na-ad-láḫ* GAR-*in* GIG-*šú* NU ZU.ZU NA BI *ka-šip* NU.MEŠ-*šú* DÙ.MEŠ-*ma ina* KI GUL.MEŠ *ana* ^{d}EREŠ.KI.GAL *pa-aq-du* (*BAM* 214 i 1–9)

**If a person's face seems continually to be spinning, his ears roar, his flesh is continually numb, his heart is continually troubled, (and) the appearance of his illness is mysterious, that person is *kišpu*'d, figurines of him were manufactured and in a place of desolation they were entrusted to Ereškigal.

In the remaining cases attributed by the *āšipu* to "cutting of the breath," we are just as mystified as they were. For more details, see the Unsolved Puzzles Appendix (Ap. 73).

Syndromes Assigned in Accordance with Known Predilections of Specific Gods/Goddesses or Demons

Ninurta and the twin gods were associated with specific internal organs.

NINURTA

19.365 *ta-kal-tu*$_4$ ŠU ^{d}NIN.IB *aḫ-ḫ*[*a-z*]*u* ŠU ^{d}[NIN.IB] (DPS XXXIII:107 [AOAT 43.358])

**Liver (problems are caused by) "hand" of Ninurta; ⌜*aḫḫāzu*⌝-jaundice (is caused by) "hand" of [Ninurta].

Ninurta's association with the liver probably has to do with a play on words between "liver" (*takaltu*),[312] the verb *to trust* (*takālu*), as in "the god in whom I put my trust," and "weapon" (^{GIŠ}TUKUL). Although the epithet *tukulti* ("one in whom one trusts") is attested for other gods, Ninurta appears fairly frequently with it in personal names and in the phrase "one in whom Anu and Enlil trust," in deference to his role as hero-god and slayer of the bird-monster Anzu.

In the following sequences of references, Ninurta appears to be associated specifically with liver problems attributable to alcoholism (see Chapters 6 and 15).

19.366 DIŠ INIM-*šú* KÚR.[KÚR-*i*] *r* MÚD *ina* KA-*šú* ŠUB.ŠUB-*a u* ŠÀ.MEŠ-*šú* ÍL-*ú ana* U$_4$.10.[KÁM . . .] / DIŠ INIM-*šú* KÚR.[KÚR-*i*] *r* IM *ina* DÚR-*šú* È.MEŠ-*a u ú-ga-aš-ši ana*

U$_4$.10.[KÁM . . .] / DIŠ INIM-*šú* K[ÚR.KÚR-*i*]*r u* KÚM ŠUB.ŠUB-*su* ŠU ^{d}MAŠ *ana* U$_4$.10.[KÁM . . .] (DPS VII B r. 10–12 = *TDP* 66:66′–68′)

**If his words are ⌜unintelligible⌝, he continually produces blood from his mouth, his insides are puffed up, (and he has been sick) for ten days, [he will die]. If his words are ⌜unintelligible⌝, he constantly emits "wind" from his anus, he belches, (and he has been sick) for ten days, [he will die]. If his words are ⌜unintelligible⌝ and fever continually falls upon him, "hand" of Ninurta. (If he has been sick) for ten days [he will die].

19.367 DIŠ INIM-*šú* KÚR.[KÚR-*i*]*r u* KAŠ APIN.MEŠ-*iš ana* U$_4$.10.[KÁM . . .] / DIŠ INIM-*šú* K[ÚR.KÚR-*i*]*r u* ⌜^{GIŠ}GEŠTIN⌝ APIN.MEŠ-*iš ana* U$_4$.DUG$_4$.GA-[*šu ana* U$_4$.10.KÁM . . .] / DIŠ INIM-*šú* [KÚR.KÚR-*i*]*r u* ⌜*i-ram*⌝*-mu-um*[313] *ana* [U$_4$.10.KÁM . . .] / DIŠ INIM-*šú* [KÚR.KÚR-*ir* . . .] *u*ʾ*-i* ŠÀ *u*ʾ*-i*[314] ŠÀ-*bi* GÙ.GÙ-*si* x [. . .] / ⌜DIŠ INIM⌝-[*šú* KÚR.KÚR-*ir* . . .] *lu* ŠU ^{d}MAŠ x [. . .] (DPS VII B r. 13–17 = *TDP* 66:69′–73′)

If his words are ⌜unintelligible⌝ and he continually asks for beer (and he has been sick) for ten days [he will die]. If his words are ⌜unintelligible⌝ and he continually asks for wine at regular intervals (and he has been sick) [for ten days, he will die]. If his words are ⌜unintelligible⌝, he drones, (and he has been sick) for [ten days, he will die]. If his words are [unintelligible . . .] he continually cries out: "Woe, my heart," "Woe, my heart" [. . .]. If his words [are unintelligible . . ., "hand" of . . .] or "hand" of Ninurta [. . .]

TWIN GODS

The twin gods seem to have been associated with organs of the body that look like a pair of identical twins, namely, the kidneys.[315]

19.368 DIŠ ÉLLAG 15-*šú* KÚ-*šú-ma ina* UGU-*šú* NÁ-*al* ŠU ^{d}MAŠ.TAB.BA DIN (DPS XII D iii 13 = *TDP* 104 iii 13)[316]

**If his left kidney (costophrenic angle) hurts him so that he can lie on it, "hand" of the twin gods; he will get well.

ANU, ENLIL, AND EA

These three gods are often represented on Middle Babylonian *kudurrus* (boundary stones) as a group of three miniature temple facades surmounted by horned crowns. Together, they governed the three "paths" or vertical bands into which the eastern horizon was divided and which were used to locate the eighteen constellations recognized by ancient astronomers. In addition, Anu ruled the highest of the ancient Mesopotamian heavens, which overlay the second heaven of Enlil (later usurped by Marduk). Below the last heaven and the first earth, Ea ruled the sweet waters of the middle earth, which rested on the fundament of the netherworld. A reference in the diagnostic series seems to indicate that this system of heavens and earths could also be imagined to exist in miniature within the head of a patient.

19.369 DIŠ UGU UGU GÙ.GÙ-*si* ŠU ^{d}60 AŠ DINGIR *šá* ŠÀ (DPS III A obv. 17//C obv. 8 = *TDP* 18:8)

**If he keeps crying out: "the top of my head, the top of my head!" "hand" of Anu because he is the god inside.

Imagining the human head as a microcosmos would place Anu in the upper and forward part of the brain (frontal lobes), Enlil just below and behind his colleague (temporal, parietal, and occipital lobes), with Ea in the cerebellum just above the "netherworld" brain stem. Although there is no reason to suppose that the *āšipu* regularly dissected human brains, we know that he was very careful to observe which part of the head had been struck in cranial trauma. This means that it should have been possible to correlate specific symptoms with injury to the top of the head as opposed to the base of the skull, and so on. Interestingly, many of the symptoms attributed to the *šedûs* of Anu, Enlil, and Ea in references that appear in sequence in *CTN* 4.72 would not be incompatible with the suggested arrangement of gods inside the head.

Patients with lesions in one or both frontal lobes sometimes present with motor abnormalities such as decomposition of gait and upright stance, culminating in an inability to stand accompanied by abnormal postures, reflex grasping or sucking, and incontinence, as suggested by the text below.

19.370 DIŠ GIG-*ma* KA-*šú* BAD.BAD-*te* ŠU^{II}-*šú* GÌR^{II}-*šú* *i-par-ru-ra* ŠU ^{d}*mu-un-*[*ni*]*-ši* ^{d}ÀLAD *šá-né-e* ^{d}*A-nim* / DIŠ *ina* ŠU DINGIR *mu-un-ni-ši* KAR-[*šú*] . . . (*CTN* 4.72 vi 1–4 = DPS XXX:1–4)[317]

**If (he) is sick and he continually opens his mouth,[318] and his hands and his feet become disconnected from one another, "hand" of "weakener," a *šedû* deputized by Anu; if (you want) to save [him] from "hand" of "weakener" . . .

The name of the god responsible for the condition described below is restored, but is reasonably certain due to the close association of the god Enlil with Zaqiqu (a folk etymology of his name made him lord [EN] of *zaqīqu*-spirits [LÍL]). Zaqiqu was not just a *šedû* of Enlil but also the god of dreams, and it is not surprising to see him associated with vision problems. Patients with lesions in occipital lobes are generally partially or completely blinded in the affected eye(s) but may also complain of changes in the form and contour of visually perceived objects and be unable to recognize colors.

19.371 DIŠ GIG-*ma* IZI.ŠUB.[BA IGI]-*ma ú-ta-ni-u* BABBAR-*ti* NU ⌜TUKU ŠU⌝ ^{d}*Za-qí-qí* ^{d}ÀLAD *šá-né-e* ^{d}[EN.LÍL] DIŠ *ina* ŠU ^{d}*Za-qí-qí* KAR-*šú* . . . (*CTN* 4.72 vi 9–11)

**If (he) is sick and [he sees] a lightning bolt and it (looks) altered (and) has no whiteness, "hand" of Zaqiqu, a *šedû* deputized by [Enlil]; if (you want) to save him from "hand" of Zaqiqu . . .

Most of the symptoms described below would appear to relate to Ea's fever (see 19.242–19.246). It is, however, possible that the attribution of the *šedû*: "stiff" (and of the fever associated with stiffness) to Ea is connected with his role inside the head. The cerebellum is needed to perform fine voluntary movements such as those needed for writing, dressing, and eating. These can be performed in the absence of cerebellar function, but the movements are clumsy and disorganized.

19.372 DIŠ MIN-*ma* IR *la-ba-ṣi ma-at-tú* TUKU.TUKU-*ši u ḫur-ba-šu* ŠUB.ŠUB-*su* ŠU ^{d}*aš-ṭi* ^{d}ÀLAD *šá-ni-e* ^{d}*É-a* DIŠ *ina* ŠU DINGIR *aš-ṭi* KAR-*šú* . . . (*CTN* 4.72 vi 14–16)

**If (he is sick) and he continually has much sweat (as in) Labaṣu and chills keep falling upon him, "hand" of "stiff," a *šedû* deputized by Ea; if (you want) to save him from "hand" of "stiff" . . .

IŠTAR

A great variety of different syndromes were attributed to Ištar, but most can be related directly or indirectly to this multifaceted goddess's personality and/or functions. When attributing syndromes to specific causal agents, there were several different manifestations of Ištar for the *āšipu* to choose from. Of these, Ištar of Aššur seems never to have been blamed for disease (nor, for that matter, was her father Aššur, chief god of the Assyrian pantheon). Ištar of Harran was the daughter of the mood-god Sîn and the twin sister of the sun-god Šamaš with whom she cooperated in causing fevers and variously colored skin lesions. Ištar of Babylon is difficult to distinguish, but may be the referrent in cases involving sexually transmitted diseases where her boyfriend Marduk is also prominently mentioned.[319] Ištar of Uruk was the "daughter of Anu" held responsible for infantile spasms, and Ištar of Arbela is specifically mentioned in connection with Strachan's syndrome[320] and with "shuddering."[321]

This leaves only Ištar of Nineveh, who was originally the Hurrian goddess Šaušga, the daughter of a completely otiose and essentially irrelevant Anu and the brother of the head of the Hurrian pantheon, Tešub, who was syncretized with the Mespotamian weather-god, Adad. This last Ištar seems to have been invoked (alongside her brother Adad) to explain abdominal pain, perhaps a reference to the sometimes severe but essentially harmless cramps that may accompany menstruation. As befitted a goddess notorious for killing her lovers, however, Ištar's abdominal pain was usually expected to result in fatality.

19.373 DIŠ *ina* ŠÀ-*šú* Á 15/150-*šú* ^{GIŠ}GIDRU GAR-*su-ma u* MÚD $BURU_8$/*i-ḫa-ḫu* ŠU ^{d}15 GAM (DPS XIII B ii 26–27//G_2 25+G_1 8 = *TDP* 120 ii 26–27)[322]

**If a burning pain[323] is firmly established in his abdomen on the left/right side and he vomits blood, "hand" of Ištar;[324] he will die.

The list of possibilities for the preceding reference is quite long, but it includes bleeding peptic ulcers and gastric cancer. Where the abdominal pain was right-sided, and jaundice is also mentioned, hepatitis is a possibility, as in the following reference. For more details, see Chapter 6.

19.374 DIŠ *ina* ŠÀ-*šú* Á 150-*šú* ^{GIŠ}GIDRU GAR-*su-ma* IGI^{II}-*šú* GU.MEŠ SIG_7.MEŠ DIRI.MEŠ ŠU ^{d}15 GAM (DPS XIII B ii 29–30 = *TDP* 120 ii 29–30)

**If a burning pain[325] is firmly established in his abdomen on the right side and his eyes are full of yellow threads, "hand" of Ištar; he will die.

It may be Ištar's propensity for causing liver pain and bleeding that produced the following reference to her alongside her "deputy," namely, "hand" of ghost-headache and severe abdominal discomfort.

19.375 DIŠ NA SAG.KI.DIB.BA-*ma* ŠÀ ŠÀ-*bi* GÙ.GÙ-*si* ŠU.GIDIM.MA *šá-né-e* ^{d}*Iš-tar* ÚŠ (*BAM* 482 iv 47′//*AMT* 19/1 iv! 30′)[326]

**If a person has a headache and he keeps crying out: "My insides, my insides!" "hand" of ghost, deputy of Ištar; he will die.

Although in some sense distinct, the various manifestations of Ištar overlap to a significant degree. Thus, a syndrome caused either by Ištar of Harran or by her father Sîn involved severe pain on the right side of the abdomen and the production of colored mucus by the lips. Possibly also to be connected with this syndrome is a second reference in which the colored mucus is described as being of abdominal origin and the patient is jaundiced and dies.

19.376 DIŠ *ina* ŠÀ-*šú* Á 150-*šú* MIN-*ma* NUNDUN.MEŠ-*šú ši-ga* ŠUB-*a* ŠU ^{d}30 *lu* ŠU ^{d}15 GAM (DPS XIII B ii 31//G_2 28+G_1 11 = *TDP* 120 ii 31)

**If in his abdomen on the right side (a burning pain[327] is firmly established) and his lips produce *šīqu* (colored mucus), "hand" of Sîn or "hand" of Ištar; he will die.

19.377 DIŠ *ina* ŠÀ-*šú ši-qu ina* ŠÀ IGI^{II}-*šú* GU.MEŠ SIG$_7$.MEŠ *ip-ri-ku* GAM (DPS XIII B ii 34 = *TDP* 120 ii 34)

**If there is *šīqu* (colored mucus) in his abdomen (and) yellow threads cross in his eyes, he will die.

If it may be allowed that fever was also present (since both Sîn and Ištar can cause fever and since this symptom is frequently omitted as obvious), one possibility for a combination of upper right quadrant pain and colored sputum is hepatic amoebiasis with extension into the right pleural cavity and perforation into the bronchus. In hepatic amoebiasis, the affected part of the liver is liquified, producing a pus that varies from thick and dark "anchovy paste" to thin and yellow or green in color. When rupture occurs, the patient expectorates large amounts of this material. Jaundice is rare, but when it is present, the prognosis is grave.

Ištar is usually known as the "goddess of love." A more accurate description would be "goddess of lust," since she was the patroness of prostitutes and a notoriously disobedient and unfaithful wife with a nasty tendency to do her husbands in when they did something to displease her. Not surprisingly, she caused what we call venereal diseases. By herself, she seems to have caused gonococcal urethritis (see 4.6–4.7) and gonococcal arthritis (see 11.49–11.53). In concert with her brother Šamaš and her father Sîn, she produced the characteristic vesicles of sexually transmitted HSV (see 10.130–10.131). She was also closely associated with two other causers of venereal diseases. The *lilû* class of demon (teenage demons) inflicted what may have been secondary and tertiary syphilis (see 4.26–4.31), whereas practices of sorcery of the type described as "laying somebody's semen with a corpse" was the ancient Mesopotamian diagnosis for reactive arthritis associated with sexually transmitted urethritis (see 11.54–11.56).

A disease that might connect right-sided abdominal pain with a sexually transmitted disease is either gonorrhea or chlamydial urethritis. These infections occasionally spread to the abdomen to infect the capsule of the liver (perihepatitis), causing not only painful urination and urethral discharge but also abdominal pain in the area of the liver. This is known as the Fitz-Hugh Curtis syndrome (see Chapter 4), and it appears also to have been attributed to Ištar.

19.378 DIŠ NA GÌŠ-*šú u* SAG ŠÀ-*šú* KÚM *ṣar-ḫa ú-kal* TÙN ŠÀ-*šú* KÚ-*šú u* ŠÀ-*šú ma-ḫu* Á^{II}-*šú* GÌR^{II}-*šú u* ŠÀ-*šú* KÚM-*im* NA BI GIG *na-a-ki* GIG ŠU ^{d}15 (DPS XXII:14–15 [AOAT 43.252])

**If a person's penis and his upper abdomen (epigastrium) hold burning fever, his liver[328] hurts him and his stomach goes crazy, (and) his arms, his feet, and his stomach are feverish, that person is sick with a disease of intercourse; "hand" of Ištar.

GHOST

As with the goddess Ištar, a great variety of different syndromes were attributed to ghosts. The fact that syndromes attributed to "hand" of ghost were not all treated with the same set of drugs[329] shows that the *āšipu* knew that some of the syndromes that he had grouped together were actually separate problems. Nonetheless, these syndromes still made sense to him as a single diagnostic category because they all could be made to fit (if for different reasons) with what a particular spirit might be expected to do.[330]

Strange noises were made by ghosts in nonmedical contexts, so it is hardly surprising that strange noises perceived by patients would have been classified as ghost problems. Ringing, roaring, or buzzing in the ears was, therefore, routinely diagnosed as "hand" of ghost.[331] The first two references below are probably cases of eustachian tube inflammation causing popping sounds as air tried to get through the narrow opening; for more details, see Chapter 9. The final reference, which combines ringing in the ears with pulsating ghost headache, may be due to cranial trauma, which was attributed to ghosts (see 19.169).

19.379 [DI]Š GEŠTU^{II}-*šú i-az-za-za* ŠU GÍDIM (DPS VIII 17b = *TDP* 70:17b)

**⸢If⸣ his ears make strange noises, "hand" of ghost.

19.380 DIŠ NA *ina* DIB-*it* ŠU.GIDIM.MA GEŠTU^{II}-*šú i-šag-gu-ma* . . . (*SpTU* 1.49:33)[332]

**If, as a result of affliction by "hand" of ghost, a person's ears roar . . .

19.381 GEŠTU^{II}-*šú iš-ta-na-as-sa-a* . . . ŠU.GIDIM.MA (*SpTU* 3.100:12–13; *SpTU* 1.49:34)

**(If) his ears continually ring, . . . "hand" of ghost.

19.382 [DIŠ N]A SAG.KI-*šú šá* ZAG *u* GÙB *ki-ma* DIB-*bat* GIDIM ZI-*ma uz-na-šú i-ša-sa-ma* [IGI^{II}-*šú*] ÍR DIRI-*a* . . . (*AMT* 14/5:6–7)

**[If] a ⸢person's⸣ left and right temples (feel like they) are pulsating as in affliction by a ghost, his ears ring, and [his eyes] are full of tears . . .

Although medically unrelated (and treated with different medicines), strange noises made by intestines also seemed to be a sign of a ghost.

19.383 DIŠ NA ŠÀ.MEŠ-*šú* MÚ.MEŠ-*ḫu ir-ru-šú* GIN$_7$ *šá* MAR.GAL *ma-gal* GÙ.GÙ-*ú* NA BI *ni-kim-tú* IM *u* UD.DA GIG KIN-*šú i-la-bir-ma* ŠU.GIDIM.MA *ana* TI-*šú* . . . (*BAM* 52:66–67//*BAM* 471 ii 3′–4′//*BAM* 88:17′–20′//*BAM* 168:1–3; *AMT* 52/4:2′–3′)

**If a person('s) insides are continually bloated (and) his intestines continually make a (loud) noise like an *iṣ̌qippu*(-bird), that person is sick with pent-up "wind" (or) *ṣētu* (enteric fever). If his attack is prolonged, "hand" of ghost, to cure him . . .[333]

Another sign of ghostly affliction was particularly sharp and unpleasant pains occurring in various parts of the body. The first reference below appears to describe otitis media (see Chapter 9) and the second and third severe abdominal pain, possibly in an alcoholic patient (see above).

19.384 DIŠ NA *ina* ŠÀ GEŠTU^{II}-*šú* GIN$_7$ GAR ŠU.GIDIM.MA KÚ.MEŠ-*šú ù* SÌG.MEŠ-*šú* . . . (*BAM* 3 iv 12//*BAM* 503 ii 63′//Labat, *RA* 53.12–13 r. 18; *RA* 53.12–13 r. 22)

**If inside a person's ears it continually hurts him and continually gives him a jabbing pain like (an attack of) "hand" of ghost . . .

19.385 [DIŠ] ŠÀ ŠÀ *rab-biš* : *rap-diš* GÙ.GÙ-*si* ŠU GIDIM$_7$ *šag-ga-ši* [GAM] (DPS XIII G$_2$ r. 20 = *TDP* 124 iii 27)

**[If] he keeps crying out softly (var. intermittently?): "My insides, my insides," "hand" of a murderous ghost; [he will die].

19.386 [DIŠ SAG Š]À-*šú* DIB.DIB-*su* DIB GIDIM$_7$ (DPS XIII B i 7′ = *TDP* 110 i 11′)[334]

**[If] his ⌜epigastrium⌝ continually afflicts him, affliction by a ghost.

When upper abdominal fever is specifically mentioned in connection with ghosts, as in the reference below, one possible diagnosis is epidemic myalgia (Bornholm disease), an enteroviral illness characterized by fever, severe chest and abdominal pain (aggravated by the patient's attempts to breathe), and frontal headache. Abdominal pain, shortness of breath, and frontal headache were all independently signs of the presence of a ghost.[335]

19.387 [DIŠ NA *ina*] DIB ŠU.GIDIM.MA SAG ŠÀ-*šú* KÚM-*im* KÚM ŠÀ TUKU-*ši* SAG ŠÀ-*šú* [*i-k*] *a-as-sa-su* . . . (*AMT* 76/1:11–12)[336]

**[If, as the result of] affliction by "hand" of ghost, [a person]'s upper abdomen (epigastrium) is hot; he has feverish intestines, (and) his upper abdomen (epigastrium) gnaws at him . . .

19.388 DIŠ SAG ŠÀ-*šú* KÚM *u* ŠÀ.MEŠ-*šú* MÚ.MEŠ-*ḫu* DIB GU$_4$ / DIŠ SAG ŠÀ-*šú* KÚM-*ma* SA SAG.KI^{II}-*šú* ŠU^{II}-*šú u* GÌR^{II}-*šú* ZI.ME IGI^{II}-*šú* DUGUD-*šú* (DPS XIII B i 26′–27′ = *TDP* 112 i 30′–31′)

**If his epigastrium is hot and his insides are continually bloated, affliction by a ghost. If his epigastrium is hot and the blood vessels of his temples, his hands, and his feet continually (feel like they) are pulsating (and) his eyes bother him (affliction by a ghost).

In view of the distribution of ghost noises, it is not surprising to find ghost pains in the ears and abdomen, but the neck and heels were also prone to spectral attack.

19.389 *ina* GÚ-*šú* TAG-*su* ŠU.GIDIM.MA (*SpTU* 3.100:13)[337]

**(If) it hurts him intensely in his neck, "hand" of ghost.[338]

19.390 [DIŠ] NA GIDIM DIB-*su* MUD-*su šá-gi-ig* [SA] MUD-*šú u* SA.SAL-*šú šu-u*[*p*]-*šu-ḫi* . . . (Scheil, *RA* 14.88 i 3′–4′)

**[If] a ghost afflicts a person (and) his heel is stiff, in order to relax the muscles of his heel and Achilles tendon . . .

Particularly diagnostic of a ghost were one-sided pains. In addition to migraine headaches (see 13.156–13.163), ghosts were responsible for pains in the armpit as well as what we call sciatica. For more details on the latter, see Chapter 11.

19.391 [DIŠ S]U.GAM-*šú šá* 150 KÚ-*šú* KÚM NU TUKU *ár-da-na-an* ÚŠ DIB-*su* GAM (DPS XII D iv 20//E iv 27 = *TDP* 108 iv 20; cf. DPS XV:31 [AOAT 43.152])

**[If] his right ⸢armpit⸣[339] hurts him (but) he does not have a fever, the "double" of a dead man afflicts him; he will die.

19.392 [DIŠ N]A ŠU.⸢GIDIM$_4$⸣.MA DIB-*su-ma* Á ZAG/GÙB-*šú* TAG.TAG-*su* . . . (*BAM* 197:1–2, 8–9; *AMT* 97/4:2)[340]

**[If] "hand" of ghost afflicts a person (so that) his left/right side continually hurts him intensely . . .

Cases where severe aches and pains coincided with severe headaches (both of which were separately caused by ghosts) were, not surprisingly, also attributed to ghosts. The first reference below is probably to be connected with the flulike illness or illnesses described in Chapter 19.247–249 and especially with references in a number of texts in which "hand" of ghost, deputy of Ištar is blamed for a complex of headache and swollen or stinging eyes.[341] The headache and myalgia of influenza are particularly marked.

19.393 DIŠ NA SAG.KI.DIB.BA *ina* NU *a-dan-ni-šú* ÚS-*šú u mim-ma ina kal* UZU.MEŠ-*šú* TAG.TAG-*su* ŠU.GIDIM$_7$.MA *šá-né-e* ᵈ*Iš-tar ana* DIN-*šú* . . . (*BAM* 3 iii 7–9)[342]

**If a headache bothers a person to an abnormal extent and something continually hurts him intensely all over, "hand" of ghost, deputy of Ištar; to cure him, . . .

19.394 DIŠ TA MURUB$_4$ UGU-*šú* TAG-*su-ma šu-ru-ʾ-šú* SAG.KI-*šú* IGI-*šú* ÚNU-*šú* GÚ-*su* GABA-*su* ⸢*tu*⸣-[*l*] *u*??-[*šú* . . .] *kìn-ṣa-a*!-*šú ki-ṣal-la-šú* 1-*niš* KÚ.ME-*šú u ina* IGI MAŠ.MAŠ NU DU$_8$ GIDIM$_7$ DIB-*su-ma* ⸢ÚS⸣.[ÚS-*su*] (DPS III A obv. 22–23//C obv. 13–14 = *TDP* 18/20:13–14; cf. *AMT* 94/5:1–5)

**If from the middle of his skull it hurts him intensely and his eyelid,[343] his forehead, his eye, his cheek, his neck, his breast, his ⸢nipples⸣(?) [. . .] his legs, (and) his ankles all hurt him continually and (the pain) does not let up despite (lit. "in the face of") the *āšipu*('s efforts), a ghost afflicts him and [continually] pursues [him].

Problem Syndromes Due to Insufficient Information

The gods/goddesses some or all of whose syndromes fall into this category are Adad, Uraš, Ninurta, the "great gods," Ningeštinanna, the "god of the quay," the (mistress) of steppe and open country" and DINGIR.MAḪ. The number of texts and their length or details are limited, making interpretation difficult; see the Unsolved Puzzles Appendix.

Summary

It is hoped that, in the future, more references will be identified to clarify these ancient syndromes and that we will acquire a better understanding of the nature of the gods/goddesses and demons, permitting us to provide additional syndrome identifications. However, it is clear from our present analysis that ancient Mesopotamian physicians were motivated to understand the disease process as manifested by recurring patterns of signs and symptoms. Despite the presence of a plethora of gods/goddesses and demons, externally acting spiritual forces were not invariably blamed for illnesses. Even when they were, review of the ancient medical records makes it clear that the ancestor of the *āšipu* began by defining groups of disease characteristics that he observed in his patients and only afterward attempted to assign those groups of disease characteristics to divine or demonic causal agents. It is this empirical rather than theoretical approach to the practice of medicine that most strongly divides the ancient Mesopotamian from the ancient Greek physician. It is one of the ironies of history that it is the *āšipu*, and not the Hippocratic physician, who would better understand the basic foundations of the discipline as it is practiced today.

CHAPTER 20

Prognostics

If his mouth is warm, he will get well;
if his mouth is [cold, he will die].

—DPS VII A obv. 29 = *TDP* 62:29

The importance of correct diagnosis looms large in both ancient and modern medicine. It guides therapy and patient management, and can be the foundation for approaches to preventive measures. Prognosis is an allied skill that can require as much medical knowledge and intuition. The art of prognosis in the modern era, however, gets less recognition and attention, even though it can be important to the mental and emotional well-being of the patient and his or her family.

In ancient Mesopotamia, prognosis had a significant impact on therapy. When the case was considered to be hopeless,[1] the *āšipu* did not continue therapy, as do modern physicians.[2] This seems less strange when we realize that the *āšipu*'s treatments consisted not merely of medicine but also of what we consider "magic" and that continuing therapy could potentially have meant engaging in expensive sacrifices and elaborate magical rituals when it was certain that the patient was going to die. We should also remember that the ancient Mesopotamians had many medicines that were not hallmarked for specific diseases but designed instead to alleviate specific symptoms (such as pain). Any of these treatments could have been applied to terminal cases without violation of the "no treatment" rule.[3]

This "no-treatment" rule has interesting implications when the "signs and symptoms" and prognoses listed in the ancient Mesopotamian diagnostic/prognostic handbook are put back into their original context. At first glance, there is a superficial resemblance between ancient Mesopotamian diagnostic and prognostic texts and omens. In both cases, there was an enumeration of "signs" derived from observations of everyday life followed by a positive or negative prediction, and in both cases there was a treatment or ritual to be performed in order to avoid death or disaster.

If what a person observed while walking in the street (or what the *āšipu* observed on his way to the patient as is outlined in the first two tablets of the diagnostic/prognostic handbook) contained a favorable omen ("his house will prosper"; "the patient will live"), all was well, and the pedestrian or *āšipu* needed to do nothing in order to benefit. If, however, the observation was of something ill-omened ("his house will be scattered"; "the patient will die"), the pedestrian or *āšipu* was well advised to perform a special type of apotropaic magic ritual called a NAM.BÚR.BI in order to avert the portended evil.

Due to the rule that forbade the *āšipu* from treating hopeless cases, however, observations taken at the patient's bedside (Tablets III to LX of the diagnostic/prognostic handbook) operated by a completely contrary principle; it was precisely those medical "signs and symptoms" with a *favorable* prognosis ("he will get well") that received treatment, magical or otherwise. As if to underline this difference, the verbal tenses used to describe patients' signs and symptoms in Tablets III to LX of the diagnostic and prognostic handbook are the same as those used in the therapeutic texts and are different from those used in Tablets I to II and in the omen literature generally.[4]

This inverted relationship between ancient Mesopotamian medicine and ancient Mesopotamian omens is most clearly evident in those medical conditions that were also considered ominous (i.e., they had both a prediction for the future and a prognosis). Although one might expect a treatable ailment to have a good prediction and vice versa, there are some quite dramatic examples of bad predictions attached to treatable conditions and of good predictions paired with "he will die" or at least with "he will die unless you treat him right away."

20.1 [DIŠ *ina* MU].⌜3⌝.KÁM ŠUB-*su* AD-*šú* DINGIR TUKU-*ši* LÚ.TUR BI *ina* MU BI ÚŠ *ana* ZI-*ḫi*... (DPS XXIX:25 [AOAT 43.320])

**[If] (spawn of Šulpaea) falls on him [in] the third[5] [year], his father will obtain a personal god; that infant will die in the same year; to remove it...

In short, the condition was potentially fatal but a good omen for the victim's father. By contrast, a ringing left ear was treatable but nonetheless portended ill for the patient after cure.

20.2 DIŠ GEŠTU 15-*šú* GÙ.GÙ-*si* DIN (DPS VIII 8a = *TDP* 68:8a)

**If his left ear continually rings, he will get well.

20.3 DIŠ NA GEŠTU ZAG-*šú* GÙ.GÙ-*si me-si-ru* DIB-*su* (*BAM* 155 ii 5′//Labat, *RSO* 32.112 iii 10′; cf. *BAM* 506:8′; DPS VIII 10a = *TDP* 68:10a)[6]

**If a person's left ear continually rings, hard times will afflict him.

If you had this or any other medical problem with a favorable prognosis but one that was ill-omened, both the ghost NAM.BÚR.BI and the relevant treatment (in this case maximally the rather elaborate ghost-laying ritual for ringing in the ears) would have been in order. If your problem had a bad outcome and was fatal, you could skip the medical treatment, but still needed to perform the NAM.BÚR.BI, and if it had a good outcome but was fatal, nothing needed to be done on either account. If your problem had a good outcome and a reasonably favorable prognosis, you could skip the NAM.BÚR.BI but would still receive treatment for your condition, as in the following example. The appended medical treatment comes almost as a shock. Would we be eager to remove something that we believed would make us rich?

20.4 [DIŠ *ina* MU].20.KÁM ŠUB-*su* NÍG.TUKU NÍG.GA DAGAL.ME *ana* ZI-*ḫi*... (DPS XXIX:15 [AOAT 43.319])

**[If] (^{d}LUGAL.ÙR.RA) falls on him [in] the twentieth [year], he will become rich (and) his possessions will be numerous; to remove it . . .

This chapter will focus on individual signs or symptoms and how they influenced the prognosis expressed by the *āšipu*. For this reason, the prognoses rendered by the *āšipu* for specific diseases or syndromes have not been discussed here but in the chapters dealing with particular diseases. Insofar as possible, those references that have more than one sign or symptom have been avoided to prevent confusion as to which sign or symptom led the *āšipu* to render a particular prognosis.

Mental Status Change

The *āšipu* described changes in mental function by a variety of statements and phrases, including "not in full possession of his faculties," difficulty speaking, "he wanders about (in a confused fashion)," "does not know where he is," mumbling and talking nonsense, lack of awareness, memory deficit, purposeless movements, abnormal emotional behavior, and loss of consciousness.

"NOT IN FULL POSSESSION OF HIS FACULTIES"

20.5 [DIŠ U]Š$_4$-*šú šá-ni-šu-ma* UŠ$_4$-*šú* NU DIB ŠU GIDIM *mur-tap-pi-du* GAM (DPS XXII:47a [AOAT 43.255])

**[If] his ⌜mentation⌝ is altered so that he is not in full possession of his faculties, "hand" of a roving ghost; he will die.

DIFFICULTY SPEAKING

20.6 DIŠ GIG MURUB$_4$ *u* ŠÀ GIG-*ma* ZI-*bi u* DU$_{10}$.GAM *rit-ta-šú paṭ-rat* KA-*šú ana* INIM.INIM *da-an* GAM (DPS XVII:56 [AOAT 43.200])

**If he is sick with an illness of the hips and abdomen and he gets up and (has to) squat down, his hand will open (but) his mouth is too strong for the words, he will die.

MUMBLING AND TALKING NONSENSE

20.7 [DIŠ UŠ$_4$]-*šú* MAN.MAN-*ni* DUG$_4$.DUG$_4$-*šú* KÚR.KÚR *mim-mu-ú i-qab-bu-ú i-ma-áš-šú* IM *ku-tal-*[*l*] *i* DIB-*su* 1-*ma* KÚR-*iš* GAM (DPS XXII:49–50 [AOAT 43.255])

**[If] his [mentation] is continually altered, what he says is continually unintelligible and he forgets whatever he says, a wind from behind afflicts him; he will die alone like a stranger.

The causes of mental change are multiple, such as shock from blood loss or sepsis syndrome, infections including meningitis and enteric fever, head trauma, and metabolic abnormalities such as that caused by liver failure. In many of the reviewed references, it is clear that the patients suffered wounds, infections, head trauma, or heart or lung disease.

WANDERING ABOUT AND "DOES NOT KNOW WHERE HE IS"

20.8 DIŠ KI.MIN-*ma ina* ÉLLAG-*šú šá* 15 SÌG-*iṣ* UŠ$_4$-*šú* NU DIB *ina* NU ZU *ú-rap-pad* ŠU ^{d}MAŠ.TAB.BA GA[M] (DPS XV:39 [AOAT 43.152]; cf. DPS XII D iii 21//E iii 22 = *TDP* 104 iii 21)

**If (it is the first day he is sick) and he was wounded on his left kidney, he is not in full possession of his faculties (and) he wanders about without knowing (where he is), "hand" of the twin gods; he will die.

Some of the conditions causing mental status change would be reversible with the aid of modern medicine, but the treatments available in ancient Mesopotamia would have had little chance of success. The *āšipu*, therefore, predicted a fatal outcome in almost all situations where these mental changes occurred.

LACK OF AWARENESS

20.9 DIŠ TA *re-še-ti ana še-pe-ti* TA *še-pe-ti ana re-še-ti ina* NU ZU BAL.BAL GAM (DPS XVII:63 [AOAT 43.201])

**If he keeps turning round from the head end to the foot end of the bed (and) from the foot end to the head end without realizing it, he will die.

MEMORY DEFICIT

20.10 DIŠ *ina* U$_4$-*mi šá* GIG GIG-*su* DUGUD-*su-ma* ZU-*šú* NU *ú-ád-da* GAM (DPS XVII:73 [AOAT 43.202])

**If on the day he becomes ill, his illness becomes so difficult that he does not recognize person(s) known to him, he will die.

PURPOSELESS MOVEMENTS

20.11 [DIŠ ŠU^{II}-*šú*] AD$_6$-*šú ma-gal* TAG.MEŠ GIN$_7$ TAG.MEŠ NU ZU [GAM] (DPS XI A obv. 30//B 29 = *TDP* 92:30//*SpTU* 1.34:29)[7]

**[If his hands] continually rub his ⌜body⌝ a lot (and) he does not realize that they are continually rubbing (it), [he will die].

Of eighty-eight texts mentioning some type of mental status change, eighty-six of the patients were predicted by the *āšipu* to die. The two texts that predicted survival indicated that the patients were tested and shown to be conscious.

20.12 DIŠ SA SAG.KI^{II}-*šú* ŠU^{II}-*šú* GÌR^{II}-*šú* GÚ-*šú pa-pan* ŠÀ-*šú* DU.MEŠ *u* SU-*šú* ŠED$_7$ *za-mar* IGI DU$_8$ DUL-*ma ni-š*[*i*] (DPS IV A r. 1//B r. 14 = *TDP* 42 r. 34)[8]

**If the blood vessel(s) of his temples, his hands, his feet, his neck, and his umbilical area[9] "go" and his body is cold, (if) he occasionally opens and closes his eyes, there may be a recovery.

Seizures

Seizures can occur at any time but are most common at night, especially when the patient is falling asleep or waking up. It is apparent that the ancient Mesopotamian physician understood this pattern. It is also clear from the following texts that when seizures began to appear more frequently and during the day, the patient's prognosis was worse. This conclusion is compatible with our current knowledge of the problem.

20.13 [DIŠ ŠUB-*ti* ŠUB]-*su-ma* MU.1.KÁM ŠUB-*šú-ma ana* GIZKIM-*šú-ma* LÁ-*šú na-kid* AN.TA.ŠUB.BA *ina ma-šal* U$_4$-*mi uš-ta-qar-rab-šú-ma* DUGUD-*su* (DPS XXVI:8′ [AOAT 43.279])

** [If a falling spell falls] upon him and it has been falling upon him for one year and as its sign it comes over him, it is worrisome. (If) the AN.TA.ŠUB.BA (seizures) come closely spaced (and) in the middle of the day, it will be difficult for him.

20.14 DIŠ UB.NÍGIN.NA-*šú i-tar-ru-ra i-ṭa-ma-a u* IGI.MEŠ-*šú* NIGIN.MEŠ-*du* AN.TA.ŠUB.BA *ina ma-šal* U$_4$-*mi* DUGUD-*su* (DPS XXVI:71′ [AOAT 43.284])

**If his limbs tremble (and) twist and his face seems continually to spin, AN.TA.ŠUB.BA (seizure). (If this happens) in the middle of the day, it will be difficult for him.

Core Body Temperature

The temperature of deep tissues of the body is called core temperature. When it falls below normal, it is referred to as hypothermia, and this generally indicates a potentially lethal cold exposure or shock (low blood pressure). Shock has multiple causes, and all can result in death. Assessment of body temperature was a major preoccupation of the *āšipu*. He assessed the skin temperature in many areas; however, surface temperature may be a poor indicator of core temperature. Much of the body surface can be affected by local vascular tone that can make the skin feel warm or cold, depending on the level of blood circulating through the skin.

20.15 DIŠ KI.MIN ŠU^{II}-*šú u* GÌR-*šú* ŠED$_7$?! GIG-*su* KÚR-*šum-ma* UGU-*šú i-sap-pi-du-ma* DIN (DPS XVI:93′ [AOAT 43.180])

**If (he is in his seventies and) his hands and feet are cold,[10] (even if) his illness changes so that they beat their breasts over him, he will get well.

Local infections and the need to conserve or dissipate body heat can also influence skin temperature. The *āšipu* would have learned from experience that certain parts of the body were more reliable indicators of prognosis. Modern physicians have determined that temperatures measured in the mouth, ear canal, and rectum approximate the core temperature because they are less subject to local vascular changes. It seems clear from the texts below that ancient Mesopotamian physicians associated poor prognosis with low temperatures at body sites that reflect core temperature.

20.16 [DIŠ ŠÀ]-*š*[*ú*] KÚM *r*[*uq-q*]*í* GEŠTU^{II}-*šú* ŠED$_7$.MEŠ *ḫaṭ-ṭu* ŠED$_7$.MEŠ *ina* KA-*šú* DU.MEŠ GÍD-*ma* GAM / [DIŠ ŠÀ-*šú*] KÚM.MEŠ *ruq-qí* GEŠTU^{II}-*šú* KÚM.MEŠ *ḫaṭ-ṭu* KÚM.MEŠ *ina* KA-*šú* DU.MEŠ *ni-ši* (DPS XIII B i 52′–55′//F 11–12//G$_2$ 2–3 = *TDP* 116 i 56′–59′ [coll.])

**[If] ⌜his⌝ [abdomen] is hot (and) his ear⌜canals⌝ are cold (and) the scepter of the cold goes to his mouth, (if) it is prolonged, he will die. [If his abdomen] is continually hot (and) his ear canals are hot (and) the scepter of the heat goes to his mouth, (there will be a) recovery.

20.17 DIŠ KA-*šú* KÚM DIN : DIŠ KA-*šú* [ŠED$_7$ GAM] (DPS VII A obv. 29 = *TDP* 62:29)

**If his mouth is hot, he will get well; if his mouth is [cold, he will die].

Nose temperature generally approximates core body temperature.

20.18 [DIŠ KIR$_4$-*šú* KÚM DI]N : DIŠ KIR$_4$-*šú* ŠED$_7$ GAM (DPS VI A obv. 3 = *TDP* 54:3)

** [If his nose is hot], ⌜he will get well⌝. If his nose is cold, he will die.

Other surfaces, however, did not have a consistent relationship between low temperature and poor prognosis.

20.19 DIŠ SAG.KI-*su ka-ṣa-at* DIN (DPS IV B r. 22//E iv 6a = *TDP* 44 r. 45//*SpTU* 3.88 iv 6a)

**If his forehead is cold, he will get well.

20.20 DIŠ IGI.MEŠ-*šú* ŠED$_7$.MEŠ GAM (DPS IX A 36//B obv. 35 = *TDP* 74:36)

**If his face is continually cold, he will die.

20.21 DIŠ SA SAG.KI^{II}-*šú* ŠU^{II}-*šú* GÌR^{II}-*šú* GÚ-*šú pa-pan* ŠÀ-*šú* DU.MEŠ *u* SU-*šú* ŠED$_7$ *za-mar* IGI DU$_8$ DUL-*ma ni-š*[*i*] (DPS IV A r. 1//B r. 14 = *TDP* 42 r. 34)

**If the blood vessel(s) of his temples, his hands, his feet, his neck, and his umbilical area[11] "go" and his body is cold,[12] (if) he occasionally opens and closes his eyes, there may be a recovery.

Pulses

As previously discussed (see Chapter 8), the *āšipu* used the term "*go*" in relation to blood vessels in various parts of the body. We have concluded that this term means an arterial pulse that could not be felt for some reason, that is, a very rapid pulse making detection of individual pulses difficult, a drop in blood pressure causing a weak pulse, or (least likely) atherosclerosis causing arterial rigidity that would make it difficult to feel the pulse. The *āšipu* determined that in most cases when pulses were difficult to feel the patients had a poor prognosis (seven of eight references). The following text is quite likely to be a patient with low blood pressure (shock), and death would be a probable outcome.

20.22 DIŠ SAG ŠÀ-*šú ana em-ši-šú* DU-*ak u* AD$_6$-*šú* ŠED$_7$ GAM (DPS XIII B i 31′//D 5 = *TDP* 114 i 35')

**If (the blood vessels of) his upper abdomen (epigastrium) or his lower abdomen (hypogastric region) "go"[13] and his body is cold, he will die.

In other texts, the underlying problems are less clear, but the outcomes are usually grave.

20.23 [DIŠ S]A ⸢SAG⸣.KI^{II}-*šú šá* 15 *u* 150 DU.ME-*ma u* IGI^{II}-*šú ú-rat-ta* GAM (DPS IV A$_2$ r. 23+A$_2$ r. 7//B r. 4 = *TDP* 40 r. 23; cf. *SpTU* 3.86 obv. 1–2)

**[If] the ⸢blood vessel(s)⸣ of his ⸢temples⸣, the ones on the left and the ones on the right, "go" and he fixes his eyes, he will die.[14]

20.24 [DIŠ SA] ⸢SAG⸣.KI^{II}-*šú šá* 15 *u* 150 DU.ME-*ma* ŠÀ-*šú* DIB-*su* GAM / [DIŠ SA] ⸢SAG⸣.KI^{II}-*šú šá* 15 *u* 150 DU.ME-*ma* DUL.DUL *u* BAL.BAL GAM (DPS IV A$_2$ r. 24–25+A$_2$ r. 8–9//B r. 5–6 = *TDP* 40 r. 24–25)

**[If the blood vessel(s)] of his temples, the ones on the left and the ones on the right, "go" and his abdomen afflicts him, he will die. [If the blood vessel(s) of] his temples, the ones on the left and the ones on the right, "go" and he veils himself (i.e., withdraws from social intercourse) and has changes of mood, he will die.

20.25 [DIŠ SA SA]G.KI^{II}-*šú* ⸢*šá*⸣ 15 *u* 150 *ina* DU-*ki im-taḫ-ru* SÌG-*iṣ* [MA]ŠKIM SÌG-*iṣ* ^{LÚ}MAŠ.MAŠ DÙ-*uš* DIN⸣ [: GAM] / [DIŠ SA] ⸢SAG⸣.KI^{II}-*šú šá* 15 *u* 150 DU.MEŠ-*ma*[15] SAG.KI-*šú ú-sa-dar-šu* GAM (DPS IV A$_2$ r. 20–22+A$_5$ r. 4–6//B r. 2–3 = *TDP* 40 r. 20–22; cf. Labat, *Syria* 33.125–126 r. 13–14)

**[If the blood vessel(s)] of his ⸢temples⸣, the ones on the left and the ones on the right, "go" to an equal extent, he was struck with the blow of a ⸢*rābiṣu*⸣ (see 19.115–19.120). You may do his medical treatment; he will get well [or die]. [If the blood vessel(s)] of his temples, the ones on the left and the ones on the right, "go" and his temple does this to him several times in a row, he will die.

Slow pulses also were viewed by the *āšipu* with concern. It is quite possible that the slow pulse rates were due to a conduction defect in the heart.

20.26 [DIŠ DIB-*su-ma* SA.MEŠ?] *nu-uḫ-ḫu-ú* DIB DINGIR-*šú* GAM (DPS XIX/XX:109′a [AOAT 43.232])

**[If it afflicts him and the blood vessels(?)] are slow, affliction by his god; he will die.

20.27 [DIŠ] SA GÌR^{II}-*šú* DU-*ku-ma šá* ŠU^{II}-*šú ne-e-ḫu ár-ḫiš* ÚŠ : AL.TI (DPS XIV A iv 23 = *TDP* 144 iv 58′)

**[If] the blood vessel(s) of his feet "go" and those of his hands are slow, he will speedily die (var. he will get well).

Excessively rapid heart rates can also be a sign of serious cardiac abnormality that can have poor prognosis. Pulsating, trembling, and fluttering heart are terms used to describe very rapid heart rates.

20.28 DIŠ GABA-*su* DU$_8$.MEŠ-*át* SAG.KI-*šú* ŠUB-*ut* MÚD *ina* KA/KIR$_4$-*šú pi-qam la p*[*i-qam*] ⌜DU⌝-*k*[*a*] ŠÀ-*šú pi-qam la pi-qam* MUD-*ud* ŠU ^{d}AMAR.UTU *a-dir-ma* BA.ÚŠ (DPS XII A 2–3 = *TDP* 100 i 2–3)

**If his chest is clear,[16] (the blood vessels of) his temple have collapsed, blood incessantly flows from his mouth/nose, (and) his heart incessantly shudders, "hand" of Marduk; he will be worried and die.

20.29 DIŠ KUŠ *šá* KI.TA-*nu* GÌR^{II}-*šú te-bi* SAG.DU-*su* DIB.DIB-*su u* ŠÀ-*šú tur-ru-ur* GAM (DPS XIV A iv 19–20 = *TDP* 144 iv 54′–55′)[17]

**If the skin on the bottom of his feet continually (feels like it) is pulsating, his head continually afflicts him, and his abdomen trembles, he will die.

Breathing

The importance of breathing to sustain life was certainly known by the ancient Mesopotamians. Twenty-three texts were reviewed that mentioned some type of abnormal breathing. Death was the predicted outcome in all references. The texts describe airway obstruction in the following ways: "grabbing of the throat," "larynx makes croaking noises," "choking," and "lungs sing like a reed flute," as in the following examples.

20.30 DIŠ ZI.ḪA.ZA SAG.ÚS DIB.DIB-*su u* ÍR ÚŠ-*ma* EGIR-*šú* AD-*šú* [GAM] (DPS X A obv. 38 = *TDP* 84:38)

**If persistent "grabbing of the throat" continually afflicts him and he wails, if he dies, afterward his father [will die].

20.31 DIŠ GÚ.MUR-*su i-ḫar-ru-ur* GAM (DPS X A obv. 29//B obv. 33 = *TDP* 84:29)[18]

**If his larynx makes a croaking noise he will die.

Physicians also mentioned the nose being blocked off, breath seized in the nose,[19] and rapid breathing.[20]

20.32 DIŠ KIR$_4$-*šú* BAD.BAD-*ir* GAM (DPS VI A obv. 4b = *TDP* 54:4b)

**If his nose is completely blocked off, he will die.

20.33 DIŠ ^{NA4}KIŠIB GÚ-*šú* DU$_8$ SA.MEŠ-*šú* GAR-*nu u* PA.AN.BI *ina* KIR$_4$-*šú* DIB.DIB GIG BI NU DIN (DPS X A obv. 24//B obv. 27 = *TDP* 82:24; cf. *SpTU* 3.86 obv. 3–4)[21]

**If his vertebra was (cut) open (and) his blood vessels are present but his breath is "seized" in his nose, that patient will not get well.

20.34 DIŠ ZI-*šú* GU$_4$.UD.ME *u* SA.MEŠ-*šú šap-ku* GAM / DIŠ ZI-*šú i-tar-rak-ma qit-ru-bat* [G]AM (DPS X A obv. 31//B obv. 35–36 = *TDP* 84:31)[22]

**If his breath becomes rapid[23] and his muscles are tense, he will die. If his breath throbs and comes closely spaced, ⌜he will die⌝.

Ḫūqu is another term the *āšipu* used to indicate a specific breathing pattern (see p. 340). In the following reference, we believe that it refers to a terminal respiratory pattern secondary to brain damage.

20.35 DIŠ U$_4$.5.KÁM U$_4$.10.KÁM GIG *dan-na* GIG-*ma uš-tar-di-ma* GI$_6$ IGI^{II}-*šú uš-ter-di-a* U$_4$.2.KÁM *ḫu-qu* DIB.DIB-*su ina* U$_4$.3.KÁM GAM (DPS XVI:53′–54′ [AOAT 43.177])

**If he has been sick with a mighty sickness for five or ten days and the pupils of his eyes persist in (moving) downward, (and) *ḫūqu* continually afflicts him for two days, he will die on the third day.

Skin Color Changes

DARK

Forty-seven texts were reviewed that mentioned dark skin in some part of the body. This color change was probably due to either cyanosis or gangrene or both. Cyanosis indicates inadequate oxygen supply to the blood, while gangrene is tissue death due to the interruption of the blood supply by trauma or blood vessel disease. Diseases causing either of these problems are serious, and a poor prognosis is understandable in either case. In all forty-seven of the reviewed references, the *āšipu* considered the prognosis to be bad, and most often the patients died. Below are some examples.

20.36 [DIŠ GIG KIR$_4$-*šú* SA$_5$ DI]N : DIŠ KIR$_4$-*šú* GI$_6$ ⌜GAM⌝ (DPS VI A obv. 1 = *TDP* 54:1)

**[If the patient's nose is red],[24] ⌜he will get well⌝. If his nose is dark, he will die.

20.37 DIŠ ŠIR^{II}-*šú* GI$_6$.MEŠ GAM (DPS XIV A$_2$ ii 6//C ii 24 = *TDP* 136 ii 56)

**If his testicles are black, he will die.

20.38 [DI]Š ÚR.MEŠ-*šú tar-ka na-ḫi-id* (DPS XIV G iii 8a = *TDP* 138 iii 10)

**⌜If⌝ (both) of his thighs are dark, it is worrisome.

DARK RED

There were sixteen texts that referred to some skin surface as dark red. This description probably does not apply to gangrenous areas since this usually looks quite black. Instead, it probably indicates tissue that has a lower than normal oxygen level. There are many possible causes, and most are serious conditions with high fatality rates. Again, the *āšipu* recognized the seriousness of this sign, and indicated a poor prognosis in all sixteen references.

20.39 DIŠ ŠIR^{II}-*šú du-ʾ-um-ma* GIG-*su* DUGUD (DPS XIV A_2 ii 8//C ii 25 = *TDP* 136 ii 58)

**If his testicles are dark red, his illness will be difficult.

20.40 [DIŠ GU].⌜DU 150⌝-*šu du-ʾ-ú-mat* GIG-*su* MAN-*ni* (DPS XIV C i 6′ = *TDP* 130 i 45)

** [If] his right ⌜buttock⌝ is dark red, his illness will change (for the worse).

RED

When the *āšipu* described areas of skin as red, he was probably indicating inflamed skin. This inflammation could be due to local infection, trauma, or chemical irritation. These conditions could be serious illnesses, but others might be mild, self-limited diseases. Of the eighteen texts reviewed, four were given a poor prognosis by the ancient physicians. Below are some examples.

20.41 DIŠ ŠIR^{II}-*šú* SA_5.MEŠ DIN (DPS XIV A_2 ii 4//C ii 23 = *TDP* 136 ii 54)

**If his testicles are red, he will get well.

20.42 DIŠ IGI.MEŠ-*šú ṣar-pu u i-ša-ap-pu-ú* ŠU ^{d}IM GAM/DIN (DPS IX A 28/B 26 = *TDP* 74:28)

**If his face is bright red and swells up like a cloud, "hand" of Adad; he will die (var. B: live).

YELLOW (JAUNDICE)

When the skin takes on a yellow color, it is often due to some type of liver disease. Even at the present time, this finding often indicates a serious and potentially fatal disease. However, some forms of viral hepatitis can cause transient, nonfatal jaundice.

Another cause of yellow skin is the result of bleeding under the skin. Initially the skin color is blue or purple, but with time the color evolves to yellow before it disappears completely. In this case the yellow color is localized, and the cause of bleeding can be either serious or benign. In reviewing twenty-three ancient texts that described yellow skin, twenty-one indicated a poor prognosis and often death. Some of these texts are shown below.

20.43 [DIŠ] TI 15-*šú* SIG_7 SILIM!-*ma* DIN (DPS XII C 9′ = *SpTU* 1.35:9′)

** [If] his left rib is yellow, he is safe and will get well.

20.44 DIŠ SAG KIR$_4$-*šú* SIG$_7$ GAM (DPS VI A obv. 25a = *TDP* 56:25a)

**If the bulb of his nose is yellow, he will die.

20.45 DIŠ IGI.MEŠ-*šú* KÚR.KÚR-*ru* EME-*šú* SIG$_7$: SU-*šú* SIG$_7$ TÙN.GIG *ana* U$_4$.3.KÁM GAM (DPS IX A 31 = *TDP* 74:31)

**If his face continually alters (and) his tongue is yellow (var. his body is yellow), "sick liver"; (if he has been sick) for three days, he will die.

20.46 DIŠ KI.MIN-*ma* IGI^{II}.MEŠ-*šú* GIN$_7$ *si-ka-a-ti ana* GA.RAŠ^{SAR} SIG$_7$.ME GAM (DPS XVI:91′ [AOAT 43.180])

**If (he is in his seventies) and his eyes are as yellow as the "peg" on a leek, he will die.

Blood Loss

Ancient societies including Mesopotamia certainly made the association between major blood loss and death. Therefore, it should be no surprise that ancient Mesopotamian physicians often viewed blood loss in their patients as a bad sign. The *āšipu*, however, understood that some types of blood loss were not as serious. For instance, uncomplicated nosebleed was considered to be benign.

20.47 DIŠ KI.MIN MÚD *ina* KIR$_4$ DU-*ku* DIN (DPS XVI:96′ [AOAT 43.180])

**If (he is in his seventies and) blood flows from his nose, he will get well.

20.48 DIŠ KI.MIN-*ma* MÚD *ina* KIR$_4$/KA-*šú* DU-⸢*ku*⸣-*ma* U$_4$ *u* [GI$_6$ . . .] ŠU ^{d}MAŠ BÚR-*ma* DIN (DPS XXI:6–7 [AOAT 43.246]; cf. StBoT 36.34 obv. 8′)

**If (his blood vessels are healthy) but blood flows from his nose/mouth and it [does not stop(?)] day or [night], "hand" of Ninurta; if it lets up, he will get well.

Nosebleeds associated with other complicating problems, however, were not so benign.

20.49 [DIŠ D]IRI.MEŠ-*pú* ŠÀ.MEŠ-*šú* MÚ.MEŠ-*ḫu* PIŠ$_{10}$ IGI^{II}-*šú* MÚ.MEŠ-*ḫu* MURGU GÌR^{II}-*šú* MÚ.MEŠ *u* MÚD *ina* KIR$_4$-*šú šá* GÙB DU-*ku* ŠU NAM.ÉRIM.MA GAM (DPS XXII:19–20 [AOAT 43.253])

**[If (his eyes)] drift downstream (horizontal nystagmus; see Chapter 13), his insides are bloated, the rims of his eyes are swollen, the soles of his feet are swollen, and blood flows from his right nostril, "hand" of curse; he will die.

The most serious source of blood loss appears to have been the vomiting of blood. All twenty-one texts that mention this received a poor prognosis, usually death. In some cases, the bleeding was due to an abdominal war wound. It is our belief that other cases represent bleeding from esophageal varicose veins (see Chapter 15) and peptic ulcers (see Chapter 6). Cancers of the esophagus and stomach are additional causes. In the absence of modern transfusion therapy, all these conditions would commonly lead to the death of the patient.

20.50 DIŠ *ina* ŠÀ-*šú* SÌG-*ma u* MÚD MUD ŠUB.ŠUB-*a* DIB-*it* ^{d}MAŠ.TAB.BA GAM (DPS XIII B ii 20 = *TDP* 118 ii 20)

**If he was wounded on his abdomen and, consequently, he continually produces dark blood, affliction by the twin gods; he will die.

20.51 DIŠ *ina* SAG ŠÀ-*šú* ^{GIŠ}NÍG.GIDRU GAR-*su-ma u* MÚD MUD ŠUB.ŠUB-*a* GAM (DPS XIII B i 36′ = *TDP* 114 i 43′)

**If a burning pain[25] is firmly established in his upper abdomen (epigastrium) and he continually produces dark blood, he will die.

20.52 DIŠ *ina* SAG ŠÀ-*šú di-ik-šú u* ^{GIŠ}NÍG.GIDRU GAR-*nu-šum-ma* MÚD *i-ḫa-ḫu ana* U_4.2.KÁM *ana* U_4.3.KÁM GAM (DPS XIII B i 39′ = *TDP* 114 i 43′)

**If a needling pain or burning pain is firmly established in his upper abdomen (epigastrium) and he vomits blood (and he has been sick) for two or three days, he will die.

20.53 DIŠ *ina* GIG-*šú* 1-*šú* 2-*šú ina* IGI ZÉ *i-ḫa-ḫu* EGIR-*nu* MÚD *i-ḫa-ḫu* GAM (DPS XVII:27 [AOAT 43.197])

**If once or twice during (the course of) his illness, he first vomits bile and afterward vomits blood, he will die.

Bleeding into the urinary tract (hematuria), like nosebleed, could represent either a serious or benign problem. One usually benign although painful cause of hematuria was kidney stones. Another condition that can be either benign or serious is hematuria from *Schistosomiasis hematobium* (see Chapter 5). This is such a common infection in the Middle East today that many people there consider hematuria a quasi-normal state of affairs. Such attitudes may well have existed in ancient Mesopotamia.

20.54 DIŠ KÀŠ.MEŠ-*šú* SA_5.MEŠ ŠU DINGIR-*šú* DIN (DPS XIV A ii 39//C ii 14 = *TDP* 134 ii 39)

**If his urine is reddish, "hand" of his god; he will get well.

20.55 DIŠ KI.MIN-[*m*]*a ina* KÀŠ-*šú* MÚD *iš-tin ana* KI GIG GAM (DPS XVI:7 [AOAT 43.172])

**If (it is the first day he is sick) and he urinates blood in his urine, he is at an acute stage of the illness;[26] he will die.

The eyes represent a bleeding site that provoked a uniformly bad prognosis. All nine references with bleeding into the eyes had serious outcomes, often death. It seems likely that bleeding into the eyes in most cases was due to some generalized clotting defect such as reduced levels of clotting factors seen in patients with advanced liver failure (see Chapter 6). In some references the patients had multiple bleeding sites, as would be expected with clotting factor defects.

20.56 DIŠ U_4.5.KÁM GIG-*ma* UZU.MEŠ-*šú* SIG_7 ŠUB-*ú* IGI^{II}-*šú* MÚD DIRI.MEŠ GAM (DPS XVI:47′ [AOAT 43.176])

**If he has been sick for five days and his flesh is unevenly colored with yellow (and) his eyes are full of blood, he will die.

20.57 [DIŠ . . . S]IG$_7$ DIRI IGI^{II}-*šú* MÚD DIRI.MEŠ NINDA *šá* KÚ *ina* ŠÀ-*šú* NU *ina-aḫ is-ḫur-ma* DUB-*ka* GAM (DPS XVIII:42′ [AOAT 43.219])

**[If his abdomen?] is full of ⌜yellow spots⌝, his eyes are full of blood, the bread that he eats does not rest easy in his stomach but it turns about and pours (it) out, he will die.

Pain

20.58 DIŠ U$_4$.5.KÁM U$_4$.6.KÁM GIG-*ma uš-tar-di-ma ia-ú ia-ú la ú-kal-la* GAM (DPS XVI:48′ [AOAT 43.176])

**If he has been sick for five or six days and he persists in not being able to stop (crying out): "Yow, Yow!" he will die.

20.59 DIŠ *ina kal* USU-*šú* GÙ-*si* U$_4$.1.K[Á]M U$_4$.2.KÁM GIG-*ma* GÙ-*šú im-ṭi* GAM (DPS XXII:60 [AOAT 43.256])

**If he cries out with all his force, he is sick for one or two days, and his crying gets softer, he will die.

Most modern physicians would agree that the more severe the pain, the greater the chance of a serious medical problem. There are some conditions, however, such as kidney stones and labor, that can cause severe pain but that generally have a benign outcome. The ancient Mesopotamian physician seems to have appreciated that severe pain was a sign of poor prognosis. In the following references, the patient who could not lie on his back had more severe pain and a poorer prognosis.

20.60 DIŠ ÉLLAG.MEŠ-*šú* KÚ.ME-*šú na-ḫi-id* (DPS XII D iii 12 = *TDP* 104 iii 12)

**If (both) his kidneys hurt him, it is worrisome.

20.61 DIŠ ÉLLAG.ME-*šú* KÚ.ME-*šú-ma ina* UGU-*ši-na* NÁ-*al* DIN PA NU TUKU (DPS XII D iii 15 = *TDP* 104 iii 15)

**If (both) his kidneys hurt him so that he can lie on them, he will get well; it is of no consequence.[27]

20.62 DIŠ ÉLLAG.MEŠ-*šú* KÚ.ME-*šú-ma ina* UGU-*ši-na* N[U N]Á-*al ana* U$_4$.15.KÁM GAM (DPS XII D iii 18//F 17 = *TDP* 104 iii 18)

**If (both) his kidneys hurt him so that he ⌜cannot⌝ lie on them (and he has been sick for) fifteen days, he will die.

There are forty-two additional texts that mention conditions causing severe pain in various parts of the body. This pain is variously described, "(sensation of being) broken in pieces," "viselike," "burning" or "needling," as in the following examples.

20.63 DIŠ SAG.KI-*šú* DIB-*su-ma* KI.MIN SA SAG.KI-*šú ma-gal* ZI.MEŠ *u e-li* SAG.DU-*šú ḫa-biš* GAM (DPS IV B obv. 9//D 9 = *TDP* 32:9)

**If his temple afflicts him so that (he continually cries out), his temporal blood vessels (feel like they) are pulsating greatly, (and) the upper part of his head (feels like it) was broken in pieces, he will die.

20.64 DIŠ SAG.KI *ḫe-si-ma* GEŠTU.MEŠ-*šú* NU ŠE.GA-*a* ŠU DINGIR-*šú* UGU-*šú um-mu-da* GAM (DPS IV B obv. 4 = *TDP* 32:4)

**If he has a viselike headache,[28] and his ears do not hear, the "hand" of his god has been imposed on him; he will die.

20.65 DIŠ *ina* SAG ŠÀ-*šú di-ik-šú u* ^{GIŠ}NÍG.GIDRU GAR-*nu-šum-ma* MÚD *i-te-zi* GAM (DPS XIII B i 38′ = *TDP* 114 i 42′)

**If a needling pain or burning pain is firmly established in his upper abdomen (epigastrium) and he excretes blood, he will die.

The texts below are similar except for the character of the pain (needling versus burning) and the outcome (survival versus death).

20.66 DIŠ *ina* ŠÀ-*šú* Á 15-*šú di-ik-šu* GAR-*nu-ma u* BURU$_8$.MEŠ-*šú* ŠU ^{d}15 DIN (DPS XIII B ii 22 = *TDP* 118 ii 22)

**If a needling pain is firmly established in his abdomen on the left side and he continually vomits, "hand" of Ištar; he will live.

20.67 DIŠ *ina* ŠÀ-*šú* Á 15-*šú* ^{GIŠ}GIDRU GAR-*su-ma u* BURU$_8$ ŠU ^{d}15 GAM (DPS XIII B ii 24 = *TDP* 118 ii 24)

**If a burning pain is firmly established in his abdomen on the left side and he vomits, "hand" of Ištar; he will die.

In other examples, the severity of the pain was inferred from the patient's vocalization and gnashing of teeth. In all cases, the prognosis was poor, often resulting in death. In many of the examples, however, there were other signs or symptoms that could have driven the *āšipu* to predict a poor outcome. Some of these references are shown below.

20.68 DIŠ *ina* GIG-*šú* ʾ*ua* GÙ-*si ina ban-ti-šú ana* GÍR *ṣa-líl-ma* NU BAL-*it* ŠU ^{d}MAŠ.TAB.BA GAM (DPS XVII:19 [AOAT 43.196])[29]

**If during his illness he cries out: "Ua" (and) he sleeps briefly[30] on his thorax and will not turn over, "hand" of the twin gods; he will die.

20.69 DIŠ ZÚ.MEŠ-*šú* ZÚ.GUZ ŠU^{II}-*šú u* GÌR^{II}-*šú* GI$_6$ D[IB] ⸢GIDIM$_7$⸣ GAM (DPS VI A r. 11//B$_1$ r. 8+B$_2$ r. 12 = *TDP* 60 r. 42′)

**If he gnashes his teeth (and) his hands and feet are dark, ⸢affliction⸣ by a ghost; he will die.

20.70 DIŠ SAG.KI-*šú* DIB-*su-ma* KI.MIN *ma-gal i*$_{16}$-*à-ru u* KI.NÁ NU ÍL ŠU GIDIM$_7$ GAM (DPS IV B obv. 11 = *TDP* 32:11; cf. *BAM* 482 iv 48′//*AMT* 19/1 iv! 31′)

**If his temple afflicts him and (he keeps crying out: "my insides, my insides!"), he vomits a lot and cannot stand the bed, "hand" of ghost; he will die.

Weakness

Seventeen texts have been reviewed that indicate that the patient had significant weakness. This is conveyed by statements such as "he gets up but has to squat down," "he is very sluggish," "his arms are continually weak," and "he does things slowly." All seventeen of these references are given a poor prognosis, usually death. Most of the cases are complex conditions with other signs and symptoms listed, such as blood loss, wounds, and neurologic complaints. Of the three references that list only weakness, all resulted in poor outcomes.

20.71 DIŠ ZI-*bi u* DU$_{10}$.GAM-*is* ŠU-*su* LAL-*át* GAM (DPS XXII:64b [AOAT 43.256])

**If he gets up and (has to) squat down (and) his hand is stretched out, he will die.

20.72 [DIŠ . . .]-⌜*šu* U$_4$.31.KÁM⌝ ŠU ^{d}*Iš-ḫa-ra* DU$_6$.DU$_6$-*ma* : NU DIN : DIN (DPS XVIII:38′ [AOAT 43.219])

**[If . . .] thirty-one days, "hand" of Išḫara. (If) he is continually overwhelmed,[31] he will not get well (var. he will get well).

20.73 DIŠ [*u*]*š-ta-na-aḫ u i-na-iš* GAM : DIŠ [N]A BI *it-ta-bi-ik* GAM (DPS XXII:73 [AOAT 43.257])

**[If he] is continually exhausted and shakes, he will die. If that ⌜person⌝ falls over in a heap, he will die.

20.74 DIŠ *ú-rap-pad ú-ma-aq it-ta-na-an-di* : ŠUB.ŠUB-*ut* GAM (DPS XXII:57 [AOAT 43.256])

**If he wanders about, he does things slowly, (and) he is continually thrown down (var. falls down), he will die.

In the following three references, the *āšipu* appears to be recognizing some of the physiological changes that occur during a prolonged illness and how they can influence the ultimate outcome. Certainly, patients often become very weak as a result of a long bed rest. The ancient Mesopotamian physician also seems to have realized that getting out of bed after an illness needs to be opportunely timed. Returning to normal activities can be harmful if done too soon or delayed too long.

20.75 DIŠ *ina* GIG-*šú lu* ŠU-*su lu* GÌR-*šú a-ku-tam* DU-*ak ul mi-šit-ti* GIG-*su* DIB-*iq-šu-ma* DIN (DPS XVII:31 [AOAT 43.198]; cf. DPS XI A r. 5 = *TDP* 94 r. 5)

**If during (the course of) his illness, either his hand(s) or his feet become weak, it is not a stroke; his illness will pass and he will get well.

20.76 DIŠ GÍR-*iš* ZI-*bi* GIG-*su* GÍD-*ma* GAM (DPS XXII:66 [AOAT 43.256])

**If he gets up (too) quickly,[32] (if) his illness was prolonged, he will die.

20.77 DIŠ SAL.KALAG.GA IGI-*ma ib-luṭ* EGIR *ib-lu-ṭu* GÌR^{II}-*šú it-te-né-eb-ṭa-ni* GIG.BI *šum-ma*[33] É.MEŠ EN LÍL-*šú i-qat-tu-ú* EN.TE.NA RI-*šum-ma* NU DIN (DPS XXII:69–70 [AOAT 43.257])

**If he experiences a mighty illness and then gets well (and) after he gets well, his feet are continually cramped, if the summer finishes before his illness does, the cold season will fall upon him so that he will not get well.

Dehydration

The *āšipu* wrote about patients with severe and continuous vomiting as well as severe diarrhea, and all ten of these references had very bad outcomes. Seven other references listed signs of significant dehydration, such as shriveled tongue and dry mouth, and these cases also had poor prognoses. It is well known by modern physicians that dehydration can cause death, but fortunately patients today can be treated for this condition by intravenous fluid replacement.

20.78 [DIŠ KI.MI]N-*ma mim-ma* KÚ *ina* ŠÀ-*šú* N[U *ina-aḫ is-ḫur-ma* DUB-*ka* GAM] (DPS XXI:22 [AOAT 43.247])

**[If (his blood vessels are healthy)] but whatever he eats does ⌜not rest easy⌝ in his stomach [but it turns about and pours out, he will die].

20.79 DIŠ GIG-*su* DU_8-*ma* $BURU_8$ NU KUD-*us* GAM (DPS XVII:33 [AOAT 43.198]; cf. *PBS* 2/2.104:2)

**If his illness lets up (but) he cannot stop vomiting, he will die.

20.80 DIŠ IGI.MEŠ-*šú* SIG_7.MEŠ *u* IGI^{II}-*šú šap-la* GAM (DPS IX A 12 = *TDP* 72:12)

**If his face is yellowish and his eyes are sunken, he will die.

20.81 DIŠ ŠÀ.MEŠ-*šú i-tab-lu* GAM (DPS XIII B ii 43 = *TDP* 120 ii 43)

**If his insides have dried up, he will die.

Urine Flow (Absent/Excessive)

The *āšipu* understood the importance of normal urine flow. It was clear that the complete absence of urine production was incompatible with life (see Chapter 4). Excessive urine flow also carried a poor prognosis, as the text below indicates. There are many causes of excessive production of urine, with early renal failure and uncontrolled diabetes being the most common.

20.82 DIŠ KÀŠ.MEŠ-*šu* DU.MEŠ GAM (DPS XIV A ii 44//C ii 16b = *TDP* 136 ii 44)[34]

**If his urine continually flows, he will die.

Duration of Illness

There is a general trend in ancient Mesopotamian medical texts to view a medical problem that persists as having a poorer prognosis. Modern physicians would certainly agree with this idea. The references below convey the poorer prognosis of prolonged diseases, with only the final text serving as an exception.

20.83 DIŠ KI.MIN-*ma* SAG ŠÀ-*šú* ÍL-*ma* IGI.ME-*šú nu-up-pú-ḫu ina* IGI^{II}-*šú* ÍR DU-*ak* GÍD-*ma* GAM (DPS XV:34 [AOAT 43.152]; cf. DPS XIII B i 18′ = *TDP* 112 i 22′)

**If (it is the first day he is sick) and his upper abdomen (epigastrium) is puffed up and his face is swollen (and) tears flow from his eyes, (if) it is prolonged, he will die.

20.84 DIŠ KI.MIN-*ma* GÚ.MURGU-*šú* GÚR-*ma* LAL NU ZU-*e* GÍD-*ma* GAM (DPS XV:47 [AOAT 43.153]; cf. DPS XII D iii 33 = *TDP* 106 iii 33)

**If (it is the first day he is sick) and his spine is curved so that he cannot straighten it out, (if) it is prolonged, he will die.

20.85 DIŠ KI.MIN-*ma ina* GÌR-*šú šá* 150 SÌG-*iṣ* ŠU ^{d}15 GÍD-*ma* GAM (DPS XV:62 [AOAT 43.154]; cf. DPS XIV C$_2$ iv 5′b)

**If (it is the first day he is sick) and he was wounded on his right foot, "hand" of Ištar. (If) (his illness) is prolonged, he will die.

20.86 DIŠ KI.MIN-*ma* GÌR-*šú šá* 15 *i-maš-šar* KA-*šú ṣu-dur mi-šit-ti* MAŠKIM GÍD-*ma* GAM (DPS XV:63 [AOAT 43.154]; cf. DPS XIV A$_2$ iv 3′–4′//C$_2$ iii 30 = *TDP* 142 iv 3′–4′)[35]

**If (it is the first day he is sick) and he drags his left foot (and) his mouth twitches, stroke of a *rābiṣu*; (if) it is prolonged, he will die.

20.87 DIŠ GABA.MEŠ *šá* GÌR^{II}-*šú* GI$_6$.MEŠ ŠU ^{d}15 GÍD-*ma* GAM (DPS XIV A iv 16//K10 = *TDP* 144 iv 51′; cf. DPS XV:65 [AOAT 43.154])

**If the "breasts" of his feet are dark, "hand" of Ištar; (if) it is prolonged, he will die.

20.88 DIŠ U$_4$.5.KÁM U$_4$.10.KÁM GIG *dan-na* GIG-*ma uš-tar-di-ma* GIG *dan-na ka-a-a-na* U$_4$.5.KÁM DIB.DIB-*su ba-liṭ* PA NU TUKU (DPS XVI:52′ [AOAT 43.176–177])

**If he has been sick with a mighty sickness for five or ten days and the mighty sickness persists in continually afflicting him for five (more days), he will get well; it is of no consequence.[36]

Another exception to this rule appears related to the time that it takes for some patients with an acute infectious disease to develop immunity. If the patient dies in a few days, the immune system would not have had time to fight the infection. It takes about five to seven days for immunity to develop; therefore, patients who live that long would have a better chance of survival.

20.89 DIŠ *ina taš-rit* GIG-*šú* SAG.⌜KI^{II}⌝-*šú um-ma* ⌜*ub*⌝*-la-nim-ma* EGIR KÚM *u* IR *it-tab-la-ni* LÍL-*ti* UD.DA U$_4$.2.KÁM U$_4$.3.KÁM LÍL-*ma* DIN (DPS XVII:8–9 [AOAT 43.195])

**If at the beginning of his illness his temples produce heat so that afterward it has brought fever and sweat, an illness of *ṣētu* of two days; (if) he is ill for three (more) days, he will get well.

20.90 DIŠ *ina taš-rit* GIG-*šú* TA TAG-*šú* EN *ik-lu-ú* 1-*is-su* KÚM 1-*is-su* ŠED$_7$ *a-ḫu ma-la a-ḫi* TUKU.MEŠ-*ši* EGIR KÚM *u* IR *ip-ṭú-ru* UB.NÍGIN.NA-*šú um-ma ub-la-nim-ma um-ma* *ma-la um-mi maḫ-ri-i ir-ši-ma ip-ta-ṭar* EGIR-*nu* ŠED$_7$ *u* IR *ir-ta-ši di-ḫu e-ri-bu wa-ṣú-ú* UD.DA TAB.BA U$_4$.7.KÁM LÍL-*ma* DIN (DPS XVII:4–7 [AOAT 43.195])

**If at the beginning of his illness from the time it "touches" him until it stops, he continually has now fever, now chills in equal proportions, (and) after the fever and sweat have left, his limbs produce heat so that he has a fever to the same degree as the previous fever and it leaves (and) afterward he has chills and sweat, *di'u* coming in and going out[37] (or) he burns with *ṣētu* (enteric fever; see Chapter 3); (if) he is ill for seven days, he will get well.

20.91 DIŠ *kal* U$_4$-*mi* ŠED$_7$-*ma kal* GI$_6$ *e-em* U$_4$.7.KÁM GIG-*ma* D[IN] (DPS XVII:76 [AOAT 43.202])

**If he is cold all day and hot all night, (if) he has been sick (for) seven days, he will get ⌜well⌝.

20.92 DIŠ *ina šèr-ti* GIG-*ma ina kin-zi-gi* GIG-*su* TA[K$_4$]-*šú-ma*[38] *za-mar-ra-nu-um-ma* GUR-*šú niš-rat* GIG-*šú ina* U$_4$.2.KÁM EN UD.SA$_9$.ÀM *ina* U$_4$.3.KÁM EN *kin-zi-gi ina* U$_4$.4.KÁM EN *ši-mi-tan ina* U$_4$.5.KÁM EN *a-dan-ni-šú ina* U$_4$.6.KÁM EN BAR EN.NUN *ina* U$_4$.7.KÁM EN EN.NUN.MURUB$_4$.BA *ina* U$_4$.8.KÁM [E]N *šat ur-ri ina* U$_4$.9.K[ÁM] EN *na-mir ina* U$_4$.10.KÁM ZI-*ma* DIN (DPS XVII:95–99 [AOAT 43.204–205]; cf. Labat, *Syria* 33.121 obv. 10–12)

**If he is sick in the morning and in the late afternoon his illness leaves him and then suddenly it returns (and he has) a reduced form of his illness the second day until noon, the third day until late afternoon, the fourth day until evening, the fifth day until its normal term,[39] the sixth day until the middle of the (first) watch (of the night), the seventh day until the middle watch (of the night), the eighth day until the dawn watch, (and) the ninth day until it is light, (if) he gets up on the tenth day, he will get well.

Patient's Age

Modern physicians understand that old age in general leads to a worse prognosis for any given disease, and the changes in the aging patient that are responsible are at least partially understood. The *āšipu* had no knowledge of the immunological and biochemical abnormalities of old age, but he knew from observation that age affects outcome, as borne out by the following texts.

20.93 DIŠ U$_4$.MEŠ-*šú* GÍD.DA.MEŠ-*ma* ŠÈ *ma-ru-ti-šú iz-zi*[40] GAM (DPS XVI:90′ [AOAT 43.180])

**If he is in his seventies[41] and he excretes the excrement of his body fat, he will die.

20.94 DIŠ KI.MIN SU-*šú* GIN$_7$ KI.MIN SIG$_7$ ŠÀ.MEŠ-*šú nap-ḫu* SA ŠÀ-*šú* SIG$_7$ GIB.MEŠ GAM (DPS XVI:92′ [AOAT 43.180])

**If (he is in his seventies and) his body is as yellow as (the "peg" on a leek), his insides are bloated, (and) yellow crosses the muscles of his abdomen, he will die.

20.95 DIŠ KI.MIN KÚ *u* NAG NU ZU ŠUK KI.MAḪ-*šú* (*ḫi-pi*) (DPS XVI:97′ [AOAT 43.180])

**If (he is in his seventies and) he is unable to eat or drink, [he has eaten] the provisions for his grave; [he will die].

20.96 DIŠ KI.MIN-*ma* DÍLIM NINDA APIN-*ma* Ì KÚ GAM / DIŠ KI.MIN-*ma* GA APIN-*ma* Ì KÚ *ana* KI GIG GAM (DPS XVI:100′–101′ [AOAT 43.180])

**If (he is in his seventies) and he asks for a spoonful of bread and eats fat (with it), he will die. If (he is in his seventies) and he asks for milk and eats the cream, he is at an acute stage of the illness; he will die.

Elderly patients, however, tolerate some illnesses well and experience excellent outcomes. The first reference below may be osteoarthritis and the second a simple nosebleed, both generally benign conditions.

20.97 DIŠ KI.MIN ŠU^{II}-*šú u* GÌR-*šú ik-tap-pá* GIG-*su* KÚR-*šum-ma* UGU-*šú* KI.MIN DIN (DPS XVI:94′ [AOAT 43.180])

**If (he is in his seventies and) his hands and feet have become bent, (even if) his illness changes so that they (beat their breasts) over him, he will get well.

20.98 DIŠ KI.MIN MÚD *ina* KIR$_4$ DU-*ku* DIN (DPS XVI:96′ [AOAT 43.180])

**If (he is in his seventies and) blood flows from his nose, he will get well.

Very young patients also can be more susceptible to certain infections as a consequence of an immature immune system. The following texts indicate that the *āšipu* realized the greater vulnerability of newborns.

20.99 DIŠ LÚ.TUR *it-ta-na-as-ḫur it-ta-na-as-la-*ʾ ŠU [^{d}*Gu-la*] (DPS XL A 82 = *TDP* 226:82)

**If an infant is repeatedly[42] (and) continually sick, "hand" of [Gula][43] (kala azar; see Chapter 19).

20.100 DIŠ LÚ.TUR *mit-ḫar-riš em-ma u* SAG ŠÀ-*šú za-qir* ŠU ^{d}*Kù-bi* / DIŠ LÚ.TUR SA.MEŠ ŠÀ-*šú* SA$_5$ *u* SIG$_7$ ŠUB-*ú* ŠU ^{d}*Kù-bi* / DIŠ LÚ.TUR ŠÀ.MEŠ-*šú eb-ṭú-ma* SIG$_7$ ŠUB-*ú* ŠU ^{d}*Kù-bi* / DIŠ LÚ.TUR *ik-ta-na-aṣ-ṣa u* ZÚ.MEŠ-*šú i-gaṣ-ṣa-aṣ* GIG-*su ir-ri-ik ṣi-bit* ^{d}*Kù-bi* (DPS XL A 31–34 = *TDP* 220:31–34)

**If an infant is equally hot (all over) and his upper abdomen (epigastrium) protrudes, "hand" of Kūbu. If the muscles of an infant's abdomen are unevenly colored with red and yellow, "hand" of Kūbu. If an infant's insides are cramped and he is unevenly colored with yellow, "hand" of Kūbu. If an infant is continually cold and he gnashes his teeth, his illness will be prolonged; affliction by Kūbu (leptospirosis; see 19.335–19.342).

Difficulty in Arousing the Patient

Patients who cannot be aroused by loud noises or other strong stimuli, such as cold water, are likely to be suffering from coma brought on by trauma, bleeding, or metabolic abnormalities. It is unlikely that the *āšipu* could have helped these patients, therefore, the poor prognosis is understandable.

20.101 DIŠ KI.MIN-*ma i-*[*na* KI.NÁ-*šú* G]Ù.GÙ-*si u de-ki-šu la ip-pal* ŠU DINGIR-*šú* GAM (DPS XV:89 [AOAT 43.155])

**If (it is the first day he is sick) and he continually cries out ⌜in⌝ [his sleep] and does not answer the one trying to wake him, "hand" of his god; he will die.

20.102 DIŠ U_4.6.KÁM LÍL-*ma ina* U_4.7.KÁM NU PA.AN-*uš* A *ana* IGI.MEŠ-*šú i-sal-la-ú-ma šum*$_4$*-ma* IGI^{II}-*šú* NU BAD GAM *šum*$_4$*-ma* IGI^{II}-*šú* BAD *u* DUL-*tam ana* A *šá is-lu-ḫu-šú* ÍR DIN (DPS XVI:63′–64′ [AOAT 43.177–178])[44]

**If he has been sick for six days and he does not get a respite[45] on the seventh, they throw water on his face and if he does not open his eyes, he will die. If he opens and closes his eyes at the water that they throw over him (and) wails, he will get well.

Premonition of Death

Modern physicians with significant clinical experience will often remember patients who thought that their death was impending even though the doctor was not aware of a life-threatening illness. With experience, physicians learn not to ignore these premonitions of death, since death often occurs. Ancient Mesopotamian physicians clearly had similar experiences, as the following references suggest.

20.103 DIŠ KI.MIN-*ma ana* É-*šú* ÍR GAM (DPS XVI:4 [AOAT 43.172])[46]

**If (it is the first day he is sick) and he wails for his household, he will die.

20.104 DIŠ U_4.MEŠ-*šú* GÍD.DA.MEŠ-*ma i-siḫ-ti* KI.MAḪ-*šú i-siḫ* GAM (DPS XVI:89′ [AOAT 43.180])

**If he is in his seventies and he makes the assignments for his tomb, he will die.

20.105 DIŠ EGIR.MEŠ-*šú ú-ḫa-as-sa-as* ŠUK-*su* APIN-*ma* KÚ GAM (DPS XXII:43 [AOAT 43.255])

**If he thinks seriously about arranging his affairs, asks for his travel provisions (to the netherworld), and eats them, he will die.

Summary

The frequent inclusion of a prognosis in medical writings indicates that the ancient Mesopotamian physician spent considerable time in making these predictions. He used them to help guide therapy and probably also in counseling patients and their families. His predictions in most cases are quite appropriate when considering the treatment options that were available.

Conclusion

In many of the previous books and articles on the subject of ancient Mesopotamian medicine, little credit has been given to the medical knowledge and skills of these early physicians. Although the roles of viruses and bacteria were played by gods/goddesses, ghosts, and demons, it does not follow that diagnosis was "irrational" and treatment "pure magic."

The problem presented by the divine language of what we still call medical signs and symptoms was to determine which combinations of animal products, minerals, and plants and which recitations were effective for which medical problems. To answer this question, the ancestor of the *āšipu* began by carefully observing his patients and deriving a vocabulary to describe their signs and symptoms so that any treatments that might subsequently be devised could be applied consistently, past successes reproduced, and repetition of past failures avoided. Gradually, it was noted which individual signs and symptoms tended to occur together, and these were grouped into syndromes.

Only after the process of gathering information was more or less complete did the ancient Mesopotamian physician attempt to assign syndromes to causal agents. In other words, he did not ask "What combinations of signs and symptoms would these gods/goddesses cause?" but "Which of these gods/goddesses, if any, would cause this combination of signs and symptoms?" This pattern of nomenclature is analogous to the use of syndromes in modern medicine with the exception that the modern physician has the luxury of being better able to correct his classification system by reference to invisible causal agents identified by laboratory analysis.

There were magical rituals, but they were intended as a supplement to, and not a replacement for, treatment with medicines and surgery. Medicines were evaluated by clinical trials, although not as rigorously controlled as in current practice. There is no evidence that Mesopotamian physicians constructed improbable and untested theoretical principles to explain illnesses, as did too many premodern physicians. Instead, they evaluated possible causes pragmatically, and systematically tested plants and minerals for useful therapies.

That ancient Mesopotamians should have produced a sophisticated medical system should come as no surprise. They also invented the potter's wheel and chariots, refined irrigation to an art, and developed the first architectural arch, the first written language, a system of measurement of time still employed by us today, as well as a sophisticated system of mathematics and astronomy.

The practice of medicine in ancient Mesopotamia had an organization that is similar to that of modern medicine. A team approach to patient care was evident, with the *āšipu* primarily responsible for diagnosis, and the *asû* for collecting and compounding the components of medicines. The *āšipu* followed a logical and organized process in describing and recording diseases. The diagnostic/prognostic handbook included all areas of medicine, listing them in head-to-toe order with special sections for pediatrics, obstetrics and gynecology, and neurology. Some recurring combinations of signs and symptoms were considered to be syndromes much as is the current practice. The exact process that was used to train physicians is unknown, but the medical literature certainly played a vital role. The organization of the diagnostic/prognostic handbook makes it clear that the object was not merely to describe specific diseases or syndromes but to function as medical textbooks do in the present era. There were series of references that compared varying presentations of the same disease and contrasted them with different diseases that may have some overlapping signs and symptoms. Also included were entries that attempted to explain the etiology of specific diseases. It seems likely that experienced senior physicians would have been preceptors to physicians-in-training.

The *āšipu* used the same general approach to the work-up of patients that is currently practiced. He obtained medical histories from the patient and family members that established past exposure to contagious diseases, important geographical and travel information, and any familial diseases. Physical examinations were performed thoroughly, and described with an extensive medical vocabulary that indicates the importance that physicians placed on these observations in understanding the disease process. The *āšipu* used touch, sound, sight, and smell as he pushed, prodded, felt, sniffed, and looked at his patients. Breathing patterns, pulse rates at many body sites, temperature, the smell of wounds and urine, and the feel of muscles, joints, and abdomen were all important factors in reaching a correct diagnosis.

In addition to direct physical findings, the ancient Mesopotamian physician also devised clinical diagnostic tests, some of which are still in use today. It is also clear from the descriptions of chronic diseases that the *āšipu* often followed his patients for long periods of time. The *āšipu* also played a significant role in preventing diseases and maintaining public health by his recognition that certain human and animal diseases were contagious and could be prevented by cleanliness and avoiding contact with infected individuals.

Of particular interest is the realization that Mesopotamian physicians followed some of the same practices as modern physicians in describing physical signs by analogies to materials and actions in everyday life. A body fluid might look like milk, a foot drop looked like the toes were "licking the ground," and a bulging abscess looked like a leech engorged with blood. A pubic louse looked like a crab then, just as it does to modern physicians.

The social significance of diseases was considered and described. An incontinent man who visits a tavern with his wife will certainly have cause for embarrassment.[1] Dementia is known to commonly cause patients to lose their social moorings, and the *āšipu* realized that they would become "strangers" in their community.[2]

The focus of this book is diagnosis; subsequent volumes will deal with therapies. The references quoted, however, should make it clear that medical and surgical therapies were the goal of the diagnostic workup, and therapy was often long-term and exhaustive in detail. Bandages and topical wound treatments were described, surgeries specified, and medicines were administered by inhalation, orally, rectally, transdermally, and by direct installation into body cavities such as the bladder. Always practical, however, the ancient Mesopotamian physician understood that some conditions were beyond his therapeutic skills, and in these cases he did not recommend futile therapy or placebos.

There were infrequent but unmistakable references to euthanasia in patients with hopeless conditions that followed a familial pattern, in the futile hope of preventing the problem from affecting other members of the family. These events, although disturbing, were rare when compared with the frequent and often long-term therapies that were provided.

It seems evident from a number of references to "internal" abnormalities that could not have been detected by external examination that at least a limited number of autopsies were performed. Additional knowledge of anatomy and pathology would have been acquired by animal dissection for omens and from the observation of war wounds and surgery.

It appears beyond reason to believe that these careful observers of medical signs and symptoms and anatomy and pathology have been considered for so long to be "mere magicians" and "conjurers." The *āšipu* was undoubtedly cognizant of the physical cause-and-effect relationships that are understood today, even though the primary cause was not always clear. It is a wonderful and ennobling experience to have sufficient information about the physicians of this era that similarities can be seen between their practice of medicine and ours. They demonstrate a level of social understanding, imagination, and humor that clearly connects them to the humanity of present-day medicine.

Unsolved Puzzles Appendix

This appendix lists all the references that have defied our abilities to suggest a probable diagnosis. This may be due to changes in the diseases that occurred in the past. However, the problem might also be due to insufficient clinical information, difficulty in understanding the clinical descriptions, or our lack of knowledge in some areas of medicine. We hope that this appendix will stimulate our readers to help solve these medical mysteries.

Mysterious References Without Helpful Attributions

The signs and symptoms in the following references do not suggest an identifiable diagnosis. Adding to the difficulty in interpreting these texts is the failure to mention a god/goddess, ghost, or demon as cause of the disease in the preserved section of the text.

Ap.1 DIŠ *i-na* IGI [^{II}-*šú* . . .]x *i-te-ni-ṭa-a* NA BI KIN-*šú* TIL-*ma* IGI^{II}-*šú* *ip-pa-a ana* TI-*šú* . . . (*BAM* 515 i 54′–55′; cf. *BAM* 22:1′)

**If (there are) [. . .] in [his] ⌜eyes⌝, they continually become darkened (and if) that person's work is prolonged, his eyes become clouded, to cure him . . .

Ap.2 DIŠ NA NINDA KÚ KAŠ NAG-*ma la i-še-eb-bi* ŠÀ-*šú* MÚ.MÚ-*ḫ*[*u* . . .]xx GIN$_7$ *it-ta-šu* KAŠ.SIG-*tú* GIG . . . (*BAM* 575 iii 37)

**If a person eats bread (and) drinks beer and is not sated, his insides are continually bloated, and [. . .] as its sign, he gets sick from (drinking) watered beer . . .

Ap.3 DIŠ SAG.DU-*su i-ṣa-ád u kìn-ṣa-a*(coll.)-*šú ka-ṣa-a* ŠU ^{d}[. . .] (DPS III C obv. 25 = *TDP* 20:25)

**If his head seems to spin and his legs are cold, "hand" of [. . .]

Ap.4 DIŠ *ú-ru-uḫ* SAG.DU-*šú bé-e-er* ŠU ^{d}[. . .] / DIŠ *ú-ru-uḫ* SAG.DU-*šú bé-e-er ṣi-bit* [. . .] (DPS III A obv. 28–29//C obv. 19–20[1] = *TDP* 20:19–20)[2]

**If his head hair is fine (lit. select), "hand" of [. . .]. If his head hair is fine (lit. select), affliction by [. . .]

Ap.5 DIŠ EME-*šú u* KA-*šú* IM DIRI [. . .] (DPS VII A obv. 11 = *TDP* 62:11)

**If his tongue and his mouth are full of "clay" [. . .]

Ap.6 DIŠ *is-sa-a-šú ḫe-sa-a-m*[*a* GEŠTU^{II}-*šú* . . .] (DPS VIII 22 = *TDP* 70:22)

**If his jaws are pressured and, ⸢consequently⸣, [his ears . . .]

Ap.7 DIŠ ŠU^{II}-*šú* SIG$_{7}$.MEŠ *u* U.MEŠ-*šú pu-ṣa* ŠUB [. . .] (DPS XI A obv. 12 = *TDP* 90:12)

**If his hands are yellow and his fingers are unevenly colored with white spots [. . .]

Ap.8 DIŠ ŠU^{II}-*šú* SIG$_{7}$.MEŠ *u* IGI^{II}-*šú pu-ṣa* ŠU[B . . .] (DPS XI B 11 = *SpTU* 1.34:11)

**If his hands are yellow and his eyes are ⸢unevenly colored⸣ with white spots [. . .]

Ap.9 [DIŠ MURU]B$_{4}$ ŠU^{II}-*šú* SIG$_{7}$ ŠUB-*di u* U.MEŠ-*šú* ÚḪ!.MEŠ [. . .] (DPS XI A r. 30 = *TDP* 96 r. 30)

** [If] the ⸢middle part⸣ of his hands is unevenly colored with yellow and his fingers feel burning hot, [. . .]

Ap.10 DIŠ *kar-ši* U.MEŠ-*šú sa-am-ta im-t*[*aḫ-ṣa* . . .] (DPS XI A r. 58, 59 = *TDP* 98 r. 58, 59)

**If the "bellies" of his fingers are ⸢streaked⸣ with redness, [. . .]

Ap.11 DIŠ ŠÀ.MEŠ-*šú* ŠU^{II}-*šú u* GÌR^{II}-*šú it-te-nen-bi-ṭu* U$_{4}$.32.KÁM *lu* NÍTA *l*[*u* MUNUS . . .] (DPS XIII G$_{2}$ r. 9 = *TDP* 122 iii 16)

**If his insides, his hands, and his feet are continually cramped (and he has been sick for) thirty-two days, either a man ⸢or⸣ [a woman . . .]

Ap.12 DIŠ ŠÀ.MEŠ-*šú* GIN$_{7}$ ŠU.SI.MEŠ-*šú it-te-nen-ṣi-la ana* U$_{4}$.31.KÁM [. . .] (DPS XIII G$_{2}$ r. 12 = *TDP* 124 iii 19)

**If his insides are as sluggish as his fingers (and he has been sick) for thirty-one days, [. . .]

Ap.13 DIŠ ŠÀ ŠÀ GÙ.GÙ-*si u gi-lid-su* KÚ-*šú* ŠU ⸢^{d}⸣[. . .] (DPS XIII G$_{2}$ r. 17 = *TDP* 124 iii 24)

**If he keeps crying out: "My insides, my insides" and his hip socket hurts him, "hand" of [. . .]

Ap.14 DIŠ *e-mir u tu-*[*l*]*im-šú* KÚ.MEŠ-*šú* ŠU [. . .] (DPS XIII D r. 10 = *TDP* 126 iv 19′)

**If he is colicky and his spleen continually hurts him, "hand" of [. . .]

Ap.15 [DIŠ SU-*šú* K]ÚM NU TUKU SA SAG.[DU-*šú* . . . -*š*] *ú šal-mu-ma* IGI.MEŠ-*šú i-sim-mu* [. . .] as sa bat [. . . KIR$_{4}$-*šú ú*]-⸢*gan*⸣-*na-aṣ* SAG.KI-*su ú-sa-ʾ-ár* [. . .]x ^{LÚ}A.ZU ^{LÚ}MAŠ

^{LÚ}ḪAL ^{LÚ}ENSI *šu-ud-di* (DPS XVIII:12–14 [AOAT 43.218]; cf. DPS XXI:15 [AOAT 43.246])

**[If his body] does not have ⸢fever⸣, the blood vessels of his ⸢head⸣ (and) ⸢his⸣ [. . .] are healthy, but his face flushes, [. . .], he wrinkles [his nose] (and) wipes his forehead [. . .] inform the *asû* (pharmacist), the *āšipu*, the diviner, (and) the dream interpreter.

Ap.16 DIŠ GIG GAR-*šú ina ši-mi-ti* ŠUB-*su-ma la ú-ta-ša*[*r-m*]*a šim-ma-tum ka-la pag-ri-šú* ⸢*ṣa-ba-tu*⸣ [. . .] (DPS XXXIII:34 [AOAT 43.355])

**If the nature of the sore is that it falls on him in the evening and will not ⸢let up and⸣ numbness afflicts(?) his whole body, [. . .]

Ap.17 DIŠ NA SA.MEŠ ŠÀ-*šú* KÚ.MEŠ-*šú* SAG.KI GÙB-*šú* TAG.TAG-*su im-ta-nag-ga-ag* KA.DIB SU-*šú* KÚM-*im u ši-ḫat* UZU.MEŠ TUKU-*ši* NA BI GIG *na-a-ki* GIG (DPS XXII:10–11 [AOAT 43.252]; cf. DPS XIII A 6–7//B i 3′–4′ = *TDP* 110 i 7′–8′)

**If the muscles of a person's abdomen continually hurt him, his right temple continually hurts him intensely, he is continually stiff/rigid, (he has) inability to eat, his body is feverish, and he has wasting away of the flesh, that person is sick with a venereal disease.[3]

The text immediately above, although difficult to interpret on its own, appears in a section with two other references[4] that describe liver problems thought to be related to a venereal disease. This illness may be a similar condition, possibly hepatitis B, but one cannot be sure. Fincke[5] believes that the following reference describes a patient with Crohn's disease. That disease, however, primarily involves the intestines and the major complaints are gastrointestinal. The only gastrointestinal complaint in the reference below is a "bloated stomach," a symptom that is not common in Crohn's disease. The "tired" and "tense" knees may be describing arthritis, and arthritis may occur in Crohn's disease, but this finding is not sufficient to establish the diagnosis as Crohn's disease.

Ap.18 DIŠ NA SAG.KI.DIB.[BA TU]KU.TUKU IGI^{II}-*šú i-bar-ru-ra* UZU^{II}-*šú i-šam-ma-mu-šu* GÍR.GÍR-*šú* ŠÀ-[*šú* MÚ.M]Ú ŠU^{II}-*šú u* GÌR^{II}-*šú ú-šam-ma-ma-šú ú-zaq-qa-ta-šú bir-ka-šú an-*[*ḫa tab-k*]*a e-ta-ta-na-aḫ* NA BI GIG *là-zi* DIB-*su i-dan-nin-šú* [*ana* G]IG-*šú* NU GÍD.DA . . . (*BAM* 482 iii 60′–63′)

**If a person ⸢continually⸣ has headaches, his eyes become dimmed, his flesh goes numb and stings him, [his] stomach is [continually] ⸢bloated⸣, his hands and his feet go numb and sting him, his knees are ⸢tired⸣ and ⸢tense⸣[6] (and) he is continually tired, a persistent illness afflicts that person and has become too strong for him; [in order that] his ⸢illness⸣ not be prolonged . . .

Some of these mystery references were intended as prognoses rather than diagnoses, which means that more than one medical condition was potentially intended to be included.

Ap.19 [DIŠ TA SAG].⸢DU-*šú*⸣ EN MURUB$_4$-*šú* SIG$_7$ TA MURUB$_4$-*šú* EN GÌR^{II}-⸢*šu*⸣ [SA$_5$?] ŠU^{II}-*šú* KÚM-*ma* PAP.ḪAL-*ma* GAM(coll.) / [DIŠ TA SAG].⸢DU⸣-*šú* EN MURUB$_4$-*šú* GIG TA MURUB$_4$-*šú* EN GÌR^{II}-*šú* DIN ITU GIG GIG-*su* GÍD-*ma* DIN /

[DIŠ TA SAG].⌜DU⌝-*šú* EN MURUB$_4$-*šú* TI TA MURUB$_4$-*šú* EN GÌR^{II}-*šú* GIG *e-reb* GIG GIG-*su* GÍD-*ma* DIN (DPS III A r. 5′–7′//C r. 28–30//F 12–13 = *TDP* 28:88–90)[7]

**[If] he is pale (greenish) [from] his ⌜head⌝ to his hip region (and) [flushed(?)] from his hip region to his feet [and] his hands are hot, (if) he has a difficult time, he will die. [If] he is ill [from] his ⌜head⌝ to his hip region (but) well from his hip region to his feet, he has been sick for a month;[8] his illness may be prolonged (but) he will get well. [If] he is well [from] his ⌜head⌝ to his hip region (but) ill from his hip region to his feet, entrance of the illness; his illness may be prolonged (but) he will get well.

Ap.20 DIŠ TA MUD Á-*šú* EN MURUB$_4$-*šú* KÚM TA MURUB$_4$-*šú* EN GÌR^{II}-*šú* ŠED$_7$ PAP.ḪAL.ME-*ma* SUR-*ma* DIN (DPS X B r. 14 = *TDP* 88 r.14)

**If he is hot from his arm socket to his hip (and) cold from his hip to his feet, (if) he has a difficult time of it and (if) he comes through, he will get well.

Ap.21 [DIŠ IGI-*šú šá* 15 *i*]*-la-wi u i-su-šú nu-*⌜*šá*!*-át* DIN⌝[9] / [DIŠ NA IGI-*šú šá* 150 *u i-su-šú* K]I.MIN GIG-*su* DUGUD-*ma* DIN (DPS V D i 3–4 = *TDP* 48 E i 3–4)

**[If his left eye] ⌜goes round⌝ and his jaw shakes, he will get well. [If his right eye] (⌜goes round⌝) [and his jaw] (⌜shakes⌝), his illness may be difficult (but) he will get well.

Ap.22 DIŠ SA IGI^{II}-*šú* GIN$_7$ ŠU.GUR *kup-pu-*[*pu* . . .] *na-kid* [. . .] (DPS V G 9–10 = *TDP* 50/52: G 9–10; cf. Labat, *Syria* 33.125 r. 7)

**If the blood vessel(s) of his eyes are ⌜curved⌝ like a ring[10] [. . .] it is worrisome [. . .]

Ap.23 [DIŠ] ⌜*ina* KIR$_4$-*šú* MÚD (coll.) DU⌝-*k*[*u* ZI-*šú pa*]*-áš-qa-a*[*t*] GEŠTU^{II}-*šú* BAB-BAR-*at u* GÌR^{II}-*šú nu-up-pu-ḫa* GAM (DPS VI A obv. 18//B$_2$ obv. 5//D 1 = *TDP* 56:18)

**[If] blood flows from his nose, [his breathing?] is labored, his ears are white, and his feet are swollen, he will die.

Ap.24 DIŠ IGI.MEŠ-*šú* NIGIN.ME *ina* SAG GI$_6$ TAG-*it* (DPS IX A 53 = *TDP* 76:53; cf. StBoT 36.53:2′)

**If his face seems continually to be spinning, (and) he is particularly affected at the beginning of the night <he will get well/die>

Ap.25 DIŠ ZÚ.MEŠ-*šú pu-uḫ-*[*ḫu*]*-ra* GAM : DIŠ ZÚ.MEŠ-*šú* [. . .] ⌜É⌝ BI BIR-*aḫ* (DPS VI A r. 8//B$_1$ r. 5+B$_2$ r. 9 = *TDP* 60 r. 39′)

**If his teeth are ⌜"gathered together"⌝, he will die;[11] if his teeth [are "scattered"], that household will be scattered.

Ap.26 DIŠ ZÚ.MEŠ-*šú* ZÚ.GUZ *šu-ú-ra-šú* DU$_8$.MEŠ IGI.ME-*šú šu-*[*ú-ra*]*-šú tar-ra* GAM (DPS VI A r. 10//B$_1$ r. 7+B$_2$ r. 11′ = *TDP* 60 r. 41′)

**If he gnashes his teeth, his eyelids are continually open, (and) his face (and) his ⌜eye-lids⌝ tremble, he will die.

Ap.27 DIŠ EME-*šú ina* ŠU^{II}-*šú ú-mar-*[*raṭ* . . .] / DIŠ EME-*šú ú-qar-ra-aš* ⌜NÍG.GIG⌝[12] [IGI-*ma* DIN] (DPS VII A obv. 14–15 = *TDP* 62:14–15)

**If he ⌜rubs⌝ his tongue with his hands [. . .] If he kneads his tongue, [(even if) he has] a hard time of it, [he will get well(?)].

Ap.28 DIŠ IGI.MEŠ-*šú* SA_5.MEŠ *u* GI_6.MEŠ SUMUN-*ma* EGIR-*šú* MAN-*ma* GAM (DPS IX A 5–7//B obv. 5–7 = *TDP* 72:5–7)

**If his face flushes and turns black, (if) he lingers and afterward (if) he makes a change (for the worse), he will die.

Ap.29 DIŠ IGI.MEŠ-*šú* GI_6.MEŠ EME-*šú* SA_5 GIG-*su* GÍD-*ma* GAM (DPS IX A 16 = *TDP* 72:16)

**If his face is dark (and) his tongue is red, (if) his illness is prolonged, he will die.

Ap.30 DIŠ IGI.MEŠ-*šú ma-aq-tu-ma su-qat-su ṣab-ta-at u* $UŠ_4$-*šú* NU DIB GAM (DPS IX A 38//B obv. 37 = *TDP* 74:38)

**If his face (looks) terrible[13] and his chin is "seized" and he is not in full possession of his faculties, he will die.

Ap.31 DIŠ *pur-qí-dam* ŠUB-*ma* BIR-*iḫ* GÚ-*su* 15 *u* 150 ŠUB.ŠUB-*di* GAM (DPS X A obv. 26//B obv. 29 = *TDP* 82:26)

**If he falls backward and (lies) stretched out (and) he continually lets his neck drop to the left and right, he will die.

Ap.32 DIŠ *r*[*i-biti r*]*i-biti* GÙ.GÙ-*si ina* DÚR-*šú* ZÉ *i-te-eṣ-ṣi u* ŠIR-*šú ze-ra*⌜GAM⌝ (DPS XIV A iii 14–15//C_2 iii 5//I 10 = *TDP* 140 iii 48′–49′)

**If he continually cries out: ⌜"the side of my abdomen, the side of my abdomen!"⌝, he excretes bile from his anus, and his testicle(s) are twisted, he will die.

Ap.33 DIŠ GÌR^{II}-*šú i-*[*nap-p*]*a-ṣa* ŠU^{II}-*šú ne-e-ḫa na-ḫi-id* (DPS XIV A_2 iv 17′//G iv 7′ = *TDP* 142 iv 17′)

**If his feet ⌜thrash around⌝ and his hands are quiet, it is worrisome.

Ap.34 DIŠ KI.MIN-*ma* UZU.MEŠ-*šú i-šam-ma-mu-šú* IGI^{II}-*šú* MÚD D[IRI.MEŠ GAM] (DPS XV:67 [AOAT 43.154])

**If (it is the first day he is sick) and his flesh goes numb (and) his eyes are ⌜full⌝ of blood, [he will die].

Ap.35 DIŠ KI.MIN-⌜*ma*⌝ ⌜UZU⌝.MEŠ-*šú ug-gag* GIN_7 *ug-ga-gu* [NU ZU GAM] (DPS XV: 68 [AOAT 43.155])

**If (it is the first day he is sick) and he scratches his flesh (and) [he does not realize] that he is scratching (it), [he will die].

Ap.36 DIŠ *a-di-na* ITU NU GIG-*ma iṣ-lim-ma kir-ra-šú šu-uḫ-ḫu-ṭa* GIG-*ma* GAM (DPS XVI:76′ [AOAT 43.179])

**If he has not yet been sick for a month and he turns black[14] and his throat (looks) skinned, (if) he worsens, he will die.

Ap.37 DIŠ KI.MIN-*ma iṣ-lim-ma* IGI^{II}-*šú rab-ṣa* GIG-*ma* GAM (DPS XVI:77′ [AOAT 43.179])

**If (he has not yet been sick for a month) and he turns black and his eyes "lie down,"[15] (if) he worsens, he will die.

Ap.38 DIŠ *ú-te-eṭ-ṭe* ZI.IR.MEŠ SÍG UGU-*šú it-ta-na-az-qap ina* GI$_{6}$ GAM (DPS XXII:68 [AOAT 43.256])

**If he continually becomes darkened (i.e., passes out), (his stomach) is continually upset, (and) the hair of his scalp continually stands on end, he will die in the night.

Ap.39 DIŠ MUNUS ⸢*ina* GI$_{6}$⸣ GIG-*ma ina šèr-ti it-te-bi* GIG-*sà i-sa-dir-ši* BA.ÚŠ (DPS XXXVII A obv. 18 = *TDP* 214:18)

**If a woman is sick in the night and gets up in the morning (and) her illness (afflicts) her time after time, she will die.

Ap.40 DIŠ TU S[AG] KA *šá* ZAG ZI-*ma u* GI$_{6}$ *šà*-ŠÀ-*šà* Ú[Š] / DIŠ *šá* GÙB ZI-*ma u* GI$_{6}$ *šà*-ŠÀ-*šà* ÚŠ : TI / [DIŠ] T[U x K]A *šá* KI.TA-*nu* 15 SA$_{5}$ *šà*-ŠÀ-*šà* ÚŠ . . . [DIŠ] KI.TA-*nu* 15/150 GÙN.A *šà*-ŠÀ-*šà* DIN (DPS XXXVI A 16–18, 20–21 = *TDP* 202:16–18, 20–21)

**If the ⸢head⸣ of a woman of childbearing age's "tip" rises to the left and is dark, her fetus will ⸢die⸣. If it rises to the right and is dark, her fetus will die (var. will live). [If the base?] of a ⸢woman of childbearing age's "tip"⸣ is reddish from below to the left, her fetus will die . . . [If] it is multicolored from below to the left/right, her fetus will live.

Ap.41 DIŠ BABBAR NU SI.SÁ PEŠ$_{4}$-*at*. . . DIŠ SIG$_{7}$ *šà*-ŠÀ-*šà* ŠUB (DPS XXXVI A 30, 32//B 17, 19 = *TDP* 202:30, 32)

**If (the tip of a woman of childbearing age's breast) is white, she is pregnant with a fetus that will not do well . . . If it is yellow/tan, she will abort her fetus.

Ap.42 DIŠ TU *mu-úḫ* UBUR-*šá* SA.MEŠ SA$_{5}$.MEŠ *pur-ru-ku* SAL PEŠ$_{4}$-*at* / DIŠ GI$_{6}$.MEŠ *pur-ru-ku* NITA PEŠ$_{4}$-*at* / DIŠ (TU *mu-úḫ* UBUR-*šá* SA.MEŠ) BABBAR.MEŠ *pur-ru-ku* NU SI.SÁ PEŠ$_{4}$-*at* / DIŠ SIG$_{7}$.MEŠ *pur-ru-ku šà*-ŠÀ-*šà* NU SI.SÁ (DPS XXXVI A 52–55 = *TDP* 204:52–55)

**If on top of the breast of a woman of childbearing age red muscles cross, she is pregnant with a female. If dark ones cross, she is pregnant with a male. If white ones cross, she is pregnant with a fetus that will not do well. If yellow/tan ones cross, her fetus will not do well.

Ap.43 DIŠ SA SAG ZI-*šú šá* 15 *u* 150 DU-*ku-ma šá pu-ti-šú* GAR-*nu* ÚŠ (DPS XII A 7 = *TDP* 100 i 7)[16]

**If the blood vessel(s) of the "head" of his neck, the ones on the left and the ones on the right, "go" but those of his forehead are present, he will die.

The references below describe blood vessels in the temple that either "cross/block each other" or "are parallel/in tandem." In either case, the patient seems able to recover.

Ap.44 DIŠ *ina* SAG.KI 15-*šú* SA.MEŠ GIB.MEŠ DIN (DPS IV A obv. 69+A$_{6}$ 4//E ii 13 = *TDP* 38:69//*SpTU* 3.88 ii 13)[17]

**If in his left temple, the blood vessels cross, he will get well.

Ap.45 DIŠ *ina* SAG.KI-*šú* SA.MEŠ SA$_{5}$.MEŠ GIB.MEŠ DIN (DPS IV E ii 16 = *SpTU* 3.88 ii 16)

**If in his temple, the blood vessels are red and cross, he will get well.

Ap.46 DIŠ SA SAG.KI^{II}-*šú tal-lu la ip-rik-u* TAB-*su ra-mu-ú* ÉN ŠUB-*šum-ma* DIN (DPS IV A r. 4+A_4 3//B r. 16 = *TDP* 42 r. 37)[18]

**If the blood vessels of his temples are parallel (and) do not cross (and) his burning (fever)? has slackened, (if) you cast a spell over him, he will get well.

One possibility that might explain the following sequenced references is that the liquid flowing from the nose represents spinal fluid leakage secondary to trauma. If so, then the patient will have died from a resulting infection.

Ap.47 DIŠ *ina* KIR_4-*šú* A DU-*ku-ma* KÚM-*mu u* SAG KIR_4-*šú na-ši* GAM / DIŠ *ina* KIR_4-*šú* A SA_5.MEŠ DU-*ku* GAM (DPS VI A obv. 20–21//C i 4–5//D 3 = *TDP* 56:20–21)

**If fluid flows from his nose and it is hot and the bulb of his nose is puffed up, he will die. If red fluid flows from his nose, he will die.

In the following sequenced references, the patient expresses a desire for particular foods. These cravings are often related to the color of the patient's forehead or face, but no prognosis is given, and there is not enough other clinical information provided to permit us to make a diagnosis.

Ap.48 DIŠ SAG.KI-*su* BABBAR *u i-riš-tú* ŠÀ TUKU-*ši ina* U_4-*me-šú-ma bi-bil* ŠÀ APIN-*iš* / DIŠ SAG.KI-*su u pa-nu-šú* BABBAR *ina* U_4-*me-šú-ma* A.GEŠTIN.NA APIN-*iš* / DIŠ SAG.KI-*su* SIG_7-*at ina* U_4-*me-šú-ma* ^{GIŠ}NU.ÚR.MA APIN-*iš* / DIŠ SAG.KI-*su* SA_5 *u* SIG_7 *ina* U_4-*me-šú-ma* KU_6 APIN-*iš* / DIŠ SAG.KI-*su* SA_5 *ina* U_4-*me-šú-ma* ZAG.ḪI.LI APIN-*iš* / DIŠ SAG.KI-*su* GI_6 *u* SA_5 *ina* U_4-*me-šú-ma* UZU *u* ZAG.ḪI.LI APIN-*iš* / DIŠ SAG.KI-*su* GI_6 *ina* U_4-*me-šú-ma* ^{GIŠ}GEŠTIN *u* ZAG.ḪI.LI APIN-*iš* / DIŠ SAG.KI-*su bar-mat ina* U_4-*me-šú-ma* ^{GIŠ}GEŠTIN APIN-*iš* / DIŠ SAG.KI-*su šal-mat ina* U_4-*me-šú-ma* ^{GIŠ}GEŠTIN APIN-*iš* / DIŠ SAG.KI-*su* GIN_7 *si-ka-a-t*[*i*. . .]⌜x-*ma*?⌝ ZÚ.LUM.MA APIN-*iš* (DPS IV B r. 24–33 = *TDP* 44 r. 47–56)

**If his forehead is white and he has some craving, on that same day, he will ask for what he wants. If his forehead and his face are white, on that same day, he will ask for vinegar. If his forehead is greenish, on that same day, he will ask for pomegranate. If his forehead is red and greenish, on that same day, he will ask for fish. If his forehead is red, on that same day, he will ask for *saḫlû*. If his forehead is dark and red, on that same day, he will ask for meat and *saḫlû*. If his forehead is dark, on that same day, he will ask for wine and *saḫlû*. If his forehead is multicolored, on that same day, he will ask for wine. If his forehead is healthy, on that same day, he will ask for wine. If his forehead is [. . .] like brewer's yeast, he will ask for dates.

Only slightly less mysterious are the following unsequenced references to requests for specific foods. A craving for bread (as in the first and second examples) might indicate that the patient was starving.

Ap.49 DIŠ KI.MIN-*ma* DÍLIM NINDA APIN-*ma* Ì KÚ GAM / DIŠ KI.MIN-*ma* GA APIN-*ma* Ì KÚ *ana* KI GIG GAM (DPS XVI:100′–101′ [AOAT 43.180])

**If (he is in his seventies) and he asks for a spoonful of bread and eats fat (with it), he will die. If (he is in his seventies) and he asks for milk and eats the cream, he is at an acute stage of the illness; he will die.

Ap.50 DIŠ IGI.MEŠ-*šú* GI_6.MEŠ ŠÀ.MEŠ-*šú nap-ḫu* GAM / DIŠ IGI.MEŠ-*šú* GI_6.MEŠ NINDA APIN-*ma* KÚ GAM (DPS IX A 18–19 = *TDP* 72:18–19)

**If his face turns black (and) his insides are bloated, he will die. If his face turns black (and) he asks for bread and eats it, he will die.

Ap.51 DIŠ GA UGU-*šú* DÙG-*ab* GIG-*su* GÍD.DA-*ma ni-kit-tam* T[UKU] (DPS XXIII:18′ [AOAT 43.273])

**If milk seems good to him (and if) his illness is prolonged, he ⌜will have⌝ a cause for worry.

The two following references appear to contradict one another. In the first, asking for dates is not a good sign. In the second, however, it is. Possibly the second reference is to be taken as the patient using the language of omens to signal a preference for living or a desire to die (the *āšipu* was well aware that the patient's attitude in such matters could be of great importance; see Chapter 20). Pomegranates were associated with love magic, and a request for them at this juncture could have been seen to represent a courtship of death. Dates were used as baby food and were associated with the goddess Ištar whose job it was to bring human souls up from the netherworld to be born. Since those who recovered from an illness were often said metaphorically to have returned from the netherworld, a request for dates could have been seen as a wish to recover.

Ap.52 DIŠ IGI.MEŠ-*šú* DAR_4 ZÚ.LUM.MA APIN-*ma* KÚ GAM (DPS IX A 26 = *TDP* 72:26)

**If his face is dark red, he asks for dates and eats them, he will die.

Ap.53 DIŠ KI.MIN *ḫu-qu* DIB.DIB-*su* ^{GIŠ}NU.ÚR.MA APIN-*iš* GAM / DIŠ KI.MIN ZÚ.LUM.MA APIN-*ma* KÚ DIN (DPS XVI:98′–99′ [AOAT 43.180])

**If (he is in his seventies[19] and) *ḫūqu* (gasping respiration) continually afflicts him (and) he asks for pomegranates, he will die. If (he is in his seventies and) he asks for dates and eats them, he will get well.

The following reference appears in a Mari letter. Since this letter was written by a non-physician, the accuracy of the observations might be questioned. Durand, *ARM* 26/1.553 suggests that Sumḫurapi died of a "cardiac crisis." However, the only information given (apart from his sudden death) is that the patient experienced foot and abdominal pain, neither of which is common in heart attacks. Deep vein thrombosis involving the lower extremeties (blood clots in the veins of the legs) may lead to pulmonary embolis and sudden death. This is commonly associated with leg pain, not foot and abdominal pain, as in this passage.

Ap.54 U_4-*um ṭup-pí an-né-e-em a-na ṣe-er be-lí-ia ú-ša-bi-lam* ^{m}*Su-um-ḫu-ra-pi ki-ma la li-ib-bi i-la la* U_4.1.KAM *la* 2.KAM [*i*]*m-ra-aṣ i-na* U_4-*mi-im-ma ša-a-ti um-ma-mi še-pí mar-ṣa-at-m*[*i*] *a-di-ma še-pí-šu* x *um-ma-mi ri-b*[*i-bi-ti*] *mar-ṣa-a*[*t-m*]*i ù qa-tam a-na qa-tim-ma na-pí-iš*$_7$*-ta-am iš*$_7$*-ta-ka-an* (*ARM* 26/1.275:5–18)

**Unfortunately, the day I sent this letter to my lord, Sumḫurapi—he was sick not one day, not two days—on that very same day (he said) "My foot hurts." As soon as (he had complained about) his foot, (he said) "My ⸢abdomen⸣[20] hurts." And shortly afterward he put down his life.

Mysterious Curses

Ancient Mespotamian curses are a good example of a set of syndromes where the organizing principle that inspired grouping the attested references under one diagnosis is relatively clear (see 19.307–19.318). Ten references, however, defied our diagnostic efforts.

Of these, six (of which four are quoted below) were too vague to be suggestive of any particular modern disease. The second reference below is from the ancient commentary to the first reference. It would appear that some of these descriptions of symptoms were as opaque to ancient Mesopotamian physicians as they are to us.

Ap.55 DIŠ *taš-⸢li⸣-ma-ti* DUG$_4$.DUG$_4$-*ub* GIG *ma-mit* GIG (DPS XXII:17 [AOAT 43.253])[21]

**If he continually says greetings, he is sick with an illness of curse.

Ap.56 [*taš-l*]*i-ma-a-ti* DUG$_4$.DUG$_4$-*ub* . . . [*taš-li-ma*]-*ti* : *nu-ul-lat ina ṣa-a-tú* E (*SpTU* 1.38:15, 17)

**He continually says ⸢"greetings"⸣ . . . in the commentary it says that ⸢"greetings"⸣ means "untruths."

Ap.57 DIŠ *ina* GI$_6$ GIG-*su* DIB.DIB-*su u* LUḪ.LUḪ NAM.ÉRIM DIB-*su* : DIB x[. . .] (DPS XVII:80 [AOAT 43.203])

**If his illness afflicts him in the night and he continually jerks, a curse afflicts him (var. affliction by [. . .]).

Ap.58 DIŠ *ina* ŠÀ-*šú* KI.MIN-*ma* EME-*šú ú-na-áṭ-ṭa* ÁŠ-*át* AD-*šú* KUR-*su* PÚŠ.ME-*ma* GAM : DIN (DPS XIII B ii 33//G$_2$ obv. 30+G$_1$ obv. 13 = *TDP* 120 ii 33)

**If in his abdomen (a needling pain or burning pain[22] is firmly established) and he licks(?) (with) his tongue,[23] the curses of his father have "gotten" him. (If) he has a difficult time of it, he will die (var. even if he has a difficult time of it, he will get well).

The remaining three references have many of the characteristics of other curse references, including apparent chronicity and findings compatible with infections. Some of the diagnoses that were considered but which were inadequately supported by the texts include miliary tuberculosis or bacterial endocarditis for the first reference, nephrotic syndrome for the second and third references, and *kala-azar* for the last.

Ap.59 [DIŠ NA . . .] *piṭ-ru-šú ir-ta-nam-mu-u šit-tú ir-te-ni-ḫi-šú* [. . .] KÚM ŠÀ TUKU-*ši* A.MEŠ *iṣ-ṣa-nam-ma* NINDA.MEŠ *u* KAŠ SAG LAL *bir-di im-ta-na-al-la* [. . .] *ik-ka-šú ik-ta-na-ru* GAZ ŠÀ-*bi* TUKU.MEŠ *ana* MUNUS DU-*ka* LAL [. . . ŠU] NAM.ÉRIM DIB-*su ana* TI-*šú* . . . (K 2426 i 9′–12′)

**[If a person. . .] his internal organs[24] are consistently relaxed (i.e., the lungs are clear, the stomach is not upset, and the liver is not tender), sleep keeps flowing over him, [. . .]

he has internal fever, he is continually thirsty for water (and) his appetite for bread and beer is diminished, he is continually full of *birdu*-nodules, [. . .], he is continually short of breath, he continually has a crushing sensation in his chest, his desire to go to a woman is diminished [. . . "hand"] of curse afflicts him, to cure him . . .

Ap.60 DIŠ IGI^{II}-*šú nu-up-pu-ḫa ma-mit* DIB-*su* BÚR-*ma* T[I-*uṭ*] *ana* NITA *u* MUNUS 1-*ma* (*STT* 89:203–204)

**If his eyes are swollen, a curse afflicts him; (if) it lets up, he will get ⸢well⸣. It is the same for a man and a woman.

Ap.61 DIŠ ⸢*za*⸣-*mar* KÚM-*em za-mar* ŠED$_7$ UZU.ME-*šu* SIG$_7$ ŠUB-*ú ga-ṣu u qá-ti-ir* ŠU *ma-mit* GAM (DPS XXII:21 [AOAT 43.253])

**If he is sometimes hot and sometimes cold, his flesh is unevenly colored with yellow, he (looks white as) whitewash and (dark as) the color of smoke,[25] "hand" of curse; he will die.

Ill-defined Syndromes of the Sort Gods/Goddesses Might Cause

The following reference is fragmentary and somewhat confusing, but appears to refer to a sudden-onset problem, perhaps trauma, accompanied by fainting spells and unusual sensations in the extremities (parasthesias) that result in the patient's sucking his fingers. The "darkened" presumably refers to the loss of consciousness and the "continually can get up afterward" to the absence of postseizure confusion and weakness (postictal state). "'Hand' of his god" indicates that the ancient physician had a general sense that this was the sort of thing that a god might have caused but did not feel that there was enough information available to make a firm diagnosis. For more examples of "hand" of his (personal) god, see above, 19.347–19.363.

Ap.62 DIŠ KI.MIN-*ma* U.MEŠ-*šú ú*-[. . .] ⸢*ú*⸣-*te-né-eṭ-ṭe* : ZI.ZI-*bi* ŠUB AN-*e* TAG-⸢*su* ŠU⸣ DINGIR-*šú* GAM (DPS XV:25 [AOAT 43.151])

**If (it is the first day he is sick) and he [sucks?] his fingers [. . .], he continually becomes darkened[26] (and) he continually can get up (afterward), *miqit šamê* (AN.TA.ŠUB.BA-seizure?) has "touched" him; "hand" of his god; he will die.

Possibly also to be classed with this reference is the following text, which attributes the problem to an unfulfilled vow.

Ap.63 D[IŠ U]$_4$ LÁ-*šú a-šiš-tum* DIB-*su* ÚḪ *ina* KA-*šú* DU-*ak* ŠÙD AD-*šú* DIB-*su* GAM (DPS XXVI:17′ [AOAT 43.279])

**⸢If when⸣ (a confusional state) comes over him, depression afflicts him (and) spittle flows from his mouth, a vow made by his father afflicts him; he will die.[27]

Mysterious Sorcery

Another set of categories used by the *āšipu* was various forms of sorcery (*kišpu*) including "inability to eat-magic" (KA.DIB.BI.DA) and "cutting of the breath" (ZI.KU$_5$.RU.DA). Ancient Mesopotamian physicians apparently used this diagnosis or rather set of diagnoses to designate syndromes that had specific signs and symptoms but seemed bizarre and mysterious. The first of these references, at least, could be a case of poisoning (see Chapter 15).

Ap.64 DIŠ NA SAG.DU-*su iṣ-ṣa-na-bat-su šit* x [. . .] MAŠ.GI$_6$.MEŠ-*šú par-da ina šit-ti-šú ig-d*[*a-na-lu-ut*] *bir-ka-šu ka-si-a ba-ma-as-su šim-ma-*[*tu* . . .] UZ[U]-*šú ru-ṭi-ib-*[*tu*] *im-ta-na-al-lu-*⌜*šú*⌝ LÚ BI *ka-ši-ip* . . . (*AMT* 86/1 ii 3–7)[28]

**If a person's head continually afflicts him, [his] ⌜sleep⌝ [. . .], his dreams are troubled, he [continually] ⌜jerks⌝ in his sleep, his knees are "bound," his chest is numb, [. . .] (and) his flesh is continually filled with "dampness," that person is *kišpu*'d. . .

Ap.65 DIŠ NA SAG.KI-*šú* RA!-⌜*su*⌝-*ma* DÙ ⌜UZU⌝.MEŠ-*šú* KÚ.MEŠ-*šú sà-li-ʾ qá-te-er* SAG ŠÀ-*šú* [K]Ú-*šú* KÚ NAG-*ma ut-ta-nar-ra* NA BI UŠ$_{11}$.ZU DIB-*šú* (*BAM* 193 i 8′–11′)[29]

**If a person's temple "strikes" him, all of his flesh hurts him, he is gloomy and depressed, his upper abdomen (epigastrium) ⌜hurts⌝ him, (and) when he eats or drinks, he continually vomits, *kišpu* afflicts that person.

Ap.66 [DIŠ N]A SAG.DU-*su* DIB.DIB-*su pa-nu-u-šú* NIGIN.MEŠ-[*du*] [*kal š*]*e-ra-šú* KÚ.MEŠ-*šú* ÚḪ-⌜*šu*⌝ *i-šal-*[*lu*] INIM.INIM.MEŠ-*šú im-ta-na-*⌜*áš*⌝-*ši* ŠÀ.MEŠ-*šú* MÚ.MÚ-[*ḫu*] Á.MEŠ-*šú ú-šam-ma-*[*mu-šú* ŠU]^{II}!-*šú e-te-né-ṣi-la-*[*šú*] GÌR^{II}.BI *ú-kan-*[*ni-na*] *u ki-ṣal-la-šú up-ta-na-ṭa-*[*ra*] LÚ BI EN D[UG$_4$].DUG$_4$-*šú kiš-pi* NIGIN-[*šú*] *kip-di-šú* [*ik-p*]*u-du-šú ana kiš-pi-šú-nu-ti* BÚR-⌜*ri*⌝ . . . (*KAR* 80 obv. 1–7)

**[If] a ⌜person's⌝ head continually afflicts him, his face seems continually to be spinning, [all] his ⌜flesh⌝ continually hurts him, he sprays his spit, he continually forgets his words, his insides are continually bloated, his arms go ⌜numb⌝, his [hands] continually become sluggish, he ⌜bends⌝ his feet but his ankles continually (feel) ⌜supple⌝, that person's adversary in court has surrounded him with *kišpu* (or) ⌜plotted⌝ his schemes against him; in order to dispel their sorcery . . .

Ap.67 [DIŠ N]A ⌜IGI^{II}⌝-*šú* [*iṣ*]-*ṣa-na-*[*p*]*ar* IGI.MEŠ NIGIN-*du* KA-*šu e-ta-*[*na-ba*]*l* KA-*šú it-ta-na-as-ḫar* UZU.[ME-*šú*] ŠUB.ŠUB-*šú* UZU.ME-*šú iṣ-ṣa-na-li-mu* GABA.ME [*i-k*]*aṣ-ṣa-su-šú* GABA.MEŠ-*šu ir-ta-na-m*[*u*] *ḫur-ba-šú* [ŠUB.Š]UB-*su* SAG.DU-*su* ŠU^{II}-*šú* GÌR^{II}-*šú* [. . .] *šá* NA BI KA.DIB.BI.DA ⌜DÙ⌝-*su* NU.MEŠ-*šú šá* DUḪ.LÀL x [. . .] (*STT* 89:96–101)

**[If] a ⌜person⌝'s eyes continually flutter, his eyes (feel like they) are spinning, his mouth [continually] ⌜dries up⌝, his mouth is continually turned to one side, [his] flesh continually (looks) terrible, his flesh continually turns black, the breasts give him a ⌜gnawing⌝ pain, both sides of his chest are continually ⌜relaxed⌝, chills [continually] ⌜fall⌝ upon him, his head, his hands, (and) his feet [. . .], KA.DIB.BI.DA ("inability to eat-magic") has been performed against that person, his figurines of wax [. . .]

Ap.68 [. . .] SÌG-*iṣ* SAG.KI.M[U. . .] *ina* GÚ.MU ta-na-ra x [. . .] *ina* GEŠTU^{II}-*ia taš-gu-*[*ma* . . .] *liq pi-ia ub-bu-la* [. . . NU.MEŠ-*ia a-šar* ANŠE *i*] *t-tag-ru-ur šu-nu-lu* [. . .] (*BAM* 484 obv. 1–5)

**[. . .] you struck my forehead [. . .] you(?) turned in my neck [. . .] you roared in my ears [. . .] they dried out my palate [. . . my figurines] were made to lie (by sorcerers) [where an equid had] rolled.[30] . . .

In some cases of "cutting of the breath," we believe that we know what it is the *āšipu* was trying to describe (see 19.364 with discussion). In the remaining cases attributed by the *āšipu* to "cutting of the breath" (ZI.KU$_5$.RU.DA), we are just as mystified as they were. Some of these conditions as, for example, the second reference below were at least treatable.

Ap.69 DIŠ NA SA ÚR ZAG-*šú* TAG.TAG-*su ši-ḫat* UZU TUKU.TUKU *mi-na-tu-šú ma-an-ga* UŠ$_4$-*šú* KÚR.KÚR *ma-la* DÙ-*šú i-ma-aš-ši* ÚḪ-*su pe-ṣa-a-at ana* NA BI *ana* IGI ^{d}*Gu-la ep-šú ep-šú-šú ina* U$_4$.27.KÁM U$_4$.28.KÁM DUG$_4$.BI AL.TIL ŠU ZI.KU$_5$.RU.DA BA.ÚŠ (*BAM* 449 iii 24′–27′; cf. *STT* 89:23–27)

**If the muscles of a person's left thigh continually hurt him intensely, he continually has wasting of the flesh, his limbs are stiff, his mentation is altered (and) he forgets whatever he does, (and) his phlegm is white, rituals have been performed against him before Gula. (If) on the twenty-seventh or twenty-eighth day he stops talking, "hand" of ZI.KU$_5$.RU.DA ("cutting of the breath"); he will die.

Ap.70 DIŠ NA KI.MIN *it-ta-na-*[*a*]*d-la-aḫ it-te-nen-biṭ* IGI^{II}-*šú ir-ru-ru* UZU.MEŠ-*šú i-šam-ma-mu-šú ši-in-na-šu ka-li-ši-na* KÚ.MEŠ-*šú* NINDA KÚ KAŠ NAG-*ma i-li-ḫi-ib ana* LÚ BI ZI.KU$_5$.RU.DA *ša* GA.ḪAB DÙ-*su šum-ma* KIN-*šú il-ta-bir* ÚŠ *la-ma* TE-*šu-ma* BA.ÚŠ . . . (*BAM* 449 iii 13′–16′//*BAM* 455 iii 4′–10′//*BAM* 467 i 1′–6′; cf. *STT* 89:18–22)

**If a person is continually troubled and cramped, his eyes tremble, his flesh goes numb, all of his teeth continually hurt him, (if) he eats bread (and) drinks beer, (his lungs) make a loud growling noise, ZI.KU$_5$.RU.DA ("cutting of the breath") with soured milk has been performed against that person. If his attack persists, he will die. Before it approaches him so that he dies . . .

The hurting teeth of the last reference above suggests something wrong with the gums. The three references below also demonstrate bleeding that could be from the gums ("blood flowing from the mouth").

Ap.71 DIŠ LÚ ^{UZU}SA ZAG *u* GÙB *uš-tab-ba-lum* MÚD *ina pi-i*-⸢*šú*⸣ x [. . .] *mi-iḫ-ḫa* U$_4$.3.KÁM DU-*ku ana* LÚ BI *ana* IGI MUL *e-pu-u*[*š* . . .] DIŠ U$_4$.10.KÁM GÍD.DA-*ma* BA.ÚŠ ŠU ZI.KU$_5$.RU.DA [. . . *a-n*] *a* ⸢ŠU⸣ ZI.KU$_5$.RU.DA KAR-*šú* . . . (*AMT* 44/4:1–4)

**If a person's muscles to the left and right are made to dry out, blood flows from his mouth, [. . .] (and) (what looks like) frothy beer (for) three days, (a ritual) has been performed against that person before the star(s) [. . .] If it lasts for ten days, he will die; "hand" of ZI.KU$_5$.RU.DA ("cutting of the breath") [in order] to save him from "hand" of "cutting of the breath". . .

Ap.72 DIŠ NA *ta-lam* 15-*šú e-em ta-lam* 150-*šú ka-ṣi*? IGI^{II}-*šú i-bar-ru-úr* MÚD *ina* ⸢KA-*šú*⸣ DU-*ku ana* NA BI [*ina*] ITI.ZÍZ x x *ana* IGI MUL x x x lum *ep-šú* [. . .] ZI.KU$_5$.<RU>.DA ÚŠ (*STT* 89:48–51)[31]

**If a person's left buttock is hot (and) his right buttock is cold, his eyes become dimmed, (and) blood comes from his nose/mouth, rituals have been performed against him in Šabaṭu before the [. . .] star; ["hand" of] ZI.KU$_5$.RU.DA ("cutting of the breath"); he will die.

Ap.73 DIŠ LÚ ŠÀ-*šú* x[. . .]x MÚD *ina* KA-*šú* DU-*ku* UZU^{II}-*šú i-gaṣ-ṣa-ṣ[u]-šú* ZI.KU$_5$.RU.DA ^{GIŠ}SAG.KUL DÙ-*su ana* KAR-*šú* . . . (*BAM* 461 iii 14′–16′)

**If a person's stomach [. . .], blood flows from his mouth, his flesh gives [him] a gnawing pain, ZI.KU$_5$.RU.DA ("cutting of the breath") has been practiced against him over the door bolt, to save him . . .

HAND OF MANKIND

This was a variety of *kišpu*-sorcery (see 19.121–19.122). Some of the examples are possibly to be classed with the *kišpu* references compatible with pneumonia discussed in Chapter 3 with 3.82–3.85 since they mention fever, coughing, and pain (groaning), which can be associated with pneumonia.

Ap.74 DIŠ GIG *ina še-re-e-ti il-te-né-eb-bu u* A *ma-gal* NAG *li-ʾ-bu* DIB-*su* GIG-*su* ŠU.NAM.LÚ.U$_{18}$.LU (DPS XXII:1 [AOAT 43.250])

**If the patient continually groans in the mornings and drinks a lot of water (and) *liʾbu*-fever afflicts him, his illness is "hand" of mankind.

Ap.75 DIŠ *i-reš-ti* ŠÀ APIN-*ma* NU KÚ *ú-gan-na-aḫ u* KÚM DIB.DIB-*su* GIG-*su* ŠU.NAM.LÚ.U$_{18}$.LU (DPS XXII:4 [AOAT 43.251])

**If he asks for something he has a craving for and then does not eat (it), he *guḫḫu*-coughs and fever continually afflicts him, his illness is "hand" of mankind.

DIRTY SUBSTANCES

Yet another variety of sorcery involved bringing the victim in contact with "dirty substances." A few of the examples accounted for drooling and speech problems in Parkinson's (see 13.263). None of the remaining descriptions is sufficiently complete to determine whether the ingested substance was a poison, a chemical irritant, or infectious in nature.

Ap.76 [DIŠ NA NINDA KÚ *u*] KAŠ NAG-*ma ina* ŠÀ-*šú la ina-aḫ* [. . .] *is!-sàl-la-a* A.MEŠ *ir-ta-na-muk ik-ka-šú ik-ta-na-ru* [. . .]-ka-ak NA BI *lu-a-te* KI NINDA KÚ *u* KAŠ [NAG *lu*]-*a-te* KI A.MEŠ NAG(!) . . . (AMT 48/2:11–14//*BAM* 90:3′–5′)

**[If a person eats bread and] drinks beer and then in his stomach he is not at ease, [. . .], he becomes ill, he continually bathes in water, he is continually short of breath, [. . .], that person has eaten or drunk dirty substances[32] with the bread he ate and the beer [he drank] or ⌜dirty⌝ substances with the water he drank . . .

Ap.77 DIŠ U$_4$ *u* G[I]$_6$ NAM.ÉRIM DIB-*su* : *lu-ʾa-ti* DIB-*su* (DPS XXII:24 [AOAT 43.253])

**If (it afflicts him) day and night . . . dirty substances afflict him.

Ap.78 [SAG.DU-*s*] *ú qá-ta-a-šu še-pa-a-[šu] m[i]-⌜it-ḫa-ri⌝-iš ik-kà-la-a-šú pu-šu a-na at-m[e-e la i-te-né]-⌜el⌝-la-a*[33] *lu-ʾa-⌜a⌝-[tu] ⌜šu⌝-[ku]l* (StBoT 36.23 r. 10′–11′)[34]

**(If) his [head(?)], his hands, (and) his feet all hurt at once (and) [he is continually unable] to ⌜raise⌝ his mouth to the ⌜words⌝, he has been made to ⌜eat⌝ dirty substances.

Ap.79 [DIŠ] ŠU^{II}-*šú ana* KA-*šú ú-ḫab-bat* TÚG-*su it-ta-na-suk u* UŠ$_4$-*šú* NU [DIB *lu-ʾ-a-tú šu-kul* GAM] (DPS XI A obv. 28//B 27 = *TDP* 92:28//*SpTU* 1.34:27; cf. DPS XV:16 [AOAT 43.151])

**[If] he moves his hands across his mouth,[35] he continually throws off his garment (and) he is not in full [possession] of his faculties, [he has been made to eat dirty substances;[36] he will die].

Ap.80 DIŠ MUNUS *ina* GIG-*šá* ŠU^{II}-*šá ú-na-aš-šak* ŠU.MEŠ *lu-ʾ-a-ti* TAG-*ši* (DPS XXXVII A obv. 16 = *TDP* 214:16)

**If a woman during her illness chews on her hands, dirty hands have touched her.

Mysterious References Attributed to Gods/Goddesses or Demons/Demonesses

The spirits in this category fall into two groups, gods/goddesses or demons/demonesses that are well known, such as the ghost, *rabīṣu*, Ištar, Lamaštu, Marduk, Sîn, and Šulpaea, and those where we have very limited information such as Adad, Uraš, Ninurta, the "great gods," Ningeštinanna, "the (mistress) of steppe and open country," and Ningizzida. In both categories, the number of texts and their length or details are limited, making interpretation difficult. Moreover, what can be puzzled out does not fit in with syndromes attributed to these spirits in other better-preserved texts (for which see Chapter 19).

GHOST

Ghosts were part of the Sîn family of fevers in connection with which they produced a benign fever or fevers involving the upper respiratory tract (19.247–19.249) and a serious neurologic illness or illnesses that included roaring in the ears plus fever (19.273–19.282). The following fever ghost references are too vague or too fragmentary to be placed definitely in one of these two categories.

Ap.81 [DIŠ . . .] *iš-tu* SAG.DU-*šú a-di* GÌR^{II}-*šú* [. . .] *ḫur-ba-šu* ŠUB.MEŠ-*su* [. . .] ŠU.^{d}INNIN ŠU.GIDIM.MA IM.RI.A-*šu* . . . (*AMT* 27/3:1–3)

**[If . . .] from his head to his feet, [. . .] chills continually fall upon him [. . .], "hand" of Ištar (or) "hand" of his family ghost . . .

Ap.82 [DIŠ SU-š] *ú* ⌜KÚM⌝-*im* ⌜ŠED$_7$⌝ *u* IR NU TUKU ŠU [GID]IM$_7$? DUMU *šip-ri* DINGIR-*šú* (DPS XVIII:2 [AOAT 43.218])

**[If] ⌜his⌝ [body] is hot (and then) cold but he does not have sweat, "hand" of ⌜ghost⌝(?) messenger of his god.

Ap.83 DIŠ GEŠTU^{II}-*šú u* SIG$_4$ GÌR^{II}-*šú* 1-*niš* [37] ŠED$_7$.MEŠ GIDIM *šu-ru-bat* EDIN DIB-*su* / DIŠ GEŠTU^{II}-*šú* GIN$_7$ GEŠTU MÁŠ.TUR *sa-al-ḫa* ŠU GIDIM DIŠ U$_4$.3.KÁM *ni-kit-tú* : LÍL TUKU (DPS VIII 15–16 = *TDP* 70:15–16)

**If his ears and the soles of his feet are cold at the same time, a ghost, one brought into the steppe, afflicts him. If his ears wiggle like the ears of a young goat, "hand" of ghost. If it is the third day (he has been sick), there will be cause for worry.

The texts below describe the prodromes of ghost-induced fevers. In the first, the patient has a brief illness followed by apparent recovery connected with an epidemic (note the comments about the ghosts of relatives). In the second, the patient has an apparently mild illness for several days before the fever sets in with a vengeance. These descriptions are suggestive, respectively, of viral meningitis and viral encephalitis, both of which are included among the possibilities for ghost-fevers with neurologic symptoms (see 19.273–19.282). Although sudden onset is characteristic, in some patients with viral meningitis, there is a prodromal "minor illness" followed by a short period of apparent recovery before the reappearance of fever and the development of signs of central nervous system involvement. In viral encephalitis, there may be a prodrome with headache, fever, myalgia, and sometimes sore throat, all symptoms associated with benign ghost-fevers. This prodrome lasts for several days before the more typical neurologic signs appear. All this is very suggestive; however, there is not enough evidence in the quotes themselves to be sure.

Ap.84 DIŠ U$_4$.1.KAM GIG-*ma* U$_4$.1.KAM *ba-liṭ* GIDIM AD *u* AMA DIB-*su* (DPS XVI:16 [AOAT 43.173])

**If he is sick for one day and then he is well for one day, the ghost of his father or mother afflicts him.

Ap.85 DIŠ U$_4$.1.KAM U$_4$.2.KAM *i-re-eḫ-ḫi-šum-ma ina* U$_4$.3.KAM DIB-*su* DIB GIDIM$_7$ (DPS XVI:17 [AOAT 43.173])

**If it flows over him for one or two days and afflicts him on the third day, affliction by a ghost.

Ghosts were often blamed for dizziness and for noisy intestines and abdominal pain (see 19.43, 19.383), so the fact that the following set of symptoms received a treatment directed against a ghost is no surprise. What is unsure is exactly what it was that the *āšipu* was attempting to treat.

Ap.86 DIŠ NA IGI.MEŠ-*šú* NIGIN-*du ù*ʾ-*a* ŠÀ-*bi i-qab-bi* ŠÀ.MEŠ-*šú i*-ʾ*a-ru-ru* SAG ŠÀ-*šú it-ta-na-az-qar* NINDA *u* KAŠ LAL *la-am ú-za-bi-lu*-«TU»-*ma* BA.ÚŠ . . . (*LKA* 85 obv. 1–4)

**If a person's face seems to spin (and) he says: "Oh, my insides!" his insides rumble, his upper abdomen (epigastrum) continually protrudes (and) he has no appetite for bread or beer; before he lingers and dies . . .

RĀBIṢU

The following references do not seem to fit any of the syndromes attributed to this demon (see Chapter 19). What is described in the first reference is excessive thirst without apparent fever. Excessive thirst is a characteric feature of some forms of untreated diabetes, and it is possible that a diabetic coma, particularly in an elderly patient who was also having strokes, might have looked to the *āšipu* like something a *rābiṣu*-demon might do, but in the absence of other suggestive signs and symptoms, this reference is not sufficient to suggest a diagnosis. The second quote is from a series of sequenced references preserved in a Middle Babylonian text from the Hittite capital of Ḫattušaš. The immediately following section discusses strokes attributed to Šulak, *rābiṣu*-demon of the toilet (see Chapter 13). The passage is suggestive of hyperthyroidism, a condition that was attributed to the *rābiṣu* (see Chapter 7), but the description is rather too vague and too heavily restored to be sure.

Ap.87 DIŠ ŠÀ-*šú* DIG-*ub* A UL$_4$-*gal* APIN-*eš* KÚM-*šú mit-ḫar* TA *taš-ri-ti* EN SAG GI$_6$ DIŠ GIG-*su id-da-lip* SÌG-*iṣ* MAŠKIM : GIDIM SÌG-*iṣ* GAM (DPS XIII B ii 13–14 = *TDP* 118 ii 13–14)

**If his abdomen is soft, he asks for a lot of water (but) his temperature is normal, (and) his illness has kept him awake from the beginning to the middle of the night, he was stricken with the blow of a *rābiṣu*-demon . . . he will die.

Ap.88 *mu-ru-us*!-*sú i-na ši-mi-ta-a-an* [. . . *ṣa*]-*bi-is-s*[*ú* [MAŠKIM] *ma-ḫi-iṣ* [BA.ÚŠ] / *pa-nu-šu iṣ-ṣa-nu-un-du* [. . . *i-na re-e*]*š mu-ši la-p*[*í-it* . . .]-⌜*e*⌝-*pa ù iš*-[*tu*] U$_4$.5.KAM U$_4$.10.KAM *i-na zu-u*[*m-ri-šu* . . .] *ma-ḫi-iṣ zu-ú-ta i*[*r-ta-na-aš-ši* MAŠKIM] ⌜*it*⌝-*t*[*i*]-⌜*šu*⌝ [*ra-ki-is i-n*]*a* U$_4$.3.KAM [BA.ÚŠ] / [. . .]x bi *ù ma-gal i-dáb-bu-ub* ŠU KI ⌜*i*⌝[. . .] / [*ina mu-ši ma-ru-u*]*ṣ i-na še-er-ti* ⌜*bá*⌝-*li-iṭ ú-ša-an-ša šu-le-e* [*mu-ur-ṣi*] (StBoT 36.21 obv. 4–9)

**If his illness [continually] afflicts him in the evening, a [*rābiṣu*] has struck (him);[38] [he will die]. If his face seems continually to be spinning (and) he was ⌜touched⌝ [at] the ⌜beginning⌝ of the night, he is [. . .] and he was struck five to ten days ⌜ago⌝ in [his] ⌜body⌝ [and his . . .] (and) he [continually has] sweat, [a *rābiṣu* is bound] with him; [he will die] ⌜on⌝ the third day. [. . .] and he talks a lot, "hand" of the netherworld; [. . .] If he is ⌜sick⌝ [in the night] and well in the morning and it keeps him up all night, [the illness] is culling (him) out.

IŠTAR

The following reference does not seem to fit any of the syndromes attributed to this goddess of sexual love and war (see Chapter 19).

Ap.89 DIŠ MUD Á-*šú šá* 15 *ú-za-qat-su* ŠU ^{d}1[5] (DPS X B r. 13 = *TDP* 88 r.13)

**If his left arm socket stings him, "hand" of Ištar.

LAMAŠTU

This demoness was responsible for a fever that may be typhus or typhoid as well as for a category of trauma (see Chapter 19).

Ap.90 [DIŠ SU].GAM-*šú šá* 15 KÚ-*šú u* IGI^{II}-*šú ur-ru-pa* ŠU ^{d}DIM$_{11}$.ME (DPS XII D iv 21//E iv 28 = *TDP* 108 iv 21)

**[If] his left ⸢armpit⸣ hurts him and his eyes are clouded, "hand" of Lamaštu.

Ap.91 DIŠ LÚ.TUR IM KA-*šú šá* 15 ŠED$_{7}$-*ma šá* 150 KÚM-*im* ŠU ^{d}DIM$_{9}$.ME (DPS XL A 54 = *TDP* 224:54)

**If the air of an infant's left nostril gets cold and that of the right gets hot, "hand" of Lamaštu.

MARDUK

This head of the Babylonian pantheon was generally held responsible for chest pain and for illnesses, including one variety of hemorrhagic fever, in which heart symptoms were prominent (see Chapter 19).

Ap.92 DIŠ NA SA.SAL.LA-*šú* KÚM.KÚM ŠU^{II}-*šú* GÌR^{II}-*šú* ⸢IR⸣ ŠUB.MEŠ-*a* GÌR^{II}-*šú ú-zaq-qa-ta-šu* ŠU ^{d}ALAD GAR!-*ni* ^{d}AMAR.UTU *ina* ŠU ^{d}ALAD KAR!-*šú* . . . (*STT* 95 i 13–14)

**If a person's upper back is continually hot, his hands and his feet continually produce sweat, (and) his feet sting him, "hand" of a *šēdu*, deputy of Marduk, to save him from the "hand" of a *šēdu* . . .

SÎN

This god of the moon and of divination is commonly associated with neurologic abnormalities (see Chapter 19).

Ap.93 DIŠ KI.MIN-*ma* ⸢Á-*šú šá* 15 GI$_{6}$⸣-*át* EME-*šú kaṣ-rat ina* EGIR-*šú* SÌG-*iṣ* GAM (DPS XV:9 [AOAT 43.151])

**If (it is the first day he is sick) and his left arm is dark (and) his tongue is tied in knots, he was wounded from behind; he will die.

Ap.94 DIŠ KI.MIN-*ma* ⸢Á⸣-*šú šá* 150 GI$_{6}$-*át i-ṭa-mu* [SÌG-*i*]*ṣ* ^{d}30 *u uš-te-zeb* [: GAM] (DPS XV:10 [AOAT 43.151]; cf. DPS X B r. 1 = *TDP* 86 r. 1)

**If (it is the first day he is sick) and his right arm is dark (and) he twists, ⸢blow⸣ of Sîn but he will get through [(var. he will die)].

ŠULPAEA

Ap.95 [DIŠ SU].GAM-*šú šá* 150 KÚ-*šú u* IGI^{II}-*šú ur-ru-pa* ŠU ^{d}*Šul-pa-è-a* (DPS XII D iv 22//E iv 29 = *TDP* 108 iv 22)

**[If] his right ⸢armpit⸣ hurts him and his eyes are clouded, "hand" of Šulpaea.

ADAD

Apart from trauma references, discussed in Chapter 19 under 19.139–19.149, Adad was associated with only a few vague and unhelpful descriptions of symptoms.

Ap.96 DIŠ GÚ-*su u* MURUB$_4$.MEŠ-*šú* 1-*niš* KÚ.MEŠ-*šú* ŠU ^{d}IM (DPS X A obv. 9//B obv. 9 = *TDP* 80:9)

**If his neck and hips continually hurt him at once, "hand" of Adad.

Ap.97 DIŠ *ina* SAG ŠÀ-*šú d*[*i-ik-šú* GAR-*su-ma* NU D]U$_8$-*ir ana* U$_4$.31.KÁM ŠU ^{d}IM GAM (DPS XIII B i 41′//F 3 = *TDP* 114 i 45′)

**If a ⌜needling pain⌝ [is firmly established] in his upper abdomen (epigastrium) [and will not] ⌜let up⌝ (and he has been sick) for thirty-one days, "hand" of Adad; he will die.

Ap.98 DIŠ *ina* ŠÀ-*šú* Á 150-*šú* ^{GIŠ}GIDRU GAR-*su-ma u* MÚD SUR ŠU ^{d}IM GAM (DPS XIII B ii 28//G$_2$ obv. 26+G$_1$ obv. 9 = *TDP* 120 ii 28)

**If a burning pain is firmly established in his abdomen on the right side and he drips blood, "hand" of Adad; he will die.

Probably the most distinctive sign is the attribution to Adad of a potentially fatal bright red and puffy face, as in the first reference below. It may be for this reason that Adad's "deputy" was "the angry one," anger being frequently associated, in more benign contexts, with turning red in the face. Whatever the problem was, the deputy was treatable, as is shown by the second reference below.

Ap.99 DIŠ IGI.MEŠ-*šú ṣar-pu u i-ša-ap-pu-ú* ŠU ^{d}IM GAM/DIN (DPS IX A 28 // B obv. 26 = *TDP* 74:28)[39]

**If his face is bright red and swells up like a cloud, "hand" of Adad; he will die (var. B: live).

Ap.100 *ana ez-zi* A.[RÁ *šá-né*]-*e* ^{d}IM SIG$_5$ (*STT* 93:60′; cf. *BAM* 379 ii 55′ [*Šammu šikinšu*])[40]

**(The plant) is good for "the angry one," a ⌜*šedû*-demon deputized⌝ by Adad . . .

URAŠ

Uraš, according to some traditions, is male and an ancestor of AN (the Sumerian version of Anu) but, according to others, female and AN's wife. The references to this divinity are equally hard to pin down, but whichever of the Uraš's it was, she/he had no mercy on adulterers.

Ap.101 DIŠ *in*[*a* KIR$_4$-*šú* U$_4$ *u* GI$_6$ MÚD *la i*] *k-kal-lu-ú* ŠU ^{d}*Uraš* MU DAM LÚ GÍD-*ma* GAM (DPS VI A obv. 16//B$_2$ obv. 2 = *TDP* 56:16; cf. StBoT 36.34 obv. 6′)

**If [day and night blood does not] ⌜stop⌝ (flowing) ⌜from⌝ [his nose], "hand" of Uraš on account of a man's wife. (If) it is prolonged, he will die.

Ap.102 DIŠ GIG-*su ina* EN.NUN MURUB$_4$.BA ZI.ZI-*šú ana* DAM LÚ TE-*ḫi* ŠU ^{d}*Uraš* (DPS XVII:32 [AOAT 43.198])

**If his illness rises in the middle watch of the night, he approached (another) man's wife; "hand" of Uraš.

Ap.103 DIŠ *ina* GI$_6$ GIG-*ma ina ka-ṣa-a-ti ba-liṭ* ŠU ^{d}*Uraš* MU D[AM LÚ] (DPS XVII:79 [AOAT 43.202])

**If he is sick in the night and well in the early morning, "hand" of Uraš on account of [(another) man's] ⌜wife⌝.

The "on account of another man's wife" in the preceding Uraš references occurs also with "hand"s of Šamaš and Ninurta (see below). Here, and in the other references, this supplementary diagnosis seems to be associated with bleeding. Perhaps what was envisiged was the adulterer suffering as if invisibly stabbed by the outraged husband.

NINURTA

In the following references, Ninurta is blamed for bleeding problems combined with neurologic symptoms and fever. It is possible that these patients' problems were attributed to Ninurta because of his association with the liver (see 19.365–19.367). Liver problems can be chronic processes, and can cause both bleeding and hepatic encephalopathy (see Chapter 6). None of the following references, however, is particularly convincing as a definite liver problem. Since Ninurta was also blamed for plague (see 3.226), it is also possible that some or all of them may be references to complications of plague. It might have helped if any of them (other than the first reference) had been completely preserved.

Ap.104 DIŠ *kal* U$_4$-*mi* TI-*ma ina* GI$_6$ GIG UD.DA GIG-*su* U$_4$.27.KÁM ŠU ^{d}MAŠ (DPS XVII:75 [AOAT 43.202])

**If he is well all day and sick in the night . . . (If he has been sick for) twenty-seven days, "hand" of Ninurta.

Ap.105 [DIŠ . . . KÚM]-*im* IGI^{II}-*šú it-te-né-ep-rik-ka-a* [. . . ŠU] ^{d}MAŠ MU DAM LÚ (DPS XVIII:15–16 [AOAT 43.218])

**[If . . .] he is ⌜feverish⌝ (and) his eyes are continually crossed [. . . "hand"] of Ninurta on account of (another) man's wife.

Ap.106 DIŠ KI.MIN-*ma* MÚD *ina* KIR$_4$/KA-*šú* DU-⌜*ku*⌝-*ma* U$_4$ *u* [GI$_6$ . . .] ŠU ^{d}MAŠ BÚR-*ma* DIN (DPS XXI:6–7 [AOAT 43.246]; cf. StBoT 36.34 obv. 8′)

**If (his blood vessels are healthy) but blood flows from his nose/mouth and it [does not stop(?)] day or [night], "hand" of Ninurta; (if) it lets up, he will get well.

"GREAT GODS"

It has been suggested that what appears to be "great gods" is possibly a writing for AN.GAL or Ištaran, serpentine god of Der.[41] His associations were with Ištar and the netherworld; neither connection sheds any light on the syndromes associated with him.

Ap.107 DIŠ KI.MIN-*ma ina* ŠÀ-*šú* ŠU^{II}-*šú* GAR.GAR U.MEŠ-*šú ú-na-ṣab* ŠU DINGIR *rab-bu-ti* GAM (DPS XVI:3 [AOAT 43.172])

**If (it is the first day he is sick) and his hands are continually placed on his abdomen (and) he sucks his fingers, "hand" of the great gods; he will die.

Ap.108 DIŠ KI.MIN-*ma a-a* GÙ.GÙ-*si-ma* NU NAG ŠU DINGIR.GAL.GAL GAM (DPS XVI:9 [AOAT 43.172])

**If (it is the first day he is sick) and he cries out "Ah" and will not drink, "hand" of the great gods; he will die.

Ap.109 DIŠ U_4.1.KÁM TAG$_4$-*šú-ma* U_4.1.KÁM LÁ-*šú* NÍG.KÚ ^{d}DIM$_{11}$.ME.LAGAB ŠU DINGIR.GAL.MEŠ GAM (DPS XVI:12 [AOAT 43.173])

**If it leaves him for one day (and then later) (febrile confusional states) come over him for one day, "eating" of *aḫḫāzu* (relapsing fever with jaundice; see Chapter 3) (or) "hand" of the great gods, he will die.

NINGEŠTINANNA

Ningeštinanna was the sister of Ištar's lover, Dumuzi. As a result of her efforts to get her brother released from the netherworld, she was given the job of scribe to Ereškigal. It was she who enrolled new entrants to the nether world and checked to make sure that no living persons were inadvertently admitted. The only reference attributed to her which is well preserved appears to be describing congenital nystagmus (see 13.109).

Ap.110 [DIŠ . . .]x-*tú sa-⌜li-iḫ⌝* ŠU ^{d}NIN.GEŠTIN.AN.NA : [DIŠ . . .]-*tú s*[*a-li-iḫ liq* K]A-*šú šá-bul* ŠU ^{d}NIN.GEŠTIN.AN.NA (DPS XVIII:43′–44′ [AOAT 43.219])

**[If. . .] shakes[42] [. . .], "hand" of Ningeštinanna. [If. . .] ⌜shakes⌝ [. . .] (and) his ⌜palate⌝ is dried up, "hand" of Ningeštinanna.

MISTRESS OF STEPPE AND OPEN COUNTRY

The one-sided viselike headache of this reference is the only attribution to the mistress of steppe and open country. Labat[43] suggests that what may have been contemplated was a form of curse or witchcraft that put the victim in the power of the goddess.

Ap.111 U_4 GIG *na-kap-ti* 150-*šu* GAT-*at* ŠU EDIN *ù ba-ma-a-ti* (*MDP* 57.11 iii 6–7)

**If the patient's left temple (feels) pressured, "hand" (of the mistress) of steppe and open country.

NINGIZZIDA

Ningizzida's only other attested reference is to abdominal ileus due to trauma (see 19.203), which might suggest that trauma was the cause of the shortness of breath mentioned in the text below.

Ap.112 DIŠ ZI-*šú* GIN_7 *šá* TA A E_{11}-*a* LÚGUD.MEŠ ŠU [d][. . .] ŠU [d]*Nin-giz-zi-da* : ŠU GIDIM *šá ina* A [ÚŠ DIB-*su*] (DPS X A obv. 32b–33 = *TDP* 84:32b–33)

**If his breath is short like one who has just come up from the water, "hand" of [. . .], "hand" of Ningizzida or "hand" of the ghost of one who [died] in the water [afflicts him].

Chart Showing the Arrangement of Entries in the Diagnostic/Prognostic Series

In studying the organization of the diagnostic/prognostic series, much can be learned about the teaching and practice of medicine in ancient Mesopotamia. Anatomy is the dominant structure, especially visible in Tablets III to XIV.[1] Listing texts in head-to-toe order facilitated the physician's search for relevant texts. Modern medical texts all have an index to help find items of interest, but indices are a relatively recent invention. Other principles of organization include ordering entries in accordance with the number of days a patient had been sick. This facilitated the addition of later material, as in Tablet XVI, where a section organized by the number of five-day weeks a patient had been sick (lines 52′–60′) was apparently inserted, set off by paragraph lines, into the approprate slot (between lines 46′–51′ [more than five days] and lines 61′–75′ [more than six days]).

Within each category, there are other types of organization. Texts that refer to a single disease are clustered together (sequenced references; see Introduction) for the likely purpose of providing the physician with an understanding of the variations in signs and symptoms that may be seen in a particular disease. Modern textbooks of medicine typically provide detailed information about the frequency and severity of signs and symptoms of a specific disease. It must be remembered, of course, that the *āšipu*'s syndromes or diseases are in some cases groups of diseases that modern physicians subdivide. Some passages in the diagnostic/prognostic handbook were apparently intended as a differential diagnosis for spirits, as, for example, Tablet IV, lines 7–18, which attempts to sort out all the different types of headaches attributed to ghosts.

Another important use of this ancient "textbook" is for comparisons between different diseases with overlapping signs or symptoms. By placing these references side-by-side (contrasted references; see Introduction), the physician and physician-in-training were able to easily make comparisons and to understand significant differences. Particularly interesting in this regard are sections discussing the progression of arthritis from pain to swelling and sluggishness to immobilization of the joints (Tablet XI, lines 99′–102′) or attempting to explain the difference between gastrointestinal ulcers and obstruction on the one hand (Tablet XIII, lines 42–43) and between bleeding ulcers and liver problems on the other (Tablet XIII, lines 82–92).

Texts with differing signs and symptoms and degrees of severity were also juxtaposed to illustrate how these differences affected prognosis. For example, Tablet XII, lines 70–81, shows how varying degrees of back (kidney) pain influence the outcome of the illness, and Tablet XVI, lines 65′–72′, explains which signs and symptoms in biphasic fever are grave and which are not. Particularly interesting are references appearing in one section of Tablet XVII which might be subtitled: "it's not what you think!" Examples include not a true seizure (lines 15–16), not a coma (line 18), and not a stroke (lines 30–31).

These same approaches are used in all modern medical texts. There can be no serious doubt that the diagnostic/prognostic series constitutes the earliest recorded medical textbook.

Key to the Chart

In the following tables, the left-hand column indicates the line number on the original tablet of the diagnostic/prognostic handbook. For Tablets XV to XXXIII, the numbers are those given in the edition in Heeßel, AOAT 43. For the remaining tablets, the number given is the actual line number of the main text as cited in the body of the book. The second column contains the ancient diagnosis, if any. Broken entries are indicated by [. . .]. The third column contains the modern diagnosis where this has been ascertained. Justification for the attribution is to be found in the cited chapters. The central column contains an abbreviated description of symptoms. The fifth column contains the ancient prognosis, if any. The last column tells where in the body of the current work this entry is cited. The first number is the number of the chapter. The number that follows the period is the number of the quoted passage within the chapter. For example, 20.26 would be the twenty-sixth quoted passage in Chapter 20. An "n" after the number indicates that the entry is cited in an endnote attached to the relevant quoted passage; "d" indicates that the entry is cited in the text that discusses the quoted passage; "dn" indicates that it is cited in an endnote to this discussion; "pn" indicates that the entry is cited in an endnote in the general discussion preceding and "fn" in an endnote in the general discussion following the quoted passage. A single horizontal line across the chart indicates subsections marked by paragraph lines on the original tablets. To aid the reader in appreciating the way in which the diagnostic/prognostic handbook was used to train students of medicine, we have made the organizing principles explicit and have marked sequenced or contrasting references off from the body of the text and from one another by blank lines.

DPS Tablet III

ORGANIZING PRINCIPLE: USES THE VERB POUR/CAST

A ob.1		preparations	cast a spell		3.222dn
A ob.2	[...]	water test: coma	water poured over face; no shuddering; no recognition of known persons	no recovery	13.286n 20.102n
A ob.3		water test: peritonitis	water poured over patient; epigastrium softens	[recovery]	17.164dn
A ob.4		water test: coma	water poured in mouth; patient can hold it there	[recovery]	13.289

ORGANIZING PRINCIPLE: TOP OF HEAD/SKULL

A ob.5		evolution of fever	skull hot; temporal blood vessels calm; 1 day	[...]	3.12 14.24dn 20.22n
A ob.6		evolution of fever	skull hot; temples lukewarm; 1 day	[...]	3.12
A ob.7		evolution of fever	skull hot; temples hot; 2 or 3 days	[...]	3.12
A ob.8		evolution of fever	skull hot; temples hot and sweaty; 3 days	[...]	3.12
A ob.9		evolution of fever	skull hot; temples and region between the arms hot and sweaty; 5 days	[...]	3.12n
A ob.10	Nusku	fever in infants	skull hot		19.346n
A ob.11	*kišpu*	pneumonia	skull hot; breast and back also hot		3.83n
A ob.12	Ardat lilî	adolescent angst	headache and libido; persistent erection		12.73
A ob.13–14	Ardat lilî	adolescent angst	headache and libido; tossing and turning; persistent erection		12.74
A ob.15–16	Ištar of Arbela	Strachan's syndrome	headache; reddish mouth; burning pubic region with loss of libido; paralysis and trembling		7.17 19.373dn
A ob.17	Anu		cries of "my skull"		19.369
A ob.18	Anu's vizier	wound	wound to the top of the head		19.204
A ob.19	Ištar	wound	wound to the top of the head with hearing loss		9.93 13.101 13.131 19.156 19.206dn
A ob.20	Ištar's vizier?	wound	wound to the top of the head with trembling legs and hurting stomach		13.134dn 19.206
A ob.21	Ištar's vizier?	wound	wound to the top of the head with bloated stomach		13.134dn 19.206
A ob.22–23	ghost	pain	nonfatal but severe pain from middle of the head down		19.394

A ob.24		fatal headache	seam of the skull feels open	[death]	13.166
A ob.25		fatal headache	seam of the skull seems to tremble	[death]	13.166n
A ob.26		nonfatal headache	seam of the skull feels normal	[recovery]	
A ob.27–30	[. . .]		head hair is fine	[. . .]	Ap.4
A ob.31–32			head hair is normal	recovery	
A ob.33		kwashiorkor	hair on crown of head frizzes	death	7.6
C ob.23b	"touched in the steppe"	kwashiorkor	hair on central part of head turns red		7.8

ORGANIZING PRINCIPLE: THE HEAD

C ob.24	[. . .]	Strachan's syndrome	head shakes; reddish mouth; burning pain; loss of sleep		7.18
C ob.25	[. . .]		head seems to spin; legs cold		3.39n Ap.3
C ob.26–27	[. . .]	dystonic movement	head twists; left or right foot paralyzed in bent position		13.63 13.63n 13.77 13.77n
C ob.28	ghost	encephalitis?	head stings and roars; fingers sting		19.276n
C ob.29–30			presence or absence of blood vessels (pulse)	[. . .]	
C ob.31	*šaššaṭu*	tetanus (physical pain)	hurting head, neck, and back		3.198
C ob.32–33	Ištar	psychosomatic pain	afflicting head; intensely hurting neck; hurting breast; chest pain but no vomiting		19.5
C ob.34	Ištar	benign fever	afflicting head with fever		19.254
C ob.35	Ištar	psychiatric	afflicting head without fever		3.3n; 13.5 19.12
C ob.36–37	Lamaštu	typhoid?	afflicting head; all-over fever, dizziness, and alteration of mentation	survival	3.25 19.227
C ob.38	Mukīl rēš lemutti	headache	afflicting head (and sometimes also alteration of mentation) but no fever		13.151
C ob.39–40		Parkinson's	head, hands, legs, and feet tremble; patient is stooped and cannot walk very well; cannot stick out tongue; drooling	no recovery	13.262
C ob.41		Parkinson's	head, hands, and feet tremble; patient cannot articulate		13.263
C ob.42	dirty substances	Parkinson's	head, hands, and feet tremble (*tarāru*); patient has scanning speech		13.85 13.263
C ob.43	[. . .]	high fever	head, hands, and feet tremble (*ra'ābu*); patient cannot articulate		13.86
C ob.44	Šamaš?	high fever	head, hands, and feet tremble (*ra'ābu*); patient is vomiting		13.86 19.252n
C ob.45	dirty substances	Parkinson's	head, hands, and feet tremble (*ratātu*); patient cannot articulate and has scanning speech		13.87 13.263n

C ob.46–47	[. . .]	biphasic fever	feverish head; relapse with hurting limbs and thirst		3.7n 3.28
C ob.48–49	*aḫḫāzu*	biphasic fever	feverish head; relapse with cold feet; leaves with crisis	[fatal] in elderly	3.7n 3.30n
C ob.50	personal god	*li'bu*-fever	feverish head and racing pulse in head		3.7 19.360
C ob.51	*ṣibit šadî*	*li'bu*-fever	feverish head and cold extremeties		3.1; 3.11n 3.15 19.216
C ob.52–54	[. . .]	encephalomyelitis	feverish head; racing pulse; cold feet; cyanosis; yellow spots and vagus nerve paralysis	death	8.41n 10.50n 13.219
C ob.55	"hand" of god	nonspecific fever	just feverish head and racing pulse; flushing	[recovery]	8.41 19.133 19.361
C ob.56	[. . .]	nonspecific fever	feverish head and abdomen; racing pulse	[. . .]	6.79n 8.41n
C ob.57	[. . .]	peritonitis	ditto with abdominal swelling and rigidity	[. . .]	3.202 6.40 8.41n
C ob.58	[. . .]		feverish head, lukewarm or [. . .] high temperature;		
C ob.59	[. . .]		feverish head and white lips; [. . .]		
C r.1	[. . .]		head burns with fever; face is flushed; [. . .]		3.8n
C r.2	[. . .]		head burns with fever; face is flushed; [. . .]		3.8n
C r.3–4	ghost	dehydration	jabbing pains in head and body; babbling; upset stomach		3.110 19.295n
C r.5–6	ghost	dehydration	jabbing pains in head and body; babbling; no upset stomach		3.110 19.295n
C r.7	twin gods	fever with possible DIC	head and body burn with fever; upset stomach	recovery unless dripping blood from anus	3.8n 19.136 19.240
C r.8	twin gods	fever with possible DIC	head burns with fever; jerking	recovery unless dripping bile and vomiting bile or blood	3.8n 19.241
C r.9	Sîn?	encephalitis?	head burns with fever; leaves at midday (i.e., worse in morning and evening); wants to bathe		3.8n 19.260n
C r.10–11	*aḫḫāzu*	biphasic fever	head burns with fever; relapse with cold feet; leaves with crisis	[recovery] if course is regular	3.8n; 3.30 6.130n

C r.12	[. . .]	wound	wound to the head		
C r.13	Adad	wound	wound to left side of the head		19.139dn 19.142
C r.14	Šamaš	wound	wound to right side of the head	death	19.190
C r.15	Ningirsu	cranial nerve injury	wound to the head with heavily clouded eyes		9.2; 13.89 19.167
C r.16	Ištar	wound	wound to the head with hurting limbs	recovery possible	19.157
C r.17	Ištar to twin gods	wound	wound to the head with twisting		13.122 19.158 19.185
C r.18	twin gods	wound	wound to the head; produces dark blood	death	13.134 19.180
C r.19	twin gods	wound	wound to the head; vomits blood	death	6.31 13.135 19.180
C r.20	"hand" of god	cranial nerve injury	wound to the head with loss of hearing; ears [. . .]	death	9.94 13.132 19.213
C r.21	"hand" of god	infected scalp wound	wound to the head with racing pulse; flushed and feverish	recovery	8.43 13.128 19.132
C r.22–23	*aḫḫāzu*	skull fracture	wound to the head with fever and twisting	death	3.40n 13.127 19.187
C r.24	Ištar	wound	wound to head and hip		7.1dn 19.164n

ORGANIZING PRINCIPLE: FROM HEAD TO MIDREGION OR FEET

C r.25		tetanus (physical illness)	shaking from head to toes	no recovery	3.200
A r.3–4	god of the quai	psychosomatic illness	heat from head to hip region and rest cold; jabbing headache; [. . .]	recovery	16.27
A r.5			pallor from head to hip region; [flushing?] from hip region to feet; hot hands	if difficult, death	Ap.19
A r.6	illness of 1 month		illness from head to hip region and rest well	recovery	Ap.19
A r.7	beginning of illness		illness from hip region to feet and rest well	recovery	Ap.19
A r.8	Sîn	HSV2	red *bubu'tu* from head to feet; body white; sexually transmitted		2.18n 3.233 4.18 10.85

A r.9	Sîn	HSV2	red *bubu'tu* from head to feet; body dark; sexually transmitted		3.233n 4.18n 10.85
A r.10	Ištar		*bubu'tu* from head to feet; body yellow; sexually transmitted		3.233n 4.18n 10.86
A r.11	Šamaš		white *bubu'tu* from head to feet; body dark; sexually transmitted		4.18n 10.87 19.106
A r.12	Šamaš		dark *bubu'tu* from head to feet; body red; sexually transmitted		3.233n 4.18n 10.87 19.106
A r.13–14	Gallû	cataplexy	healthy blood vessels from head to midpoint; paralysis and unresponsiveness		13.212n
A r.15		comatose patient	blood vessels run parallel and are present; does not open his eyes	recovery possible	2.7n Ap.46n

ORGANIZING PRINCIPLE: CENTRAL AREA OF THE HEAD

A r.16	"touched in the steppe"	kwashiorkor	hair abnormal	worrisome	7.1n
A r.17	"touched in the steppe"	kwashiorkor	hair stands on end	worrisome	7.4n 10.189dn
A r.18	"touched in the steppe"	kwashiorkor	hair brittle		7.2n
A r.19	"touched in the steppe"	kwashiorkor	hair trembles		7.5

ORGANIZING PRINCIPLE: HAIR OF THE HEAD

A r.20	"touched in the steppe"	kwashiorkor	hair frizzes	worrisome	7.6n
A r.21a		frizzies	hair chopped-looking	survival	7.3
A r.21b		kwashiorkor	hair brittle	death	7.3
A r.22a	"touched in the steppe"	kwashiorkor	hair brittle	worrisome	7.2
A r.22b	"touched in the steppe"	kwashiorkor	hair abnormal	worrisome	7.1
A r.23	"touched in the steppe"	kwashiorkor	hair stands on end	[worrisome]	7.4 10.189dn
A r.24	"touched in the steppe"	kwashiorkor	hair of head and body stands on end	death	7.4n 10.189dn

A r.25	"touched in the steppe"	kwashiorkor	hair stands end on end	[death]	7.4n 10.189dn
A r.26		kwashiorkor	hair easily pulled out	death	7.7
A r.27	[. . .]	kwashiorkor	hair turns bright red	[. . .]	7.9n
A r.28		kwashiorkor	hair turns red and/or frizzes	death	7.9
A r.29			rubs the hair of head and [. . .] his garment		

DPS Tablet IV

ORGANIZING PRINCIPLE: TEMPLES

B i 1	Kūbu	leptospirosis?	viselike headache; fever		19.339
B i 2	Kūbu	leptospirosis?	viselike headache; loose bowels		13.13 19.339
B i 3	Kūbu	leptospirosis?	viselike headache; cramped insides		13.13n 13.18dn 19.339
B i 4	personal god	meningitis?	viselike headache with loss of hearing	death	13.14 19.212 19.292 20.64
B i 5a			temples normal	recovery	14.24
B i 5b		shock	temporal blood vessels have collapsed	death	3.12dn 14.24 20.22n
B i 6		shock	temporal blood vessels have collapsed; eyes blurred	death	3.12dn 14.25 20.22n
B i 7	ghost	alcoholism	severe headache with bleeding from the mouth		15.23
B i 8	ghost	fatal headache	severe headache; racing pulse; seam of head feels open	death	13.167
B i 9	ghost	fatal headache	severe headache; racing pulse; seam of head feels broken into pieces	death	13.168 20.63
B i 10	ghost	alcoholism?	severe headache with hurting insides	if prolonged, death	19.301n 19.375n
B i 11	ghost	alcoholism?	severe headache with hurting insides; vomiting; sleepless nights	death	6.28 19.302 20.70
B i 12		fatal headache	headache all night	death	13.165
B i 13	ghost	tension headache	headache all day		13.154n
B i 14	ghost	alcoholism	headache with bleeding from the mouth		15.23n
B i 15	ghost	tension headache	headache with hurting neck muscles		13.152n
B i 16	ghost	benign fever	headache with hurting eye muscles		9.56n 19.247

B i 17	ghost	benign fever	headache with fever and swollen eyes		9.56n 19.247
B i 18	ghost		headache with vertigo		13.104n 19.43
B i 19	ghost	alcoholism	headache and low-grade fever with numbness		15.22n
B i 20–21	Ardat lilî	syphilis?	headache and low-grade fever with epigastric pain and patchy hair loss		3.4n 4.26
B i 22	ghost	migraine	left temple feels hot and right temple feels cold (genuinely one-sided heat sensation)		13.158
B i 23	*rābiṣu*'s footsteps	rheumatic fever?	left temple feels hot and right temple shakes (figure of speech; way of saying that heat and rapid pulse are in proportion to one another)	recovery	3.202dn 19.82
B i 24	Sîn	encephalitis?	right temple hurts plus nystagmus; 5 days	[death]	13.113n 19.263dn
B i 25	Šamaš	benign fever	left temple hurts	recovery	19.253
B i 26	Ištar	benign fever	right temple hurts	recovery	19.253
B i 27	city god	nutritional? optic neuropathy	left temple hurts and left eye makes a "shadow"	may go away by itself	9.91n 19.206dn 19.350n
B i 28	Šulpaea	retrobulbar? optic neuropathy	right temple hurts and right eye makes a "shadow"	may go away by itself	9.90n 19.86 19.206dn
B i 29	city god	nutritional? optic neuropathy	both temples hurt and both eyes make a "shadow"	may go away by itself	9.91 19.206dn 19.350
B i 30–31	ghost, deputy of Ištar	benign fever	left or right temple hurts and left or right eye swollen and tearing		9.54n 19.247dn 19.393dn
B i 32	personal god	stress headache	both temples hurt but no fever	recovery	3.3 13.164 16.6 19.35 19.211
B i 33	city god	nonspecific fever	both temples hurt and fever present	recovery	3.3n 13.164 19.363dn
B i 34	ghost	benign fever	temple hurts and jabs; eyes sting; neck muscles hurt		9.52
B i 35a	Kūbu	wound	wound to the temple		19.188
B i 35b	[. . .]	wound	wound to left temple	recovery	
B i 36a	personal god	wound	wound to right temple		19.210
E i 18b	ghost or "hand" of god	wound	wound to left temple	recovery	19.169 19.210

A ob.40	[Sîn]	petrous bone fracture	wound to left or right temple with [tearing] eyes		19.200
A ob.41	[Sîn]	petrous bone fracture	wound to right temple with moist eyes		19.200
A ob.42	[. . .]	wound	wound to left temple with twisting		13.123
A ob.43	[. . .]	wound	wound to right temple with twisting		13.123
A ob.44	[Ereškigal]	wound	wound to temple, epigastrium, and rib	[death]	19.173n
A ob.45	[. . .]	wound	wound to temple with intestinal [cramping?]		13.134dn
A ob.46	[. . .]	infected wound	wound to temple; racing pulse; [. . .]	recovery	8.43n 13.128n
A ob.47	[. . .]	infected wound	wound to temple; racing pulse; [. . .]	recovery	8.43n 13.128n
A ob.48	[. . .]	wound	wound to temple and hip region; [. . .]	recovery	
A ob.49		pregnancy, etc.	small webs on temple and [. . .]	recovery	6.153
A ob.50	Šamaš		small webs on temple, mouth, and abdomen		6.153
A ob.51		cirrhosis	small webs on temple, frontside, hands, and [. . .]	death	6.153
A ob.52	[. . .]		hot temples and cold ears; [. . .]	death	3.2n
A ob.53	[. . .]		hot ears and cold temples; [. . .]	death	3.2n
A ob.54–55	Marduk		warm temples and [. . .] ears; [. . .]		3.4n
A ob.56–57	Sîn or Šamaš	encephalitis?	warm temples and ears; clear [lungs]; headache		3.4n 19.263dn 19.270
A ob.58	personal or city god	encephalitis?	warm temples and ears	if severe, death	3.4n 19.292n
A ob.59	Sîn or Šamaš	encephalitis?	hot temples and ears		19.261n 19.270n
A ob.60	Sîn's deputy	encephalitis?	hurting temples and ears; hot body	(if only 3 days, survivable)	3.5 19.261n
A ob.61	"hand" of god	encephalitis?	hurting temples and ears; hot body; 3 days	death	19.292n
A ob.62	Azu	ear infection	hurting temples and continual chills		19.343
A ob.63	Azu	ear infection	hurting temples and ears and continual chills; 5 days		19.343
A ob.64	personal god or Kūbu	nonspecific fever or leptospirosis?	temples are hot but ears are not		3.2 19.335 19.360dn
A ob.65	Ištar or Šamaš	benign fever	both temples "go"; heavy sweating; vomiting		3.12dn 19.252
A ob.66–67	Ištar or Šamaš	benign fever	both temples shake or "go"; heavy sweating; 5 days		19.257

A ob.68		septic shock	temporal blood vessels have collapsed; photophobia	death	9.16 14.25n

ORGANIZING PRINCIPLE: BLOOD VESSELS/MUSCLES

A ob.69			they cross in left temple	recovery	Ap.44
A ob.70			they cross in right temple	recovery	Ap.44n
A ob.71			they cross in both temples	prolonged	Ap.44n
E ii 16			blood vessels red and cross in the temple	recovery	Ap.45
E ii 17		infected wound	temporal blood vessels are cut through; fever	recovery	14.4
E ii 18	wound from in front	wound	temporal blood vessels are cut through and dark	difficult	14.4
E ii 19–20	ghost	migraine	afflicting blood vessels in left or right temple; left or right eye contains blood		9.35n 13.160n
E ii 21	ghost	migraine	afflicting blood vessels in both temples; both eyes contain blood		9.35n 13.162n
E ii 22–23	ghost	migraine	afflicting blood vessels in left or right temple; left or right eye contains tears		13.159n
E ii 24	[ghost]	migraine	afflicting blood vessels in both temples; both eyes contain tears		13.161n
E ii 25	ghost	alcoholism	afflicting blood vessels in the temples; vomiting blood		15.23n
E ii 26	ghost	alcoholism	afflicting blood vessels in the temples; vomiting blood; nausea		6.56n 15.23n
E ii 27	ghost	benign fever	muscles of left temple swollen over left eye		9.55 19.247n
E ii 28	ghost	benign fever	muscles of right temple swollen over right eye		9.55 19.247n
E iii 1	holding fast of illness	head wound	blood vessels of left temple dark	death	14.4n
E iii 2		head wound	blood vessels of right temple dark	weakening	14.4n
A_2 r.1		head wound	blood vessels of temples dark	death	14.4n
A_2 r.2		head wound	blood vessels of temples red; left temple dark	worrisome	14.4n
A_2 r.3		head wound	blood vessels of temples red; right temple dark	recovery	14.4n
A_2 r.4	wound from in front	head wound	blood vessels of temples red; both temples dark	recovery	14.4n
A_2 r.5	wound from in front	head wound	temporal blood vessels "go" on left and are present on right	if difficult, death	8.58
A_2 r.6	wound from behind!	head wound	temporal blood vessels "go" on right and are present on left	recovery	8.59
A_2 r.7		shock	temporal blood vessels "go" on left	death	14.24n

			and are slow on right; temporal blood vessels have collapsed		
A_2 r.8		shock	temporal blood vessels pulse rapidly on right; [gangrene?] in fingers	death	8.9n
A_2 r.9		shock	temporal blood vessels vomit forth	death	14.30
A_2 r.10		shock	temporal blood vessels collapse	death	14.24n
A_2 r.11		shock	temporal blood vessels water the ground with blood	death	14.31
A_2 r.12			temporal blood vessels dark; [. . .]	death	
A_2 r.13			temporal blood vessels partially present; [. . .]	recovery	
A_2 r.14			temporal blood vessels [. . .]	worrisome	
A_2 r.15			temporal blood vessels [. . .]	death	
A_2 r.16			temporal blood vessels on both sides are present; [. . .]	death	
A_2 r.17			temporal blood vessels on both sides pulsate; [. . .]	death	
A_2 r.18			temporal blood vessels on both sides pulsate and are dark; [. . .]	worrisome	
A_2 r.19			temporal blood vessels on both sides pulsate; epigastrium [. . .]	[. . .]	
A_2 r.20–21	*rābiṣu*	tachycardia	temporal blood vessels on both sides"go" to an equal extent; treatment allowed	recovery possible	19.116 20.25
A_2 r.22		tachycardia	temporal blood vessels on both sides "go" several times in a row	death	20.25
A_2 r.23		tachycardia	temporal blood vessels on both sides "go"; eyes fixed	death	20.23
A_2 r.24		tachycardia	temporal blood vessels on both sides "go" plus afflicting abdomen	death	20.24
A_2 r.25		tachycardia	temporal blood vessels on both sides "go"; is withdrawn and has changes of mood	death	20.24
A_2 r.26–27	*rābiṣu*	tachycardia	temporal blood vessels on both sides "go" at same time plus afflicting epigastrium; treatment allowed	recovery possible	19.117
A_2 r.28	*rābiṣu*	tachycardia	temporal blood vessels on both sides "go" at same time plus changes of mood	death	19.118
A_2 r.29			blood vessels of temples, hands, and feet continually "go"	death	8.55
A_2 r.30	city god or Šamaš	atherosclerosis	blood vessels of temples, hands, or feet "go" on right and are present on left		19.124
A_2 r.31–32	Šamaš	claudication	ditto on either side plus muscles of feet on left or right become stiff and shift under him; feet have viselike pain but patient can lift them; gazes at his body		16.55 19.125

A_2 r.33			blood vessels of temples, hands, feet, neck, and epigastrium "go";	7 days > no recovery	8.56
A r.1			blood vessels of temples, hands, feet, neck, and umbilical area "go"; body is cold but eyes open and close	recovery possible	8.57 20.12 20.21
A r.2–3			blood vessels of temples and hands run parallel and are present but he doesn't open his eyes	recovery possible	2.7
A r.4			blood vessels of temples run parallel and the fever lets up	recovery possible	Ap.46
A r.5	ghost	benign fever	pulsating temples; hurting body		19.26dn 19.393n
A r.6	ghost	alcoholism	pulsating temples, numb hands and feet		15.22 19.26dn
A r.7	ghost	alcoholism	pulsating temples, numbness, and limpness		15.22n 19.26dn
B r.20	*rābiṣu*	Graves' disease	hair of temples fine; pulsating blood vessels; afflicting abdomen and rumbling epigastrium	death	7.27 19.115

ORGANIZING PRINCIPLE: THE FOREHEAD

B r.21a			forehead holds fever	recovery	
B r.21b			forehead holds sweat	recovery	
B r.22			forehead cold	recovery	3.39n 20.19
B r.23			forehead white; tongue is white	recovery	18.38
B r.24–32		food cravings	forehead is various colors; he asks for various foods		Ap.48
B r.33			forehead is [. . .] like brewer's yeast; patient asks for dates	[. . .]	Ap.48
B r.34			forehead is [. . .] like brewer's yeast; eyes are crossed	death	13.92 Ap.48

DPS Tablet V

ORGANIZING PRINCIPLE: THE EYES

IVB r.35	father's god	fever	left eye hurts	recovery	19.222n
A 1′–2′	[. . .]		[. . .]	[. . .]	
A 3′		wound	left eye was smashed and [. . .]	[. . .]	14.5n
A 4′		wound	right eye was smashed and [. . .]	[. . .]	14.5n
A 5′		wound	both eyes were smashed and [. . .]	[. . .]	14.5n
A 6′		wound	left eye was smashed and is full of sediment	[. . .]	9.85n 14.5n

A 7′		wound	right eye was smashed and is full of sediment	[. . .]	9.85n 14.5n
A 8′		wound	both eyes were smashed and are full of sediment	[. . .]	9.85 14.5
A 9′		pinguecula	left eye has light yellow spots; [. . .]	[. . .]	9.41n
A 10′		pinguecula	right eye has light yellow spots; [. . .]	[. . .]	9.41n
A 11′		pinguecula	both eyes have light yellow spots; [. . .]	[. . .]	9.41
A 12′		periorbital ecchymosis	left eye dark; [. . .]	[. . .]	9.25n 10.37n
A 13′		periorbital ecchymosis	right eye dark; [. . .]	[. . .]	9.25n 10.37n
A 14′		periorbital ecchymosis	both eyes dark; [. . .]	[. . .]	9.25n 10.37n
A 15′		periorbital ecchymosis	left eye dark and will not open; [. . .]	[. . .]	9.25 10.37
A 16′		periorbital ecchymosis	right eye dark and will not open; [. . .]	[. . .]	9.25n 10.37n
A 17′		periorbital ecchymosis	both eyes dark and will not open; [. . .]	[. . .]	9.25n 10.37n
B i 1′–9′	[. . .]		[. . .]	[. . .]	
C i 1′–3′	Ištar		[. . .]	[. . .]	
C i 4′–8′	[. . .]		[. . .]	[. . .]	
D i 1′–2′	[. . .]		[. . .]	[. . .]	
D i 3′–4′			left or right eye goes round; jaw shakes	recovery	Ap.21
D i 5′	Sîn	encephalitis?	right eye droops; jaws shake		13.97n 19.259n
D i 6′–7′	[. . .]	stroke	left eye droops; left lip is slippery; [. . .]		13.235
D i 8′–15′	[. . .]		[. . .]	[. . .]	
B ii 1′	[. . .]		[. . .]	[. . .]	
B ii 2′			eyes full of sediment; [. . .]	[. . .]	9.86n
B ii 3′			eyes full of sediment; [. . .]	[. . .]	9.86n
B ii 4′–5′			eyes full of sediment; [. . .]	recovery	9.86n
B ii 6′			eyes full of blood; [. . .]	[. . .]	9.84n
B ii 7′			eyes full of blood; [. . .]	[. . .]	9.84n
B ii 8′			eyes full of blood; [. . .]	[. . .]	9.84n
B ii 9′–10′			eyes full of blood and slime; [. . .]	[. . .]	9.84n
B ii 11′	[. . .]		[. . .]	[. . .]	
C ii 1–3′	[. . .]		[. . .]	[. . .]	
C ii 4′			eyes "confused"; pupil [. . .]	[. . .]	
C ii 5′		onchocerciasis	eyes "confused"; *birdu*-nodules; [. . .]	[. . .]	3.279 10.76
C ii 6′			eyes have tears; [. . .]	[. . .]	9.42n
C ii 7′			eyes shed tears; [. . .]	[. . .]	9.42n
D ii 2–3′	[. . .]		[. . .]	[. . .]	

D ii 4′			eyes are dilated; [. . .]	[. . .]	13.95n
D ii 5′			eyes are dilated; [. . .]	[. . .]	13.95n
D ii 6′		seizure	eyes are opened wide; [. . .]	[. . .]	13.117n
D ii 7′		seizure	eyes are opened wide; [. . .]	[. . .]	13.117n
D ii 8′		Parinaud's syndrome?	he lets his eyes fall; [. . .]	[. . .]	13.119n
D ii 9′		Parinaud's syndrome?	he lets his eyes fall; [. . .]	[. . .]	13.119n
D ii 10′		Parinaud's syndrome?	he lets his eyes fall; [. . .]	[. . .]	13.119n
D ii 11′		Parinaud's syndrome?	he lets his eyes fall; [. . .]	[. . .]	13.119n
D ii 12′		Parinaud's syndrome?	he lets his eyes fall; [. . .]	[. . .]	13.119n
D ii 13′–14′		Parinaud's syndrome?	he lets his eyes fall; [. . .]	[. . .]	13.119n
F 1′–4′	[. . .]		[. . .]	[. . .]	
F 5′			eyes are crossed?; [. . .]	[. . .]	
F 6′			eyes are crossed?; [. . .]	[. . .]	
F 7′			eyes are crossed?; [. . .]	[. . .]	
F 8′–9′			eyes seem to spin; limbs move; [. . .]	[. . .]	
F 10′			eyes seem to spin; [. . .]	[. . .]	
F 11′		Hansen's disease?	eyes are continually constricted; [. . .]	[. . .]	3.216 13.94n
F 12–13′			eyes stare fixedly; [. . .] flows from his mouth; [. . .]	[. . .]	
F 14′		ectropion	eyes leave a space between (the lids); [. . .]	[. . .]	9.51
F 15′			eyes feel heavy; [. . .]	[. . .]	
F 16′–19′	[. . .]		[. . .]	[. . .]	
G 1′–2′	[. . .]		[. . .]	[. . .]	

ORGANIZING PRINCIPLE: WHITES OR PUPILS OF THE EYES

G 3′		seizure	whites of the eyes roll; [. . .]	[. . .]	13.118n
G 4′		seizure	whites of the eyes roll; [. . .]	[. . .]	13.118n
G 5′			whites of the eyes roll; feet are cold [. . .]	[. . .]	3.39n 13.118n
G 6′			whites of the eyes roll; feet are raised [. . .]	[. . .]	13.118n
G 7′			pupils roll; [. . .]	[. . .]	13.93n
G 8′			pupils roll so eyes look inward; [. . .]	[. . .]	13.93

ORGANIZING PRINCIPLE: BLOOD VESSELS/MUSCLES OF THE IRIS

G 9′–10′	[. . .]		blood vessels curved like a ring; [. . .]	worrisome	Ap.22
G 11′–12′	city god	iritis	blood vessels like a web; [. . .]		9.73 19.353n

G 13′			blood vessels "go" in eyes and in temples are [. . .]	[. . .]	
G 14′			black lesions on the muscles of left iris; [. . .]	[. . .]	9.71
G 15′			black lesions on the muscles of right iris; [. . .]	[. . .]	9.71
G 16′			black lesions on the muscles of both irises; [. . .]	[. . .]	9.71n
G 17′			dark lesions on the muscles of left iris; [. . .]	[. . .]	9.72
G 18′			dark lesions on the muscles of right iris; [. . .]	[. . .]	9.72
G 19′			[. . .] lesions on the muscles of left iris; [. . .]	[. . .]	9.71dn
G 20′			[. . .] lesions on the muscles of right iris; [. . .]	[. . .]	9.71dn
G 21′			[. . .] lesions on the muscles of both irises; [. . .]	[. . .]	9.71dn

ORGANIZING PRINCIPLE: RIMS OF EYES/EYELIDS

G 22′–23′			rims swollen; [. . .] swollen; [. . .]	[. . .]	
G 24′–27′			eyelids [. . .]	[. . .]	

DPS Tablet VI

ORGANIZING PRINCIPLE: THE NOSE

A ob.1a			nose red	recovery	20.36
A ob.1b			nose dark	death	20.36
A ob.2a			[nose. . .]	death	
A ob.2b			nose dark red	death	
A ob.3			[nose hot]	recovery	3.39n 20.18
A ob.4			nose cold	death	3.39n 20.18
A ob.4		wound	nose blocked off	death	14.7n 20.32
A ob.5		wound	nose knocked in	death	14.7
A ob.6–7		wound	left or right nostril closed in	death	14.7n
A ob.8			nose full of [red *ramīṭu*-lesions]	recovery	
A ob.9			nose full of [white *ramīṭu*-lesions]	recovery	
A ob.10			nose full of [black *ramīṭu*-lesions]	death	
A ob.11–15	[. . .]		[. . .]	[. . .]	

ORGANIZING PRINCIPLE: BLEEDING FROM THE NOSE/MOUTH

A ob.16	Uraš		bleeding from nose/mouth	if prolonged, death	Ap.101

A ob.17		liver failure	bleeding from nose/mouth; shuddering; yellow spots	death	6.125n 6.142n
A ob.18			bleeding from nose/mouth; labored [breathing]; white ears; swollen feet	death	8.25n 20.32dn Ap.23
A ob.19	Gula	viral hemorrhagic fever	bleeding from nose, eyes, and ears at the same time	death	3.239
A ob.20			fluid from the nose; fever; bulb of nose puffed up	death	Ap.47
A ob.21			red fluid from the nose	death	Ap.47

ORGANIZING PRINCIPLE: BULB OF THE NOSE

A ob.22	personal god		bulb of the nose soft; fever	recovery	19.215 19.360n
A ob.23	personal god		bulb of the nose hot and then cold		19.360n
A ob.24			bulb of the nose lukecold	recovery	3.37
A ob.25			bulb of the nose yellow or looks terrible	death	20.44
A ob.26			red *ramīṭu*-lesions on the bulb of the nose	of no consequence	10.165n
A ob.27			white *ramīṭu*-lesions on the bulb of the nose	recovery	10.165n
A ob.28			red or white *ramīṭu*-lesions on the bulb of the nose	of no consequence	10.165
A ob.29			black *ramīṭu*-lesions on the bulb of the nose	3 days → death	10.169
A ob.30			black *ramīṭu*-lesions on the bulb of the nose; eyes full of blood	death	10.170
A ob.31a	personal god	wound	wound to the bulb of the nose		19.214
A ob.31b	Papsukkal	wound	wound to the base of the nose; 15 days		19.205

ORGANIZING PRINCIPLE: BREATH OF THE NOSE

A ob.32			breath of nose comes out the mouth	3 days → death	20.32dn
A ob.33	illness gores him		breath of nose violent	death	20.32dn
C i 21			breath of nose rises up; illness has fever	death	20.32dn
C i 22			breath of nose stiffled and hot; fever	death	20.32dn

C i 23–24			breath of nose massive, long and hot; [. . .]; attack comes at the beginning of the night	[death]	20.32dn
B_5 6–11	[. . .]		[. . .]	[. . .]	
B_3 1–9	[. . .]		[. . .]	[. . .]	
B_4 2–3	[. . .]		[. . .]	[. . .]	
C ii 3			blood vessels of the nose [. . .]	[. . .]	
C ii 4–5			middle part of the nose [. . .]	[. . .]	

ORGANIZING PRINCIPLE: NOSTRILS

C ii 6			right nostril stings; [. . .]	[. . .]	13.25n
C ii 7			nostrils joined together; [. . .]	[. . .]	
C ii 8			nostrils cleft; [. . .]	[. . .]	
C ii 9			nostrils stiff; [. . .]	[. . .]	
C ii 10			nostrils [. . .]	[. . .]	
C ii 11			nostrils stopped up; [. . .]	[. . .]	9.120
C ii 12			nostrils stopped up; [. . .]	[. . .]	
C ii 13–14	[. . .]		[. . .]	[. . .]	
B_4 r.3–4	[. . .]		[. . .]	[. . .]	
B_3 r.1	[. . .]		[. . .]	[. . .]	

ORGANIZING PRINCIPLE: LIPS

B_3 r.2–14	[. . .]		[. . .]	[. . .]	
B_3 r.15	[. . .]		lips [. . .]; palate hot	will not go away	
B_5 r.1	[. . .]		lips [. . .]; palate dry; 37 days		
B_5 r.2a			lips [. . .]	recovery	
B_5 r.2b			lips and palate hot; [. . .]	[. . .]	
B_5 r.3a			lips [. . .]	death	10.51
B_5 r.3b		Osler-Rendu-Weber	lips have dark red spots	[. . .]	10.51
B_5 4–6	[. . .]		[. . .]	[. . .]	
B_5 7			rubs lips together; [. . .]	[. . .]	
B_5 8–11	[. . .]		[. . .]	[. . .]	
B_2 1	[. . .]		[. . .]	[. . .]	
A r.1–3	[. . .]		[. . .]	[. . .]	

ORGANIZING PRINCIPLE: TEETH

A r.4			tooth hurts; saliva falls; [. . .]	[. . .]	18.3
A r.5			teeth shine	recovery	18.21
A r.6			teeth tremble	prolonged	
A r.7			teeth dark	prolonged	18.20
A r.8a			teeth gathered	death	Ap.25
A r.8b			teeth [scattered]	household scattered	Ap.25
A r.9			gnashes teeth [and loses consciousness]	prolonged	
A r.10			gnashes teeth; eyelids open; face and eyelids tremble	death	Ap.26
A r.11	ghost	septic shock	gnashes teeth; hands and feet dark	death	14.41n 19.130 20.69
A r.12	Sîn	encephalitis?	gnashes teeth; hands and feet shake	death	18.27 19.264dn
A r.13	Ištar	meningitis?	gnashes teeth; lets head drop		19.283
A r.14	Ištar	meningitis?	gnashes teeth; lets hand drop		19.284
A r.15	Ištar	meningitis?	gnashes teeth; lets foot drop	death	19.285
A r.16	Ištar	meningitis?	gnashes teeth; cold face; afflicted		19.286

DPS Tablet VII

ORGANIZING PRINCIPLE: THE TONGUE

A ob.1			tongue red	recovery	18.39
A ob.2–8	[. . .]		[. . .]	[. . .]	
A ob.9	[. . .]		licks? with tongue	[. . .]	Ap.58n
A ob.10	[. . .]		tongue full of black *ramūṭu*-lesions	[death]	10.168
A ob.11			tongue and mouth full of "clay"	[. . .]	Ap.5
A ob.12		dehydration	tongue dries out	[. . .]	3.104
A ob.13		dehydration	tongue and palate [dry out]	[. . .]	3.104
A ob.14			he rubs his tongue	[. . .]	Ap.27
A ob.15			he kneads his tongue	[. . .]	Ap.27
A ob.16	[. . .]	psychiatric	he habitually bites his tongue	[. . .]	16.64
A ob.17	top of the head was struck	wound	he bites his tongue once	[. . .]	14.10
A ob.18	[. . .]		he is tongue-tied	[. . .]	16.39n

A ob.19–20	kissed his mother	psychiatric	he is tongue-tied and cannot open his mouth		16.39
A ob.21		panting	his tongue hangs out	recovery	18.35
A ob.22		mental retardation	his tongue hangs out and he is not in full possession of his faculties; [...]	[...]	18.34
A ob.23	wound to the tongue	wound	tongue is black	[...]	14.8 18.32 18.42
A ob.24	[...]	wound	tongue is too swollen to fit in the mouth	[...]	14.8n 18.32
A ob.25	[...]	wound	tongue hurts; saliva falls	[...]	14.8n 18.32
A ob.26	Adad	wound	wound to the tongue	[...]	19.139dn 19.143

ORGANIZING PRINCIPLE: THE MOUTH

A ob.27			mouth red	recovery	18.46
A ob.28			mouth dark	death	18.46
A ob.29a			mouth hot	recovery	3.39n 20.17
A ob.29b			mouth [cold]	[death]	3.39n 20.17
A ob.30-32	[...]		[...]	[...]	
B ob.1′	[...]		[...]	[...]	
B ob.2′	city god	cranial nerve malfunction	mouth is seized; patient cannot eat; [...]		13.98 19.353dn
B ob.3′	[...]	stuttering	mouth is seized; patient cannot say certain words		18.48
B ob.4′	[*buʾšānu*]	herpetic stomatitis	mouth full of *bubuʾtu*; saliva flows		3.65; 4.17 10.81 18.47
B ob.5′	[...]		mouth hurts; saliva flows; [...]		18.44

ORGANIZING PRINCIPLE: IN/FROM THE MOUTH

B ob.6′–7′	sorcerous spittle	Parkinson's	patient has scanning speech; head [trembles]		13.263n
B ob.8′		wound	mouth crushed; black blood produced; [...]	[...]	14.9
B ob. 9′			vomits stomach fat; [...]	[...]	6.24n
B ob.10′			vomits black bile; [...]	[...]	6.5dn
B ob.11′			vomits red bile; [...]	[...]	6.5dn
B ob.12′			vomits yellow bile; [...]	[...]	6.5dn
B ob.13′			vomits white bile	3 days → [...]	6.5dn 6.32

ORGANIZING PRINCIPLE: PALATE

B ob.14′	[. . .]		palate hot; epigastrium protrudes; [. . .]		6.35n
B ob.15′	[. . .]	dehydration	palate dry and dotted with slag		3.105
B ob.16′	[. . .]	dehydration	palate dry; insides bloated; [. . .]		3.105
B ob.17′	[. . .]	dehydration	palate dry; insides bloated and cramped; [. . .]		3.105n
B r.1	[. . .]	dehydration	palate dry; insides bloated; patient exhausted; [. . .]		3.105n
B r.2	[. . .]		[. . .]	[. . .]	

ORGANIZING PRINCIPLE: WORDS

B r.3–4		post-traumatic stress syndrome	unintelligible words; wandering about	3 days → [. . .]	14.34 16.48
B r.5		liver failure	unintelligible words; vomits yellow stuff; flesh yellow	3 days → [. . .]	6.140
B r.6	[. . .]	delirium	unintelligible words; fever; wandering about; 3 days		3.124
B r.7	[. . .]		unintelligible words; nausea; 3 days		
B r.8	[. . .]	post-traumatic stress syndrome	unintelligible words; regular depression; 3 days		14.36 16.85
B r.9	[. . .]	post-traumatic stress syndrome	unintelligible words; regular weeping; 3 days		14.36n 16.85
B r.10	[. . .]	alcoholic liver failure	unintelligible words; produces blood; puffed up insides; 10 days	[death]	6.141 19.366
B r.11	[. . .]	alcoholism	unintelligible words; farting; belching; 10 days	[death]	19.366
B r.12	Ninurta	alcoholic liver failure	unintelligible words; fever; 10 days	[death]	19.366
B r.13	[. . .]	alcoholism	unintelligible words; craving for beer; 10 days	[death]	15.14 16.82n 19.367
B r.14	[. . .]	alcoholism	unintelligible words; regular craving for wine; [10 days]	[death]	15.14 16.82 19.367
B r.15	[. . .]	alcoholism	unintelligible words; droning; [10 days]		16.41 19.367
B r.16	[. . .]	alcoholism	unintelligible words; cries of woe; [. . .]	[. . .]	19.367
B r.17	Ninurta	alcoholic liver failure	unintelligible words; [. . .]	[. . .]	19.367
A r.1′–10′			unintelligible words; [. . .]	[. . .]	
A r.11′–17′			his cry resembles [. . .]	[. . .]	

DPS Tablet VIII

ORGANIZING PRINCIPLE: EARS

1			left ear dark	difficult	
2			right ear dark	worrisome	
3			both ears dark	death	
4		endocarditis	left ear looks sprinkled	prolonged	10.52
5		endocarditis	right ear looks sprinkled	worrisome	10.52
6a		endocarditis	both ears look sprinkled	death	10.52
6b		wound	left ear was broken open	recovery	9.95n 14.6n
7a		wound	right ear was broken open	prolonged	9.95n 14.6n
7b		wound	both ears were broken open	death	9.95; 14.6
8a			left ear rings	recovery	9.116n 20.2
8b			right ear rings	prolonged	9.116n
9			both ears ring	difficult	9.116
10a			left ear rings	bad omen	9.116n 20.3
10b			right ear rings	good omen	9.116n
11a			both ears ring	bad omen	9.116n
11b		ear wax	left ear obstructed	recovery	9.100n
12a		ear wax	right ear obstructed	difficult	9.100n
12b		ear wax	both ears obstructed	bad omen	9.100n
13	Ištar	meningitis?	ears roar; skull numb		19.287
14		meningitis	ears heavy; mentation altered; scanning speech	death	13.220
15	ghost	fever	ears and soles of feet cold		Ap.83
16	ghost	fever	ears wiggle	3 days → worrisome	Ap.83
17a	ghost	mastoiditis	ears stand up		9.112
17b	ghost	eustachian tube inflammation	ears make strange noises		9.113 19.379
18–21		strep throat	ears, throat, and elbows hurt; keeps coming back; [. . .]	if only one relapse survivable	3.54 11.38
22			jaws pressured; ears [. . .]	[. . .]	Ap.6
23			ears, neck, and [. . .]	[. . .]	
24	[. . .]	wound	wound to left ear; [. . .]		9.95n
25	[. . .]	wound	wound to right ear; [. . .]		9.95n
remainder of obv. and all of rev. = [. . .]					

DPS Tablet IX

ORGANIZING PRINCIPLE: FACE

A					
1–2	twin gods	fevers with possible DIC	face holds sweat; patient is withdrawn	recovery with treatment	19.239
3			[. . .]; face red	death	
4			face red and swells like a cloud	death	Ap.99n
5		epilepsy	face flushes and turns pale	treatable, but illness will return	13.187n
6			face flushes and turns black	potentially fatal	Ap.28
7		fainting	face turns white	recovery	
8–9		Wilson's disease?	face has light yellow spots; mouth and lips glazed; right eye flutters	death	6.149 10.50n 13.115n 18.30
10			face has white, black, red, or yellow spots	recovery	10.49 10.50n
11	Lamaštu	typhoid?	face yellow		3.26 19.223
12		dehydration	face yellowish; eyes sunken	death	3.106 20.80
13	*aḫḫāzu*	liver disease	face and eyes yellow; base of the tongue black		6.117
14		liver disease	face yellow and black	death	6.117n
15		cyanosis	face dark	if prolonged, death	
16		cyanosis	face dark; tongue red	if prolonged, death	Ap.29
17		*kala-azar*?	face turns black and white	death	19.321 Ap.61n
18		starvation?	face dark; insides bloated	death	Ap.50
19		starvation?	face dark; patient asks for bread and eats it	death	Ap.50
20	wound from in front	wound with cyanosis	face dark; vomits blood	death	8.92
21–24		cyanosis	face turns dark like a corpse; frowning; thick lips; face changes	death	8.91 10.38
25			face dark red	death	
26			face dark red; patient asks for dates and eats them	death	Ap.52

27			face swells up like a cloud	death or recovery	
28	Adad		face is bright red and swells up like a cloud	death or recovery	19.139dn 20.42 Ap.99
29		Wilson's disease?	face has light yellow spots; lips glazed; yellow discoloration in the eyes; left eye flutters	death	6.148 10.50n 13.115n 18.29
30			face alters	death	6.138n
31	TÙN.GIG	liver failure	face alters; tongue or body yellow	3 days → death	6.138 18.41 20.45
32			face is full	recovery	
33			face holds sweat	recovery	3.24n
34			face holds fever	recovery	3.2n
35		Graves' disease	face warm; eyes prominent; attack comes in the dead of night	death	7.25
36			face is cold continually	death	3.39n 20.20
37			face looks terrible	death	Ap.30n
38			face looks terrible; chin "seized"; not in full possession of faculties	death	Ap.30
39			face healthy	recovery	
40			face healthy; tongue red	recovery	18.40
41			face mournful	recovery	16.30
42		seborrhea	face oily	recovery	10.9
43			face full of red *ramīṭu*-lesions	recovery	10.161
44			face full of white *ramīṭu*-lesions	recovery	10.162
45	Marduk		face full of yellow *ramīṭu*-lesions	recovery	10.163 19.102
46			face full of black *ramīṭu*-lesions	death	10.164
47	Sîn	HSV1	face full of red *bubuʾtu*	recovery	3.232 4.16 10.82 19.105dn
48	Šamaš		face full of white *bubuʾtu*	recovery	10.83 19.105dn
49	Ištar		face full of black *bubuʾtu*	death	10.84 19.105dn
50	personal god or father's god	benign fever	face full of *birdu*	recovery	10.72 19.222n 19.353dn
51	Marduk	acne	face full of *ziqtu*	recovery	10.109 19.97dn 19.98dn 19.139dn

52a	*rišûtu*		face full of "redness"	recovery	10.13
52b	*išītu*		face full of *išītu*	recovery	10.174
53			face seems to spin; attack comes at the beginning of the night	<recovery>	Ap.24
54	city god	meningitis?	face seems to spin; keeps him up all night	death	19.293n
55	father's god	benign fever	face seems to spin; eyes heavily clouded		19.222n
56		facial wound	face seems to spin; chin cut open	death	13.133
57–58	Lugalgirra and Meslamtaea	cerebral malaria	face seems to spin; head, hands, and feet tremble (*tarāru*)		3.45 13.82
59	Dapinu	multiple sclerosis?	face seems to spin; hands and feet tremble (*raʾābu*); 59 days		13.82 13.102 19.88
60	ghost	encephalitis?	face seems to spin; ears roar; tense limbs		19.278
61	ghost	encephalitis?	face seems to spin; ears roar; temples jab and shake		19.278
62	ghost	alcoholism	face seems to spin; respiratory distress		8.78 19.303n
63	ghost	vertigo	face seems to spin; gets up and falls down		13.104
64–65	Lugalgirra and Meslamtaea	cerebral malaria	face seems to spin; limbs tremble and twist		3.46 13.76
66		congestive heart failure	face and eyes swollen or face and insides swollen	death	8.24
67	TÙN.GIG	cirrhosis	face and insides swollen	3 days → death	6.150
68	Šamaš	glomerulonephritis?	face, insides, hands, feet swollen		5.39n 19.104
69–70	wound from in front; Ninurta	wound to the penis	face and eyes swollen; rims of eyes red; breath of nose hot; cannot urinate		5.38 19.138
71		stroke	face twitches; torso is powerless; cannot hold up right hand; drags one foot	death	13.50 13.242n
72–73		stroke	face twitches; torso is powerless; cannot hold up right hand; drags one foot	will never fully recover	13.80 13.242 19.306dn
74		throat tumor or abscess	face looks like strangled sheep; keeps him up all night; vomits blood	death	8.90
75	drowned ghost	river toxins (physical illness)	massages his face		19.46n
76	burned ghost	battle fatigue? (psychiatric)	strikes his face and screams		16.63 19.27

77			red *ramīṭu*-lesions erupt on upper part of the face	recovery or death	10.166
78			black *ramīṭu*-lesions erupt on upper part of the face	death	10.167
79	"touched in the steppe"	kwashiorkor	face falls flat against the skull	death	7.10

DPS Tablet X

ORGANIZING PRINCIPLE: NECK

A 1–3	AN.TA.ŠUB.BA	seizure	head turns to left; hands and feet immobilized; eyes close and roll; spittle flows; rumbling noises	if heart is awake, recovery; if he does not know who he is, death	8.5 13.118 13.193
A 4–6	AN.TA.ŠUB.BA; Sîn	encephalitis?	head turns to right; hands and feet stretched out; eyes turned upward; spittle flows; rumbling noises; does not know who he is before the confusional state comes over him		13.116 13.194 19.266
A 7	personal god or Šamaš	arthritis	neck hurts	recovery	11.42 19.353dn
A 8	wound to neck; Ištar	wound	neck hurts; continually thirsty	death	13.138 19.150
A 9	Adad	arthritis	neck and hips hurt		11.18n 19.139dn Ap.96
A 10	*šaššaṭu*	tetanus	neck, hips, hands, and feet stiff		3.199
A 11	*šaššaṭu*	tetanus	neck twists; eyes jerk; he jerks or shudders incessantly		3.197 13.68 13.107
A 12–13	Ardat lilî	tabies dorsalis?	neck throbs; lets head drop; stiff hands and feet; patient rubs them against the ground		4.30 16.65
A 14a		spasmodic torticollis	head returns to left or right	death	13.251 13.283
A 14b		spinal muscular atrophy	lets head drop to left or right	death	13.246 13.283
A 15		spinal muscular atrophy	head falls to left or right; and/or head falls when turned from left to right	death	13.246 13.284
A 16	Adad	wound	wound to the neck		19.139dn 19.148

A 17	Ištar	wound	wound to the neck with hurting breast		7.1dn 13.138n 19.157n 19.274
A 18	Ištar	wound	wound to the neck with loss of virility	death	5.68 13.139 19.149 19.274
A 19	ghost	wound	wound to the neck with cramped insides and raised feet		13.140 19.171n
A 20	ghost	wound	wound to the neck with cramped insides and trembling feet		13.83 13.140n 19.171
A 21	Gallû	hemophilia with wound	wound to the neck with pain in the upper part of the eyes; produces blood from nose/ mouth; sluggish hands and feet		13.46 13.141 19.176
A 22a		wound	vertebra is cut open	death	13.143
A22b		wound	vertebra is cut open; nostrils are "seized"	death	13.143
A 23		wound	vertebra is cut open; blood vessels are present; nostrils are "seized"	death	13.144n
A 24		wound	vertebra is cut open; blood vessels are present; breath is "seized" in the nose	no recovery	13.144 20.33
A 25		wound	vertebra is cut open; nose twitches; [does not recognize friends]	[death]	13.144n
A 26			falls backward and stretched out; lets neck drop to left and right	death	Ap.31
A 27	*šaššaṭu*	tetanus	muscles stiff from neck to heel; eyebrows knitted; jaws pressured		3.196

ORGANIZING PRINCIPLE: LARYNX

A 28	tabooed food	choking	larynx constricted	recovery	8.88; 16.26 19.353dn
A 29		epiglottitis	larynx croaks	death	3.58; 20.31

ORGANIZING PRINCIPLE: BREATH

A 30		coma in congestive heart failure	rapid breath; cramped insides	death	8.18 13.278 20.34n
A 31a		coma in congestive heart failure	rapid breath; tense muscles	death	8.19 13.278 20.34

A 31b		coma in congestive heart failure	breath throbs and is closely spaced	death	8.19 13.278 20.34
A 32a		congestive heart failure	breath goes up	no recovery	8.20 20.32dn
A 32b–33	[. . .], Ningizzida or ghost	respiratory distress	breath is continually short		8.77 19.202dn 19.303n Ap.112
A 34a		epiglottitis	larynx croaks when he breathes	death	3.57 20.31n
A 34b		epiglottitis	chokings closely spaced; not in full possession of faculties	death	3.57

ORGANIZING PRINCIPLE: GRABBING OF THE THROAT/BREATH

A 35	emnity of the gods		grabbing of the throat; [. . .]	[. . .]	3.59n
A 36	[. . .]		grabbing of the throat; scratching; [. . .]	[. . .]	3.59n
A 37	Ištar	meningitis?	grabbing of the throat; shuddering	death	3.59n 19.288
A 38		epiglottitis	grabbing of the throat; wailing	if death, then father dies	2.11n 3.60n 20.30
A 39		epiglottitis	grabbing of the throat; twisting	if death, mother dies	2.11 3.59
A 40		epiglottitis	grabbing of the throat; roaring	if death, then brother dies	2.11 3.60

ORGANIZING PRINCIPLE: THROAT

A 41			left or right side of the throat red	recovery	
A 42a			both sides of the throat red	recovery	
A 42b			left or right side of the throat yellow	prolonged or death	
A 43a			both sides of the throat yellow	if prolonged, death	
A 43b			left side of the throat black	alters for the worse	
A 44a			right side of the throat black	prolonged	
A 44b			both sides of the throat black	death	

A 45			left or right side of the throat dark	illness weakens him or death	
A 46a			both sides of the throat dark	death	
A 46b–c			left or right side of the throat swollen	recovery or death	3.56n
A 47a			both sides of the throat swollen	death	3.56n
A 47b		epiglottitis	left side of the throat continually swollen	death	3.56n
A 48a		epiglottitis	right side of the throat continually swollen	difficult	3.56
A 48b		epiglottitis	both sides of the throat continually swollen	death	3.56
A 49		pharyngitis	left side of the throat appears skinned	recovery with difficulty	3.50
A 50a		pharyngitis	right side of the throat appears skinned	death	3.50n
A 50b		pharyngitis	both sides of the throat appear skinned	death	3.50n
A 51		pharyngitis	both sides of the throat appear skinned; flesh is normal	recovery	3.51
A 52		scarlet fever	both sides of the throat appear skinned; flesh is spotted with red dye spots	worrisome	3.52 10.59
A 53	city god	meningitis?	throat looks terrible, feet are flexed, sleepless nights	death	19.293
A 54a	ghost	benign fever	throat looks terrible and hurts		19.248
A 54b	twin gods	wound	wound to the throat		14.11 19.182

ORGANIZING PRINCIPLE: ARMS

B r.1	Sîn	septic shock	right arm dark; twisting	death	19.201 Ap.94
B r.2		wound	unable to turn arms; drips blood and excrement	death	13.136n
B r.3	wound from behind	wound	unable to turn arms; blood excreted	death	13.136
B r.4	Ištar	wound	unable to turn arms; blood vomited	if prolonged, death	19.160

B r.5	Ištar	meningitis?	gazing at arms; chills		3.40n 7.1dn 19.283dn
B r.6	ghost	psychiatric	chews on his arms		16.79 19.28
B r.7	twin gods	shock	continually cold arms		3.39n 19.134 19.237
B r.8–10	*kišpu*	mushroom poisoning	tired arms and knees, fluttering heart, flowing saliva; sluggishness; internal fever		8.10 15.4n
B r.11	twin gods	wound	wound to the arm		19.135
B r.12	Ištar	wound	wound to the arm and elbow		19.164n

ORGANIZING PRINCIPLE: ARMPIT

B r.13	Ištar		left armpit stings		Ap.89
B r.14			hot from the armpit to the hip region and cold from the hip region to the feet	recovery possible	Ap.20

ORGANIZING PRINCIPLE: FOREARM/ELBOW

B r.15	Šamaš	psychiatric	forearms kept away from body		19.3
B r.16	Šamaš	arthritis	forearms, legs, and feet hurt		11.43
B r.17	Ištar	arthritis	forearms, hips, and feet hurt		11.52
B r.18	Šamaš	psychiatric	elbows placed on the head; sprays spit	recovery	19.4

DPS Tablet XI

ORGANIZING PRINCIPLE: HANDS

A ob.1	Šamaš	arthritis	left hand hurts	recovery	11.44
A ob.2		arthritis	right hand hurts	[recovery]	11.17n
A ob.3		arthritis	both hands hurt	[recovery]	11.17n
A ob.4	[. . .]		top part of the hands [. . .]; 5 days		
A ob.5	Šamaš	arthritis	left hand hurts		11.44n
A ob.6	[Ištar?]	arthritis	right hand hurts		11.49n
A ob.7	[. . .]	arthritis	cannot touch his nose with left hand and right does it stiffly		11.26

A ob.8	[...]	arthritis	cannot touch his nose with right hand and left does it stiffly		11.26
A ob.9	wound to navel; Ištar	hemorrhagic shock	hands placed on the navel; hands and feet cold; talks without knowing what he is saying; gets up and sits down		3.39 14.26 19.64 19.129 19.151
A ob.10			hands red; flesh bright red	[...]	
B 9		palmar erythema in liver failure	hands red; flesh yellow	[...]	6.146
A ob.11		jaundice	hands yellow; flesh yellow	[...]	6.147
A ob.12	[...]		hands yellow; fingers have white spots; [...]	[...]	10.50n 10.54; Ap.7
B 11	[...]		hands yellow; eyes have white spots; [...]	[...]	10.50n 10.55; Ap.8
A ob.13	*rābiṣu*	cyanosis due to heart failure?	hands dark	[...]	19.119n
A ob.14	*rābiṣu*	cyanosis due to heart failure?	hands dark; loses consciousness	[...]	19.119n
A ob.15	[...]	septic shock	hands dark; body hot; [...]	[...]	14.40
A ob.16	[...]	shock in jaundiced patient	hands dark; flesh yellow; [...]	[...]	
A ob.17	"hand" of god	nonspecific fever	hands tremble	recovery	19.363dn
A ob.18	Ištar	neuropathy	hands sluggish and contorted	[...]	13.268
A ob.19	Šamaš	psychiatric	hands kept away from body		19.3n
A ob.20	Šamaš	encephalitis?	hands immobilized in bent position; not in full possession of faculties	[death]	19.271
A ob.21	*rābiṣu* of the river	river toxins	hands never leave the face		15.28n 19.46n
A ob.22	*rābiṣu* of the roof	thyrotoxicosis	hands never leave the skull		19.42n
A ob.23	Lamaštu	typhoid?	hands never leave the head	[...]	19.227n
A ob.24	Lugalgirra and Meslamtaea	cerebral malaria	hands continually over the head	[...]	3.49n 19.41
A ob.25	[wound to epigastrium]	peritonitis	hands continually over the head; insides puffed up; burns with fever	[death]	3.8n 3.210
A ob.26		primitive reflex	hands placed in mouth and if you take them out, he returns them to his mouth	[death]	16.61
A ob.27	[...]	septic shock	hands in mouth; he sucks them; burns with fever; insides puffed up; wanders about	[...]	3.8n 14.37n

A ob.28	[dirty substances]	mental status change	hand moves across mouth; throws off garment; not in full possession of faculties	[death]	16.59 16.62 Ap.79
A ob.29		mental status change	hands continually rub body	if prolonged, [death]	16.60n 20.11n
A ob.30		mental status change	hands continually rub body without his being aware of this	[death]	16.60 20.11
A ob.31	[...]		hands continually rub head; [...]	[...]	16.60n 20.11n
A ob.32	[...]		hands bound; feet pulled taut; [...]		13.60
A ob.33	[...]	arthritis	hands stiff; [...]		11.15
A ob.34	[...]	arthritis	hands stiff; feet swollen; [...]		11.15n 11.18n
A ob.35	[...]	arthritis	hands stiff, sluggish, and swollen; [...]		11.16
A ob.36	[...]		rubs hands; licks? with tongue; drools?; [...]		Ap.58n
A ob.37	[...]	congenital heart disease	gazes at his hands; changes of mood; [...]		8.29n 16.54n
A ob.38		congenital heart disease	gazes at his hands; changes of mood; gets up and squats down; attack comes at the beginning of the night	[...]	8.29 16.54
A ob.39		congenital heart disease	hands and feet dark; changes of mood; gets up and squats down; [...]	[...]	8.29 10.39
A ob.40	ghost	psychiatric	chews on his hands		16.79n 19.28n
A ob.41	[twin gods?]	shock?	chews on his hands		16.78n

ORGANIZING PRINCIPLE: HANDS AND FEET

A ob.42	[...]		hands hot; feet sluggish; [...]		
A ob.43	[...]	fever	hands hot; feet cold; [...]		3.2n
A ob.44	[...]	fever	hands cold; feet hot; [...]		3.2n
A ob.45		poor circulation	hands and feet cold	[recovery]	2.42n 3.39n 20.15n
A ob.46			hands and soles of feet cold; [...]	[...]	3.39n
A ob.47			hands cold; [...]	[...]	3.39n
A ob.48	[...]		hands thrash around; feet hot; [...]		
A ob.49	[...]		hands and feet thrash around; feet immobilized?; [...]		
A ob.50	[...]		hands and feet thrash around; soles of feet [...]		

A ob.51	[...]		hands and feet thrash around; body cold; [...]		3.39n
A ob.52	[...]		[...]		
A ob.53	[...]		hands and feet swollen; [...]		
A ob.54	[...]		hands and feet swollen; lukewarm temperature; [...]		3.4n
A ob.55	[...]	arthritis	hands and feet sluggish; [...]		11.19n
A ob.56	[...]		[...]		
A r.1′	[...]		[...]		
A r.2′	[...]		twists his hands and feet; spittle flows [...]		
A r.3′–5′	[...]		[...]		

ORGANIZING PRINCIPLE: BLOOD VESSELS/MUSCLES

A r.6′			muscles of the hands red; [...]	[...]	
A r.7′			muscles of the hands yellow; [...]	[...]	
A r.8′			blood vessels of the hands take up blood; [...]	[...]	8.33
A r.9′			blood vessels of the hands afflict him; [...]	[...]	
A r.10′			blood vessels of hands, ones above "go" and ones below [...]	[...]	
A r.11′			blood vessels of hands, ones below "go" and ones above [...]	[...]	
A r.12′			blood vessels of hands, ones above and ones below "go" [...]	[...]	
A r.13′	[...]	atherosclerosis	blood vessels of hands tense; those of feet pulsate; eyes [...]		8.49
A r.14′	[...]	atherosclerosis	blood vessels of hands on the left side tense/"go"; [...]		8.49
A r.15′	[...]		blood vessels of hands on the left "go"; epigastrium hurts		
A r.16′			blood vessels of hands "go"; those of feet slow; [...]	[...]	8.53n
A r.17′			blood vessels of hands "go"; those of feet present; [...]	[...]	8.54n
A r.18′			blood vessels of hands "go"; those of forehead present; [...]	[...]	Ap.43n
A r.19′	[...]	atherosclerosis	blood vessels of hands or feet on the left "go"; those on the right are present; [...]		19.124n
A r.20′	[...]		blood vessels of hands and feet, ones above "go" and ones below are slow [...]		8.53n

A r.21′	*rābiṣu*	tachycardia	blood vessels of hands and feet, ones above and ones below "go"	recovery possible	19.116n 20.25n
A r.22′	[. . .]	dehydration	blood vessels of hands and feet "go" at the same time [. . .]		8.52n
A r.23′	[. . .]	fever with dehydration	blood vessels of hands and feet "go" at the same time; burns with fever; head [. . .]		3.8n 8.51n
A r.24′	[. . .]	fever with dehydration	blood vessels of hands and feet "go" at the same time; burns with fever; body [. . .]		3.8n 8.52n
A r.25′	[. . .]	fever with dehydration	blood vessels of hands and feet "go" at the same time; burns with fever; head [. . .]		3.8n 8.51
A r.26′	[. . .]	fever with dehydration	blood vessels of hands and feet "go" at the same time; burns with fever; body [. . .]		3.8n 8.52n
A r.27′	[. . .]	fever with dehydration	blood vessels of hands and feet "go" at the same time; burns with fever; body [. . .]		3.8n 8.52
A r.28′	[. . .]	fever with dehydration	blood vessels of hands and feet "go" at the same time; burns with fever; bottoms of feet [. . .]		8.52n
A r.29′	[. . .]	fever	blood vessels of hands and feet pulsate; eyes feel heavy; head [. . .]		8.42n 19.338n

ORGANIZING PRINCIPLE: PARTS OF THE HAND

A r.30′	[. . .]		middle part of hands unevenly colored with yellow; fingers burning hot; [. . .]		10.50n Ap.9
A r.31′	[. . .]		middle part of hands unevenly colored with yellow; hands were cut open; [. . .]		10.50n

ORGANIZING PRINCIPLE: FINGERS

A r.32′	[. . .]	Hansen's disease	fingers rubbed off [. . .]		3.215
A r.33′	[. . .]	cyanosis	fingers dark [. . .]		
A r.34′	[. . .]	cyanosis	fingers dark [. . .]		
A r.35′	[. . .]	arthritis	fingers sluggish [. . .]		11.19
A r.36′	[wound to neck; Bau]	septic shock	sucks his fingers; burns with fever; abdomen [bloated; wanders about]	[death]	3.8n 14.37 19.166
A r.37′	[. . .]	Raynaud's phenomenon	left hand's fingers full of blood and continually hurt	[. . .]	8.60
A r.38′	[. . .]	Raynaud's phenomenon	right hand's fingers full of blood and continually hurt	[. . .]	8.61

A r.39′	[...]	Raynaud's phenomenon	both hands' fingers full of blood and continually hurt	[...]	8.62
A r.40′	[...]	Raynaud's phenomenon	all fingers and toes full of blood and continually hurt	[...]	8.63
A r.41′	[...]	snake bite	one hand's fingers full of venom and continually hurt	[...]	15.39
A r.42′	[...]	snake bite	one hand's fingers full of venom and continually hurt	[...]	15.39n
A r.43′	[...]	arthritis	fingers and toes hurt [...]		11.27
A r.44′	[...]	arthritis	fingers and toes swollen [...]		11.28
A r.45′	[...]	arthritis	fingers and toes sluggish [...]		11.29
A r.46′	[...]	arthritis	fingers and toes stiff; pelvis [...]		11.7n
A r.47′	[...]		yellow spots on fingers and toes; pelvis [...]		10.50n
A r.48a′	Išḫara		yellow spots on fingers	no recovery	10.50n 19.289
A r.48b′	[...]		yellow spots on [fingers; ...]	[...]	
A r.49′	[...]		fingers dark; breasts of fingers were cut open [...]	[...]	
A r.50′		primitive reflex	fingers placed in mouth and if you take them out, [he returns them to his mouth]	[if death; then another death in household]	2.11n 16.61n
A r.51′	[...]	Hansen's disease?	twists his fingers; constricts the pupils of his eyes; [...]	[...]	3.216n 13.94n
A r.52′	[...]	Lesch-Nyhan syndrome	chews his fingers; eats his own lips; [...]	[...]	7.31

ORGANIZING PRINCIPLE: PARTS OF THE FINGERS

A r.53′			tips of fingers red	death	
A r.54′		gangrene	bellies of fingers look terrible and dark	death	14.41n
A r.55′			bellies of fingers yellow	death	
A r.56′		endocarditis	bellies of fingers sprinkled with dark spots	death	10.53
A r.57′			bellies of fingers red [...]		
A r.58′			bellies of fingers streaked with red; [...]	[...]	Ap.10
A r.59′			bellies of fingers streaked with red; [...]	[...]	Ap.10
A r.60′			nails [...]	[...]	

DPS Tablet XII

ORGANIZING PRINCIPLE: BREAST/CHEST

A 1	personal god	stress	breast hurts; [. . .]	[. . .]	19.36n 19.209
A 2–3	Marduk	viral hemorrhagic fever	chest clear; blood vessels of temple collapsed, blood flowing from mouth/nose; shuddering heart; patient worried	death	3.237 8.6 19.235 20.28
A 4	wound from in front; Nergal	wound	wound to the chest; blood pours out; wanders about	death	14.32 19.174
A 5	Šamaš	psychiatric	sprinkles water on breast; makes gestures of supplication		19.2
A 6		liver failure	muscles of breast turn yellow	no recovery	6.144n
A 7			blood vessels of head and neck to left and right "go"; those of forehead present	death	Ap.43
A 8	river hoist water		hair of breast twines		15.30n
A 9a			left nipple red	recovery	10.45dn
A 9b			right nipple red	death	10.45dn
A 10a			both nipples red	no consequence	10.45dn
A 10b			left nipple yellow	worsens	10.45dn
A 11a			right nipple yellow	difficult	10.45dn
A 11b			both nipples yellow	worrisome	10.45dn
A 12a			left nipple black	worrisome	10.45dn
A 12b			right nipple black	if prolonged, death	10.45dn
A 13a			both nipples black	speedy death	10.45dn
A 13b			left nipple dark	worsens	10.45dn
A 14a			right nipple dark	if lingering, death	10.45dn
A 14b			both nipples dark	death	10.45dn
A 15a			left nipple dark red	illness lasts long	10.45dn
A 15b			right nipple dark red	worsens	10.45dn
A 16a			both nipples dark red	worrisome	10.45dn
A 16b			left nipple swollen	worsens	10.45dn
A 17a			right nipple swollen	[. . .]	10.45dn
A 17b			both nipples swollen	[. . .]	10.45dn

A 18	left nipple bruised	[...]	10.45dn
B 11	right nipple bruised	[...]	10.45dn
B 12	both nipples bruised	[...]	10.45dn
B 13	left nipple cut open	[...]	10.45dn
B 14	right nipple cut open	[...]	10.45dn
B 15	both nipples cut open	[...]	10.45dn
B 16	[left ?] sluggish	[...]	
B 17	[right ?] sluggish	[...]	
B 18	[both ?s] sluggish	[...]	
C 0′	[left ? twitches]	[...]	
C 1′	[right ?] twitches	[...]	
C 2′	[both ?s] twitch	[...]	
C 3′	[left ?] relaxed	[...]	
C 4′	right [?] relaxed	[recovery]	
C 5′	both [?s] relaxed	no consequence	

C 6′	left [rib] red	prolonged	10.45dn
C 7′	right rib red	difficult	10.45dn
C 8′	both ribs red	recovery	10.45dn
C 9′	left rib yellow	if heals, recovery	10.45dn 20.43
C 10′	right rib yellow	worrisome	10.45dn
C 11′	both ribs yellow	[...]	10.45dn
C 12′	left rib black	[...]	10.45dn
C 13′	right [rib] black	[...]	10.45dn
[C 14′]	[both ribs black]	[...]	
D i 2–8	[...]	[...]	
F 0′	[left kidney black]	[...]	10.45dn
F 1′	[right kidney black]	if prolonged, death	10.45dn
D ii 1′	[both kidneys black]	[...]	10.45dn
F 2′	left [kidney] dark	difficult	10.45dn
D ii 3′	[right kidney dark]	[...]	10.45dn
D ii 4′	both [kidneys] dark	death	10.45dn
D ii 5′	[left] kidney [dark red]	[...]	10.45dn
D ii 6′	right kidney dark red	worsens	10.45dn
D ii 7′	both kidneys dark red	worrisome	10.45dn
D iii 1	left kidney swollen	worsens	10.45dn
D iii 2	right kidney swollen	[...]	10.45dn
D iii 3	both kidneys swollen	worrisome	10.45dn
D iii 4	left kidney bruised	[...]	10.45dn
D iii 5	right kidney bruised	prolonged	10.45dn
D iii 6	both kidneys bruised	no consequence	10.45dn

D iii 7			viselike pain in left kidney	difficult	13.15n
D iii 8			viselike pain in right kidney	worrisome	13.15n
D iii 9			viselike pain in both kidneys	death	13.15
D iii 10	twin gods		left kidney hurts	worrisome	19.368n
D iii 11	twin gods		right kidney hurts	recovery	19.368n
D iii 12			both kidneys hurt	worrisome	20.60
D iii 13	twin gods		left kidney hurts but he can lie on it	recovery	5.57n 19.368
D iii 14			right kidney hurts but he can lie on it	recovery	5.57
D iii 15			both kidneys hurt but he can lie on them	recovery; of no consequence	5.57n 20.61
D iii 16			left kidney hurts so he cannot lie on it	7th day → death	5.56
D iii 17			right kidney hurts so he cannot lie on it	recovery or death	5.56n
D iii 18			both kidneys hurt so he cannot lie on them	15 days → death	5.56n 20.62
D iii 19	Adad or Kūbu	wound	wound to the kidney		19.139dn 19.141 19.189
D iii 20	Šamaš	wound	wound to left kidney; 14 days		19.191
D iii 21	twin gods	hemorrhagic shock	wound to left kidney; not in full possession of faculties; wanders about	death	14.33 19.179 20.8
D iii 22	Sibitti	hemorrhagic shock	wound to right kidney; not in full possession of faculties; vomits blood	death	14.27 19.178
D iii 23	city god	hemorrhagic shock	wound to left side of back; wanders about	death	14.33n 19.207
D iii 24	personal god	hemorrhagic shock	wound to right side of back; wanders about	death	14.33n 19.207
D iii 25			spine red	[...]	10.45dn
D iii 26			spine yellow	prolonged	10.45dn
D iii 27			spine black	death	10.45dn
D iii 28			spine dark	worrisome	10.45dn
D iii 29			spine dark red	prolonged	10.45dn
D iii 30			spine skinned	death	10.45dn
D iii 31			spine intact	recovery	
D iii 32		spondylitis	spine curved	worrisome	11.23
D iii 33		spondylitis	spine curved and he cannot straighten it out	if prolonged, death	11.24 20.84
D iii 34		spondylitis	spine curved and he cannot straighten it out; not in full possession of faculties	if prolonged, death	11.25

D iii 35	ghost	wound	wound to spine; no excretion	[death]	5.40 6.155 13.142 19.172
D iii 36	Šamaš	arthritis	hips hurt	if goes away, [recovery]	11.47
D iii 37	city god	arthritis	hips hurt; no fever	[. . .]	3.3n 11.17n 19.353dn
D iii 38	[. . .]		hips hurt; fever; [. . .]	[. . .]	
D iii 39	[. . .]		hips hurt; feet [. . .]	[. . .]	
D iii 40	[. . .]		lets pelvic region drop and cannot lift it; [. . .]	[. . .]	
D iii 41		opisthotonus	raises pelvic region and does not know he is doing this	death	13.88
D iii 42	[. . .]		hips [. . .]	[. . .]	
D iii 43	Ištar	wound	wound to hips, [. . .], elbows		19.164n
D iii 44	Ištar	wound	wound to hips, arms, elbows		19.164n
E iv 4–5	wound complications	wound	wound to hips and elbows; [. . .]		13.121dn
D iv 1–2		encephalyomyelitis	pelvic region and abdomen sick; gets up and kneels down; does not remember dreams; mouth too strong for words	death	13.216
D iv 3–4		encephalyomyelitis	pelvic region and abdomen sick; gets up and kneels down; does not eat or drink; eyes shudder	death	6.50n 13.105 13.216
D iv 5			ill from hips to head; well from hips to feet	recovery	Ap.19n
D iv 6			well from hips to head; ill from hips to feet	recovery	Ap.19n
D iv 7			coccyx red	recovery	10.45
D iv 8			coccyx yellow	worsens	10.45
D iv 9			coccyx black	death	10.45
D iv 10			coccyx dark	worrisome	10.45
D iv 11			coccyx dark red	worsens	10.45
D iv 12			coccyx swollen	difficult	10.45
D iv 13			coccyx bruised	no consequence	10.45
D iv 14			coccyx skinned	worrisome	10.45
D iv 15			coccyx cut open	death	10.45
D iv 16	Gula	shingles	coccyx hurts; yoke-shaped lesion rises and curves round		10.102 19.328
D iv 17	Šulak or incest or Sîn		wound to coccyx	if prolonged, death	19.196dn 19.198n
D iv 18	*maškadu*		muscles hurt from coccyx to feet		11.60

D iv 19	wound from in front	wound	left armpit hurts; wanders about	death	14.32n
D iv 20	ghost		right armpit hurts; no fever	death	3.3n 19.391
D iv 21	Lamaštu		left armpit hurts; eyes clouded		Ap.90
D iv 22	Šulpaea		right armpit hurts; eyes clouded		Ap.95
D iv 23	Dapinu	wound	wound to [left femoral crease]; unconscious	death	14.16 19.197
D iv 24–25	Ištar	wound	wound to [right femoral crease]; leg immobilized	death	14.18 19.153
D iv 26	twin gods		[. . .] dried up	[. . .]	
D iv 27	[. . .]		[. . .]	[. . .]	

DPS Tablet XIII

ORGANIZING PRINCIPLE: EPIGASTRIUM (UPPER ABDOMEN)

A 1			epigastrium red	recovery	
A 2		dehydration	epigastrium dark; tongue shriveled	acute stage; death	3.103n 18.37
A 3	[. . .]		[. . .]	[. . .]	
A 4–5	netherworld		yellow spots on the epigastrium; neck [. . .]; breath of nostrils cold	death	
A 6–7	disease of intercourse		epigastrium hurts; one-sided headache; rigidity; fever; wasting away		2.18n Ap.17
B i 5–6	disease of intercourse	hepatitis	epigastrium burns; fever; food and drink do not taste good; jaundice		4.35 6.51n 6.128dn 13.27 Ap.17dn
B i 7	ghost	alcoholism	afflicting epigastrium		19.297n 19.386
B i 8		dehydration	afflicting epigastrium; shriveled tongue	death	3.103 18.36
B i 9–10	great gods	chronic peritonitis	afflicting epigastrium; bloated insides; 31 days	prolonged	3.211 6.33n
B i 11	personal god	fever	afflicting epigastrium; hurting insides, forearms, shins, and feet	recovery	19.363
B i 12	ghost	alcoholism	epigastrium cramped; hurting back		6.46n 19.297 19.386n
B i 13a			epigastrium stiff	no recovery	3.208n 6.33n
B i 13b			epigastrium bloated	worrisome	3.208n 6.33n
B i 14	ghost	alcoholism	epigastrium bloated		6.33 19.298

B i 15			epigastrium protrudes; insides bloated	prolonged	6.35n
B i 16–17	*agannutillû*	congestive heart failure	epigastrium protrudes; no fever; mentation altered	death in cold weather	3.3n 6.35n 8.22
B i 18		congestive heart failure	epigastrium puffed up; face swollen; tears flow	if prolonged, death	6.36 8.21 20.83
B i 19	great gods	chronic peritonitis	epigastrium puffed up; hypogastric region hard; 27 days		3.212 6.41n
B i 20–21	incest	acute peritonitis?	epigastrium puffed up; hypogastric region hard; fever	if under 31 days, recovery	6.41
B i 22	great gods	chronic peritonitis	epigastrium puffed up; hypogastric region soft		3.213 6.37n
B i 23	great gods	chronic peritonitis	epigastrium clear; hypogastric region hard; 27 days		3.213 6.41n
B i 24	great gods	chronic peritonitis	epigastrium clear but rumbles		3.213 6.44n
B i 25	personal god	nonspecific fever	epigastrium soft; fever; same for adults and children		6.42n 19.362
B i 26	ghost	Bornholm disease	epigastrium hot; insides bloated		6.76n 19.388
B i 27	ghost	Bornholm disease	epigastrium hot; blood vessels of temples, hands, and feet pulsate; eyes feel heavy		6.79; 8.42 19.338 19.388
B i 28	goddess	peritonitis	epigastrium puffed up; hypogastric region hard; fever	no recovery	6.41n 19.347
B i 29	river hoist water	river toxins	feverish epigastrium; mentation altered		15.31
B i 30	ghost	Bornholm disease	epigastrium sore; short of breath; brother or sister was also sick		19.387dn
B i 31		shock	loss of epigastric or hypogastric pulse; body cold	death	3.12dn 3.39n 8.57n 20.21n 20.22
B i 32	Adad or Šamaš to twin gods	wound	wound to the epigastrium		3.206n 19.139dn 19.139 19.183
B i 33	Ištar	wound	wound to the epigastrium; hands and feet immobilized		3.206n 19.159
B i 34	adultery	wound	wound to the epigastrium and armpit		
B i 35	Ereškigal	wound	wound to the epigastrium, temple, and rib	death	19.173
B i 36		peptic ulcer	burning pain in epigastrium; produces dark blood	death	6.93 20.51

B i 37		peptic ulcer	burning pain in epigastrium; vomits dark blood; viselike headache	death	6.93n
B i 38		peptic ulcer	needling or burning pain in epigastrium; excretes blood	death	6.94 20.65
B i 39		peptic ulcer	needling or burning pain in epigastrium; vomits blood	2 to 3 days → death	6.95 20.52
B i 40		obstruction	needling or burning pain in epigastrium; constipated	death	6.91
B i 41	Adad		needling pain in epigastrium; 31 days	death	19.139dn Ap.97
B i 42	Marduk or Ištar		needling pain in epigastrium; yellow spots	death	10.50n 19.113 19.373dn
B i 43	rainbow		[. . .]	recovery or death	

ORGANIZING PRINCIPLE: ABDOMEN

B i 44			abdomen bloated on left side	worsens	6.33n
B i 45			abdomen bloated on right side	difficult	6.33n
B i 46	Kūbu	leptospirosis?	abdomen bloated on both sides	recovery	6.33n 19.337n
B i 47	Ištar		abdomen [. . .]		
B i 48	Damu		abdomen [. . .]		
B i 49	Šamaš		abdomen hurts		13.3n
B i 50	Bau	wound	[afflicting] abdomen; cannot lift his hand		19.166n
B i 51	Gula	shingles	afflicting abdomen; yoke curving round on the neck		10.103 19.329
B i 52–53			abdomen hot; ear canals and mouth cold	if prolonged, death	3.39n 14.45 20.16
B i 54–55			abdomen hot; sweat; ear canals and mouth hot	recovery	14.46 20.16
B ii 1			abdomen hot; epigastrium protrudes	recovery	6.35n
B ii 2–3			abdomen burning hot; toes cold	if survives 3 to 4 days, recovery	3.2n 3.8n
B ii 4			abdomen hot; sweat as in *lubāṭu*; stomach upset	death	6.80n 10.26n
B ii 5–6	Šamaš	benign fever	abdomen hot; sweat as in *lubāṭu*; stomach upset	recovery, if treated	6.80 10.26n 19.256
B ii 7–8			abdomen hot; sweat as in *lubāṭu*;	if survives	3.2n; 3.8n

			stomach upset; abdomen burning hot; toes cold	three days, recovery	6.80n 10.26
B ii 9	Šamaš	benign fever	abdomen hot; sweat as in *lubāṭu*; cold; 31 days		6.80n 10.26n 19.193 19.258
B ii 10	wound from in front; Šamaš or Šulak	infected wound	abdomen hot; sweat		6.80n 19.192 19.196dn
B ii 11	Lamaštu	typhoid?	abdomen hot and cold; asks for lots of water and drinks it		19.230
B ii 12	Lamaštu	typhoid?	abdomen hot and cold; asks for lots of water to bathe in		19.231
B ii 13–14	*rābiṣu* or ghost	excessive thirst or cholera	abdomen soft, asks for lots of water; no fever; illness keeps him awake from beginning to middle of the night	death	3.3n 3.102n 6.42 19.296n Ap.87
B ii 15–16	ghost	encephalitis?	heart flutters; epigastrium pulses rapidly; photophobia		8.9, 9.15 13.215
B ii 17–18	twin gods	wound	9-day wound to the abdomen		19.139dn 19.146
	Adad	wound	2-day wound to the abdomen		
	Ea	wound	3-day wound to the abdomen		
	Dingirmaḫ	wound	4-day wound to the abdomen		
	Papsukkal	wound	5-day wound to the abdomen		
B ii 19a		wound	wound to the abdomen; colicky and constipated	death	3.204 6.156n
B ii 19b	twin gods	wound	wound to the abdomen; upset stomach	death	3.204 19.137
B ii 20	twin gods	wound	wound to the abdomen; produces dark blood	death	3.205n 19.181 20.50
B ii 21	Nergal	wound	wound to the abdomen or right side of abdomen; vomits dark blood; 31 days	death	3.205n 19.175
B ii 22	Ištar	ulcer?	needling pain in abdomen on left side; vomiting	recovery	19.373n 20.66
B ii 23	Ištar	liver?	needling pain in abdomen on right side; no vomiting	death	19.373n
B ii 24	Ištar	peptic ulcer	burning pain in abdomen on left side; vomiting	death	6.95n 19.373n 20.67
B ii 25	Ištar	peptic ulcer	burning pain in abdomen on right side; vomiting	death	6.95n 19.373n
B ii 26	Ištar	peptic ulcer	burning pain in abdomen on left; vomiting blood	death	6.95n 19.373

B ii 27	Adad or Ištar	peptic ulcer	burning pain in abdomen on right; vomiting blood	death	6.95n 19.139dn 19.373
B ii 28	Adad	cirrhosis	burning pain in abdomen on right side; dripping blood	death	6.152 19.139dn Ap.98
B ii 29–30	Ištar	hepatitis	burning pain in abdomen on right side; yellow threads in eyes	death	6.126 9.38 19.374
B ii 31	Sîn or Ištar	hepatic amoebiasis?	burning pain in abdomen on right side; lips produce colored mucus	death	19.376
B ii 32		peptic ulcer	needling or burning pain in abdomen on either side; produces dark blood	death	6.7 6.93n
B ii 33	curse	liver?	needling or burning pain in abdomen; licks? with tongue	death or recovery	Ap.58
B ii 34		hepatic amoebiasis?	produces colored mucus; yellow threads in eyes	death	3.73n 9.37 19.377

ORGANIZING PRINCIPLE: CHEST AND ABDOMEN/INSIDES

B ii 35			chest and abdomen red	recovery	
B ii 36			chest and abdomen yellow	worrisome	
B ii 37			chest and abdomen black	death	3.208n
B ii 38–39		wound to the abdomen	chest and abdomen black; muscles of abdomen pulled taut; belches wind from mouth	3 days → death	3.208
B ii 40			chest and abdomen dark	worrisome	
B ii 41			chest and abdomen dark red	prolonged	
B ii 42		thin	chest and abdomen flat	no consequence	7.16
B ii 43		dehydrated	chest and abdomen dried up	death	3.109 20.81
B ii 44	Damu	intestinal artresia	insides blocked off		6.89n 17.120
B ii 45			insides bloated	prolonged	6.33n
B ii 46	Ištar	infected wound	insides bloated; muscles of abdomen pulled taut	no recovery	3.208n 19.152
B ii 47–48		liver failure	insides bloated; muscles of abdomen pulled taut; yellow spots/streaks on muscles; no fever; comes back	death	3.3n 6.144 10.50n
B ii 49–50	Išḫara		insides bloated; yellow spots on abdomen; 31 days	[. . .]	10.50n 19.290n
B ii 51	[. . .]		insides bloated; [yellow spots] on abdomen; [. . .]	[. . .]	
B ii 52	[. . .]		insides bloated; [. . .]; rims of eyes [. . .]	[. . .]	

B ii 53–58	[...]		[...]		
I 1′	[...]		[...]		
I 2′	[...]		insides bloated and full of wind; [...]		6.33n
I 3′–4′	personal god		insides bloated and full of wind		6.33n 19.363dn
I 5′	[...]		insides bloated and full of wind; fever; [...]		3.3n 6.33n
I 6′	[...]		insides bloated; shoulders [...]		6.33n
I 7′	Kūbu	leptospirosis?	insides bloated		6.33n 13.18dn 19.337
I 8′	Kūbu	leptospirosis?	insides bloated; wails		13.18dn 19.337
I 9′	Kūbu	leptospirosis?	insides bloated; eyes bother him		13.18dn 19.337
G_2 2′	Kūbu	leptospirosis?	insides bloated; eyes bother him	recovery	19.337n
G_2 3′	[...]		insides cramped; patient cannot eat; [...]		6.46n
G_2 4′	[...]		insides cramped; arms tense; [...]		
G_2 5′	[...]		insides cramped; eyes bother him; [...]		
G_2 6′	[...]		chest and abdomen soft; thirst; [...]		6.42n
G_2 7′	[...]		chest and abdomen soft; thirst; no fever; keeps him awake from middle of the night to [...]		3.3n 3.102n 6.42n 19.296n
G_2 8′	[...]		chest and abdomen soft; thirst; no fever; keeps him awake from beginning of the night to [...]		3.3n 3.102n 6.42n 19.296n
G_2 9′	[...]		insides, hands, and feet cramped; 32 days	[...]	Ap.11
G_2 10′	[...]		rubs chest and abdomen, hands and feet; utters *šigu*-prayer	[...]	16.60n
G_2 11′	[...]		rubs chest and abdomen, hands and feet; tendons limp	[...]	16.60n
G_2 12′	[...]		insides and fingers sluggish; 31 days	[...]	11.19n Ap.12
G_2 13′	[...]	dehydration	insides purged; cannot urinate		5.28 5.38n
G_2 14′	[...]		cries "my insides"		
G_2 15′	personal god	psychiatric	cries "my insides"		19.36n
G_2 16′	wound to thorax	wound	cries "my insides"; tears hair	[death]	14.12
G_2 17′	[...]		cries "my insides"; hip socket hurts		11.17n Ap.13
G_2 18′	[Ardat lilî]	Gilles de la Tourette	cries "my insides"; hips raised up; confusional states; talks in a frightful manner		13.264

G_2 19′	ghost	psychiatric	cries "my insides"; gets up and runs		19.30
G_2 20′	ghost	alcoholism	cries "my insides" softly or intermittently	[death]	19.385
G_2 21′	Šamaš		cries "my insides" [. . .]		
G_2 22′	personal god	stress	cries ["my insides"]; [*x*] days		19.36n
G_2 23′	[. . .]		[. . .]		
J 1′	[. . .]		[. . .]		
J 2′	[. . .]	alcoholism?	cries "my insides"; [. . .]		
J 3–4	[. . .]	alcoholism?	cries "my insides"; [. . .]		
J 5–6	curse	chronic meningitis?	[cries "my insides"]; hearing difficult; neck "falls"; one-sided headache	death [death]	13.222 19.314
J 7′		wound to epigastric region?	[cries "my insides"]; epigastrium protrudes	[death]	6.35n
J 8′		chest wound	[cries "my insides"]; diaphragm breaks	[death]	14.13
J 9′	Ištar	wound to hypogastric region	[cries "my insides"]; impotent	acute stage; [death]	5.66n 19.162
J 10′	[. . .]		[. . .]	[. . .]	
J 11′	Ištar	psychiatric	[cries "my insides"]; crushing sensation in chest		19.13n

ORGANIZING PRINCIPLE: BLOOD VESSELS/MUSCLES

J 12′	[. . .]	shock	blood vessels of umbilical area "go"		8.57n
J 13′	[Kūbu]	leptospirosis?	petechial rash on muscles of abdomen		19.336n
J 14–15′	curse	wasting	muscles of abdomen drawn taut		19.307
J 16–17′	[. . .]		[. . .]	[. . .]	
D r.1′	[. . .]		[. . .]	[. . .]	

ORGANIZING PRINCIPLE: HYPOGASTRIC REGION (LOWER ABDOMEN)

D r.2′	[. . .]		[. . .]	[. . .]	
D r.3′	twin gods	wound	wound to the hypogastric region	[. . .]	3.206n
D r.4′	[Ištar]	wound	wound to the hypogastric region with loss of virility	[. . .]	3.206n 5.69 19.161
D r.5′	[. . .]	wound	wound to the hypogastric region; feet [. . .]	[. . .]	3.206n

ORGANIZING PRINCIPLE: COLIC

D r.6′	[. . .]		colicky and constipated; [. . .]		6.67n
D r.7′	[. . .]		colicky and constipated; insides cramped; [. . .]		6.67n
D r.8′	[. . .]		colicky and constipated; insides cramped; [. . .]		6.67n
D r.9′	[. . .]		colicky; loss of virility; [. . .]		
D r.10′	[. . .]		colicky; spleen hurts; [. . .]		Ap.14
D r.11′	[. . .]		sluggish; dysentery; [. . .]		3.118n

ORGANIZING PRINCIPLE: BOWELS

D r.12′	[. . .]		bowels rumble; arms [. . .]		
D r.13′	[. . .]		bowels rumble; abdomen [. . .]		
D r.14′	[. . .]		bowels rumble; [. . .]		
D r.15′	[. . .]		bowels rumble; [. . .]		
D r.16′	[. . .]		bowels vomit forth; [. . .]		
D r.17′		abdominal wound	bowels cut loose	worrisome	3.203
D r.18′		diarrhea	bowels loose; arms [. . .]	[. . .]	3.115n 6.69n
D r.19′		diarrhea	bowels loose; insides [. . .]	[. . .]	3.115n 6.69n
D r.20′–21′	[. . .]		[. . .]	[. . .]	

DPS Tablet XIV

ORGANIZING PRINCIPLE: HIP SOCKETS

A i 1	left hip socket red	recovery	2.34dn 10.46dn
A i 2	right [hip socket] red	illness lasts long	2.34dn 10.46dn
A i 3	both [hip sockets] red	no consequence	2.34dn 10.46dn
A i 4	left hip socket yellow	worsens	10.46dn
A i 5	right hip socket yellow	difficult	10.46dn
A i 6	[both hip sockets yellow]	worrisome	10.46dn
A i 7	[left hip socket black]	difficult	10.46dn
A i 8	[right hip socket black]	worrisome	10.46dn
A i 9	[both hip sockets black]	death	10.46dn
A i 10	[left hip socket dark]	worsens	10.46dn
A i 11	[right hip socket dark]	difficult	10.46dn
A i 12	[both hip sockets dark]	worrisome	10.46dn
A i 13	[left hip socket dark red]	illness lasts long	10.46dn
A i 14	[right hip socket dark red]	worsens	10.46dn
A i 15	[both hip sockets dark red]	difficult	10.46dn

A i 16			[left hip socket swollen]	worsens	10.46dn
A i 17			[right hip socket swollen]	difficult	10.46dn
A i 18			[both hip sockets swollen]	worsens	10.46dn
A i 19			[left hip socket bruised]	recovery	10.46dn
A i 20			[right hip socket bruised]	worsens	10.46dn
A i 21			[both hip sockets bruised]	worrisome	10.46dn
A i 22			[left] hip socket [cut open]	difficult	10.46dn
A i 23			[right] hip socket [cut open]	worrisome	10.46dn
A i 24			both hip sockets [cut open]	[difficult]	10.46dn
A i 25			left hip socket [sluggish]	difficult	11.19n
A i 26			right hip socket [sluggish]	[. . .]	11.19n
A i 27			both hip sockets sluggish	[. . .]	11.19n
A i 28			woman's hip sockets sluggish	[. . .]	11.19n
A i 29			hip sockets normal	recovery	
A i 30–31	*kiṣṣatu*	myalgia	muscles [. . .] from hip socket to toes		3.129

ORGANIZING PRINCIPLE: BUTTOCKS

A i 32			left buttock red	[recovery]	10.46dn
A i 33			right buttock red	illness lasts long	10.46dn
A i 34			both buttocks red	no consequence	10.46dn
A i 35			left buttock yellow	worsens	10.46dn
A i 36			right buttock yellow	difficult	10.46dn
A i 37			both buttocks yellow	worrisome	10.46dn
A i 38			left buttock black	difficult	10.46dn
A i 39			right [buttock] black	worrisome	10.46dn
A i 40			both [buttocks] black	death	10.46dn
A i 41			left buttock dark	recovery	10.46dn
C i 5a			right buttock dark	[. . .]	10.46dn
C i 5b			both buttocks dark	death	10.46dn
C i 6a			[left buttock dark red]	[illness lasts long]	10.46dn
C i 6b			right buttock dark red	worsens	10.46dn
C i 7a			[both buttocks dark red]	[difficult]	10.46dn
C i 7b			left buttock swollen	worsens	10.46dn
C i 8a			[right buttock swollen]	[difficult]	10.46dn
C i 8b			both buttocks swollen	worsens	10.46dn
C i 9a			[left buttock bruised]	[. . .]	10.46dn
C i 9b			right buttock bruised	prolonged	10.46dn
C i 10a			[both buttocks bruised]	worrisome	10.46dn
A_2 i 1′			left buttock skinned	worsens	10.46dn
A_2 i 2′			[right buttock] skinned	difficult	10.46dn

A_2 i 3′			both buttocks skinned	worrisome	10.46dn
A_2 i 4′			left buttock cut open	worsens	10.46dn
A_2 i 5′			right buttock cut open	worrisome	10.46dn
A_2 i 6′			both buttocks cut open	death	10.46dn
A_2 i 7′			buttocks normal	recovery	
A_2 i 8′–9′	wound from behind	wound	buttocks dark; no excretion; no urination	death	5.41 13.142n
A_2 i 10′	Ištar	wound	wound to hip socket and buttock		19.163
A_2 i 11′	Ištar	wound	wound to hip socket and leg		19.163

ORGANIZING PRINCIPLE: INGUINAL REGION

A_2 i 12′			inguinal regions shift under him	worsens	19.272
A_2 i 13′	Šamaš		inguinal regions shift under him; nature of disease alters	recovery	19.272
A_2 i 14′			[. . .]; patient tries to stand	death	
A_2 i 15′		wound	wound to left inguinal region; not in full possession of faculties; wanders about	death	14.14
A_2 i 16′		wound	wound to right inguinal region; cries out without knowing it	death	14.15
A_2 i 17′		plague?	blood vessels of left inguinal region pulsate and are dark	2 or 3 days → death	3.230
A_2 i 18′		plague?	blood vessels of right inguinal region pulsate and are dark	speedy death	3.231

ORGANIZING PRINCIPLE: ANUS

A_2 i 19′		ileus	anus stands still	death	6.154
A_2 i 20′		ileus	anus stands still; wind; [. . .]	if difficult, death	6.154n
A_2 i 21′		obstruction	anus blocked off	death	6.89
A_2 i 22′			anus twitches(?); [. . .]	death	
C_2 i 11a			red liquid flows from anus	prolonged	6.14
C_2 i 11b			yellow liquid flows from anus	[. . .]	6.21
C_2 i 12a			red bile flows from anus	recovery	6.15
C_2 i 12b			yellow bile flows from anus [. . .]	death	6.22
A ii 6			black bile flows from anus	death	6.18
A ii 7			body fat flows from anus	death	6.23
A ii 8			produces material from insides from anus	death	6.19n
A ii 9			produces flesh from anus	[. . .]	6.19
A ii 10			produces dark red blood from anus	death	6.16n
A ii 11			produces blood and wind from anus	[. . .]	6.16n

A ii 12			excretes blood from anus	[...]	6.16
A ii 13			excretes dark blood from anus	[...]	6.16
A ii 14			excretes blood and pus from anus	[...]	6.16
A ii 15		obstruction	anus blocked off	death	6.89n

ORGANIZING PRINCIPLE: EXCREMENT

A ii 16			excrement red	recovery	6.13
A ii 17			excrement yellow	[...]	6.20
A ii 18			excrement [black]	death	6.13
A ii 19			excrement dark red	[...]	6.13
A ii 20			excrement [...]	prolonged	
A ii 21			excrement [...]	[...]	
C ii 4	ḪAR.GIG		scratches? [his anus]	[...]	

ORGANIZING PRINCIPLE: PENIS

C ii 5a			[penis red]	recovery	10.46dn
C ii 5b			penis yellow	[...]	10.46dn
A ii 25			[penis black]	death	10.46dn
A ii 26			penis dark	worrisome	10.46dn
A ii 27			[penis dark red]	will exhaust him	10.46dn
A ii 28			penis swollen	worrisome	10.46dn
A ii 29			[penis] bruised	recovery	10.46dn
A ii 30			penis skinned and does not heal	death	10.46dn
A ii 31			[penis normal]	recovery	
A ii 32		obstruction	penis blocked off	death	5.35
A ii 33			penis [...]	death	
A ii 34–36	disease of intercourse; personal god or goddess	Fitz Hugh Curtis	penis and epigastrium hold burning fever; liver hurts; stomach goes crazy; arms, feet, and stomach hot		2.18; 3.8n 4.34 6.74n 19.348 Ap.17dn
A ii 37	Šamaš as punishment for illicit sexual intercourse	urethritis	blood drips from penis	death	4.4 5.18 19.108
A ii 38	Ištar		penis and testicles swollen; sexually transmitted		2.18n; 4.1 5.76

ORGANIZING PRINCIPLE: URINE

A ii 39	personal god	hematuria	urine red	recovery	5.2 19.353dn 20.54
A ii 40	*ṣētu*	fever with dehydration	urine yellow	prolonged	3.168 5.4

A ii 41		black water fever or alkaptonuria	urine black	death	5.5 7.32
A ii 42		black water fever	urine dark	death	5.7
A ii 43		obstruction	urine blocked off	death	5.36
A ii 44		excessive urine flow	urine continually flows	death	20.82
A ii 45		excessive urine flow	urine and semen continually flow	death	4.8; 5.22n 20.82n
A ii 46			urine is like [. . .]	death	
A ii 47			urine is like water	recovery	5.6
A ii 48			urine is like *kasû* juice	recovery	5.9
A ii 49		porphyria	urine is like wine	recovery	5.3
A ii 50		filariasis	urine is like milk	recovery	5.11
A_2 ii 1			urine normal	recovery	5.1
A_2 ii 2	"touched in the steppe"	diabetes	*lipištu* in the urine		5.27n 7.30
A_2 ii 3	"touched in the steppe"	diabetes	flesh in the urine		5.27 7.29

ORGANIZING PRINCIPLE: TESTICLES

A_2 ii 4			testicles red	recovery	5.84 10.46dn 20.41
A_2 ii 5			testicles yellow	[. . .]	10.46dn
A_2 ii 6			testicles black	death	5.84 10.46dn 20.37
A_2 ii 7			testicles dark	[. . .]	10.46dn
A_2 ii 8			testicles dark red	difficult	10.46dn 20.39
A_2 ii 9			testicles bruised	[. . .]	10.46dn
A_2 ii 10			testicles skinned	death	10.46dn
A_2 ii 11			testicles intact	[recovery]	
A_2 ii 12	incest		testicles twisted	death	5.83 19.198dn
A_2 ii 13–14	[. . .]		testicles twisted; stammers; [. . .] his lips	[. . .]	5.86n
A_2 ii 15	incest		testicles swollen	worrisome	4.28n 5.76n 19.198dn
A_2 ii 16	incest		testicles swollen; penis full of *sikkatu*		4.28 5.76n 10.149 19.198dn
A_2 ii 17	incest	wound	wound to testicles		5.87 19.198dn

A_2 ii 18		wound	wound to testicles; [. . .]	[. . .]	5.87n
A_2 ii 19–20			testicles crushed; umbilical area [. . .]; retention of urine	[. . .]	5.86
A_2 ii 21	[. . .]	congestive heart failure	lower parts of the body swollen	[. . .]	8.26

ORGANIZING PRINCIPLE: CROTCH/THIGHS

A_2 ii 22			left thigh red	[. . .]	10.46dn
A_2 ii 23			right thigh red	[. . .]	10.46dn
A_2 iii 1			both thighs red	worrisome	10.46dn
A_2 iii 2			left thigh [yellow]	[. . .]	10.46dn
A_2 iii 3			right thigh yellow	[. . .]	10.46dn
A_2 iii 4			both thighs yellow	worrisome	10.46dn
A_2 iii 5			left thigh black	[. . .]	10.46dn
G iii 6a			right thigh black	worrisome	10.46dn
G iii 6b			both thighs black	[. . .]	10.46dn
G iii 7a			left thigh dark	worsens	10.46dn
H 3			right thigh dark	[. . .]	10.46dn
G iii 8a			both thighs dark	worrisome	10.46dn 20.38
H 4			left thigh dark red	[. . .]	10.46dn
G iii 9			right thigh dark red	weakens him	10.46dn
G iii 10			both thighs dark red	worrisome	10.46dn
G iii 11			left thigh swollen	illness will linger	10.46dn
G iii 12			right thigh swollen	[. . .]	10.46dn
G iii 13a			both thighs swollen	worrisome	10.46dn
H 9			left thigh [bruised]	[. . .]	10.46dn
G iii 14			right thigh bruised	[. . .]	10.46dn
G iii 15			both thighs bruised	[. . .]	10.46dn
G iii 16			left thigh skinned	[. . .]	10.46dn
G iii 17			right thigh skinned	[. . .]	10.46dn
G iii 18			both thighs [skinned]	[. . .]	10.46dn
A iii 1–2	twin gods	fevers with possible DIC	[strikes crotch]; chews [hands if not prevented]	death	16.78 19.238
A iii 3–4	*maškadu*	sciatica	[muscles of thigh] hurt from [hip sockets] to ankles; [can stand and walk]		11.59
A iii 5	*sagallu*	sciatica	[muscles of thigh all hurt at once]; cannot [stand] or walk		11.58
A iii 6		wound	wound to [left thigh]; constipated	death	14.19
A iii 7		wound	[wound to right thigh; stomach cramped]; viselike headache	death	14.20

ORGANIZING PRINCIPLE: SIDE OF THE ABDOMEN

A iii 8	personal god	stress	[left side of abdomen hurts]	recovery	19.36n
A iii 9	personal goddess	stress	[right side of abdomen hurts]	recovery	19.36n
A iii 10–11	[Adad]	septic shock	[left side] of abdomen swollen and dark; wanders about	death	3.206n 14.38 19.139dn 19.144
A iii 12–13	[Ištar]	septic shock	right [side of abdomen] swollen and dark; wanders about	death	3.206 14.38n 19.155
A iii 14–15			cries "the side of my abdomen"; excretes bile; testicles twisted	death	5.86n Ap.32
A iii 16	Adad	wound	wound to the side of the abdomen		3.206n 19.139dn 19.140n
A iii 17	Adad	wound	wound to the side of the abdomen; produces dark blood	death	3.205 19.139dn 19.140 19.183dn
A iii 18	Ningizzida	wound	wound to the side of the abdomen; constipation		3.209 6.156 19.203
A iii 19	Ningizzida	wound	wound to the side of the abdomen; subdued countenance; "touched in the steppe"		3.209 19.203n
A iii 20	[. . .]	wound	wound to the side of the abdomen; withdrawn countenance; trembles on legs; [. . .]		3.206n
A iii 21–22	[. . .]	wound	wound to the side of the abdomen; cries out; vomits bile from [. . .]		3.206n
A iii 23	[. . .]	wound	wound to the side of the abdomen and armpit		

ORGANIZING PRINCIPLE: KNEES

A iii 24	Šamaš	arthritis	knees continually hurt		11.17 11.45n
A iii 25–26	Šamaš	arthritis	knees and hips continually hurt in the night; no fever		3.3n 11.17n 11.45

ORGANIZING PRINCIPLE: ANAL OPENING

C_2 iii 16			anal opening continually opened	death	6.162
C_2 iii 17			anal opening continually constricted	recovery	6.161

ORGANIZING PRINCIPLE: LEG

C_2 iii 18	Ištar	arthritis	left leg hurts; no fever		3.3n 11.53
C_2 iii 19			right leg hurts; fever	recovery	3.3n
C_2 iii 20	personal god	fever	both legs hurt; fever	will let up	3.3n 19.363dn
C_2 iii 21	city or personal god	arthritis	legs hurt		19.353dn
C_2 iii 22	Šamaš	arthritis	legs hurt	recovery	11.46
C_2 iii 23–24			legs full of gnawing; salivation	lets up unless patient lies there with mouth open	3.129n
C_2 iii 25			legs full of gnawing; flesh hot; vomits whatever he eats	[. . .]	3.129n
C_2 iii 26a	[. . .]	wound	wound to the leg		
C_2 iii 26b		wound	wound to left leg; vomits blood	[if prolonged, death]	14.17
C_2 iii 27		wound	wound to right leg; produces dark blood	[death]	14.17

ORGANIZING PRINCIPLE: FEET

A_2 iv 1	Ištar	arthritis	left foot hurts		11.50
A_2 iv 2a	[Šamaš]	arthritis	right foot hurts		11.50
A_2 iv 2b	[. . .]	arthritis	both feet hurt	recovery	11.50
A_2 iv 3–4	*rābiṣu*	stroke	drags left foot; mouth twitches	if prolonged, death	13.55 13.79 13.243 20.86
A_2 iv 5	wound of Bau	wound simulating stroke	drags right foot	death	19.165
A_2 iv 6	Ištar	arthritis	left foot shrunken	if ghost, death	11.20n 11.51 19.392n
A_2 iv 7	Ištar	arthritis	right foot shrunken		11.20n 11.51
A_2 iv 8	evil god	arthritis	both feet shrunken		11.20 11.51n 19.353dn
A_2 iv 9	[. . .]		left [foot] stretched toward the right		13.64
A_2 iv 10	[. . .]		unable to turn his feet		
A_2 iv 11			feet immobilized in bent position; not in full possession of faculties	[death]	19.271n
A_2 iv 12	Šamaš	arthritis	feet twisted		11.21 11.48

A_2 iv 13–14	[. . .]	neuropathy	feet sluggish and contorted		13.269
A_2 iv 15	*rābiṣu*	rheumatism	feet stiff	recovery	11.15n 11.40 19.83
A_2 iv 16	dirty bath water	neuropathy	feet numb		3.249n 13.266n
A_2 iv 17			feet thrash around; hands quiet	worrisome	Ap.33
A_2 iv 18			feet hot; hands cold	if illness goes away, recovery	
G iv 10–13	[. . .]		[. . .]	[. . .]	
C_2 iv 3a		arthritis	feet stiff	worsens	11.6n
C_2 iv 3b	Ištar	arthritis	[feet so stiff patient cannot] stand		
C_2 iv 4a	[. . .]		[. . .]	[. . .]	
C_2 iv 4b	twin gods	wound	wound to foot		19.186n
C_2 iv 5a	Šamaš	wound	wound to left [foot]	[3 days → death]	19.186 19.194
C_2 iv 5b	Ištar	wound	wound to right foot	if prolonged, death	19.154 19.186 19.194dn 20.85
C_2 iv 6	Šamaš to twin gods	wound	wound to [left] foot; cries out		19.186
A iv 1–2	Ištar to twin gods	wound	wound to right foot; cries out		19.186
A iv 3	to twin gods	wound	wound to foot; cries out		19.186n
A iv 4–5	Ištar	wound	wound to foot, hips, arms, and neck; 41 days		19.164

ORGANIZING PRINCIPLE: PARTS OF THE FOOT

A iv 6			toes dark	if prolonged, death	
A iv 7	Išḫara	arthralgia	toes sluggish		11.19n
A iv 8–9	Nergal	trauma	toes split to pieces	death	19.175n
A iv 10–11		rat bite fever	toes full of blood and hurt; develops Labaṣu	death	3.35
A iv 12		yellow nail syndrome	toenails yellow	death	10.204
A iv 13			toenails red	recovery	10.205
A iv 14		gangrene	bellies of toes dark; twists	death	14.42 19.131n
A iv 15		shock	tips of toes cold	death	3.39n 14.26n

A iv 16	Ištar	gangrene	breasts of feet dark	if prolonged, death	14.44 19.128 20.87
A iv 17–18	curse	sickle cell anemia	soles of feet cold; rims of eyes swollen; penis stiff; navel supple	if lingers, death	3.39n 5.59 19.316
A iv 19–20			skin on bottom of feet throbs; headache; trembling abdomen	death	20.29
A iv 21–22			difficult to bend and straighten out left or right foot	death	13.64n 13.285n

ORGANIZING PRINCIPLE: BLOOD VESSELS

A iv 23			blood vessels of feet "go"; those of hands slow	recovery or death	8.53 20.27
A iv 24–25			blood vessels of feet "go"; those of hands present	recovery	8.54
A iv 26–27	Šamaš	benign fever	blood vessels of feet pulsate; cannot raise eyes; head and epigastrium hot	recovery	8.42n 19.255
A iv 28	[...]		blood vessel pulsates; ankles not hot; [...]	[...]	
A iv 29–30			blood vessel pulsates; ankles hot; lungs [sick]; mouth roars	recovery unless prolonged	8.83

DPS Tablet XV

ORGANIZING PRINCIPLE: PATIENT SICK ONE DAY

1–3	[...]		[...]	[...]	
4	death-demon	neck wound	[twists; vomits blood]	death	
5	wound from in front	neck wound	face dark; [vomits blood]	death	8.92
6	wound to neck; Ištar	neck wound	neck hurts; [continually thirsty]	death	13.138 19.150
7	tabooed food	choking or food allergy	larynx constricted	death	8.89
8		epiglottitis	chokings closely spaced; not in full possession of faculties	[death]	3.57
9	wound from behind	septic shock	left arm dark; tongue-tied	death	13.125dn Ap.93
10	Sîn	septic shock	right arm dark; twisting	death	19.201 Ap.94
11		wound to back	unable to turn arms; blood drips from [anus]	[death]	13.136n

12		wound to back	unable to turn arms; [. . .]	[death]	
13–14	wound to navel; Ištar	hemorrhagic shock	hands placed on the navel; hands and feet cold; [talks] without knowing what he is saying; gets up and sits down	[death]	3.39 14.26 19.64 19.129 19.151
15	[wound] to epigastrium	peritonitis	hands continually over the head; insides puffed up; burns with fever	[death]	3.8n 3.210
16	dirty substances	mental status change	hand moves across mouth; throws off garment	[death]	16.59 16.62 Ap.79
17		mental status change	hands continually rub body	if prolonged, [death]	16.60n 20.11n
18	Šamaš	encephalitis?	hands immobilized in bent position; not in full possession of faculties	[death]	19.271
19		encephalitis?	hands or feet immobilized in bent position; not in full possession of faculties	acute stage; [death]	19.271n
20	city god	acute arterial occlusion	hands or feet immobilized in bent position without confusion	[death]	19.126
21	Adad	wound	hands and feet [. . .]; speech wanders about	[death]	14.38 19.139dn 19.145
22	Nergal	wound	hands and feet [. . .]; vomits blood	death	19.175n
23	*bennu*	cysticercosis?	hands and feet [. . .]; it itches	death	3.267n
24a			hands and [feet rub?]; thirsty; not in full possession of faculties	death	16.60n
24b			hands and feet rub each other	if prolonged, death	16.60n
25	*miqit šamê* has "touched" him; personal god		[sucks?] his fingers; [. . .]; continually passes out; can get up afterward	death	Ap.62
26	wound to neck; Bau	septic shock	sucks his fingers; burns with fever; abdomen bloated; wanders about	death	3.8n 14.37 19.166
27		primitive reflex	fingers placed in mouth and if you take them out, he returns them to his mouth	if death; then another death in the household	2.11n 16.61n
28	city god	gangrene	breasts of hands dark	death	14.43 19.127
29	ghost	gangrene	bellies of fingers dark; twists	death	14.41 19.131
30	wound from in front	wound	left armpit hurts; wanders about	death	14.32n
31	ghost		right armpit hurts; no fever	death	3.3n 19.391

32	wound from in front; Nergal	wound	wound to the chest; blood pours out; wanders about	death	14.32 19.174
33		dehydration	epigastrium dark; tongue shriveled	acute stage; death	3.103n 18.37
34		congestive heart failure	epigastrium puffed up; face swollen; tears flow	if prolonged, death	6.36; 8.21 20.83
35		wound	wound to the abdomen; colicky and constipated	death	3.204 6.156n
36	twin gods	wound	wound to the abdomen; upset stomach	death	3.204 19.137
37		wound to the abdomen	chest and abdomen black; muscles of abdomen pulled taut; belches wind from mouth	3 days → death	3.208
38	wound to thorax	wound	cries "my insides"; tears hair	death	14.12
39	twin gods	hemorrhagic shock	wound to left kidney; not in full possession of faculties; wanders about	death	14.33 19.179 20.8
40	Sibitti	hemorrhagic shock	wound to right kidney; not in full possession of faculties; vomits blood	death	14.27 19.178
41	Sîn	wound	wound to coccyx or testicle	if prolonged, death	19.198
42	wound to kidney; Damu	hemorrhagic shock	left rib dark; mouth continually dry; rolls over and over	death	10.36 14.28 19.202
43	Damu	hemorrhagic shock	right rib dark; vomits blood; stomach upset	death	10.36n 14.29
44	city god	hemorrhagic shock	wound to left side of back; wanders about	death	14.33n 19.207
45	personal god	hemorrhagic shock	wound to right side of back; wanders about	death	14.33n 19.207
46	ghost	wound	wound to spine; no excretion	death	5.40 6.155 13.142 19.172
47		spondylitis	spine curved and he cannot straighten it out	if prolonged, death	11.24 20.84
48		opisthotonus	raises pelvic region and does not know he is doing this	death	13.88
49	Šulpaea	wound	wound to left femoral crease; unconscious	death	14.16 19.197
50	Ištar	wound	wound to right femoral crease; leg immobilized	death	14.18 19.153
51	wound from behind	wound	buttocks dark; no excretion; no urination	death	5.41 13.142n

52	Adad	septic shock	left side of abdomen swollen and dark; wanders about	death	3.206n 14.38 19.139dn 19.144
53	Ištar	septic shock	right side of abdomen swollen and dark; wanders about	death	3.206 14.38n 19.155
54		wound	wound to left thigh; constipated	death	14.19
55		wound	wound to right thigh; stomach cramped; viselike headache	[death]	14.20
56	twin gods	fevers with possible DIC	strikes crotch; chews hands if not prevented	[death]	16.78 19.238
57		wound	wound to left inguinal region; not in full possession of faculties; [wanders about]	[death]	14.14
58		wound	wound to right inguinal region; cries out without knowing it	[death]	14.15
59		wound	wound to left leg; vomits blood	[if prolonged, death]	14.17
60		wound	wound to right leg; produces dark blood	[death]	14.17
61	Šamaš	wound	wound to left foot	3 days → [death]	19.186 19.194
62	Ištar	wound	wound to right foot	if prolonged, [death]	19.154 19.186 19.194dn 20.85
63	[*rābiṣu*]	stroke	drags left foot; mouth twitches	[if prolonged, death]	13.55 13.79 13.243 20.86
64a	wound of Bau	wound simulating stroke	drags right foot	death	19.165
64b			feet immobilized in bent position; [not in full possession of faculties]	[death]	19.271n
65	[Ištar]	gangrene	breasts of feet dark	[if prolonged, death]	14.44 19.128 20.87
66		gangrene	bellies of toes dark; [twists]	death	14.42 19.131n
67			flesh goes numb; eyes full of blood	[death]	9.36n Ap.34
68			scratches his flesh without realizing it	[death]	Ap.35
69–75	[. . .]		[. . .]	[. . .]	
76	[. . .]		wails; [. . .]	[. . .]	
77	[. . .]		laughs [. . .]	[. . .]	

78	[. . .]		does not answer one trying to wake him; [. . .]	[. . .]	
79	[. . .]		continually falls down; [. . .]	[. . .]	
80	[. . .]		withdraws from social intercourse; [. . .]	[. . .]	
81	[. . .]		continually cries out; [. . .]	[. . .]	
82	[. . .]		continually shudders; [. . .]	[. . .]	
83	[. . .]		continually jerks; [. . .]	[. . .]	
84	[. . .]		continually twists; [. . .]	[. . .]	
85–87	[. . .]		[. . .]	[. . .]	
88			[. . .]; continually cries out	death	
89	personal god		continually cries out in his sleep; does not answer one trying to wake him	death	19.294 20.101
90		status epilepticus	continually cries out in his sleep like a bird; continually jerks	3 days → death	13.208
91	Lamaštu or Adad	wound	wounded; makes assignments for his tomb	death	19.139dn 19.147
92	Ištar to twin gods		[. . .]	worrisome/ death	19.158n 19.184

DPS Tablet XVI

ORGANIZING PRINCIPLE: PATIENT SICK ONE DAY

1	*ṣētu* or father's god	enteric fever	1 day; head hurts	recovery or death	3.142 19.222
2			1 day; hands placed on abdomen; utters *šigu*-prayer; supplicates	death	
3	great gods		1 day; hands placed on abdomen; sucks fingers	death	Ap.107
4			1 day; wails for his household	death	20.103
5			1 day; wails for his children	death	20.103n
6			1 day; excretes body fat	death	6.24
7			1 day; urinates blood in urine	acute stage; death	5.19; 5.52 20.55
8			1 day; groans and cries out	death	
9	great gods		1 day; cries out "ah"; will not drink	death	6.50n Ap.108
10	Gallû	bleeding	1 day; excretes dark blood	death	6.17 19.177n
11		dehydration	1 day; does not recognize people he knows	death	3.112

ORGANIZING PRINCIPLE: PATIENT SICK MORE THAN ONE DAY

12	*aḫḫāzu* or great gods	biphasic fever	1 day leaves him; (later) comes over him 1 day	death	3.30n 6.131 Ap.109
13	oath by a god	remittent fever	1 day afflicts him; 1 day releases him		3.20n 19.225n
14–15	Lamaštu	remittent fever	1 day afflicts him; 1 day releases him; confusional state with hurting limbs, fever, and trembling; sweating, then relief; thirst	recovery	3.20 13.84 19.225
16	ghost	prodrome of of viral meningitis?	sick one day; well 1 day; father or mother was also sick		Ap.84
17	ghost	prodrome of viral encephalitis?	flows over 1 or 2 days; afflicts on 3rd day		Ap.85
18		fatal fever	1 or 2 days; abdomen afflicts him; affliction continually falls on him	death	
19–20		fatal fever	1 to 3 days; burning fever; lets up in body but not in head; 3 more days	6th day → death	3.8

ORGANIZING PRINCIPLE: PATIENT SICK TWO DAYS

21–22	Dapinu	retrobulbar? optic neuropathy	2 days; left or right temple hurts; left or right eye makes a "shadow"	may go away by itself	9.90 19.87
23–24	city god	nutritional? optic neuropathy	2 days; both temples hurt; both eyes make a "shadow"	may go away by itself	9.91n 19.349

ORGANIZING PRINCIPLE: PATIENT SICK MORE THAN TWO DAYS

25–27	*ṣibit šadî*	regular pattern	falls on him 2 days; afflicts him the 3rd day; affliction with rigidity followed by trembling; limbs hurt; hands and feet cold; afterward fever rides/flows over him everywhere at once; sweating, then relief		3.10 19.218
28	*ṣibit šadî*	irregular pattern	afflicts him 2 days; flows over him the 3rd day	death	3.11n 3.21 19.220
29	*kiṣṣatu*	fever with myalgia	2 to 3 days; persistently afflicting abdomen; produces blood from nose		3.129n
30		coma	2 to 3 days; persistent gasping respiration	7th day → death	8.84n 13.280n
31–32	[. . .]	fever	2 to 3 days; burning fever; lets up in body but not in head; [. . .]	[. . .]	3.8n

33	[. . .]	fever	2 to 3 days; fever; sweat as in *lubāṭu*; [. . .]	[. . .]	10.26n
34	[. . .]	fever	2 to 3 days; continuously falls on him; fever and sweat; [. . .]	[. . .]	
35	[. . .]	fever	2 to 3 days; [. . .]; fever and sweat; [. . .]	[. . .]	
36	[. . .]	fever	2 days; 3rd day [. . .]	[. . .]	
37	[. . .]	fever	2 days; 3rd day gets up; [. . .]	[. . .]	

ORGANIZING PRINCIPLE: PATIENT SICK MORE THAN THREE DAYS

38′	[. . .]	fever	3 days; 4th day gets up; [. . .]	[. . .]	
39′	[. . .]	fever	3 days; 4th day blood flows from nose; [. . .]	[. . .]	
40′		fever	3 days; gets up in evening	illness lets up	
41′		biphasic fever	3 days; flesh normal; illness returns	death	3.27n
42′			3 days; cries out "my insides"; insides bloated	death	

ORGANIZING PRINCIPLE: PATIENT SICK MORE THAN FOUR DAYS

43′		liver failure	4 days; hands placed on abdomen; yellow spots/streaks on face	death	6.143 10.50n
44′–45′	*aḫḫāzu*	biphasic fever with jaundice	4 to 5 days; sweat continually falls on him	illness lets up	3.31 6.132

ORGANIZING PRINCIPLE: PATIENT SICK MORE THAN FIVE DAYS

46′	*ṣētu*	enteric fever	5 days; 6th day blood flows from nose	illness lets up	3.138n
47′		liver failure	5 days; yellow spots; eyes full of blood	death	6.123 9.36 10.50n 20.56
48′			5 or 6 days; persistent crying of "yow, yow"	death	20.58
49′		coma	5 to 10 days; persistent gasping respiration	death	8.84 13.280n
50′–51′	*ṣētu*	enteric fever	mighty sickness for 5 to 10 days; persistent bleeding from nose for 5 days then stops	illness lets up; recovery; of no consequence	3.138

ORGANIZING PRINCIPLE: PATIENT SICK ONE TO TWO FIVE-DAY WEEKS

52′		fever	mighty sickness for 5 to 10 days; persists for 5 more days	recovery; of no consequence	20.88
53′–54′		coma	mighty sickness for 5 to 10 days; pupils persistently move downward; gasping respiration for 2 days	3rd day → death	8.84n 13.119 13.279 20.35
55′		fever	5 to 10 days; afterward blood flows from nose	recovery	
56′	Sîn	encephalitis?	5 to 10 days; no fever or sweat	death	3.3n 19.262

ORGANIZING PRINCIPLE: PATIENT SICK ONE TO FOUR FIVE-DAY WEEKS

57′		coma	5, 10, or 15 days; on and off gasping respiration	if difficult, death	8.84n 13.280n
58′		coma	5, 10, or 15 days; pupils move upward; continuous gasping respiration for 3 days	death	8.84n 13.120 13.280
59′–60′	Ištar	arthritis:	5, 10, 15, or 20 days; digits of hands and feet immobilized and too stiff to open or stand on	chance of recovery	11.6 11.49 13.40

ORGANIZING PRINCIPLE: PATIENT SICK MORE THAN SIX DAYS

61′		biphasic fever	6 days; flesh normal; illness returns; illness worsens and abdomen continually afflicts him	death	3.27 3.32
62′		biphasic fever	6 to 10 days; illness returns; epigastrium afflicts him	death	3.27n 3.32
63′–64′		coma test	6 days; no respite on 7th; water thrown on face; if eyes not opened	death	13.286 20.102
			if eyes opened and closed in response to water	recovery	13.286 20.102
65′–66′		biphasic fever	6 days; 7th day chills continually fall on him; after chills, sweat from head to shins	illness lets up; recovery	3.29 3.33 3.40
67′–68′		biphasic fever	[6 days; 7th day gets well but after recovery gets sick again]; sweat from head [to shins; abdomen afflicts him]	death	3.34n
69′		biphasic fever	[6 days]; 7th day gets well but after recovery gets sick again; epigastrium afflicts him	death	3.34
70′		biphasic fever	[6 days]; 7th day gets well [but after recovery gets sick again]; turns dark; excretes bile from anus	death	

71′		biphasic fever	6 days; [7th day gets well but after recovery gets sick again]; forgets what he has said; excretes bile from anus	death	
72′		biphasic fever	6 days; 7th day [gets well but after recovery gets sick again]; eyes full of sediment; blood flows from nose	recovery	9.86
73′–74′		malaria	6 days; 7th day well; 8th day sick; 9th day well; 10th day sick; 11th day well; illness takes turn for worse	recovery not predicted	3.44

ORGANIZING PRINCIPLE: PATIENT SICK UNDER A MONTH

75′			15 days; illness falls on him	diminution caused by the illness	
76′			not yet a month; turns black; throat looks skinned	if it worsens, death	Ap.36
77′			not yet a month; turns black; eyes "lie down"	if it worsens, death	Ap.37

ORGANIZING PRINCIPLE: PATIENT SICK A MONTH OR MORE

78′–79′	*kiṣṣatu*	fever with myalgia	1 or 2 months; illness leaves; afflicting abdomen; produces red blood from nose	recovery	3.129n
80′	Ištar's shuddering	hysterical seizure	falls on him in the night; 1 to 2 months; cries out; can get up afterward		19.15

ORGANIZING PRINCIPLE: PATIENT SICK A LONG TIME

81′–82′	*ṣētu*'s confusional state	febrile seizure	daily at expected time comes over him and leaves him; when coming over him, becomes hot and muscles continually hurt; sweating, then relief		3.123 3.148n 13.173
83′–84′	*ṣētu*	enteric fever	sick a long time; red liquid flows from anus	illness lets up; recovery; of no consequence	3.139 3.151
85′		liver failure	sick a long time; yellow spots/streaks on muscles; eyes full of blood	death	6.123n 9.36n 10.50n
86′		liver failure	sick a long time; yellow spots; red spots in eyes	no recovery	6.124 9.36n 10.50n

ORGANIZING PRINCIPLE: PATIENT IN HIS SEVENTIES

87′		premonition	wails for household	death	2.40n
88′		premonition	wails for household and children	death	2.40
89′		premonition	makes arrangements for funeral	death	2.40n 20.104
90′			excretes body fat	death	6.25 20.93
91′		jaundice	eyes yellow	death	2.41 6.136 20.46
92′		liver failure	body yellow; insides bloated; yellow streaks on abdomen	death	2.41n 6.145 20.94
93′		poor circulation	hands and feet cold	recovery	2.42 20.15
94′		arthritis	hands and feet become bent	recovery	2.43n 11.30 20.97
95′		arthritis	hands and feet become shrunken	recovery	2.43 11.31
96′			blood flows from nose	recovery	2.44 20.47 20.98
97′			unable to eat or drink	[death]	2.44 20.95
98′			persistent gasping respiration; asks for pomegranates	death	2.44n 8.84n Ap.53
99′			asks for dates and eats them	recovery	2.44n 8.84n Ap.53
100′			asks for a spoonful of bread and eats fat with it	death	2.44n 20.96 Ap.49
101′			asks for milk and eats the cream	acute stage; death	2.44n 20.96 Ap.49

DPS Tablet XVII

ORGANIZING PRINCIPLE: BEGINNING OF ILLNESS

1–3	illness of 2 days	fever	sweat; fever blisters; sweat not reaching from shins to ankles and soles of feet	3 more days → recovery	10.79
4–7	*diʾu* or *ṣētu*	enteric fever	fever and chills in equal proportions; after fever and sweat, limbs produce heat leading to fever of same degree as previous fever; leaves but afterward chills and sweat	7 days → recovery	3.163 20.90

8–9	*ṣētu* of 2 days	enteric fever	temples produce heat leading to fever and sweat	3 more days → recovery	3.122n 3.143 20.89
10–13	*rābiṣu* in the food	hepatitis A	burns with fever, eats much bread, beer, and fruit but cannot keep it down and pours it out; none of normal symptoms of *rābiṣu*; stomach upset; face turns yellow	5 or 7 days → recovery	3.8n 6.71n 6.127 19.233

ORGANIZING PRINCIPLE: DURING ILLNESS

14		non-life-threatening pain	groans; illness with ice cold	recovery	3.41
15	illness of limbs	pseudo-seizure	cries out	recovery	19.14dn
16	illness of limbs	pseudo-seizure	can get up afterward	recovery	19.14dn
17	ghost	psychiatric problem	continually talks	recovery	16.45 19.29
18		not a coma	does not respond to shouting; not afflicted by fever	recovery	
19	twin gods	life-threatening pain	cries out "wah"; sleeps briefly on thorax and will not turn over	death	19.368n 20.68
20	twin gods	life-threatening pain	cries out "wah"; sleeps on thorax and will not turn over; makes him ill		19.368n 20.68n
21	river hoist water	river toxins	dizziness		15.29
22	river hoist water	river toxins	twisting		15.30
23		congestive heart failure	shudders; gets up and squats down	death	8.30
24		congestive heart failure	jerks; gets up and sits down; eats and drinks	death	8.30
25–26	Sibitti	hemorrhagic fever	does not raise eyes; blood comes out of eyes, nose, mouth, ears, and penis all at the same time		3.236 9.26 19.234
	twin gods	fever with DIC	31 days		3.236 9.26 19.236
27			once or twice vomits bile and afterward blood	death	6.5 20.53
28			inguinal regions? hurt and afterward vomits blood	death	
29			insides alternate between being relaxed and upset	illness leaves	6.48
30		not a stroke	mouth seized; hands and feet become shrunken	illness passes	

31		not a stroke	hand or foot becomes weak	illness passes; recovery	20.75

ORGANIZING PRINCIPLE: ILLNESS ENTERS AND LEAVES

32	Uraš		illness rises in middle of night		Ap.102
33			illness lets up; cannot stop vomiting	death	6.62 20.79
34	Šamaš	postictal state	illness enters and leaves; confusional state with difficulty lifting eyes		13.189
35–36	Šamaš	postictal state	illness enters and leaves; confusional state with difficulty lifting eyes; cannot talk for 1 to 2 days		13.190
37	Šamaš	postictal state	illness enters and leaves; confusional state with hurting limbs		13.191
38–39	Šamaš	postictal state	illness enters and leaves; confusional state with difficulty lifting eyes; insides bloated; muscles in legs all hurt at once		13.191n
40	Ardat lilî	Gilles de la Tourette	illness enters and leaves; confusional state with frightful talk		13.265

ORGANIZING PRINCIPLE: USES PHRASE "PATIENT IS SICK"

41–42	*di'u*	enteric fever	during sickness talks with wife and family as if well but does not eat bread	recovery	3.22 3.162 6.50
43			illness falls on him; red blood sprays from mouth	death or recovery	
44–45			illness flows over him; lot of blood found in bed	3 days → death	
46		biphasic fever	illness returns; afflicting epigastrium	death	3.27n
47		reinfection	gets well; illness returns	no recovery	
48–49	[...]		gets well; diarrhea 3 to 4 days; gets no rest	5 to 6 days → [...]	3.113
50			stupor	prolonged	
51			body very cold	if prolonged, death	3.38
52–53			food will not stay in stomach; projectile vomiting	death	6.61
54–55		polio	illness of the hips; gets up and squats down; chest clear; mouth too strong for words; eyes stand still	death	13.90 13.217

56		polio	illness of hips and abdomen; gets up and squats down; hand open; mouth too strong for words	death	13.218 20.6
57–58		polio	illness of hips and abdomen; stops eating and drinking; mouth too strong for words; face swollen	death	6.50n 13.218n

ORGANIZING PRINCIPLE: USES PHRASE "AFTER FALLING ILL"

59	"trembler"		moistens lips while sleeping		15.14n 19.370n
60		fly test	vomits; flies will not go near vomit	death	6.12
61			gets up 1 to 2 days and walks about	if illness returns, death	
62			dreams of lovemaking; ejaculates in sleep	illness lets up	
63		mental status change	turns round from head end to foot end of bed and back again without realizing it	death	20.9
64	river hoist water	river toxins	bloated insides on leaving water		6.33n 15.32
65–66	river hoist water	river toxins	soles of feet cold; ear canals hot; nostrils feverish	31 days → death	15.31n

ORGANIZING PRINCIPLE: USES THE PHRASE "THE DAY HE BECOMES ILL"

67			continually pulls himself taut(?)	entrance of illness	
68			does not open mouth	entrance of illness	
69			continually opens mouth	entrance of illness	
70			continually opens eyes and mouth	illness falls on him	
71			continually lifts eyes	illness lets up	
72			continually lifts eyes and mouth/ tongue	illness lets up	
73		mental status change	does not recognize people he knows	death	3.112n 20.10

ORGANIZING PRINCIPLE: ALL DAY

74	*ṣētu*		sick all day; well at night		
75	*ṣētu* Ninurta		well all day; sick at night 27 days		
76			cold all day; hot all night	7 days → recovery	20.91

77	[...]		cold all day; chills; eyes full of red threads	[...]	3.39n 3.40n 9.17

ORGANIZING PRINCIPLE: NIGHT, MORNING, EVENING

78	Lilû	psychiatric problem	sick in the night; well in the morning; keeps her up all night		19.18n
79	Uraš		sick in the night; well in early morning		Ap.103
80	curse		illness afflicts him in the night; continually jerks		Ap.57
81	*rābiṣu*		illness afflicts him in the night		
82	*rābiṣu*		illness afflicts him in the evening		Ap.88n
83–85	ghost	nightmare	in the evening, sees someone living or dead, known or unknown, or anybody or anything and becomes afraid; turns around but unable to cry out to one sleeping next to him		16.19 19.32
86	Kūbu?		in the evening, continually wails		
87	Kūbu	leptospirosis?	in the evening, continually wails and will not drink milk		6.49n 19.340
88	Kūbu	leptospirosis?	before bed, shakes		19.340
89	Kūbu	leptospirosis?	wails and shakes		19.340
90	Sîn	encephalitis?	morning hot; evening cold; trembles		3.23n 19.261
91–92	Sîn	encephalitis?	morning hot; evening cold; middle of night says "wah"	brother dies too	2.12 19.261
93	Sîn	encephalitis?	morning hot; evening cold		19.261
94	Sîn	encephalitis?	morning hot; hands and feet tremble		3.23 19.261
95–99			sick in the morning; the late afternoon illness leaves and then suddenly returns; reduced form of illness the 2nd day until noon, the 3rd day till late afternoon, the 4th day until evening, the 5th day until its normal term, the 6th day until the middle of the first watch of the night, the 7th day until the middle watch of the night, the 8th day until the dawn watch, and the 9th day until it is light	if gets up on 10th day, recovery	20.92
100–105	*ṣētu* of 1 day		from morning until evening, *di'u* starts leading to illness of the stomach; on defecation, wind belches from mouth and emits wind from anus		3.164
	ṣētu going down and up		seems over but next morning, so sick hands thrash around; feet hot		3.164

DPS Tablet XVIII

ORGANIZING PRINCIPLE: FEVERS AND ACCOMPANYING SIGNS AND SYMPTOMS

1	Sîn	encephalitis?	body feverish	affliction worsens	
2	ghost or personal god		body feverish; no sweat		19.362n Ap.82
3–4	ghost	encephalitis?	body feverish; attacks numerous; confusional states close together; no rest; cry like goat		19.275dn
5–6	Ištar or Kūbu	benign fever	body burns with fever; hands and feet sore and sluggish, legs hurt; feet [. . .]		19.250 19.341
7	Lamaštu	typhoid?	body not feverish but a lot of sweat		19.231n
8–9	love-sickness		no fever; loss of appetite; short temper; excessive talking, upset stomach; same for a man and a woman		6.83n 16.24n
10–11	[. . .]	psychiatric problem	no fever; can eat and drink; blood vessels of head and abdomen healthy but says "my heart, my head"; withdraws from social intercourse		
12–14	no clue		no fever; blood vessels healthy but face flushes; [. . .]; wrinkles nose; wipes forehead		Ap.15
15–16	Ninurta		[. . .]; fever; eyes crossed; [. . .]		13.92n Ap.105
17–18	ghost		[. . .] cold; eyes crossed; [. . .]		13.92n 19.279
19	Ištar		[. . .]		
20	Ištar		[. . .]; white bile? mixed with yellow		
21	Šamaš		white *bubu'tu* from head to feet; body is dark; sexually transmitted	recovery	3.233n 4.18n 10.87n 19.106n
22	Sîn	HSV2	red *bubu'tu* from head to feet; body is dark; sexually transmitted	recovery	3.233n 4.18n 10.85n
23	Ištar		*bubu'tu* from head to feet; body is yellow; sexually transmitted	recovery	3.233n 4.18n 10.86n
24	*amurriqānu*	liver disease	body yellow; eyes yellow; wasting of the flesh		6.114dn 6.121
25–26		liver disease	[. . .]; eyes full of blood; diarrhea	will not last 3 days	6.61n 6.125n

27			[. . .] cold	death enters him	
28			[. . .] cold	illness worsens	
29	Ištar		[. . .]		
30	Ištar		[. . .]; same for a man and a woman	[. . .]	
31	scepter of Šamaš		[. . .]		
32′–34′	[. . .]		[. . .]	[. . .]	
35′	[. . .]		[. . .]	death	
36′	[. . .]		[. . .]	recovery	
37′	Lilû or personal god		[. . .]	death	
38′	Išḫara		[. . .] 31 days	if continually overwhelmed, no recovery	19.64n 19.290n 20.72
39′	*ṣētu*	enteric fever	[. . .]; afflicting head		3.125n
40′–41′		stones	stone in urethra; drinks beer	stone falls out	5.25n 5.34
			does not drink beer but water	death	
42′		liver disease	[flesh?] full of yellow spots; eyes full of blood; diarrhea	death	6.71n 6.125 20.57
43′	Ningeštinanna		[. . .] shakes		Ap.110
44′	Ningeštinanna		[. . .] shakes; palate dried up		3.105n Ap.110
45′			gets hot, then cold; [. . .]	recovery	

DPS Tablets XIX/XX

ORGANIZING PRINCIPLE: PATIENT HAS A FEVER

1′–4′	[. . .]		[. . .]	[. . .]	
5′	[. . .]		[. . .]; insides cramped; yellow spots on abdomen		10.50n
6′	[. . .]		[. . .]	[. . .]	
7′	[. . .]		[. . .]; asks for water to drink		
8′	Lamaštu		[. . .]; fever		
9′	Lamaštu or Sîn		[. . .]; asks for water to bathe in		19.231n 19.261n
10′	Lamaštu		[. . .]	recovery	
11′	Sîn	encephalitis?	[sick 1 to 2 days]; fever but no sweat; same for adults and children	recovery	19.263
12′	Sîn	encephalitis?	[. . .]; illness worsens; 5 days	[death]	19.262n

13′	Sîn	encephalitis?	[. . .]; illness worsens/mentation altered		19.264dn
14′	[. . .]		unintelligible words; 3 days		
15′	Ningirsu		[. . .]; eyes clouded; 12 days		9.2n 19.168
16′	[. . .]		[. . .]; eyes clouded; confusional state twice in 1 day		
17′	Ištar		[. . .]; gets up and sits down; 59 days		19.64n
18′	personal god		[. . .]; left side of abdomen hurts; [. . .]		19.36n
19′	personal goddess		[. . .]; right side of abdomen hurts; [. . .]		19.36n
20′	[. . .]		[. . .]	[. . .]	
21′	[. . .]		[. . .]; does not recognize people he knows; [. . .]		
22′	[. . .]		[. . .]; not in full possession of faculties; [. . .]		
23′	[. . .]		[. . .]; rubs his body; [. . .]		
24′	[. . .]		[. . .]; rubs left foot; [. . .]		
25′	[. . .]		[. . .]; chokes; "touched" at beginning of night	[. . .]	
26′	daughter of Anu		[. . .]; soles of feet cold		
27′	daughter of Anu		[. . .]; buttocks and hips cold		
28′	ghost		[. . .]; buttocks cold; [. . .]		
29′	Sîn	encephalitis?	[. . .]; hands and feet cold; [. . .]		3.39n 19.261n
30′–36′	Lamaštu		[. . .]		
37′	[. . .]		[. . .] look terrible; insides [. . .]		
38′	[. . .]		[. . .] insides cramped; yellow spots on chest and abdomen; gets up at night to [. . .]		10.50n
39′	[. . .]		[. . .] in the evening; affliction of feet [. . .]		
40′	[. . .]		[hot from armpit to hip region]; cold from hip region to feet; [. . .]		
41′	[. . .]		[. . .]; 1 day afflicts him; 1 day falls on him; [. . .] lot of bread and beer [. . .]		
42′	[. . .]		[. . .]; continually says greetings; [. . .] his garment [. . .]		
43′	[. . .]		[. . .]		
44′	[. . .]		[. . .]; forearms cold		
45′a	personal god		[. . .]	recovery	

45′b	Lamaštu	typhoid?	no apparent fever but left side of buttocks and ears cold		19.231n
46′	Lamaštu	typhoid?	[. . .]; hands and feet cold		19.231n
47′a	personal god		[. . .]		
47′b	[. . .]		[. . .]; 31 days		
48′	personal god or goddess		[. . .]; drinks water; water tastes good; illness falls on him		
49′	[. . .]		[. . .]; no fever; [drinks water]; water tastes good		
50′	[. . .]		[. . .]; [water] does not taste good; [. . .]		6.51n
51′	[. . .]		[. . .] bathes in water; makes him feel worse; stomach upset		
52′	personal god		[. . .]		
53′	personal god		[. . .] feel tied together; insides bloated		
54′–56′	[. . .]		[. . .]		
57′–62′	[. . .]		[. . .]		
63′–87′	[. . .]		[. . .]		
88′–93′		hemerology	ominous significance of fevers beginning each month		
94′–99′		hemerology	ominous significance of fevers beginning each day		
100′	a god		afflicting head or afflicting temple		16.5 19.35n 19.211n 19.363dn
101′–103′		medical omens			
104′–105′	[. . .]		[. . .]		
106′a	*ṣētu*	enteric fever	when afflicted, he asks for water		3.165n
106′b	[. . .]	alcoholism	when afflicted, he asks for beer		
107′a			when afflicted, can still excrete	recovery	5.37
107′b			when afflicted, can still urinate	recovery	5.37
108′a	a god		when afflicted, diarrhea		6.69n 19.363dn
108′b	personal god		when afflicted, vomiting	death	6.62n 19.363dn
109′a	personal god		when afflicted, slow pulse	death	8.53n 19.353dn 20.26
109′b	personal god		when afflicted, trembles	death	19.294n
110′–111′	Lamaštu		all day: afflicts him at sunrise, after the sun has gotten high, at noon, in the evening		3.25dn
112′–113a′	Lamaštu, messenger of Sîn		all night: afflicts him in the early evening watch, middle watch of the night, last watch of the night		3.25dn

113′b	Labaṣu		all day: afflicts him daily as above		3.29dn
114′	Sîn and Šamaš or father's god		sweat; bouts of fever		19.256n 19.270n
115'			[...]; illness falls on him; sweat dries out	prolonged	
116′			no sweat from head to feet	worrisome	
117′	*rābiṣu*		[...] afflicts him, flows over him, and pulls him taut	death	19.120
118′–124′	[...]		[...]		

DPS Tablet XXI

ORGANIZING PRINCIPLE: PATIENT HAS NO FEVER

1		kwashiorkor	blood vessels healthy but hair of head stands on end at ear	death	7.4n 10.189
2		kwashiorkor	blood vessels healthy but hair red; [no flesh] on forehead	death	7.9n
3	[...]	annular posterior synechia	blood vessels healthy but grapes of eyes pulled taut	[...]	9.74
4	[...]		blood vessels healthy but mouth twitches	[...]	
5	[...]		blood vessels healthy but bleeding from nose/mouth; [...]	[...]	
6–7	Ninurta		blood vessels healthy but bleeding from nose/mouth does not stop day or night	if lets up, recovery	20.48 Ap.106
8	[...]		blood vessels healthy but bleeding from nose/mouth day and night; [...]	[...]	
9	[...]		blood vessels healthy but bleeding from nose/mouth day and night; [...]	[...]	
10	[...]		blood vessels healthy but teeth dusky	[...]	18.20n
11	[...]		blood vessels healthy and teeth shine	[...]	18.21n
12	[...]		blood vessels healthy but excretes black bile	[...]	
13	[...]		[blood vessels healthy] but [face full of black] *ramīṭu*-lesions	[death]	10.164n
14	[...]		blood vessels healthy but face yellow	[...]	
15	[...]		[blood vessels] healthy and face flushes	[...]	Ap.15
16	[...]		blood vessels healthy but vertebra was cut open	[death]	13.143
17	[...]		blood vessels healthy but hands and feet paralyzed	[...]	

18			blood vessels healthy but feet swollen	death	8.25n
19			blood vessels healthy but testicles twisted	death	5.83
20		fly test	blood vessels healthy but vomits blood from anus; flies will not go near vomit	[death]	6.12n
21	[...]		blood vessels healthy but illness draws him taut	[...]	
22			blood vessels healthy but diarrhea	[death]	6.71n 20.78
23			blood vessels healthy and he can eat bread and fat and drink beer	[recovery]	

DPS Tablet XXII

1	hand of mankind	lungs?	groans in the morning and drinks a lot of water; *li'bu* afflicts him		3.83n Ap.74
2–3	hand of mankind	heart?	limpness; afflicting epigastrium; sluggishness		19.122
4	hand of mankind	lungs?	asks for things but won't eat them; *guḫḫu*-cough; fever		3.83n Ap.75
5	*kišpu*	Parkinson's	scanning speech		13.85n 13.263n
6–7	love-sickness		flutters about; insolent; talks to himself; laughs for no reason; same for a man and a woman		16.23
8–9	love-sickness	depression	short temper; food does not agree with him; says "oh my heart"		6.83 16.24
10–11	disease of intercourse		muscles of abdomen hurt; right temple hurts intensely; continually stiff/rigid; cannot eat; body hot; wasting away of flesh		2.18n Ap.17
12–13	disease of intercourse	hepatitis B	burning pain in epigastrium; fever; epigastrium; food does not agree with him; water does not taste good; body yellow		2.18n 4.35 6.51n 6.128dn 13.27 Ap.17dn
14–15	disease of intercourse or Ištar	Fitz-Hugh Curtis syndrome	burning fever in penis and epigastrum; liver hurts; stomach goes crazy; arms, feet and stomach hot		2.18 3.8n 4.34 6.74n 19.347dn 19.378 Ap.17dn
16	curse	liver disease	spittle flows in talking, *aḫḫāzu*-jaundice fills face; diarrhea	death	19.312
17	curse		continually says greetings		Ap.55

18			continually says greetings; gets well and then sick again	death	Ap.55n
19–20	curse	liver disease	nystagmus; insides bloated; rims of eyes swollen; soles of feet swollen; bleeding from right nostril	death	6.141n 13.113n 19.313 20.49
21	curse		sometimes hot and sometimes cold; yellow spots; white as whitewash and dark as smoke	death	10.50n Ap.61
22–23	curse	Hansen's disease	flesh thickens and not through eating; smell of garlic/*saḫlû* bothers him; tips of fingers and toes appear to dissolve		3.214
24	curse or dirty substances		afflicts him day and night		2.20n Ap.77
25	curse	pneumonia	fever; stomach nauseous; *guḫḫu*-cough; dark, thick sputum		3.79 3.85d 8.69n
26–27	curse	pneumonia	fever; no rest; deep breathing; *su'ālu*-cough; stomach nauseous to point of vomiting		3.80 6.54 8.66
28	curse or wrongdoing	pneumonia	breast and back hurt him; dark, thick sputum; stomach nauseous		3.81n 3.89n 19.309n
29–30	curse or wrongdoing	pneumonia	abdomen hot; *guḫḫu*-cough after eating; epigastrium and shoulders hurt him; *su'ālu*–coughs; breathes deeply; sprays saliva		3.81n 3.88n 8.69n 19.309
31–32	curse	pneumonia	gnawing pain in epigastrium; fever grips stomach; temperature lukewarm; produces dark phlegm and continually vomits		3.4 3.81 3.85d 19.309n
33	*li'bu*-fever		epigastrium dried out and hurts; temperature lukewarm; urinates blood	illness lets up	3.4n 5.19n
34–35	Marduk	viral hemorrhagic fever	limbs supple; needling pain in epigastrium; incessant bleeding from nose; arms weak; depressed; eyes suffused with blood	worries and dies	3.238 9.24 19.235n
36–37	Marduk	viral hemorrhagic fever	limbs supple; temporal blood vessels collapsed; throat looks skinned; insides cramped; sick day and night	worries and dies	3.238 19.235n
38	wound from behind	wound	limbs limp; excretes blood	death	13.51 13.137
39a	Ištar	arthritis	limbs hurt	recovery	11.52n

39b	death demon	neck wound	twists; vomits blood	death	
40	*rābiṣu* of the road	chorea	twists; continually asks for water and beer		19.82dn
41			frequent changes of mood; withdraws from social intercourse; continually falls down	death	
42a			frequent changes of mood; asks for lots of food	no recovery	
42b			arranges affairs	recovery	
			illness worsens and "touches" him	death	
43		premonition of death	arranges affairs; asks for last meal and eats it	death	20.105
44	Šulpaea	chorea	tears his garment; limbs twist		13.258
45	Šulpaea	chorea	tears his garment; limbs raised up		13.74 13.258
46	twin gods	mental status change	takes off and puts on garments	death	16.57 19.238n
47a	ghost	mental status change	mentation altered; not in full possession of faculties	death	16.35 19.33 19.281 20.5
47b	a god		mentation continually altered		16.34 19.38dn
48			mentation altered; tongue roves about	death	16.40 19.281
49–50	wind from behind		mentation altered; words unintelligible; forgets what he says	death alone like a stranger	13.252 20.7
51–52	ghost or Ardat lilî or Lilû		mentation altered; scanning speech		16.36 19.22 19.34n 19.282
53–54	ghost or Lilû		mentation altered; [. . .]; scanning speech		16.37 19.34 19.282n
55a	Šamaš	loses his mind	mentation continually alters		16.38 19.1
55b			loses consciousness; [. . .]	death	
56		mental status change	does not recognize people he knows; words unintelligible	death	16.42
57		mental status change	wanders about; does things slowly; falls down	death	16.50 20.74
58	oath by a god		groans; fever rides him/cries out	death	19.291
59	ghost deputy of Ea		cries out; feverish		19.242
60			cries out as loud as he can; 1 to 2 days; crying gets softer	death	20.59

61			brays; hands and bottoms of feet cold	death	3.39n
62	*Mukīl rēš lemutti* or Ištar		continually laughs	death	16.74 19.7 19.63
63	*Mukīl rēš lemutti* or Ištar		rejoices and is terrified	death	16.75 19.9 19.63
64a	*Mukīl rēš lemutti*		feels harassed	death	19.63
64b		polio	gets up and squats down; hand stretched out	death	13.218n 20.71
65			gets up and shakes hands	if he dies, will be another patient after him	2.16
66			gets up too quickly	if prolonged, death	20.76
67	touch of *di'u*	enteric fever	lies down and becomes rigid		3.158
68			passes out frequently; stomach upset; scalp hair stands on end	death in the night	19.59n Ap.38
69–70		cold weather	mighty illness; gets better but feet cramped; goes into winter; cold falls on him	no recovery	2.8 20.77
71–72		cold weather	mighty illness; loss of appetite; lungs sing like reed flute; fever daily in winter	death	6.53n 8.98
73		weakness	exhausted and shakes or falls in a heap	death	20.73
74a		sleep	curled up	recovery or death	
		sleep	lying flat	death	
74b–75a		sleep	powerless	death	
		sleep	tossing and turning	recovery	
75b		sleep	falls out of bed or snores	recovery	
76		mentally alert	asks questions and answers them	recovery	20.12n
77			[. . .]; feels better and belches	illness diminishes	
78		Words of Wisdom	If they have a long history of sinning against the god[s of the city], they (the gods) will leave.		

DPS Tablet XXIII

ORGANIZING PRINCIPLE: INTO AND OUT OF THE MOUTH

1	father's god	enteric fever	vomits bile; burns with *ṣētu*		3.133 19.222n

2	curse		continual vomiting		6.29n 19.315n
3	[curse]		[vomits]; rolls to left and gets up; [...]		6.29n
4	ghost	wound	[vomits?]; wounded on left or right side	[death]	19.170
5		fly test	[vomits]; flies will not go near vomit	death	6.12n
6	[...]		[spittle] flows; eyes dilated/roll	[...]	13.95n 13.118n
7	[...]		[...]; [blood] flows; face/flesh dark; [...]	[...]	
8		wound	wound to right temple; [blood] continually flows	death	
9			[...]; produces red blood from nose/mouth	death	
10			[...]; produces dark blood from nose/mouth	death	
11	personal god		[...]; body hot	32 days → death	19.362n
12	[...]		[...] afflicts him	[...]	
13–14′	[...]		[...]	[...]	
15′	[...]		[...]; asks for lots of water	[...]	
16′	personal god		[...]; asks for lots of water and drinks it	[...]	19.362n
17′	[...]		withdrawn; asks for lots of water/ groans; [...]	[...]	
18′			milk tastes good	prolonged; worrisome	Ap.51
19′	[...]		patient asks for an apple; [...]	[...]	

DPS Tablet XXVI

ORGANIZING PRINCIPLE: GENERAL DISCUSSION OF SEIZURES

1′	[...]		[...]	[...]	
2′	[...]		[...]	[...]	
3′	Ardat lilî	complex partial seizure	face flushes and turns pale		19.58
4′	spinning *bennu*	complex partial seizure	aura	comes through	3.269 13.202
5′	AN.TA.ŠUB.BA	grand mal seizure	generalized flushing and pallor; 2 or 3 times a day		13.188 19.57
6′		grand mal seizure	2 or 3 times a day; generalized pallor grows out of the falling spell		13.187
7′		status epilepticus	7 in one day; comes through	8 → does not come through	13.207
8′		brain tumor	for a year; closely spaced in middle of day	difficult	13.224 20.13

9′–10′	ghost	status epilepticus	7 very closely spaced; feels better afterward	death	13.209
11′–13′	ghost	complex partial seizures with status epilepticus	opens and closes his eyes; jaws shake;hands and feet stretched out; can see one who afflicts him	death	9.34n 13.81 13.204
14′	Lilû	gelastic seizure	generalized pallor; laughing; hands and feet contorted		13.206 19.56

ORGANIZING PRINCIPLE: CONFUSIONAL STATE

15′	AN.TA.ŠUB.BA	grand mal seizure	confusional state; spittle flows		13.171
16′	AN.TA.ŠUB.BA	grand mal seizure	confusional state; bends hands and feet toward neck		13.172
17′	father's vow		confusional state; depression; spittle flows	death	Ap.63
18′	Lilû	grand mal seizure	confusional state; spittle flows		13.171n
19′	ghost	cholera	confusional state; wasting; afflicting abdomen; diarrhea		3.101 3.116 19.296
20′–21′	ghost	cholera	confusional state; numb limbs; dizziness; wasting; extreme diarrhea		3.111 19.296
22′–25′	infectious Lilû	neurosyphilis?	confusional state; aura of numb limbs; "wind-blasted" eyes; face flushes; racing pulse; groans; tips of fingers and toes cold; patient can repeat things but does not remember what he said afterward		4.29 13.290
26′–27′	AN.TA.ŠUB.BA	complex partial seizure	confusional state; aura of heaviness and stinging in torso	in middle of day, difficult	13.201
28′–29′	falling spell of Ištar	pseudo-seizure	confusional state; headache; chest pain; rubbing of limbs; rolls over and over; no spit		13.42 16.66 19.14
30′	Lilû or Lilītu	pseudo-seizure?	confusional state; gazing at hands; rolls whites of eyes; blood runs from nose		13.118n 19.21

ORGANIZING PRINCIPLE: COMPLEX PARTIAL SEIZURES VERSUS ENCEPHALITIS, NEUROTOXINS, PSEUDO-SEIZURES, ALCOHOLIC CONFUSIONAL STATE; NEUROSYPHILIS

31′	ghost	encephalitis?	worse in the evening		0.2 19.273
32′	ghost	encephalitis?	worse in the evening; bloating; curled up in a ball		0.2 6.33n 19.273
33′	ghost	encephalitis?	worse in the evening; bloating; difficulty getting to sleep		0.2 6.33n 19.273

34′	ghost	encephalitis?	worse in the evening; eyes clouded; ears roar		0.2 19.273
35′	ghost	encephalitis?	worse in the evening; ears roar		0.2 19.273
36′	ghost	encephalitis?	worse in the evening; ears numb		0.2 19.273
37′	ghost	encephalitis?	worse in the evening; temples hurt		0.2 19.273
38′	ghost	encephalitis?	worse in the evening; fever keeps him up at night		0.2; 3.9 19.273
39′	Ardat lilî	complex partial seizure	worse in the evening; aura		13.203 19.55
40′	Ardat lilî	complex partial seizure	face flushes and turns pale		19.58n
41′	Lilû	complex partial seizure	hands and feet turn pale		19.58n
42′	*rābiṣu* of the river or drowned ghost	river toxins	rubs hands and face	in middle of day, difficult	15.28n 19.46
43′–44′	"binder"	complex partial seizure	closely spaced; wrings hands as if cold; stretches out feet; jerks, then quiet; gazes at one who afflicts him		13.69 13.199
45′–47′	Ardat lilî or Lilû or Lilītu	complex partial seizure	in the middle of the night; hands and feet cold; passes out; continually opens mouth, face flushes and turns pale; no pelvic thrusting	if prolonged, death	3.39n 19.59
48′–49′	false Lilû	pseudo-seizure	in bed; he gazes at the one who afflicts him, loses consciousness, shudders like one awakened/groggy; can get up afterward		12.71 13.73 16.51 19.19
50′	ghost	hypoglycemia	in late afternoon; temperature not very high but sweat presses down on temples and eyes; abdomen hurts		13.3n 15.17
51′–52′	ghost	complex partial seizure with status epilepticus	visual aura; neck muscles hurt; chest [. . .]; continual falling spells	death	13.205
53′–55′	infectious Lilû	neurosyphilis?	aura?; hands and feet immobilized; limbs twist; [. . .]	[. . .]	4.31

ORGANIZING PRINCIPLE: GRAND MAL SEIZURES VERSUS CHOREA, SEIZURES IN CARDIAC ARREST, ETC.

56′–57′	[. . .]		[. . .]	[. . .]	
58′	[. . .]	chorea	[. . .] jump; hands and feet [. . .]	[. . .]	
59′–60′	[. . .]		[. . .]	[. . .]	

61′	ghost		[. . .] hurts him so badly he cannot sleep		
62′–63′	AN.TA.ŠUB.BA	grand mal seizure	afflicts him as he is sitting; eye flutters; lips come apart; spittle flows; hand, foot, and right side of torso thrash around like a slaughtered sheep; if during affliction heart is awake	can be removed	8.4 13.114n 13.185n
		seizure due to cardiac arrest	heart is not awake	cannot be removed	

ORGANIZING PRINCIPLE: LILÛ

64′–65′	Lilû		cries out "my insides, my insides!"; opens and shuts eyes; has *li'bu*-fever; rubs bulb of nose; tips of fingers and toes cold; does not answer questions		19.25
66′–68′	infectious Lilû		cries out "my insides, my insides!"; opens and shuts eyes; has *li'bu*-fever; rubs bulb of nose; tips of fingers and toes cold; can see the illness that afflicts him; talks with it and answers himself as if he were another person		16.92 19.24

ORGANIZING PRINCIPLE: TYPES OF SEIZURES AND ATTENDANT SIGNS AND SYMPTOMS

69′–70′	AN.TA.ŠUB.BA	grand mal seizure	stupor flows over him; fingers and toes thrash around; afflicted in an abandoned place or in a corner		13.186 13.275n 13.198dn
71′	AN.TA.ŠUB.BA	simple partial seizure	limbs tremble and twist; dizzy	in middle of day, difficult	13.198 20.14
72′	AN.TA.ŠUB.BA	simple partial seizure	limbs go numb and sting; dizzy	in middle of day, difficult	13.198
73′–74′	Lilû	psychiatric problem	limbs still; opens eyes and when he sees the one who afflicts him, talks with him and answers himself as if he were another person		16.69 16.90 19.23
75′	ghost	psychiatric problem	limbs still but cannot talk		16.46 19.31
76′	ghost	psychiatric problem	limbs still but silent and does not take any food		16.22 16.47 19.31n
77′	AN.TA.ŠUB.BA	focal seizure	cries out "Oh woe!"; groans; spittle flows; neck twisted to right		13.192 13.198dn

ORGANIZING PRINCIPLE: COMA AND ATTENDANT SIGNS AND SYMPTOMS

78′–79′	Ištar	psychiatric problem	puts on and throws off garments; cries out; talks a lot; not vomiting so can eat; cannot sleep	recovery	16.56 16.88 19.6
80′		coma	makes motions of putting on and throwing off clothing; pupils constrict	death	13.94n 13.276
81′		coma	continually trembles; pupils constrict	death	13.94n 13.277

ORGANIZING PRINCIPLE: SHUDDERING

82′–83′	Lilû or Lilītu	pseudo-seizure	shudders but can get up afterward; talks a lot; jerks; can get up afterward		12.72 16.44 19.20
84′	*bennu*	cysticercosis?	shudders/jerks in his bed and raises his pelvis; Ardat lilî "touches" him		3.273
85′	Ištar of Arbela		shudders		19.15n 19.373dn

ORGANIZING PRINCIPLE: NARCOLEPSY AND ATTENDANT SIGNS AND SYMPTOMS

86′–87′	*muttillu*		hears mournful cry and answers it with: "Who are you?"	death	16.71
88′	*rābiṣu* of the wastes	narcolepsy	hears mournful cry and answers it; gets up and squats down		13.211n 16.72 19.61n
89′–90′	roving *rābiṣu*	narcolepsy	hears mournful cry and answers it; behaves like trapped animal; gets up and feels exhausted; gets up and squats down	comes through	13.211 16.72 19.61 19.62d

DPS Tablet XXVII

ORGANIZING PRINCIPLE: STROKE

1		stroke	stroke affects face; torso goes numb; is result of the stroke		13.241
2–3		stroke	has stroke; gets better but frontal headache and shuddering; is lingering effect of stroke		13.231
4		stroke	has stroke; frontal headache; visual hallucinations	death	16.70
5–7	ghost	transient ischemic attack	has stroke; left or right side affected; shoulder not released but can straighten out fingers and can lift hand and stretch it out; can bend his foot and stretch it out again;	recovery in 3 days	13.227 13.285

8		stroke	can eat and drink difficult for him to bend hand or foot; has had stroke	recovery	13.239
9	stroke of a *rābiṣu*	stroke	left side tense	recovery	13.228
10	stroke of a *rābiṣu* or wound from behind	stroke or wound similating stroke	left side of body tense		13.126 13.228n 19.196
11	Šulak	stroke	right side tense		13.229
12–13	Šulak or wound from in front	stroke or wound simulating stroke	right side of body tense	recovery not predicted	13.125 13.229n 19.195

ORGANIZING PRINCIPLE: *GALLÛ* (CATAPLEXY INCLUDED)

14–15	*gallû*	hemophilia	appearance worsens; eyes disconnected from one another; rubs lips and chin; they cannot stop the blood that flows from his nose/mouth	19.177
16–17	*gallû*	cataplexy	walking along and falls down; opens eyes wide and does not know how to turn them back; cannot move hands and feet by himself; flows over him like a seizure (AN.TA.ŠUB.BA)	13.117n 13.212
18	*gallû*	cataplexy	something like a seizure (AN.TA.ŠUB.BA) flows over him; cannot move his hands and feet by himself	13.213
19	*gallû*	psychiatric problem	sees; throws off garment; wanders about and strikes his eyes	16.77 19.26

ORGANIZING PRINCIPLE: *ALÛ* (COMA)

20	*alû*	coma	drags his [. . .]; fever; does not know who he is; when you recite a recitation over him, constricts pupils	13.94n 13.277n
21–22	*alû*	coma	something like a stupor afflicts him; limbs tense; ears roar; cannot talk	13.59 13.273
23	*alû*	coma	something like a stupor afflicts him; ears roar; cannot talk	13.274 19.306

ORGANIZING PRINCIPLE: *RĀBIṢU* OF THE RIVER (NEUROTOXINS)

24	*rābiṣu* of the river	river toxins	when bathing, when coming up from the river, dizzy and falls down	15.27 19.45n

25	*rābiṣu* of the river	river toxins	when coming up from the water, body paralyzed; dizzy and falls down	13.41 15.28 19.45

ORGANIZING PRINCIPLE: GHOST (CONFUSIONAL STATES; ALCOHOLIC WITHDRAWAL SEIZURES)

26	ghost	confusional state of cholera	powerless and dazed	3.102
27–28	ghost	cholera	keeps asking for more and more water; no fever; blood vessels of hands "go"; groans from beginning to middle of night	3.3n 3.102 8.50 19.296n
29–31	ghost	hypoglycemia	worried; makes frequent supplication; limbs hot; sweats every day; big appetite at unpredictable times; until they bring him what he wants, vomits but when they bring it to him, looks at it and does not eat it	15.16
32–34	ghost	delirium tremens	headband seems to sting; ears roar; hair of head stands on end; whole body crawls as if there were lice but nothing there; may also bend and stretch out feet as in the scepter of Sîn	10.186 15.18 16.68
35–36	ghost	alcoholic withdrawal seizures	scepter of Sîn placed on him; bends and stretches out foot; drones; saliva flows from mouth	15.19

DPS Tablet XXVIII

ORGANIZING PRINCIPLE: PROGRESSION IN SEIZURE DISORDERS

1–3	city god	aura followed by seizure	ghost → AN.TA.ŠUB.BA	treatable	19.65 19.353dn
4–6	*rābiṣu*	cataplexy followed by narcolepsy	AN.TA.ŠUB.BA → ghost plus *Mukīl reš lemutti*, Ištar, and *rābiṣu*	treatable	19.60 19.63d 19.64d
7–10	city god or goddess	seizures followed by prostration	AN.TA.ŠUB.BA → Ištar	treatable	19.68 19.353dn
11–13	Sîn or Ištar	prostration followed by generalized seizures (= encephalitis or meningitis)	Ištar → AN.TA.ŠUB.BA	treatable	19.71 19.267

14–16	Šamaš	prostration followed by focal seizures (= encephalitis)	Ištar → Lugalurra	treatable	19.72 19.268
17–18	Ištar	focal seizures progress to generalized seizures followed by prostration	Lugalurra → AN.TA.ŠUB.BA → Ištar	treatable	19.69
19	city god	focal seizures progress to generalized seizures	Lugalurra or spawn of Šulpaea → AN.TA.ŠUB.BA	treatable	19.66 19.353dn
20		Huntington's chorea	Lugalurra → Ištar or spawn of Šulpaea → ghost	does not do well	19.62 19.65dn 19.70
21		brain tumor	inappropriate emotions; paralysis of upward gaze	does not do well	13.225
22–32		medical dream omens	stag, gazelle, ox, donkey, wild boar good; other animals bad		
33			turns into "hand" of god	recovery	
34			turns into "hand" of Ištar	recovery	19.17
35–43		medical dream omens	people, forests, canebrakes, and gardens good; rivers and mountains bad		

DPS Tablet XXIX

ORGANIZING PRINCIPLE: LUGALURRA AT VARIOUS AGES

1–3	Lugalurra	Huntington's disease; Wesphal variant	from moment of birth; wails, twists, and continually rigid	bad omen	13.261
4–5	Lugalurra	focal seizures	begin in 3rd year	potentially fatal but treated	19.73
6–7	Lugalurra	focal seizures	begin in 7th year	potentially fatal but treated	19.73
8–10	Lugalurra	focal seizures	begin in 10th year	survival; treated	19.74
11–12	Lugalurra	focal seizures	begin in [15th] year	survival; treated	19.74n
13–14	[Lugalurra]		[. . .]	[. . .]	

15–17	Lugalurra	focal seizures	begin in 20th year	survival; treated	19.74 20.4
18–19	Lugalurra	focal seizures	begin in 30th year	bad omen; treated	19.75
20	Lugalurra	focal seizures	begin in 50th year	bad omen; does not do well	19.75
21	Lugalurra of *bennu*	cysticercosis?	[. . .]	[. . .]	3.269n

ORGANIZING PRINCIPLE: SPAWN OF ŠULPAEA AT VARIOUS AGES

22–24	spawn of Šulpaea	floppy baby syndrome	from moment of birth; does not wail, cry, or stiffen up	bad omen	13.247
25–28	spawn of Šulpaea	Werndig-Hoffman	begins in 3rd year	potentially fatal but treated	13.248 20.1
29	spawn of Šulpaea	Werndig-Hoffman	begins in 7th year	survival; treated	13.249
30–33	spawn of Šulpaea	Werndig-Hoffman	begins in 10th year	survival; treated	13.250
34	spawn of Šulpaea	Werndig-Hoffman	begins in [. . .] year	survival; treated	
35′–48′	[. . .]		[. . .]	[. . .]	

ORGANIZING PRINCIPLE: LOCATION/TIME OF DAY OF SEIZURE

49′–51′	Sîn or Nergal		falls on him in/while [. . .]		
52′–54′	[. . .]		falls on him while sleeping		
55′–59′	[. . .]		[. . .]		
60′–61′	[Namtar]		falls on him in the evening		
62′	[. . .]		falls on him in the morning		
63′–64′	[quay of Šamaš]		seizure while on a journey	potentially fatal but treated	19.76
65′–66′	city god		falls on him on way down to river	potentially fatal but treated	19.78
67′–69′	Marduk or [. . .]		falls on him while going about where he pleases	[. . .]	19.77

70′		label			
71′–80′	[. . .]		[. . .]	[. . .]	

ORGANIZING PRINCIPLE: DEPUTIES

81′–82′	"trembler"		[. . .]		
83′–84′		recitation			
85′–86′	Šulak		[. . .]		
87′ (catch-line)	["weakener," *šedû* of Anu]		sick; continually opens mouth; [hands and feet powerless]		

DPS Tablet XXX

ORGANIZING PRINCIPLE: DEPUTIES

1–8	"weakener," *šedû* of Anu		sick; continually opens mouth; hands and feet powerless		19.370
9–13	Zaqīqu, *šedû* of Enlil		sick; lightning bolt looks altered and has no whiteness		19.371
14–20	"stiff," *šedû* of Ea		sick; lot of sweat as in *labaṣu*; chills		19.372

DPS Tablet XXXI

ORGANIZING PRINCIPLE: *ṢĒTU* (ENTERIC FEVER)

1–2	3rd day	enteric fever	the day you see him, chills	treated	3.126n 3.144
3–5	7th day	enteric fever	the day you see him, blood flows from nose	treated	3.138n 3.146
6–8	14th day	enteric fever	head throbs; knocked down; burning fever	treated	3.122n 3.147
9–11	25th day	enteric fever	the day you see him, blood flows from mouth	treated	3.139n 3.151n
12–14	1 month along	enteric fever	sometimes hot, sometimes cold; *li'bu*-fever but no sweat	treated	3.18 3.122n 3.152
15	14th day	enteric fever	the day you see him [. . .]	treated	3.147n
16′–18′	[. . .]	enteric fever	[. . .]	treated	
19′–22′	persistent	enteric fever	great deal of sweat; drips sweat like water	treated	3.122

23′–24′	[*x*]th day	enteric fever	a lot of sweat	treated	3.122n
25′–27′	21st day	enteric fever	face very red like one who drinks beer; [. . .]	treated	3.149
28′–31′	[*x*]th day	enteric fever	*bubu'tu*-vesicles like those of *ašû*	treated	3.122n 10.79n
32′–34′	[*x*]th day	enteric fever	skin reddish and he scratches	treated	3.128
35′–39′	21st day	enteric fever	daily, at the expected time, comes over him and leaves him; burning fever; muscles hurt; sweat, then relief	treated	3.8n 3.123n 3.148 13.173n
40′	[. . .]	enteric fever	[. . .]	treated	
41′–42′	[. . .]	enteric fever	[. . .]	treated	
43′–45′	52nd day	enteric fever	[. . .]; a lot of trembling	treated	3.156
46′–49′	44th day	enteric fever	nausea; food cravings but [cannot eat]	treated	3.133n 3.154 6.59n
50′–51′	21st day	enteric fever	groans all day and all night	treated	3.150
52′–56′	1 month along	enteric fever	groans all day and all night; cannot sleep; nauseous but can eat fruit and drink water	treated	3.133n 3.153 6.59
57′	[. . .]		"wind blasting"; he is very hot; [. . .]	[. . .]	10.17n

DPS Tablet XXXIII

ORGANIZING PRINCIPLE: SKIN LESIONS IN CROPS

1	*ašû*	measles or chickenpox etc.	clustered	10.89
2	*ašû*		clustered; skin reddish; itches; contains fluid	10.90
3	*ašû*		clustered; fluid sticky; skin reddish; gets scratched until it bleeds	10.91
4	*ašû*		swollen face and eyes; difficulty seeing; red eyes	9.31 10.96
5	*ašû*		swollen face; difficulty seeing; body full of *birdu*-lesions; afflicting abdomen	10.92
6	fleeting *ašû*		body full of louse bitelike lesions	2.23n 10.101
7	*kullaru*		body full of dark spots	10.64
8	*kullaru*		dark and dry; skin reddish; itches	10.65
9	*kullaru* of *ašû*		stiff; surrounded by clusters; [. . .]	10.94

10	*ekketu*	"scratchies"	clustered; goes round the hips		10.34
11	*rišiktu*	"dry patches"	fish scales; predictable course		10.2 10.10dn

ORGANIZING PRINCIPLE: PIGMENTED SKIN LESIONS

12	*rišûtu*	"redness"	hot; [. . .]		10.10
13	*girgišu*	"strawberry"	hot; no fluid; [. . .]		10.142
14	*bubuʾtu*	vesicle	hot; fluid		4.11 10.77
15	*išītu*		hot; no fluid; contains lots of little *bubuʾtu*		10.173
16	*nipištu*		hot; full of clusters; redness		10.181
17	*nipištu*		clustered; swelling blocks its exit		10.182
18	*ruṭibtu*	"dampness"	clustered; itches; fluid flows from [. . .]		10.5
19	*ruṭibtu*	"dampness"	red or white; hurts; contains fluid		10.6
20	*ḫarasu*	onchocerciasis	black		3.280 10.74
21	*ḫarasu*	onchocerciasis	body full of *birdu*-lesions; stinging and redness		3.281 10.75
22	*ruṭibtu*	tinea	on foot or testicle; skin reddish; itches		3.257 10.7
23	*samānu*	soft tissue infection	red; hot; swollen; flows		3.172
24	*samānu*	soft tissue infection	red; patient has fever and vomits		3.173
25	*midru/ samānu*	soft tissue infection	hard; burns; [. . .]; unresponsive		3.192
26	"wind blasting"		like a *bubuʾtu*; body full of them		4.12 10.17 10.80n
27	*pindû*		red; granular		10.126
28	*šadānu*	swollen lymph nodes	like obsidian; goes around the neck		3.228
29	*šadānu*	plague	hard; patient has a red rash		3.229
30	*šadānu*, Marduk, and Ninurta	plague	hard; patient burns with fever; speen enlarged; loss of appetite		3.8n 3.225
31	*šadānu*, Marduk, and Ninurta	plague	hard; under the surface of the skin; makes it difficult for him to move his legs		3.226 19.100 19.114
32		plague	hard; in neck or armpit or groin	3 days → death	3.227
33	[. . .]	bleeding wound			14.21
34	[. . .]	scorpion sting?	in evening; produces numbness		Ap.16
35	[. . .]	scorpion sting?	mysterious origin; stings		

36	*epqēnu*		[. . .]		
37	[. . .]		[. . .]; divided		
38	*kirbānu*	lumpy jaw	surrounded by "silt"; afflicts the neck		3.240 10.146
39	*kirbānu*	lumpy jaw	hard; on the surface; hot		3.240 10.146
40	*ziqtu*	whitehead	compact; tip deeply incised		10.108
41	*ziqtu*	whitehead	*ibāru*-like; tip dotted white		10.108
42	*ziqtu*	whitehead	red, white, small; hurts		10.108
43–44	[. . .]		[. . .]		

ORGANIZING PRINCIPLE: DIFFICULT SKIN LESIONS

45	[. . .]		red; hurts; puffed up; hot		
46	[. . .]		hurts; goes away; [. . .]		
47	*abābu*?		does not hurt; [. . .]		10.184fn
48	*abābu*?		does not hurt; [. . .]		10.184fn
49	[. . .]		does not hurt; flows or keeps coming back		
50	[. . .]		infected wound: serous fluid flows; persistent		3.178
51	[. . .]		[. . .]		
52	*abiktu*		hurts day and night		10.184fn
53	*miqtu*		like [. . .]; puffed up; hot	simple enough for *asû* to treat	10.44n
54	*miqtu*		[. . .]; swelling goes down but still has liquid	simple enough for *asû* to treat	10.44n
55	Bau		[. . .]; swelling goes down but does not recover; [. . .]		
56	*gallû*	infected wound	like a growth; coated; coating dotted with black		3.176
57	[. . .]	infected wound	[. . .] contains pus		
58	*šaḫšaḫḫu*	infected wound	red or white; produces pus; [. . .]		3.177
59	*ni-lu-gu*$_4$	guinea worm track	red or white; hurts; no fluid; gets bigger		3.276 10.69pn
60	*ni-lu-gu*$_4$	guinea worm track	gets bigger; what eventually comes out is a *guzallu*		3.278
61	*ni-lu-gu*$_4$	guinea worm	comes up to the thighs; [. . .] what eventually comes out is a *guzallu*		3.275n
62	[. . .]		accompanies pneumonia		
63	*sikkatu*		has a red [. . .]		
64	*sagbānu*		its [. . .] is linked; dark		10.104n
65–66	*ṣinnaḫ tiri*	diarrhea	with fever and [. . .]		

67–68	*ṣiriptu*	"bright red"	has fluid and flows; [. . .]	10.60n
69–70	[. . .]		[. . .]	
71–74	[. . .]		[. . .]	

ORGANIZING PRINCIPLE: SKIN LESIONS PART OF SYNDROMES CAUSED BY GODS

75–79	[. . .]		[. . .]	
80	Sîn	HSV2	red *bubuʾtu* from head to foot; body is white/whitish	3.233n 4.18n 10.85n
81	Ea		[. . .] on the middle of the cheek	19.245
82	[. . .]		[. . .] on the throat and middle of [. . .]	
83	Išḫara		[. . .] on epigastrium; appearance worsens	19.290
84	personal goddess		[. . .] on inguinal region and base of testicle; appearance worsens	19.348n
85	[. . .]		[. . .] and a black hair grows out of it	10.125
86	[. . .]		[. . .] and a white hair grows out of it	10.125

ORGANIZING PRINCIPLE: SKIN LESIONS/SKIN COLOR CHANGES PART OF THE NAMED SYNDROMES

87	*buʾšānu*		mouth full of *bubuʾtu*; saliva flows	3.64 4.17 10.81 18.47
88	*buʾšānu*		infant's spittle contains blood	17.157
89	*buʾšānu*		infant's insides cramped; mouth feels heavy	17.157
90	*buʾšānu*		infant's skull, breast, and back feverish	17.157
91	*buʾšānu*		infant has lukewarm temperature; insides cramped	3.4n 17.157
92	*amurriqānu*	liver disease	body yellow; face yellow; eyes yellow; wasting of the flesh	6.121
93	*aḫḫazu*	liver disease	face and eyes yellow; base of tongue black	6.117

ORGANIZING PRINCIPLE: TETANUS AND LEG PAIN THAT IS NOT TETANUS

94	*šaššaṭu*	tetanus	head, neck, and inguinal regions hurt at same time	3.198
95	*šaššaṭu*	tetanus	neck, hips, hands, and feet are stiff	3.199

96	*šaššaṭu*	tetanus	neck twists; eyes jerk; he jerks or shudders incessantly		3.197 13.68 13.107
97	*šaššaṭu*	tetanus	muscles stiff from neck to heel; eyebrows knitted; jaws pressured		3.196
98	*sagallu*	sciatica	muscles of thigh hurt; cannot stand or walk		11.58
99	*maškādu*	sciatica	muscles of thigh hurt from hip sockets to ankles; can stand and walk		11.59
100	*maškādu*	sciatica	muscles hurt from coccyx to toes		11.60
101	*kiṣṣatu*	myalgia	hurts from hip sockets to opening of ankles	no consequence	3.129n
102	*kiṣṣatu* of *šētu*	myalgia	muscles sluggish from hip sockets to toes		3.129

ORGANIZING PRINCIPLE: GODS AND SKIN LESIONS THEY CAUSE

103	Gula		*samānu*; *ašû*		3.172n 10.103dn 19.98dn 19.328dn
104	Gula		growths; [. . .]		19.98
105	Gula		proliferating sores; *šadānu*		19.98
106a	Gula	diarrhea	diarrhea		19.327dn
106b	Ninurta		*šadānu*		19.99
107	Ninurta		liver problems; *aḫḫazu*		19.99 19.365
108	Marduk		needling pain; [. . .]		19.101
109a	Marduk		"contagious"?		
109b	Ea		*ummedu*		19.91 19.246
110	Šamaš		[. . .]; *girgišu*		10.144 19.103
111	Šamaš		[. . .]; *ekketu*		10.32n 19.103
112	Šamaš		[. . .]; *quliptu*		10.68n 11.42d
113	Šamaš		[. . .]; white *bubu'tu*	recovery	10.84n 19.105
114a	Ištar		[black *bubu'tu*]	death	10.84n 19.105
114b	Sîn		red *bubu'tu*	recovery	3.233n 4.18n 10.84n 19.105
115a	Šamaš		[left foot . . .]		
115b	Ištar		right foot [. . .]		

116a	Sîn	[...]
116b	personal god?	[falls] on his back
117a	Ištar	[...]
117b	[...]	falls on his front
118	[...]	[...]; insides cramped; flesh [...]
119	[...]	[...]; flesh wastes away
120	Šulpaea	upper [...] hurts so badly he cannot sleep
121	Ištar	upper [...] hurts so badly he cannot sleep
122–123	[...]	[...]

DPS Tablet XXXVI

ORGANIZING PRINCIPLE: PREGNANT FEMALE PATIENT; PREDICTIONS OF OUTCOME

A

1	baby male	chloasma	top of (mother's) forehead yellow/tan	(fetus) fully formed	12.91 12.108
2	baby female		top of forehead white and shines	fattens	12.92 12.107
3	baby female		top of forehead dark	healthy	12.104
4	baby male		top of forehead reddish	dies	12.105
5		cerebral palsy	top of forehead multicolored	child that "lies down"	12.114
6	baby male		top of forehead full of "grains"	fattens	10.154 12.101 12.109
7			top of forehead full of red "grains"	fattens	10.155 12.109n
8	baby male		past normal childbearing age		12.106
9	baby male		muscles of forehead reddish		12.87n
10	baby female		muscles of forehead white		12.88n
11	baby female		blood vessels of temple, the lower ones to the left pulsate		12.79
12	baby male		blood vessels of temple, the lower ones to the right pulsate		12.79
13	baby male		muscles of temple reddish		12.87
14	baby female		muscles of temple white		12.88
15	baby male		tip twitches/protrudes; [...]	[...]	12.95

16			head of tip rises to the left and is dark	fetus dies	Ap.40
17			head of tip rises to the right and is dark	dies/lives	Ap.40
18			base of tip reddish from below to the left	fetus dies	Ap.40
19	baby male		base of tip reddish from below to the right		
20			base of tip multicolored from below to the left	fetus lives	Ap.40
21			base of tip multicolored from below to the right	fetus lives	Ap.40
22	baby male		base of tip rises from below to the left		12.81
23	baby female		base of tip rises from below to the right		12.81
24	baby male		*umṣātus* look peeled; face yellow/tan		10.121n 12.91n
25	baby female		*umṣātus* look peeled; face reddish		12.92n
26		inverted nipples	tip of breast twisted shut	fetus does not do well	12.27
27			tip of breast open	fetus does well	12.28
28	baby male		tip of breast dark		12.90
29	baby female		tip of breast reddish		12.89
30			tip of breast white	fetus does not do well	Ap.41
31	baby male		tip of breast blood-red		12.90
32			tip of breast yellow/tan	aborted	Ap.41
33			tip of breast full of white *umṣatus*	delivery easy	10.120
34			tip of breast full of reddish *umṣatus*	delivery not easy	10.121
35	baby male		tip of breast full of dark *umṣatus*		10.121n
36			tip of breast has 3 dimples	thin	
37			tip of breast has 4 dimples	thin	
38			tip of breast has 5 dimples	dies	
39			tip of breast has 6 dimples	does not do well	
40			tip of breast has 7 dimples	lives	
41			tip of breast has 8 dimples	lives	
42			tip of breast has 9 dimples	bad omen	
43			tip of breast has 10 dimples	brings children to term	
44			tip of breast has 14 dimples	does not bring children to term	
45	baby male		tip of breast has 15 dimples; their . . . are reddish		
46	baby female		tip of breast has 15 dimples; their . . . are dark		

47	baby male		tip of breast has 5 dimples; their . . . are reddish		
48	baby female		tip of breast has 5 dimples; their . . . are dark		
49	baby female		blood vessels of breast run in straight line		12.77
50	baby male	Mondor's disease?	blood vessels of breast held by threads		12.78
51	baby male	Mondor's disease?	blood vessels of breast red		12.78
52	baby female		top of breast red muscles cross		22.35n Ap.42
53	baby male		top of breast dark muscles cross		22.35n Ap.42
54			top of breast white muscles cross	fetus does not do well	Ap.42
55			top of breast yellow/tan muscles cross	does not do well	Ap.42
56		stria	muscles of epigastrium unevenly colored yellow/tan	does well	10.50n 12.93
57	baby male		insides feel balled up?		12.97
58			insides protrude/slither	. . .	
59			insides slither toward the hypogastric region	. . .	
60			insides protrude toward the hypogastric region	. . .	
61			insides packed into the hypogastric region	child deaf/retarded	12.111
62			insides poured into the hypogastric region	child deaf/retarded	12.112
63	baby male		insides protrude toward the hypogastric region		12.83n
64	baby female		insides protrude from above toward the hypogastric region		12.82n
65	baby male		insides protrude/turned from below toward the hypogastric region		12.83n
66	baby male		insides cramped		12.99
67	baby female		insides bloated		12.100
68	baby female		insides large		12.103
69		stria	chest and abdomen unevenly colored with yellow/tan	completely formed	10.50n 12.94
70	baby female		insides pointed as her nose		12.103n
71	twins		insides large; both feet and both ankles swollen; steps to left and right		12.110
72	baby male		holds insides with hands		12.96
73	baby female		muscles protrude toward epigastrium		12.82
74	baby male		muscles protrude toward hypogastric region		12.83

75	baby female		insides large		12.103n
76	baby male		insides bloated		12.98
77			face changes for the worse	mother dies	12.25
78			face calm	fetus brought to term	12.26
79		lupus	face full of what looks like oxhide treated with depilatories	fetus dies	12.65
80		lupus	face full of what looks like oxhide treated with depilatories; both eyes spotted	mother and fetus die	12.66
81			continually vomits	not brought to term	6.62n 12.55 17.5
82		endometritis	dark blood flows from womb's mouth	mother does not recover	12.47
83		endometritis	pus produced from womb's mouth	mother and fetus die	12.48
84	no clue	arthritis	hands and feet sluggish	21 possible prognoses	11.19n
85			head of navel unraveled	brought to term	12.29
86			head of navel twisted	does not live	12.30
87		endometritis	dark blood flows from womb's mouth to left	fetus dies	12.47n
88		endometritis	dark blood flows from womb's mouth to right	fetus dies	12.47n
89		epileptic mother; child with hare-lip	continually rolls eyes	carries a hare; fetus dies	12.115 13.118n 17.63
90	baby female		blood vessels of left ankle pulsate		12.80
91	baby male		blood vessels of right ankle pulsate		12.80
92	twins		blood vessels of both ankles pulsate	will not do well	12.110n
93	baby male	varicose veins	blood vessel of ankle continually full of blood		12.102
94		cerebral palsy	steps consistently to left	child that "lies down"	12.113
95	baby female		steps consistently to right		12.84
96	baby male/ female		steps to left; foot feels heavy		12.85
97	baby female		steps to right; foot feels heavy		12.86
98	twins		steps to left and right		12.110n
99		swollen ankles	feet seem small	brings children to term	
100	baby male		womb? red		12.2
101	baby male		womb? bright red		12.2
102			womb? shining	child will not do well	12.3

103			properly respectful of pregnancy	mother lives	12.23
104			careless of pregnancy	mother dies	12.24
105			[stomach] continually upset	fetus dies	12.56
106			approached at 5 months, 3 days	life	12.40
107			approached at 5 months, 4 days	life	12.40n
108			approached at 5 months, 5 days	bleeding	12.41
109			approached at 5 months, 6 days	bleeding	12.41n
110			approached at 5 months, 7 days	life	12.39 12.40n
111			approached at 5 months, 8 days	father's evil	12.42
112			approached at 5 months, 9 days	mother dies	12.43
113			approached at 5 months, 10 days	life	12.40n

DPS Tablet XXXVII

ORGANIZING PRINCIPLE: FEMALE PATIENT

A					
1			pregant woman approached in 3rd month	recovery	12.31
2			4th month	recovery	12.32
3			5th month	worrisome	12.34
4			6th month	worrisome	12.35
5			7th month	worrisome	12.36
6			8th month	recovers or father's curse	12.37
7			9th or 10th month	does not recover or give birth	12.38
8–9		septic shock	burning fever or collapse and fever; coldish hands	death	3.8n 3.37n 14.37n
10		thyrotoxicosis?	head hair fine	2 or 3 days → death	19.42
11	lord of roof or *rābiṣu* of roof		cradles head in hands	death	19.42
12	Lilû	hysteria	afflicted in the night		12.69 19.18n
13	Lilû	hysteria	afflicted in the evening; takes her clothes off		12.70 16.58 19.18
14	Lilû	hysteria	afflicted in the night		12.69n 19.18n
15	[...]	eclampsia	continual jerking; [...]	[...]	12.115dn
16	dirty hands		chews on hands		Ap.80
17	Ištar	hysteria	thinks abdomen is too short	recovery	12.68 19.16
18		eclampsia?	sick in night; gets up in morning; time after time	death	Ap.39

19		wound	wound to hip region; epigastrium takes up wind	death	3.208n
20	incest		cannot sleep at night whether sick or not		16.28
21	incest		cannot sleep at night; either hands or feet hurt; bed throws her off		16.29
22–r.1′	[. . .]		[. . .]	[. . .]	

DPS Tablet XL

ORGANIZING PRINCIPLE: INFANT EATS BUT DOES NOT GET FAT

A 1–2	"dust"	failure to thrive	suckling eats but does not get fat; diarrhea and wasting		7.14n 17.146
A 3	"dust"	failure of Moro test	does not jerk and straighten out arms when suspended		13.281
A 4	"dust"	seizures interfering with nutrition	3 months old; wasting; extremities contorted/rigid		13.183
A 5	*bu'šānu*	kala azar with superinfections?	petechial rash; no fever; collapsed temporal blood vessels; something in the nose that is bothersome but is not snot		3.3n 10.50n 19.331
A 6–7	*meḫru*	gastroenteritis	plentiful flesh before illness; flesh looks terrible; fever 3 or 4 days; cramping; diarrhea		3.120n
A 8–9	*meḫru*	gastroenteritis	1 to 3 months old; cannot sleep; flesh looks terrible, cramping; diarrhea; looks crushed		3.120
A 10–12		teething	fever in head; body lukewarm; no sweat; hands and feet hot; drooling; diarrhea	recovery after 15 to 20 days	3.4n 6.71n 17.147
A 13	abdomen "broken"	abdominal injury	always sick; fails water test		17.164
A 14	abdomen "broken"	abdominal injury	eats but not sated; drooling		17.163n

ORGANIZING PRINCIPLE: INFANT DOES NOT WANT TO EAT

A 15	*kišpu*		bloated insides; refuses to eat		6.49n
A 16	*kišpu*	seizures	turns round in sleep; shuddering		13.184n
A 17	*kišpu*	seizures	continual shuddering and wailing		13.184n
A 18–19	*kišpu*	seizures interfering with nutrition	3 months old; contorted limbs; wasting		13.184
A 20	vow	benign fever	restless and sick or wailing and fever		19.357
A 21–23	Šulpaea	cerebral palsy	1 to 4 years old; writhes in contortion; unable to eat solid food or talk	will not straighten up	13.244

A 24–25	Ištar	seizures	jerking and wailing or restless, jumping and wailing		13.179n 19.50dn
A 26–27	Ištar	seizures	2 or 3 days old; nausea; continual falling spells	death	13.178 19.50dn
A 28	Ištar	simulated epilepsy	wailing and screaming		19.54n
A 29	"hand" of god	congenital syphilis	petechial rash, cramped insides; swollen hands and feet; *li'bu*-fever; "sick lungs"	recovery	3.18dn 4.23 10.50n 19.96
A 30	Ištar or "hand" of god	simulated epilepsy or colic	bloated insides and wailing	recovery	6.33n 17.161n 19.54n
A 31	Kūbu	leptospirosis?	fever; epigastrium protrudes		19.336 20.100
A 32	Kūbu	leptospirosis?	petechial rash		10.50n 19.336 20.100
A 33	Kūbu	leptospirosis?	cramping; petechial rash		10.50n 19.336 20.100
A 34	Kūbu	leptospirosis?	chills; gnashing of teeth [shaking chills]	prolonged	3.39n 19.336 20.100
A 35	Sîn	seizures	jerking and restlessness		13.179 19.47
A 36–37		nursing problems	wasting; disinterest in the breast	if moved to another breast, recovery	6.49 7.13 17.143
A 38	*ašû* or *samānu*			if moved to another breast, recovery	17.144
A 39–40	[. . .]		cough; [. . .]	[. . .]	8.66n

ORGANIZING PRINCIPLE: BONY STRUCTURES

A 41		spina bifida	transverse processes of neck and spine open	death	17.70
A 42–43	Sîn	respiratory distress	whole abdomen shudders	may recover	8.79
A 44		meningitis with open fontanelles	head bulges for only a week	may recover	17.151
A 45		meningitis with open fontanelles	head bulges	death	17.152

ORGANIZING PRINCIPLE: INFANT IS VOMITING

A 46	Sîn	seizures	jerking and restless; wailing and shuddering; continual raising of hands and feet	death	13.181 19.48
A 47	Sîn or Ištar	seizures	jerking; restless; shuddering		13.67 13.179n 19.50
A 48	promise to Sîn	simulated epilepsy	vomiting or diarrhea leading to sluggish hands and feet		3.107 19.53

A 49		seizures		if prolonged, death	13.176
A 50	Dingirmaḫ or "hand" of god		colic and projectile vomiting	recovery	6.58 19.344 19.354
A 51	Lamaštu	typhoid?	*li'bu*-fever; cold		3.16 19.224
A 52	Lamaštu	typhoid?	fever with thirst		19.229n
A 53	Lamaštu	typhoid?	feverish abdomen with thirst		19.229
A 54	Lamaštu	typhoid?	feverish nostrils		Ap.91
A 55	Sîn or Ištar	similated epilepsy	screaming, jerking, and restless; wailing and shuddering; projectile vomiting		6.58n 19.52
A 56	scepter of Sîn or Ištar	congenital syphilis	swollen hands and feet; constricted pupils		4.24 13.94n 19.51 19.95
A 57	Sîn	encephalitis?	cold buttocks and ears		3.3n 19.259n
A 58	Lamaštu	typhoid?	continuous as in adult version		19.228
A 59a	*aḫḫāzu*	biphasic fever with jaundice	no fever but a lot of sweating		3.3n 6.126n
A 59b	[. . .]		[. . .]		
A 60	Sîn or Ištar	seizure	falling spell after eating		13.177 19.50n

ORGANIZING PRINCIPLE: NUTRITIONAL PROBLEMS

A 61	*bu'šānu*	kala-azar with superinfections?	dark/terrible-looking flesh; something in the nose that bothers; tearing eyes		19.332
A 62		hypotonia	fisted thumb; laughing; wasting	death	17.167
A 63	"hand" of god	colic	colicky insides; heavy eyes	recovery	17.161
A 64	"hand" of god	colic	bloated insides and wailing	recovery	6.33n 17.161
A 65	"hand" of god	colic	bloated insides	recovery	6.33n 17.161
A 66	"hand" of god	colic	cramped insides	recovery	17.161
B 68	"hand" of god		sweating; flushes and turns pale	recovery	19.355
B 69	"hand" of god		vomiting	recovery	6.29n 19.356
B 70	"hand" of god		vomiting; dry palate; [. . .]	[. . .]	3.105n 19.356
B 71	"hand" of god		vomiting; [. . .]	[. . .]	6.29n 19.356
B 72a	Ningeštinanna	nystagmus	oscillating eyes		13.109
B 72b	[. . .]		dry eyes; [. . .]	[. . .]	
B 73a	Damu	intestinal artresia	insides blocked off		6.89n 17.120

B 73b	[...]		[...]	[...]	
B 74	abdomen "broken"	abdominal injury	refuses to eat		6.49n 17.163
B 75	[...]		refuses to eat; insides [...]	[...]	6.49n
A 75	Gula	kala-azar?	petechial rash; insides [...]		10.50n 19.320n
A 76	Gula	kala-azar?	petechial rash		10.50n 19.320
A 77	Gula?	kala-azar?	petechial rash on the abdomen		10.50n 19.320n
A 78	Gula	kala-azar?	protruding epigastrium		19.323
A 79	Gula?	kala-azar with dysentery?	fever and cramped insides		19.327
A 80	Gula?	kala-azar with dysentery?	cramped insides		3.3n 19.327n
A 81	Gula?	superinfection?	firmly planted		19.327dn
A 82	Gula?	kala-azar?	always sick		19.319 20.99
A 83	Gula?	superinfection?	restless		19.327dn
A 84	Gula?	superinfection?	stretching with arms turned		19.327dn
A 85	Gula	kala azar?	wasting in some places; getting fatter in others		19.325
A 86	Gula	kala azar?	flushing and pallor		19.324n
A 87	Gula	kala azar?	anemia and dark color		19.322 22.54n
A 88	Gula	kala azar?	thining and getting fatter		19.326
A 89	Gula	kala azar?	fever and wasting		19.324
A 90	Gula	kala azar?	burning fever		3.8n 19.324n
A 91	Gula	superinfection?	constricted larynx		0.3 19.333
A 92	Gula	superinfection?	choking and jaundice		0.3 19.320dn 19.334n
A 93	Gula	superinfection?	choking, refusal to eat; jaundice		0.3; 6.49n 19.320dn 19.334
A 94	Gula	superinfection?	choking and refusal to eat		0.3; 6.49n 19.334n
A 95	Gula	superinfection?	cramped insides and constricted anus		19.327n
A 96	Gula	superinfection?	cramped insides; jaundice; *bu'šānu*		19.320dn 19.327n 19.330
A 97	*bu'šānu*	diphtheria?	cramped insides; something in the nose		17.157
A 98	*bu'šānu*	herpes stomatitis?	spittle flows		17.157
A 99	*bu'šānu*	herpes stomatitis?	spittle contains blood		17.157

A 100	*bu'šānu*	diphtheria?	feverish head, chest, and back		17.157
A 101	*bu'šānu*	diphtheria?	warm temperature; cramped insides		3.4n 17.157
A 102		green stools	wailing at the breast; excreted bile	death	17.162
A 103	vow		restless at the breast		19.358
A 104	vow		drinks; drools		19.358
A 105	vow		refusal to eat; bloated insides		6.49n 19.358
A 106	Ištar	simulated epilepsy	no fever; cramped insides; wailing		3.3n 19.54
A 107	Ištar	simulated epilepsy	wailing; rigid		19.54
A 108	Ištar	simulated epilepsy	nonstop wailing		19.54
A 109	vow		groaning; refusal to eat		6.49n 19.359
A 110	congenital "hand" of god	meningitis?	seizures developing after 1 to 2 months; immobilized hands and feet	family members expected to die	13.221
A 111		meningitis?	seizures; immobilized hands and feet; soaked eyes		13.39 13.221n
A 112	Ištar	nightmares	screaming in bed; cannot remember		17.165 19.10
A 113	Ištar or vow	nightmares	screaming in bed; can remember		17.166 19.10
A 114	*bu'šānu*	diphtheria?	cry stifled but no snot		17.158
A 115		teething	head hot; body lukewarm; drooling	after 14 to 20 days, recovery	3.4n 17.148
A 116		teething	fever in the head but not yet in body	after 21 days, recovery	3.3n 17.149
A 117	Nusku	fever in infants	skull is hot		19.346
A 118	Gula	superinfection with *kala-azar*?	choking and jaundice		19.320dn 19.334n
A 119	curse		choking; fever; loss of appetite		6.52 19.315n
A 120	Sîn	seizures	no fever; eyes dilated; hands and feet tremble	recovery	3.3n 13.95 13.180 19.49
A 121	Sîn	seizures	no fever but trembling		3.3n 13.180n 19.49
A 122	Sîn	seizures	no fever but continual trembling		3.3n 13.180n 19.49
B 117	promise to Sîn	simulated epilepsy	vomiting leading to sluggish hands and feet		3.107n 19.53n

Notes

CONCORDANCE OF SIGLA

1. Readings of this text are based on the author's transliteration from the original as modified on the basis of a copy subsequently provided by M. Geller.

TRANSLATOR'S NOTES

1. A convention of ancient Mesopotamian scientific texts in general is the use of Sumerian word-signs (Sumerograms) to render Akkadian vocabulary words. Compare the Arabic numeral "2" which would be read as "two" by an English-speaking reader.

2. The accuracy with which they worked is remarkable, as is the care which they took not to introduce mistakes where the text they were copying was lost or illegible. The usual convention in the latter case was to omit the missing sections and to write instead simply *ḫe-pí*: "broken."

3. See, for example, Labat, *TDP* 113:22′; Stol, *JEOL* 32.53.

INTRODUCTION

1. Assyriology is the study of those civilizations of the ancient Near East that wrote their languages using syllabic cuneiform scripts.

2. For the arrangement of entries on the original tablets, see the set of charts on the Diagnostic and Prognostic Series (DPS) in the back of this book.

3. As, for example, Volk, *OrNS* 68.13.

4. As, for example, Cadelli, *Ktèma* 22.17, who argues that the *āšipu* arrived at his prognoses by making an accounting of good and bad signs, the outcome being determined by a summation with two negative signs yielding a positive outcome. This assertion is directly contradicted by literally thousands of examples.

5. See Chapter 1.

6. For the actual relationship between genuine omens and the prognoses in the diagnostic/prognostic handbook, see Chapter 20.

7. See Heeßel, AOAT 43.13–17,105–107.

8. For a complete listing of the entries in the diagnostic/prognostic handbook in their original order, see the set of charts on the Diagnostic and Prognostic Series (DPS) in the back of this book.

9. See Parpola, AOAT 5/2.230–236.

10. An example is the recitation published in Nougayrol, *RA* 41.31, 41–42, which was designed to elicit the support of NIN.DIN.UG$_5$.GA in curing a number of possible diseases, including various types of fever and worms.

11. This is certainly the case with the recitation republished in Kämmerer, *UF* 27.140–143. As may readily be seen from *YOS* 11.7:3–8 (see Chapters 10.148 and 2.26), the section referring to transmission of the disease from animals to human babies originally applied only to *sikkatu*. The other skin conditions mentioned were originally part of a separate multiuse recitation describing ills that descended from heaven (A10) and for which assistance was required from the seven and seven daughters of Anu (A13–20), a well-known spell type (see W. Farber, *JNES* 49.299–321). This multiuse recitation was apparently combined with the *sikkatu* spell (A1, 11–12) by the simple expedient of cutting and pasting the two together. To judge from the ritual oath that occurs atypically after the "spell is not mine" formula (B26–33), *šuruppû*, *epqēnu*, and *bu'šānu* were also once the subjects of a separate recitation.

12. See, for example, Kämmerer, *UF* 27.147; Kinnier Wilson, *Diseases in Antiquity* 199.

13. Kämmerer, *UF* 27.129–168 and *RA* 94.79–81; Kinnier Wilson, *Diseases in Antiquity* 195 and *JNES* 27.243–244.

CHAPTER 1. THE ANCIENT MESOPOTAMIAN CONTEXT

1. GIG A.<<NU>>.ZU NU.ME.A ŠÀ.GAR.RA KÚ.E NU.ME.A

2. On this point, see also Volk, *OrNS* 68.12–13.

3. For example, Rose, *Cephalalgia* 19.1–3, after summarily dismissing "Babylonian literature," gives credit to the Egyptians for the first description of unilateral headaches accompanied by vomiting and then asserts that Hippocrates was the first to distinguish different types of headache. In fact, the ancient Mesopotamian physician had already distinguished different types of headache, and described various features of classic migraine, including flashes in the eyes, unilateral pain, and vomiting (see Chapter 13).

4. The Shatt-al-Arab did not form until classical antiquity, and the head of the Persian Gulf was somewhat farther north than it is today.

5. For a lively account of these texts, see Kramer, *Sumerians* 237–248.

6. Indo-European horse nomads are first mentioned in the annals of the Neo-Assyrian king Shalmaneser III in connection with a campaign of 835 B.C.E. Under the influence of the Assyrians, who incorporated them into their provincial system, the Medes settled down in a region of the Zagros (near modern Hamadan) that came to be known as Media. It is probably through their intermediation that techniques of rulership and other elements of Mesopotamian civilization were passed to the Medes' kinsmen and southern neighbors, the Persians.

7. The latest known dated cuneiform text is an astronomical almanac dated to 74/75 C.E. (see Edzard, *RLA* 5.559).

8. For the third century as the terminal date for the cuneiform tradition, see Geller, *ZA* 87.43–95.

9. In Laws of Ḫammurapi § 278, it is stated that a slave who has just been bought can be returned to the seller if the slave suffers from an attack of *bennu*. See Chapter 3.

10. The expression commonly appears as a colophon in Middle Assyrian texts; for examples, see *CAD* M/1.400a s.v. *mašû* mng. 1d.

11. Kinnier Wilson, "Medicine in the Land and Times of the Old Testament" 347–348, pl. 5 suggests that there is an illustration of forceps on the seal of an AZU. Other scholars (as, e.g., Stol, *Childbirth* 72–73) believe that the instrument in question was used to deliver calves.

12. Archi, *Fs von Soden*^{2} 10.

13. See Heeßel, AOAT 43.72. For an illustration of such a lens, found by Layard in Nineveh, see Fales and Postgate, SAA 7.86 fig. 20.

14. For example, LB 2126, an Old Babylonian diagnostic and prognostic text (see Geller, *AfO* 48/49.73–74), bears little resemblance to the later diagnostic/prognostic handbook. For specific examples of improvements and additions, see Finkel, *Fs. Lambert* 140.

15. For more details on the respective roles of these two healing specialists, and their professional relationship, see Scurlock, "Physician," in *Mesopotamian Magic* 69–79. Finkel argues (Fs. Lambert 146) that a collection of texts used to instruct medical students can readily be divided into *asûtu* (texts intended for the use of the *asû*) and *āšipūtu* (texts designed for the use of the *āšipu*) by the simple expedient of examining to see whether they are in vertical (portrait) or horizontal (landscape) format. In fact, his texts are by no means in full concord with this distinction, as he himself admits: "The result is a little arbitrary, but it is hardly possible to force all such texts into a modern straight jacket" (Finkel, Fs. Lambert 147). Thus, nine of the texts

that Finkel classes as *asûtu* (his nos. 1, 9, 10, 15, 21, 23–24, 25, and 28) are actually in what he argues to be the vertical *āšipūtu* format, and this is ignoring borderline exemplars. (A number of texts are sufficiently square that they could be classified either way.) What is worse, one of these texts actually has a colophon indicating that it belonged to a known *āšipu* (Finkel, Fs. Lambert 186–187). Conversely, all but three of the texts that Finkel classes as *āšipūtu* (nos. 34 copy B, 36, and 49) are actually in what he argues to be horizontal *asûtu* format. Included among these texts in horizontal format are several examples of astrological medicine (Finkel, Fs. Lambert 212–217) which nobody doubts fell under the purview of the *āšipu*.

We would argue that the real reason for the difference in formats is to be sought elsewhere. All but one of what Finkel argues to be school texts on internal grounds are in the unusual horizontal format. In other words, the most logical suggestion is that this format marks the work of students or, to be more precise, of beginning students, an interesting discovery in its own right.

16. A colophon is a paragraph appearing at the end of a tablet and containing such information as the name of the work, the number of the tablet in the series, the first line of the next tablet, and the name of the scribe and/or owner.

17. Brown, *Planetary Astronomy-Astrology* 211.

18. See ibid. 218–220, 223, 230.

19. That is, the text may be assigned to that date because the scribe or owner of the text is known to have been active in that period.

20. On the dating of BM 56605, see my "A Weakness for Hellenism," *Fs. Leichty*, forthcoming.

21. For references, see *CAD* G 130b s.v. *gullubu* mng. 2.

22. See Charpin, *Clergé* 251–269; for actual examples of such sales see, for example, 174–175, 178–179, 180–182, 190–191.

23. See McEwan, *Priest and Temple* 1–23.

24. The diviner was responsible for determining the will of the gods, most usually by posing a question to them in the form of a prayer that was recited over a sacrificial animal. The sheep was then slaughtered and its internal organs examined. Using manuals of extispicy, the diviner translated the various lumps and bumps on the liver and other internal organs, the number of turns of the intestines, irregularities in the bones, and the like into specific messages that were totaled to produce a yes or no answer.

25. On this point, see also Heeßel, AOAT 43.43.

26. We have receipts of *āšipus* for plants to be used for the treatment of specific patients (W. Farber and Freydank, *AOF* 5.256–258).

27. "If the ⸢sore⸣ [. . .], he will die; (the *āšipus*) shall not make a prognosis (as to his recovery). If [the sore . . .], (the *āšipus* may make a prognosis as to his recovery; to remove it . . ." (*BAM* 580 iii 3′–5′).

28. Köcher, *Fs. Goerke* 19 argues that there was a therapeutic companion to the diagnostic/prognostic handbook that consisted of forty-five tablets arranged in head-to-toe order. Stol, *JEOL* 32.49 agrees on the number of tablets and the arrangement but wishes to disassociate this from the diagnostic/prognostic handbook.

29. A true index is a surprisingly modern invention.

30. Medical (and other) texts could be borrowed from palace or temple libraries but could not be kept out overnight (*BAM* 1 iv 34). For other references, see *CAD* Š/3.283b s.v *šumšû* mng. 2 (note that the colophons in question are dated to the Assyrian king Aššurbanipal [Abp.] and not Aššurnaṣirpal II [Asn.] as in the *CAD*).

31. The chance omens observed by the *āšipu* were considered to be medically significant only if they were seen when he was on his way to the patient's house (DPS I obv. 1–2; DPS II obv. 1). Compare also Geller, *Udug-Ḫul* 20:4–11; 24:74–86; cf. 93:180–185 (recitations to protect the *āšipu* when he enters a patient's house in order to examine him).

32. A set of such jars that originally contained plant mixtures intended for use as fumigants has been found in excavation (Walker, *Iraq* 42.84–86).

33. Laws of Ḫammurapi §§ 215–223.

34. Note: "If a man is sick with *aḫḫāzu* and his head, his face, his whole body, and the base of his ⸢tongue⸣ [are affected], the *asû* is not to lay his hands on that patient; that man will die; he will not [live]" (*BAM* 578 iv 45–46).

35. Although the final elaboration of this system awaited the works of Galen, the core (i.e., the belief that the body is made up of the four humors of blood, phlegm, bile, and black bile) is already present in the late fifth-century Hippocratic treatise, *The Nature of Man*. For an English translation of this treatise, see Chadwick and Mann, *The Medical Works of Hippocrates* 202–213.

36. A little known archaic language of northern Mesopotamia used to communicate with ghosts and similar spirits. It has been suggested that this is actually an archaic form of Hurrian (see Prechel and Richter, *Fs. Haas* 333–372).

37. For more on this subject, see Scurlock, *Magico-Medical Means*, Chapter 7.

38. Particularly valuable in this regard is the work of Franz Köcher, whose six published volumes of hand copies of cuneiform texts are referred to in this book under the abbreviation *BAM* (short for *Die babylonisch-assyrische Medizin in Texten und Untersuchungen* [Berlin, 1963–1980]).

39. First in this category is *TDP* (short for R. Labat, *Traité Akkadien de diagnostics et pronostics médicaux* [Paris, 1951]), an edition of what survives of the ancient Mesopotamian Diagnostic Handbook, referred to in the current book under the abbreviation DPS. Since the publication of *TDP*, more pieces of this ancient medical handbook DPS have been discovered; especially important for the neurology chapter (Chapter 13) are Tablets XXVI–XXX, for which see Stol, *Epilepsy* 55–90. A new edition of DPS XIV–XXXV is to be found in Nils P. Heeßel, *Babylonisch-assyrische Diagnostik*, Alter Orient und Altes Testament 43 (Münster: Ugarit Verlag, 2000), referred to in the current book as AOAT 43. An edition of the remaining tablets of DPS by Heeßel is also planned.

40. We concur with the conclusion of Haussperger, *ZA* 87.196–218 that ancient Mesopotamian physicians deserve our respect and that it is high time that their accomplishments be seen in the right light: "Die Ärzte von damals verdienen unsere uneingeschränkte Hochachtung, und es ist an der Zeit, ihre Leistungen ins rechte Licht zu setzen" (217). Note also the comments of Brown, *Astronomy-Astrology* 228: "Science in modern parlance is recognized by some to have more specific meanings and it so happens that these in some cases correspond closely with the approaches undertaken by the Mesopotamian scholars . . . if it so happens that elements akin (and possibly ancestral) to modern science happen to be recorded in the ancient sources, they cannot be ignored."

CHAPTER 2. GENERAL HEALTH AND PUBLIC HEALTH PRACTICES

1. See Renfrew, *BSAg* 2.67–71.

2. See ibid. 3.157–161.

3. See Englund, *AOF* 22.37–55; cf. Heimpel, *RLA* 7.605–609.

4. Illustrations may be seen on Assyrian reliefs as, for example, Gadd, *Shalmaneser III to Sennacherib* pl. 59.

5. For references, see *CAD* Š/3.99–100 s.v. *šiqqu*.

6. See Stol, *BSAg* 7.99–113.

7. On this point, see also Ellison, *Iraq* 43.35–45.

8. These are published in Bottéro, *Textes culinaires*.

9. *Emar* VI.3 no. 388:7–10. For a complete recipe for bisteeya (including the manufacture of the requisite leaves of dough), see Wolfert, *Couscous* 101–115.

10. For references to stockpiles, and issues and thefts from such stockpiles, see *CAD* K 226–229 s.v. *karû* A.

11. Admiralty Handbook *Mesopotamia*, vol. 1 (August 1916) 28–29, 32–33.

12. So ubiquitous was the practice that hemerologies needed to warn "(on such and such a particularly ill-omened day), the person, on account of Bau should not sweep his house (or) wash his feet" (*KAR* 178 ii 70–72).

13. Lit. "turning away," that is, intended to ward off evil.

14. For other references, see *CAD* Š/3.387 s.v. *šūšurātu*: "sweepings."

15. There were exceptions—one apotropaic ritual instructs that the sweepings of the house were to be collected into a reed basket and burned (see Maul, *Zukunftsbewältigung* 500:28–30).

16. For references, see *CAD* K 69–70 s.v. *kalbu* mng. 1b.

17. For references, see *CAD* S 402b s.v. *sūqu* mng. 1a2′.

18. For references, see *CAD* K 69b s.v. *kalbu* mng. 1a.

19. For references, see *CAD* M/2.234–235 s.v. *musâtu*.

20. For a description of such bathrooms and drains, see Mallowan, *Nimrud and its Remains* 1.40–42 and Thureau-Dangin and Dunand, *Til-Barsib* 34–40.

21. A sump pit consists of a hollowed-out area at the bottom of a shaft for collecting waste.

22. "If a woman water drawer who carries a jar scoops in a fish and brings it into a man's house" (*CT* 41.14:15).

23. See also Fincke, *Augenleiden* 70 w/n. 538.

24. The connection is that the pupil was described as the "protective spirit" (^{d}LAMMA) of the eye.

25. One section of the omen series *Šumma ālu* detailed every conceivable time and place that a person might wash himself or herself (see W. Farber, *OrNS* 58.86–101). For more references, see *CAD* M/2.29–33 s.v. *mesû*: "washed" and *mesû*: "to wash."

26. For references, see *AHw* 948–949, 985–986 s.v. *ramāku* and *rimku*.

27. Even gods/goddesses expected this courtesy: "When day dawns, the door is unlocked and what has spent the night is cleared away and he brings water for washing. Oil is taken out. The big meal of the morning is offered" (Thureau-Dangin, *Racc.* 92 r. 11–12).

28. See Thureau-Dangin and Dunand, *Til-Barsib* 19.

29. For more details on this and other practices relating to childbirth, see Stol, *Birth* 141–142; Scurlock, *Incognita* 2.137–185; and Chapter 12.

30. Labat read this sign as *ú* followed by *u*. He also read the following *ina* KI (coll.) as BAD DIB and interpreted it as referring to a wrestling contest between the patient and death. This is very poetic, but seems out of place in this context.

31. See also DPS III A r. 15′//C r. 38–39 = *TDP* 30:98–99.

32. See Heeßel, AOAT 43.187 ad line 7.

33. See Mallowan, *Nimrud and its Remains* 1.106.

34. Heeßel, AOAT 43.257, 261 interprets this as TAG-*ma* and translates "that patient was touched."

35. ⸢KI.TAG.GA⸣ = *la-a-bu* (5R 16 i 37 w. *ASKT* p. 198).

36. On this point, see also Neufeld, *JANES* 18.52.

37. The term literally means "one that continually causes (someone else) to get it." See also Finet, *AIPHOS* 14.129; Durand, *MARI* 3.144; Neufeld, *JANES* 18.52–66; Biggs, *History of Science* 8.96. Note also Durand, *MARI* 3.143–149; Labat, *MDP* 57, p. 257.

38. BM 64526 is a medical text that forms part of the Sippar collection. The authors would like to thank the Trustees of the British Museum for permission to quote from this unpublished material.

39. See also DPS X A obv. 38 = *TDP* 84:38; DPS XV:27 (AOAT 43.151); cf. DPS XI A r. 50 = *TDP* 98 r. 50.

40. See Chapter 3.

41. The Sumerian has as a consequence having wind in the insides.

42. Lit. "it will be ignited (like a fire)."

43. For other references to sexual transmission, see DPS III A r. 8′//C r. 31 = *TDP* 28:91; DPS XIII A 6–7//B i 3′–6′ = *TDP* 110 i 7′–10′ (cf. DPS XXII:10–13 [AOAT 43.252]); DPS XIV A ii 38//C ii 13//F 4 = *TDP* 134 ii 38.

44. The epigastrium is the midline region of the abdomen between the navel and the lower rib cage.

45. That this organ is the liver may be seen from Izbu comm. 203 (Leichty, *Izbu* 218): *ta-kal-tú* = *ga-bi-du*: "liver." See also Nougayrol, *RA* 44.3 and Goetze, *YOS* 10 p. 7. Note also *CAD* N 376a.

46. DPS XIV A ii 34–36//C ii 10–11 = *TDP* 134 ii 34–36 has "hand" of his god (var. "hand" of his goddess).

47. See also *BAM* 318 ii 38–39.

48. See also DPS XXII:24 (AOAT 43.253).

49. Note *STT* 403:44: *lu*ʾ*-tum* = *kiš-pu*.

50. See also *BAM* 494 i 32′; Labat, *RA* 53.10–11 obv. 38. Note also DPS XXXIII:6 [AOAT 43.353].

51. The commentary (*SpTU* 1.51:2) adds: *šá* SAG.DU-*su kal-ma-tu ú-nak-ki-*[*is*]: "whose head lice have ⸢bitten⸣."

52. Kämmerer, *UF* 27.166–167 believes that orf is a type of variola (smallpox) virus that can be spread to humans and cause smallpox. Orf is not a type of variola virus and, more importantly, smallpox virus is known to infect only humans and no other animals.

53. See Collins, *Natural Illness* 291–292, Various Illnesses 5.

54. See Kinnier Wilson, *Diseases in Antiquity* 205.

55. Pierce, *Cuneiform Cryptography* 168–169 suggests that the mysterious 6,40 might be a substitution cipher for *ašar*.

56. See also *CT* 14.23 [K 9283]:11//*STT* 92 i 11; Scheil, *RA* 15.76:11.

57. There is no reason to suppose that this disease originated in ancient Mesopotamia simply because it is first attested there (differently Adamson, *JRAS* 1977.140–144).

58. See also Stol, *Birth* 128–129.

59. Fincke, *Augenleiden* 74, 109 suggests a number of further possibilities for rabies but we do not concur. For further discussion of the relevant passages, see Chapter 13 under TRAUMA TO THE SPINAL CORD, NYSTAGMUS, and SENSORY SEIZURES.

60. See Chapter 13.

61. Lit. "cutting of the breath," *zikurudû* describes a form of sorcery intended to kill the victim.

62. Stol, *Mesopotamian Magic* 66 characterizes this text as "nothing but fear (of being murdered by witches)." Although these symptoms could indeed be hysterical, this would not be an adverse reaction to the discovery of an act of witchcraft, but pseudohydrophobia (hysterical reaction to animal bites). Biggs, *RLA* 6.211 considers this text to be describing a stroke. This seems particularly unlikely given the references to fever and the absence of any of the classical neurological abnormalities seen in stroke.

63. See, for example, DPS XII A 13–14 = *TDP* 102 i 13–14 (quick versus lingering death) and DPS XIV A i 1–3 = *TDP* 128 i 1–3 (persistent problem versus recovery).

64. See above, Chapter 2.18n.

65. See *AHw* 775a s.v. *neḫsu* I.

66. Note Dandamayev, *Death in Mesopotamia* 183–186, who argues that detailed studies of prosopography might ultimately provide answers to these questions, at least for the later periods.

67. "40 = *lalûtu* (prime); 50 = *ūmū kurūtu* (short life); 60 = *bēlūtu* (maturity); 70 = *ūmū arkūtu* (long life); ⌜80⌝ = *šībūtu* (old age); 90 = *littūtu* (extreme old age) (*STT* 400:45–47). Note also *CAD* D 115b s.v. *dāru* A: "generation" (= 70 years).

68. See Stol, *CANE* 487.

69. See J. Oates, *CAH*² 3/2.167–168.

70. Dandamayev, *Death in Mesopotamia* 184–185.

71. See also DPS XVI:87′ (AOAT 43.180); DPS XVI:89′ (AOAT 43.180).

72. References in the diagnostic/prognostic handbook to people with "long days"and the like are oblique references to the age of the individual, in this case, seventy years ("70 = *ūmū arkūtu*" [*STT* 400:46]). For similar usages in the physiognomic omens, see Böck, *Morphoskopie* 30–31.

73. See also DPS XVI:92′ (AOAT 43.180).

74. Heeßel, AOAT 43.185, 193 suggests interpreting this as *sīku*, which would have to mean "powdered part." The "peg" could be the long stem; it is difficult to imagine what the "powdered part" of a leek would be.

75. The interpretation is based on restoration of the passage from DPS XI A obv. 45 = *TDP* 92:45 as suggested by Heeßel, AOAT 43.193.

76. See also (DPS XVI:94′ [AOAT 43.180]).

77. Lit. "they become shorter (than they were)."

78. See also (DPS XVI:98′–101′ [AOAT 43.180]).

79. ⌜80⌝ = *šībūtu* (*STT* 400:47).

80. See Chapter 3.

81. It is regrettable that no scientific records have survived from the Minoans and Myceneans, whose expertise in draining Lake Copais and providing drainage systems in cities suggest a similarly technical orientation.

CHAPTER 3. INFECTIOUS DISEASES

1. A similar problem is faced by scholars who study another medical tradition of the ancient world, the Hippocratic corpus. This has not, however, prevented many passages from being positively identified (see especially Grmek, *Diseases in the Ancient Greek World*). Many of the infectious diseases described by ancient Mesopotamian physicians also appear in the various treatises attributed to the "father of medicine." The omissions may be due to the loss of data in the Roman and later periods. However, diseases that were not common in Greece and Asia Minor and of which Greek physicians consequently had little knowledge may

have been deliberately omitted. Finally, it is possible that some diseases present in the ancient world have simply not been recognized in the descriptions given by ancient Greek physicians.

2. The Akkadian is from *emēmu,* "to be hot."

3. For similar references, see DPS IV A obv. 52, 53 = *TDP* 38:52, 53; DPS IV A obv. 64//E ii 9 = *TDP* 38:64//*SpTU* 3.88 ii 9; DPS IX A 34 = *TDP* 74:34; DPS XI A obv. 43, 44 = *TDP* 92:43, 44; DPS XIII B ii 2–3, 7–8 = *TDP* 116 ii 2–3, 7–8.

4. The attempt by Adamson, *JRAS* 1979.3 to apply temperature levels to "fever" as recognized by the *āšipu* ignores the existence of more than one level of fever.

5. For other references to normal temperature, see DPS XII D iii 37 = *TDP* 106 iii 37; DPS XIII B ii 13–14 = *TDP* 118 ii 13–14; DPS XIII B ii 47–48//G_2 38+G_1 21 = *TDP* 120 ii 47–48; DPS XIII G_2 7, 8 = *TDP* 122 iii 14, 15; DPS XIV C_2 iii 18//F 6//J 6 = *TDP* 142 iii 63′; DPS XXVII:27–28 (AOAT 43.299); DPS XL A 57 = *TDP* 224:57; *BE* 17/1.32:8–14, apud Parpola, *LAS* 2.493. Compare also DPS IV B obv. 33//E i 13 = *TDP* 36:34//*SpTU* 3.88 i 13; DPS XII D iii 38 = *TDP* 106 iii 38; DPS XIII I 5 = *TDP* 122 iii 5; DPS XIV C_2 iii 19, 20//F 7, 8//J 7 = *TDP* 142 iii 64′ (not normal); DPS III C obv. 35 = *TDP* 22:35; DPS XII D iv 20///E 27/G_2 iv 18 = *TDP* 108 iv 20 (cf. DPS XV:31 [AOAT 43.152]); DPS XIII B i 16′–17′ = *TDP* 112 i 20′–21′; DPS XIV A iii 25–26//F 3//J 3 = *TDP* 142 iii 59′–60′; DPS XVI:56′ [AOAT 43.177]; DPS XL A 5//B 5–6 = *TDP* 218:5; DPS XL A 59a = *TDP* 224:59a; DPS XL A 80 = *TDP* 226:80; DPS XL A 106 = *TDP* 228:106; DPS XL A 116, 120, 121, 122 = *TDP* 230:116, 120, 121, 122 (the patient does not have a fever).

6. For other references, see *BAM* 145:1–17//*BAM* 146:29′–38′; *BAM* 174 r. 29–31; DPS IV B obv. 20–21 = *TDP* 34:20–21; DPS III A obv. 6//B 6; DPS IV A obv. 54–58//E ii 1–3//G obv. 8–11 = *TDP* 38:54–58//*SpTU* 3.88 ii 1–3//*LKU* 94:8–11; DPS XI A obv. 54 = *TDP* 94:54; DPS XXII:33 (AOAT 43.254); DPS XL A 10–12 = *TDP* 218:10–12; DPS XL A 101 = *TDP* 228:101 (cf. DPS XXXIII:91 [AOAT 43.357]); DPS XL A 115 = *TDP* 230:115.

7. For other references, see *BAM* 147 obv. 12, 13, 22//*BAM* 148 obv. 12, 13, 22.

8. The passage has been collated.

9. For other references, see DPS III C obv. 46–47, 48–49 = *TDP* 22/24:46–47, 48–49.

10. For similar references, see DPS III C r. 1, 2//E_1 r. 2, 3 = *TDP* 24:61, 62; DPS III C r. 7–11 = *TDP* 26:67–71 (cf. *KAR* 211 obv. 4–6); DPS XI A obv. 25//B 24 = *TDP* 90:25//*SpTU* 1.34:24 (cf. DPS XV:15 [AOAT 43.151]); DPS XI A obv. 27//B 26 = *TDP* 92:27//*SpTU* 1.34:26; DPS XI A r. 23–27 = *TDP* 96 r. 23–27; DPS XI A r. 36 = *TDP* 96 r. 36 (cf. DPS XV:26 [AOAT 43.151]); DPS XIII B ii 2–3, 7–8 = *TDP* 116 ii 2–3, 7–8; DPS XIV A ii 34–36//C ii 10–11 = *TDP* 134 ii 34–36 (cf. DPS XXII:14–15 [AOAT 43.252]); DPS XVI:31–32 (AOAT 43.175); DPS XVII:10–13 (AOAT 43.195–196); DPS XXXI:35′–37′ (AOAT 43.343); DPS XXXIII:30 (AOAT 43.354; cf. *BAM* 409 obv. 26′–28′); DPS XXXVII A obv. 8–9 = *TDP* 212/214:8–9; DPS XL A 90 = *TDP* 228:90; *MDP* 57.11 iii 4–5; StBoT 36.35 r. 2–3//StBoT 36.57 r. 9′–10′; Meier, *ZA* 45.208 v 15–20; BM 64371 iii 8′; *BAM* 66 obv. 21–22; *BAM* 201:23′–25′.

11. ÚḪ is usually "phlegm." However, when used with KÚM ("fever") it is to be read as a form of *ṣarāḫu,* as has now been demonstrated by Heeßel, AOAT 43.162–163. Previously, Labat, *TDP* 25 n. 44 had suggested and then rejected the correct reading in favor of *nuppuḫ*: "it is swollen," an interpretation that is followed by Biggs, *RLA* 6.210 and *CAD* N/1.268b s.v. *napāḫu* mng. 7b, but which makes no sense in this context.

12. See also DPS XVI:31–32 (AOAT 43.175).

13. See also DPS XVI:28 (AOAT 43.175). Note also DPS III C obv. 51 = *TDP* 24:51; K 2581 obv. 20′–21′// *AMT* 53/7+K 6732:1; BM 64526:2, 5.

14. The text has "the temples are calm." The *āšipu* liked to use the absolute minimum of words; in this case it was obvious that the temporal blood vessels were meant, so why mention them? Compare DPS IV A obv. 65//E ii 10 = *TDP* 38:65//*SpTU* 3.88 ii 10 and DPS XIII B i 31′//D 4 = *TDP* 114 i 35′ (temples and abdomens that "go," meaning blood vessels that "go" in these locations; see Chapters 19.252 and 20.22), DPS IV B obv. 5b–6 = *TDP* 32:5b–6 ("collapsed temples," meaning collapsed temporal blood vessels; see Chapter 14.24), and the relatively common expression "pulsating temples," meaning a sensation of pulsation in the temporal arteries (see Chapter 13.149).

15. Note also DPS III A obv. 9.

16. For references, see *CAD* L 6.

17. See also Stol, *Epilepsy* 68; Volk, *OrNS* 68.24; Cadelli, *Ktèma* 22.28 w/ n. 122.

18. See *SpTU* 1.30 obv. 8, 38:10; cf. *AHw* 1530a s.v. *ziʾpu* III mng. 4.

19. See also *BAM* 240:59′–60′; DPS XL A 29 = *TDP* 220:29.
20. Lit. "one day" . . . "one day" . . .
21. For similar references, see DPS XVI:13 (AOAT 43.173); K 2581 obv. 7′.
22. See also DPS XVII:90 (AOAT 43.204).
23. For other references, see DPS IX A 33 = *TDP* 74:33; *SpTU* 3.65 r. 12; cf. *SpTU* 2.2:58, 165.
24. See DPS XIX/XX:110′–113′ (AOAT 43.232–233).
25. The passage has been collated.
26. The passage has been collated.
27. The passage has been collated.
28. UNU = *šubtu*; see *CAD* Š/3.172b s.v. *šubtu* A lex. section.
29. For other references, see DPS XVI:41′ (AOAT 43.176); DPS XVI:62′ (AOAT 43.177); DPS XVII:46 (AOAT 43.199).
30. Adamson, *JRAS* 1979.3 w/ n. 22 considers this pattern to be a description of tertian malaria, interpreting this phrase as: "the fever leaves him one day and on the second day . . ." However, "on the second day" is invariably represented by *ina* U_4.2.KÁM. Without the *ina*, the text must be taken to mean "it leaves him one day and then later (*-ma*) it overpowers him and flows over him two days." There is nothing to indicate that this was a repeating pattern, but even if it was, it does not fit any of the known forms of malaria. For example, Vivax and Ovale malaria alternate between days with fever and days with no fever. *Plasmodium malaria* produces febrile days separated by two days without fever.
31. The passage has been collated and the "*ḫaš*" is unusual, but is listed as Fossey no. 900.
32. The term is often used in enumerations of febrile diseases, typically contrasted with *liʾbu* or alongside Lamaštu and *aḫḫāzu* as a triad. For references, see *CAD* L 16–17. Note also "If . . . he continually has much sweat (as in) Labaṣu and chills keep falling upon him" (*CTN* 4.72 vi 14′–16′ [Kinnier Wilson, *Iraq* 19.40–49 (ND 4368)]) and "If it continually afflicts him daily as in affliction by Lamaštu (i.e., all day), "hand" of Labaṣu (DPS XIX/XX:113′b [AOAT 43.233]).
33. The reading follows *CAD* K 374b.
34. The sign looks more like an ID.
35. See also *KAR* 211 obv. 4–6; DPS XVI:12 (AOAT 43.173).
36. ÚḪ is usually "phlegm." However, when used with KÚM ("fever") it is to be read as a form of *ṣarāḫu* as the parallel between DPS III C r. 10–11//E_1 r. 11–12+E_2 r. 7–8 = *TDP* 26:70–71 (DIŠ *ina* SAG.DU-*šú* KÚM ÚḪ) and *KAR* 211 obv. 4–6 ([DIŠ *i-na*] SAG.DU-*šú* KÚM *ṣa-ri-iḫ*) shows and has now been demonstrated by Heeßel, AOAT 43.162–163. Previously, Labat, *TDP* 25 n. 44 had suggested and then rejected the correct reading in favor of *nuppuḫ*: "it is swollen" (followed by Biggs, *RLA* 6.210 and *CAD* N 268b), which makes no sense in this context.
37. For the interpretation of KI.TA as "plantar surface," see Adamson, *JRAS* 1981.128.
38. Note also a similar reference to *aḫḫāzu* (DPS III C obv. 48–49 = *TDP* 22/24:48–49). Labat, *TDP* 24:49 has Labaṣu (^{d}DIM$_{10}$.ME.A); Goetze's copy, however, has ^{d}DIM$_{10}$.ME.LAGAB or *Aḫḫāzu*, and this reading has been confirmed by collations (Heeßel and Scurlock). The prognosis given in this latter text is: ⌜(If)⌝ he is an old man (lit. "if his days are near"), [he will die].
39. For a discussion of this term, see Heeßel, AOAT 43.191.
40. The reading follows *CAD* K 374b.
41. On the reading and interpretation, which can be slightly strengthened by reading his GIG TI-*uṭ-ma* TI GIG as GIG TI U_4-*ma* TI GIG, see Heeßel, AOAT 43.191.
42. See also DPS XVI:67′–68′ (AOAT 43.178).
43. See also *BAM* 3 ii 27–28//*BAM* 480 iii 8//*BAM* 9:23–24.
44. That is, falling out; for the expression, see *CAD* A/1.347b s.v. *āliku* mng. c.
45. See *CAD* Š/3.371–373. Goetze, *JCS* 9.12–13 quotes Landsberger, *ZA* 42.159 to the effect that *šuruppû* means "ice cold" and that it therefore identifies tetanus or meningitis (cerebrospinal fever). However, there is nothing about a sensation of "ice cold" that specifically identifies either of these diseases. Kämmerer, *UF* 27.165 argues that *šuruppû* refers specifically to the fever of smallpox. However, this and many other of Kämmerer's identifications are predicated on the assumption that an Old Babylonian recitation originally published by A. Goetze is a systematic description of an epidemic outbreak of smallpox. Although a few recitations do describe single diseases, many, including this one, were clearly intended for multiple uses (see Introduction under Retrospective Diagnosis).
46. See also DPS XXXVII A obv. 8–9 = *TDP* 212/214:8–9.

47. That is, lukecold, so to speak.

48. For other references to cold (without explicit mention of heat or fever), see *BAM* 231 i 1–18; *LKA* 102 obv. 18–22; DPS III C obv. 25 = *TDP* 20:25; DPS IV B r. 22//E iv 6a = *TDP* 44 r. 45//*SpTU* 3.88 iv 6a; DPS V G 5 = *TDP* 50 G 5; DPS VI A obv. 3 = *TDP* 54:3; DPS VII A obv. 29 = *TDP* 62:29; DPS IX A 36//B obv. 35 = *TDP* 74:36; DPS X B r. 7 = *TDP* 88 r. 7; DPS XI A obv. 45, 46 = *TDP* 92:45, 46; DPS XI A obv. 47, 51 = *TDP* 94:47, 51; DPS XIII B i 31′//D 4 = *TDP* 114 i 35′; DPS XIII B i 52′–53′//F 11//G_2 2 = *TDP* 116 i 56′–57′; DPS XIV A iv 15, 17–18//K 9 = *TDP* 144 iv 50′, 52′–53′; DPS XVII:77 (AOAT 43.202); DPS XXII:61 (AOAT 43.256); DPS XL A 34 = *TDP* 220:34; DPS XIX/XX:29′ (AOAT 43.228); DPS XXVI:45′–47′ (AOAT 43.282).

49. The reading follows *CAD* K 374b.

50. For other references, see *BAM* 66 r. 10′//*AMT* 45/1:6′//*AMT* 14/7:7; *AMT* 27/3:1–3; *BAM* 315 iii 39//*BAM* 314 obv. 4′–5′//*STT* 95 ii 63; *BAM* 232 i 1′–23′; *BAM* 438 obv. 5–14; *BAM* 445:10–16; *CTN* 4.72 vi 14–16 (Kinnier Wilson, *Iraq* 19.40–49 [ND 4368]); *LKA* 88 obv. 1–9//*LKA* 87 obv. 1′–10′; StBoT 36.40 obv. 3′–5′; *STT* 89:96–101, 196–198 (Stol, *Epilepsy* 97); DPS III C r. 22–23 = *TDP* 28:82–83 (cf. *KAR* 211 obv. 7–10); DPS X B r. 5 = *TDP* 88 r. 5; DPS XVII:77 (AOAT 43.202).

51. For other references, see *BAM* 344:6; *STT* 273 iii 6′–7′//*BAM* 358 ii 17′–18′ (cf. *SpTU* 4.129 ii 10–11, iii 21, 34, iv 13–14); *BAM* 183:31; *BAM* 377 iii 7; *SpTU* 3.106 i 4.

52. Adamson, *JRAS* 1979.3–4 nn. 22, 25 has a number of further suggestions for malaria with which we do not concur. For discussion of the relevant passages, see above under BIPHASIC FEVER and below under ENTERIC FEVER, in Chapter 4 under SECONDARY SYPHILIS, in Chapter 9 under EXTRAOCULAR MUSCLES: Periorbital Cellulitis, in Chapter 13 under MIGRAINE HEADACHE and TRAUMA TO THE HEAD: skull fracture, in Chapter 17 under TEETHING, in Chapter 19 under *li*ʾ*bu* fevers (typhus or typhoid).

53. Newton and Warrell, *Ann. Neurol.* 43.695–702.

54. Interesting in view of the presence of fever blisters in malaria is the fact that Nergal's name is written ^{d}Ù/U_4.BU.BU.UL: "god of *bubu*ʾ*tu*-blisters," in several god lists [*CAD* B 301a s.v. *bubu*ʾ*tu* mng. c].

55. Compare *STT* 89:120–123 (Stol, *Epilepsy* 93).

56. Compare *STT* 89:128–132 (Stol, *Epilepsy* 93). For other references, see DPS XI A obv. 24//B 23 = *TDP* 90:24//*SpTU* 1.34:23.

57. For probable cases of chronic malaria in Coptic mummies found in Egypt, see Ruffer, *J. Path. Bact.* 18.149–162.

58. See also DPS X A obv. 50 = *TDP* 86:50.

59. The Akkadian word, like the English, refers to the outside as well as the inside. In addition to the throat proper, the *kirru* appears to extend as far as the clavicles. For references, see *CAD* K 410–411 s.v. *kirru* B.

60. Lit. "fallen" or "attacked (by something)."

61. According to the commentary *SpTU* 1.31:27, this is because of the cold.

62. See also DPS X A obv. 46, 47 = *TDP* 86:46, 47.

63. See *AHw* 734a s.v. *napāqu*.

64. See also DPS X A obv. 35, 36, 37 = *TDP* 84:35, 36, 37.

65. See also DPS X A obv. 38 = *TDP* 84:38.

66. Adamson, *JRAS* 1984.4–5 argues that this and the preceding reference are to problems caused by diphtheria. We believe, however, that these texts are describing stridor, and the struggles to breathe in a patient with epiglottitis. Diphtheria, with its oral lesions and odor, appears to fall under the term *bu*ʾ*šānu* (see below).

67. See *SpTU* 1.44:62, 68, 75; *BAM* 543 iii 40′, 53′, 63′, iv 3; *SpTU* 1.44:40; *BAM* 379 iv 18; *BAM* 543 iv 6, 11; BM 66560 r. 7′; *SpTU* 1.44:51, cf. 48; BM 66560 r. 3′.

68. *SpTU* 1.44:69–70//*BAM* 28 r. 3′–5′//*BAM* 29:18′–22′//*BAM* 533:77–80//*BAM* 543 iii 65′–67′. The interpretation of *nurzu* and *nurbu* as "hard and soft palates" is preferable to W. Farber's, *JNES* 49.315 "soft cheek pockets."

69. *SpTU* 1.44:65–66//*BAM* 29:6′–10′//*BAM* 543 iii 58′–59′//*BAM* 533:50–52. See also *BAM* 538 ii 52′–55′; BM 67158 obv. 9′; BM 66560 obv. 1, r. 7′; *STT* 279:10.

70. Kämmerer, *UF* 27.157 argues that *bu*ʾ*šānu* refers to nasal infections encountered in smallpox. However, unlike *bu*ʾ*šānu*, smallpox does not cause loose teeth. This and many other of Kämmerer's identifications are predicated on the assumption that an Old Babylonian recitation originally published by Goetze is a systematic description of an epidemic outbreak of smallpox. Although a few recitations do describe single diseases, many, including this one, were clearly intended for multiple uses (see Introduction under Retrospective Diagnosis). *CAD* B 350–351 (followed by Volk, *OrNS* 68.27–28) identifies *bu*ʾ*šānu* as leprosy, citing

the same Old Babylonian multiuse recitation that Kämmerer uses to argue for smallpox, as well as others in which *girgiššu* (erysipelas; see Chapter 10) also appears, as well as a "group vocabulary." The "group vocabulary" is a lexical text whose purpose is to list three different ancient syndromes which (because they stink) can all be referred to with the Sumerogram for "stinking" (on this point see also Köcher, "Lepra" 30). *CAD* B 350–351 also mentions the "stark description of the symptoms" in a text whose untranslated section makes explicit reference to the hard and soft palates, and both of the cited references to "secretions from the ravaged nostrils" are clearly talking about salivation from the mouth. In fact, as with other references not cited by the *CAD*, the major areas affected by *bu'šānu* are the mouth and throat, sites that are seldom if ever infected by Hansen's bacillus. On these points, see also Köcher, *Fs. Goerke* 20–21 and Volk, *OrNS* 68.27–28.

71. Pangas, *Bull.Hist.Med.* 73.205–206 believes that all *bu'šānu* references are to scurvy. Kinnier Wilson, *Diseases in Antiquity* 193–194 and *RA* 60.52–54 also interprets *bu'šānu* as scurvy. He notes the lung symptoms (*Diseases in Antiquity* 199), but attributes them to pneumonia secondary to scurvy. Although this is possible, Köcher's suggestion of "diphtheria" (Köcher, Fs. Goerke 20–21) for these references seems more likely. See also Cadelli, *Ktèma* 22.32. Kinnier Wilson, *Jour.Roy.Soc.Med.* 89.138 defers to Köcher on diphtheria, but suggests bronchiectasis as an alternative possibility. However, although bronchiectasis may be associated with fetid breath, it lacks the grayish membrane or grayish coloration of the gums that seems to be associated with *bu'šānu.*

72. See also *SpTU* 1.44:20; *BAM* 543 ii 11, 61', iv 10; BM 66560 obv. 4'; *BAM* 159 v 31; *SpTU* 1.44:35, cf. 42, 44, 46.

73. See also *BAM* 558 i 14'//*BAM* 44:14'.

74. See also *BAM* 543 ii 24; *SpTU* 1.44:16.

75. See also BM 67158 obv. 4', 7'//BM 66560 obv. 3, 5//*SpTU* 1.44:48, 50.

76. See *CT* 14.23 (K 259):4//*BAM* 1 i 4.

77. See *AHw* 303a s.v. *ḫabāru* II.

78. Fincke, *Augenleiden* 211 interprets this text as referring to a disease of the eyes characterized by pus. However, this is based on a radically differing, and probably incorrect, transliteration (Scurlock, *AfO* 48/49.242–244).

79. See *BAM* 1 ii 25; *CT* 14.31 [D.T. 136]:5; Labat and Tournay, *RA* 40.116 obv. 15; *STT* 92 ii 8, 20–22; *BAM* 379 iv 11; *BAM* 36:5'; *BAM* 44:18'; *BAM* 558 i 23'; *AMT* 54/1 obv. 8'; BM 78963:36; cf. *BAM* 556 ii 67'//*BAM* 42:10.

80. See also *AMT* 50/3:1–2; *AMT* 52/9:6'; BM 76515 r. 11'; *BAM* 549 iv 12; *AMT* 81/1 iii 17'–18'//*BAM* 551 iii 2'.

81. See also *BAM* 554 i 3'; BM 78963:25; *BAM* 549 iv 6–8//*ABRT* 2.11 obv.! ii 21–24//*BAM* 553 obv. 1'–2'; *BAM* 548 iv 14'.

82. The word used to describe this, *kiṣirtu*, is from a verb which means "to concentrate" (*CAD* K 260–261 s.v. *kaṣāru* mng. 3). Formally, it is an adjective modifying an unexpressed feminine substantive, presumably *ru'tu*: "phlegm." With Heeßel, AOAT 43.266, this is a form of sputum and not oliguria, as Adamson, *JRAS* 1981.126, maintains.

83. See also *BAM* 1 ii 37–40; *BAM* 379 iv 6; *BAM* 421 i' 38'; *BAM* 423 i 2'; *STT* 92 ii 15–19; *STT* 93:28; BM 78963:50, 52.

84. "⌜From⌝ the lungs (come). . . *šīqu*" (*SpTU* 1.43:20–21). Note also that in *BAM* 1, Ú *ši-qí* (ii 37–40) appears between Ú *su-a-lim* (ii 27–33) and Ú NA *šá sah-ḫa* GIG (ii 41), a good indication that a lung problem is indicated. A hemerological text warns "he should not eat *bišru* or *saḫlû* (or else) *šīqu* will afflict him" (Labat, *Hémérologies* 170:42–43, 178:24–25; ND 5545:25 [Hulin, *Iraq* 21.46–53]). The analogy is presumably between the color of the phlegm and the color of the plants in question. The *CAD* translates *šīqu* as "eczema" based on DPS XIII B ii 34 = *TDP* 120 ii 34. The reference in question is, however, to phlegm *in* the abdomen, as the next cited reference to *šīqu* being produced by the lips (DPS XIII B ii 31//G_2 28+G_1 11 = *TDP* 120 ii 31) shows. Note also Fincke, *Augenleiden* 148, who suggests "bronchitis."

85. Note also *BAM* 1 ii 42–45; *BAM* 2 obv. 7'–8'; *BAM* 575 iii 21; *STT* 92 ii 12–14; *BAM* 550 iv 8//*BAM* 549 iv 19.

86. This term is derived from a verb that means "to vomit blood" (see Chapter 6). Labat, *RLA* 4.523 agrees that *ḫaḫḫu* means a wet cough, although he does not mention blood as the source of the wetness. Adamson, *JRAS* 1979.4 argues that *ḫaḫḫu* was a nonproductive cough. However, this argument presupposes that the term *ḫaḫḫu* was meant to be contrasted with *su'ālu*, which Adamson believes to be a productive cough, and

that the reference quoted above is to coughing accompanying pulmonary edema in left-sided cardiac failure. In fact, there is a very clear reference to a nonproductive "dry" cough, and that uses the term *suʾālu* (see 8.70). Moreover, the idea that *BAM* 547 iv 13′ is a reference to pulmonary edema is based on a transliteration that omits the word *bread*. For our suggestion of a reference describing pulmonary edema that mentions a persistent *suʾālu*-cough, see Chapter 8 with 8.93.

87. IM could potentially mean "wind" as well as "clay"; however, it was noted by ancient observers that "solidified" lungs did not take in "wind." [DIŠ ḪAR] *up-pu-uq-ma* IM NU IGI-*ḫar*: "If the lung is solidified so that it will not accept wind" (*KAR* 151:37, 39).

88. The translation of KAK.TI/*sikkat ṣēli* follows *CAD* S 246–247. *AHw* 1042a s.v. *sikkatu* I mng. b translates "breastbone," which is rather strange since references clearly indicate that there were more than one of them in any given animal.

89. See also *BAM* 571 ii 16′//*AMT* 64/3:6′; BM 78963:47, 78; *BAM* 42:56 (cf. *SpTU* 1.64:1); BM 79308:17.

90. We cannot concur with Adamson's position (*JRAS* 1981.126) that *kiṣirtu* ("thick sputum") when applied to symptoms of the chest fits in "quite satisfactorily" with a clinical condition of the kidneys (low output, oliguria). He further argues that when the *kiṣirtu* is described as "dark," as in this reference, it is a reference to blackwater fever, a severe kidney complication of malignant malaria. There is nothing in this reference to suggest malaria.

91. The Aramaic cognate means "to sigh."

92. See also DPS XXII:28, 29–30 (AOAT 43.254).

93. See also *BAM* 434 i 13′–15′.

94. Compare also "[If his skull], his ⌜breast⌝ and his upper back are continually feverish, *kišpu* afflicts him" ([DIŠ UGU-*šú* GA]BA-*su u ša-šal-la-šu* KÚM.KÚM ⌜UŠ$_{11}$.ZU⌝ DIB-*su* [DPS III A obv. 11]).

95. Note also DPS XXII:1, 4 (AOAT 43.250/251).

96. See also *BAM* 564 ii 14′–15′; *AMT* 45/6:6–7, 9; *BAM* 575 iv 11; *BAM* 174 obv. 28′–29′; *BAM* 579 i 40–41, 44//*BAM* 52:39–40, 44//*BAM* 67:1′–4′, 9′.

97. See also *AMT* 45/6:6–7; *CTN* 4.114 r. 7′–9′; DPS XXII:29–30 (AOAT 43.254).

98. See also *BAM* 44:9′–10′//*BAM* 165 ii 7′–8′; DPS XXII:28 (AOAT 43.254). Note also *AMT* 45/6:5.

99. See also *AMT* 51/2:7–8; *AMT* 51/5 r. 7.

100. See also *BAM* 557:20′–21′.

101. Restored on the basis of *BAM* 520 ii 9′–10′.

102. For the term, see also BM 78963:53. *Bitqu* is from the verb *batāqu*: "to cut through," and can refer to the cut made in the bank of a canal to let the water flow into a field as well as to the canal that carries the diverted water. For references, see *CAD* B 277–279.

103. The idea that incense was to "swirl" through the house prior to the operation (Kinnier Wilson, *Journ.Roy.Soc. Med.* 89.136) is based on a mistranslation of this term.

104. This is counting from the top down. Labat, *Journal Asiatique* 242.246–248 argues that the ribs were counted from the bottom up. This is, however, based on the erroneous assumption that the text refers to a liver abscess (an interpretation followed, inter alia, by Kinnier Wilson, *Diseases in Antiquity* 195, *Journ.Roy.Soc.Med.* 89.136 and *JNES* 27.244). The liver at this level is very deep, and draining an abscess through the chest wall would involve going into the pleural space and lungs, a very difficult and extremely dangerous maneuver.

105. See Krafeld-Daugherty, *Fs Dietrich* 257.

106. Salo et al., *Proc.Nat.Acad.Sci.* (USA) 91.2091–2094.

107. On the identification of this text as bronchitis, see also Sigerist, *A History of Medicine* 480–481 and Adamson, *JRAS* 1974.103. Adamson further argues that the "windpipe" (GI.GÍD ḪAR.MEŠ) of this text, which Labat transcribed as *malīl ḫašê*, refers specifically to the trachea in contrast to the *embūb ḫašê* which he argues to be the bronchus on grounds of its association with the lungs. However, *malīl ḫašê*, is simply an alternative (and incorrect) transcription of GI.GÍD ḪAR.MEŠ: *embūb ḫašê*. All of the texts cited use the same term and even if they did not, *malīl ḫašê* would still mean "flute of the lungs" and should thus have encountered the same objections as *embūb ḫašê* for "trachea."

108. See also K 3010+K 6187+K 13346+DT 86 v 8′–9′//*BAM* 361:37–38; cf. *BAM* 372 iii 14′.

109. Kinnier Wilson, *Medical History* 34.187, 190, 195 suggests that this text is describing a patient with a nocturnal grand mal seizure with bowel incontinence. As Kinnier Wilson also notes, bowel incontinence is unusual in grand mal seizures, and this text describes not simple incontinence but diarrhea and wasting of the limbs, problems that are not associated with seizures.

110. Compare also DPS XIII B ii 13–14 = *TDP* 118 ii 13–14; DPS XIII G_2 r. 7, 8 = *TDP* 122 iii 14, 15.

111. The suggested reading is based on collation of the text.

112. Geller, *RAI* 28.193 interprets this as "he constantly needs to urinate." We find no basis for this interpretation.

113. See also DPS XV:33 (AOAT 43.152); cf. DPS XIII A 2.

114. See Heeßel, AOAT 43.187.

115. See also DPS VII B obv. 17′, r. 1 = *TDP* 64:56′, 57′; DPS XVIII:44′ (AOAT 43.219); DPS XL B 70 = *TDP* 226:69.

116. See also Fincke, *Augenleiden* 166.

117. See also DPS XL B 117 = *TDP* 230:123(!).

118. See Volk, *OrNS* 68.21.

119. Lit. "his heart does not rise in him."

120. Restored from DPS III C r. 5–6//E_1 r. 6–7+E_2 r. 2–3 = *TDP* 26:65–66.

121. The restoration is suggested by the commentary *STT* 403:51, which explains this as meaning *ik*-[*ki*]-*lu* ŠUB.ŠUB-*di*: "he continually lets out a ⌜mournful cry⌝."

122. In medical texts, this expression is used of the stomach (with or without explicit mention) and means simply "upset." There is no justification (differently *CAD* A/2.423–424 s.v. *ašāšu* A mng. 3a) for seeing what would literally mean "worried" or "disturbed" as a synonym for pain, let alone "spasms."

123. See Stol, *Epilepsy* 61; Köcher, *Fs. Goerke* 29.

124. Kinnier Wilson, *Medical History* 34.190, 195 interprets this text as a reference to Todd's paralysis. It is difficult to understand how he could have reached this conclusion.

125. Compare also DPS XVII:73 (AOAT 43.202).

126. For this interpretation of *redû*, see *CAD* R 239a s.v. *redû* A mng. 7.

127. See also *BAM* 240:33′, 36′; *BAM* 395:1, 5; Beckman and Foster, *Mem. Sachs* 19 no. 17 ii 5′; DPS XIII D r. 18, 19 = *TDP* 128 iv 27′, 28′.

128. For this interpretation of *redû*, see *CAD* R 239a s.v. *redû* A mng. 7.

129. Labat, *RLA* 3.231 believes that this term means ptosis abdominalis (sagging of the abdominal wall), but provides no evidence to support this opinion.

130. See also *BAM* 145:1–17//*BAM* 146:29′–38′.

131. Note also *BAM* 240:34′ and DPS XIII D r. 11 = *TDP* 128 iv 20′ which appears to say "flowing of blood."

132. Kinnier Wilson, *Jour.Roy.Soc.Med.* 89.135–136; *JNES* 27.244 interprets this and similar texts as amoebic dysentery. We agree that it may include an amoebic etiology, but there is nothing that excludes other causes of dysentery.

133. See also *BAM* 159 iii 10–11.

134. See also DPS XL A 6–7//B 7–8//C 8–9 = *TDP* 218:6–7.

135. The commentary, *SpTU* 1.41:6 explains that this is because Lamaštu has "married" him.

136. See Heeßel, AOAT 43.186–188 for previous attempts to identify UD.DA = *ṣētu*. The most commonly suggested identification is "heat stroke" (see, e.g., Köcher, *Fs. Goerke* 24; Stol, *Epilepsy* 80–81; Kinnier Wilson, *Iraq* 18.144; Heeßel, AOAT 43.186–188). Adamson, *JRAS* 1984.11–12 offers heat stroke with possible concomitant malaria (in the wet season) and severe sunburn (in the dry season) to explain *ṣētu*. However, the relative importance in the references of gastrointestinal and pulmonary complaints (diarrhea, cough, sputum production, etc.) does not fit any of these diagnoses. Kinnier Wilson, *Jour.Roy.Soc.Med.* 89.136 is of the opinion that *ṣētu* has a single cause, namely, tuberculosis. Although it would not be surprising if some cases of gastrointestinal tuberculosis were included, it seems highly unlikely that tuberculosis, a disease that is primarily pulmonary in location, would be the sole cause of *ṣētu*, a condition that is primarily gastrointestinal in nature. Geller and Cohen (*Kidney International* 47.1815 n. 11) suggest an alternative diagnosis of liver disease due to worms for *ṣētu*, but typical liver signs and symptoms are not found in the references. Kämmerer, *UF* 27.164 believes that *ṣētu* is dehydration associated with smallpox. Although there may be dehydration in smallpox, dehydration is more commonly associated with conditions that cause vomiting and diarrhea. This and many other of Kämmerer's identifications are predicated on the assumption that an Old Babylonian recitation originally published by Goetze is a systematic description of an epidemic outbreak of smallpox. Although a few recitations do describe single diseases, many, including this one, were clearly intended for multiple uses (see Introduction under Retrospective Diagnosis).

137. See also *BAM* 146:43′–46′.

138. *CAD* S 340 restores *BAM* 145:13 as "*su'ālu*-cough" but note that *BAM* 146:36′ appears to have *ina a-la-li-šú*: "when he tries to ululate."

139. Kinnier Wilson, *Journ.Roy.Soc.Med.* 89.136 suggests a diagnosis of pulmonary tuberculosis for this text, with secondary tuberculosis of the intestines as cause for the diarrhea. This reference could be describing pulmonary tuberculosis with secondary tuberculosis of the intestines, but since the process seems more acute than chronic, we favor enteric fever with secondary pneumonia as the explanation. What Kinnier-Wilson translates as "fire-scorch" and interprets as cyanosis is a reference to burning internal fever. For references in ancient Mesopotamian medical texts to cyanosis, see Chapter 8 with 8.91–8.92.

140. See also DPS XXXI:23′–24′ (AOAT 43.343); DPS XXXI:6–7 (AOAT 43.342); DPS XVII:8–9 (AOAT 43.195); *BAM* 174 obv. 21′//*BAM* 66 r. 6′//*AMT* 14/7:3; *BAM* 66 obv. 21–22; DPS XXXI:12–13 (AOAT 43.342)//*BAM* 66 obv. 10–11); cf. *ARM* 26/1.261:13–16. Note also DPS 28′–29′, 30′–31′ (AOAT 43.343) (fever blisters).

141. See also DPS XXXI:35′–37′ (AOAT 43.343); *BAM* 66 r. 12′//*AMT* 45/1:8′//*AMT* 14/7:9.

142. TAB.BA might be expected in this context, but the copies of *BAM* 3 and *BAM* 9 both show a very clear *-ma*.

143. See also DPS XVIII:39′ (AOAT 43.219); *BAM* 66 obv. 13–14; *BAM* 66 r. 4′//*AMT* 14/7:1; *BAM* 578 iv 47.

144. See also DPS XXXI:1–2 (AOAT 43.342); *SpTU* 3.106 i 18.

145. See also DPS XXXIII:101 (AOAT 43.357); cf. DPS XIV G 13 = *TDP* 144 iv 22′); DPS XIV C_2 iii 23–24, 25//F 11–12, 13; *SpTU* 1.36 obv. 6–7; cf. DPS XVI:29 (AOAT 43.175); DPS XVI:78′–79′ (AOAT 43.179).

146. The term employed refers to the femur head and adjacent soft tissue (see Adamson, *JRAS* 1979.2).

147. "Body hurting" (is Sumerian) for "gnawing" (SU.GÚ : *ki-iṣ-ṣat* [*SpTU* 1.51 r. 5). "Sore muscle" (is Sumerian) for "gnawing" (SA.GIG : *ki-iṣ-ṣa-tum* [*GCCI* 4.406:17]).

148. See also *BAM* 52:72 (cf. *BAM* 403 r. 7); *AMT* 45/6:12–13.

149. See also DPS XXXI:52′–54′ (AOAT 43.344); DPS XXXI:46′–47′ (AOAT 43.344); *BAM* 146:43′–46′; *BAM* 174 obv. 23′//*BAM* 66 r. 8′//*AMT* 14/7:5.

150. See also *BAM* 564 ii 14′–15′; *AMT* 45/6:6–7; *BAM* 579 i 40–41, 44//*BAM* 52:39–40, 44//*BAM* 67:1′–4′, 9′.

151. See also *AMT* 45/6:9; *BAM* 575 iv 11.

152. See also DPS XVI:46′ (AOAT 43.176); DPS XXXI:3–4 (AOAT 43.342). Kinnier Wilson, *Journ.Roy.Soc.Med.* 89.136 believes *TDP* 150:40′ to refer to hemoptysis in tuberculosis.

153. For the reading, see Heeßel, AOAT 43.190. The expression *ḫīṭu laššu* or *ḫīṭu yānu* appears not infrequently in Neo-Assyrian and Neo-Babylonian letters; it means something on the order of "no harm done" or "it is of no consequence." For references, see *CAD* Ḫ 210 s.v. *ḫīṭu* A mng. 1. For the interpretation, see also Ritter, *AS* 16.302 (quoting Landsberger).

154. See also DPS XXXI:9–10 (AOAT 43.342).

155. For the reading, see Heeßel, AOAT 43.190. The expression *ḫīṭu laššu* or *ḫīṭu yānu* appears not infrequently in Neo-Assyrian and Neo-Babylonian letters; it means something on the order of "no harm done" or "it is of no consequence." For references, see *CAD* Ḫ s.v. *ḫīṭu* A mng. 1. For the interpretation, see also Ritter, *AS* 16.302 (quoting Landsberger).

156. See also *BAM* 416 obv. 10′–11′; *BAM* 480 ii 26, 35.

157. See also *BAM* 3 i 20//*BAM* 480 ii 19//*AMT* 5/3 i 8′; *BAM* 516 ii 6′//*AMT* 18/4:6′; *BAM* 515 i 9.

158. Adamson, *JRAS* 1979.4 n. 25 cites this text as "evidence of fevers associated with chills, rigors, and cold sweats," suggesting the presence of endemic malaria in ancient Mesopotamia. He also argues (Adamson, *JRAS* 1981.126 n. 20) that "burning of *ṣētu*" refers to the "onset of malaria." With neither assertion do we concur. For possible descriptions of malaria in ancient texts, see Chapter 3 under MALARIA.

159. Note also DPS XXXI:15 (AOAT 43.343).

160. Restorations are based on DPS XVI:81′–82′ (AOAT 43.179); see Heeßel, AOAT 43.350.

161. See Heeßel, AOAT 43.349.

162. See also DPS XXXI:9–10 (AOAT 43.342).

163. For the reading, see Heeßel, AOAT 43.190. The expression *ḫīṭu laššu* or *ḫīṭu yānu* appears not infrequently in Neo-Assyrian and Neo-Babylonian letters; it means something on the order of "no harm done" or "it is of no consequence." For references, see *CAD* Ḫ s.v. *ḫīṭu* A mng. 1. For the interpretation, see also Ritter, *AS* 16.302 (quoting Landsberger).

164. For the link between *liʾbu*, *ziʾpu*, and *diʾu*, see *SpTU* 1.38:10.

165. Jensen, KB 6/1.542–543 suggests that *diʾu* is malaria, but we disagree since *diʾu* presents with more gastrointestinal complaints than are normally associated with malaria. Moreover, *diʾu* is closely associated with *ṣētu*, which can be excluded as malaria because not only gastrointestinal complaints but also dehydration are prominent problems in this disease.

166. Note also *CAD* D 165–166.

167. The translation assumes an otherwise unattested form of *itūlu*. Heeßel, AOAT 43.270–271 takes this from *eṭēlu* the Dt of which *CAD* takes to mean "rejuvenate" and AHw "to become a fully powerful person" and which Heeßel interprets to mean "to reach puberty" (i.e., he has grown up and he is still becoming rigid). The interpretation is interesting, but seems a bit forced.

168. Adamson, *JRAS* 1979.4 n. 25 cites this text as "evidence of fevers associated with chills, rigors, and cold sweats," suggesting the presence of endemic malaria in ancient Mesopotamia. Adamson, *JRAS* 1984.11–12 w/ n. 90 narrows his diagnosis of this text to heat stroke with concomitant malignant malaria. However, nothing in this text provides information that would support either diagnosis, and it would be highly unlikely for a patient with malignant malaria to recover in seven days. For possible descriptions of malaria in ancient Mesopotamian texts, see Chapter 3 under MALARIA.

169. With *CAD* Q 183 B the *uq-ta-ta*$_5$ is not to be removed from this sentence and inserted into the previous line. Not only does this rearrangement of the text not improve the sense, but it disagrees with *both* text exemplars. Heeßel, AOAT 43.216–217 takes the opposite position.

170. It would appear from this that Labat's suggestion that the ideogram UD.DA should be translated "sécheresse" and TAB UD.DA, conventionally: "burning of *ṣētu*" as "fièvre de sécheresse" (*Manuel* no. 175) was probably correct. See also Goetze, *JCS* 9.13.

171. See also DPS XIX/XX:106′ (AOAT 43.232).

172. See also BM 78963:66; *SpTU* 1.63:8.

173. Note also *BAM* 114:5 (the urine is like *kasû* juice).

174. Restorations are based on *BAM* 579 i 40–41//*BAM* 52:39–40//*BAM* 67:1′–4′. See also *BAM* 112 ii 6′–7′; *BAM* 111 ii 15′–17′//*BAM* 159 i 15–17; *BAM* 396 i 14′.

175. Majno, *Healing Hand* 37–38 argues that ancient Mesopotamians could not possibly have understood the relationship between "wounds and symptoms." His evidence for this is the fact that Labat, *RLA* 3.231–233 has a single entry for "bumps" and "holes." The reason for the single entry is, however, that the German word *Geschwür* means "boil" or "abscess" as well as "ulcer." Akkadian clearly distinguishes ulcers from tumors (see Chapter 10). Moreover, the article cited, although technically on skin diseases (*Hautkrankheiten*), includes a discussion of body swelling, again because German has a single word (*Geschwulst*) to describe tumors and ascites or anasarca, and not because of any deficiencies in ancient Mesopotamian medicine.

176. Kinnier Wilson, *JNES* 53.111–115 argues that *samānu* is mycetoma, which he believes to be a fungal infection affecting the head and hands as well as the feet. In fact, mycetoma may be caused either by a fungus or by a specialized bacterium, *Actinomycosis*. Carrying firewood on the head (*JNES* 53.114) is an exclusively female task, whereas the typical victim of mycetoma is an adult male and, although lesions can occur on the leg, torso, hand, and face, the characteristic site for the disease is the foot. Since *samānu* is not typically associated with the foot, it is unlikely to be mycetoma. There is, in any case, already an excellent candidate for mycetoma in ancient texts, namely *muruṣ kabbarti* (see Chapter 3). *CAD* S 112b interprets *samānu* to mean ergotism on the grounds that there was also a *samānu* of grain (rejected by Biggs, *AuOr* 9.20). However, with Finkel, *Fs. Borger* 71–72, *samānu* simply means "red-like" which, in grain, refers to rust, and in people to a reddish coloration of the skin. *Samānu* cannot possibly be ergotism, since the characteristics of *samānu* (redness, heat, swelling, and pus) have no relationship to the findings in ergotism (gangrene). Labat, *RLA* 3.233 believes that *samānu* means heat rash. This seems unlikely since the description of *samānu* includes swelling and drainage, characteristics that would not usually be part of heat rash. Also, some texts describe wounds, where cellulitis would be a likely complication and heat rash would not. Kämmerer, *UF* 27.159–160 argues that *samānu* is the exanthem of smallpox. However, this and many other of Kämmerer's identifications are predicated on the assumption that an Old Babylonian recitation originally published by Goetze is a systematic description of an epidemic outbreak of smallpox. Although a few recitations do describe single diseases, many, including this one, were clearly intended for multiple uses (see Introduction under Retrospective Diagnosis).

177. See also *BAM* 1 ii 12–14, 16–20; *BAM* 324 i 8′, 15′; *BAM* 422 iii 8; BM 38583:3′, 11′; *KUB* 4.49 iii 4; Cavigneaux and al-Rawi, *Iraq* 55.104 A 7′; cf. DPS XXXIII:103 (AOAT 43.357).

178. See also *BAM* 494 i 38′.

179. Compare *BAM* 583 i 7′.

180. *CAD* M/1.351b, followed by Attia, *Histoire des sciences Médicales* 34.8, interprets this as a stroke, but the blood vessels in this example are not themselves "going" but making some sort of fluid (A.MEŠ) "go"; it should also be noted that this entry appears in a text that collects treatments for skin problems.

181. Landsberger, *MSL* 2.113–115 argued that *samānu* was a condition resulting from the bite of a homophonous *samānu*-insect, which he interpreted as a "tick" (*Argas persicus*). Tick bites, however, have a punctate appearance that does not fit with the description of *samānu*.

182. The Sumerian has SA.GÚ.

183. See Adamson, *RA* 84.31–32.

184. Cited in *CAD* N/2.248b s.v. *nipšu* A mng. 2.

185. Note *ABL* 392 obv. 8–r. 8 (Parpola, SAA 10 no. 319).

186. See also *BAM* 1 ii 53; *BAM* 421 i′ 24′; *CT* 14.37 (Rm 357):6; *STT* 92 iii 9′.

187. "His ear" (UZU.GIŠ-*šú*) with *CAD* B 4b s.v. *ba'āšu*. Read as ^{UZU}*giš-šú* by Labat, *RLA* 3.231b and translated "boil" and by *AHw* 94a s.v. *ba'āšu* and 288b s.v. *gilšu* and translated "hip (socket)."

188. Note also *BAM* 480 iv 1.

189. Haussperger, *Mem. Cagni* 446 considers this text to be describing angioneurotic edema. This seems an unlikely diagnosis since pain is not a common symptom in this disease and applied heat, although beneficial for an abscess, would be likely to worsen the lesions of angioneurotic edema.

190. Heeßel, AOAT 43.354, 360 interprets these signs as MÚD ŠUB: "it produces blood."

191. Note also *CTN* 4.116 obv. 27.

192. Fader and McGinnis, *Inf. Dis. Clinics of North America* 2/4.925–937.

193. See also *BAM* 32:18′ (with a white surface).

194. See also Fincke, *Augenleiden* 109; Attia, *Histoire des sciences Médicales* 34.7–8.

195. Goetze, *JCS* 9.13 believes, on the basis of the fact that *šaššaṭu* and *bennu* share a common Sumerogram, that *šaššaṭu* is a form of epilepsy. *Bennu* is not actually epilepsy but does refer to seizures of infectious origin (see below). *Šaššaṭu* has a wide variety of possible Sumerograms, some of which it shares with two other terms that have nothing to do with epilepsy, namely, *rapādu* and *samānu*. All that a common Sumerogram can tell us is that the terms have something important in common. With *šaššaṭu* and *bennu* that something is rather obviously the fact that the texts describe in *šaššaṭu* movements that resemble the tonic contractions of epileptic seizures but without any of the other symptoms that are normally associated with epilepsy (see Chapter 13). With *rapādu* ("wandering about", i.e., shock; see Chapter 14) and *samānu* (soft tissue infection; see above), the only obvious connection is that all three were known to result from trauma.

196. Labat, *RLA* 3.199 believes that *šaššaṭu* means rheumatism. Although some of the texts mention pain that could possibly be associated with the joints, this diagnosis fails to explain the jerking and spasms that are a prominent part of this illness. Kämmerer, *UF* 27.164–165 argues that *šaššaṭu* means "bedridden with pains in the legs" in the context of smallpox. He fails to explain what would cause "bedridden" patients to suffer from muscular spasms and contractions. This and many other of Kämmerer's identifications are predicated on the assumption that an Old Babylonian recitation originally published by Goetze is a systematic description of an epidemic outbreak of smallpox. Although a few recitations do describe single diseases, many, including this one, were clearly intended for multiple uses (see Introduction under Retrospective Diagnosis).

197. The parallel passage in Tablet XXXIII has *šá-aš-*[*šá-ṭu*].

198. DPS XXXIII:94 (AOAT 43.357) has "inguinal regions" instead of "back."

199. For other references, see *BAM* 129 iv 3′; *BAM* 129 iv 6′–7′; *BAM* 129 iv 14′–15′//*AMT* 31/2 r. 5′; *BAM* 129 iv 19′; *BAM* 131 obv. 1; *BAM* 171:14′; *BAM* 1 iii 22–23; *BAM* 379 iv 17//*SpTU* 3.106 iv 5; *BAM* 422 ii 10′.

200. Sign looks more like DU (coll.).

201. The passage has been collated.

202. Lit. "to his completion."

203. This is presumably a pun, since *rabû* ("great") is phonetically similar to *ra'ābu* ("to tremble").

204. Compare the "shaking" left temple and hot right temple in DPS IV B obv. 23 = *TDP* 34:23 (19.82).

205. The commentary *STT* 403:48 explains this term as KI.TA LI.DUR-*sa re-di*: "abutting the lower part of her navel."

206. See also DPS XIII B ii 20,21 = *TDP* 118 ii 20, 21.

207. For other references to abdominal wounds, see DPS XV:52 (AOAT 43.153); cf. DPS XIV A iii 10–11//C_2 iii 3//I 6–7 = *TDP* 140 iii 44′–45′); DPS XIII B i 32′, 33′//D obv. 5, 6 = *TDP* 114 i 36′, 37′; DPS XIII D r. 3, 4, 5 = *TDP* 126 iv 12′, 13′, 14′; DPS XIV A iii 16 = *TDP* 140 iii 50′ (cf. *MDP* 57.11 ii 2); DPS XIV A iii 20, 21–22 = *TDP* 140 iii 54′, 55′–56′.

208. The term *ḫašû* almost always refers to the lungs (see AHw 335a s.v. *ḫašû* II) but can sometimes refer more generally to the complex of lungs, liver, and spleen (for lexical references, see *CAD* Ḫ 143b).

209. See also DPS XXXVII A obv. 19 = *TDP* 214:19. Note also DPS XIII B i 13′ = *TDP* 112 i 17′.

210. See also DPS XIII B ii 37 = *TDP* 120 ii 37.

211. See also DPS XIII B ii 46//G_2 37 + G_1 20 = *TDP* 120 ii 46.

212. This expression was apparently sometimes used to describe untreated diabetes (see Chapter 7). Diabetic ketoacidosis, a metabolic complication of untreated diabetes, may cause severe abdominal symptoms that resemble the picture of acute peritonitis.

213. ÚḪ is usually "phlegm." However, when used with KÚM ("fever") it is to be read as a form of *ṣarāḫu* as the parallel between DPS III C r. 10–11//E_1 r. 11–12 + E_2 r. 7–8 = *TDP* 26:70–71 (DIŠ *ina* SAG.DU-*šú* KÚM ÚḪ) and *KAR* 211 obv. 4–6 ([DIŠ *i-na*] SAG.DU-*šú* KÚM *ṣa-ri-iḫ*) shows and has now been demonstrated by Heeßel, AOAT 43.162–163. Previously, Labat, *TDP* 25 n. 44 had suggested and then rejected the correct reading in favor of *nuppuḫ*: "it is swollen" (followed by Biggs, *RLA* 6.210 and *CAD* N 268b), which makes no sense in this context.

214. The translation assumes a direct connection with the Arabic cognate that means "to become thick or dense" (Lane, *Arabic-English Lexicon* 2591). *CAD* K 304b s.v. *katātu* mng. 1b interprets this as the patient's flesh collapsing. Von Soden *AHw* 465a, followed by Heeßel, AOAT 43.259 translates "vibrate."

215. The translation assumes a D-stem from *ḫâlu*.

216. See also DPS XI A r. 51 = *TDP* 98 r. 51.

217. Tsukimoto, *Priests and Officials* 199–200:53–54 and 58–59.

218. See *CAD* G 46a under *garābu*, lex. section.

219. A recitation of this sort (DPS III A obv. 1) was cast over the ancient physician before commencing the diagnosis of illnesses to protect him, since the *āšipu* was going to have to touch his patients.

220. Kinnier Wilson, *RA* 60.49–51; *Diseases in Antiquity* 206–207; "Medicine in . . . Old Testament (times)" 354–355. We agree that the white lesions could be the depigmented skin of tuberculoid leprosy. However, we have reached no conclusions on the suggestion that the punctate lesions are in patients with lepromatous leprosy, since the characteristic lesions can be small but are not typically tiny. Kinnier Wilson, *Journ.Roy.Soc. Med.* 89.139 proposes an alternative suggestion that the "white spots" might be due to leukoderma (see Chapter 10). He proposes no alternative for the punctate lesions.

221. Gorbach, Bartlett, and Blacklow, *Infectious Diseases* 1568.

222. Adamson, *RA* 82.167–169 believes that the term *ṣiḫḫu* means "lymph node." However, the term was applied to lesions on the liver, gall bladder, and forehead, locations that lack lymph nodes.

223. The text has been collated.

224. Heeßel, AOAT 43.368 tentatively suggests restoring Ningeštinanna. However, the sign that precedes the NA on *BAM* 409 obv. 29′ does not look at all like a GEŠTIN. Instead, it appears to be a RIN, suggesting a restoration of either "curse" (NAM.RIN.NA), or more probably an ingredient in the treatment such as *kurkānû* (KUR.GI.RIN.NA).

225. Heeßel, AOAT 43.360 translates: "he (the patient) is raised up and is unable to get himself up, etc." However, the verb is active (with direct object) and not passive as this translation would require.

226. Restorations are based on *BAM* 409 obv. 33′–36′.

227. On this reference as a description of bubonic plague, see also Köcher, *AUWE* 10.212.

228. See Heeßel, AOAT 43.368 but note that the passage has been collated.

229. See also *BAM* 1 i 40; *BAM* 423 i 31′.

230. See also *KAR* 211 obv. 19–20; DPS III A r. 9′–12′//C r. 32–35 = *TDP* 28:92–95; DPS XVIII:21–23 (AOAT 43.219); DPS XXXIII:80 (AOAT 43.357); DPS XXXIII:114 (AOAT 43.358); *BAM* 584 ii 25′–26′, 29′.

231. This is the ancient Mesopotamian god of the moon.

232. See Dunham, *ZA* 75.234–264.

233. The Sumerian has KA/KIR_4.BI.

234. See *CAD* S 1a s.v. *saʾālu*, mng. b.

235. See Chapter 8.

236. Fincke, *Augenleiden* 169 suggests Behçet's syndrome for this text. However, although eye problems are an important part of Behçet's syndrome, bleeding is not. Also, the text specifically mentions the absence of arthritis, whereas arthritis is commonly present in Behçet's syndrome.

237. As is now obvious from Text C, Labat was confused by the fact that Text D omits line 21 and thus miscombined Text D with Text A so that the actual beginning of line 19 is listed in *TDP* as belonging to line 20. Labat also mistook a partially effaced DINGIR sign for a *qa* and thus did not recognize "hand" of Gula. Fincke's (*Augenleiden* 75) diagnosis of petrous bone fracture explains bleeding from the ears, but fails to explain bleeding from the nose and eyes. It is more likely that the patient had a clotting abnormality causing this multifocal bleeding.

238. The reference to white spots on the tongue quoted by Adamson, *WO* 16.9 is describing an animal, not a human being.

239. Lit. "sickness of the *kabbartu*." For the part of the foot involved, see Adamson, *RA* 87.158–159. The Akkadian term literally means "thick" or "heavy" part (see *CAD* K 18–20).

240. On this point, see also Müller, *AGM* 18.189. Kinnier Wilson, *JNES* 53.111–115 suggests that *samānu* is mycetoma. Against this however, in addition to the fact that *samānu* is associated with the head rather than the foot is the fact that, unlike mycetoma, *samānu* is painful.

241. See also *BAM* 380:18//*BAM* 381 iii 10.

242. See also *BAM* 124 i 15//*AMT* 73/1+ i 20; *BAM* 124 i 17//*AMT* 73/1+ i 22; *AMT* 73/1+ i 26; *BAM* 124 ii 19; *BAM* 124 ii 36//*AMT* 74/1 ii 12; *AMT* 74/1 ii 15; *AMT* 100/3 i 3+*AMT* 32/2 i 13.

243. See also *AMT* 73/1 i 6+*AMT* 15/3 i 16.

244. See also *BAM* 124 i 26//*AMT* 73/1 i 29+*AMT* 18/5 i 3.

245. Note also DPS XIV A_2 iv 16′//G iv 6′ = *TDP* 142 iv 16′.

246. With Attia, *Histoire des Sciences Médicales* 34.7, we agree that IM in this context is to be interpreted as "clay," but for a different reason. She thinks, following Ebeling, *AGM* 13.131 n. 1 and Campbell Thompson, *JRAS* 1937.279 w. n. 6, that this reference refers to ankle swelling (pitting edema) since pressure on wet clay can produce an indentation (see Chapter 8). However, *muruṣ kabbarti* does not mean edema, nor is edema included among its signs.

247. See Chapter 10.

248. See also *AMT* 74/1 ii 24, ii 25.

249. See also *BAM* 120 iii 6.

250. See Chapter 10.

251. See also *BAM* 156:25; *BAM* 494 iii 24′; cf. *BAM* 33:9; *BAM* 494 iii 42′.

252. Labat's (*RA* 53.7 n. 5) collation had *gu-*⌈*reš*⌉*-tú*. However, Labat later (*RA* 55.95) thought he saw *gu-r*[*a-á*]*r-tú*. The original reading has been confirmed by collation by Scurlock.

253. See also *BAM* 480 i 1–3//*BAM* 3 i 1–3; cf. *BAM* 379 i 37′//*SpTU* 3.106 i 13.

254. Fincke, *Augenleiden* 197 n. 1470 cites an ancient commentary that explains *quqānu* as a "small worm."

255. For a description of loiasis, see ibid. 211. Fincke rejects the equation of *quqānu* with loaisis (p. 197) on the grounds that the latter is the *tultum*-worm mentioned in an Old Babylonian recitation (*YOS* 11.5:1–8). However, the recitation in question is a reference to the imaginary "tooth worm" and has nothing to do with diseases of the eye (for a full citation, see 3.70).

256. This, or some other insect vector, is presumably the NIM.BAR.ḪUZ: "BAR.ḪUZ fly" with which *quqānu* is lexically equated (see Fincke, *Augenleiden* 196). Adamson, RA 87.156, interprets *quqānu* as the "eye-fly" that transmits *amurdinnu*, a condition of the eyes that he believes to be trachoma (see Chapter 9). *Amurdinnu* ("pink eye") has no connection with *quqānu* (apart from appearing with it in one treatment good for a number of different eye conditions). Moreover, understanding *quqānu* as a fly ignores ancient commentaries that explain it as meaning "worm" (see above) as well as the Sumerogram, which indicates something that is threadlike and actually visible in the eyes.

257. See also *BAM* 2 r. 1′, 2′; *BAM* 159 ii 25, ii 43–44; *BAM* 379 ii 12′; *CTN* 4.196+195 ii 20′; *YOS* 11.29:4; BM 113970+ ii 10; cf. *BAM* 172:15′, 16′.

258. See also *BAM* 159 ii 46; *AMT* 31/4:7; cf. *AMT* 57/5+ r. 1–2; *AMT* 29/3:7′.

259. For references, see *AHw* 1428b s.v. *urbatu* II.

260. Kinnier Wilson, *Diseases in Antiquity* 195; cf. *JNES* 27.243–244, quotes a recitation designed to elicit the support of NIN.DIN.UG_5.GA in curing a number of possible diseases, including various types of fever, jaundice, and worms (Nougayrol, *RA* 41.31). Kinnier Wilson believes that the presence of a worm plus jaundice

permits the diagnosis of ascaris infestation. However, although the adult ascaris may migrate up the biliary tree, causing jaundice, this is an uncommon event. Moreover, the many different types of fever listed strongly suggest that the recitation is describing multiple conditions (see Introduction under Retrospective Diagnosis).

261. Stol, *Epilepsy* 5–7, 20–21 (followed by Volk, *OrNS* 68.17–18) argues that *bennu* is Akkadian for "epilepsy" and that all neurological syndromes presenting with seizures, whatever the ancient diagnosis, are simply synonyms of *bennu* on the grounds that lexical texts appear to equate various neurological syndromes with *bennu*. When discussing "leprosy," however, Stol, *JEOL* 30.29 denies the lexical equation of *saḫaršubbû* with *garābu* on the grounds that these texts are treacherous for the uninitiated. He should have applied his salutary caution in this instance as well. The problem is that in some cases, we can prove that two words that are equated in lexical texts are synonyms and in others we can prove that they are not. This is for the simple reason that equations in lexical texts have multiple meanings. For example, in the plant lists, some plant equations represent alternative names for a plant (in different languages or dialects) whereas others indicate medicines that could be substituted for the plant in certain uses. With medical terms that appear in astrological or other omens, there is another possible explanation why two terms that are not synonyms might be equated. The word *nuballu* means "wing of an army" but is lexically equated with another term, *ašarēdu*, which means "vanguard of an army." The reason for this equation is that there is a common omen prediction, "the vanguard of the army will fall" and another, relatively rare, omen prediction which says "the wing of the army will fall." What the equation means is that these two predictions are essentially the same (i.e., that no significance is to be attached to the fact that one passage says "vanguard" and the other "wing"). Given that this is the case with lexical texts, the final decision as to whether the ancients considered two terms to be synonyms or not is whether the definitions given for these two terms in other contexts are the same or different. In medical texts, *bennu* is clearly differentiated from AN.TA.ŠUB.BA, which is also clearly differentiated from A.RI.A ŠUL.PA.È.A. It follows that these three terms are not synonyms, lexical equations to the contrary notwithstanding.

262. Fincke, *Augenleiden* 218 does not believe that the ancient Mesopotamian physician knew the difference between shaking chills and seizures. She bases this on Stol, *Epilepsy* 38, where the association of "ice cold" with *bennu* is explained as Fieberfrost (shaking chills), which he believes to be a prodrome of grand mal seizures. However, although patients with falciparum malaria may display spectacularly abnormal eye movements, the shaking chills characteristic of the disease are in no sense a prodrome of the neurological signs. In these matters, the confusion rests with the modern researcher and not the *āšipu*. The latter, unlike the former, clearly knew the difference between shaking chills (see Chapter 3 under FEVER), the abnormal eye movements of cerebral malaria (see Chapter 13 under NYSTAGMUS), and grand mal seizures (see Chapter 13 under SEIZURES).

263. The restoration is based on DPS XV:23 (AOAT 43.151).

264. Köcher, *Fs. Goerke* 35 suggests that this might be hysteria, but we have better candidates for hysterical seizures (see Chapter 19 with 19.14–19.15, 19.19–19.21).

265. Note also DPS XXIX:21 (AOAT 43.320), which speaks of the [LUGAL].⌜ÙR.RA⌝ (focal? seizures; see p. 447) of ⌜*bennu*⌝.

266. See also *BAM* 183:32; *BAM* 377 iii 7.

267. See above.

268. For references, see *CAD* B 206c s.v. *bennu* A, mng. c.

269. For other references to *bennu* in medical texts, see *STT* 286 ii 9; *BAM* 423 i 22′; *CT* 14.23 [K 9283]:17–18; *BAM* 344:1, 14; *SpTU* 4.129 iii 15; *BAM* 356 ii 13//*BAM* 376 ii 25′.

270. After Köcher, apud Stol, *Epilepsy* 97.

271. Kinnier Wilson's (*Diseases in Antiquity* 202) diagnosis of angina pectoris or coronary thrombosis is based on a defective translation in which only the presence of breast pain is clear. Köcher, *Fs. Goerke* 35 suggests that this text describes a petit mal seizure. However, jerking and shuddering do not occur with this type of seizure. For TÚR/*tarbaṣu* as "courtyard," see *AHw* 1327–1328.

272. Durand, *ARM* 26/1.553 w/ n. 87 attributes the mutilated fingers to a "crisis of hemiplegia" associated with a "crisis of epilepsy" (*bennu*). Since hemiplegia is not commonly associated with epilepsy and since hemiplegia does not result in "mutilation" of the fingers, we favor our explanation.

273. Heeßel, AOAT 43.356, 369, 370 interprets this as "ox fat." It seems more likely that this is simply a foreign loanword into Akkadian.

274. See also DPS XXXIII:61 (AOAT 43.356).

CHAPTER 4. SEXUALLY TRANSMITTED DISEASES (STDS)

1. This is the ancient Mesopotamian god of the moon.

2. The notion that sex was some sort of religious duty for Mesopotamians and that virgin priestesses (actually nuns) were "sacred prostitutes" may appeal to romantic notions of free love in ancient times, but have no basis in reality.

3. See below.

4. Kinnier Wilson, *Diseases in Antiquity* 196; "Medicine in . . . Old Testament (times)" 358; and *JNES* 27.245 does not believe that gonorrhea existed in ancient Mesopotamia since it is "a communicable disease and not a nutritional, or known endemic, disease." We do not find this a sufficient basis for excluding this condition, especially when many of the translated references are consistent with this disease.

5. The word *mūṣu* is probably related to a verb that means "to come out." In all cases where symptoms are given, reference is made to some unusual color or consistency to the urine, suggesting to the ancient physician the presence of a discharge (see Chapter 5).

6. See also *AMT* 32/1:11′.

7. This interpretation of KI NU GI (usually "land of no return") follows the ancient commentary *SpTU* 1.36:23–24.

8. See Chapter 13 with 13.57–13.59.

9. Lit. "just like that."

10. For this term, see the discussion in Chapter 8 with 8.1.

11. J. V. Kinnier Wilson, *Iraq* 18.144–145 interprets "wind blasting" as trachoma, but we do not concur. For possible descriptions of trachoma in ancient texts, see Chapter 9.

12. See also *BAM* 1 ii 9–11; cf. *BAM* 421 i′ 28′; *BAM* 52:58–59.

13. Adamson, *Medical History* 14.314 suggests herpes genitalis as the diagnosis for this reference. However, the text describes stomatitis that is caused by HSV1 and not HSV2, the virus responsible for herpes genitalis.

14. See also *KAR* 211 obv. 19–20; DPS III A r. 9′–12′//C r. 32–35 = *TDP* 28:92–95; DPS XVIII:21–23 (AOAT 43.219); DPS XXXIII:80 (AOAT 43.357); DPS XXXIII:114 (AOAT 43.358); *BAM* 584 ii 25′–26′, 29′.

15. This is the ancient Mesopotamian god of the moon.

16. See also Adamson, *Medical History* 14.314.

17. The translation is from context; see *CAD* N/2.133b; *AHw* 768a.

18. Excavations at a medieval friary at Hull in northern England have uncovered skeletons dated to between 1300 and 1450 that show signs of syphilis or possibly yaws.

19. Volk, *OrNS* 68.24 believes this reference to be describing a "parasitic infection of the liver and lungs" (presumably amoebiasis). However, although amoebiasis can rarely cause jaundice, it does not cause the petechial rash described in the reference. Also, amoebic hepatitis is not likely to occur in a nursing infant.

20. Fincke, *Augenleiden* 184 suggests porphyria and erythema multiform for this reference. However, only swelling of the extremities is described.

21. The text adds the note that, if the patient has "wind blasting," the twin gods are responsible. The "wind blasting" may be describing a concurrent HSV2 infection (see above) or simple redness and inflammation surrounding the ulcer.

22. Labat, *RLA* 3.231–232 believes that this text is describing a tuberculous cold abscess (a draining tuberculous lymph node). We favor a syphilitic chancre but a cold abscess is also possible.

23. The reading is indicated by the commentary *SpTU* 1.30 obv. 6: [*ina ma-rak*] U_4-*mi* = *ina*? [*a-r*] *a-ku* U_4-*mu*.

24. For the translation of *šāpulu* as "inguinal region," see Heeßel, AOAT 43.168 ad line 57′. Adamson, *JRAS* 1984.7 proposes an alternative translation of "scrotal sac." However, in this passage, the hair of the *šāpulu* is described as falling out. Since the scrotal sac usually has minimal or no hair, "inguinal region" appears to be the preferable translation.

25. Adamson, *JRAS* 1979.4 n. 25 cites this text as "evidence of fevers associated with chills, rigors and cold sweats," suggesting the presence of endemic malaria in ancient Mesopotamia. Although we believe that malaria occurred in ancient Mesopotamia (see Chapter 3), we do not believe that this text is describing that condition.

26. See also DPS XIV A_2 ii 15//C ii 29 = *TDP* 136 ii 65.

27. On the translation of this particular symptom, see Fincke, *Augenleiden* 187. Note also Heeßel, AOAT 43.293 n. 17.

28. Kinnier Wilson, *Medical History* 34.190, 195 believes that this text is describing Todd's paralysis but we believe that there is a better candidate for this condition elsewhere (see Chapter 13).

29. The text adds the note that, if the patient has "wind blasting," the god Pabilsag is responsible. The "wind blasting" may be describing a concurrent HSV2 infection (see above) or simple redness and inflammation surrounding the ulcer.

30. Labat, *RLA* 3.231–232 believes that this text is describing a tropical ulcer (cutaneous leishmaniasis). However, although tropical ulcers can be large and may leave a permanent scar, they typically produce little or no pain.

31. That this organ is the liver may be seen from Izbu comm. 203 (Leichty, *Izbu* 218): *ta-kal-tú = ga-bi-du*: "liver." See also Nougayrol, *RA* 44.3 and Goetze, *YOS* 10 p. 7. Note also *CAD* N 376a.

CHAPTER 5. GENITOURINARY TRACT DISEASES

1. This chapter deals with all aspects of the genitourinary tract with the exception of pregnancy-related problems (see Chapter 12) and sexually transmitted diseases (see Chapter 4).

2. Zakaria, *J.Fac.Med.Baghdad* N.S. 1.2.

3. Gorbach, Bartlett, and Backlow, *Infectious Diseases* 2475. See also Krafeld-Daugherty, *Fs Dietrich* 256.

4. The text (*BAM* 114:9–10//*BAM* 161 iv 4′–7′//*AMT* 58/4:5′–6′) is translated by Geller (*Kidney International* 47.1813) as "If his urine is normal, the loins and epigastrium (upper abdomen) are [. . .]; that man suffers from stricture of the rectum." It actually reads: "If his urine is like that of one whose pelvic region and epigastrium [continually] hurt [him], that person (has) the constriction of DÚR.GIG (var. is sick with constriction of the urethra), to cure him . . ."

5. Labat's edition has [G]IG-*su* GÍD-*ma* [DIN] in this line. However, this phrase does not appear in Reisner's copy (*SBH* 148 ii 19′) and is not currently visible on the tablet.

6. Mujais, *Am.J.Nephrology* 19.136 suggests that wine-colored urine could be due to acute glomerulonephritis, and we agree.

7. Text A has "prolonged."

8. See also Kämmerer, *RAI* 44.169.

9. See also *BAM* 114:6.

10. Mujais, *Am.J.Nephrology* 19.136 agrees that watery urine could be due to renal failure, and lists two possible causes.

11. Whatever is missing must be masculine plural, which makes *mû*: "liquid" the most reasonable restoration.

12. See also *BAM* 114:5.

13. Mujais, *Am.J.Nephrology* 19.136 suggests severe nephrosis as the source of the milky urine in this reference.

14. Lit. "falling out." "Dissolving" is also possible; see *CAD* Š/1.95b.

15. Ancient Mesopotamians knew how to produce chamois (oil-treated skins), tawed leather (alum and salt-treated skins) and tanned leather (gall nut- and sumac-treated skins). As in the later Islamic Middle East, tawed skins were dyed bright red (*ṣarāpu*) with madder (*ḫurātu*), producing what came to be known in Europe as "Moroccan" or "Cordoba" leather.

16. For this term, see below.

17. See Chapter 13 with 13.57–13.59.

18. *CAD* K 74b, followed by Adamson, *RA* 87.154–155 reads this passage as ÉLLAG *bir-ki-šú* and interprets the expression as meaning specifically "testicles." However, there is no necessary connection between hematuria and testicular pain, which makes "testicles" less likely in this context. It is, in any case, curious, that the word for "testicle" (ŠIR) was not used.

19. For the expression, see also *BAM* 112 i 2′–3′; *BAM* 396 i 23′–24′//*AMT* 66/7:18–19.

20. This expression is sometimes mistakenly taken to refer to anal stricture (see Kinnier Wilson, *Journ.Roy.Soc.Med.* 89.136; Adamson, *JRAS* 1979.5–6; note that Adamson also mistakes a graphic variant for a separate syndrome). For our interpretation, see Chapter 6.

21. See also *BAM* 112 ii 17′–18′.

22. See also *BAM* 112 ii 17′–18′.

23. So the commentary *SpTU* 1.36 obv. 23–24.

24. See also *AMT* 58/5:6′; DPS XXII:33 (AOAT 43.254).
25. See Heeßel, AOAT 43.187.
26. See also BM 42406+:1 (Finkel, *Fs. Lambert* 208).
27. See also *BAM* 112 i 13′; *BAM* 114:1.
28. For this term, see below. The commentary to this passage, 11 N-T 4:22 (Civil, *JNES* 33.336–337), explains *mu-ṣa* as *ḫi-níq-tum*: "constriction."
29. See also Farber, *BID* 227–234:1–14, 84′; 234–235:*23–*26; *AMT* 32/1:11′; *AMT* 61/1:9′–10′; *BAM* 396 iv 6–8//*AMT* 61/1:5′–6′; DPS XIV A ii 45//C ii 17 = *TDP* 136 ii 45.
30. See also *AMT* 61/1:12′.
31. For the term, see below.
32. Usually, after the first of a series of treatments for the same condition, subsequent examples are marked by ditto (KI.MIN = KI.2); in this text however, "ditto" is followed by KI.3, KI.4, KI.5, and so on.
33. On this point, see also Geller and Cohen, *Kidney International* 47.1813 correcting, inter alia, Kinnier Wilson, *Diseases in Antiquity* 195–196; Biggs, *RLA* 7.628 and *CAD* M/2.247a. Since *mūṣu* can refer to a discharge of any kind, we agree with Kinnier Wilson, *Diseases in Antiquity* 195–196; *Studies in the Period of David and Solomon* 357–358; and *JNES* 27.245–246 and Herrero, *RA* 69.49–51, that the term could be applied to patients with *Schistosomiasis hematobium* and hematuria; however, we also agree with Campbell Thompson, *Proc.Roy.Soc.Med. Hist.* 19/3.38–39 n. 2 (followed by Labat, *RLA* 3.221–222, Biggs, *SÀ.ZI.GA* 3 n. 16, and Sigerist, *History of Medicine* 1.482) that some of the references could be describing gonorrhea.
34. See also *AMT* 66/11:3–5+K 11230:6–8, cf. *AMT* 66/11:2+K 11230:5; *BAM* 114:7//*BAM* 161 iv 1′–2′//*AMT* 58/4:3′; *AMT* 30/12 ii 2′; *AMT* 39/6:7′; *AMT* 89/4:2; *BAM* 396 ii 22′, 25′; BM 38583:25′; DPS XVIII:40′–41′ (AOAT 43.219).
35. See also *KAR* 73 obv. 1–5 (reading NA_4! *dan-nu* as suggested by Haussperger, *ZA* 87.208); *BAM* 396 ii 21′–22′.
36. See also DPS XIV A_2 ii 2//C ii 21 = *TDP* 136 ii 52.
37. Note that in BM 78963:66 "sick kidneys" are associated with stricture and other urinary tract problems.
38. As in *AMT* 59/1 i 19, 22, 23; *BAM* 1 i 21; *BAM* 111 ii 25′–26′; *BAM* 112 i 19′, 22′, 25′–26′//*AMT* 58/6:4, 6, 8; *BAM* 112 i 28′–29′, 31′–32′; *BAM* 159 i 8; *BAM* 237 iv 12; *BAM* 396 i 28′–29′//*AMT* 66/7:20; *BAM* 396 ii 10′//*BAM* 111 iii 12′//*AMT* 66/11:22+*AMT* 65/6:10; *BAM* 396 ii 17′, iv 10.
39. See, for example, *BAM* 161 vi 20//*BAM* 431 v 25′; Herrero, *RA* 69.42 i 5; cf. *BAM* 163 obv. 9′; *BAM* 164 obv. 9//*BAM* 431 v 32′//*BAM* 162:4′//*BAM* 163 obv. 4′ ("plants for the kidneys").
40. *CAD* Ṣ 45b puts this under "to soak" and translates "flow out" but based on this passage alone. Lambert's suggestion of "purge" is based on etymological connection with Syriac *ṣebᶜ*.
41. See also *BAM* 96 ii 18–19; *BAM* 96 iii 8′//*AMT* 53/1 iv 6; *BAM* 114:9–10//*BAM* 161 iv 4′–7′//*AMT* 58/4:5′–6′; *AMT* 40/5 iii 14–16; *AMT* 56/1 obv. 1–3//*BAM* 88:1′–2′; *BAM* 95:23.
42. See Chapter 6.
43. The tablet and copy have ḪI.
44. Mujais, *Am.J.Nephrology* 19.137 correctly points out that the mental status changes mentioned in this reference could be secondary to advanced kidney failure.
45. See also *AMT* 59/1 i 14, 18, 46; *AMT* 40/5 iii 9//*BAM* 106 r. 1′//*STT* 101:3′; *BAM* 1 i 21, 22; *AMT* 89/4:7, 10; *AMT* 60/1 ii 2, 8, 10; *BAM* 422 ii 32′; BM 42342:45 (Finkel, *Fs. Lambert* 163).
46. Both translations are possible; for references, see *CAD* Š/1.75–77.
47. Lit. "(going) to his fate is established for him."
48. Mujais, *Am.J.Nephrology* 19.136 also notes this point.
49. See also *BAM* 414 obv. 8–9.
50. For the expression, see also DPS XIII G_2 13 = *TDP* 124 iii 20.
51. Fincke, *Augenleiden* 141 offers ophthalmic herpes zoster or blepharitis as the diagnosis for this text, but fails to explain the patient's inability to urinate.
52. See also DPS IX A 68//B r. 14 = *TDP* 78:68.
53. The reference is presumably to positional vertigo.
54. See Chapter 13 with 13.57–13.59.
55. For the reading, see Stol, *Epilepsy* 91–92.
56. Lit. "he was struck on the back side." The commentary to DPS XIV A_2 i 8–9 = *TDP* 132 i 60, *SpTU* 1.36 obv. 11, indicates that the "striking" in question was done with a weapon.

57. See also "[If a man and a] woman lie down on the bed and the man ⌜pours out⌝ his urine/excrement . . ." (*AMT* 66/2:7′–8′; cf. *CT* 28.41 [K 8821]:10′–11′).

58. For the reading, see Campbell Thompson, *Babylonaica* 14.119.

59. See also *AMT* 62/1 ii 9′; *BAM* 396 i 10′; *KAR* 73 obv. 1–5.

60. Labat, *RLA* 3.222 and Mujais, *Am.J.Nephrology* 19.137 believe that this reference describes prostatic hypertrophy (an enlarged prostate), and we agree that this is a possibility.

61. See Labat, *RLA* 3.222.

62. Geller, *Am.J.Nephrology* 22.104, 106 argues that this term, which he interprets as *maṣraḫ ušāri*, "duct of the penis," refers specifically to the seminal duct. However, Köcher's copy clearly indicates that the term *maṣraḫu* in this text refers not to the "duct" of the penis (GÌŠ/*ušāru*) but to the "duct" for the urine (KÀŠ.MEŠ/*šinātu*). Nonetheless, the specification that this "duct" was the one that carried the urine does suggest, with Geller, that a distinction was made between this *maṣraḫ šināti* or urinary tract and a **maṣraḫ reḫūti* or seminal duct.

63. See also *BAM* 182 obv. 2′, 5′; *BAM* 112 i 17′–19′//*AMT* 58/6:2–3; *BAM* 112 i 34′–36′; *AMT* 62/1 ii 9′; *AMT* 63/1:4.

64. See Chapter 6.

65. See Heeßel, AOAT 43.187.

66. See also *BAM* 114:9–10//*BAM* 161 iv 4′–7′//*AMT* 58/4:5′–6′; *BAM* 95:23; *AMT* 40/5 iii 9//*BAM* 106 r. 1′//*STT* 101:3′.

67. See Chapter 13 with 13.57–13.59.

68. For this term, see above.

69. See Chapter 13 with 13.57–13.59.

70. *CAD* K 74b s.v. *kalīt birki*, followed by Adamson, *RA* 87.154–155 reads this passage as ÉLLAG *bir-ki-šú* and interprets the expression as meaning specifically "testicles." However, there is no necessary connection between hematuria and testicular pain, which makes "testicles" less likely in this context. It is, in any case, curious that the word for "testicle" (ŠIR) was not used.

71. Mujais, *Am.J.Nephrology* 19.136.

72. See also DPS XII D iii 17, 18 = *TDP* 104 iii 17, 18.

73. See also DPS XII D iii 13, 15 = *TDP* 104 iii 13, 15.

74. "If while walking down the street a person continually has an erection . . ." (*CT* 39.45:21).

75. See also *BAM* 161 v 24//*BAM* 159 i 14; *BAM* 111 ii 15′–17′//*BAM* 159 i 15–17; *BAM* 379 ii 15′–16′//*CTN* 4.195 iii 11′; *BAM* 396 i 14′; *BAM* 115 obv. 13′.

76. See also *BAM* 205:7′–10′//Biggs, *ŠÀ.ZI.GA* 68–69:9′–13′; W. Farber, *BID* 227–234:1–14; *BAM* 112 i 17′–19′//*AMT* 58/6:2–3; *BAM* 112 i 34′–36′.

77. Some form of stiffness; see Chapter 11.

78. As with the English "courage," the reference is to inability to have an erection.

79. A reddish root vegetable, possibly the beet; apparently the saltpeter of ancient Mesopotamia.

80. See also DPS XIII J 9 = *TDP* 126 iii 41; *STT* 92 ii 31–34; *STT* 93:52′; *KADP* 1 v 2, 11.

81. Lit. "his heart does not rise in him."

82. ⌜80⌝ = *šibūtu* (*STT* 400:47).

83. For this interpretation of ^{GIŠ}NÍG.GIDRU/*ḫaṭṭu*: "scepter" as a pun for *ḫaṭṭu* from *ḫamāṭu*: "to burn," see *CAD* D 137b s.v. *dikšu* mng. 1a1′.

84. These cases were attributed, inter alia, to the machinations of sorcerers. See Abusch, *Mesop. Witchcr.* 82 n. 14, but note that some of his examples are actually cases of sexually transmitted disease in which impotence is only one of the findings.

85. For details, see Biggs, *ŠÀ.ZI.GA.*

86. The term is almost always used to describe fertile semen; for references, see *CAD* Z 93–94.

87. For eunuchs in Mesopotamia and surrounding lands, see most recently Hawkins, RAI 47.217–233. For references to *ša ziqni*, see *CAD* Z 126–127.

88. Middle Assyrian Laws A § 15.

89. For a discussion of this and other skin lesions, see Chapter 10.

90. See also DPS XIV A_2 ii 15–16//C ii 29–30 = *TDP* 136 ii 65–66.

91. Adamson, *RA* 87.154–155 argues that the term here translated "testicle" should instead be understood to refer to benign tumors of the spermatic cord. However, this is a relatively uncommon abnormality, and would not have appeared in so many references to diverse problems within the scrotal sac.

92. The Mesopotamian equivalent of our "his father's son" was the "son of his god." The *ēntu* was a virgin priestess who was envisaged as the wife of a god and therefore forbidden to have sexual intercourse with men. The woman with whom you may not have sex because she is married to your "god" is, therefore, your mother. The point is that this condition was thought to be a divine punishment for incest.

93. See also DPS XIV A_2 ii 13–14//C ii 28 = *TDP* 136 ii 63–64; DPS XIV A iii 14–15//C_2 iii 5//I 10 = *TDP* 140 iii 48′–49′.

94. See also DPS XIV A_2 ii 18//C ii 32 = *TDP* 138 ii 68.

CHAPTER 6. GASTROINTESTINAL DISEASES

1. In its broadest sense, the Sumerian term ŠÀ (= Akkadian *libbu*) refers to the heart and to the outer surface of the abdomen and all of the internal organs contained in it. Ancient physicians used a special set of terminology to describe signs and symptoms of the heart (see Chapter 8), which allows us to translate ŠÀ in those contexts specifically as "heart." The remaining references are either to the outer surface of the abdomen or to the stomach, and so on. These two possibilities may to some extent be distinguished since there are also terms for signs and symptoms that apply only to the internal organs of the abdomen or only to the external surface. Stomachs get upset; abdomens do not. Conversely, abdomens turn red; stomachs might, but not visibly in intact patients. Otherwise, the use of ŠÀ is close to modern doctors' use of the term *abdomen* (i.e., the external surface plus the organs inside). As in modern usage, there were terms in Akkadian for the individual internal organs (e.g., *karšu* for stomach), which were used when the ancient physician felt it necessary to avoid confusion.

2. In this connection, it is interesting to compare the use of the German word *Netzhaut:* "retina" for "omentum."

3. The tablet and copy have a clear TE.

4. *Emar* VI/1.109:1–3 confirm that this is from *arāku:* "to become long," and not *arāqu:* "to be yellow." On this point, see also W. Farber, *JNES* 49.310.

5. "Vessels of blood" is quite literally the meaning of the Akkadian term *pursīt dāme.*

6. Fincke, *Augenleiden* 144, 180 understands this text to refer to conjunctival injection. However, what are being described are not the patient's eyes but the "eyes" of the digestive system, namely, the omentum and mesenteries.

7. Malfunctioning organs are not infrequently said to have "turned over."

8. For a diagram of a sheep's liver and the Akkadian names for various parts of livers and lungs, see Star, *SAA* 4.xl–lv.

9. For references, see *CAD* I 192b. Adamson, *JRAS* 1984.6–7 argues that the *išiltu* refers to the right and left hepatic ducts on the grounds that the sphincter is small and would therefore inevitably have been missed. However, the *āšipu* was a keen observer, as Adamson himself admits (Adamson, *Medical History* 14.313, 316), and the presence of a magnifying glass would have made such observation easier.

10. There are similar references to colored vomitus that specify black, red, yellow, and white bile (DPS VII B obv. 10′–13′ = *TDP* 64:49′–52′). Since stomach acids also have a bitter taste, it is likely that only the yellow bile (DPS VII B obv. 12′ = *TDP* 64:51′) is actually bile, the remaining references representing a combination of stomach acids with other substances found in the gastrointestinal tract (see below). See also Kämmerer, *RAI* 44.167; cf. Michalowski, *ZA* 71.8–9; Biggs, *RLA* 7.628.

11. The same interpretation holds for references to colored vomitus that specify red and black bile as the substance vomited (DPS VII B obv. 10′, 11′ = *TDP* 64:49′, 50′).

12. Kämmerer, *RAI* 44.167, confused by the conventional translation of Akkadian "red" as "brown" or "red-brown," takes the red bile as representing "coffee grounds."

13. Kämmerer, *RA* 94.69 correctly indicates yellow fever as a condition in which black vomitus also occurs.

14. For this interpretation of ^{GIŠ}NÍG.GIDRU/*ḫaṭṭu:* "scepter" as a pun for *ḫaṭṭu* from *ḫamāṭu:* "to burn," see *CAD* D 137b s.v. *dikšu* mng. 1a1′.

15. The same interpretation holds for references to colored vomitus that specify white bile as the substance vomited (DPS VII B obv. 13′ = *TDP* 64:52′).

16. The term *rupuštu* is one of many words for phlegm (for references, see *CAD* R 414–415). Modern physicians call the phlegm-like substance in the gastrointestinal tract *mucus.*

17. See also *BAM* 190:22–24//*STT* 102:7–9//*BAM* 193 ii 2′–5′; *BAM* 90:9′–11′//*BAM* 434 iii 10–13.

18. See Chapter 10 with 10.19.

19. For other similar references, see DPS XXIII:5 (AOAT 43.272); *PBS* 2/2.104:1; DPS XXI:20 (AOAT 43.247).

20. Compare also DPS XIV A ii 10–11//C_2 i 15 = *TDP* 132 ii 10–11; *BAM* 159 ii 49–50.

21. Note also DPS XIV A ii 8//C_2 i 14a = *TDP* 132 ii 8, which appears, according to the copy provided by Geller, to describe the excretion of "material removed from his insides."

22. Kämmerer, *RAI* 44.168 suggests typhus as the specific cause of yellow stools ("pea-soup" diarrhea). However, diarrhea and yellow stools are not common problems with this disease. Moreover, Kämmerer claims that the excrement of patients with diarrhea was used as medicine. The reference that he cites is not, however, to human excrement but to gazelle pellets. Like Yemeni Arabic (Dan Varisco, personal communication), Akkadian distinguishes between the excrement of various types of animals and that of humans). Moreover, the word that Kämmerer takes to be "yellow" means "fresh" in this context, and the dung is baked before being applied (externally).

23. Ibid. takes this to be a specific reference to infants, but if that were so, it would have begun with DIŠ LÚ.TUR.

24. Readings of this text are based on the author's transliteration from the original as modified on the basis of a copy subsequently provided by Geller.

25. The ancient physician also noted the presence of fat in vomit: DIŠ *ina* KA-*šú* Ì.GIŠ ŠÀ-*šú i*-[*ú-a* . . .]: If he ⌜vomits⌝ his stomach fat from his mouth [. . .] (DPS VII B obv. 9′ = *TDP* 64:48′).

26. Lit. "fattening" (for references to the expression used of animals at Mari, see *CAD* M/1.321a; for references to the verb, see *CAD* M/1.307–308). Heeßel, AOAT 43.187 tentatively suggests reading instead *ba-ru-ti-šú*: "hunger??."

27. 70 = U_4.MEŠ GÍD.ME[Š] (*STT* 400:46).

28. For other references, see *BAM* 95:29; *BAM* 94 r. 7′; *BAM* 96 iii 2′–4′//*BAM* 104:42; *BAM* 99:1; *BAM* 575 iv 11; *AMT* 101/3 i 21. See also *BAM* 96 iii 10′; *BAM* 579 iv 32.

29. See also *BAM* 482 iv 48′//*AMT* 19/1 iv! 31′.

30. Note also DPS XL B 69, 71 = *TDP* 226:68, 70; DPS XXIII:2, 3 (AOAT 43.272).

31. The text has been collated.

32. Fluid accumulation can also result from severe famine (Kinnier Wilson, *Diseases in Antiquity* 193), but in the irrigated croplands of ancient Mesopotamia, which were renowned in antiquity for their fertility, ascites from famine would have been a much less common occurrence.

33. See also *AMT* 43/6:3; DPS XIII B i 9′–10′, 13′ = *TDP* 112 i 13′–14′, 17′; DPS XIII B i 44′, 45′, 46′//F 6, 7 = *TDP* 116 i 48′, 49′, 50′; DPS XIII B ii 45//G_2 36+G_1 19 = *TDP* 120 ii 45; DPS XIII I 2, 3–4, 5, 6, 7 = *TDP* 122 iii 2, 3–4, 5, 6, 7; DPS XVII:64 (AOAT 43.201); DPS XXVI:32′, 33′ (AOAT 43.281); DPS XL A 30//B 31 = *TDP* 220:30; DPS XL A 64, 65//B 65, 66 = *TDP* 224:64, 65; *BAM* 73 ii 1–3; *BAM* 393 r. 11, 26; *BAM* 401:33; *BAM* 574 i 21; *BAM* 575 ii 48–50; BM 64371 ii 12′; *STT* 100 r. 3′, 11′–12′; *AMT* 42/2:1.

34. See also *BAM* 240:25′, 26′.

35. Note also DPS VII B obv. 14′ = *TDP* 64:53′; DPS XIII B i 15′, 16′–17′ = *TDP* 112 i 19′, 20′–21′; DPS XIII B ii 1//F 13//G_2 4 = *TDP* 116 ii 1; DPS XIII J 7 = *TDP* 126 iii 39; StBoT 36.48 D 2 r. 5 (with *zaqāru*).

36. See also DPS XIII B i 22′ = *TDP* 112 i 26′.

37. That this organ is the liver may be seen from Izbu comm. 203 (Leichty, *Izbu* 4.218): *ta-kal-tú* = *ga-bi-du*: "liver." See also Nougayrol, *RA* 44.3 and Goetze, *YOS* 10 p. 7. Note also *CAD* N 376a.

38. See also *BAM* 578 iii 4–5.

39. The commentary *STT* 403:48 explains this as KI.TA LI.DUR *re-di*: "abutting the lower part of the navel."

40. For other references, see DPS XIII B i 19′, 23′, 28′ = *TDP* 112 i 23′, 27′, 32′.

41. That is, his mother.

42. For other references, see DPS XIII G_2 6, 7, 8 = *TDP* 122 iii 13, 14, 15.

43. See also DPS XIII B i 25′ = *TDP* 112 i 29′.

44. The copy has KI.

45. See also DPS XIII B i 24′ = *TDP* 112 i 28′; BM 64371 ii 7′–9′; cf. *BAM* 159 ii 20–22.

46. See also *BAM* 85:2′–4′//*BAM* 86:3′–4′//*BAM* 159 vi 26–28; cf. *BAM* 575 ii 20, 57, iii 27, iv 48; *BAM* 52:77; *BAM* 158 iv 14//*BAM* 575 iii 25; *BAM* 54:14–15, 17; *BAM* 93:16; *BAM* 95:7; *BAM* 152 iii 7//*BAM* 95:4; *BAM* 168:80//*BAM* 95:9//*BAM* 54:19; Labat, *RA* 54.172 [AO 17624] r. 6; BM 32277++ ii 16.

47. See also *BAM* 52:72; cf. *BAM* 403 r. 7.

48. See also DPS XIII B i 12′ = *TDP* 112 i 16′; DPS XIII G_2 3; *BAM* 575 ii 20, 22, 24, 26.
49. See also *AMT* 48/1:10+*AMT* 78/3:7; *AMT* 48/1:12+*AMT* 78/3:9; *AMT* 44/6:1–2; cf. *BAM* 575 ii 50.
50. See *AHw* 839b.
51. See also DPS XL A 15 = *TDP* 218:15; DPS XL B 74, 75 = *TDP* 226:73, 74; DPS XL A 93, 94 = *TDP* 228:93, 94; DPS XL A 105, 109 = *TDP* 228:105, 109; DPS XVII:87 (AOAT 43.203).
52. For refusal to eat or drink, see also DPS XII D iv 3–4//E iv 8–9 = *TDP* 106 iv 3–4; DPS XVII:57–58 (AOAT 43.200–201); DPS XVI:9 (AOAT 43.172).
53. See also *BAM* 556 ii 70′–71′; DPS XIX/XX:50′ (AOAT 43.229); DPS XXII:12–13 (AOAT 43.252); cf. DPS XIII B i 5′–6′ = *TDP* 110 i 9′–10′).
54. See also *BAM* 575 ii 38; DPS XXII:71–72 (AOAT 43.257); *AMT* 48/2:1–3; *BAM* 190:22–24//*STT* 102:7–9//*BAM* 193 ii 2′–5′; *BAM* 434 i 13′–15′.
55. See also *BAM* 575 iii 7; *LKA* 85 obv. 1–4; *LKA* 102 obv. 18–23//*BAM* 369:2′–5′; *AMT* 40/5 iii 9//*BAM* 106 r. 1′//*STT* 101:3′; *STT* 100 obv. 9′–10′.
56. See also DPS XXII:25, 28 (AOAT 43.253–254).
57. The Arabic cognate means "to sigh."
58. See also *BAM* 174 obv. 23′, 28′–29′.
59. See also *BAM* 155 i 4′; *BAM* 407:6′–8′//*CTN* 4.72 ii 1′–2′; *BAM* 482 ii 14; *BAM* 575 iii 4–5, iv 48; DPS IV E ii 26 = *SpTU* 3.88 ii 26; cf. *BAM* 49:9′–14′//*BAM* 50 obv. 11–15//*BAM* 51:2′–3′; *BAM* 96 iii 15′–16′//*AMT* 58/2:1–2//*BAM* 88:13′–15′; *AMT* 58/2:8; *BAM* 579 i 8 [bread and water]; *BAM* 575 iii 6 [just bread].
60. See also *BAM* 574 i 26–27; *BAM* 575 iv 37//*BAM* 58:8–9; *BAM* 575 iv 43; *BAM* 578 iii 4–5, iv 43–44; cf. *BAM* 89:1–3; *BAM* 575 ii 57, 60, 63 [bread and water]; *KUB* 4.49 ii 4–5 [bread]; BM 78963:64 [liquid]; *BAM* 193 i 8′–11′ [unspecified].
61. Kinnier Wilson, *Journ.Roy.Soc.Med.* 89.137–138 believes that this reference is describing esophageal reflux disease. We agree that this is a possible interpretation.
62. See also DPS XL A 55 = *TDP* 224:55.
63. See also DPS XXXI:46′–47′ (AOAT 43.344).
64. Note also *BAM* 578 i 1–2.
65. *CAD* E 188b (cf. Š/1.371a) takes this as "dry matter," but the basic meaning of SAḪAR is "earth" or "dirt."
66. See also DPS XVIII:25–26 (AOAT 43.219).
67. See also *PBS* 2/2.104:2; DPS XXXVI A 81 = *TDP* 208:81; DPS XIX/XX:108′b (AOAT 43.232).
68. For other references, see K 2426 iv 1.
69. See also *BAM* 380:65//*BAM* 381 iv 20; *BAM* 422 iii 28′; *BAM* 575 iii 1, 3; *STT* 93:67′; DPS XIII D r. 6, 7, 8 = *TDP* 126 iv 15′, 16′, 17′. Cf. *BAM* 380:62–63//*BAM* 381 iv 17–18; *AMT* 45/5 r. 2′; *ABRT* 2.11 r.! iii 3′; *CTN* 4.196+195 ii 12′; *BAM* 379 i 29′//*SpTU* 3.106 i 7//*CTN* 4.196+195 ii 28′; *BAM* 379 i 31′; *SpTU* 3.106 i 22 (treatments to produce bowel movements).
70. See W. Farber, *JNES* 49.319–320.
71. See also BM 59626:1, 11–12; *BAM* 240:33′, 36′; *BAM* 395:1, 5; Beckman and Foster, *Mem. Sachs* 19 no. 17 ii 5′; cf. DPS XIII D r. 18, 19 = *TDP* 128 iv 27′, 28′; DPS XIX/XX:108′a (AOAT 43.232).
72. See also *BAM* 145:1–17//*BAM* 146:29′–38′.
73. Emendations are courtesy of an anonymous reviewer.
74. See also DPS XVII:10–13 (AOAT 43.195/196); DPS XVIII:42′ (AOAT 43.219); DPS XXI:22 (AOAT 43.247); DPS XL A 10–12 = *TDP* 218:10–12; cf. *BAM* 575 i 25.
75. See also *BAM* 90:3′–5′//*AMT* 48/2:11–14.
76. For the rest of this passage, see below, Chapter 6.109.
77. See also *BAM* 579 i 20, 25, 27, 29.
78. See also BM 76515 r. 7′; *BAM* 579 i 1, 6, 11, 13, 15, 46, 51, 59; *BAM* 579 i 61//*BAM* 174 r. 4; *BAM* 579 ii 1//*BAM* 174 r. 7; *BAM* 168:62//*BAM* 169b:16′//*BAM* 108 obv. 8//Beckman and Foster, *Mem. Sachs* 16 no. 12 ii 1; *BAM* 1 iii 28//*CT* 14.43 [S. 60]:5′; DPS XXII:14–15 (AOAT 43.252); cf. DPS XIV A ii 34–36//C ii 10–11 = *TDP* 134 ii 34–36); cf. *BAM* 421 i′ 30′; *BAM* 3 iv 3.
79. See also DPS XIII B i 26′ = *TDP* 112 i 30′.
80. See also *BAM* 49:21′–24′.
81. Cf. also *BAM* 579 i 8; *BAM* 575 iii 4–5.
82. See also DPS III C obv. 56 = *TDP* 24:56.

83. See also DPS XIII B ii 4, 7–8, 9, 10 = *TDP* 116/118 ii 4, 7–8, 9, 10.

84. See also *BAM* 508 ii 11′; *AMT* 45/5 obv. 10′; *AMT* 52/1:7, 15; *BAM* 575 i 51; cf. i 37; *BAM* 574 iv 51; *KUB* 4.49 ii 1.

85. See also DPS XVIII:8–9 (AOAT 43.218).

86. Note also BAM 574 i 42, ii 10, 15; *KBo* 36.29 iv 22; cf. 30′.

87. See also *BAM* 89:1–3.

88. See above, Chapter 6 n. 37.

89. Restoration is based on *BAM* 575 iv 48. The "limp flesh" refers to the absence of skin lesions (see Chapter 10).

90. See also *BAM* 574 i 1, 4, 11; ii 28, 33, 43; iv 52; *AMT* 58/5:9′.

91. See also *BAM* 575 iv 37//*BAM* 58:8–9.

92. The text is published in Leichty, *Mem. Sachs* 263–264 (BM 59623).

93. See also *BAM* 575 iii 55–56.

94. Fincke, *Augenleiden* 168 w/ nn. 1262–1263 suggests that this text might be describing asthma. However, it is clearly a gastrointestinal illness. Shortness of breath, the only respiratory finding in the reference, may occur with esophageal reflux.

95. Note also DPS XIV A ii 15//E 3′ = *TDP* 134 ii 15; DPS XL B 73 = *TDP* 226:72; DPS XIII B ii 44 = *TDP* 120 ii 44.

96. The verb employed literally means "to dam up, close, or clog" (said of canals, drainpipes, and the like), which implies total and relatively permanent closure.

97. For this interpretation of GIŠNÍG.GIDRU/*ḫaṭṭu*: "scepter" as a pun for *ḫaṭṭu* from *ḫamāṭu*: "to burn," see *CAD* D 137b s.v. *dikšu* mng. 1a1′.

98. See also DPS XIII B i 37′//D 11 = *TDP* 114 i 41′; DPS XIII B ii 32 = *TDP* 120 ii 32.

99. For this interpretation of GIŠNÍG.GIDRU/*ḫaṭṭu*: "scepter" as a pun for *ḫaṭṭu* from *ḫamāṭu*: "to burn," see *CAD* D 137b s.v. *dikšu* mng. 1a1′.

100. Kinnier Wilson, *Diseases in Antiquity* 195 suggests hookworm as the diagnosis for this text. Although this is a possibility, hookworm seldom causes grossly visible bleeding.

101. Note also DPS XIII B ii 24–25 = *TDP* 118 ii 24–25; DPS XIII B ii 26–27//G_2 25+G_1 8 = *TDP* 120 ii 26–27.

102. On the surface of it, this would appear to mean "water (and) milk come up."

103. See also Adamson, *JRAS* 1974.106.

104. For other references, see *STT* 96:16.

105. For other references, see *BAM* 73 i 2′; *BAM* 74 iii 1–2; *BAM* 76:11–12; *BAM* 72:9′; *BAM* 176:8′.

106. For other references, see BM 78963:19, 56–57; BM 101569:5′.

107. See also BM 42398:11 (Finkel, *Fs. Lambert* 162).

108. See also *STT* 96:1.

109. Lit. "marsh water"; see below. If there is gastric outlet obstruction, fluid and air may collect in the distended stomach.

110. For other references, see BM 78963:19, 56–57; BM 101569:5′.

111. If related to the *saḫḫu*, which means "marsh," this should refer to liquid vomited from the stomach (see Chapter 8). Note also *BAM* 578 ii 7 (with bile). *CAD* Q 251a reads this as *qidḫu* but admits that *saḫḫu* is also possible.

112. For references, see *AHw* 874a.

113. *JCS* 21.178–182.

114. See also Adamson, *JRAS* 1974.105–106.

115. See also *BAM* 164:12; *BAM* 431 v 46′; *BAM* 431 v 49′//*BAM* 430 vi 7; *BAM* 305:4′.

116. See also *BAM* 1 i 30–34; *BAM* 61:5; *BAM* 429:6′–12′; *BAM* 578 i 20–26, ii 11, 23, 56, 67; *BAM* 578 i 14//*BAM* 60:1′ (without symptoms).

117. See also *BAM* 578 i 46–47.

118. See Chapter 10 with 10.19.

119. See Köcher, *Fs. Goerke* 35–36. Labat and Tournay, *RA* 40.115, 117 suggest that *pašittu* is "bilious regurgitation" and interpret the Sumerogram as referring to subsequent irritation to the teeth. ZÚ.MUŠ does not however, mean "dental nerve" but "snake bite," presumably a reference to the quality of the pain.

120. See also *BAM* 578 ii 9, 13, 14, 18; Labat and Tournay, *RA* 40.116 obv. 1; *BAM* 183:39.

121. See Collins, *Natural Illness* 230–231 *mārtu* 1. Note also *BAM* 578 ii 45–50 and its Sumerian parallel (Michalowski, *ZA* 71.4).

122. Parpola, AOAT 5/2.139–140 interprets this as a case of baby diarrhea.

123. Pangas, *Bull.Hist.Med.* 73.200 was puzzled by what he believed to be a reference to "sparkling" teeth in this text. The "sparkling" is, however, a mistranslation of *ḫâlu*, which means "to ooze (blood)."

124. That this organ is the liver may be seen from Izbu comm. 203 (Leichty, *Izbu* 218): *ta-kal-tú* = *ga-bi-du*: "liver." See also Nougayrol, *RA* 44.3 and Goetze, *YOS* 10 p. 7. Note also *CAD* N 376a.

125. See *BAM* 1 ii 47–52; cf. *BAM* 421 i′ 32′; *BAM* 426 ii 6′–12′; *CT* 14.37 [Rm 357]:1–5; *STT* 92 ii 24–30; *BAM* 92 ii 22′.

126. Haussperger, *Fs. Spycket* 130.

127. Adamson, *RA* 87.157–158 suggests that *aḫḫāzu* refers specifically to obstructive jaundice and that *amurriqānu* means infectious hepatitis. We see no reason to restrict *aḫḫāzu* to a single specific entity, and it seems clear from two references, *BAM* 578 iii 7 and DPS XVIII:24 (AOAT 43.219) (see below), that wasting is linked to *amurriqānu*. Although some cases of infective jaundice may have associated wasting, cirrhosis and liver cancer would be more common causes. Kämmerer, *RAI* 44.166 announces that he is seeking evidence in ancient Mesopotamia for cases of jaundice with the following symptomology: yellow skin and eyes, itching skin, circulatory problems, light-colored stools, yellow or brownish urine, night blindness, and wounds that no longer bleed. It seems unlikely that he will find a medical condition that incorporates all of these findings. Biliary tree obstruction would fit most of them, but it is difficult to understand either "night blindness" or "wounds that no longer bleed" in this context.

128. See also *BAM* 52:91.

129. Note also *BAM* 389:5′.

130. See above, Chapter 6 n. 37.

131. See also DPS IX A 14 = *TDP* 72:14; *BAM* 578 iii 6, iv 26.

132. See also *BAM* 52:97//*BAM* 62:1//*BAM* 578 i 70; cf. *BAM* 189 iv 15–16; *BAM* 1 ii 46; *BAM* 426 ii 5′; *BAM* 431 vi 42′//*BAM* 430 vii 3; *BAM* 159 ii 11//*BAM* 160:2′; *BAM* 578 iv 28, 30, 31, 35 (just *aḫḫāzu*); *BAM* 1 ii 56; *BAM* 423 i 11′; *BAM* 426 ii 2′–4′; *BAM* 429:13′–14′; *BAM* 431 vi 45′–46′//*BAM* 430 vii 7; *CT* 14.37 [Rm 357]:9; *STT* 92 ii 1–4, 6–7; *BAM* 52:87, 88, 94; *BAM* 171:58′–59′; *BAM* 393 obv. 4; *BAM* 578 iii 25, 42′, iv 37; BM 38583:12′; BM 78963:16 (just *amurriqānu*).

133. See also *BAM* 578 iv 16.

134. See also *BAM* 515 ii 43, 44; *BAM* 578 iv 5, 6, 17.

135. See also BM 64371 ii 7′–9′.

136. On this point, see also Kämmerer, *RA* 94.65.

137. See also DPS XVI:85′ (AOAT 43.179).

138. Fincke, *Augenleiden* 138 suggests cirrhosis of the liver for this reference.

139. See also DPS XVIII:25–26 (AOAT 43.219).

140. See also DPS VI A obv. 17//B_2 obv. 3–4 = *TDP* 56:17.

141. Kämmerer, *RAI* 44.169 appears to regard yellow fever as the major cause of hepatitis in ancient Mesopotamia. He seems to base this interpretation on the presence in the texts of references to the vomiting of black bile (Kämmerer, *RA* 94.69). We agree that yellow fever could have been present in this area, but the vomiting of black bile can have other causes and is not in itself sufficient evidence for a major presence of yellow fever in ancient Mesopotamia. He further argues (Kämmerer, *RA* 94.79–81) that the Babylonian Job experienced a viral infection of the liver which is, according to him, clinically described in *Ludlul bēl nemeqi*. However, this is a literary text that does not intend to describe a single disease but to put forward a laundry list of possible ills. To transform it into an *Epikrisenmüster* requires the retranslation of innumerable Akkadian terms in directions suggested neither by etymology nor by any real context. For a discussion of similar methodological problems displayed in an earlier article by Kämmerer, see the Introduction.

142. For other examples of hepatitis, see *BAM* 87:14–17; *BAM* 92 iii 10–13; cf. possibly also DPS XL A 59a = *TDP* 224:59a.

143. For this interpretation of ^{GIŠ}NÍG.GIDRU/*ḫaṭṭu*: "scepter" as a pun for *ḫaṭṭu* from *ḫamāṭu*: "to burn," see *CAD* D 137b s.v. *dikšu* mng. 1a1′.

144. ÚḪ is usually "phlegm." However, when used with KÚM ("fever") it is to be read as a form of *ṣarāḫu* as the parallel between DPS III C r. 10–11//E_1 r. 11–12+E_2 r. 7–8 = *TDP* 26:70–71 (DIŠ *ina* SAG.DU-*šú* KÚM ÚḪ) and *KAR* 211 obv. 4–6 ([DIŠ *i-na*] SAG.DU-*šú* KÚM *ṣa-ri-iḫ*) shows and has now been demonstrated by Heeßel, AOAT 43.162–163. Previously, Labat, *TDP* 25 n. 44 had suggested and then rejected the correct reading in favor of *nuppuḫ* "it is swollen" (followed by Biggs, *RLA* 6.210 and *CAD* N/1.268), which makes no sense in this context.

145. The *rābiṣu* can, in other contexts, cause strokes (see Chapter 13 with 13.228).

146. The *rābiṣu* can, in other contexts, cause narcolepsy (see Chapter 13 with 13.211).

147. DPS XXII:12–13 (AOAT 43.252); cf. DPS XIII B i 5′–6′ = *TDP* 110 i 9′–10′.

148. See also *AMT* 43/1 ii 12; *BAM* 92 iii 10–13.

149. See above, Chapter 6 n. 37.

150. See above, Chapter 6 n. 37.

151. See Chapter 10 with 10.19.

152. See Chapter 13 with 13.57–13.59.

153. For the interpretation of KI.TA as "plantar surface," see Adamson, *JRAS* 1981.128.

154. See above, Chapter 6 n. 37.

155. See above, Chapter 6 n. 37.

156. Heeßel, AOAT 43.185 suggests interpreting this as *sīku* which would mean "powdered part." The "peg" could be the long stem of the leek; it is difficult to imagine what the "powdered part" of a leek would be.

157. See also *AMT* 43/1 ii 12.

158. See above, Chapter 6 n. 37.

159. Note also DPS IX A 30 = *TDP* 72:30.

160. See above, Chapter 6 n. 37.

161. See also DPS XXII:19–20 (AOAT 43.253).

162. See above, Chapter 6 n. 37.

163. See also DPS VI A obv. 17//B_2 obv. 3–4 = *TDP* 56:17.

164. Yellowish-brown is within the range of colors indicated by the Akkadian word *arqu*. For a chart of Akkadian colors, see Kämmerer, *RA* 94.61.

165. See also DPS XII A 6 = *TDP* 100 i 6.

166. 70 = U_4.MEŠ GÍD.ME[Š] (*STT* 400:46).

167. Fincke, *Augenleiden* 139, 159, 180.

168. For possible ancient descriptions of Parkinson's disease, see Chapter 13.

169. Labat, *RLA* 3.232 believes that this term means "blister" or "vesicle." However, *šišitu* is also used to describe something visible in the eyes, where neither "blister" nor "vesicle" would be appropriate. See also *CAD* Š/3.125–126.

170. Cf. also *BAM* 84:5′–6′; *AMT* 43/6:1.

171. See above, Chapter 6 n. 37.

172. See above, Chapter 6 n. 37.

173. For this interpretation of ^{GIŠ}NÍG.GIDRU/*ḫaṭṭu*: "scepter" as a pun for *ḫaṭṭu* from *ḫamāṭu*: "to burn," see *CAD* D 137b s.v. *dikšu* mng. 1a1'.

174. See also DPS XIV A_2 i 20//C_2 i 9b = *TDP* 132 i 71.

175. Note also *BAM* 575 iii 47.

176. See also *PBS* 2/2.104:6–9; DPS XIII B ii 19a = *TDP* 118 ii 19a; cf. DPS XV:35 (AOAT 43.152).

177. For other references, see *BAM* 1 iii 12; *BAM* 425:8′, 10′.

178. Heeßel, AOAT 43.30 n. 48 argues against *AHw* 880a that this is a part of the knee on the grounds that the word literally means "constricted/narrow place" or "split." However, both of these meanings are eminently appropriate to the anal opening. It is, moreover, hard to imagine any part of the knee being either "constricted" or "open." That anal opening would be slightly out of the normal head-to-toe order is not sufficient argument against the interpretation. As with a number of anatomical terms in Akkadian, the word actually refers to one side of the anal opening (compare *ribītu*: "one side of the abdomen"). When in the dual, as here, it refers to both sides, that is, the entire opening.

179. Kinnier Wilson, *Diseases in Antiquity* 195 considers this text to be describing intestinal parasites because of the rectal itching. Although some intestinal parasites can cause rectal itching (see Chapter 3 under WORMS), the "choking" that we believe to be tenesmus would not occur with intestinal parasites.

180. See also *BAM* 94 r. 16′.

181. Lit. "falling out of the intestines."

182. Geller, *Am.J.Nephrology* 22.105 interprets this and the preceding reference as renal disease. This interpretation is apparently based on the Akkadian description of (parts) of the intestines "dropping" or "falling" out and the assumption that this expression is identical with English "dropsy," which can be a manifestation of renal disease. However, "dropsy" has nothing to do with "drop" but is short for "hydropsy" from the Greek *hydor*: "water."

183. See also *BAM* 96 iii 2′–3′//*BAM* 104:42.
184. See also *BAM* 95:14//*STT* 97 iii 15; *AMT* 17/5:1; *AMT* 40/4:3′; *KADP* 1 v 35.
185. See also *BAM* 168:66//*BAM* 108 obv. 1–2//*BAM* 110:3′–4′; *BAM* 182 r. 7′–8′; *AMT* 101/3 i 4′.
186. See Nougayrol, *RA* 66.191 no. 17; *CAD* M/1.324.
187. See *AHw* 1434b.
188. See Chapter 13 with 13.57–13.59.
189. *CAD* K 74b, followed by Adamson, *RA* 87.154–155 reads this passage as ÉLLAG *bir-ki-šú* and interprets the expression as meaning specifically "testicles." However, there is no necessary connection between hematuria and testicular pain, which makes "testicles" less likely in this context. It is, in any case, curious that the word for "testicle" (ŠIR) was not used.
190. This expression is sometimes mistakenly taken to refer to anal stricture (see Kinnier Wilson, *Journ.Roy.Soc.Med.* 89.136; Biggs, *RLA* 7.628; Adamson, *JRAS* 1979.5–6; note that Adamson also mistakes a graphic variant for a separate syndrome).
191. For similar references, see *BAM* 94 r. 2′–3′; *BAM* 96 ii 18–19 (cf. *AMT* 58/3 + K 2960 i 1–2); *BAM* 96 iii 8′//*AMT* 53/1 iv 6; *BAM* 114:6. For the association of this syndrome with stones, discharge (*mūṣu*), incontinence, gross hematuria, "sick" kidneys, and priapism ("burning" of *ṣētu*), see *KAR* 73 obv. 1–5 (restored from 18–20) and BM 78963:66. For bloating and loss of appetite, see *STT* 100 obv. 9′–10′, r. 3′, 11′–12′; *AMT* 40/5 iii 9//*BAM* 106 r. 1′//*STT* 101:3′ (restored from *BAM* 95:23; *AMT* 42/2:1//*AMT* 57/3 r. 1; cf. *AMT* 53/1 ii 2′).
192. For similar references, see *AMT* 43/5:7–8//*AMT* 7/7:11–12//*AMT* 56/1 obv. 12–13; *AMT* 43/5:13; *AMT* 56/3+*AMT* 84/7:3–4; AMT 57/5+ obv. 9–10, 13//*AMT* 43/5:5, 11//*AMT* 7/7:9//*BAM* 95:21//*BAM* 182 r. 9′; *BAM* 49:32′–34′//*BAM* 579 iv 33–35//*BAM* 50 r. 7–10; *BAM* 94 r. 12′–13′; *BAM* 182 r. 13′.
193. This section is restored from *AMT* 58/1+*AMT* 56/5:8.
194. For similar references, see *BAM* 95:19–20//*AMT* 53/9:5′–6′; *BAM* 95:29; *BAM* 94 r. 7′; *BAM* 99:19–20//*BAM* 100:2′–4′; *BAM* 99:25//*BAM* 95:27; *BAM* 99:42–43//*AMT* 43/1 iii 3′–4′; *BAM* 159 iii 10–11.
195. The translation is from context; see *CAD* N/2.133b; *AHw* 768a.
196. Kämmerer, *UF* 27.163 argues that *nīṭu* refers specifically to bloody diarrhea in smallpox. However, this and many other of Kämmerer's identifications are predicated on the assumption that an Old Babylonian recitation originally published by Goetze is a systematic description of an epidemic outbreak of smallpox. Although a few recitations do describe single diseases, many, including this one, were clearly intended for multiple uses (see Introduction under Retrospective Diagnosis).
197. Cf. *BAM* 96 iii 15′–16′//*AMT* 58/2:1–2//*BAM* 88:13′–15′ (phlegm).
198. See also *STT* 100a:1–2; *AMT* 56/1 obv. 8//*BAM* 182 r. 11′–12′.
199. Note also *BAM* 174 obv. 36′–37′//*BAM* 175:1′–2′.
200. See above, Chapter 6 n. 37.
201. For similar references, see *BAM* 89:8–9; *BAM* 96 ii 1//*BAM* 97:9′.
202. See also *BAM* 108 obv. 15–18.
203. "If a person's hips hurt him before (the age when) this would be expected, his feet are continually [tired], his shins sting him, his thighs are continually tired, and his knees give him a gnawing pain, that person was sick with DÚR.GIG in his childhood; to cure him . . ." (*BAM* 168:70–72//*AMT* 43/1 i 1–3//*BAM* 95:16–17; *BAM* 108 obv. 15–18).

CHAPTER 7. METABOLIC AND NUTRITIONAL DISEASES

1. Adamson, *JRAS* 1984.3–4 argues for the ubiquity of pellagra (niacin deficiency) in ancient Mesopotamia, citing texts that end with the diagnosis "'hand' of Ištar for egg-shaped beads." He believes that the phrase "egg-shaped beads" describes pigmentation around the neck, as first suggested by Labat, *RLA* 3.232–233. Cf. *CAD* A/2.470a, which interprets the beads as "carbuncles." Adamson further interprets these lesions as being caused by pellagra. However, two of the texts in question (DPS X A obv. 17//B obv. 19 = *TDP* 82:17 [cf. StBoT 36.35:15′//StBoT 36.57:5′] and now DPS III C r. 24 = *TDP* 28:84) are explicit references to wounds, and in the remaining reference (DPS X B r. 5 = *TDP* 88 r. 5) the patient gazes at his arms and has chills. None of these descriptions fits pellagra. Moreover, pellagra may be endemic among populations whose staple diet is based on "corn," but the corn is question is neither ancient Mesopotamian barley

(ŠE) nor wheat (GIG) but American corn (maize). This latter crop is native to the New World and was not grown in the Middle East as a staple crop until Lord Cromer introduced it into Egypt as part of his scheme to maximize the production of Egyptian cotton (Yapp, *Modern Near East* 232). It used to be thought that the reason that native American populations who subsist on a diet of maize did not get pellagra was because they ate vegetables. This did not, however, protect Egyptian peasants, for whom spinach has been a sort of national dish since at least the Middle Ages. It now appears that the real culprit is the milling process originally invented by Europeans to make white flour, which was substituted for the native American technique of treatment with alkali (*Harrison's Principles* 411–412).

2. See also DPS III A r. 16′//C r. 40 = *TDP* 30:100.

3. See also DPS III A r. 18′//C r. 42 = *TDP* 30:102.

4. The commentary *STT* 403:28 explains SI *se-pu-u* SI *e-ni-šú* SÍG SAG.DU-*šú en-šat*: "SI/*sepû*; SI means to be weak (as in the phrase) the hair of his head is weak." That the weakness in question refers to brittle hair is suggested by [NA_4] GAR-*šú* GIN_7 LAG MUN *sà-pi*: "the nature of the [stone] is that it is as brittle as a lump of salt" (*BAM* 378 iii 10).

5. See also DPS III A r. 17′//C r. 41 = *TDP* 30:101 (cf. StBoT 36.60:2); DPS III A r. 24′//C r. 49//G 6 = *TDP* 30:109 (cf. Labat, *Syria* 33.125 r. 5); DPS III A r. 25′//C r. 50; DPS XXI:1//DPS XIX/XX:125′ (AOAT 43.233 [catchline]).

6. Compare Labat, *Syria* 33.125 r. 3, 6. See also DPS III A r. 20′//C r. 44 = *TDP* 30:104.

7. The reading *sa-mi* ("red") is confirmed by *STT* 403:27 and *SpTU* 1.40:7.

8. Compare DPS III A r. 27′//C r. 52//G 7b = *TDP* 30:111. See also DPS XXI:2 (AOAT 43.246; restored after the commentary, Leichty, *AfO* 24.82–86:1–3). Note also Labat, *Syria* 33.125 r. 4 (the hair "rises like the mane of a lion"; i.e., it is red and standing on end). In the physiognomic omens (Köcher and Oppenheim, *AfO* 18.63–67 ii 35–38), a person with hair as red as red-dyed wool was expected to do poorly whereas one with black hair would find food to eat.

9. Adamson, *WO* 16.13 mentions hair color changes as evidence for the presence of protein malnutrition. However, the texts that he cites as evidence for a specifically "yellow" color in the hair do not actually refer to changes in hair color but to brittleness (see above). Also he asserts that aflotoxin plays some role in protein malnutrition, but this is incorrect.

10. For references, see *CAD* Ṣ 138–148.

11. *ABL* 1000:5–16.

12. "To still their hunger, they ate their sons' and daughters' flesh." (Streck, *Asb.* 36 iv 44–45).

13. Emendations are courtesy of an anonymous reviewer.

14. See DPS XL A 1–2//C 1–2 = *TDP* 216:1–2 (in infants).

15. See also *AMT* 52/5 obv. 4–5//*BAM* 139 obv. 1′–3′.

16. For the reading, see Heeßel, AOAT 43.190. The expression *ḫīṭu laššu* or *ḫīṭu yānu* appears not infrequently in Neo-Assyrian and Neo-Babylonian letters; it means something on the order of "no harm done" or "it is of no consequence." For references, see *CAD* Ḫ 210 s.v. *ḫīṭu* A mng. 1. For the interpretation, see also Ritter, *AS* 16.302 (quoting Landsberger).

17. Milk, ghee, or cheese would also have been appropriate recommendations (see Ellison, *Iraq* 43.36).

18. The referrent appears to be masculine but the previous entry has the patient having an erection like one who lays himself down on top of a woman.

19. After a suggestion by Stol, *Epilepsy* 72; cf. Heeßel, AOAT 43.296.

20. The restoration is suggested by the commentary *STT* 403:29, which has *su-uḫ-ši*: "bed."

21. Vegetables high in vitamin C include cress, which has been suggested as an identification for *saḫlû*, a condiment commonly eaten with bread in ancient Mesopotamia. A more surprising source of the vitamin, which would also have been readily available, is sprouted grain (Ellison, *Iraq* 43.36).

22. Lit. "it does not approach his flesh."

23. Adamson, *WO* 16.14 is not aware of any ancient Mesopotamian references to goiter but argues that goiter must have been "endemic" in ancient Mesopotamia on the grounds that millet was the staple crop. Millet is attested for ancient Mesopotamia, but it was never the staple crop. In any case, goiter is not "endemic" in areas where millet is grown but in areas where soil and water are deficient in iodine, most notably Switzerland and the American Great Lakes region.

24. A commentary equates *e-me-ru* with *na-pa-ḫu*. See 11 N-T 4:26 (Civil, *JNES* 33.336–338).

25. Coleman (*Thyroid* 12.799) quotes *TDP* 98:51 as a possible example of hyperthyroidism. However, we believe that the verb *zaqāpu* (mistranscribed as *ittanaqapa* and translated "protruded") refers to constriction of the pupils (see Chapter 13).

26. Fincke, *Augenleiden* 123. Ibid. 76–77 suggests a further possibility for exophthalmos with which we do not concur. For a discussion of the relevant passages, see Chapter 9 under FLOATERS.

27. Böck, *Morphoskopie* 288–289:20 reads KIR_4-*šá šá-gi-ig*, following *CAD* Š/1.72a. However, "If a woman's nose is stiff" does not make any apparent sense.

28. Fincke, *Augenleiden* 123 suggests restoring the end of the line as "she will not become (somebody's) wife." As may be seen from the illustration that she gives (pl. 2 ill. 4), victims of this condition are not terribly attractive.

29. Labat, *Syria* 33.125 mistranslates this as "white."

30. Note Šumma Izbu I:31–32 (Leichty, *Izbu* 34), where a woman gives birth to *lipištu* alongside the afterbirth and other membranous substances (I:28–29, 35). The translation of "scrotum" for *lipištu* (Landsberger, *MSL* 1.146–147; Leichty, *Izbu* 34; Stol, *Birth* 160) is inappropriate to this context.

CHAPTER 8. HEART, CIRCULATORY SYSTEM, AND LUNGS

1. Attia, *Histoire des Sciences Médicales* 34.1–10, argues that *šerʾānu* can mean "vein" but not "artery" and that the *āšipu* did not take the patient's pulse. The crux of the argument is that, in sharp contrast to Egyptian and Hippocratic physicians who also used a single word to describe muscles, veins, and arteries, the *āšipu* allegedly never attributed diseases to what we know to be internal (i.e., "natural") causes and therefore will not have had any interest in the pulse (pp. 2–3, 10). In fact, the *āšipu* attributed diseases to a combination of external and internal causes (see Chapter 19). There was also some learned speculation among *āšipus* in the late periods that "hand" of god, "hand" of goddess, and "hand" of ghost might actually be caused by the malfunctioning of internal organs such as the heart or stomach (see most recently Geller, *AfO* 48/49.61). In any case, frequent references to pulse rates clearly indicate that they did note the patient's pulse (on this point, see also Heeßel, *Medizin Historisches Journal* 36.259–260). Ironically, abnormalities in the pulse were not infrequently attributed by the *āšipu* to what we would describe as external ("supernatural") causes.

2. Both are mentioned in the Gilgamesh epic. For references and discussion, see Labat, *RLA* 4.367.

3. On this point, see also Heeßel, AOAT 43.74.

4. As, for example, Biggs, *Journal of the History of Science* 8.101, quoting Oppenheim, *OrNS* 30.27–33.

5. Text A has a mysterious gur ud.

6. Kinnier Wilson, *Medical History* 34.192,196 believes as do Labat and Stol (see next note) that the "heart is awake" and "heart is not awake" refers to consciousness. Also he believes that this reference describes a Jacksonian (focal) seizure that may or may not progress to a generalized seizure with loss of consciousness. He does not explain, however, why if that is the only difference the seizure with "heart awake" should have been removable if the one with "heart not awake" was not.

7. Labat, *RLA* 4.367 and *RLA* 3.197 defines "the heart is awake" as referring to mental lucidity and "does not know who he is" as loss of consciousness (see also Stol, *Epilepsy* 67). Labat also believes that the *āšipu* had it backward when it came to distinguishing true from false (hysterical) seizures. This is based on his interpretation that the ZI ("can/cannot be removed") is "true/false." In fact, the mistake is Labat's. The *āšipu* knew perfectly well that the patient lost consciousness in a true seizure (see Chapter 13). ZI is never read *kēnu*: "true," and "does not know who he is" implies a patient who is not unconscious but in shock or comatose.

8. See *CAD* S 1 s.v. *saʾālu*.

9. That this organ is the liver may be seen from Izbu comm. 203 (Leichty, *Izbu* 218): *ta-kal-tú* = *ga-bi-du*: "liver." See also Nougayrol, *RA* 44.3 and Goetze, *YOS* 10 p. 7. Note also *CAD* N 376a.

10. Lit. "jumps." That the reference is indeed to the pulse may readily be seen from the use of the verb to describe temporal blood vessels in DPS IV A_2 r. 8//G r. 7 = *TDP* 40 r. 8//*LKU* 94 r. 7.

11. Adamson, *JRAS* 1981.126–127 argues that *kamīt murṣi*, "a severe disease that may be fatal," refers specifically to the onset of anginal pain. However, *ka-mi-it* GIG is mentioned only once in a hemerology and is possibly a scribal error for *kimilti* GIG: "bitter wrath."

12. See Chapter 13 with 13.57–13.59.

13. See also *BAM* 316 iii 17′; *BAM* 317 r. 20, 22, 23.

14. Köcher, *Fs. Goerke* 24 suggests that *ḫuṣ ḫepi libbi* is depression, agitation, or bad temper, Labat, *RLA* 4.367 that it is "anguish," and Kinnier Wilson, *Medical History* 34.190 "emotional upset." Stol, *Epilepsy* 25, 27–32 translates *ḫuṣ ḫepi libbi* as "heartbreak" and suggests that it is grouped with "epilepsies" in a late Babylonian text for the same reasons that led Hippocrates to believe that black bile (melancholy) produced epilepsy. However, as Stol himself points out, the *āšipu* associated chest pain with stress and "bad temper, provoking strife and quarreling" (p. 29) or what would have been described by professors of humoral medicine as choleric (bilious), not melancholic, behavior. We have the *āšipu*'s description of love-sickness (see Chapter 16), but the associated depression is not described as *ḫuṣ ḫepi libbi*, as it would be if the pain in question were purely emotional. Black bile is the product of Hippocratic rationalism, not Greek folklore; it has in any case no connection with ancient Mesopotamia and the fact that the spleen was called "dark" because it is, in fact, purple, is irrelevant to the argument. Plants for the spleen are treatments for splenomegaly, and have nothing to do with either black bile or melancholy. Adamson, *JRAS* 1981.126–127 argues that *ḫuṣ ḫepi libbi* is the abdominal pain associated with angina, and in *RA* 87.154, he translates the latter term as "severe abdominal colic." We disagree, since there are other terms for abdominal colic (see Chapter 6). Moreover, since *ḫuṣu* specifically means "pain" and GAZ (*ḫepû*) means "to crush," it is difficult to interpret this symptom in any other way than "crushing pain." Modern physicians have found that patients with coronary artery disease commonly use this precise term in describing their pain.

15. See also *BAM* 388 i′ 11//*TCL* 6.34 iii 10; cf. BM 78963:83.

16. See also *BAM* 311:22′; *BAM* 375 i 11; *CTN* 4.196+195 ii 22′//*BAM* 379 i 21′; *KADP* 1 v 66; cf. BM 55251:9.

17. See also *BAM* 370 ia 3′–4′//*BAM* 372 i 2; cf. *SpTU* 2.22 i 16–21; *BAM* 316 ii 5′–13′//BM 64174:1–6//*STT* 95:130–137.

18. See also *KAR* 92 obv. 1–2, r. 1–3.

19. Lit. "jumps."

20. Lit. "jumps."

21. See Chapter 13 with 13.57–13.59.

22. See also StBoT 36.23 r. 6′–8′ (glomerulonephritis due to a strep infection—see 3.53).

23. According to the commentary *SpTU* 1.31:27, this is because of the cold.

24. Alternatively, as suggested by Attia, *Histoire des Sciences Médicales* 34.7, IM in the context of edema might mean "clay," since the *āšipu* in touching the patient's swollen ankles would have discovered that his finger left an indentation (pitting edema) such as might be produced by pressing one's thumb into wet clay.

25. See also *BAM* 380:20//*BAM* 381 iii 13; DPS VI A obv. 18//B_2 obv. 5//D 1 = *TDP* 56:18; DPS XXI:18 (AOAT 43.247); StBoT 36.60:5; cf. *AMT* 69/4:8′ (hands and feet).

26. The text has been collated.

27. Restorations are based on *BAM* 445:10–16.

28. See Chapter 13 with 13.57–13.59.

29. See also DPS XI A obv. 37 = *TDP* 92:37.

30. *BAM* 354 iii 16.

31. Restorations are based on the context provided by the surrounding entries.

32. For an edition of the relevant omens, see Böck, *Morphoskopie* 234–237, but note that she translates SA as "muscle" and ZI as "twitch." ZI means "to pulsate" (*AHw* 1343b s.v. *tebû* mng. 7), and muscles do not pulsate.

33. For similar descriptions of the pulse in fever, see DPS III C obv. 52–54, 56, 57–58 = *TDP* 24:52–54, 56, 57–58.

34. See also DPS XI A r. 29 = *TDP* 96 r. 29; DPS XIV A iv 26–27//C_2 iv 21//L 5–6 = *TDP* 146 iv 61′–62′.

35. See also DPS IV A obv. 46, 47 = *TDP* 36:46, 47.

36. See also *BAM* 66 obv. 13–14.

37. See also *BAM* 482 ii 2//*BAM* 9:61//*BAM* 11:19//Jastrow, *TCPP* r. 13; *BAM* 482 ii 4//*BAM* 9:40; Labat, *RA* 53.10–11 obv. 14; *BAM* 7:1//*BAM* 482 iii 40′//*BAM* 9:1//*BAM* 158 i 1–2//Jastrow, *TCPP* r. 19.

38. Fincke interprets many references in which this symptom occurs as referring to temporal arteritis (as, e.g., *Augenleiden* 80, 139). Temporal arteritis, an inflammatory condition of one or more branches of the carotid artery, is an uncommon disease that generally occurs after age fifty-five, especially in women. Against Fincke's interpretation are the frequency with which this symptom occurs, and the fact that this would require rejecting the now generally accepted translation of "pulsate" (*AHw* 1343b s.v. *tebû* mng. 7) in favor of "swell up." Early in the disease, the involved blood vessels may pulsate, but the cordlike thickening to

which Fincke believes this description refers is accompanied by a slowing of blood flow and obstruction of the vessels.

39. See also *BAM* 3 iii 25–26//*BAM* 35 iv 5′//*AMT* 20/1 ii! 16′.

40. Kinnier Wilson, *Iraq* 24.61 interprets "go" as normal and thinks that GAR means that the heart has stopped. Since, according to Kinnier Wilson, the absence of a pulse would mean that the patient was "either dead or very nearly so," where GAR is mentioned, "it must be assumed that the priest failed to locate the exact spot." The absence of a peripheral pulse does not necessarily mean a dead patient, the *āšipu* was not a priest, and the reasons for his not detecting a pulse do not include his inability to locate the exact spot. In any case, the references to the use of the term GAR are consistent with the translation "present," and "go" with "not present," the exact opposite of Kinnier Wilson's interpretation.

41. See Chapter 10 with 10.19.

42. See also DPS XI A r. 23 = *TDP* 96 r. 23.

43. See also DPS XI A r. 22, 24, 26, 28 = *TDP* 96 r. 22, 24, 26, 28.

44. See also DPS XI A r. 16 = *TDP* 96 r. 16; DPS XI A r. 20 = *TDP* 96 r. 20; cf. DPS XIX/XX:109′a (AOAT 43.232).

45. See also DPS XI A r. 17 = *TDP* 96 r. 17.

46. Labat, *Syria* 33.125 r. 8 interprets passages in which blood vessels are said to "go" and "present" as referring to muscles "moving" and "being immobile." We do not concur. For the ancient Mesopotamian terms used to describe muscle spasms and paralysis, see Chapter 13.

47. See Adamson, *RA* 84.27–28.

48. See also DPS XIII B i 31′//D 4 = *TDP* 114 i 35′; DPS XIII J 12 = *TDP* 126 iii 44.

49. The text repeats the GABA.RI of the preceding reference.

50. For details, see McEwan, *RLA* 7.170–171.

51. Kinnier Wilson, *Diseases in Antiquity* 199–200 suggests pneumonic plague or tuberculosis for *suʾālu*-cough. However, we believe this term to be a sign and not a specific disease. Moreover, most of the references do not mention death, a probable outcome in pneumonic plague and a likely outcome in tuberculosis.

52. See also DPS XXII:29–30 [AOAT 43.254].

53. The Arabic cognate means "to sigh."

54. See also *BAM* 1 ii 27–28, 34; *BAM* 2 obv. 6′; *CT* 14.31 [D.T. 136]:7; *STT* 92 ii 9–11; *AMT* 80/1 i 1//*BAM* 548 i 1; *AMT* 80/1 i 8//*BAM* 548 i 8; *BAM* 548 i 25; *BAM* 548 iv 2′//*BAM* 552 iv 4′; *BAM* 549 i 10′//*BAM* 550 i 1′; *BAM* 550 i 8′//*AMT* 80/1 ii 8; *BAM* 567 ii 2′, 3′; *CTN* 4.113 iii 8′; BM 78963:44; *AMT* 80/1 i 17//*BAM* 548 i 17; *BAM* 552 iii 3′//*AMT* 81/1 iii 10′; DPS XL A 39 = *TDP* 222:39; BM 78963:45; cf. *BAM* 567 ii 4′.

55. Labat, *RLA* 4.523 interprets this as a "fit of coughing."

56. See also Labat and Tournay, *RA* 40.116 obv. 8–9; *BAM* 575 ii 43; *BAM* 575 iii 12; BM 78963:40; DPS XXII:25 [AOAT 43.253]; DPS XXII:29–30 [AOAT 43.254].

57. Cf. also *CTN* 4.113 iii 4′.

58. See also *AMT* 50/3:6–7; *AMT* 52/9:6′; cf. *BAM* 555 iii 55′ (blood).

59. See also *BAM* 549 iv 19; *BAM* 550 iv 8.

60. See also *BAM* 575 iii 65–67.

61. Labat read DINGIR.MAḪ, but there is nothing after the DINGIR on the tablet or in the copy.

62. For a treatment, see *BAM* 216:59′–63′//*BAM* 470 obv. 12′–15′.

63. For a treatment, see *BAM* 216:55′–58′//Scheil, *RA* 14.88 ii 6′–10′//Labat, *RSO* 32.112 v 1′–5′. Note that Labat, *RSO* 32.117, 121 misrestores and consequently mistranslates this passage.

64. Geller, *RAI* 28.193 interprets this as the throat contracting. However, ZI.ME is plural and must, therefore, refer to the breath and not the throat.

65. Note the instruction GABA-*su te-še-ʾi*: "You examine his chest" (BM 78963:37).

66. See also *BAM* 575 iii 30–32//*BAM* 55:1–7//*BAM* 56 r. 8′–10′//*BAM* 57:1′–5′.

67. See also DPS XVI:30 (AOAT 43.175); DPS XVI:53′–54′, 57′, 58′ (AOAT 43.177); DPS XVI:98′–99′ (AOAT 43.180).

68. See Chapter 13 with 13.57–13.59.

69. For this interpretation of *paṭāru*, said of the chest, see *CAD* S 1a s.v. *saʾālu*.

70. An anonymous reviewer suggested that these references may be not to the sides of the chest (GABA) but to the joints (DU_8/*pitru*). Although DU_8 certainly has a reading of *pitru*, the generally accepted interpretation of this latter term is "abdominal wall" (*AHw* 870b) and not "joint." The new reading may have merit in some passages, but in these references, we prefer our interpretation.

71. *CAD* M/2.165a takes this as a statement rather than a question, but this would imply that there is nothing wrong with him when, in fact, he dies.
72. The text has been collated.
73. See also *STT* 92 ii 23.
74. See also Adamson, *JRAS* 1979.4.

CHAPTER 9. EYES, EARS, AND NOSE

1. See *BAM* 19:8′; *BAM* 156:48; *BAM* 194 vii 6′; *BAM* 307:7; *BAM* 379 iii 38′; *BAM* 393 obv. 21; *BAM* 510 i 5′; *BAM* 510 i 7′//AMT 20/2:5′; *BAM* 510 i 27′//*BAM* 19:3′; *BAM* 510 i 29′//*BAM* 19:11′; *BAM* 510 i 30′; *BAM* 510 ii 33′//*BAM* 513 ii 46′//*BAM* 514 ii 44′; *BAM* 510 iii 6, 14, 22//*BAM* 513 iii 7′, 15′, 24′//*BAM* 514 iii 11′, 19′, 27′; *BAM* 513 iii 31′//*BAM* 514 iii 38′; *BAM* 513 iv 4, 6//*BAM* 514 iv 3, 5; *BAM* 510 iv 4, 22, 26//*BAM* 513 iv 10, 32//*BAM* 514 iv 9, 27, 31; *BAM* 515 ii 52; *KADP* 1 v 45, 46; *STT* 279:22, 51; cf. *BAM* 15 obv. 10′–11′; *BAM* 379 iv 8; BM 42610+:26 (Finkel, Fs. Lambert 164–165).
2. Fincke, *Augenleiden* 78–81 argues for *apû* as a description of blepharospasm. However, the literal translation of "clouded" seems to yield perfectly good sense.
3. *CAD* E 279–280 translates the verb *erēpu* as "dark" (see also Fincke, *Augenleiden* 178–179). However, with *AHw* 238a, it actually means "clouded," as the derivatives *erpu* and *erpitu* show.
4. Note also *BAM* 423 i 28′; *BAM* 482 iv 35′–36′.
5. See also DPS XIX/XX:15′ (AOAT 43.227); cf. *BAM* 23:15; BM 42419:4′ (Finkel, *Fs. Lambert* 161–162, but reading IGI *er-pu* instead of *ši-ir-pu*).
6. This term should not be confused with the skin disease *ašû,* for which see Chapter 10.
7. See also *BAM* 510 iv 31//*BAM* 514 iv 36; *BAM* 515 iv 45′; *BAM* 516 i 1; *SpTU* 2.50:24; BM 54641+BM 54826 r. 9. Fincke, *Augenleiden* 92 suggests a diagnosis of keratitis for *BAM* 522:6′. However, although keratitis may produce a gray-red color, this passage suggests that frank bleeding has occurred.
8. On this point, see also Fincke, *Augenleiden* 87 and Stol, *JNES* 45.296.
9. See also *BAM* 3 iii 47; *BAM* 3 i 20//*BAM* 480 ii 19//*AMT* 5/3 i 8′; *BAM* 382:2; *SpTU* 2.50:4, 7; BM 132097 obv. 12′ (Geller, *AfO* 35.22–23); *BAM* 351:7//*STT* 111:8′; *BAM* 352 i 13–14, ii 14–15; *SpTU* 2.22 i 5+*SpTU* 3.85 i 10; *SpTU* 3.85 i 2, 6, 14.
10. *CAD* A/2.204b interprets this phrase to mean "when that person finishes his work." *CAD* Š/3.84a interprets KIN as "affliction" and the TIL as SUMUN, which would yield "if his affliction is prolonged." The best sense would appear to lie in a combination of the two suggestions, that is, taking KIN as "work" and reading TIL as SUMUN.
11. Fincke, *Augenleiden* 87, 91.
12. After a suggestion by Stol, *Epilepsy* 94.
13. Haussperger, *Mem. Cagni* 442–445 has a number of suggestions for interpreting this text, namely, onchocerciasis, glaucoma, and trachoma. We agree that the early stages of trachoma are compatible with *amurdinnu* (pink eye), but we have other suggested references for onchocerciasis (see Chapter 3) and glaucoma (see below).
14. See Fincke, *Augenleiden* 240–241.
15. See also ibid. 91.
16. See also ibid. 92.
17. Ibid. 92 suggests *synchysis scintillans* as another possible cause of flashes. *Synchysis scintillans* causes a condition in older individuals where liquified vitreous and the presence of crystals can cause silvery showers when the eyeball is moved. However, *Synchysis scintillans* does not scintillate for the patient; it can be observed only by the ophthamologist after dilation of the pupil (observation courtesy of A. Attia).
18. Possibly also referring to a flash of light is a *ṣirāḫu* that is attested once: DIŠ NA *ṣi-ra-ḫu ina* IGI-*šú it-tab-šu-ú* (BM 76515 obv. 1).
19. See also *AMT* 87/3 ii 6′; *SpTU* 2.22 i 13 (without explicit diagnosis).
20. Note also *AMT* 87/3 ii 6; *BAM* 351:13; *BAM* 344:9.
21. See also *BAM* 516 i 9–10. Compare: DIŠ NA *ina pa-an* IGI^{II}-*šú* ⌜*lu*⌝ [. . .] *lu* GIN$_7$ *ḫi-mi-te* ⌜*lu*⌝ [. . .] GAR.GAR-*an* ⌜*it-ta*⌝-[. . .] KIN-*šú* x x [. . .] (K 13239:1′–4′) (with frost).
22. For this interpretation of the phrase, see also Fincke, *Augenleiden* 103–104.
23. See ibid. 91–92.

24. The passage has been collated.

25. Fincke, *Augenleiden* 130 suggests that the red threads are mucus found in chronic conjunctivitis. We believe that prominent conjunctival blood vessels are a far more likely explanation.

26. See also ibid. 210–211.

27. Note also BM 132097 obv. 4′ (Geller, *AfO* 35.22–23) (with *ṣarāḫu*).

28. The reading follows a suggestion by Stol, *Epilepsy* 94.

29. Fincke, *Augenleiden* 91–92 n. 70 believes this text to be describing glaucoma. This interpretation is, however, based on a mistranslation of "it flutters" as "it kills (him)," that is, it is extremely painful.

30. For the join, see Geller, *ZA* 74.293.

31. For a complete translation, see Collins, *Natural Illness* 203–205 (Eyes 2).

32. Fincke, *Augenleiden* 127–128 suggests that the phrase "like a sheep with its throat cut" refers to a bright red color (as of fresh blood).

33. Heeßel, AOAT 43.254 reads *qan* but the copy and *TDP* 180:34 have *qam.*

34. Note also *BAM* 40 obv. 12–14.

35. See also DPS V A 12′–14′, 16′–17′ = *TDP* 46 B 12–14, 16–17.

36. This is related to the Arabic word for "rose"; see *AHw* 45–46 and Stol, *JNES* 45.296.

37. Fincke, *Augenleiden* 192–193 identifies *amurdinnu* as rosacea. However, this condition is not commonly associated with "pink eye." Adamson, *RA* 87.156 identifies *amurdinnu* as trachoma. Although in its early stages, trachoma may have "pink eye," there are many other causes of this condition (see below). Haussperger, *Mem. Cagni* 444 also identifies *amurdinnu* as trachoma but thinks that *amurdinnu* refers to the nodes that are often present on the eyelids in trachoma. *Amurdinnu,* however, refers specifically to the color "rose."

38. See also *BAM* 382:15; *BAM* 515 i 9; BM 132097 obv. 9′–10′ (Geller, *AfO* 35.22–23).

39. See *CAD* Z 63b s.v. *zaqtu* mng. 4.

40. Heeßel, *AOAT* 43.359, 366 interprets this as DIRI/*neqelpû,* which he translates as "unsteady."

41. See also *BAM* 510 i 40′//*BAM* 514 i 48′; *BAM* 510 ii 5′, 8′, 14′//*BAM* 514 ii 16′, 19′, 25′//*BAM* 513 ii 20′, 23′, 29′.

42. Note also *BAM* 516 ii 6′//*AMT* 18/4:6′; *BAM* 18:20; Labat, *RA* 53.12–13 r. 33.

43. See Chapter 3.

44. Restored from *STT* 89:103–108 (Stol, *Epilepsy* 91). Note also DPS XXVI:11′–13′ (AOAT 43.279).

45. See also *BAM* 3 iii 28//*BAM* 482 ii 26//*AMT* 20/1 ii! 3′; *BAM* 3 iii 31//*BAM* 482 ii 28//*AMT* 20/1 ii! 5′; *BAM* 3 iii 34//*AMT* 20/1 ii! 7′; DPS IV E ii 19–21 = *SpTU* 3.88 ii 19–21.

46. See also DPS XVI:85′, 86′ (AOAT 43.179); cf. DPS XV:67 (AOAT 43.154).

47. See also Fincke, *Augenleiden* 190–192.

48. Compare *BAM* 578 iii 4–5 (with *amurriqānu*-jaundice; see 6.122).

49. See Chapter 6, pp. 138–139.

50. See also *BAM* 515 ii 43, 44; *BAM* 578 iv 5, 6.

51. See Chapter 6, pp. 138–139.

52. See also DPS V A 9′–10′ = *TDP* 46 B 9–10.

53. Fincke, *Augenleiden* 137 also suggests corneal ulcers as a possibility.

54. This is by the Middle Chronology.

55. See also *BAM* 14:5//*BAM* 18:14 (cf. BM 54641+BM 54826 r. 6); *BAM* 159 v 5; *SpTU* 2.50:22; DPS V C ii 6′//E ii 6′ = *TDP* 48 D ii 6; DPS V E ii 7′//D ii 1′ = *TDP* 48 D ii 7.

56. Note also *BAM* 14:1; *BAM* 382:11.

57. Note also *BAM* 159 iv 23′–24′.

58. See also Fincke, *Augenleiden* 235–236.

59. For the transliteration, see Geller, *ZA* 74.296–297. See also Landsberger, *JNES* 17.58; cf. Nougayrol, *Ugaritica* 5.64–65 no. 19.

60. Miller, *NABU* 1989 no. 10 suggests that this is a threat to (a) botch an operation or (b) remove damaged conjunctival tissue after a trachomal infection. Given the clear mention of a foreign body in the eye, neither suggestion has anything to recommend it.

61. Note also *BAM* 510 iv 5//*BAM* 513 iv 11//*BAM* 514 iv 10; *BAM* 510 iv 23–25//*BAM* 514 iv 28–30.

62. See also Kinnier Wilson, *Diseases in Antiquity* 198; Adamson, *RA* 87.156 w/ n. 26.

63. See also Fincke, *Augenleiden* 182.

64. For the interpretation of *merḫu* as sty, see Landsberger, *JNES* 14.16; cf. Fincke, *Augenleiden* 199–200. Adamson, *WO* 16.9–10 misinterprets Landsberger's argument that the *merḫu* on wheat or barley is "ergot"

(see Chapter 15) and that the *merḫu* in a person's eye is the similarly appearing sty to mean that the fungus that infects wheat and rye to produce the ergot toxin can actually infect a person's eye. There is no evidence to support this contention. On this point, see also Stol, *Fs. Finet* 165. Stol argues that *merḫu* could mean sty or trachoma. He bases the latter argument on the fact that the ancient Greek word for trachoma was "barley grain." However, *merḫu* does not mean "barley grain" and in any case the description is not particularly apt since trachoma typically produces diffuse thickening and scarring of the lids.

65. Fincke, *Augenleiden* 221–222.

66. The commentary (*SpTU* 1.31:30–31) confirms that this expression means that the eyes are (partially) open.

67. See also *AMT* 19/1 iv! 9′–10′.

68. Fincke, *Augenleiden* 124–125 suggests a diagnosis of urticaria or periarteritis nodosa for this reference. However, none of the signs listed in the text corresponds to the findings normally associated with either of these conditions. Fincke further suggests that "soaked" refers to swelling of the eyes. However, as she points out, the term *maḫāḫu* in other contexts means "to soften" or "to make pliable." Swelling would have exactly the opposite effect.

69. See also DPS IV B obv. 30–31//E i 10–11 = *TDP* 36:31–32//*SpTU* 3.88 i 10–11; cf. *BAM* 482 iii 1.

70. Fincke, *Augenleiden* 140 suggests epidemic keratoconjunctivitis for these references. However, the swelling described in the text would appear to be periorbital rather than just conjunctival in nature.

71. See also DPS IV B obv. 17 = *TDP* 34:17; cf. DPS IV B obv. 16 = *TDP* 34:16 (headache with hurting eye muscles). Fincke, *Augenleiden* 73–74 suggests that *TDP* 34:16 might be describing iridocylitis. However, in the absence of redness, this seems unlikely. Kinnier Wilson, *Diseases in Antiquity* 200–201 interprets *TDP* 34:16–17 as meningitis, but we do not concur. For possible ancient descriptions of meningitis, see Chapter 13 under MENINGITIS. Adamson, *JRAS* 1979.4 n. 25 cites *TDP* 34:17 as "evidence of fevers associated with chills, rigors, and cold sweats" suggesting the presence of endemic malaria in ancient Mesopotamia, but again we do not concur. For possible descriptions of malaria in ancient texts, see Chapter 3 under MALARIA.

72. See also Stol, *JNES* 45.295–299; Fincke, *Augenleiden* 200–202; Kinnier Wilson, *Diseases in Antiquity* 192; Pangas, *Am.Journ.Med.Gen.* 91.320; Ebeling, *RLA* 1.314.

73. This has been missed by previous editors of *BAM* 516 ii 32′–iii 3//*BAM* 25:4′–10′ (Stol, *JNES* 45.297; Geller, *BiOr* 43.742) who wish to see in this treatment nothing more than "ritual and magic." However, the parallel *BAM* 25:9′ (of which Stol was aware) follows the instruction to cut off a chunk of liver ([*ta-ḫar-r*] *a-aṣ*) with a very clear KÚ ("he eats (it)").

74. As Stol, *JNES* 45.296–297 and Fincke, *Augenleiden* 201 note, Greek, Aramaic, and Hebrew also use the same term for "day" and "night" blindness. German distinguishes the two terms but they are apparently used somewhat interchangeably in common parlance.

75. See *CAD* Š/3.125–126; *AHw* 1250. *BAM* 515 i 16 also mentions another type of membraneous substance, *lipištu*. The translation of "scrotum" for *lipištu* (Landsberger, *MSL* 1.146–147; Leichty, *Izbu* 34; Stol, *Birth* 160) is inappropriate to this context.

76. Labat, *RLA* 3.232 believes that *šišītu* means blisters or vesicles. This seems unlikely, since neither blisters nor vesicles commonly occur on the conjunctiva.

77. See also *BAM* 23:6; *BAM* 578 iv 15.

78. We concur with Fincke, *Augenleiden* 202–203 that the translation of "shadow" is to be preferred to "slime" (Veldhuis, *NABU* 1991 no. 106). Note also Kinnier Wilson, *Diseases in Antiquity* 198–199 ("shadow") versus Stol, *JNES* 45.296 ("slime").

79. See also Fincke, *Augenleiden* 202–208.

80. For the join, see Geller, *ZA* 74.293.

81. See Collins, *Natural Illness* 203–205 (Eyes 2).

82. On the identification of some *ṣillu* references with pterygium, see also Miller, *NABU* 1989 no. 10.

83. See also *BAM* 3 iv 46; *BAM* 15 obv. 6′; *BAM* 382:6; *BAM* 423 i 9′; *BAM* 515 iv 3, 4, 6, 11.

84. The term is variously written *zi-iḫ-ḫu*, *zi-ḫu*, and even *di-ḫu*. For references, see *CAD* Ṣ 176–179.

85. Fincke, *Augenleiden* 164 suggests that *šīlu* might be referring to extreme wasting (cachexia). Although the *āšipu* describes eye changes in extreme wasting (see 3.106), he does not use this expression to describe it.

86. *Augenleiden* 163–165.

87. See the illustration ibid. 164.

88. See ibid. 163–165.

89. The *di-kal* is present in both versions (the passage has been collated).

90. The interpretation of this and the following BE sign as BAD: "either" rather than MÚD: "blood" follows *CAD* Š/1.371a. This seems preferable to interpreting a term that normally refers to an aromatic plant (*baluḫḫu*) as some sort of strange excretion from the eye (Geller, *BiOr* 43.741).

91. For the translation of ᵈLAMMA IGI: "guardian spirit of the eye" as "cornea," see also Kinnier Wilson, *Diseases in Antiquity* 199.

92. See also *BAM* 15 obv. 4′.

93. See Fincke, *Augenleiden* 231–232.

94. Ibid. 232 suggests siderosis for the "dark" color in the iris. However, iron deposits generally produce spots of a yellow/brown color, which would have been described by the *āšipu* as SIG_7: "yellow." The following lines, DPS V G 19–21 = *TDP* 52 G 19–21, are formatted in such a way as to suggest that other colors (now lost in lacunae) were originally mentioned, so it is conceivable that siderosis was indeed originally described.

95. See also DPS V G 16 = *TDP* 52 G 16 (both eyes).

96. *Kakkulti īni* is sometimes translated as "eyeball." Fincke, *Augenleiden* 231–232, 257 translates it as "iris" and we agree (see also Adamson, *JRAS* 1974.104–105; *AHw* 423a). Attia questions the ability of the *āšipu* to see these muscles with the naked eye. However, the *āšipu* had a low-powered magnifying glass.

97. *Augenleiden* 138–139.

98. The text has been collated. Labat read "hand of his goddess."

99. *Augenleiden* 163–164.

100. For helpful illustrations, see ibid.

101. The restoration is based on the commentary (see below). The traces in Falkenstein's copy (*LKU* 78) are not compatible with a KUR (*šad*) sign but could represent a partially broken MU (*šád*).

102. Fincke, *Augenleiden* 163 suggests "flattened."

103. See ibid. 163 n. 1239, correcting Adamson, *JRAS* 1974.105.

104. Fincke, *Augenleiden* 257.

105. Fincke further suggests (ibid. 257) the Brushfield spots of Down syndrome and nevi of the iris, but the color and/or consistency of these lesions make them unlikely possibilities.

106. See also *BAM* 382:4; cf. *BAM* 515 i 12.

107. Previous suggestions for the meaning of "moving tissue" include eye tumors (Kinnier Wilson, *JNES* 27.244), pterygium (Stol, *JNES* 45.296), and exophthalmus (Fincke, *Augenleiden* 76–77). In none of these diagnoses, however, is there true movement of the tissue, whereas movement is characteristic of floaters. Also favoring the diagnosis of floaters is their benign nature, which is not always the case in the other diagnoses.

108. See also *BAM* 522:3′, 5′, 6′, 10′.

109. See Fincke, *Augenleiden* 176.

110. See also DPS V B ii 6, 7, 8 = *TDP* 48 C ii 6, 7, 8; StBoT 36.23 r. 5′a; cf. DPS V B ii 9–10 = *TDP* 48 C ii 9–10.

111. See also DPS V A 6′–7′ = *TDP* 46 B 6–7.

112. See also DPS V B ii 2, 3, 4–5 = *TDP* 48 C ii 2, 3, 4–5; cf. *BAM* 382:8.

113. Fincke, *Augenleiden* 193–195.

114. For an illustration, see ibid. pl. 2 ill. 5.

115. See *CAD* D 67b for the suggestion that this is a euphemistic reference to the red eyes of an albino. We believe Fincke's suggestion to be preferable. Since congenital glaucoma often leads to blindness, Stol, *JNES* 45.295 w/ n. 8 is not far off the mark when he translates the term as "blind."

116. See Fincke, *Augenleiden* 193; cf. also *CAD* Ṣ 236a, which quotes another commentary equating "pressed" with "wide open eyes."

117. See also DPS IV B obv. 28//E i 8 = *TDP* 36:28//*SpTU* 3.88 i 8.

118. See also DPS IV B obv. 27//E i 7 = *TDP* 34:27//*SpTU* 3.88 i 7; DPS XVI:23–24 (AOAT 43.174).

119. Powell, *ZA* 62.165–221.

120. The text has been collated. Ritter, AS 16.303 n. 13 restored [*uk-ta-at*]*-ta-at* against the traces. The meaning is the same.

121. See also DPS VIII 6b, 7a = *TDP* 68:6b, 7a; cf. DPS VIII 24, 25 = *TDP* 70:24, 25.

122. Labat, *RSO* 32.116, 121 takes this to mean that the man's ear feels heavy when the wind happens to be blowing, but the word order would seem to indicate that the ear is the object of the verb.

123. Livingstone, SAA 3.39:2, 3, 11, 14, 18.

124. See also DPS VIII 11b, 12 = *TDP* 68/70:11b, 12.

125. See also *AMT* 105/1 iv 10//*AMT* 35/5:3′.

126. Haussperger, *Mem. Cagni* 448 agrees with the diagnosis of otitis media.

127. See also *BAM* 503 ii 54′//Labat, *RSO* 32.112 ii 14′–15′. Note also *BAM* 503 ii 61′//*BAM* 3 iii 50; *BAM* 503 iii 48′; *BAM* 3 iv 28//*BAM* 503 iv 29; *RSO* 32.112 iii 4′; *BAM* 503 iv 11//*CTN* 4.113 ii 4//*RSO* 32.112 iv 10′; *BAM* 503 iv 20; *CTN* 4.113 ii 9.

128. See also DIŠ NA GEŠTU[II]!-*šú neš-ma-a he-sa-a* (BM 76023+83009 obv. 6′).

129. See also *BAM* 379 i 25′//*SpTU* 3.106 i 4//*CTN* 4.196+195 ii 25′.

130. See also *BAM* 503 iii 12; *BAM* 327 i 7′.

131. See also BM 32277++ iii 9–10.

132. See also *BAM* 503 ii 67′–68′.

133. See also *CTN* 4.113 ii 28//BM 76023 + 83009 obv. 10′–11′.

134. Note also *BAM* 480 iv 12.

135. See also *SpTU* 1.49:33; *BAM* 503 i 17′, 20′, 28′, 30′ (cf. *BAM* 503 i 11′); *STT* 281 i 21; BM 76023+83009 r. 2′; Labat, *RSO* 32.112 v 13′; *BAM* 506:4′//*CT* 51.199 obv. 1; *BAM* 503 ii 3, 7, 13; *BAM* 506:34′//*BAM* 508 iv 31//*CT* 51.199 obv. 17; *BAM* 507:12′; *BAM* 506:2′; *BAM* 506:6′//*BAM* 508 iv 8//*CT* 51.199 obv. 10. Cf. *BAM* 3 ii 47, iv 31; *KAR* 22 obv. 1.

136. Labat, *MDP* 57, p. 254 ad ii 12′, followed by *CAD* Š/1.63–65 suggests "buzz" as a translation for this term. Outside of medical contexts, the verb is mostly used to describe the storm-god's thunder.

137. Labat, *MDP* 57 p. 254 ad ii 12′ suggests "hiss" as a translation for this term. *CAD* Š/2.151b s.v. *šasû* mng. 1 i translates "ring." Outside of medical contexts, this common verb is used to describe human shouts and calls, bird and reptile calls, and thunder.

138. See also DPS VIII 8 = *TDP* 68:8; *BAM* 155 ii 5′//Labat, *RSO* 32.112 iii 10′; *BAM* 506:8′; DPS VIII 10a–b = *TDP* 68:10a–b; *BAM* 506:10′; *RSO* 32.112 iii 16′; DPS VIII 11a = *TDP* 68:11a; *BAM* 3 iv 25//Labat, *RA* 53.12–13 r. 31; *STT* 281 i 17.

139. Note also *BAM* 159 v 25.

140. Köcher suggests that this expression is short for *na-piš* KIR_4-*šú* DUGUD: "it is difficult for him to breathe (through) his nose" (*BAM* 6 p. xxi).

141. Note also *BAM* 393 r. 3.

142. *CAD* Ṣ 35 cites this passage as an example of the Gt of *ṣabātu* and interprets it to mean that the nostrils are "grown together." However, the other examples of the Gt of *ṣabātu* (with snakes and hair) refer to temporary and reversible "interwinings." It seems probable that the reference is to a temporary blockage of the nasal passages. For treatments of nasal problems, see *SpTU* 1.45:7, 16, 18.

143. See also K 1452 obv. 8′; BM 42634+:1 (Finkel, *Fs. Lambert* 166); *BAM* 530 iv 2′; *AMT* 27/9:3′; *KADP* 1 v 20; cf. *STT* 93:6; *SpTU* 1.45:19.

144. See also *SpTU* 4.129 vi 10; K 4782:8′, 12′–13′. Cf. *ABL* 111+:8–15 (Parpola, SAA 10.321) and *ABL* 108 r. 1–17 (Parpola, SAA 10.322).

CHAPTER 10. SKIN AND HAIR

1. For references, see *CAD* B 332b.

2. *TCL* 3 + Weidner, *AfO* 12 pl. 11:102.

3. For references, see *CAD* Z 154–155.

4. Lyon, *Sar.* 7:41.

5. Gilg. P iii 24. For these and other references, see *CAD* Š/1.325.

6. Durand, *ARM* XXVI/1.552 proposes a similar interpretation but then translates *simmu* when used to describe infectious processes as "anthrax" (552, 578–579) and when used to describe wounds (as in Laws of Ḫammurapi § 206) as "hematoma" (552 n. 83). Both of these translations are far too specific.

7. See also *STT* 92 iii 19′, 24′. Note also *BAM* 1 iii 24//*CT* 14.43 [S. 60]:1′; *BAM* 380:4–5; *BAM* 379 i 33′, 35′//*SpTU* 3.106 i 9, 11 (for a persistent sore).

8. See *AHw* 989a; *CAD* R 377a gives no translation.

9. Heeßel, AOAT 43.353, 367 restores *ri-*[*šu*]*-tum* (following von Weiher, *SpTU* 4 p. 81; cf. Finkel, *Fs. Lambert* 152; see below).

10. Note also *BAM* 3 i 49//*BAM* 152 i 14.

11. See *AHw* 997b; *CAD* R 437–438. Adamson, *RA* 82.163–164 argues that *ruṭibtu* is restricted to a pathological condition of the feet (*muruṣ kabbarti*), and represents an allergic reaction to wheat dust. *Muruṣ kabbarti* is one of the most readily diagnosable conditions among the skin diseases, namely, mycetoma (see Chapter 3), and *ruṭibtu* is by no means restricted to this condition. The idea of wheat allergy is based on the prediction in hemerologies that he who stands behind a mortar on a particular ill-omened day will have trouble with *ruṭibtu* (Hulin, *Iraq* 21.50:28). Hemerologies are not medical texts but omens and, as with our own "Step on a crack, break your mother's back," the medical information contained in them is only rarely to be taken at face value. In this example, the obvious suggestion is that the person standing behind the mortar was apparently getting ready (*raṭābu*) to pound, thus suggesting a punning reference to "dampness" (*ruṭibtu*). In any case, barley was not merely pounded but also ground in a hand quern before use which should have brought wheat dust into contact with the hands and chest as well as the legs and feet. Hulin, *Iraq* 21.49–50:28 w/ n. 36 (followed by Labat, *Iraq* 23.90–91:16–18) translates *ruṭibtu* as "gangrene" because "dampness" suggests suppuration. Infected gangrene can be "wet," but this is not the only skin condition that can be "wet" (infected), and uninfected gangrene is dry.

12. Heeßel, AOAT 43.354 reads GÁL? GIG.

13. For *rušumtu* "oozing," see *AHw* 997a; *CAD* R 432–433; Hulin, *Iraq* 21.49 n. 36.

14. *CAD* N/1.278b adds an extra NI sign and reads the UD of UD.DU (È) as PER to yield a reading: "his face glistens like oil." In either case, the patient clearly has oily skin.

15. See *AHw* 989–990. *CAD* R 207a translates "itch" based on context alone, ignoring etymology and lexical equations with *ezzu*: "angry." However, the contexts will fit "redness" quite easily. Heeßel, *AOAT* 43.353, 367 (following von Weiher, *SpTU* 4 p. 81; cf. Finkel, *Fs. Lambert* 152) restores *ri-*[*šu*]*-tum* instead of *ri-*[*šik-t*]*um* in DPS XXXIII:11 [AOAT 43.353] and, on this basis translates *rišûtu* as "scales" (359, 360). However, fish scales are more appropriate to dry skin (*rišiktu*) than to reddened skin (*rišûtu*) which, according to BM 43171+:15–16 (Finkel, *Fs. Lambert* 152; see below), can produce fluid.

16. See *CAD* R 381–382.

17. Campbell Thompson, *PRSM* 17.2 n. 5 suggests "lice" for *rišūtu*. Although redness may accompany lice infestation, Akkadian has a separate word for lice, UḪ/*kalmatu* (see Chapter 2). Goetze, *JCS* 9.12 and Kinnier-Wilson, *Iraq* 24.59 translate *rišūtu* as "itch, scabies." Finkel, *Fs. Lambert* 152 suggests "eczema" or "psoriasis." This is, however, based on an incorrect restoration of DPS XXXIII:11 (AOAT 43.353) (see above). Adamson, *RA* 82.164–165 considers this term to be synonymous with impetigo, a potentially serious infection if untreated. The texts do not suggest a serious condition and it appears more likely that the term was used as a sign (redness) rather than a specific disease. The alleged association of *rišūtu* with Nergal, god of the netherworld (Adamson, *RA* 82.164 w/ n. 9; cf. also von Weiher, AOAT 11.86 n. 3) is based on a misinterpretation of *CT* 24.41:70 as referring to a Nergal of "skin redness" (*šá ri-šú-ti*). Incongruous as it may seem, the reference is actually to a Nergal "of exultation" (*šá ri-šá-ti*); see *CAD* R 379b. Compare "Emeslam (Nergal's temple in Kutha), sanctuary of exultation" (Böllenrücher, LSS 1/6 no. 3:7) and note VAB 7/2.266:14–15 (von Weiher, AOAT 11.68), where Nergal is said to depart the Emeslam "in joy and exultation." Kämmerer, *UF* 27.159 argues that *rišūtu* refers specifically to the scarlet exanthem of smallpox. However, this and many other of Kämmerer's identifications are predicated on the assumption that an Old Babylonian recitation originally published by Goetze is a systematic description of an epidemic outbreak of smallpox. Although a few recitations do describe single diseases many, including this one, were clearly intended for multiple uses (see Introduction under Retrospective Diagnosis).

18. Note also *BAM* 391:24–25//BM 42404 r. 5′–6′ (Finkel, *Fs. Lambert* 155); BM 42576+:21 (Finkel, *Fs. Lambert* 160); *AMT* 30/1 obv. 5′, 9′; *STT* 93:112′.

19. See also *BAM* 120 iii 1.

20. Note also *BAM* 1 ii 9–11; *BAM* 421 i 28′; *BAM* 580 vi 8′; *BAM* 52:58–59; DPS XXXI:57′ (AOAT 43.344).

21. See *AHw* 987a; *CAD* R 365a does not translate this term.

22. Note also *BAM* 578 i 27–30.

23. See also DPS XIII B ii 4, 5–6, 9 = *TDP* 116 ii 4, 5–6, 9; DPS XVI:33 (AOAT 43.175). Note also Herrero, *RA* 69.42 i 6, 11; *BAM* 151:50′.

24. So also *AHw* 489b; *CAD* K 443 does not translate this term.

25. Labat's (*RA* 53.7 n. 5) collation had *gu-*⌜*reš*⌝*-tú*. However, Labat later (*RA* 55.95) thought he saw *gu-r*[*a-á*]*r-tú*. The first reading has been confirmed by collation of Scurlock.

26. See also *BAM* 33:1–3; *AMT* 18/3:1; Labat, *RA* 53.10–11 obv. 25; cf. *BAM* 422 ii 11′; *RA* 53.10–11 obv. 34.

27. Labat, *RLA* 3.126 interprets *kiṣṣatu* in this passage as "cracks and fissures" but gives no justification for his translation, which is accepted by neither dictionary.

28. Goetze, *JCS* 9.12 considers *ekketu* to be a festering sore. This seems unlikely, since infected sores are typically painful rather than itchy. Von Soden's suggestion (*AHw* 195a; also Labat, *RLA* 3.233; Haussperger, *Mem. Cagni* 446) of "scabies" as a possible cause of this condition seems reasonable. Kämmerer, *UF* 27.158 dismisses von Soden's and embraces Goetze's interpretation because it seems to him to sort better with smallpox. However, this and many other of Kämmerer's identifications are predicated on what we believe to be a false premise. See above, n. 17.

29. See also Beckman and Foster, *Mem. Sachs* 19 no. 18:3′, 10′, cf. 2′; DPS XXXIII:111 (AOAT 43.358).

30. See also DPS XV:43 [AOAT 43.152].

31. See also DPS V A 12′–14′, 16′–17′ = *TDP* 46 B 12–14, 16–17.

32. This seems a more likely explanation than Sturge-Weber's syndrome, a condition in which a port wine facial nevus is present on the first division of the trigeminal nerve and a hemangioma on the cerebral cortex (Fincke, *Augenleiden* 247). The obvious interpretation of "his face has been burned" is simply that his face has been burned. Nevi of all colors were described by the *āšipu* as *umṣātu*-lesions. Moreover, Sturge-Weber's produces exophthalmus that causes a widening rather than a narrowing of the ocular opening.

33. See *CAD* M/2.103 s.v. *miqtu* mng. 1a1′ for other references to *miqtu* appearing in enumerations of skin conditions such as *sikkatu*, burns, and *ziqtu*. In the discussion of *miqtu* in Stol, *Epilepsy* 9–12, some of these references are cited in full. Kämmerer, *UF* 27.162 argues that *miqtu* refers to the onset of smallpox. However, this and many other of Kämmerer's identifications are predicated on what we believe to be a false premise. See above, n. 17.

34. Note DPS XXXIII:53–54 [AOAT 43.356], which are unfortunately fragmentary and partially incomprehensible but which tell us that swelling was involved and that the *asû* was responsible for treating it.

35. This interpretation for *rapaštu* was first suggested and then rejected by Labat, *TDP* 108 n. 192. The Sumerogram literally means "tail" or "thigh tail" for which the human tail bone and the immediately surrounding area would be appropriate. The suggested alternatives to this translation, "pelvis" (*AHw* 955a) and "loins" (*CAD* R 152–153) already have perfectly good candidates in MURUB$_4$.MEŠ and *birku*, respectively.

36. For the reading, see Heeßel, AOAT 43.190. The expression *ḫīṭu laššu* or *ḫīṭu yānu* appears not infrequently in Neo-Assyrian and Neo-Babylonian letters; it means something on the order of "no harm done" or "it is of no consequence." For references, see *CAD* Ḫ 210 s.v. *ḫīṭu* A mng. 1. For the interpretation, see also Ritter, *AS* 16.302 (quoting Landsberger).

37. See, for example, DPS XII A 9–18//B 1–15 = *TDP* 100 i 9–18 (nipples); DPS XII C 6′–13′ = *SpTU* 1.35:6′–13′ (ribs); DPS XII D ii 1′–iii 6//F 1–7//G$_2$ ii 1′–iii 3 = *TDP* 102 ii 52′–iii 6 (lower back); DPS XII D iii 25–30 = *TDP* 104 iii 25–30 (spine); DPS XIV A i 1–24 = *TDP* 128/130 i 1–24 (hip socket); DPS XIV A i 32–41, C i 5′–10′, A$_2$ i 1–6 = *TDP* 130/132 i 32–58 (buttock); DPS XIV A ii 23–30//C ii 5–8 = *TDP* 134 ii 23–30 (penis); DPS XIV A$_2$ ii 4–10//C ii 23–26 = *TDP* 136 ii 54–60 (testicles); DPS XIV A$_2$ ii 22–23, iii 1–5//G iii 2′–18′//H 1–10 = *TDP* 138 ii 72–iii 22 (thigh).

38. For the reading, see Heeßel, AOAT 43.190. The expression *ḫīṭu laššu* or *ḫīṭu yānu* appears not infrequently in Neo-Assyrian and Neo-Babylonian letters; it means something on the order of "no harm done" or "it is of no consequence." For references, see *CAD* Ḫ 210 s.v. *ḫīṭu* A mng. 1. For the interpretation, see also Ritter, *AS* 16.302 (quoting Landsberger).

39. *SpTU* 1.36 obv. 4.

40. For references, see *CAD* A/2.300–301 s.v. *arqu* mng 1a.

41. See also Šumma Izbu IV 13 (Leichty, *Izbu* 67).

42. For other references to this use of ŠUB/*nadû*, see DPS III C obv. 52–54 = *TDP* 24:52–54; DPS IX A 8–9, 10 = *TDP* 72:8–9, 10; DPS IX A 29//B obv. 27–28 = *TDP* 74:29; DPS XI A obv. 12 = *TDP* 90:12; DPS XI B 11 = *SpTU* 1.34:11; DPS XI A r. 30, 31 = *TDP* 96 r. 30, 31; DPS XI A r. 47, 48 = *TDP* 98 r. 47, 48; DPS XIII B i 42′//F 4 = *TDP* 114 i 46′; DPS XIII B ii 47–48, 49–50//G$_2$ 38, 39+G$_1$ 21, 22 = *TDP* 120 ii 47–48, 49–50; DPS XVI:43′, 47′ (AOAT 43.176); DPS XVI:85′, 86′ (AOAT 43.179); DPS XIX/XX:5′ (AOAT 43.227); DPS XIX/XX:38′ (AOAT 43.228); DPS XXII:21 (AOAT 43.253); DPS XXXVI A 56 = *TDP* 204:56; DPS XXXVI A 69 = *TDP* 206:69; DPS XL A 5//B 5–6 = *TDP* 218:5; DPS XL A 29, 32, 33 = *TDP* 220:29, 32, 33; DPS XL A 75, 76, 77//B 76, 77 = *TDP* 226:75, 76, 77.

43. Kinnier Wilson, *RA* 60.49–51; *Diseases in Antiquity* 206–207; "Medicine in . . . Old Testament (times)" 354–355. This position was critized by Stol, *JEOL* 30.23–24 on the grounds that physiognomic omens generally describe "relatively innocent marks, traits, habits, tics, etc." (cf. Köcher, "Lepra" 30) and that the com-

mentators to the passages in Leviticus describing Hebrew *ṣaraʿat* insist that "white lesions are not a symptom of leprosy." Convinced by these arguments, Kinnier Wilson withdrew his suggestion. Kinnier Wilson, *Journ.Roy.Soc. Med.* 89.139 proposes no alternative for the punctate lesions, but suggests that the "white spots" might instead be due to the leukoderma "common in native races" and supports his suggestion by pointing to the theory that the Sumerians were originally (Dravidian) blacks from southern India. In the first place, leukoderma is not a disease, but a general term meaning loss of pigmentation caused by a number of different diseases. This problem, although more easily seen in darker-skinned individuals, is no more common in one race than in another. Second, although physiognomic omens do generally refer to relatively benign conditions, this does not exclude tuberculoid leprosy from consideration. Tuberculoid leprosy is usually a very mild disease compatible with long life. Its main manifestation, commentators to Leviticus to the contrary notwithstanding, is the presence of depigmented (white) lesions that have reduced sensation due to nerve involvement.

44. Labat, *RLA* 3.232 translates this term as redness (erythema).

45. For the term, see below.

46. Note also DPS XXXIII:67–68 [AOAT 43.356].

47. Adamson, *JRAS* 1984.9 suggests that *terku* refers to hairy moles, which can develop into malignant melanoma. However, there is nothing to suggest that a *terku* was either hairy or elevated. Ebeling, *RLA* 1.321 lists this (interpreted as "yellow") as one of many alleged terms for "leprosy" in ancient Mesopotamian texts. Most of these identifications are based on the descriptions given of Hebrew *ṣaraʿat* in Leviticus 13. However, the latter term is not actually leprosy and is in any case irrelevant to the argument (see below, n. 139). Holma, *Kleine Beiträge* 25 offers "vesicle." However, there is nothing to suggest that *terku* lesions contained fluid.

48. See *AHw* 1357b.

49. See *AHw* 1530a.

50. See *CAD* Š/3.72.

51. For references, see *CAD* Q 296–297.

52. Note also DPS XXXIII:112 (AOAT 43.358).

53. Kinnier Wilson, *JNES* 53.113 interprets both verb and noun as referring to "discharge." However, the expression "if a sore comes out on a person's body" is simply the conventional way of describing rashes, and does not refer to discharge. This may readily be seen from *BAM* 417 obv. 25–26//DPS XXXIII:59 (AOAT 43.356; see 3.276, above) which has: [If a sore] comes out on a person's body (and it is) red (or) white (and) it hurts him, there is no fluid (in it but) it is swollen (and) it ⸢grows larger⸣ on contact, it is called *nilugu*. By Kinnier Wilson's interpretation (*JNES* 53.113), this passage would read: "If a sore is discharging red or white discharge . . . and there is no fluid in it," which is clearly contradictory.

54. The reading of the signs is uncertain. The name is probably simply *nilugu* (a foreign loanword).

55. Adamson, *JRAS* 1984.12 w/ n. 94 interprets the word *ṣētu* as "wheal" and takes it to refer to severe sunburn. It seems difficult to imagine how the boy could have had sunburn restricted to such a small (and comparatively sheltered) area of his head. In any case, the term *ṣētu* does not otherwise refer to sunburn (see Chapter 3 under enteric fever).

56. Adamson, *JRAS* 1969.12 suggests that the term *birdu* was applied to two lesions: pockmarks that may follow skin infections and (after Labat, *TDP* 76 n. 138) abdominal stretch marks that often follow pregnancy. Both of these lesions are flat or depressed, whereas *birdu*-lesions appear to be elevated.

57. Labat, *TDP* 76 n. 138 interprets the *birdu* in this reference as abdominal stretch marks. However, in Labat, *RLA* 3.232 he retracts this explanation. See previous note.

58. Holma, *Kleine Beiträge* 3 n. 4 suggests that *bubuʾtu* might mean "slime" or "filth." Other suggestions tend to assume the possible presence of pus (*AHw* 135; *CAD* B 300–301; Labat, *RLA* 3.232). Adamson, *JRAS* 1969.10–12, cf. *Medical History* 14.314, identifies *bubuʾtu* as a vesicle, and we agree. Herpetic lesions, which is what many of the references to *bubuʾtu* appear to be describing, contain clear fluid rather than the opaque white pus of a pustule. The word is also used to describe bubbles in a river (see *CAD* B 301a), which again seems more appropriate to a vesicle.

59. Adamson, *Medical History* 14.317 suggests that internal *bubuʾtu* involving the liver and lungs of sheep are the cysts of *Echinococcus*. If so, some of the references to right-sided abdominal pain and vomiting might possibly be due to hydatid cysts, since humans are also susceptible to this parasitic infection. Kinnier Wilson, *Diseases of Antiquity* 196–197 suggests another lesion (*erištu*: "wish mark") for the cysts of *Echinococcus*, but their small size and numbers (see *CAD* E 299–300) seem incompatible with this diagnosis.

60. Collated *CAD* B 300; the collation is confirmed by the quotation of this line by incipit in ND 4358:5 (Kinnier Wilson, *Iraq* 18.133:17) and by the catchline of *SpTU* 2.44 r. 23.

61. Compare DPS XXXI:28′, 30′ (AOAT 43.343).

62. Kinnier Wilson, *Iraq* 18.134 interprets this as "prickly heat." However, "prickly heat" is the lay term for miliaria rubra. This is a benign transient skin condition of most infants that produces small raised white spots with surrounding redness and is caused by blocked sweat glands. There is nothing in our reference to suggest "prickly heat."

63. See also DPS XXXIII:26 [AOAT 43.354]//K 3526 r. 8; cf. *BAM* 580 vi 8′.

64. Compare also BM 76515 obv. 11–12. Heeßel, *AOAT* 43.357 restores an *ina* at the beginning of the line.

65. See also DPS XXXIII:113–114 (AOAT 43.358).

66. See also Adamson, *JRAS* 1969.11.

67. Ibid. considers this to be a papule. However, a papule is a raised and red lesion that contains no fluid, and being fluid-filled is an essential requirement for a *bubu'tu.*

68. Adamson, ibid. suggests "pustule" (small skin abscess) for the white and black lesions. However, this translation assumes that the infection being described is smallpox, which is the diagnosis proposed by Adamson, *Medical History* 14.314–316 for all of the *TDP* references to *bubu'tu* attributed to "hands" of gods. We believe that these references describe HSV1 or HSV2 infections because smallpox does not produce vesicles restricted to the face and mouth, nor is it sexually transmitted, and stomatitis or a sexually transmitted infection is indicated in all cases.

69. See also *KAR* 211 obv. 19–20; DPS XVIII:22 (AOAT 43.219); *BAM* 584 ii 25′–26′; DPS XXXIII:80 (AOAT 43.357).

70. See also *DPS* XVIII:23 (AOAT 43.219): *BAM* 584 11 25′–26′.

71. See also StBoT 36.40 obv. 9′–10′; DPS XVIII:21 (AOAT 43.219); *BAM* 584 ii 29′.

72. Köcher has suggested (*BAM* vol. 5.xxix) that the Sumerogram for *ašû* was MAŠ.TAB.BA, lit. "twin" (see *BAM* 494 ii 35//*BAM* 500 i 11′; *BAM* 495 ii 4′//*BAM* 494 ii 39; cf. *BAM* 494 ii 55). The fact that prescriptions for *ašû* and MAŠ.TAB.BA are frequently intermixed on the same tablet (as in *BAM* 494) would seem to support this suggestion. Moreover, the idea of "twins" would not be inappropriate to *ašû,* which is typically characterized by a number of more or less identical lesions appearing together in clusters.

73. Heeßel, AOAT 43.359 takes this to mean that the patient's eye produces fluid.

74. Ibid. 353, 359 reads *e-bíṭ* and translates "swollen."

75. On this point, see also Fincke, *Augenleiden* 99–103 correcting Labat and Tournay, *RA* 40.115, 117; cf. Goetze, *JCS* 9.11–12 who interprets *ašû* as "vertigo." Haussperger, *Mem. Cagni* 442–445 interprets *ašû* as an eye disease under the mistaken impression that *BAM* 480 i 1–3//*BAM* 3 i 1–3 is a reference to *ašû.* For our interpretation of this text, see 9.9.

76. Kämmerer, *UF* 27.161–162 adopts Labat and Tournay's suggestion of "vertigo" for *ašû,* now effectively refuted by Fincke (see previous note).

77. Heeßel, AOAT 43.353, 359, 366 interprets this as DIRI/*neqelpû,* which he translates as "unsteady."

78. See also *BAM* 481 obv. 11′; *BAM* 494 ii 4, 7, 10, 23; *BAM* 3 i 35.

79. Note also *BAM* 1 i 67; *BAM* 426 ii 40′, 41′; *AMT* 1/3:8′.

80. DPS XXXIII:103 (AOAT 43.357); see Chapter 19, n. 88.

81. Kämmerer, *UF* 27.160 argues that *sagbānu* refers to the painful nature of smallpox lesions. However, this and many other of Kämmerer's identifications are predicated on what we believe to be a false premise. See above, n. 17. Adamson, *Medical History* 32.206, followed by Miller, *NABU* 1988 no. 45, suggests Dracunculiasis. However, an important part of the justification for this is the idea that *sagbānu* affects the joints. Adamson bases this idea (and the idea that *rapādu* is "migratory arthritis"; see *RA* 82.165 w/ n. 14d) on a lexical list that groups *sagbānu* and *rapādu* with *ṣidānu, šaššaṭu,* and *maškādu,* all of which Adamson believes to be joint diseases (*Medical History* 32.206 w/ n. 13). In fact, this sort of grouping is relatively common in lexical texts, and seems to have been motivated by the fact that the listed words have Sumerograms that are confusingly similar (they all begin with SAG or SA, sometimes both). *Ṣidānu* (SAG.NIGIN or SA.NIGIN) means "dizziness," *šaššaṭu* (SA.DUGUD) "tetanus," and *maškādu* (SA.GIG) "sciatica," none of which are joint diseases. Other similar lists include also *samānu:* "cellulitis," which does not even involve the muscles (SA) but which has a pseudo-Sumerogram SA.MA.NUM (see *CAD* R 147a lex. section). For an alternative suggestion for Dracunculiasis, see Chapter 3, pp. 85–86.

82. See also DPS XXXIII:64 (AOAT 43.356); cf. *AMT* 75/1 iii 24, 26.

83. For references, see Holma, *Kleine Beiträge* 4; *CAD* E 13b s.v. *ebēru* B, lexical section. Note also *AMT* 98/3:5, where the patient's hand is rubbed with a salve until the surface contains *ibāru*-lesions.

84. For references, see *CAD* I 1.

85. For references, see *AHw* 363a; *CAD* I 1; Böck, *Morphoskopie* 210.

86. Kinnier Wilson, *Diseases in Antiquity* 197 and *JNES* 27.244, suggests scars from what he calls "Baghdad boil" for *ibāru*. However, cutaneous leishmaniasis is not actually a boil, but an ulcer (see below).

87. For treatments, see *CT* 44.36:4, 10; *BAM* 417 r. 6′.

88. Heeßel, AOAT 43.356, 369, 370 interprets this as a Sumerogram meaning "ox fat." It seems more likely that this is simply a foreign loanword into Akkadian.

89. See also *BAM* 417 r. 9′–11′.

90. Labat, *RLA* 3.232 translates *ziqtu* as "pimple." The word is also used for scorpion stings (see *CAD* Z 132–133; Goetze, *JCS* 9.12). Kämmerer, *UF* 27.161 is prepared to understand *ziqtu* as referring to smallpox, whether it is to be translated as "scorpion sting" or "pustule." However, this and many other of Kämmerer's identifications are predicated on what we believe to be a false premise. See above, n. 17.

91. Heeßel, AOAT 43.361, 369 (also *CAD* Z 132b) mistakes this passage as referring to the skull or nose of the patient.

92. Heeßel, AOAT 43.361, 369 (also *CAD* Z 132b) mistakes this passage as referring to the nose of the patient.

93. Heeßel, AOAT 43.361, 369 reads the "white" and the "small" as *ut-tur* and interprets this as "exceedingly."

94. See *CAD* L 68b.

95. For references, see *CAD* L 68b.

96. For the suggestion that the primary meaning of *lamṣātu*-lesion is a sore produced by the bite of a *lamṣātu*-fly, see *AHw* 533b.

97. Note also *BAM* 581:6′; *STT* 93:87′.

98. The text adds the note that, if the patient has "wind blasting," the god Pabilsag is responsible. The "wind blasting" may be describing a concurrent HSV2 infection (see Chapter 4) or simple redness and inflammation surrounding the ulcer.

99. Labat, *RLA* 3.231–232 believes that this text is describing a tropical ulcer (cutaneous leishmaniasis). However, although tropical ulcers can be large and may leave a permanent scar, they typically produce little or no pain.

100. The text adds the note that, if the patient has "wind blasting," the twin gods are responsible. The "wind blasting" may be describing a concurrent HSV2 infection (see Chapter 4) or simple redness and inflammation surrounding the ulcer.

101. Labat, *RLA* 3.232 believes that this text is describing a tuberculous cold abscess (a draining tuberculous lymph node). We favor a syphilitic chancre but a cold abscess is also possible.

102. For references, see *AHw* 1090b; *CAD* Ṣ 127; cf. W. Farber, *ZA* 71.61–63.

103. Goetze, *JCS* 9.12 (following Holma, *Kleine Beiträge* 17–20; cf. Ebeling, *RLA* 1.321) suggests "leprosy" as a translation for *ṣennītu* on the basis of an alleged etymological connection with Hebrew *ṣaraʿat*. However, although the latter term has often been translated as "leprosy," a careful examination of the relevant passages in Leviticus reveals that the object of the rulings was not to define a single disease entity but to describe a number of different skin diseases, all of which shared an element of cultic impurity (for a full discussion, see Levine, "Leviticus" in *The JPS Torah Commentary* 76–84). Kämmerer, *UF* 27.160 argues that *ṣennītu* refers to some undefined sign or symptom of smallpox. However, this and many other of Kämmerer's identifications are predicated on what we believe to be a false premise. See above, n. 17.

104. Compare NUMUN-*šú* GIN$_7$ ^{Ú}*túb-ba-qi* 3.TA!.ÀM *um-mu-ud*: "its seed resembles (that of) ^{Ú}*tubāqu*, clustered (into clusters) of three (seeds) each" (*KADP* 33:15–16).

105. Labat, *RLA* 3.231 translates this term as "tumor," but gives no justification for the translation.

106. For an edition of the relevant omens, see Böck, *Morphoskopie* 124, 184–193, 296–305. Other lesions, such as *liptu*, *pindû*, *terku*, and ŠE, are attested as being located on the penis but not at the opening of the penis.

107. Šumma Izbu IV 2 (Leichty, *Izbu* 66).

108. Ebeling, *RLA* 1.321 lists this as one of many alleged terms for "leprosy" in ancient Mesopotamian texts. Most of these identifications are based on the descriptions given of Hebrew *ṣaraʿat* in Leviticus 13.

However, the latter term is not actually Hansen's disease (leprosy) and is in any case irrelevant to the argument (see nn. 103, 139–140). Adamson, *JRAS* 1984.8 believes that *umṣātu* must be translated as "pigmented nevus." This interpretation will not, however, account for the uses of this term in many of the references to this lesion in medical texts. A *black umṣātu* could be a pigmented nevus, but this was given a separate name (*ḫalû*; see below). In any case, the *umṣātu*-lesion appears to have been solid, making Labat's (*RLA* 3.232) suggestion of blister or vesicle unlikely. Holma's suggestion (*Kleine Beiträge* 4–6) of burn scar is based on an insecure Arabic etymology.

109. Note also *BAM* 96 iii 3′–4′//*BAM* 104:42; *AMT* 17/5:1; *AMT* 40/4:3′.

110. Adamson, *JRAS* 1984.8 suggests Paget's disease for *umṣātu* lesions on the nipples.

111. Lit. "she is pregnant with a delivery that will be easy."

112. See also DPS XXXVI A 24, 35 = *TDP* 202:24, 35.

113. Lit. "she is pregnant with a delivery that will not be easy."

114. See also *BAM* 152 iii 16//*BAM* 182 r. 4′; *AMT* 101/3 i 4; cf. *BAM* 95:12, 14//*STT* 97 iii 10, 15; *BAM* 168:66//*BAM* 108:1–2//*BAM* 110:3′–4′; *BAM* 182 r. 7′–8′.

115. For references, see *AHw* 1418a.

116. Šumma Izbu IV 9 (Leichty, *Izbu* 67).

117. For references, see *AHw* 314b; *CAD* Ḫ 53b.

118. Adamson, *JRAS* 1984.9–10 suggests and then rejects this possibility in favor of a junction nevus on the grounds that this lesion commonly develops into a malignant melanoma. However, there is nothing in any of the references to suggest that *ḫalû*-lesions ever had a fatal outcome. For what are more probably texts describing malignant melanomas, see below.

119. For an edition of the relevant omens, see Böck, *Morphoskopie* 194–202.

120. Šumma Izbu IV 8 (Leichty, *Izbu* 66).

121. For references, see *AHw* 854b; *CAD* Ṣ 114a s.v. *ṣarpu* B. Labat, *RLA* 3.233 points out that *pindû* also means "glowing coal," which is an appropriate comparison to a red skin lesion.

122. See also Böck, *Morphoskopie* 29; cf. Adamson, *JRAS* 1979.2–3.

123. See *CAD* A/2.450–452 s.v. *ašnan*.

124. Kinnier Wilson, *RA* 60.57–58 proposes "leprosy" for *garābu* in this passage. Rather confusingly, on page 55 he argues that the white *pindû* with which *garābu* are equated must be referring to vitiligo on the grounds that Hansen's disease (leprosy) was considered by the ancient Mesopotamians to be incurable. This argument is of questionable logic, and in any case, *pindû* is an elevated granular lesion, whereas vitiligo is flat. Köcher, "Lepra" 32 argues that this text proves that *garābu* are pustules since the lesions are described as white. A pustule is not, however, a lesion that is white but one that contains pus. Moreover, *garābu* are granular and pustules are not.

125. Kinnier Wilson, *RA* 60.51–57 argues that *buʾšānu* is scurvy and that, since *garābu* "joins forces" with it, the latter can represent the lesions of pellagra. *Buʾšānu* does not, in fact, "join forces" with *garābu* (*RA* 60.57); the two terms appear in consecutive entries in a lexical text whose purpose is to distinguish three different ancient syndromes which (because they stink) can be referred to with the Sumerogram for "stinking" (on this point, see also Köcher, "Lepra" 30). In any case, the pellagra ring is hyperpigmented, whereas *garābu* is definitionally hypopigmented. Pellagra is a nutritional disease common in populations whose staple diet is American maize that has been milled using European techniques, a combination extremely unlikely to have occurred in ancient Mesopotamia (see Chapter 7, n. 1). Stol, *JEOL* 30.30 argues that *garābu* means favus, a chronic fungal infection of the scalp. Since, however, *garābu* is defined as occurring "on a man's body" and not just his scalp, this conclusion seems unwarranted. For our suggestion for favus, see under *Kibšu*.

126. This interpretation of *garābu* is accepted by *CAD* G 46 and *AHw* 281–282. They also suggest scabies in sheep (*Räude*) for the references to animals with these lesions (see next note). Holma, *Kleine Beiträge* 8, Ebeling, *RLA* 1.321, Labat, *RLA* 3.233, and Goetze, *JCS* 9.13 understand *garābu* as scabies in humans (*Krätze*) and Ebeling also asserts that the ancients only associated *garābu* with *saḫaršubbû* because they had a "deficient knowledge of medicine." In fact, the problem lies not with the *āšipu* but with the modern identification of *garābu* as scabies in humans. *Garābu* is a cognate of Syriac *garbā*, which means Hansen's disease (leprosy; Stol, *JEOL* 30.30). Moreover, *garābu*-lesions were white and granular like the lesions of lepromatous leprosy, whereas the lesions of scabies are typically small, red, and nongranular.

127. See *CAD* G 90a and *AHw* 285a.

128. Scott, *Large Animal Dermatology*.

129. A legal case from mid-second-millennium Nuzi involves a person who accused another of being "full of *epqu*" (for references, see *CAD* E 246).

130. For references, see *CAD* E 246a; *AHw* 230b. Kinnier Wilson, *RA* 60.57 accepts *epqu* as Hansen's disease (leprosy) but takes *epqēnu* ("the leprosy-like disease") to mean pellagra on the grounds that the eighteenth-century physician Thiéry was not sure of the difference between pellagra and leprosy (*RA* 60.57–58). However, pellagra is not "like" leprosy, and the twists and turns taken by eighteenth-century European physicians in coming to grips with unfamiliar diseases are of no relevance to the issue.

131. Stol, *JEOL* 30.30 argues that *epqu* is specifically a scale and refers to psoriasis. However, there is already a word for scale (see QULIPTU), which requires that the two terms be seen as synonyms. The text that is cited to prove the identity of *epqu* with *quliptu* is not a lexical text that equates the two but an omen (*SpTU* 2.38:21–22). Stol, *JEOL* 30.29 makes the point that lexical equations do not always mean what they seem to mean. This is true enough, but omens are even more treacherous than lexical texts. In *SpTU* 2.38.21–22, the presence of scales (*quliptu*) covering the body of a dead infant like a carp or a snake predicts that Sîn is angry and that, consequently, the person for whom the prediction is being made will be full of *epqu*. That the *epqu* of the *saḫaršubbû* inflicted by Sîn can cover the body like the scales of a carp or snake is the most that should be inferred from this passage. This is in itself, however, enough to exclude psoriasis from consideration, since the scales of this skin condition primarily involve the scalp, elbows, and knees. Kämmerer, *UF* 27.158 argues that *epqu* refers specifically to the scaling of smallpox lesions. However, this and many other of Kämmerer's identifications are predicated on what we believe to be a false premise. See above, n. 17.

132. Köcher, "Lepra" 31–32 uses this text to argue that *saḫaršubbû* consists of generalized blisters. However, this is based on a mistranslation of passages (*BAM* 35 ii 9′–10′, cf. 7′–8′) which instruct that treatment is to be applied until blisters "come out" (È-*a*). In other words, there is every reason to suppose that there were no blisters before the patient was treated. In any case, the *āšipu* already had a term for generalized blisters, namely, *ašû* (see above).

133. Many scholars (Stol, *JEOL* 30.29; Labat, *RLA* 3.233; Kinnier Wilson, *RA* 60.52; Biggs, *History of Science* 8.102) maintain that *saḫaršubbû* was considered to be incurable and that no treatments for *saḫaršubbû* are ever found in the medical texts. In fact, several treatments each for *garābu* (see above) and *saḫaršubbû* (*BAM* 35 ii 5′–10′; see Köcher, "Lepra" 30) have long been known to exist. Stol, *JEOL* 30.29 deals with this problem by arguing that the treatments could not really have worked. Whether the treatments worked or not, however, is immaterial; the issue is not whether *we* think they could have cured *saḫaršubbû* but whether *the ancient physician* thought so. Since the *āšipu* clearly thought he had treatments, he cannot have considered the disease to be incurable. The issue has now been settled with the publication of A. Tsukimoto, *Priests and Officials* 187–200, which contains no less than twelve treatments for *saḫaršubbû* and a purificatory ritual for those who have been cured.

134. With Borger, *AfO* 23.25 this is not to be emended away.

135. For other references, see *CAD* S 36–37.

136. Other references make it clear that the moon-god Sîn is the god usually held responsible for this condition; see *CAD* S 36–37.

137. Shaffer, *Tablet XII* 96 obv. 5–7 (see Stol, *JEOL* 30.28).

138. Kinnier Wilson, *Journ.Roy.Soc.Med.* 89.137 suggests inability to bear children as a result of hookworm as the wife's problem, but we see no basis for this attribution. Abusch, *Underst.Witchcr* 68–73 (accepted by Stol, *JEOL* 30.31) interprets this passage as referring to a skin disease involving both skin eruptions and puslike secretion covering the body "like a garment" and caused by "the anger of god and man." Part of his argument is based on the definition of all passages in which the term *to infect* (*la*ʾ*ābu*) or *li*ʾ*bu* fever appears as a single disease. The alleged "puslike secretion" is further based on his interpretation of Šurpu VII 25–26 ("they infected his body and sprinkled gall on him") as referring to a body "covered with a yellow-green liquid substance." We do not find these arguments convincing.

139. The yeas include Oppert, Belser, Delitsch, Zimmern, Holma, Meissner, Ebeling, Ungnad, Nougayrol, Lambert, Oppenheim, and Labat (for references, see Köcher, "Lepra" 27–31 and Kinnier Wilson, *RA* 60.48–49) as well as the *CAD* (S 36–37) and *AHw* 1005a. It should be noted that Oppert's original translation of "leprosy" was based on the equation of the Akkadian *saḫaršubbû* with Hebrew *ṣara*ʿ*at* on the grounds that both were incurable and that therefore the two must be the same (see Köcher, "Lepra" 27). That two diseases are incurable does not mean that they are the same disease. In any case, there is no reason to believe that *ṣara*ʿ*at* was incurable simply because it was not treated by the priests and because the sufferer was made

to live outside the camp. The doctor could have gone to the patient or the two could have met at the outer gate as was apparently the case with the treatment of *saḫaršubbû* (Tsukimoto, *Priests and Officials* 199–200:64). An entire chapter of Leviticus (chap. 14) is, in fact, devoted to priestly purification of those who have recovered or been cured. *Ṣaraʿat* was, then, potentially curable, as was *saḫaršubbû*. Both were socially stigmatizing but, again, this does not mean that they were the same. That Hebrew *ṣaraʿat* represents "several diseases all of which manifested themselves in unpleasant . . . skin conditions" (Stol, *JEOL* 30.28; cf. Neufeld, *JANES* 18.57 n. 21) is thus not at issue (see above, n. 103). The point is that *ṣaraʿat* is not a cognate of *saḫaršubbû*, *epqu*, or *garābu* and that *ṣaraʿat* is inextricably linked with concepts of cultic purity and impurity that most scholars would à priori assume to be peculiar to ancient Israel.

140. The nays include Neufeld, *JANES* 18.57, Biggs, Kinnier Wilson, Köcher, Adamson, and Stol (see references below). Oppert's original translation of "leprosy" was based on the equation of the Akkadian *saḫaršubbû* with Hebrew *ṣaraʿat* (see previous note). Curiously, although the nays deny that *saḫaršubbû* is "leprosy," they continue to base their interpretation of *saḫaršubbû* on their understanding of Hebrew *ṣaraʿat*. Kinnier Wilson, "Medicine in . . . Old Testament (times)" 355–357 argues that *saḫaršubbû* is scurvy, pellagra, or both on the grounds that Lamentations 4.5, 8 (siege of Jerusalem by Nebuchadnezzar) refers to scurvy and Job 19.7, 20 to pellagra, (*Medicine . . . Old Testament* 360). Neither Biblical passage is correctly interpreted and pellagra is, in any case, extremely unlikely to have existed in ancient Mesopotamia (see Chapter 7 n. 1). Kinnier Wilson already has another, more reasonable, suggestion for scurvy (see Chapter 3 under *buʾšānu*). Adamson, *RA* 82.169–170 argues that *saḫaršubbû* is psoriasis (also long suggested for Hebrew *ṣaraʿat*) on the grounds that the skin lesions were "scaly, well defined, and slightly elevated above the surface of the skin." However, the translation that is offered as proof of the identification of *saḫaršubbû* with psoriasis is actually based on the modern definition of psoriasis, and not on any ancient text. His argument that the lesions were "differentiated from vesicles or bullae" is based on an entry from the omen series Šumma Alu, which predicts that if a pig eats its young, the owner will have either generalized body swelling or *saḫaršubbû* all over (for a full citation, see Köcher, "Lepra" 28). This interpretation of Šumma Alu is not accepted by Köcher, "Lepra" 31, who wishes to see *saḫaršubbû* as precisely consisting of boils and pustules (see above). Stol, *JEOL* 30.30 n. 53 also points out the inadequacy of Adamson's arguments, and follows the interpretation only for *epqu* and not *garābu*, which he argues is favus (see above). Barring the fact that we accept neither Köcher's nor Stol's identifications, their interpretation of *saḫaršubbû* is actually not too far from ours, namely, that the term refers to generalized skin lesions of characteristic types. Where we disagree most is over the issue of whether Hansen's disease was *one* of the diseases that could have been included under this rubric. An attractive possibility is that Hansen's disease was the disease around which the ancient syndrome of *saḫaršubbû* was organized, just as chickenpox was probably the major cause of *ašû* (see above), another ancient syndrome involving generalized skin lesions of characteristic types.

141. An argument that is often given by skeptics is that there is no skeletal evidence from the pre-Christian Near East supporting a diagnosis of Hansen's disease (see, e.g., Biggs, *RLA* 6.605). The major skeletal changes, however, are in the small bones (digits) of the hands and feet. These bones are unfortunately seldom available for study, and in fact the primary skeletal remains from Iraq are skulls (see Biggs, *History of Science* 8.102). As Biggs also points out, patients with Hansen's disease were likely not to have been buried in the communal cemetery where they could have been discovered by excavators.

142. See *CAD* K 556b. Haussperger, *Mem. Cagni* 440 applies a similar diagnosis to this term.

143. *BAM* 494 iii 70′, iv 6.

144. For *kurāru* in physiognomic omens, see Böck, *Morphoskopie* 179–183.

145. The suggestion was originally made by Campbell Thompson, *DAB* 146 and followed by Adamson, *JRAS* 1981.125–126. The interpretation of "sty" for this lesion (Fincke, *Augenleiden* 222) depends on a translation of "carbuncle" for *kurāru*.

146. See also *BAM* 156:25; *BAM* 494 iii 24′; cf. *BAM* 33:9; *BAM* 494 iii 42′.

147. See also Wasserman, *RA* 90.3:1–2.

148. See also *BAM* 494 iii 21′; *BAM* 34:5′; cf. *BAM* 494 iii 76′.

149. See Labat, *RLA* 3.233.

150. See also *BAM* 155 iii 3′, 5′; *KADP* 1 v 37, 39; *BAM* 379 iii 47′; *BAM* 422 ii 13′. Cf. *BAM* 33:1–3; *BAM* 379 ii 18′–19′ (with other skin conditions).

151. Pierce, *Cuneiform Cryptography* 168–169 suggests that the mysterious 6,40 might be a substitution cipher for *ašar*.

152. See also Cavigneaux and al-Rawi, *Iraq* 55.104 B 1′.

153. Note also *BAM* 379 iii 45′.

154. Kämmerer, *UF* 27.158 argues that *girgiššu* refers to the scarlet-red exanthem of smallpox. However, this and many other of Kämmerer's identifications are predicated on what we believe to be a false premise. See above, n. 17.

155. Haussperger, *Fs Spycket* 131 suggests *Pityriasis versicolor*, scabies, and urticaria as possible diagnoses. The appearance of these lesions, however, do not fit with the characteristics of *girgiššu*.

156. For references, see *CAD* K 339–340; *AHw* 472b. The commentary *SpTU* 1.51:4 equates *kibšu* with *qummānu*, which is a type of mold (see *CAD* Q 305).

157. Labat's (*RA* 53.7 n. 5) collation had *gu-⌈reš⌉-tú*. However, Labat later (*RA* 55.95) thought he saw *gu-r*[*a-á*]*r-tú*. The first reading has been confirmed by collation by Scurlock.

158. Meier, *OrNS* 8.302–303 argues for a translation of *sikkatu* as "strangury" and Goetze, *JCS* 9.11 (followed by Kämmerer, *UF* 27.164) as "constipation." Neither translation has anything obvious to recommend it.

159. Ebeling, *RLA* 1.321 lists this (misread *muššu*) as one of many alleged terms for "leprosy" in ancient Mesopotamian texts. Most of these identifications are based on the descriptions given of Hebrew *ṣaraʿat* in Leviticus 13. However, the latter term is not actually leprosy and is in any case irrelevant to the argument (see above, n. 139).

160. See *AHw* 1446–1447.

161. Adamson, *JRAS* 1984.10 proposes a translation of "hemangioma" for *uṭṭeṭu*. However, since none of the references mention infants, this seems unlikely.

162. The passage has been collated.

163. See also *BAM* 35 i 11′, 12′.

164. Adamson, *JRAS* 1981.129 considers this condition to be angiokeratoma, a benign dilation of blood vessels on the tongue and scrotum. Since, as Adamson himself points out, *erimu*-lesions were not normally present on the external genitalia, this seems an inappropriate diagnosis. Labat, *RLA* 3.232–233 believes that the term refers simply to a rash.

165. See Böck, *Morphoskopie* 176–178.

166. For references, see *AHw* 241a; *CAD* E 294–295.

167. The reading follows Labat, *RLA* 3.221 and *AHw* 241a. *CAD* E 295a is skeptical.

168. See Holma, *Kleine Beiträge* 7.

169. The Sumerogram could be interpreted to mean "(sun) dried."

170. Lane, *Arabic Lexicon* 1154–1155, 1156–1157.

171. Note also DPS XXI:13 (AOAT 43.246).

172. See also DPS VI A obv. 26, 27//C i 12, 13 = *TDP* 56:26, 27.

173. For the reading, see Heeßel, AOAT 43.190. The expression *ḫīṭu laššu* or *ḫīṭu yānu* appears not infrequently in Neo-Assyrian and Neo-Babylonian letters; it means something on the order of "no harm done" or "it is of no consequence." For references, see *CAD* Ḫ 210 s.v. *ḫīṭu* A mng. 1. For the interpretation, see also Ritter, *AS* 16.302 (quoting Landsberger).

174. Curiously, Adamson, who identifies any number of other skin lesions as possible malignant melanoma (*JRAS* 1984.9–11), explains this and similar references as gangrene due to ergotism (*WO* 16.10 w/ n. 32—note that the reference is cited as "*TDP* 56:23"). Gangrene is an unlikely cause of black lesions on the bulb of the nose, and in the absence of rye cultivation, gangrene from ergotism would have been a rare occurrence (see Chapter 15 for more on ergotism).

175. Parpola, AOAT 5/2.492–496; cf. *CAD* I 233a; *AHw* 393a. *AHw* has a noncommittal "breast diseases" and *CAD* ventures "abscess."

176. Goetze, *JCS* 9.11 takes "fire" to mean "fever." Kämmerer, *UF* 27.162, argues that this term refers specifically to the "fever" of smallpox and that the Middle Babylonian letters are further references to smallpox, which the ancient Mesopotamians are supposed to have imagined as originating in the chest. However, medical texts use the term KÚM/*ummu* (see Chapter 3) for fever, and the references are not to the putative origins of the disease but to actual lesions on the chest and ribs, a region of the body not particularly favored by smallpox. Moreover, this and many other of Kämmerer's identifications are predicated on what we believe to be a false premise. See above, n. 17.

177. For treatments, see *BAM* 582 ii 1′–2′, 3′–4′.

178. Fincke, *Augenleiden* 99 w/ n. 770 translates this passage as "he is hot as if with (fever)-heat, he cannot hold his water and he is full of little pustules." However, she failed to appreciate the fact that this reference is drawn from Tablet XXXIII of the diagnostic series, which describes skin lesions, and that the phrase "does

not hold water" refers to a lesion without fluid and not an incontinent patient. In any case, incontinence is never described in this way (see Chapter 5).

179. Haussperger, *Mem. Cagni* 447 w/ n. 33 claims that she and her colleagues have tasted the secretions from impetigo lesions and asserts that they are slightly sweet. The streptococcal infections that are likely to follow such an action can in modern times be treated with antibiotics. In the absence of modern antibiotics, the *āšipu* would soon have learned not to perform such a test.

180. See also *CT* 23.50:7; cf. Cavigneaux and al-Rawi, *Iraq* 55.104 B 4′.

181. The *sí-mu mat-qu* of Goetze, *JCS* 9.10:26 is presumably a syllabic writing of "sweet" sores. Kämmerer, *UF* 27.161 suggests that this might refer to a sweet smell of the body (in a context of smallpox). To the best of our knowledge, the body does not smell sweet in smallpox.

182. Labat, *RA* 53.9 has "lice and nits," but gives no justification for this translation.

183. For an edition of the relevant omens, see Böck, *Morphoskopie* 174–176.

184. For references, see *CAD* L 202; *AHw* 554–555.

185. Labat, *RA* 53.8 tentatively suggests DIB DÙG.GA-*tú*.

186. See also *AMT* 75/1 iii 31, 32.

187. For references to *kittabru* in the physiognomic omens, see Böck, *Morphoskopie* 212–233. Note also *Morphoskopie* 88:171.

188. Kinnier Wilson, "Medicine in . . . the Old Testament" 351–352 suggests a small cyst for this lesion (almost always written ŠE), which he understands as equivalent to Akkadian *šeʾu*. The correct reading for ŠE in the physiognomic omens appears to be *kittabru* (see *AHw* 1446–1447), but the suggestion nonetheless seems reasonable. Adamson treats ŠE (*JRAS* 1984.10–11) and *kittabru* (*JRAS* 1984.11) as separate entities, apparently under the mistaken impression that *CAD* K 468 states that ŠE is only used for *kittabru* 1, meaning "side" or "arm" and not for the homophonous skin lesion. It is hard to imagine how Adamson concluded this from the entry in *CAD* which clearly indicates that *kittabru* 2 (the skin lesion) can be written ŠE in physiognomic omens (see also Böck, *Morphoskopie* 29). In any case, Adamson, *JRAS* 1984.10–11 proposes for ŠE a translation of "malignant melanoma" and for *kittabru* "lentigo" (because of its potential for malignancy). As with a number of other lesions for which Adamson has proposed malignancy, none of the references to ŠE or *kittabru* as a skin lesion indicates a fatal outcome (for ŠE *ubanāti*, see Chapter 14, n. 29). In addition, lentigo is flat and is rarely multiple on the face, which does not fit the references that Adamson has himself collected for *kittabru*.

189. For references, see *CAD* Š/2.440b; *AHw* 1235b.

190. Böck, *Morphoskopie* 202–203.

191. In *AHw* 1428a s.v. *urāšu* II mng. 2.

192. Böck, *Morphoskopie* 29.

193. DPS XXXIII:47, 48 (AOAT 43.355).

194. DPS XXXIII:52 (AOAT 43.355).

195. See also *BAM* 480 ii 26.

196. DPS III A r. 17′//C r. 41 = *TDP* 30:101 (cf. StBoT 36.60:2); DPS III A r. 23′–24′//C r. 48–49//G 5–6 = *TDP* 30:108–109) (cf. Labat, *Syria* 33.125 r. 5); DPS III A r. 25′//C r. 50.

197. The Hebrew cognate to *gubbuḫu* refers specifically to balding on the front part of the head (see Levine, "Leviticus" in *The JPS Torah Commentary* 82).

198. See also *BAM* 3 ii 27–28//*BAM* 480 iii 8//*BAM* 9:23–24.

199. For references, see *CAD* Q 319b s.v. *qurrudu*.

200. For references, see *CAD* G 157–158; *CAD* Q 319; *CAD* K 483; *CAD* Ṣ 44; *CAD* Q 99–100.

201. See also *BAM* 379 iv 23.

202. See Parrot, *Dawn of Sumer*, especially the Stele of the Vultures, pp. 134–137, and the Ur Standard, pp. 146–149.

203. See ibid, especially the votive statuary from Tel Asmar in the Diyala, p. 101.

204. As, for example, in Meier, *ZA* 45.200 i 11.

205. For references to the presence of beards as the distinguishing feature between noneunuch and eunuch courtiers, see *CAD* Z 126–127.

206. For references, see *AHw* 960b; *CAD* R 191a.

207. Haussperger, *Mem. Cagni* 445 agrees that this is a fungal infection involving the skin and hair.

208. Ebeling, *RLA* 1.321 (cf. Labat, *RLA* 3.233) suggests head leprosy on the basis of an alleged Talmudic cognate.

209. See also *BAM* 499 iii 7′.
210. See also *BAM* 499 iii 25′; cf. 22′.
211. See also *AMT* 76/6:9′.

CHAPTER 11. BONES AND JOINTS

1. For references, see *CAD* Š/2.248a.
2. H. Lewy, *HUCA* 40.52 (L29–581):8–10 = Gwaltney, *Pennsylvania Old Assyrian* no. 24:8–10 = Larsen, *Aššur-nādā* no. 127:8–10.
3. *BE* 17/1.21:27–31.
4. See also *AMT* 56/1 r. 10′//*AMT* 69/8 obv. 15; *AMT* 32/5 iv! 17+*AMT* 43/3 iv 6′//*BAM* 131 r. 8′.
5. For references, see *CAD* A/2.475–476.
6. See also *BAM* 415 r. 7; cf. *BAM* 379 iv 24//*SpTU* 3.106 r. 10 (back).
7. See also *BAM* 56:1; *AMT* 56/1 r. 5′//*AMT* 69/8 obv. 11; cf. BAM 379 iv 26; *BAM* 380:23//*BAM* 381 iii 15 (legs).
8. For *aš-ṭa-a-ma*, Heeßel, *AOAT* 43.177 reads *ina-da-a-ma*, following Labat, *TDP* 152:52′. Note also stiff feet: [DIŠ GÌR]^{II}-*šú áš-ṭa-a* GIG-*su* MAN-*ni* : DIŠ GÌ[R . . .] (DPS XIV C_2 iv 3//G iv 14′–15′ = *TDP* 144 iv 24′–25′).
9. Labat, *RLA* 3.126, 233 interprets some of the references to *šiggatu* as *šikkatu*, which he translates as "scurf" (dandruff or desquamation) and the rest as *šiggatu*, which he translates "ulcer"; *CAD* S 251 s.v. *sikkatu* A mng. 6 interprets all of the references as *sikkatu* and translates "pimple"; Campbell Thompson, *JRAS* 1937.268 read the references as *šiggatu* and translated the term as "strain, bruise, or blain." However, since *šagāgu* means "to be stiff" and since *BAM* 124, the therapeutic text in which most of the references to bandages for *šiggatu* appear, contains treatments for difficulty walking, bandages for setting fractures, and the like, it seems likely that "stiffness" is meant. On this point, see also *AHw* 1231a.
10. See also *AMT* 70/3 i 7–8//*AMT* 68/1 r. 5–6; *AMT* 68/1 r. 12; cf *BAM* 124 i 28//*AMT* 73/1 i 31+*AMT* 18/5 i 5; *BAM* 122 obv. 8–10//*AMT* 70/7 ii 7–8; DPS XI A r. 46 = *TDP* 98 r. 46.
11. Note also *AMT* 32/5 iv! 6; *AMT* 32/5 iv! 9//*BAM* 124 iii 43; *BAM* 124 iii 2//*AMT* 32/5 iv! 11//*BAM* 181:11; *BAM* 124 iii 5//*AMT* 32/5 iv! 15+*AMT* 43/3 iv 4′//*BAM* 181:15//*BAM* 131 r. 6′; *BAM* 124 iii 11; *AMT* 93/2 r. 5, 8, 11; *AMT* 51/4 iv 7; *AMT* 32/5 iv! 4; *AMT* 32/5 iv! 7//*BAM* 124 iii 41.
12. Labat, *RLA* 3.126, 233 believes that *šiggatu* caused by cold is frost bite. This interpretation is, however, predicated on the idea that *šiggatu* by itself is some sort of skin lesion (see above, n. 9).
13. See also *SpTU* 1.9:19′–21′.
14. See also DPS XI A obv. 34//B 33 = *TDP* 92:34//*SpTU* 1.34:33; cf. *AMT* 68/1 r. 16–17; DPS XIV A_2 iv 15′//G iv 5′ = *TDP* 142 iv 15′ (feet); *BAM* 124 iii 13//*BAM* 181 l.e. 2 (neck).
15. The translation assumes a denominal Dt verb from *akṣu* that is lexically equated with *aštu* (*CAD* A/1.281b). *AHw* 28a lists a verb *akāṣu* that he translates "to be stiff necked" (i.e., stubborn).
16. See also DPS XIV A iii 25–26//C_2 15//F 3//J 3 = *TDP* 142 iii 59′–60′. Note DPS XI A obv. 2, 3//B 2, 3 = *TDP* 90:2, 3//*SpTU* 1.34:2, 3 (hands); *BAM* 56 r. 5′ (feet); *BAM* 56 obv. 5′ (cf. *AMT* 40/5 iv 10′); *AMT* 52/6 + K 13425:6′; BM 41281 i 28, 32; DPS XII D iii 37 = *TDP* 106 iii 37; DPS XIII G_2 r. 17 = *TDP* 124 iii 24 (hips).
17. See also *BAM* 158 iii 9′, 16′; *BAM* 112 ii 15′; *STT* 92 iii 29′, 31′–32′; *BAM* 380:15; *KADP* 1 v 42 (sore hips); *AMT* 46/1 ii 24′–25′; *AMT* 47/3 iii 12′; *AMT* 29/4+K 2991 i 6//*AMT* 47/3 iii 7′; *BE* 31.60 i 5; *BE* 31.60 i 15, 18, 23// *AMT* 47/3 iv 5, 8, 14; *AMT* 29/4+K 2991 ii 3, 8//*AMT* 47/3 iv 20, 26 (sore neck); DPS X A obv. 9//B obv. 9 = *TDP* 80:9 (sore neck and hips); BM 43295:9–10 (Finkel, *Fs. Lambert* 153–154 with parallels) (sore leg); *BAM* 124 ii 47//*AMT* 74/1 ii 20 (sore foot and ankle); *BAM* 121:12; *BAM* 380:20//*BAM* 381 iii 13; DPS XI A obv. 34//B 33 = *TDP* 92:34//*SpTU* 1.34:33 (swollen feet); *AMT* 75/1 iv 23+*AMT* 15/3 iv 1 (sore heels).
18. See also DPS XIII G_2 r. 12 = *TDP* 124 iii 19; cf. DPS XIV A iv 7//C_2 iv 10b//K 3 = *TDP* 144 iv 42′ (toes); *BAM* 152 iv 7//*AMT* 70/5 ii 8′; *AMT* 70/5 ii 16′; *BAM* 121:18 (feet); DPS XI A obv. 55 = *TDP* 94:55; DPS XXXVI A 84 = *TDP* 208:84 (hands and feet); DPS XIV A i 25–27, 28 = *TDP* 130 i 25–27, 28; Böck, *Morphoskopie* 266:28 (hip sockets).
19. See also DPS XIV A_2 iv 6′–7′//C_2 iii 32–33a = *TDP* 142 iv 6′–7′; *BAM* 240:67′; cf. Böck, *Morphoskopie* 266:27 (bent).
20. Lit. "they continually become shorter (than they were)."
21. See also *BAM* 379 iv 24//*SpTU* 3.106 iv 10.

22. Lit. "they become shorter (than they were)."

23. See also *AMT* 53/1 iii 6′–7′, cf. 4′.

24. See also *BAM* 96 ii 1//*BAM* 97:9′.

25. See Chapter 13, p. 293.

26. *CAD* K 74b, followed by Adamson, *RA* 87.154–155 reads this passage as ÉLLAG *bir-ki-šú* and interprets the expression as meaning specifically "testicles." However, there is no necessary connection between hematuria and testicular pain, which makes "testicles" less likely in this context. It is, in any case, curious that the word for "testicle" (ŠIR) was not used.

27. Fincke, *Augenleiden* 73 interprets this text as representing reactive arthritis (*Morbus Reiter*). Since, however, sore throat is part of the description and urethritis is not mentioned, and since we also believe that the patient had congestive heart failure, rheumatic fever seems a more likely diagnosis. For what we believe to be descriptions of reactive arthritis, see below.

28. According to the commentary *SpTU* 1.31:27, this is because of the cold.

29. Adamson, *RA* 82.165–166 cites streptococcal infections as a possible cause of arthritis. In the same context, Adamson also lists erysipelothrix infections as a common cause of arthritis. However, this is an uncommon complication of this uncommon infection. Also, the evidence from lexical lists that he presents is insufficient to establish *rapādu* as "migratory arthritis." *Rapādu* is indeed grouped with *ṣidānu*, *šaššaṭu*, and *maškādu*, all of which Adamson believes to be joint diseases (*RA* 82.165 w/ n. 14). However, this sort of grouping is relatively common in lexical texts, and seems to have been motivated by the fact that the listed words have Sumerograms that are confusingly similar (they all begin with SAG or SA, sometimes both). *Ṣidānu* (SAG.NIGIN or SA.NIGIN) means "dizziness," *šaššaṭu* (SA.DUGUD), "tetanus," and *maškādu* (SA.GIG), "sciatica," none of which are joint diseases. Other, similar, lists also include *samānu:* "cellulitis," which does not even involve the muscles (SA) but which has a pseudo-Sumerogram SA.MA.NUM (see *CAD* R 147a lex. section).

30. For references, see *AHw* 935; *CAD* R 20–23.

31. Note also *BAM* 415 r. 1–2//*CT* 23.5–14 iii 50//*AMT* 19/8:3.

32. See also DPS XI A obv. 5//B 5a = *TDP* 90:5//*SpTU* 1.34:5a.

33. See also DPS XIV A iii 24//F 2//J 2 = *TDP* 140 iii 58′.

34. For *aš-ṭa-a-ma*, Heeßel, AOAT 43.177 reads *ina-da-a-ma*, following Labat, *TDP* 152:52′. Note also DPS XI A obv. 6 = *TDP* 90:6 (hands).

35. See also DPS XIV A_2 iv 8′//C_2 iii 33b = *TDP* 142 iv 8′.

36. Lit. "it continually becomes shorter (than it was)."

37. See also DPS XXII:39a (AOAT 43.255); cf. BM 47687+ (Finkel, *Mem. Sachs* 153):14 (left arm).

38. The reading follows Stol, *JEOL* 32.45, correcting *CAD* A/2.470a, which reads TAG-*te* and interprets this as a skin condition. "Touching the cheek" is presumably a prelude to seduction.

39. The term *Reiter's syndrome* has been used synonymously with *reactive arthritis,* but because of Reiter's Nazi past and involvement in involuntary human experimentation, we choose to avoid this term.

40. Fincke, *Augenleiden* 73 suggests that StBoT 36.23:6′–8′ contains a reference to the conjunctivitis of reactive arthritis (*Morbus Reiter*). We, however, interpret this text differently (see above).

41. For other references, see *BAM* 158 ii 14; *BAM* 182 obv. 7′; Herrero, *RA* 69.44 ii 38; K 2428+2548+6728 obv. 7′; *BAM* 182 obv. 11′; *BAM* 81:7′; *BAM* 379 ii 10′; *BAM* 423 ii 12′ (cf. *BAM* 1 i 36); *BAM* 182 obv. 17′, 22′; K 2428+2548+6728 obv. 11′–16′, 23′; K 9100+7964 iii 12′; *BAM* 354 iii 10//*BAM* 350:7′//*STT* 273 i 21′.

42. See also *BAM* 130:1, 22; *AMT* 42/6:2; *BAM* 350:4′; *BAM* 354 iii 3//*STT* 273 i 14′; *STT* 274:4′; K 9100+7964 iii 5′, 10′; *BAM* 124 iv 28//*BAM* 128 iv 25′; *BAM* 129 i 7//*CT* 23.5–14 ii 8′; *BAM* 129 i 17//*CT* 23.5–14 ii 17′//*CT* 23.2–4+K 2551:19′; *BAM* 129 i 24; *CT* 23.5–14 ii 39′//*BAM* 415 obv. 13′; *CT* 23.5–14 ii 47′, iii 10, 22, 29, 35, 41, 47; *CT* 23.1–2:8; *CT* 23.2–4+K 2551:15′; *CT* 23.4:5, 12; *BAM* 130:24; Böck, *Morphoskopie* 270:65.

43. Durand, *ARM* 26/1.553, 568 argues that *ARM* 26/1 no. 266 is a reference to sciatica. However, the pain as described is a stinging pain (*ziqtu*) rising from the sole of the foot and spreading to the abdomen (*ribītu*). The location of the pain as indicated in this text is not typical for sciatica, which spreads along the back of the leg. The pain that is described could be caused by many conditions and there is not sufficient information to indicate what might be the cause. Durand (*ARM* XXVI/1.568, 574) attempts to solve this problem by reinterpreting *ribītu* as "buttocks." However, this translation does not fit with other references to this term in medical texts.

44. Labat, *RLA* 3.127, 199 suggests "gout" for *sagallu*. However, the texts refer to muscle pain and stiffness rather than joint problems as would be expected with gout. Also, foot pain (podagra), a common sign of gout, is not mentioned in these texts. Müller, *AGM* 18.190 suggests *Filiaria medinensis* (guinea worm) as the cause for *sagallu*, but we do not concur. For our suggestions for guinea worm, see Chapter 3.274–277. Kinnier Wilson, *Iraq* 24.61 suggests filariasis (with accompanying elephantiasis), apparently on the grounds that *sagallu* refers to dilated (varicose) veins. He further argues that, since ancient Mesopotamia is located in the "East," varicose veins can only have been due to filariasis. However, there is no recognizable reference to elephantiasis in ancient Mesopotamian texts and nothing in the symptoms of *sagallu* to suggest either varicose veins or filariasis. In any case, filariasis does not cause varicose veins. With Attia, *Histoire des Sciences Médicales* 34.7, the most likely diagnosis for *sagallu* is sciatica.

45. See also *BAM* 216:16′//*BAM* 217:1//*AMT* 97/5:9; *AMT* 96/1:14; *AMT* 97/5:6; cf. *BAM* 197:1–2, 8–9; *AMT* 97/4:2 (intense pain in the left/right side).

46. Note also *BAM* 152 iv 16//*BAM* 158 iii 27′–28′//*AMT* 70/7 i 3; *BAM* 405:14′; *KAR* 56 r. 1 (stinging pains).

47. See also *BAM* 217:23; *AMT* 97/5:5′. For pains specific to right or left sides, see also K 2428+2548+6728 obv. 2′, 3′, 4′; BM 98584+BM 98689 i 12′–13′ (*maškādu*); Böck, *Morphoskopie* 270:65 (*sagallu*).

CHAPTER 12. OBSTETRICS AND GYNECOLOGY

1. This seems preferable to Stol's (*Birth* 200–201) interpretation of this as some sort of textile inserted into the womb. Suppositories of whatever material are usually described as such.

2. Finkel, *AfO* 27.37–52 and *CAD* N 141–142 understand *naḫšātu* to refer specifically to bleeding during pregnancy. Labat, *RLA* 3.109, however, understands this term to refer to increased menstruation and Butz, *OrAn* 21.221–226 translates "irregular bleeding."

3. For other references, see BM 42313+ obv. 26, 29; *BAM* 235:14//*BAM* 236 r. 6′; cf. *BAM* 236 obv. 17; *BAM* 237 ii 16′; K 263:37′.

4. See also *BAM* 237 i 17′, 21′, ii 5′, 15′, 22′, 33′, 40′, iii 19, 26, 32, 36. We know that *naḫšātu* refers to bleeding from the following: DIŠ NA MÚD *ina* DÚR-*šú* GIN$_7$ MUNUS *ša na-aḫ-ša-te* ŠUB.ŠUB-*a ta-ḫi-iz-zu-ma* DÚR.GIG.GA.KÁM NU TUKU-*ši tir-di-it ir-ri-šú* GIG: "If blood emits from a person's anus like a woman upon whom *naḫšātu* continually falls but he does not have DÚR.GIG, he is sick with 'flowing of the bowels'" (*BAM* 99:19–20//*BAM* 100:2′–4′; *BAM* 99:42–43//*AMT* 43/1 iii 3′–4′) and from *ša na-*[*aḫ-š*]*á-a-tú* GIG-*át* MUNUS *šá ina me-re-e-šú da-mu i-ta-nam-ma-ru*: "she who is sick with ⸢*naḫšātu*⸣ is a woman during whose pregnancy blood is continually seen" (*SpTU* 1.39:6′–7′).

5. *KBo* 28.30 (edited in Edel, *Die ägyptisch-hethitische Korrespondenz* 1 no. 75).

6. See also *BAM* 243:1′; *BAM* 244:71; BM 42333+:12//BM 42313+ r. 37 (Finkel, *Fs. Lambert* 171–172).

7. See also *STT* 98 obv. 2′; BM 42313+ obv. 5; BM 42333+:5//BM 42313+ r. 33 (Finkel, *Fs. Lambert* 171–172); BM 59710:1; BM 79061:1–2.

8. Laws of Ḫammurapi §§ 144–147. Compare Laws of Lipit-Ištar § 27 (begetting children by a prostitute); Middle Assyrian Laws A § 41 (by concubines).

9. See also Stol, *Birth* 37–48.

10. See also *BAM* 246:1.

11. *BRM* 4.12:36–37; Boissier, *DA* 220:14–15.

12. See also *CTN* 4.196+195 ii 15′.

13. For more details, see Stol, *Birth* 171–181.

14. Note this passage in a Sumerian hymn: "He (Enlil) gives her (Ninlil) the name Nintu, the Lady-who-gives-birth and the Lady-of-the-open-legs . . . The [functions of] the *qadištu*, everything pertaining to women that no man must see" (Civil, *JAOS* 103.57:152, 154; cf. W. G. Lambert's comments on p. 65).

15. It has been suggested (Jacobsen, *OrNS* 42.290 w/ n. 63) that an enigmatic passage in the Atraḫasīs (I 282) is a direct reference to the rupturing with a slender rod of the membranes of the woman giving birth. The interpretation is not entirely unreasonable. *Williams Obstetrics* 1093 describes this procedure, which is still recommended, albeit when performed with sterile instruments, as a method of inducing labor. However, it should be noted that both the reading and the interpretation of the line in question are hotly disputed (for references and discussion, see Stol, *Birth* 115).

16. This brick also appears in the myth "Enki and the World Order" as part of the birth goddesses' insignia (Jacobsen, *OrNS* 42.289 w/ n. 57). For more on the "brick of birth," see Stol, *Birth* 118–122.

17. This distribution of labor is also reflected in the divine sphere. Although female birth-goddesses were honored in the birth ritual and celebrated in hymns and prayers as divine midwives, when appeals had to be made to divinities because things were not going well, it was from male patrons of childbirth such as the Akkadian moon-god Sîn and Asalluḫi/Marduk that assistance was typically sought.

18. For references and discussion, see Sjöberg, *AfO* 24.43 ad 72 and van Dijk, *OrNS* 44.61 w/ n. 24. A GI.DUR.KU$_5$ of silver and forty-one of copper appear in an inventory of the temple of Ninḫursag (A 5834:5, 15; reference courtesy M. Civil).

19. For more on cutting the umbilical cord, see Stol, *Birth* 141–142.

20. For more details, see Scurlock, *Incognita* 2.149 w/ n. 129.

21. The context would seem to call for something that could be poured on the wound. *Immanakku*-stone was used in the manufacture of glass, and is described as being like river silt dotted with pebbles (for references, see *CAD* I 127–128; suggestion courtesy of M. Civil). Drower, *Iraq* 5.110, reports that pastes of various kinds were still being rubbed on the infant's navel in Iraq as of 1938.

22. Scurlock has personally witnessed a cut onion being rubbed over an open scratch wound—the almost immediate result was the production of a pronounced welt and the cessation of bleeding.

23. This pail appears as part of the insignia of the birth-goddess (Jacobsen, *OrNS* 42.289–290).

24. See Livingstone, SAA 3.48:15′–17′, who translates the enigmatic key word (Ì.ZUM), from context, as "phlegm." The present translation assumes a connection between this Ì.ZUM and the verb *ḫâlu* (ZUM): "to be in labor; exude liquid." Compare the term Ì.KÚM of *BAM* 237 iv 9, and Ì.RA of *BAM* 240:18′, perhaps from *emēmu* (KÚM) and *maḫāṣu* (RA), respectively. Also note the formation Ì.DAB$_5$ (*ṣibtu*: "agricultural holding") from *ṣabātu* (DAB$_5$) and Ì.DUB (*išpikū*: "storage jar") from *šapāku* (DUB). The accompanying recitation ends with: "What do you ask of me, my lady? What may they give [you]? May they give you oxen, grain, (and) fattened sheep?" "I do not eat oxen, grain, (and) fattened sheep. Let them give me the (healthy) glow of young women, the beauty of young men. Place at my disposal unlimited medical knowledge; let the amniotic fluid(?), like ball lightning from the sky, continually fall to the earth" (Livingstone, SAA 3.48:8′–14′); the following recitation mentions pregnant cows going into labor: "In the temple of Bēlit-ili, in the sheepfold of Ninegal, the pregnant ones became pregnant, the laboring ones went into labor" (ibid.: r. 1–2).

25. "Then the midwife puts her finger into the mouth of the newborn child and gently raises its uvula" (Massé, *Persian Beliefs and Customs* 14). Compare the cleansing of the mouth of the newborn described in *KBo* 17.61 obv. 12–14, edited in Beckman, StBoT 29.42. Interestingly, one of the incantations that accompanied the Hittite postpartum cleanup ritual was entitled: "Down from the sky it flowed" (*KBo* 17.61 r. 7′–8′, in Beckman, StBoT 29.44). If this was intended to accompany the cleansing of the mouth, it would almost directly parallel the Akkadian ritual whose incantation ends with the line: "let the amniotic fluid(?), like ball lightning from the sky, continually fall to the earth" (Livingstone, SAA 3.48:13′–14′). In modern American practice, the nose and mouth of the newborn baby are suctioned to remove the amniotic fluid. A failure to do so not only results in discomfort for the baby, but can cause infections as well.

26. Römer, *Lišan Mitḫurti* 295:77–78; cf. Th. J. H. Krispijn, apud Stol, *Birth* 177.

27. *SRT* 6 iii 2 = 7 obv. 12 (Jacobsen, *OrNS* 42.290 n. 59).

28. This is probably to be identified with an object that is mentioned alongside the birth brick, the cutter for the umbilical cord, and the water pail, as belonging to the paraphernalia of a midwife in the Sumerian composition "Enki and the World Order" (Jacobsen, *OrNS* 42.289–290).

29. See Stol, *Birth* 144–145.

30. Another text, *SpTU* 2.43:13–17, apud Hunger, *NABU* 1996 no. 39, explains how to calculate the size of the fetus mathematically.

31. Stol, *Birth* 12, in his discussion of this text, gives 2.7 mm as the modern equivalent for the "grain."

32. Ibid. 201 takes this as "enjoy," but the verb is *šelû*: "to be negligent."

33. Mujais, *Am.J.Nephrology* 19.137, based on a mistranslation, interprets this reference to be facial swelling secondary to eclampsia.

34. *ABL* 1405 r. 7–9. For other references to this usage of the verb "to approach," see *CAD* Q 233b s.v. *qerēbu* mng. 3b.

35. Stol, *Birth* 202 rejects the conventional interpretation in favor of Kraus's "daring" suggestion that ll. 1–7 of *TDP* 37 and the preceding ll. 106–111 of *TDP* 36 refer to the number of times sexual intercourse takes place

rather than the month of pregnancy. However, this interpretation requires omitting the word *five* from line 106 and goes against the obvious reading of the text. It also makes less sense than the original interpretation.

36. For a full discussion of the number of months in pregnancy by various systems of counting, see Stol, *Birth* 24–25.

37. See, for example, Cavigneaux and al-Rawi, *Iraq* 55.96–100.

38. Stol, *Birth* 201 asserts that "life" can only refer to the fetus. However, every explicit prognosis in this section concerns the mother and not the fetus.

39. Compare DPS XXXVI A 107//D 4 = *TDP* 210:107 (day 4); DPS XXXVI A 110//D 7 = *TDP* 210:110 (day 7); DPS XXXVI A 113//D 10 = *TDP* 210:113 (day 10).

40. The passage has been collated.

41. See also DPS XXXVI A 109//D 6 = *TDP* 210:109 (day 6).

42. See also DPS XXXVI A 87, 88 = *TDP* 208:87, 88.

43. The possessive suffix is masculine, presumably referring to the *libbu*: "womb."

44. Collation shows that BM 42313+ r. 36 ends with [*šum*$_4$]-*ma er-ri u* A.MEŠ ŠUB.ŠUB (i.e., Finkel omitted several signs from his transliteration).

45. Finkel, *Fs. Lambert* 173, interprets this passage as "she will open (reading BAD-*ma*) and will become pregnant and (her) waters will flow." He further suggests (*Fs. Lambert* 172) that the "waters" refers to the woman's "semen." Although Finkel is quite correct in his understanding that the ancient Mesopotamians interpreted a woman's sexual secretions as "semen" and as the woman's contribution to forming the fetus (see below), this substance is called "semen"; "waters" refer to amniotic fluid.

46. That such things did actually happen may readily be seen from the following, drawn from a remedy against sorcery: "If 'cutting of the breath' [has been performed against] a man by means of a roof mouse [and consequently] a slaughtered roof mouse is found in the man's house" (*BAM* 458 i 8′–9′).

47. *LKA* 9 iii 2–4, cf. 7 (see Reiner, *AfO* 19.150). For more on this subject, see Scurlock, *Incognita* 2.140–142.

48. This text consistently uses masculine-singular suffixes to refer to the pregnant woman.

49. Kinnier Wilson, *Diseases in Antiquity* 203 suggests toxemia of pregnancy for this text. However, vomiting is not a prominent finding in toxemia of pregnancy.

50. Kinnier Wilson, *Jour.Roy.Soc.Med.* 89.137 believes that difficult births in ancient Mesopotamia were most commonly caused by deficiency states resulting in pelvic deformities. Rickets (vitamin D deficiency) is the major deficiency disease that can lead to pelvic deformities. However, this is uncommonly seen except in northern latitudes where both limited sun exposure and vitamin D deficiency exist.

51. For references and discussion, see Oppenheim, *Journ.Hist.Med.* July 1960.292–294; *CAD* Š/2.447–448.

52. See also Lambert, *Iraq* 31 pl. 6:33 (the incipit of a recitation for this problem).

53. Finkel (*Fs. Lambert* 158–159) interprets this as "for by-passing child bearing and regarding whom 'agony' (menopausal back pain) hurts her." The verb is *kalû*: "to delay" and not *akālu*: "to hurt." The "bypassing" is based on interpreting the last sign of line 3′ as a KI. It is a little known fact that there is a generally observed convention among ancient scribes of the late periods of drawing the horizontal wedges of the DI (and not the KI) well out beyond the end of the sign. By this criterion alone, the sign at the end of line 3′ is a clear DI. Köcher's suggestion of ŠA!! (*Fs. Lambert* 159) is even less likely. With these difficulties removed, the "agony" becomes birth pangs. Back pain is not, in any case, a particularly diagnostic sign of menopause.

54. See also *STT* 241:7,29; *SpTU* 5.248 r. 12.

55. See also *BAM* 248 i 51,67; *BAM* 248 iii 6//K 3485+K8210+K10443 ii 6; *BAM* 248 iv 11//*AMT* 67/1 iv 4.

56. Deller, *OrNS* 54.327–330 and *NABU* 1992 no. 79.

57. Curse formulae on Neo-Assyrian contracts threaten as punishment for breach of contract having to eat a mina of the resulting "*kurru* hair" called *qerdu*, a word related to an Akkadian verb *qurrudu*, meaning "to fall out in tufts," used to describe the hair on rapidly balding heads, and to an Aramaic/Hebrew verb meaning "to scrape off."

58. This is one of the verbs used to describe the hair of someone "touched in the steppe" (i.e., affected by severe protein deficiency; see Chapter 7).

59. In more modern tanning processes, a solution of quicklime is used for this purpose (Wulff, *Crafts of Persia* 231).

60. Fincke, *Augenleiden* 173–174 does not appear to recognize the serious prognosis seen in this reference when she assigns it to a completely benign condition of the eyes that heals itself without treatment in less than two weeks.

61. See also Šumma Izbu 49 (Leichty, *Izbu* 35).

62. See also DPS XXXVII A obv. 14 = *TDP* 214:14.

63. Note that the commentary, *STT* 403:19 explains this phrase as ŠÀ-*šú ana* $BURU_8$ *e-te-ni-la-a*: "his stomach continually rises up to vomit." Although an invaluable source of information, some commentaries read as if they were the exams of substandard students. See, for example, Leichty, *AfO* 24.82–86.

64. The scribe, who made a number of other errors of this sort elsewhere in the tablet, appears to have written U.

65. The scribe, who made a number of other errors elsewhere in the tablet, appears to have written IR.

66. See previous note.

67. See Lackenbacher, *RA* 65.150–154.

68. Compare ibid.135–136 r. i 2′–9″; W. Farber, *ZA* 79.16:13–24.

69. Ancient Mesopotamian men seem to have expected to take an active role in parenting. For this and more details on *lilû* demons, see Scurlock, *Incognita* 2.150–153.

70. As, for example, in W. Farber, *Schlaf* 126–127 § 45.

71. With Stol, *Birth* 7–8 and Reiner, *ZA* 72.132–133. Biggs', *Fs. Lambert* 2, contrary assertion is based on alleged classical parallels, and overlooks ancient Mesopotamian evidence.

72. See Scurlock, *NIN*, forthcoming.

73. See also Stol, *Birth* 206–208.

74. This is the exact opposite of Hippocrates as quoted in Aetios of Amida, *Tetrabiblon* 16.9; see Ricci's commentary (Ricci, *Aetios of Amida* 124 [he is unaware of the Chinese and Mesopotamian examples]).

75. Attia, *Histoire des Sciences Médicales* 34.4 argues that this reference is to the varicose veins. However, the *āšipu* described this phenomenon using the verb GUB: "to stand up" (see Chapter 8 with 8.31–8.32) and not ZI: "to pulsate."

76. See also Stol, *CANE* 490.

77. Compare DPS XXXVI A 64 = *TDP* 206:64 (protrude from above toward her hypogastric region).

78. See also DPS XXXVI A 63 = *TDP* 206:63. Compare DPS XXXVI A 65 = *TDP* 206:65 (protrude/are turned from below towards her hypogastric region).

79. "If you want to know whether a pregnant woman will have a boy or a girl, call her over to you. If she starts off on the right foot it will be a boy; if on the left foot, a girl" (Massé, *Persian Beliefs and Customs* 10; cf. also al-Qurtʾubi, *Génération du foetus*, tr. H. Jahier and N. Abdelkader, chapter 4, p. 33 quoting Hippocrates).

80. See also DPS XXXVI A 9 = *TDP* 200:9.

81. See also DPS XXXVI A 10 = *TDP* 200:10.

82. The scribe put a vertical through the MÚD yielding what looks like a $GIDIM_2$ sign.

83. Compare DPS XXXVI A 52–53 = *TDP* 204:52–53.

84. Note also DPS XXXVI A 24 = *TDP* 202:24.

85. Note also DPS XXXVI A 25 = *TDP* 202:25.

86. Old Wives' Tales have it that male babies are more active in the womb than female ones.

87. See also DPS XXXVI A 70, 75 = *TDP* 206:70, 75.

88. Compare also al-Qurtʾubi chapter 4 quoting Galen and Aetios of Amida, *Tetrabiblon* 16.9 quoting Hippocrates; see Ricci's commentary p. 124.

89. Massé, *Persian Beliefs and Customs* 10.

90. See also DPS XXXVI A 7 = *TDP* 200:7.

91. See Kinnier Wilson, *Diseases in Antiquity* 203. Kinnier Wilson also considers an alternative diagnosis of toxemia of pregnancy. Since this seems to be a benign condition, toxemia of pregnancy is not an appropriate diagnosis.

92. See also DPS XXXVI A 98 = *TDP* 210:98; DPS XXXVI A 92//B 27′ = *TDP* 208:92.

93. Stol, *Birth* 25–26, 199 interprets this text to mean that the woman is having her menstrual period and does not realize that she is pregnant until she steps to the right. At this point, she tells her husband and they have intercourse and this awakens the child so that it is born. This interpretation seems rather forced and is, in fact, not based on any evidence from ancient Mesopotamia but on a folk tradition attested only in ancient Greece and modern North Africa of the "sleeping child" who is supposedly born years after conception. These traditions (as with the Talmudic passage also cited by Stol) are designed to allow women whose husbands are absent at sea to become pregnant without having to admit to adultery and to allow the husbands to accept the resulting children as their own. Since ancient Mesopotamians, unlike Greeks and North Africans, were not seafaring peoples, no such custom is to be expected here.

94. A possible description of this is DIŠ MUNUS *ina* GIG-*šá* LUḪ.LUḪ-*ut* bad ina su un meš-šá bad-ši: "If a woman continually jerks in her illness . . ." (DPS XXXVII A obv. 15 = *TDP* 214:15).

95. See also *BAM* 240:25′.

96. See also *BAM* 237 iv 9.

97. Note also *BAM* 240:65′.

CHAPTER 13. NEUROLOGY

1. Note also DPS XXVI:50′ (AOAT 43.282); DPS XIII B i 49′//F 8 = *TDP* 116 i 53′ (Šamaš); *BAM* 165 i 16′.

2. Note also *BAM* 574 iv 41.

3. See also DPS IV B obv. 3 = *TDP* 32:3.

4. The commentary *SpTU* 1.30 obv. 2 explains that AL.DU means *il-la-ku*: "they run."

5. See also DPS XII D iii 7, 8//F 8//G_2 iii 4, 5 = *TDP* 102 iii 7, 8.

6. Von Soden, *AHw* 182–183, 214 followed inter alia by Heeßel, AOAT 43.168 ad l. 55′. This would seem to be supported by ancient commentaries such as *CT* 51.136:9–10 and *SpTU* 1.30:3. However, what equivalents in ancient commentaries and lexical lists often mean is not that the two words are exact synonyms but that they can be interchanged in a given ominous or medical context without changing the outcome or diagnosis. In this case, the phrase being commented on is "If he has a viselike headache, and his insides are continually cramped, 'hand' of Kūbu" (DPS IV B obv. 3 = *TDP* 32:3). What the commentary is telling us is that if the equivalent form of *napāḫu* were to be substituted for *ebēṭu* to yield: "If he has a viselike headache, and his insides are continually bloated," the diagnosis would still be "hand" of Kūbu. That this is indeed a correct statement may readily be seen from a number of references in which intestinal bloating (with other supplemental symptoms) is attributed to "hand" of Kūbu (DPS XIII I 7–9 = *TDP* 122 iii 7–9; see pp. 512–514).

7. See *CAD* E 148a.

8. The term is lexically equated with *ezēḫu*: "to gird" and *kaṣāru*: "to knot." Moreover, *ebēṭu* is used to describe the brief continuation of contractions of a sheep's heart after the animal is slaughtered. See *CAD* E 13–14.

9. See also *CAD* E 148.

10. Note also *BAM* 575 iii 28//*BAM* 54:1; *BAM* 575 i 25.

11. Note also *AMT* 76/1:11–12; *AMT* 45/6:12–13.

12. Note also DPS VI C ii 6 (right nostril).

13. See also *BAM* 108 obv. 15–18.

14. See *CAD* D 34–35, 137–138. Unaccountably, *AHw* 151b, 169b translates "to swell" and "swelling" (followed by Labat, *RLA* 3.231; Köcher, *Fs. Goerke* 38).

15. See also *BAM* 434 i 13′–15′; *AMT* 48/4 r. 8–9.

16. Note also *BAM* 164:4; BM 101938:4′.

17. Compare also *šaqāru*, which should mean something similar to *dakāšu* but appears only in broken context (*STT* 89:120–123, 124–127 [Stol, *Epilepsy* 93]).

18. Haussperger, *Mem. Cagni* 446 believes that this text is describing angioneurotic edema. This seems unlikely, since pain is not a significant symptom in this disease. The error was probably caused by a mistranslation of *dikšu* as "swelling" (see above).

19. For *šimmatu* as paralysis, see, for example, Kinnier Wilson, *Diseases in Antiquity* 192–193; Herrero, *RA* 69.52; Geller, *RAI* 28.193; Attia, *Histoire des Sciences Médicales* 34.8.

20. See next note.

21. Stol, *Epilepsy* 62–63, 79 interprets this as "goose flesh." In *Fs. Borger* 344 he further argues that it is named after *ḫamītu*: "wasp." However, wasp stings do not cause goose bumps.

22. See Adamson, *RA* 84.31–32.

23. Note also *KUB* 37.9 ii 10′–12′.

24. For the translation of *šāpulu* as "inguinal region," see Heeßel, AOAT 43.168 ad 57′ and *AHw* 1177b. Adamson, *JRAS* 1984.7 proposes an alternative translation of "scrotal sac" and argues that this and similar passages are describing torsion of the testicles. Neither argument seems logical in this context.

25. Note StBoT 36.30 ad 4′; Heeßel, AOAT 43.169 ad 63.

26. The *CAD* Š/1.419a takes *šapāku* as "limp?"; however, one of the examples given is of a part of the lung that is *šapāku*'d like a staff. In this context, "limp" hardly seems appropriate.

27. See also DPS III C obv. 26 = *TDP* 20:26.

28. Note also: DIŠ *ka-bit-ma* GÌR-*šú šá* 150 : 15 *i-qan-na-an u i-tar-ra-aṣ* BA.ÚŠ: "If it is difficult (for him) to bend and straighten out his right (var. left) foot, he will die" (DPS XIV A iv 21–22 = *TDP* 144 iv 56′–57′).

29. After F. Köcher, apud Stol, *Epilepsy* 97. See further Chapter 3, n. 271.

30. Many scholars are confused by the fact that fearful people can express their fear by jerking or shuddering. They therefore tend to assume that all patients with "jerking" or "shuddering" are frightened when in fact there are other causes of this phenomenon (see, e.g., Kinnier Wilson, *Medical History* 34.192, 193; Stol, *Epilepsy* 66, 71, 72, 75, 93; Fincke, *Augenleiden* 108, 110, 147), a mistake not made by the *āšipu*.

31. See also DPS III C obv. 26 = *TDP* 20:26.

32. See also StBoT 36.23 r. 4′, 60:10.

33. See Stol, *Epilepsy* 59. Kinnier Wilson, *Medical History* 34.187, 189 interprets this expression here and in other passages as referring to a regaining of consciousness, but this seems unlikely.

34. Kinnier Wilson, *Medical History* 34.189, 194 also describes this text as a complex partial seizure.

35. Note that Adamson, *RA* 84.28–30, followed by Kämmerer, *RA* 94.70, defines *ra*ʾ*ābu* incorrectly as Parkinson's tremor.

36. The restoration is based on the commentary *STT* 403 r. 43–45. Note also DPS XXII:5 (AOAT 43.251).

37. For the reading and interpretation, see Heeßel, AOAT 43.263 ad 5.

38. See previous note.

39. See Heeßel, AOAT 43.214 ad 54–55.

40. See also K 2351+:9′.

41. For a possible example, see 19.177.

42. See also DPS XVIII:15–16, 17–18 (AOAT 43.218–219); cf. StBoT 36.60:3.

43. That *parāku* refers to crossed eyes, see also Fincke, *Augenleiden* 147–148, 233–234.

44. See also DPS V G 7 = *TDP* 50 G 7.

45. For *petû*, see also Fincke, *Augenleiden* 149–150 and for *katāmu* 115–118.

46. On this point, see also ibid. 83–86; Labat, *MDP* 57 p. 257 ad v 15′. Besides eyes, the term is used to describe what an ox does with his anus (dilates) when he raises his tail to defecate (*CT* 40.32:21).

47. Fincke, *Augenleiden* 107–108, 183–184 believes that *zaqāpu* means "to roll eyes upward until only the whites are showing." Inability to do this would indicate extraocular muscle paralysis, a finding not consistent with many of the contexts in which *zaqāpu* occurs. *CAD* Z 54a and *AHw* 512b interpret the D-stem of *zaqāpu* as meaning "to make the eyes protrude" (see also Kinnier Wilson, *Medical History* 34.193). Again, this translation is not appropriate to the contexts in which this term appears.

48. For *zaqāpu*, see also DPS V F 11 = *TDP* 50 F 11; DPS XI A r. 51 = *TDP* 98 r. 51; DPS XL A 56 = *TDP* 224:56; DPS XXVII:20 (AOAT 43.298); DPS XXVI:80′, 81′ (AOAT 43.285).

49. See also DPS V D ii 4′, 5′ = *TDP* 48 E ii 4, 5; DPS XXIII:6 (AOAT 43.272).

50. For *balāṣu*, see also *SpTU* 3.86 obv. 7–8; Lambert, *BWL* 42:71–75.

51. Note also *STT* 89:208 (Stol, *Epilepsy* 98—he translates *kapāṣu* as "bulge"); DPS V D i 5 = *TDP* 48 E i 5; *BRM* 4.32:2.

52. Fincke, *Augenleiden* 104–107 suggests blepharospasm for this reference. However, this is not a condition that would cause fatality.

53. The text has been collated.

54. On this point, see also Frans Schlessinger, apud Geller, *AfO* 48/49.57 n. 69.

55. The expression is used of applying plasters. Note Stol, *Epilepsy* 65 n. 31.

56. For this symptom, see also *BAM* 480 iv 32–33//Jastrow, *TCPP* obv. 35–37; *BAM* 578 i 46–47.

57. See also *AMT* 97/4:6′–7′. Compare DPS IV B obv. 18 = *TDP* 34:18; *BAM* 482 iv 40′ (with headache).

58. Some forty-four ancient texts contain references to *ṣâdu*. The conditions described suggest that "dizziness" would be an appropriate translation, with Stol, *Epilepsy* 61 and passim. See also Kinnier Wilson, *Diseases in Antiquity* 201, but note that on p. 192 he suggests "nystagmus" in close association with dietary deficiency for *iṣṣanundu*, apparently without realizing that this is a conjugated form of *ṣâdu*. Other suggested interpretations include Lambert, *AfO* 18.290, 295 ad. l. 13 ("tic"), Geller, RAI 28.193 ("face is contorted" for IGI.MEŠ-*šú* NIGIN.MEŠ in *TDP* 76:60 but "vertigo" for IGI.MEŠ-*šú* NIGIN.MEŠ in *TDP* 76:63), and Landsberger, *WO* 3.51 n. 26 ("chorea"). Adamson, *RA* 82.170–171 interprets *ṣâdu* and *ṣīdānu* to refer to Sydenham's chorea based on his translation of *ṣâdu* as "repetitive and involuntary twisting movements that take

place; they are usually performed in a circular manner but are of little apparent use to the performer." However, the translation that is offered as proof of the identification of *ṣâdu* and *ṣīdānu* with Syndenham's chorea is actually based on the modern definition of Sydenham's chorea, and not any ancient text. Syndenham's chorea is not likely to have been attested so frequently, and is inappropriate to many of the contexts in which *ṣâdu* occurs. For possible ancient references to chorea, see below. Sjöberg's (*JCS* 25.141) suggestion of listeriosis for Sumerian SAG.NIGIN (the Sumerogram for *ṣidānu*) was specifically meant to apply to a disease in sheep: UDU.SAG.NIGIN. Sheep infected with listeria meningitis sometimes walk in circles; humans with listeriosis, however, do not. It is, therefore, necessary to find some other explanation when *ṣidānu* is used of a human being. Fincke, *Augenleiden* 157 thinks that *ṣâdu* is a sign and refers to the eyes literally spinning round, but we believe that it refers to a sensation of spinning perceived by the patient.

59. See *AHw* 65b s.v. *arāru* II. *CAD* A/2.237–238 s.v. *arāru* C translates this term as "to rot," "to discharge a putrid liquid," and "to defecate." In all cited references, however, either "to tremble" or "to make a rumbling noise" fits the context better. Landsberger, *MSL* 9.215 believes that the lone reference to *arāru* of the eyes (see 13.106) is a scribal error for the more common *barāru*. If so, it would mean that the eyes were dimmed (see Chapter 9).

60. See also *SpTU* 1.31:9.

61. See n. 59.

62. For other examples of eyes "jerking", see also *STT* 89:133–136a (Stol, *Epilepsy* 93—he translates "jerking" as "fearful") and StBoT 36.22 r. 3′.

63. Fincke, *Augenleiden* 108–110 believes that this term refers to dilation of the pupil. Since, however, *galātu* means "to jerk" in other contexts, it seems more likely that it means "to jerk" in this context as well.

64. Ibid. 174–175 believes that this term refers to eyes that are spinning round in a circle. We agree that this is a possibility, but prefer our explanation.

65. Ibid. 121–122 believes this to be elliptical nystagmus.

66. Ibid. 109 suggests that this passage is referring to tetanus or rabies. However, this identification depends on lumping this description of ᵈLUGAL.GÌR.RA together with the following entry, which has a different ancient diagnosis. For possible ancient descriptions of rabies and tetanus, see Chapter 2 under ENVIRONMENTAL HAZARDS and Chapter 3 under TETANUS.

67. Ibid. 146 suggests that this term may refer to eye movements that occur at the beginning of a seizure. However, *neqelpû* is not used to describe eye movements in any of the descriptions of seizures that we possess at present. *AHw* 779b translates *neqelpû* as "dizzy." There is, however, a better candidate for "dizzy" in *ṣâdu* (see p. 302 with n. 58, above).

68. Ibid. 159–160, 233–234 believes that this term means strabismus (crossed eyes). Since some texts refer to *ṣapāru* in only one eye, and a single eye cannot be crossed, we reject this definition.

69. See also DPS IV B obv. 24 = *TDP* 34:24; cf. DPS XXII:19–20 (AOAT 43.253).

70. See also DPS XXVI:62′–63′ (AOAT 43.283).

71. For *ṣapāru*, see also DPS IX A 8–9 = *TDP* 72:8–9; DPS IX A 29//B obv. 27–28 = *TDP* 74:29; *STT* 89:96–101; *STT* 105:16′–17′; *BAM* 480 i 1–3//*BAM* 3 i 1–3; *AMT* 76/5:11–13+79/4:2′–4′//*SpTU* 1.46:16–19//*AMT* 35/6:5′–7′.

72. See Fincke, *Augenleiden* 145; cf. Kinnier Wilson, *Iraq* 19.47.

73. The text has been collated. The copy has ᵈ20.

74. For *napalkû*, see also DPS V D ii 6′, 7′ = *TDP* 48 E ii 6, 7; DPS XXVII:16–17 (AOAT 43.298); *CTN* 4.72 i 3–5 (Kinnier Wilson, *Iraq* 19.40–49 [ND 4368]).

75. See Fincke, *Augenleiden* 133–135.

76. *Medical History* 34.191.

77. For *nabalkutu*, see also DPS XXIII:6 (AOAT 43.272); DPS V G 3–6 = *TDP* 50 G 3–6; DPS XXXVI A 89 = *TDP* 208:89; DPS XXVI:30′ (AOAT 43.280/281).

78. Possibly also to be considered in this context is a series of fragmentary references in Tablet V (DPS V D ii 8′–13′ = *TDP* 48 E ii 8–13) which mention that the patient "lets his eyes fall."

79. See DPS XII E iv 4–5 = *TDP* 106 iii 45.

80. See Stol, *Epilepsy* 76–77.

81. See above, 13.57–13.59.

82. In DPS XV:9 (AOAT 43.151), the *āšipu* appears to have gotten confused, since he attributes what is clearly a wound to the left side of the body (the left arm is dark and the patient is having difficulty speaking) to being struck from behind.

83. See above, 13.57–13.59.

84. See above, 13.57–13.59.

85. The passage has been collated. Labat, omitting the LAGAB, read Lamaštu.

86. Adamson, *JRAS* 1979.4 n. 25 cites this text as "evidence of fevers associated with chills, rigors, and cold sweats" suggesting the presence of endemic malaria in ancient Mesopotamia, but we do not concur. For possible descriptions of malaria in ancient Mesopotamian texts, see Chapter 3 under MALARIA.

87. See also DPS IV A obv. 46–47 = *TDP* 36:46–47.

88. The text has been collated. Ritter, AS 16.303 n. 13 restored [*uk-ta-at*]-*ta-at* against the traces. The meaning is the same.

89. Note DPS III A obv. 20, 21//C obv. 11, 12 = *TDP* 18:11, 12; DPS IV A obv. 45 = *TDP* 36:45 (head wounds accompanied by abdominal pain, bloating, or cramping).

90. Note also DPS XV:11 (AOAT 43.151); DPS X B r. 2 = *TDP* 86 r. 2.

91. Note also DPS X A obv. 17//B obv. 19 = *TDP* 82:17; cf. StBoT 36.35 obv. 15′//StBoT 36.57 r. 5′.

92. Note also DPS X A obv. 20//B obv. 22 = *TDP* 82:20.

93. So *CTN* 4.72 i 17′–18′ (Kinnier Wilson, *Iraq* 19.40–49 [ND 4368]).

94. Fincke, *Augenleiden* 74 suggests meningitis or rabies to explain these findings. However, it seems clear that the *āšipu* is describing a neck wound with probable spinal cord transection. For possible ancient descriptions of meningitis and rabies, see below and in Chapter 2 under ENVIRONMENTAL HAZARDS.

95. Note also DPS XV:51 (AOAT 43.153); DPS XIV A_2 i 8–9//D obv. 5 = *TDP* 132 i 60.

96. See Stol, *Epilepsy* 92.

97. *CAD* Ṣ 35 s.v. *ṣabātu* mng. 9a2′c′ cites this passage as an example of the Gt of *ṣabātu* and translates "if the vertebrae of his neck are loose and his nostrils grown together." The translation is highly improbable.

98. Note also DPS X A obv. 23, 25//B obv. 26, 28 = *TDP* 82:23, 25.

99. Note also *BAM* 422 ii 3′; *SpTU* 4.129 iv 17, vi 42; *AMT* 103/1 ii 13; *AMT* 104/1 iii 24′, 32′, 35′, 38′, 41′; *BAM* 11:36.

100. Biggs, *RLA* 6.210 and *CAD* S 25b fail to identify SAG.KI.DIB.BA as a headache and consider it to be an unknown illness of the head. Köcher, *BAM* vol. 1, p. xiv, Herrero, *RA* 69.49, and Haussperger, *Mem. Cagni* 440 recognize SAG.KI.DIB.BA as a headache but suggest specifically "migraine." Although migraine headaches are described (see below), when "affliction of the temples" appears by itself the a priori assumption is that this is a headache of unspecified type.

101. Note *BAM* 11:16.

102. See *AHw* 1343a (following Furlani, *ArOr* 17/1.263–264). Labat, *RA* 53.4, 5 interprets this as "shooting" pain.

103. Note *AMT* 34/6:4′; *BAM* 185 v 51′; cf. K 9762 ii 15′//DT 86+ ii 20–21 (with "hand" of ghost).

104. Attia, *Histoire des Sciences Médicales* 34.5 assumes SAG.KI.DIB.BA attributed to ghosts was invariably accompanied by continual crying and blood running from the mouth. These symptoms may under certain circumstances be associated with ghost headaches (see Chapter 15 with 15.23). It does not, however, follow that these symptoms are to be "understood" whenever SAG.KI.DIB.BA and ghosts occur together.

105. See also DPS IV B obv. 15 = *TDP* 34:15. Kinnier Wilson, *Diseases in Antiquity* 200 interprets *TDP* 34:15 as meningitis, but we do not concur. For possible ancient descriptions of meningitis, see below under MENINGITIS.

106. See also DPS IV B obv. 13 = *TDP* 34:13. Kinnier Wilson, *Diseases in Antiquity* 200 interprets *TDP* 34:13 as meningitis, but we do not concur. For possible ancient descriptions of meningitis, see below under MENINGITIS. In a subsequent publication, Kinnier Wilson, *Medical History* 34.187 provides another suggested diagnosis, namely, nocturnal epilepsy. However, there is nothing in this text to suggest either epilepsy or a nocturnal problem.

107. Adamson, *JRAS* 1979.4 n. 25 mistakes these symptoms for a fever and cites this text as "evidence of fevers associated with chills, rigors, and cold sweats" suggesting the presence of endemic malaria in ancient Mesopotamia. For possible descriptions of malaria in ancient Mesopotamian texts, see Chapter 3 under MALARIA.

108. Note also *BAM* 482 ii 20//*BAM* 9 obv. 14; *BAM* 482 ii 22//*BAM* 9 obv. 16; DPS IV E ii 22–23 = *SpTU* 3.88 ii 22–23.

109. The description of pulsation is not a sign observed by the *āšipu*, but a symptom or sensation perceived by the patient. On this point, see also Attia, *Histoire des Sciences Médicales* 34.5.

110. Note also DPS IV E ii 19–20 = *SpTU* 3.88 ii 19–20.

111. Note also *BAM* 3 iii 25–26//*BAM* 35 iv 5′//*AMT* 20/1 ii! 16′; DPS IV E ii 24 = *SpTU* 3.88 ii 24.
112. Note also *BAM* 3 iii 34//*AMT* 20/1 ii! 7′; DPS IV E ii 21 = *SpTU* 3.88 ii 21.
113. See also DPS III A obv. 25//C obv. 16 = *TDP* 20:16.
114. See also *BAM* 183:31; cf. *BAM* 423 i 34′; *BAM* 344:13, 15, 16.
115. See also DPS XXVI:18′ (AOAT 43.279).
116. Kinnier Wilson, *Medical History* 34.190 translates "spittle" here and elsewhere as "foam." Stol, *Epilepsy* 8–9 translates "spittle" but believes that "foam" is correct and that the *āšipu* used "spittle" to describe drooling in epileptics for mythological reasons. In fact, the distinction is irrelevant. Foam in the mouth is the product of saliva mixed with air. Patients with seizures will have saliva, foam, or both.
117. Note also DPS XXXI:35′–37′ (AOAT 43.343); *BAM* 66 r. 12′//*AMT* 45/1:8′//*AMT* 14/7:9; *BAM* 177:12.
118. See also Volk, *OrNS* 68.16–18; Cadelli, *Ktèma* 22.23–24. It should be noted that German has a single word to describe convulsions and abdominal cramping, which is presumably why Volk includes pylorospasm in his section on infantile seizures.
119. Note also *bul-ṭi ša* LÚ.TUR AN.TA.ŠUB.BA . . . DIB-*su* (K 3628+4009 r. 20′–21′; cf. *ABL* 1289:1′–8′ (Parpola, *SAA* 10.309).
120. The restoration is based on K 3628+4009 obv. 5′, which quotes this line.
121. See also DPS XL A 24–25//B 25–26 = *TDP* 220:24–25; DPS XL A 47 = *TDP* 222:47; cf. *STT* 89:210 (Stol, *Epilepsy* 98).
122. See also DPS XL A 121, 122 = *TDP* 230:121, 122. On these three references, see also Cadelli, *Ktèma* 22.24.
123. Lit. "he will have a finishing off."
124. See also DPS XL A 16, 17//B 17, 18 = *TDP* 218:16, 17.
125. This appears to be described in the unfortunately fragmentary *STT* 89:105b–108 (Stol, *Epilepsy* 91).
126. See also DPS XXVI:62′–63′ (AOAT 43.283); *BRM* 4.32:1.
127. See also Kämmerer, *RA* 94.74.
128. Note also DPS IX A 5//B obv. 5 = *TDP* 72:5.
129. Fincke, *Augenleiden* 114 suggests that this reference could be describing myasthenia gravis. However, there is no mention of lid weakness. Also the patient is in a confused or stuporous state following a seizure. Seizures do not occur in myasthenia gravis, whereas weakness of the extraocular muscles following a seizure would not be unusual.
130. Text E (K 3706+:11′) has "two or three days."
131. Note also DPS XVII:38–39 (AOAT 43.198–199).
132. Kinnier Wilson, "Medicine in . . . Old Testament (times)," 351 and *Medical History* 34.197 has dubbed this the first reference in history to the epileptic cry.
133. See also Kinnier Wilson, *Diseases in Antiquity* 202.
134. The passage has been collated. The copy has ^{d}20.
135. In addition to epilepsy, Fincke, *Augenleiden* 145 also suggests rabies and Huntington's chorea for this text. None of the findings of these later two diagnoses are presented in this text reference. For possible ancient descriptions of Huntington's chorea and rabies, see below and in Chapter 2 under ENVIRONMENTAL HAZARDS.
136. Fincke, *Augenleiden* 109 suggests that this passage is referring to tetanus or rabies. However, this identification depends on lumping this description of AN.TA.ŠUB.BA together with the preceding entry, which has a different ancient diagnosis. For possible ancient descriptions of rabies and tetanus, see Chapter 2 under ENVIRONMENTAL HAZARDS and Chapter 3 under TETANUS.
137. Preceding is a section marked off with paragraph lines with an entry describing a grand mal seizure (DPS XXVI:69′–70′ [AOAT 43.284]; see Chapter 13.186) and following is a similarly marked section containing an entry describing a focal seizure (DPS XXVI:77′ [AOAT 43.285]; see Chapter 13.192).
138. See Stol, *Epilepsy* 59. Kinnier Wilson, *Medical History* 34.187, 191 interprets this expression here and in other passages as referring to a regaining of consciousness, but this seems unlikely.
139. Kinnier Wilson, *Medical History* 34.191, 196 considers this text to be describing tonic seizures. The difference in our interpretations is partly based on the translation of the term *hesû*. He believes that it means clenched fists as in rigor mortis, whereas we follow Stol, *Epilepsy* 65 in interpreting the motion as wringing the hands as from cold. If "wringing hands" is the correct translation, this semi-purposeful movement is better associated with complex partial seizures.

140. Kinnier Wilson, *Diseases in Antiquity* 202 also recognizes this text as describing an aura.

141. Kinnier Wilson, *Medical History* 34.189, 194 recognizes this text as describing an aura.

142. See Stol, *Epilepsy* 59. Kinnier Wilson, *Medical History* 34.187, 189 interprets this expression here and in other passages as referring to a regaining of consciousness, but this seems unlikely.

143. Kinnier Wilson, *Medical History* 34.189, 194 also describes this text as a complex partial seizure.

144. That is, the patient has a vacant expression.

145. Kinnier Wilson, *Medical History* 34.190, 195 also describes this reference as a gelastic seizure.

146. Heeßel, AOAT 43.279, 287, 292 follows Stol, *Epilepsy* 58 in reading *šum-ma* 8-*šú* NU ŠUB-*aš-šú ul uš-te-*[*zib*]: "If it does *not* fall on him eight times, he will not come through." This makes no sense at all, which led Stol to suggest omitting the "not" from the translation. However, reading instead 8-*šú-nu*: "eight of them" (von Soden, *GAG* 195 § 139j) restores the sense and makes this emendation unnecessary.

147. For the reading, see Stol, *Epilepsy* 59. Kinnier Wilson, *Medical History* 34.189 w/ n. 28 interprets the verb as *edēpu* but does not propose a translation.

148. See also DPS XXVI:88′ (AOAT 43.286).

149. The verb is otherwise used to describe the action of animals caught in a trap (see *AHw* 1025a; *CAD* S 157).

150. See also [DIŠ TA SA]G.⌜DU⌝-[š] *ú* [E]N? *meš-*⌜*li*⌝*-šú* SA.MEŠ-*šú* TI-*ma* NU DU.MEŠ *šá-pu-la-šú* (coll.) *ka-sa-a* GEŠTU^{II}-*šú mim-ma la i-šem-ma-a* NA BI ḪUL DIB-*su* (DPS III A r. 13′–14′//C r. 36–37 = *TDP* 28/30:96–97): "[If from his] ⌜head⌝ to his midpoint(?) his blood vessels are healthy and do not 'go' (but) his inguinal regions are 'bound' (and) his ears cannot not hear anything, a *gallû*-demon afflicts that person".

151. The parallel *CTN* 4.72 i 3′ (Kinnier Wilson, *Iraq* 19.40–49 [ND 4368]) adds "along the street."

152. Kinnier Wilson, *Iraq* 19.44 suggests that this text refers to "heat exhaustion" (the only possibility other than epilepsy according to "one authority whom I consulted") or "tonic epilepsy" (his own interpretation). There is nothing in this text that appears to support the diagnosis of "heat exhaustion."

153. The text has been collated.

154. Kinnier Wilson, *Diseases in Antiquity* 192 has also interpreted this sign as ocular paralysis. However, he goes on to state that this commonly occurs in dietary deficiency. The only dietary defficiency in which occular paralysis occurs is thiamine deficiency, usually secondary to alcoholism (Wernicke-Korsakoff syndrome). This syndrome is described in *BAM* 575 iii 51–52//*BAM* 59:21–24 (see 15.24).

155. Lit. "sleep."

156. Heeßel AOAT 43.200, 209, 214 interprets this as "he continually bares his chest."

157. See also DPS XXII:64b (AOAT 43.256); DPS XVII:57–58 (AOAT 43.200–201).

158. The commentary *STT* 403 r. 47 explains the "40 U.MEŠ-*šú*" as meaning TA *mu-ap-pat* ŠU.SI.MEŠ-*šú* EN SAG *ṣu-ur-ri-šú.*

159. Temporal arteritis and malaria have been suggested by Fincke for this reference (Fincke, *Augenleiden* 139). However, the diagnosis of temporal arteritis in this and other passages is based on a translation of "swollen" rather than "pulsating" for ZI.MEŠ (see Chapter 8). There are no findings in the text that would identify this condition as malaria. For possible ancient descriptions of malaria, see Chapter 3 under MALARIA.

160. See also DPS XL A 111 = *TDP* 230:111.

161. Labat, *TDP* 126 read this as "ghost." The text, however has NAM.ÉRIM: "curse."

162. Kinnier Wilson, *Diseases in Antiquity* 201 identifies this text as bacterial meningitis and in *Journ. Roy.Soc.Med.* 89.136–137 he specifies tuberculous meningitis (for a discussion of tuberculous and chronic meningitis, see Chapter 19). Fincke, *Augenleiden* 89 also suggests meningitis but does not specify tuberculous meningitis. She further suggests (*Augenleiden* 74, 109) that a number of additional texts refer to meningitis or rabies, but we do not concur. For further discussion of the relevant passages, see above, 13.111, 13.141, 13.195. Kinnier Wilson also diagnoses (*Diseases in Antiquity* 200–201) a number of other references as meningitis, but we do not agree. Some of the references describe tension headaches, others drug and alcohol poisoning, minor upper respiratory illnesses, and so on. What links them is the attribution to "hand" of ghost (See Chapter 19 with 19.379–19.394). Geller and Cohen, *Kidney International* 47.1813 w. n. 33 appear to believe that this reference is to some sort of kidney disease and that the "headache" refers to high blood pressure. Since headache is not usually associated with high blood pressure, it is difficult to follow the logic of this attribution.

163. The Sumerogram TÉŠ is equivalent to Akkadian *ba'āšu/bâšu*, "to come to shame," which is inappropriate for this context. However, nearly homophonous *ba'āšu/be'ēšu* means "to smell bad" and is not uncommonly used of the ears (see CAD B 4b s.v. *ba'āšu* A mng. 1a). Scribal word games of this sort are commonplace in ancient scholarly texts.

164. Labat, *RLA* 4.367–368 believes that *mišittu* means "heart attack." Given the frequent descriptions of neurological abnormalities in these references, heart attack seems a highly unlikely explanation.

165. For references to *mišittu* in medical texts, see *AMT* 82/2 iii! 7//*BAM* 138 ii 1–3; *AMT* 76/3:2′; *BAM* 138 ii 9–10; *AMT* 82/2 iii! 1; *BAM* 388 i′ 2; *BAM* 135:10′; Labat, *RA* 54.174 [AO 17617] obv. 11; *BAM* 372 iii 12′//*BAM* 376 iii 7 (cf. *SpTU* 4.129 iv 9, 35); *AMT* 60/3 ii 8′ and the references below.

166. See also DPS XXVII:10 (AOAT 43.297); cf. *AMT* 77/1 i 7.

167. See above, 13.57–13.59.

168. See also DPS XXVII:12–13 (AOAT 43.297); cf. *AMT* 77/1 i 9–10.

169. See above, 13.57–13.59.

170. See Stol, *Epilepsy* 76–77.

171. See above, 13.57–13.59.

172. Text B (*SpTU* 1.46) has *ur-ga-at-tú*.

173. Note also *AMT* 79/1 iv 6//*BAM* 135:15′//*BAM* 136 i 2′; *AMT* 76/5:9; *AMT* 76/5:4.

174. Note also *AMT* 78/1+ iii 5; *AMT* 78/1+ iii 6//*AMT* 23/2:14; *SpTU* 1.46:33.

175. A therapeutic tablet containing treatments for strokes mentions a slippery left [lip] as a symptom (*AMT* 77/5+K 11127 i 2′–3′).

176. Note also BM 41281 ii 11 (stones for stroke affecting the arm).

177. Geller, *AfO* 48/49.59 n. 95 translates this passage: "if a man is 'thick' and contorts either his hand or his foot." However, *kabātu* means "heavy" and not "thick" and the two verbs are in any case in hendiadys.

178. Note also *AMT* 79/1 iv 24; *AMT* 82/2 ii! 8.

179. See above, 13.57–13.59.

180. Note also *AMT* 76/2:8–9; *AMT* 77/5+K 11127 i 4′, 16′, 17′.

181. Kinnier Wilson, *Iraq* 18.134 translates this as "muscle-contracted with spasm of the face." He seems to derive this translation (143) from the further argument that we should translate *mišittu* as "stroke" because this is a less scientific term than "apoplexy" and because "apoplexy" is rarer in the East than in the West. In fact, the currently used medical term is "stroke" and strokes may be more common in the West, but not significantly so.

182. See also DPS IX A 71//B r. 17–18 = *TDP* 78:71 (with fatal outcome).

183. Note StBoT 36.30 ad. 4′.

184. See also ibid. 36.23 r. 4′, 60:10.

185. Stol, *Epilepsy* 5–7, argues that *bennu* is Akkadian for "epilepsy" and that spawn of Šulpaea is one of many synonyms for epilepsy (*Epilepsy* 14–16), but we do not concur. For our reasons, see Chapter 3 under *bennu*.

186. Volk, *OrNS* 68.19 and Cadelli, *Ktèma* 22.25 recognize this as a motor problem. Volk cites multiple conditions that can cause perinatal brain damage especially to the motor centers. We believe that he considers this to be cerebral palsy, but he does not use that term. A mistake originally made by Labat in omitting from his copy a "not" that is clear on the original tablet has led many translators of this passage to falsely assume that the child can eat (as, e.g., also Stol, *Epilepsy* 14).

187. For the reading, see Stol, *Epilepsy* 97.

188. See above, 13.57–13.59.

189. That is, because of weakness, he is unable to place his feet in a normal forward position when walking.

190. The expression is drawn from more general omen literature: the prognosis is bad, but the actual prediction differs slightly depending on the social status of the affected person.

191. Note also Šumma Izbu I 68 (Leichty, *Izbu* 38) where a woman gives birth to a "spawn" of Šulpaea.

192. The number is restored from Arnaud, *Emar* VI/4.695:6.

193. Ibid. 695:8 has "6."

194. Lit. "arrival (in due course of time) at the (netherworld) mountain."

195. Biggs, *RLA* 6.211 believes that this text is describing a patient with a stroke. We agree that there is a type of dementia (multi-infarct dementia) that is caused by recurrent strokes, but there are many other causes, the most frequent being Alzheimer's disease.

196. Note also NA_4.MEŠ *ma-ši-ti ḫa-sa-su*, "stones for remembering what one has forgotten" (*BAM* 372 iii 10′).

197. According to the commentary Á.KAM = *šeḫānu* = *maḫḫû*. A genuine ecstatic (*maḫḫû*) can only be recognized in late childhood or early adulthood; the reference here is to behavior like an ecstatic, that is, insanity.

198. This section was broken away in the original tablet that was copied by the scribe of *STT* 89; the restoration is conjectural.

199. In other words, it is not just an act.

200. A similar fate seems to have befallen a couple with congenital spinal malformations who were found buried together in the excavation of a Roman camp at Corinth (for details, see Grmek, *Diseases in the Ancient Greek World* 69–70).

201. Shaffer, *Tablet XII* 97 r. 3–4.

202. Only the beginning of the horizontal of the NU is visible. The LÁL requires interpreting subsurface traces and so is very unsure.

203. The passage has been collated.

204. See also Adamson, *RA* 84.29.

205. The restoration is based on the commentary *STT* 403 r. 43–45. Note also DPS XXII:5 (AOAT 43.251).

206. Note also DPS III C obv. 45 = *TDP* 22:45 (13.87); DPS VII B obv. 6′–7′ = TDP 64:45′–46′; DPS XXII:5 (AOAT 43.251).

207. For the reading and interpretation, see Heeßel, AOAT 43.263.

208. Kinnier Wilson, *Medical History* 34.193, 197 argues that this phrase means "lifting the spirits," but pelvic thrusting is what is obviously indicated.

209. See the commentary *GCCI* 2.406:9.

210. See also DPS XIV A_2 iv 16′//G iv 6′ = *TDP* 142 iv 16′.

211. Note also *BAM* 152 iv 16//*BAM* 158 iii 27′–28′//*AMT* 70/7 i 3; *BAM* 405:14′.

212. For the identification of this text as peripheral neuropathy, see Attia, *Histoire des Sciences Médicales* 34.7.

213. Note also *KUB* 37.9 ii 10′–12′.

214. For the translation of *šāpulu* as "inguinal region," see Heeßel, AOAT 43.168 ad 57′. Adamson, *JRAS* 1984.7–8 proposes an alternative translation of "scrotal sac" and argues that this and similar passages are describing torsion of the testicles. Neither argument seems logical in this context.

215. The involvement of this spirit is most probably due to the fact that its name is written with the Sumerogram LÁ, a term otherwise used to describe confusional states (see p. 315). Stol, *Epilepsy* 38–42 argues that *alû* is a "terror of the night" based on the fact that Greek philosophers thought nightmares and epilepsy were related. The "sacred disease" specialists criticized in the Hippocratic treatise of the same name were Greeks with a philosophy of epilepsy that bears no resemblance (and is in no way related) to that of ancient Mesopotamia (see Scurlock, "From Esagil-kin-apli to Hippocrates").

216. See above, 13.57–13.59.

217. For references to *alû*, see also *BAM* 364 i 4; *BAM* 183:30; *BAM* 356 ii 10//*BAM* 370 iv 12′//*BAM* 365 ii 6′//*BAM* 376 ii 28′//*BAM* 377 iii 15; *BAM* 311:47′; cf. K 3628+4009 r. 16′; W. Farber, *Schlaf* 128:8 (in infants).

218. Geller (as quoted in Butler, *Dreams* 62–63) attaches sexual connotations to the expression, and uses this passage as evidence that the *alû* was a succubus producing sexual dreams. However, the expression "flow over" (*reḫû*) is used in medical texts to describe the effects of fevers (see p. 31) and stupors (see DPS XXVI:69′–70′ [AOAT 43.284] above, 13.186). As this passage clearly indicates, the stupor produced by an *alû* is different from ordinary sleep, but more on the order of being knocked flat than pleasurably stimulated.

219. Kinnier Wilson, *Medical History* 34.193, 197 believes that, in 13.276–13.277 the patients' eyes are bulging due to fear. This is, however, a mistranslation of *zaqāpu*, which means "to constrict." See p. 300.

220. See also DPS XXVII:20 (AOAT 43.298).

221. Lit. "jumps."

222. Lit. "jumps."

223. See above, 13.57–13.59.

224. This term has no known roots, and is used exclusively to refer to breathing patterns. Most of the patients so described die but a few exceptions suggest that the *āšipu* used this term for similar-sounding noises in cases that were not necessarily terminal. See also Adamson, *JRAS* 1979.6.

225. See also DPS XVI:30 (AOAT 43.175); DPS XVI:49′ (AOAT 43.176); DPS XVI:57′ (AOAT 43.177).

226. See also Volk, *OrNS* 68.14–15; Cadelli, *Ktèma* 22.18–19.

227. The restoration is necessitated by the presence of the verb *našû* in the stative, which may refer to the bulb of the nose, the feet, the upper abdomen (epigastrium) or, as in this case, the innards but never the muscles/blood vessels (differently, Stol, *Epilepsy* 95).

228. The meaning of this phrase is unclear.

229. Stol, *Epilepsy* 95 suggests ḪÁD.A for the beginning of this line. The traces in the copy do not, however, look at all like a ḪÁD and possibly represent an erasure.

230. Ibid., followed by Attia, *Histoire des Sciences Médicales* 34.6 suggests "ritual scarification." Bloodletting is occasionally described in rituals, but the implement used is a knife, not a "small copper object," and the pouring out of blood is invariably mentioned. In any case, it is hard to imagine a battle-scarred ancient Mesopotamian "quivering" at the mere prospect of being bled.

231. Note DPS XIV A iv 21–22 = *TDP* 144 iv 56′–57′ (it is difficult for him to do this).

232. Compare also DIŠ *ana* IGI GIG A.MEŠ ŠUB-*ma* NU ⌜MUD⌝ [*u* ZU-*šú l*] *a ú-ád-da* Š[U? . . .] ⌜NU⌝ D[IN]: "If you pour water on the patient's face and he does not shudder [and] he ⌜does not⌝ recognize [person(s) known to him], ⌜hand⌝ of [. . .]; he will not ⌜get well⌝" (DPS III A obv. 2//B 2).

233. See Heeßel, AOAT 43.191.

234. This phrase is mistranslated in Labat, *MDP* 57 p. 250.

235. "Bad sleep" is associated with silence (*qūlu*) and stupor (*kūru*). See *CAD* Š/3.141–142.

236. Note Heeßel, AOAT 43.293 n. 17.

CHAPTER 14. TRAUMA AND SHOCK

1. Note also DPS IV A_2 r. 1–4//E iii 1–6//H 3–6 = *TDP* 38 r. 1–4//*SpTU* 3.88 iii 1–6.

2. See also DPS V A 3′–7′ = *TDP* 46 B 3–7.

3. See also DPS VIII 6b, 7a = *TDP* 68:6b, 7a

4. See also "blocked off" and "closed in" (lit. "bounded") (DPS VI A obv. 4, 6–7 = *TDP* 54:4, 6–7).

5. Note also swelling and pain (DPS VII A obv. 24, 25 = *TDP* 62:24, 25).

6. See also, inter alia, McEwan, *RLA* 7.172. Adamson, *RA* 87.154 considers this text to be describing a wound involving the chest wall. However this proposal fails to explain why the abdomen "approaches his lung."

7. See Heeßel, AOAT 43.168 ad 57′.

8. Sjöberg's (*JCS* 25.141) suggestion of listeriosis for Sumerian SAG.NIGIN (the Sumerogram for both *ṣidānu* and *rapādu*; see *CAD* R 147) was specifically meant to apply to a disease in sheep: UDU.SAG.NIGIN. Sheep with listeria meningitis sometimes walk in circles. However, humans with this condition do not. Neither do they "wander about" (*rapādu*). It is, therefore, necessary to find some other explanation when *ṣidānu* or *rapādu* is applied to human beings.

9. The restoration is based on the parallel text from Tablet XIV.

10. The restoration is based on the parallel text from Tablet XIV.

11. See Scurlock, *NABU* 1993 no. 47.

12. See ibid.

13. Lit. "his temple (feels) squeezed."

14. The text has "the temples have collapsed." Compare DPS III A obv. 5//B 5 ("calm temples," meaning calm temporal blood vessels) and the relatively common expression "pulating temples" meaning a sensation of pulsation in the temporal arteries (see Chapter 13.149).

15. See also DPS IV A_2 r. 10//G r. 9 = *TDP* 40 r. 10//*LKU* 94 r. 9 (cf. Labat, *Syria* 33.125 r. 11); DPS IV A_2 r. 7//G r. 6 = *TDP* 40 r. 7//*LKU* 94 r. 6.

16. The commentary *CT* 51.136:12 shows that even ancient scribes were unsure as to the correct reading.

17. See also DPS IV A obv. 68+A_6 obv. 3//E ii 12 = *TDP* 38:68//*SpTU* 3.88 ii 12.

18. See also DPS XIV A iv 15//K 9 = *TDP* 144 iv 50′.

19. See also DPS XII D iv 19 = *TDP* 108 iv 19; cf. DPS XV:30 (AOAT 43.152).

20. See also DPS XV:44, 45 (AOAT 43.152); cf. DPS XII D iii 23, 24//E iii 25, 26–27 = *TDP* 104 iii 23, 24.

21. Mujais, *Am.J.Nephrology* 19.136 attributes the patient's confusion to uremia secondary to obstruction of a solitary functioning kidney. However, the translation from which he was working did not correctly identify this as a reference to a wound. Given this context, blood loss is the likely cause of the patient's altered mental status.

22. See also DPS VII B r. 9 = *TDP* 66:65′.

23. See also DPS XI A obv. 27//B obv. 26 = *TDP* 92:27//*SpTU* 1.34:26; DPS XXXVII A obv. 8–9 = *TDP* 212/214:8–9.

24. ÚḪ is usually "phlegm." However, when used with KÚM ("fever") it is to be read as a form of *ṣarāḫu* as the parallel between DPS III C r. 10–11//E_1 r. 11–12+E_2 r. 7–8 = *TDP* 26:70–71 (DIŠ *ina* SAG.DU-*šú* KÚM ÚḪ) and *KAR* 211 obv. 4–6 ([DIŠ *i-na*] SAG.DU-*šú* KÚM *ṣa-ri-iḫ*) shows and has now been demonstrated by Heeßel, AOAT 43.162–163. Previously, Labat, *TDP* 25 n. 44 had suggested and then rejected the correct reading in favor of *nuppuḫ:* "it is swollen" (followed by Biggs, *RLA* 6. 210 and *CAD* N 268b), which makes no sense in this context.

25. See also DPS XV:53 (AOAT 43.153); cf. DPS XIV A iii 12–13//C_2 iii 4//I 8–9 = *TDP* 140 iii 46′–47′. Note also DPS XV:21 (AOAT 43.151) (speech wanders; wounded at noon; "hand" of Adad [coll.]).

26. In this recitation, a sorceror is blamed for the patient's condition.

27. Kinnier Wilson, *JNES* 53.111–115 interprets SA.AD.NIM as referring to *samānu* and Falkenstein, *ZA* 45.30 as *šaššaṭu*. However, while the Sumerogram SA.AD.NIM may be used for other conditions, it appears primarily to represent *rapādu* as would be indicated in any case by fact that "going about without knowing (where he is going)" is also mentioned.

28. See also Adamson, *JRAS* 1981.128.

29. See also dark hands and feet (DPS VI A r. 11//B_1 r. 8+B_2 r. 12′ = *TDP* 60 r. 42′; DPS XI A r. 54 = *TDP* 98 r. 54). Adamson, in *JRAS* 1984.11 argues that *TDP* 98 r. 54 (which uses ŠE for *kittabru*: "side") is referring to malignant melanoma of the digits and in Adamson, *WO* 16.10 n. 32 that the same text (plus *TDP* 98 r. 49 and 144 iv 49′) refers to gangrene from eating ergot-infected grain. Of these possibilities, the latter is considerably more likely, although in the absence of rye cultivation, cases would probably have been relatively rare (see Chapter 15). Kinnier Wilson, *Journ.Roy.Soc.Med.* 89.138 identifies *TDP* 98 r. 54 as gangrene but translates "looks terrible" as literally "fallen off" and considers the underlying disease to be diabetes. We are hesitant to identify the cause of the gangrene without further information.

30. See also Adamson, *JRAS* 1981.128. Heeßel, *AOAT* 43.152, 157, 165 has "rücken" and "bed of fingernails" for "bellies."

31. See Adamson, *RA* 84.31.

CHAPTER 15. POISONS

1. It was not uncommon even in relatively modern times for hungry Breton peasant children to eat wild plants and to be able to recognize which were poisonous (Hélias, *The Horse of Pride* 12).

2. This text has been diagnosed by Kinnier Wilson, *Diseases in Antiquity* 201 as bacterial meningitis. We feel that the potential for survival mentioned in the reference and the findings in general are more compatible with belladonna poisoning than meningitis.

3. See also *AMT* 21/2:1–25 (restored from *AMT* 22/2 obv. 1–5 and K 9216+17521 ii 1′–10′).

4. Lit. "his heart does not rise in him."

5. Abusch, *Mesop. Witchcr.* 79–88 interprets references to eating or drinking "witchcraft" as psychosomatic problems especially related to "socialization anxiety" experienced in childhood (i.e., weaning). There is, however, good reason to believe that many of the cases attributed to witchcraft are real poisonings. See, for example, the discussion of sorcery in Bellakhdar, *Médicine traditionelle* 142–144.

6. Note also BM 42272 obv. 23, 25–26, 28–29; *AMT* 29/13:9′.

7. See also DPS X B r. 8–10 = *TDP* 88 r. 8–10.

8. The restoration of Butler, *Dreams* 54 of *iq-b*[*i*! . . .] is unlikely (because the verb would have to be in the preterite, which is not usual in therapeutic texts) and does not fit the traces visible on the original tablet.

9. See Chapter 10 with 10.19.

10. See Chapter 10 with 10.19.

11. Landsberger, *JNES* 14.19.

12. See Bellakhdar, *Médicine traditionelle* no. 153.

13. The text has been collated.

14. *AuOr* 9.15–21.

15. Roderick, *Am.J. Physiology* 96.413–425.

16. Townsend, *Flora of Iraq* 3 no. 10.

17. al-Rawi and Chakravarty, *Medicinal Plants of Iraq* 65.

18. It is supremely ironic that modern science uses an Arabic word to describe a substance in which Muslim Arabs are forbidden to indulge.

19. See Heeßel, *Fs. Walker* 104–106.

20. Note also: "If after falling ill, he keeps moistening his lips while he sleeps, 'hand' of 'the trembler'" (DPS XVII:59 [AOAT 43.201]).

21. An example of the latter might be "getting a woman to talk" (for information or as a prelude to sex) for which there are known magical rituals. For references, see *CAD* D 13 s.v. *dabābu* mng. 9a.

22. Geller and Cohen, *Kidney International* 47.1813.

23. For other suggestions, see *BAM* 260:4, 5–6; *BAM* 414 r. 7′–8′; BM 59634:9–13 (see Heeßel, *Fs. Walker* 100–103).

24. See Stol, *Epilepsy* 66. Kinnier Wilson, *Medical History* 34.192 is unable to read these lines but thinks they have something to do with speech.

25. Kinnier Wilson, *Medical History* 34.187 believes this reference to be describing nocturnal epilepsy. However, the text does not describe a seizure, and the time specified is during the day and not the night.

26. The translation of the term follows Labat, *Manuel* (1952/1995) 175.

27. "Confusional states" or "falling spells" caused by ghosts are also mentioned in other texts. For references, see Scurlock, *Ghost-Induced Illnesses*, forthcoming, Chapter 2.

28. See also *BAM* 482 i 60′; cf. DPS IV A r. 7+A_4 r. 6//B r. 19//E iv 3 = *TDP* 42 r. 40//*SpTU* 3.88 iv 3; *BAM* 11:32//*BAM* 482 i 49′//*AMT* 20/1 i! 36′; *AMT* 20/1 i! 38′; *BAM* 11:34//*BAM* 482 i 54′; DPS IV B obv. 19 = *TDP* 34:19.

29. See also DPS IV B obv. 14 = *TDP* 34:14; DPS IV E ii 25, 26 = *SpTU* 3.88 ii 25, 26. Kinnier Wilson, *Diseases in Antiquity* 200 interprets *TDP* 34:14 as meningitis, but we do not concur. For possible ancient descriptions of meningitis, see Chapter 13 under MENINGITIS.

30. *Diseases in Antiquity* 206. See also Fincke, *Augenleiden* 112–114.

31. See Heeßel, *Fs. Walker* 104–106.

32. The passage has been collated.

33. The text has been collated.

34. For this demon, see also DPS XXVI:42′ (AOAT 43.282); DPS XI A obv. 21//B 20 = *TDP* 90:21//*SpTU* 1.34:20.

35. Stol, *Epilepsy* 79 interprets this symptom as "goosebumps."

36. Note also DPS XII A 8 = *TDP* 100 i 8.

37. The passage has been collated.

38. See also DPS XVII:65–66 (AOAT 43.201).

39. Maluszak et al., *Maryland Med J* 46.515–520.

40. Personal communication. Dr. Val Beasley, University of Illinois at Champaign, Urbana.

41. See *CAD* Z 133a s.v. *ziqtu* B.

42. See also *BAM* 176:15′; *CT* 14.23 [K 9283]:5–11//*STT* 92 i 5–11//BM 68046:5–10; *CTN* 4.194:11–15; *KADP* 1 v 10, 25, 26, 31, 62, 63; *BAM* 379 iv 7; *BAM* 422 ii 29′; cf. Scheil, *RA* 15.76:11.

43. Note also BM 53834:7′.

44. Note also *KADP* 33:17; *KADP* 34b r. 7′.

45. Note also *KADP* 1 v 13.

46. See also DPS XI A r. 42 = *TDP* 98 r. 42.

47. Kämmerer, *RAI* 44.168 believes that the substance in the patient's left hand is bile and that the patient is experiencing pain because he has gallstones. However, it is very difficult to imagine a clinical situation where bile would be present only on one side of the body. Moreover, gallstones cause abdominal colic, not pains in the extremities. The Sumerogram for "bile" (ZÉ) is the same as that for "venom," as may be seen from *BAM* 499 iii 3′ which has ZÉ MUŠ ZÉ GÍR.TAB (snake and scorpion venom), and it is easy to envision a patient having a painful bite on only the left hand.

CHAPTER 16. MENTAL ILLNESS

1. As, for example, Kinnier Wilson, AS 16.289–298 and *Diseases in Antiquity* 723–733. In addition to witchcraft and magic, the author applies his psychoanalysis to ancient Mesopotamian prayers to multiple gods,

several of the Psalms, and the Dead Sea Scrolls. The latter he dismisses as not the products of "a real religion and a real person" and asserts that they were written by "paranoiacs."

2. See also *BAM* 364 i 3; *BAM* 376 ii 16′–17′.

3. See also *BAM* 311:87′.

4. See also Kinnier Wilson, *Journ.Roy.Soc.Med.* 89.137.

5. Note also *AMT* 103/1 ii 5//*BAM* 469 r. 32.

6. Note also K 3010+6187+13346+DT 86 iii 31′–33′; *BAM* 315 iv 27–28//*BAM* 316 i 20′–21′.

7. The passage has been collated.

8. Note also BM 62397:1–4//BM 77041:13′–16′.

9. Ritter and Kinnier Wilson, *AnSt* 30.25 interpret this as "frequent nervous breakdowns." However, chest pain is not a significant symptom of nervous breakdown.

10. See also King, *BMS* 11 obv. 3–4.

11. Lit. "the desires of the mouth of the people."

12. For this meaning of *šapāku*, see Chapter 13 with 13.57–13.59. The person described is clearly under a great deal of stress, a condition to which a certain tenseness would be appropriate.

13. Ritter and Kinnier Wilson, *AnSt* 30.25 specifically interpret this as "ataxic looseness," but this interpretation seems forced.

14. Ibid. 29–30 interpret this as "stroke," on the grounds that "hand" of god is lexically equated with "affliction" (*ṣibtu*) and that the conventional phrase in guaranty clauses of slave sales against *ṣibtu* and *bennu* refers to "strokes" and "heart attacks." However, "stroke" is *mišittu* and not *ṣibtu* and *bennu* is not a "heart attack." For our interpretation of *bennu*, see 3.267–3.274.

15. Ibid. 29 interpret this as "delusions of persecution." The symptoms listed in the diagnostic handbook (see p. 565) do not support this conclusion.

16. For this phenomenon, see 19.14–15.

17. Kinnier Wilson, *Diseases in Antiquity* 725 suggests that this refers to "ecchymoses around the eyes resulting from one or more convulsions of a particularly violent nature." We feel this to be an unlikely explanation.

18. Ibid. interprets this text as epileptic psychosis, a condition that is not described in the medical literature. Personality disorders may occur with temporal lobe seizures, manifested by alterations in sexual behavior, hyperreligiosity, verbose speech, and aggressive behavior, but this is not psychosis nor does it persist after the seizures terminate. In any case, Kinnier Wilson's "evolves his own religion" is a mistranslation. The correct translation is "frightens even himself." The patient is, moreover, described as raging against the gods, not usually a sign of hyperreligiosity.

19. Heeßel, AOAT 43.251 reads GUR.MEŠ: "continually returns." However, all copies including his own have a clear LÚGUD.MEŠ and collation of Text A confirms the reading. Labat, *TDP* 178–179 reads the signs correctly but misunderstands the expression to refer to a "contracted" throat.

20. See also DPS XVIII:8–9 (AOAT 43.218).

21. Stol, "Psychosomatic suffering" 60–66 quotes under this heading a number of texts that describe the person for whom a ritual is to be performed as fearful, downcast, and socially isolated. Since *somatic* (physical) symptoms are either not listed or insignificant in these references, however, the term *psychosomatic* does not really apply. For our discussion of these texts, see under ANXIETY and PARANOIA. Also often classed as "psychosomatic" (as, e.g., in Pangas, *AuOr* 7.215–233) are references that happen to have been attributed by the *āšipu* to what modern observers believe to be "supernatural" causes (especially *kišpu*-sorcery and ghosts). We feel such blanket categorizations, which are read into rather than derived from the evidence, to be inappropriate; for the true role of gods/goddesses, ghosts, and demons/demonesses in ancient Mesopotamian medicine, see Chapter 19. Some of the references to loss of potency cited by Stol (pp. 58–59) mention symptoms that are anything but psychosomatic (e.g., urethritis and arthritis—see Chapter 4 under URETHRITIS and Chapter 11 under REACTIVE ARTHRITIS) and, as Biggs points out (*History of Science* 8.102–103), cases of impotence imputed to sorcery "are as often subjected to a purely therapeutic treatment as are those in which it is attributed to a physiological cause."

22. See Chapter 8.88.

23. See the commentary *SpTU* 1.29:3′–4′.

24. See also *BAM* 316 ii 5′–13′//BM 64174:1–6//*STT* 95:130–137.

25. Note also Labat, *Syria* 33.23; *BAM* 376 iii 3.

26. The epithet is probably intended as a pun. *Mušamšû* could also be an Š participle from *mašû*: "to forget," which would make this also the "ghost who causes forgetfulness."
27. The passage has been collated.
28. See also DPS VII A obv. 18 = *TDP* 62:18.
29. The reference is to the patient's mother. In ancient Mesopotamia kissing was a post-coital activity.
30. ⌜*i-ram-*⌝ coll. W. G. Lambert, ex-margina and again by Scurlock.
31. See *SpTU* 1.38:6–7.
32. Kinnier Wilson, *Medical History* 34.193, 197 considers this and the preceding reference to be describing postictal mutism. However, since the limbs are described as being as still as those of a healthy person, and since there is no mention of anything suggestive of a seizure, it seems unlikely that this explanation is correct.
33. Note also Labat, *RLA* 3.197.
34. For references, see *CAD* M/2.214.
35. For a discussion of *zaqāpu*, said of the eyes, see p. 300.
36. See also DPS XI A obv. 37 = *TDP* 92:37.
37. The commentary to Tablet IV, *SpTU* 1.30 explains (obv. 14–15) the supplementary diagnosis "on account of a man's wife" in this "hand" of Šamaš reference where the temples are involved by pointing out that SAG ("head") is equivalent to "man" and KI ("earth") to woman.
38. Kinnier Wilson, *Medical History* 34.193, 197 and Stol, *Epilepsy* 70 consider this text to be "clearly" describing a seizure. Part of the problem is that both scholars mistranslate the phrase that tells us that the patient can eat.
39. For the reading, see Heeßel, AOAT 43.164.
40. For the reading, see ibid. 163 (after a suggestion by Stol).
41. See also DPS XI A obv. 29, 31//B 28, 30 = *TDP* 92:29, 31//*SpTU* 1.34:28, 30; DPS XIII G_2 r. 10, 11 = *TDP* 122/124 iii 17, 18; DPS XV:24a, 24b (AOAT 43.151) = *TDP* 234:24; cf. DPS XV:17 (AOAT 43.151).
42. See also DPS XI A r. 50 = *TDP* 98 r. 50; cf. DPS XV:27 (AOAT 43.151) = *TDP* 234:27 (fingers).
43. Attia and Buisson, *Le journal des médecines cunéiformes* 4.11, suggest that this may be a primitive reflex, and we concur. There are a variety of brain diseases that can cause primitive reflexes.
44. For the reading, see Heeßel, AOAT 43.164.
45. For the reading, see ibid. 163 (after a suggestion by Stol).
46. See Stol, *Epilepsy* 69.
47. Kinnier Wilson, *Medical History* 34.193, 197 considers this text to be describing postictal mutism. Since the text explicitly states that the patient is talking, this seems unlikely.
48. Ibid. believes that the "mournful cry" described in these texts is real, but it is obvious that only the patient hears it.
49. The verb is otherwise used to describe the action of animals caught in a trap (see *AHw* 1025a; *CAD* S 157).
50. See also DPS XXII:63a (AOAT 43.256).
51. See also DPS XI A obv. 41 = *TDP* 92:41.
52. See also DPS XI A obv. 40 = *TDP* 92:40 (hands).
53. See also DPS VII B r. 13 = *TDP* 66:69′.
54. Note also *STT* 281 i 25, ii 31; *BAM* 372 ii 17//*BAM* 373 ii 5.
55. See also *BAM* 1 iii 35; *BAM* 318 iii 29. The *āšipu* was aware that certain plants could also cause depression (see *BAM* 318 iii 20, 24; cf. *BAM* 1 iii 36).
56. This section was broken away in the original tablet being copied by the scribe of *STT* 89; the restoration is conjectural.
57. In other words, it is not just an act.
58. Kinnier Wilson, AS 16.289–298 and *Diseases in Antiquity* 723–733 routinely assumes situations to be imaginary that could have been real (on this point, see also Abusch, *JCS* 37.95–96). A particularly glaring example is his interpretation of ÍD.GUR.RA, a type of magic allegedly engaged in by persons with a difficult legal case and designed to make the other party "turn away from the river," that is, lose the case. In ancient Mesopotamia, water ordeals were inverted from those of medieval Europe, that is, it was the guilty and not the innocent who was expected to drown. In practice, guilty parties facing such an ordeal were expected to "turn away from the river," that is, to refuse at the last minute to actually go through with the ordeal, thus

admitting their guilt. We know from actual examples (the É.GAL.KU_5.RA dismissed as "delusions" by Kinnier Wilson 724–725) that people did indeed attempt to influence the course of justice (as many perfectly sane people with similarly difficult cases might be sorely tempted to do today if such remedies were available). In any case, people did sue one another, and there must have been situations where, to the undisguised glee of his opponent in court, the party due to take the water ordeal found himself mysteriously unable to take the risk of being drowned even though he was, in fact, innocent. Kinnier Wilson, however, misled by W. G. Lambert into thinking that "turning back" from an ordeal meant "acquitted" and crossing this with a reference to a witchcraft trial in the Laws of Ḫammurapi that does not actually use the term produced the following analysis (p. 728): "The patient believes he has returned a free man from the river ordeal in which he and a 'witch' have been contending for life . . . The explanation of the term which one may thus suitably offer is that ÍD.GUR.RA was a delusion whereby the patient's fear of death in the ordeal, giving rise to an obsessive-ruminative psychoneurosis not finally to be tolerated, became permanently suppressed into the subconscious."

CHAPTER 17. PEDIATRICS

1. For further information and references, see Scurlock, *Incognita* 2.151–153.

2. See also *CAD* K 487–488 s.v *kūbu* A.

3. Borger, *Lišan Mitḫurti* 4 § III:13–14.

4. *CT* 23.10:16; Myhrman, *ZA* 16.178 iii 24–25//*PBS* 1/2.113 iii 12–13 (as corrected by Ungnad, *ZA* 33.71); *KAR* 330:5; cf. "just as . . . an aborted foetus never took its mother's breast" (*SpTU* 1.44:58, 67 [with duplicates—see *SpTU* 1 p. 52]).

5. *SpTU* 3.67 iii 9–12; for similar references, see *CAD* K 487–488 and Nougayrol, *Ugaritica* 6.398:10′–14′. The mention of holy women in this context has to do with their role in midwifery (for which see Stol, *Birth* 172–173).

6. See *BAM* 248 i 50, 66, ii 56, 69, iv 1, to quote only childbirth recitations.

7. See Drower, *Iraq* 5.112.

8. On this class of "demon by accident," see also Lackenbacher, *RA* 65.150–154.

9. For more on breech births, see Stol, *Birth* 132.

10. See also Šumma Izbu IV 52 (Leichty, *Izbu* 71) (identical).

11. See also Šumma Izbu IV 53 (Leichty, *Izbu* 71).

12. See also Šumma Izbu I 100a (Leichty, *Izbu* 42); Šumma Izbu IV 54 (Leichty, *Izbu* 71).

13. *Am.Journ.Med.Gen.* 91.319.

14. Reiner, *ZA* 72.133 suggests that the reference is to superfetation. However, superfetation is a purely imaginary phenomenon invented by Greek philosophers. It has no relevance to Mesopotamia, and goes against the obvious reading of the text. See also Stol, *Birth* 162 n. 102 ("we prefer the idea that twins are meant").

15. See Šumma Izbu I 113 (Leichty, *Izbu* 43) (*tak-ši-i*).

16. See also Šumma Izbu I 114 (Leichty, *Izbu* 43).

17. See also Šumma Izbu I 108 (Leichty, *Izbu* 42) (two boys and one girl).

18. See also Šumma Izbu I 120 (Leichty, *Izbu* 43) (two or three or four children).

19. See also Šumma Izbu I 123–124 (Leichty, *Izbu* 44) (four or five boys/girls).

20. See also Šumma Izbu I 126 (Leichty, *Izbu* 44) (three girls and two boys).

21. See also Šumma Izbu I 107 (Leichty, *Izbu* 42) ([six] boys).

22. See also Šumma Izbu I 47 (Leichty, *Izbu* 35).

23. Šumma Izbu I 36 (Leichty, *Izbu* 34).

24. Šumma Izbu I 37 (Leichty, *Izbu* 35). See also Šumma Izbu I 26 (Leichty, *Izbu* 34) (finger); Šumma Izbu I 38 (Leichty, *Izbu* 35) (paw).

25. Šumma Izbu I 39 (Leichty, *Izbu* 35).

26. Šumma Izbu I 80 (Leichty, *Izbu* 39). See also Šumma Izbu I 17–18 (Leichty, *Izbu* 33).

27. Šumma Izbu I 77 (Leichty, *Izbu* 38). The word for gecko (*ḫumbabītu*) indicates that a resemblance to the mythical Huwawa was imagined; see also Šumma Izbu I 78 (Leichty, *Izbu* 39).

28. Šumma Izbu I 41 (Leichty, *Izbu* 35). See also Šumma Izbu I 42–43 (Leichty, *Izbu* 35); cf. Šumma Izbu I 16, 79, IV 55 (Leichty, *Izbu* 33, 71) (snake); Šumma Izbu I 79 (Leichty, *Izbu* 39) (scepter).

29. Šumma Izbu I 40, 46 (Leichty, *Izbu* 35).

30. Šumma Izbu I 45 (Leichty, *Izbu* 35). See also Šumma Izbu I 33–34 (Leichty, *Izbu* 34); Šumma Izbu IV 39 (Leichty, *Izbu* 70) (brick).

31. Šumma Izbu I 29 (Leichty, *Izbu* 34). See also Šumma Izbu I 28, 31–32, 35 (Leichty, *Izbu* 34); cf. Šumma Izbu I 19–21 (Leichty, *Izbu* 33) (egg); Šumma Izbu I 70–71 (Leichty, *Izbu* 38).

32. Pangas, *Am.Journ.Med.Gen.* 91.321 asserts that a high rate of anomalies (meaning higher than in modern times) must have existed among "Assyro-Babylonians" on the grounds that women were expected to have many children, that birth control was unknown, and that inbreeding was the norm. That birth control was unknown and inbreeding was the norm are assumptions directly contradicted by the evidence. Moreover, higher pregnancy rates do not result in more anomalies. What does increase the risk is attempting to have children when the mother is too old or too young. In many traditional societies, women marry young, but most traditional cultures also put social pressure on couples to cease childbearing after age forty. By contrast, Western women typically marry late but, responding to the "inexorable ticking of the biological clock," many attempt to have their first child in their forties, thus balancing out the statistics. The real reason so many anomalies are described in ancient Mesopotamian texts is not that they had an unusually high rate of congenital birth defects, but because data on the subject was collected over the course of several millennia. The ancient Romans also took a great interest in malformed births; unfortunately they did not write on clay so their descriptions of these anomalies do not survive.

33. Jones, *Teratology* 48/6.552.

34. For a discussion of malformations described in ancient texts, see also Pangas, *Am.Journ.Med.Gen.* 91.320–321; Stol, *Birth* 160–165.

35. Pangas, *Am.Journ.Med.Gen.* 91.321.

36. See especially under SPOTS, AŠ.(GI$_6$) / *ṢENNĪTU, UMṢĀTU, ḪALÛ,* and *PINDÛ.*

37. *Ktèma* 22.18.

38. Böck, *Morphoskopie* 312:42–45 (see Fincke, *Augenleiden* 257 n. 1916).

39. Adamson, *JRAS* 1979.4–5 suggests that *ḫimṣu* on the skin are references to neurofibromatosis. However, the texts that he quotes refer exclusively to animals or demons in the form of animals.

40. See also Šumma Izbu IV 18 (Leichty, *Izbu* 68).

41. See also Šumma Izbu IV 20 (Leichty, *Izbu* 68) (horns). Other possible examples of neurofibromatoses are described in Šumma Izbu IX 1–6, 8–19 (Leichty, *Izbu* 115). Included in the presentations is the term *ṣibāru* (Šumma Izbu IX 8), which appears to have been a fleshy finger-like projection. Adamson, *JRAS* 1984.10 suggests that this term is describing a squamous papilloma of the skin, which is hard and hornlike. Since squamous papillomas occur typically in elderly adults, and the texts refer to malformed fetuses, this diagnosis seems inappropriate.

42· For this interpretation of *ubbuṭu,* see W. Farber, *ZA* 75.210–233.

43. Stol, *Birth* 165 suggests a caul and Fincke, *Augenleiden* 260 a congenital tumor or a hematoma for this reference. However, none of these suggestions can explain the neurological findings.

44. See also Šumma Izbu III Colophon A:1//D:1//f:1 [catchline] (Leichty, *Izbu* 65).

45. See also Fincke, *Augenleiden* 260–268; Kinnier Wilson, *Diseases in Antiquity* 204.

46. See also Šumma Izbu II 61′; IV 26; X 28′ (Leichty, *Izbu* 51, 68, 123; for the interpretation, see W. Farber, *ZA* 75.210–233).

47. See also Šumma Izbu II 51 (Leichty, *Izbu* 50).

48. See Fincke, *Augenleiden* 161.

49. See also Šumma Izbu II 60 (Leichty, *Izbu* 51).

50. See also Šumma Izbu II 53–59 (Leichty, *Izbu* 50–51).

51. See also Šumma Izbu II 62 (Leichty, *Izbu* 51) (eyes are blocked up).

52. See also Šumma Izbu IV 48 (Leichty, *Izbu* 70).

53. See also Šumma Izbu III 13, 16–17 (Leichty, *Izbu* 54, 55).

54. See also Šumma Izbu III 20–21 (Leichty, *Izbu* 55–56).

55. See also Šumma Izbu III 8–9 (Leichty, *Izbu* 54); Šumma Izbu III 10, 22 (Leichty, *Izbu* 54, 56).

56. See also Šumma Izbu III 28 (Leichty, *Izbu* 56); Šumma Izbu I 89 (Leichty, *Izbu* 40).

57. See also Šumma Izbu III 32 (Leichty, *Izbu* 57).

58. This is restored on the basis of *YOS* 10.12:1–2 (Leichty, *Izbu* 207; the Old Babylonian Forerunner). See also Šumma Izbu II 63 (Leichty, *Izbu* 52) (donkey-faced).

59. Adamson, *JRAS* 1974.102–104 argues that the term *aruppu* refers to a minor degree of hare-lip in animals on the grounds that "otherwise (the sacrificial animals) would have died soon after birth and would

have been quite unsuitable for sacrifice." In passing, he also suggests that *suḫātu* (which is lexically equated with *aruppu*) is to be translated "upper lip." However, *suḫatu* means "armpit" and the references to *aruppu* are drawn from the omen series Šumma Izbu that refers, not to animals for sacrifice, but precisely to malformed animals that died at or soon after birth.

60. Mujais, *Am.J.Nephrology* 19.137–138 suggests that references to women giving birth to a lion are describing patients with cleft lip/cleft palate and possibly hydrocephalus.

61. We agree with *CAD* B 219 that this passage demonstrates that this is the correct translation of the term. Adamson, *JRAS* 1974.102 argues that this text refers to a severe degree of hare-lip in animals, and that *bibēnu* should be translated "external nares" on the grounds that it would be too difficult for the "priest who conducted the sacrifice" to note lesions on the nasal septum of animals. However, animals with severe hare-lip would not have lived long enough to have been eligible for sacrifice, as the author himself notes apropos of *aruppu* (see previous note). Moreover, the physiognomic omens in which this passage appears refer neither to sacrifices nor to animals but to human beings. Finally, cleft lips may extend into the nose, producing a deviated or defective nasal septum, but they rarely affect the external nares.

62. See also Šumma Izbu III 38, 39, 42 (Leichty, *Izbu* 57–58).

63. See also Šumma Izbu III 33 (Leichty, *Izbu* 57).

64. See also Šumma Izbu III 35 (Leichty, *Izbu* 57) (no chin). Note also Šumma Izbu I 110–111 (Leichty, *Izbu* 42).

65. See also Volk, *OrNS* 68.20; Cadelli, *Ktèma* 22.16; Adamson, *JRAS* 1981.127; Stol, *Birth* 210–211.

66. The meaning of this term is known from extispicy, where it is used to describe parts of the vertebrae of sacrificed sheep. For references, see *CAD* K 425 s.v. *kislu*.

67. The translation is based on the assumption that the Akkadian *šappu* is related to the Hebrew *šafouf*.

68. See also Šumma Izbu III 65 (Leichty, *Izbu* 60). Note also Šumma Izbu III 64 (Leichty, *Izbu* 60) (gastroschisis: malformations where the abdomen is abnormally open; see Pangas, *Am.Journ.Med.Gen.* 91.321).

69. See also Pangas, *Am.Journ.Med.Gen.* 91.321.

70. See also Pangas, *Am.Journ.Med.Gen.* 91.319; Kinnier Wilson, *Diseases in Antiquity* 203–204; Mujais, *Am.J.Nephrology* 19.137–138.

71. See also Šumma Izbu I 74 (Leichty, *Izbu* 38).

72. In some cases, such a child can have an extra eye on the forehead; for an illustration, see Fincke, *Augenleiden* pl. 3 ill. 7.

73. See also Šumma Izbu II 22.

74. See also Šumma Izbu II 24, 26, 28 (Leichty, *Izbu* 48).

75. See also Šumma Izbu II 23 (Leichty, *Izbu* 48).

76. The following lines, Šumma Izbu II 34–41 (Leichty, *Izbu* 49–50), are fragmentary but apparently also dealt with conjoined twins.

77. See also Šumma Izbu III 97 (Leichty, *Izbu* 64) (three feet and two bodies).

78. For the restoration, see Šumma Izbu III 58–59 (Leichty, *Izbu* 60).

79. See also Šumma Izbu III 89 (Leichty, *Izbu* 63).

80. *Am.Journ.Med.Gen.* 91.321.

81. See also Šumma Izbu III 91 (Leichty, *Izbu* 63).

82. See also Šumma Izbu III 45 (Leichty, *Izbu* 58).

83. See also Šumma Izbu II 11 (Leichty, *Izbu* 47) (no forearm). Note also Šumma Izbu II 9–10 (Leichty, *Izbu* 46) (the forearm is pointed/split in two).

84. See also Šumma Izbu II 12 (Leichty, *Izbu* 47).

85. See also Šumma Izbu III 47 (Leichty, *Izbu* 58).

86. See also Šumma Izbu III 53 (Leichty, *Izbu* 59).

87. See also Šumma Izbu III 79 (Leichty, *Izbu* 62).

88. See also Šumma Izbu III 82 (Leichty, *Izbu* 62).

89. See also Šumma Izbu III 83–84 (Leichty, *Izbu* 62) (twisted).

90. See Šumma Izbu III 63 (Leichty, *Izbu* 60).

91. Four ancient skeletons of achondroplastic dwarfs were found at Tepe Hissar (see Krafeld-Daugherty, AOAT 281.262–263 with illustration on 285 no. 16).

92. See also Šumma Izbu I 65–67, IV 24–26 (Leichty, *Izbu* 37–38, 68).

93. Note also Šumma Izbu III 39, 79 (Leichty, *Izbu* 58, 62).

94. See also Šumma Izbu III 71 (Leichty, *Izbu* 61).

95. See also Mujais, *Am.J.Nephrology* 19.137–138.
96. See also Šumma Izbu III 76 (Leichty, *Izbu* 62) (no anus).
97. See also Šumma Izbu I 57 (Leichty, *Izbu* 37).
98. See also Šumma Izbu IV 49 (Leichty, *Izbu* 70).
99. According to the commentary, the Sumerogram Á.KAM is equivalent to Akkadian *šēḫānu* or *maḫḫû* (ecstatic). A genuine ecstatic can only be recognized in late childhood or early adulthood; the reference here is to behavior like an ecstatic, that is, insanity.
100. See also Šumma Izbu II 7 (Leichty, *Izbu* 46).
101. See also Šumma Izbu III 25, 26, 27 (Leichty, *Izbu* 56).
102. It was also noted that some children had unusual facial (or other) features that reminded people of the appearance of animals, as we might say, "with a face like a mule": Šumma Izbu I 5, II 1, 44′, IV 56 (lion); I 6, II 2 (wolf); I 7, II 3 (dog); II 4 (monkey); I 8, II 5, 45 (pig); I 13 (donkey); I 9, 11 (ox); I 14 (wither-sheep); I 12 (elephant); I 15 (cat); II 6 (snake). The passages in question are edited in Leichty, *Izbu* 32, 46, 50, 71 (lion); 32, 46 (wolf and dog); 46 (monkey); 32, 46, 50 (pig); 33 (donkey, ox, sheep, elephant, and cat); 46 (snake).
103. See also Pangas, *Bull.Hist.Med.* 73.198–199.
104. See also Šumma Izbu IV 30 (Leichty, *Izbu* 69).
105. See also Šumma Izbu IV 29 (Leichty, *Izbu* 69).
106. This particular hairstyle was the characteristic mark of slaves in the Old Babylonian period.
107. Guichard, *MARI* 8.306–307.
108. See also Šumma Izbu IV 51 (Leichty, *Izbu* 71).
109. See also Šumma Izbu I 81 (Leichty, *Izbu* 39).
110. See also Šumma Izbu III 90, 94–95 (Leichty, *Izbu* 63, 64).
111. For more discussion of findings in infants, see Volk, *OrNS* 68.15–16, 20–22, 24–28; Cadelli, *Ktèma* 22.22–23, 27–32.
112. See, for example, Volk, *OrNS* 68.12. Kämmerer, *RA* 94.75, 93 argues that "infant" refers specifically to a neonate in the first weeks of life. However, there are a number of references to "infants" of three months and even three years and it is quite clear that older "infants" are expected to be able to stand, to eat solid food, and to talk.
113. In a Middle Assyrian fable, the date palm boasts: "I make the infant grow with my fruit" (Lambert, *BWL* 162:28)
114. For more details, see Stol, *Birth* 181–192.
115. For references, see *CAD* M/2.265–266.
116. See also *BAM* 409 obv. 17′.
117. Labat, *RLA* 3.109 interprets this passage to mean that *samānu* caused amenorrhea (absence of menstruation) in adolescent girls and cult prostitutes. The *qadištu* and *kulmašītu* were not cult prostitutes. Even real prostitutes do not typically cease to menstruate. Amenorrhea is a rare consequence of sexually transmitted diseases and other gynecological problems that can be associated with prostitution. In any case, the demon did not prevent menstruation as such. He prevented the adolescent girl from reaching the age of menstruation, as is made quite clear by the references to the suckling infant and the adolescent boy.
118. The commentary *SpTU* 1.41:3–5 explains this as meaning that the patient has, figuratively speaking, been thrown to the earth.
119. See also Pangas, *Bull.Hist.Med.* 73.199–200.
120. Cadelli, *Ktèma* 22.30 attempts to find meanings other than "drool" for *ṣurruḫu*. However, drooling is so clearly part of the picture of a crying, teething infant that her suggestion (regurgitation) seems quite unlikely.
121. Adamson, *JRAS* 1979.4 n. 25 cites this text as "evidence of fevers associated with chills, rigors, and cold sweats" suggesting the presence of endemic malaria in ancient Mesopotamia, but we do not concur. For possible descriptions of malaria in ancient Mesopotamian texts, see Chapter 3 under MALARIA.
122. For a discussion of this text and the *TDP* passages, see Parpola, *LAS* 2.209–210.
123. The translation assumes a D-stem from *šapālu*. Volk, *OrNS* 68.9–10 argues that this text refers not to teething "against *CAD* Š/1.425b" (and also Parpola, *SAA* 10 no. 302), but specifically to the arrival of the second or third molar on the grounds that in 670 B.C.E., Aššurbanipal was no longer an infant. However, the text is undated and makes no reference to Aššurbanipal (or anyone else) by name. Denton (*JNES* 2.314–315) argues that the reference is to the fully grown Esarhaddon. However, we agree with Parpola (*LAS*

2.209–210) that the description in this letter is sufficiently close to that of the diagnostic handbook references quoted 17.147–17.149 to be clearly describing the same problem. See also Cadelli, *Ktèma* 22.20–21, 28–29.

124. Volk, *OrNS* 68.19 and Cadelli, *Ktèma* 22.16–17 opt for hydrocephalus. Cadelli also suggests brachycephaly as a further possibility. Brachycephaly (short skull), however, is a normal variant of skull configuration.

125. Fincke, *Augenleiden* 117.

126. Ibid. 81–82.

127. Ibid. 127 suggests that Šumma Izbu X 11′–12′ (a malformed birth with one eye full of blood) could be due to vitamin K deficiency, but there are other causes of ocular bleeding including trauma. Her further suggestion (*Augenleiden* 127, 259) that Šumma Izbu X 11′–12′ and 13′–14′ (a malformed birth with one eye yellow dyed red) might be ophthalmia neonatorum seems inappropriate, since ocular bleeding is not a major manifestation of that condition.

128. See also DPS XL A 30//B 31 = *TDP* 220:30.

129. See also DPS XL A 14 = *TDP* 218:14 (eats but is not sated).

130. Lit. "broken" (said of bones) or "smashed" (said of pots).

131. DIŠ *ana* UGU-*šú* A.MEŠ ŠUB-*ma* GABA-*su u* SAG ŠÀ-*šú i-nar-*⌜*ru*⌝-[*bu* DIN?] (DPS III A obv. 3//B 3) "If you pour water over him and his chest and his upper abdomen (epigastrium) become ⌜soft⌝, [. . .]".

132. The translation assumes that this is a verb related to the commonly attested noun *šēlu/šīlu*: "hole, depression."

133. Cadelli, *Ktèma* 22.17–18 interprets this and the preceding reference as describing a congenital malformation. It seems clear, however, that an injury has caused this problem.

134. Ibid. 25 argues that the laugh is a description of risus sardonicus (involuntary smiling due to facial muscle spasms), a sign of tetanus. This diagnosis appears highly unlikely since the patient was wasted. Significant weight loss would not occur in the few days that it takes tetanus to cause death.

135. See *CAD* Ṣ 65a.

CHAPTER 18. DENTAL AND ORAL DISEASES

1. Paleopathological studies of jaws found in cemeteries in Iran and Iraq indicate that there were individuals who died with teeth already missing (for references, see Pangas, *Bull.Hist.Med.* 73.204), but these teeth could have fallen out rather than having been pulled.

2. See also Pangas, *Bull.Hist.Med.* 73.201, 203.

3. See also *BAM* 1 i 1; *CT* 14.23 [K259]:1–7; *CTN* 4.194:6–8; *KADP* 1 v 7; *CT* 17.50:24//*AMT* 23/6:6′; *BAM* 538 iii 43′; *BAM* 538 iii 56′, 62′//*AMT* 24/2:7′, 16′; *BAM* 538 iii 68′, iv 49′; *AMT* 25/2:5′.

4. Kinnier Wilson, *Jour.Roy.Soc.Med.* 89.138 believes that periapical osteitis was common in ancient Mesopotamia, and that it was initiated by excessive wear of teeth from fine sand that was put into wheat to facilitate grinding. There is no evidence that this type of flour milling occurred in ancient Mesopotamia. It is certainly possible that dental osteitis occurred, but it was probably secondary to chronic gingivitis.

5. Note also *BAM* 543 i 3.

6. Note *BAM* 24 obv. 2′ (the tooth "changes" [position])

7. See Pangas, *Bull.Hist.Med.* 73.203–204.

8. For other tooth worm problems, see *BAM* 542 iii 4–7; cf. *BAM* 538 iv 40′–49′.

9. See also Pangas, *Bull.Hist.Med.* 73.202.

10. This recitation is mentioned in Kinnier Wilson, *RA* 60.53.

11. Pangas, *Bull.Hist.Med* 73.200.

12. Hojgaard, *Dilmun* 11:11–13; cf. Littleton and Frohlich, *Paleorient* 15.59–75.

13. Krafeld-Daugherty, *Fs. Dietrich* 265–269.

14. Note also *BAM* 543 i 35; DPS XXI:10 (AOAT 43.246).

15. Note also DPS XXI:11 (AOAT 43.246). Pangas, *Bull.Hist.Med.* 73.200 is puzzled by what he believes to be a reference to "sparkling" teeth connected with gall bladder disease (see Chapter 6). We believe that the reference is actually talking about the teeth oozing blood.

16. See also *BAM* 364 i 3; *BAM* 376 ii 16′–17′.

17. It is this which accounts for the sometimes grim prognosis associated with references including bruxism noted by Pangas, *Bull.Hist.Med.* 73.200–201.

18. Labat, *RLA* 3.232 believes that this term means "blister" or "vesicle." However, *šišitu* is also used to describe something visible in the eyes, where neither "blister" nor "vesicle" would be appropriate. See also *CAD* Š/3.125–126.

19. The commentary *SpTU* 1.47 obv. 1 explains: DIŠ NA EME-*šú eb-ṭe-et-ma* : *e-bé-ṭu* : *na-pa-ḫu* : *e-bé-ṭu* : *ra-bu-ú*: "If a person's tongue is cramped — to cramp means to swell; to cramp means to get large."

20. See Heeßel, AOAT 43.187. The parallel with the following reference would seem to confirm the interpretation.

21. For the reading and interpretation, see Heeßel, AOAT 43.164 (after Landsberger).

22. See the collations to *BAM* 28 in Durand, *Documents Cunéiformes* pl. 120 (= 333).

23. See also BM 47687+:10 (Finkel, *Mem. Sachs* 153).

24. The context makes it clear that "mouth" and not "tooth" was meant.

CHAPTER 19. ANCIENT ETIOLOGIES

1. On this point, see also (somewhat differently argued) Collins, *Natural Illness* 1–12.

2. See also DPS XI A obv. 19//B 18 = *TDP* 90:19//*SpTU* 1.34:18.

3. Heeßel, AOAT 43.48 suggests that *nakkamtu* refers to a storehouse that the patient has robbed and that the sickness is a punishment for having done this.

4. See Harris, "Inanna-Ishtar as Paradox and Coincidence of Opposites" in *Gender and Aging in Mesopotamia* 158–171.

5. For more details, see Scurlock, *JANER* 3:103.

6. The restoration is suggested by the commentary *STT* 403 r. 35.

7. The restoration is based on the commentary, *STT* 403 r. 40: [KI.SIKIL.B]ÀN.DA = *ba-tul-tu*.

8. Lit. "house of four"; compare "street of four" (crossroads).

9. "Place of destruction" does not seem particularly appropriate to the context; perhaps the similar-sounding *kiḫullum*: "place of mourning" was meant.

10. See also DPS XIII J 11 = *TDP* 126 iii 43.

11. See DPS XVII:15–16 (AOAT 43.196).

12. Stol, *Epilepsy* 62–63, 79 interprets this as "goose flesh." In *Fs. Borger* 344 he further argues that it is named after *ḫamītu*: "wasp." However, wasp stings do not cause goose bumps.

13. Kinnier Wilson, *Medical History* 34.190, 195 also believes this text to be describing a hysterical seizure.

14. For the reading, see Heeßel, AOAT 43.192.

15. Note also DPS XXVI:85′ (AOAT 43.285) (shuddering caused by Ištar of Arbela).

16. Although the word *hysteria* was originally applied only to women, current usage includes men.

17. For more details, see Chapter 12. They sometimes attacked children but it is clear that adolescents were the primary targets (differently Kinnier Wilson, *Medical History* 34.187).

18. See also DPS XXXVII A obv. 12, 14 = *TDP* 214:12, 14. Note also DPS XVII:78 (AOAT 43.202) (the patient is sick at night and well in the morning and is kept up all night; the end of the line reads ŠU LÍL.LÁ.[EN.NA] as suggested by Heeßel, AOAT 43.215 and confirmed by collation).

19. The variant has: "when they try to wake him, he is groggy."

20. Heeßel, AOAT 43.289 interprets this as affliction by a criminal *lilû*. However, *sarru* is not a generic term for "criminal"; it refers to someone who cheats or lives by deception.

21. Kinnier Wilson, *Medical History* 34.192, 196 believes that this reference is describing a postictal state. We believe that the phrase "he can get up afterward" is intended specifically to mean that the patient does *not* have a postictal state.

22. Kinnier Wilson, ibid. 193, 197 considers this text to be describing interictal confusion with agitation and restlessness. We do not agree.

23. Kinnier Wilson, ibid. 191, 195 believes that this reference is describing a grand mal seizure. We find it difficult to be certain about the diagnosis and cannot exclude hysterical seizures.

24. See also DPS XXII:53–54 (AOAT 43.256).

25. [*la-a*]ʾ-*bi* : *šá li-lu-ú i-zi-*⌜*bu*⌝-*uš* [*la-a*]ʾ-*bi* : *le-e-bu* : *zi-i-pi* "⌜*la*ʾ*bu*⌝ is what the *lilû* left behind; ⌜*la*ʾ*bu*⌝ = *li*ʾ*bu* = *zi*ʾ*pu* (a macular red rash; see Chapter 10)" (*SpTU* 1.30 obv. 7–8).

26. 5R 16 i 37; Haupt, *ASKT* 198 (Rm. 2,585):32, apud *CAD* L 34b.

27. Kinnier Wilson, *Medical History* 34.192, 196 believes that this and the preceding reference are describing complex partial seizures. Part of his interpretation is based on the fact that the patient is crying "my insides," which Kinnier Wilson attributes to what he calls "epigastric rising sensation." It is likely that he is referring to a syndrome called abdominal epilepsy, a condition that is no longer considered a valid diagnosis. Kinnier Wilson's interpretation also ignores the fever.

28. See Heeßel, AOAT 43.304.

29. Collation reveals that one of the copies of the fourth tablet of the diagnostic/prognostic handbook (DPS IV B rev. 17–19) contains a short section in which the GIDIM$_2$ sign at the end of each line is written as a "bar" followed at an interval by a "u."

30. See also DPS XI A obv. 40 = *TDP* 92:40.

31. The passage has been collated. The copy has AB.

32. See also DPS XXVI:76′ (AOAT 43.285).

33. The text has been collated.

34. Note also BM 62397:1–4//BM 77041:13′–16′.

35. See also DPS XXII:51–52 (AOAT 43.255), cited above as 19.22.

36. Note also DPS XIX/XX:100′ (AOAT 43.232); *AMT* 103/1 ii 5//*BAM* 469 r. 32.

37. See also DPS XIV A iii 8–9//C_2 iii 2 = *TDP* 140 iii 42′–43′ (cf. DPS XIX/XX:18′, 19′ [AOAT 43.227]); DPS XIII G_2 r. 15, 22 = *TDP* 124 iii 22, 29. Note also DPS XI A r. 61//DPS XII A 1 = *TDP* 100 i 1//*TDP* 100 r. 61 (catchline) (pain in the breast).

38. See DPS XXII:47b [AOAT 43.255].

39. For example, Stol, *Epilepsy* 16–19 conflates the two as one of many synonyms for epilepsy.

40. See also DPS XI A obv. 22//B 21 = *TDP* 90:22//*SpTU* 1.34:21 (cf. StBoT 36.62:6).

41. Von Weiher, *Nergal* 86 interprets "lord of the roof" as sonambulism, quoting Ungnad, *AfO* 14.268. The reference is, however, not to wandering about on the roof of the house in the middle of the night but to something wrong with the patient's head. In any case, walking around on the roof at night would not have been all that unusual an activity in ancient Mesopotamia, since roofs were flat and often used for sleeping.

42. Note also *MDP* 57.11 vi 20′–21′ (gazelle of the roof).

43. See also *BAM* 482 iv 40′//*AMT* 97/4:6′–7′.

44. See also DPS XXVII:24 (AOAT 43.299); cf. Ni. 470:9–10 (Kraus, *ZA* 77.197).

45. See also DPS IX A 75 = *TDP* 78:75; DPS XI A obv. 21//B 20 = *TDP* 90:21//*SpTU* 1.34:20.

46. Lit. "he will have a finishing off."

47. DPS XL A 24–25//B 25–26 = *TDP* 220:24–25; DPS XL A 26–27 = *TDP* 220:26–27.

48. Note also DPS XL A 60 = *TDP* 224:60 (cf. K 3628+4009 obv. 5′).

49. For a discussion of *zaqāpu*, said of the eyes, see p. 300.

50. See also DPS XL B 117 = *TDP* 230:123!

51. See also DPS XL A 28 = *TDP* 220:28 (cf. K 3628+4009 obv. 4′); DPS XL A 30//B 31 = *TDP* 220:30.

52. In principle, the "daughter of Anu" could be either Ištar or Lamaštu. However, Ištar is mentioned under her proper name as causing seizures in infants whereas Lamaštu is not.

53. Kinnier Wilson, *Medical History* 34.194, 196 also understands this text to be describing an aura.

54. See also DPS XXVI:40′, 41′ (AOAT 43.281).

55. Kinnier Wilson, *Medical History* 34.189, 191, 192 interprets this and similar passages as subcutaneous bleeding (ecchymosis) or red (suffused) eyes. However, neither subcutaneous bleeding nor red eyes are commonly found in patients with seizures, whereas pallor and flushing are often present (see p. 318).

56. See also DPS XXII:68 (AOAT 43.256).

57. Kinnier Wilson, *Medical History* 34.192, 196 interprets this phrase as lip smacking, a type of automatism, and we concur.

58. Kinnier Wilson, ibid. 187 interprets this text as diurnal epilepsy (AN.TA.ŠUB.BA) turning into nocturnal epilepsy ("hand" of ghost). However, "hand" of ghost is not nocturnal epilepsy and diurnal epilepsy does not "turn into" nocturnal epilepsy.

59. See also DPS XXVI:88′ (AOAT 43.286).

60. The verb is otherwise used to describe the action of animals caught in a trap (see *AHw* 1025a and *CAD* S 157).

61. The alternative diagnosis was "hand" of Ištar.

62. See also DPS XIX/XX:17′ (AOAT 43.227); cf. DPS XVIII:38′ (AOAT 43.219) (Išḫara).

63. DPS XXVIII:20 (AOAT 43.310) = 19.62, in which "spawn" of Šulpaea turns into "hand" of ghost, may be a reference to a separately described syndrome that combined symptoms more usually associated with "spawn" of Šulpaea with a "mournful cry" (i.e., "hand" of ghost by the code). For more details, see 13.260.

64. Kinnier Wilson, *Medical History* 34.187 interprets this text as nocturnal epilepsy ("hand" of ghost) turning into diurnal epilepsy (AN.TA.ŠUB.BA). However, "hand" of ghost is not nocturnal epilepsy. The only association of ghosts with seizures is in connection with alcohol withdrawal, and ghosts were implicated not because of the seizures but due to alcoholic hallucinations (see Chapter 15).

65. Kinnier Wilson, *Diseases in Antiquity* 201 suggests that this god's name, which literally means "lord of the roof (beam)," refers specifically to the upward rolling of the patient's eyes.

66. See also BM 56605:16–17 (AOAT 43.118).

67. See also DPS XXIX:11 (AOAT 43.319).

68. Lit. "arrival (in due course of time) at the (netherworld) mountain." Heeßel, AOAT 43.331 suggests that the expression *ul-tab-bar* TAS-*níq* KUR.RA GAR-*šú* is related to the disease *tašniqu* which would, in this case, have come into Mesopotamia from the East. However, a patient with *tašniqu* was spitting blood (see *BAM* 575 iv 34), not a recipe for long life. The most likely explanation is that this is *tasniqu* from *sanāqu* and refers to the "approach to the netherworld mountain" (i.e., a natural death).

69. See also BM 56605:21 (AOAT 43.118).

70. The number is restored from *Emar* VI/4.695:3; see Heeßel, AOAT 43.335.

71. Heeßel, AOAT 43.123 tries to interpret the KAR as a form of *ezēbu*, notes that the result is rather strange, and ends by translating "hand?" in each of the places where this expression occurs. However, it is always best to give what the text seems to say, and another reading of KAR, "quay," makes at least passable sense in this context. The two gods of whom the expression is used, Sîn and Šamaš, both traveled across the sky in boats.

72. It is interesting to note that infections of the mouth such as Ludwig's angina which adversely affect the patient's ability to speak were also blamed on the *rābiṣu* (see 18.43).

73. See Stol, *Epilepsy* 76–77.

74. See also *AMT* 23/2:5.

75. Severe pain and stiffness in the feet could also be due to gout; see Chapter 11. When the patient has fever, however, as in the first reference below, the diagnosis is more likely to be rheumatic fever. Note also DPS XXII:40 (AOAT 43.255), which describes "twisting" attributed to the *rābiṣu* of the road.

76. The commentary to this line (*SpTU* 1.30 obv. 9) defines *râdu* as *salāḫu.*

77. This interpretation of SAG.TUKU follows the commentary, *SpTU* 1.30 obv. 9–11.

78. The Sumerogram TÉŠ is equivalent to Akkadian *ba*ʾ*āšu*, "to come to shame," which is inappropriate for this context. However, nearly homophonous *ba*ʾ*āšu* means "to smell bad" and is not uncommonly used of the ears (see *CAD* B 4b s.v. *ba*ʾ*āšu* A mng. 1a). Scribal word games of this sort are commonplace in ancient scholarly texts.

79. See also Heeßel, AOAT 43.268–269.

80. For twenty-five examples of curse formulae in which Sîn is called upon to inflict the miscreant with *saḫaršubbû*, see the chart in Watanabe, *ASJ* 6.102–104.

81. In Tsukimoto, *Priests and Officials* 199–200:85–93, the purificatory ceremony undergone by the patient who has recovered from *saḫaršubbû* is addressed to Šamaš.

82. For two examples of curse formulae in which Ištar of Arbela is called upon to inflict the miscreant with *saḫaršubbû*, see the chart in Watanabe, *ASJ* 6.102–104 (nos. 26–27). There is also a curse that makes this request of Sîn, Šamaš, and Ištar acting in concert (no. 18).

83. For a discussion of *zaqāpu*, said of the eyes, see p. 300.

84. The reading of the signs is uncertain. The name is probably simply *nilugu* (a foreign loanword).

85. *BAM* 580 iii 2′–5′.

86. For references, see *CAD* B 301a s.v. *bubu*ʾ*tu* mng. c.

87. DPS IX A 51//B obv. 50 = *TDP* 76:51.

88. Gula also caused (DPS XXXIII:103 [AOAT 43.357]) *samānu* (cellulitis; see Chapter 3) and *ašû* (generalized macular, papular, or vesicular eruptions; see Chapter 10).

89. Šamaš also caused scales (*quliptu*; see Chapter 10), *sagbānu* (*CAD* S 22a; see Chapter 10), and "small webs" (spiders; see Chapter 6).

90. For references, see *CAD* S 277b s.v. *simmu* mng. 1b.

91. That this organ is the liver may be seen from Izbu comm. 203 (Leichty, *Izbu* 218): *ta-kal-tú* = *ga-bi-du*: "liver." See also Nougayrol, *RA* 44.3 and Goetze, *YOS* 10 p. 7. Note also *CAD* N 376a.

92. Note that DPS XXXIII:105–106 (AOAT 43.357–358) seems to be unsure whether to attribute this to Ninurta or to Gula.

93. Heeßel, AOAT 43.360 translates: "he (the patient) is raised up and is unable to get himself up, etc." However, the verb is active (with direct object) and not passive, as this translation would require.

94. For an interpretation of this reference as possible "Bright's disease," see Kinnier Wilson, *Diseases in Antiquity* 193.

95. In DPS IX A 47–49//B obv. 46–48//C 15–17 = *TDP* 74:47–49 (see 10.82–84).

96. See also StBoT 36.40 obv. 9′–10′; DPS XVIII:21 (AOAT 43.219); *BAM* 584 ii 29′.

97. So the commentary *SpTU* 1.36 obv. 23–24.

98. Note also *BAM* 316 iii 13′–14′//*BAM* 317 r. 16–17//*STT* 95 iv 145//*BAM* 447:4′; cf. BM 101938:4′ (*dikšu* and divine anger).

99. Note also BM 64174:1–5 (Geller, *AfO* 35.21).

100. For references, see *CAD* L 170b s.v. *libbu* mng. 3a.

101. Note also *BAM* 370 ia 3′–4′//*BAM* 372 i 2; cf. *BAM* 423 i 32′.

102. Heeßel, AOAT 43.360 translates: "he (the patient) is raised up and is unable to get himself up, etc." However, the verb is active (with direct object) and not passive, as this translation would require.

103. See also DPS XI A r. 21 = *TDP* 96 r. 21.

104. See Chapter 20 under Pulses.

105. Restorations are based on DPS XI A obv. 13–14//B 12–13 = *TDP* 90:13–14//*SpTU* 1.34:12–13.

106. For "hand" of mankind as a form of sorcery, see Heeßel, AOAT 43.263 with previous bibliography.

107. Heeßel, AOAT 43.263 reads *si-mu-tu* and suggests that this might be an otherwise unattested variant of *sāmūtu*: "redness." "Limpness" seems to suit the context somewhat better.

108. Restorations are based on *BAM* 445:10–16. Note also *BAM* 460:5′–10′ (with numb limbs, loss of appetite, and feeling hot at sundown).

109. See, for example, *BAM* 232 i 1′–23′ and K 9216+K 17521 ii 2′–10′.

110. See, for example, *AMT* 21/2+K 15966:1–25 (restored from *AMT* 22/2 obv. 1–5 and K 9216+).

111. See also DPS XI A r. 19 = *TDP* 96 r. 19.

112. The commentary to Tablet IV, *SpTU* 1.30 explains (obv. 14–15) the supplementary diagnosis "on account of a man's wife" in this "hand" of Šamaš reference where the temples are involved by pointing out that SAG ("head") is equivalent to "man" and KI ("earth") to woman.

113. Kinnier Wilson, *Diseases in Antiquity* 201 interprets this text as meningitis.

114. Note also DPS XIV A iv 14//K 8 = *TDP* 144 iv 49′; cf. DPS XV:66 (AOAT 43.154) = *TDP* 238:66 (with toes).

115. For references, see *CAD* M/1.71–84; *AHw* 580–582. Note especially the description of assault in the Laws of Ḫammurapi § 206: "If a man strikes another man in a brawl and inflicts a wound upon him."

116. These are: DPS III C r. 13 = *TDP* 26:73; BM 47687:10 (Finkel, *Mem. Sachs* 153); DPS VII A obv. 26 = *TDP* 62:26; DPS IX A 28 = *TDP* 74:28; DPS IX A 51//B obv. 50 = *TDP* 76:51 (cf. *BAM* 418 obv. 3′); DPS X A obv. 9//B obv. 9 = *TDP* 80:9; DPS X A obv. 16//B obv. 18 = *TDP* 82:16; DPS XII D iii 19 = *TDP* 104 iii 19; DPS XIII B i 32′//D 6 = *TDP* 114 i 36′; DPS XIII B i 41′//F 3 = *TDP* 114 i 45′; Labat, *MDP* 57.11 ii 1; DPS XIII B ii 17–18 = *TDP* 118 ii 17–18; DPS XIII B ii 27–28//G_2 25–26+G_1 8–9 = *TDP* 120 ii 27–28; DPS XV:52 (AOAT 43.153) (cf. DPS XIV A iii 10–11//C_2 iii 3 = *TDP* 140 iii 44′–45′); DPS XIV A iii 16 = *TDP* 140 iii 50′ (cf. Labat, *MDP* 57.11 ii 2); DPS XIV A iii 17 = *TDP* 140 iii 51′; DPS XV:21 (AOAT 43.151); DPS XV:91 (AOAT 43.155).

117. Compare also *MDP* 57.11 ii 1 (abdomen).

118. See also DPS XIV A iii 16 = *TDP* 140 iii 50′; cf. *MDP* 57.11 ii 2.

119. In the only text with a positive prognosis (DPS IX A 51//B obv. 50 = *TDP* 76:51 [cf. *BAM* 418 obv. 3′]), "hand" of Adad is given as a variant of "hand" of Marduk as the causal agent for a whitehead (*ziqtu*).

120. The text has been collated.

121. Note also BM 47687:10 (Finkel, *Mem. Sachs* 153) (mouth hurts).

122. The text has been collated.

123. After the reading of Heeßel, AOAT 43.151. However, ibid. 157, 164, interprets KA as "mouth" rather than "speech."

124. In other words, the goddess caused the wound because she wanted a gift.

125. Since StBoT 36.35 obv. 17′ has *a-na ú-bur-ti*, Wilhelm, StBoT 36.38 suggested reading the traces in DPS III C r. 16 as *ú*-[*u*]*r-ti* and interpreting this as *uʾʾurti*: "instruction/order" with *uburti* as an unusual vari-

ant. Collation of DPS III, however, shows that the text has *ú-qàt-ti*. Moreover, the remaining passage, StBoT 36.57 r. 5, has *ana qá-a*[*t-ti*].

126. Note also DPS X A obv. 17//B obv. 19 = *TDP* 82:17 (cf. StBoT 36.35 obv. 15′//StBoT 36.57 r. 5′).

127. Note also DPS XV:92 (AOAT 43.155).

128. The restoration is based on the surrounding entries in Tablet XIII.

129. See Heeßel, AOAT 43.187.

130. See also DPS X B r. 12 = *TDP* 88 r. 12 (arm and elbow); DPS XII D iii 43, 44//E iv 1–2, 3 = *TDP* 106 iii 43, 44 (hips, arms, and elbows); cf. DPS III C r. 24 = *TDP* 28:84 (head and hip).

131. Note also DPS XIII B i 50′//F 9 = *TDP* 116 i 54′.

132. ÚḪ is usually "phlegm." However, when used with KÚM ("fever") it is to be read as a form of *ṣarāḫu* as the parallel between DPS III C r. 10–11//E_1 r. 11–12+E_2 r. 7–8 = *TDP* 26:70–71 (DIŠ *ina* SAG.DU-*šú* KÚM ÚḪ) and *KAR* 211 obv. 4–6 ([DIŠ *i-na*] SAG.DU-*šú* KÚM *ṣa-ri-iḫ*) shows and has now been demonstrated by Heeßel, AOAT 43.162–163. Previously, Labat, *TDP* 25 n. 44 had suggested and then rejected the correct reading in favor of *nuppuḫ* "it is swollen" (followed by Biggs, *RLA* 6.210 and *CAD* N/1.268b), which makes no sense in this context.

133. See also DPS X A obv. 19//B obv. 21 = *TDP* 82:19.

134. See Stol, *Epilepsy* 92.

135. See also DPS IV A obv. 44 = *TDP* 36:44 (the restoration of "hand" of Ereškigal is confirmed by the commentary *SpTU* 1.30 obv. 2′).

136. For references, see *CAD* A/1.253–254 s.v. *akālu* mng. 5a and *AHw* 26 s.v. *akālu* mng. 6b.

137. See also DPS XV:22 (AOAT 43.151). Note DPS XIV A iv 8–9//C_2 iv 11//K 4 = *TDP* 144 iv 43′–44′.

138. So *CTN* 4.72 i 17′–18′.

139. See also DPS XVI:10 (AOAT 43.172) (excreting blood).

140. This is the literal meaning of the term; see *AHw* 829–830.

141. See DPS XIV A iii 17 = *TDP* 140 iii 51′ (see Chapter 19.183).

142. See also DPS XIV C_2 iv 4b; DPS XIV A iv 3//C_2 iv 8 = *TDP* 144 iv 38′ (cf. StBoT 36.34 obv. 4′).

143. Labat's edition gives Lamaštu but the tablet has *aḫḫāzu*.

144. Adamson, *JRAS* 1979.4 n. 25 cites this text as "evidence of fevers associated with chills, rigors, and cold sweats" suggesting the presence of endemic malaria in ancient Mesopotamia, but we do not concur. For possible descriptions of malaria in ancient Mesopotamian texts, see Chapter 3 under MALARIA.

145. See Chapter 19 with 19.335–19.342.

146. Var. G_2: fifteen days; var. E: five days.

147. DPS XV:62 (AOAT 43.154); cf. DPS XIV C_2 iv 5b (see Chapter 19.186).

148. These two references mention fever (DPS XIII B ii 10 = *TDP* 118 ii 10) and trauma to the hip region (DPS XII D iv 17//G_2 iv 15 = *TDP* 108 iv 17). The latter trauma may have to do with the fact that the hip region is mentioned in descriptions of Šulak's fever with neurologic symptoms (*MDP* 57.11 v 6′–8′).

149. The other possible reason why someone might have suffered trauma to the testicles was as punishment for incest (DPS XIV A_2 ii 17//C ii 30 = *TDP* 138 ii 67), a punishment that might also take the form of torsion of the testicles (DPS XIV A_2 ii 12//C ii 26 = *TDP* 136 ii 62) or of venereal disease producing swollen testicles (DPS XIV A_2 ii 15–16//C ii 29–30 = *TDP* 136 ii 65–66).

150. See also DPS XII D iv 17//G_2 iv 15 = *TDP* 108 iv 17.

151. See Heeßel, AOAT 43.166.

152. See also *KAR* 211 obv. 14.

153. Fincke, *Augenleiden* 124–125 suggests a diagnosis of urticaria or periarteritis nodosa for this and other references to "hand" of Sîn that describe the eyes as being "soaked." However, none of the signs listed in these texts corresponds to the findings normally associated with either of these conditions.

154. Ibid. 83.

155. The only other attestation is in DPS X A obv. 32b–33 = *TDP* 84:32b–33, where he appears alongside the more obviously appropriate drowned ghost as a causer of shortness of breath.

156. See also DPS XIV A iii 19 = *TDP* 140 iii 53′.

157. The most common pattern is to have two syndromes that need to be distinguished simply listed side by side. However, in some cases what happens instead is that one of the syndromes is sandwiched between references to the other syndrome. For example, in Tablet IV, a reference to the optical neuropathy induced by the god Šulpaea (DPS IV B obv. 28//E i 8 = *TDP* 36:28//*SpTU* 3.88 i 8) is sandwiched between two references to the optical neuropathy induced by the city god (DPS IV B obv. 27//E i 7 = *TDP* 34:27//*SpTU* 3.88

i 7 and DPS IV B obv. 29//E i 9 = *TDP* 36:29–30//*SpTU* 3.88 i 9). In this case, a reference to a head wound attributed to the goddess Ištar (DPS III A obv. 19//C obv. 10 = *TDP* 18:10; cf. StBoT 36.35 r. 1//StBoT 36.57 r. 8′) would, if this interpretation is correct, be sandwiched between a series of references to head wounds attributed to Papsukkal.

158. See also DPS XIX/XX:100′ (AOAT 43.232).

159. Lit. "his temple (feels) squeezed."

160. The text was collated. E. Ritter, AS 16.303 n. 13 restored [*uk-ta-at*]-*ta-at* against the traces. The meaning is the same.

161. For DPS III C r. 21 = *TDP* 26:81, see text 19.132, above.

162. See *CAD* Š/1.59a s.v. *šadû* A mng. 3.

163. See also DPS IV B r. 35 = *TDP* 44 r. 58 (left eye hurts); DPS IX A 50//B obv. 49 = *TDP* 76:50 (face full of *birdu*-nodules); DPS IX A 55//B obv. 55 = *TDP* 76:55 (dizziness and clouded eyes), but note DPS XXIII:1 (AOAT 43.272); DPS XXII:79 (AOAT 43.257) [catchline] (vomiting bile).

164. For treatments, see *CT* 14.23 [K 9283]:23, 25–26; *STT* 281 iv 9; Labat, *RA* 54.174 [AO 17617] r. 12; *BAM* 183:19; *STT* 281 i 7; *BAM* 183:23, 38; *STT* 275 ii 10′.

165. Stol, *Birth* 210 believes that this text refers to Rh factor incompatibility. Nothing in this reference, however, indicates that the victim is an infant.

166. Adamson, *JRAS* 1979.4 n. 25 cites this text as "evidence of fevers associated with chills, rigors, and cold sweats" suggesting the presence of endemic malaria in ancient Mesopotamia, but we do not concur. For possible ancient descriptions of malaria, see Chapter 3 under MALARIA.

167. Text B (*SpTU* 1.37) has Marduk instead of Lamaštu.

168. For similar references, see *BAM* 174 r. 29–31; DPS XVI:13 (AOAT 43.173); K 2581 obv. 7′.

169. Note also the occasional association of Lamaštu with *pašittu* (possibly cholecystitis; see Chapter 6). For references, see Köcher, *Fs. Goerke* 35–36.

170. The text has been collated.

171. The text has been collated.

172. The passage has been collated.

173. See also DPS XI A obv. 23//B 22 = *TDP* 90:23//*SpTU* 1.34:22.

174. UNU = *šubtu*; see *CAD* Š/3.172b s.v. *šubtu* A lex. section.

175. See also DPS XL A 52 = *TDP* 224:52.

176. See also DPS XIX/XX:9′ (AOAT 43.227). Note also DPS XIX/XX:45′, 46′ (AOAT 43.229) and DPS XVIII:7 (AOAT 43.218).

177. See also Kinnier Wilson, *Diseases in Antiquity* 204–205; *JNES* 27.244–245; Wiggerman in Stol, *Birth* 237. Note that Kinnier Wilson uses the outdated term *abdominal typhus* to mean typhoid.

178. Alimurung and Manahan, *J.Phillipp.Med.Assoc* 28.388.

179. The *rābiṣu*, whose name literally means "baliff demon," more normally caused strokes and heart problems involving irregularities in the pulse. Since Marduk caused chest pain (see 19.111), it is possible that the *rābiṣu* was, in these cases, acting specifically as Marduk's "baliff." However, subordinates always are, or feel themselves to be, underpaid. Was the *rābiṣu* who caused hepatitis A attempting to supplement his income by beating up and stealing food and drink from humans he was not ordered to attack?

180. On this point, see also Heeßel, AOAT 43.267.

181. See also DPS XXII:34–35, 36–37 (AOAT 43.254).

182. See *CAD* S 1a s.v. *sa'ālu* mng. b.

183. This is mentioned in a medical commentary (Civil, *JNES* 33.336–337:6–7).

184. Note also DPS XXII:46 (AOAT 43.255).

185. So Labat, *TDP* 26:68. Both C and E seem to have "u" between KÚM and LUḪ.

186. Labat reads the NAR with the rare phonetic reading *puḫ* as a phonetic complement of KÚM. Similar lines above have KÚM followed by ÚḪ which Labat also read as a phonetic complement. We, however, prefer to read the ÚḪ as a Sumerogram. Therefore, the NAR is probably also a Sumerogram. The sign lists give no usable reading. However there is a *ṣarāḫu*, which means "to cry or lament." Since the Sumerogram usually used for this *ṣarāḫu* (ŠÌR) means "to sing," it is conceivable that NAR (which also means "to sing") could be read *ṣarāḫu*. If so, then what we have here is a scribal pun of a sort surprisingly common in scholarly texts whereby *ṣarāḫu*: "to be burning hot" would have been written with the Sumerogram for *ṣarāḫu*: "to lament."

187. The commentary *STT* 403 r. 52 has "he continually vomits blood."

188. Kinnier Wilson, *Iraq* 19.44 interprets this text as a reference to malaria, but feverish sweating and chills are by no means exclusive to that disease. For possible examples of malaria in ancient Mesopotamian texts, see Chapter 3.

189. These are *BAM* 482 ii 62′–63′, iii 1; cf. DPS IV B obv. 30–31//E i 10–11 = *TDP* 36:31–32//*SpTU* 3.88 i 10–11).

190. See also DPS IV E ii 27–28//H 1–2 = *SpTU* 3.88 ii 27–28.

191. Kinnier Wilson, *Diseases in Antiquity* 200 interprets this text as meningitis. However, this is based on a misinterpretation of "his throat looks terrible" as "his neck is retracted." For possible ancient descriptions of meningitis, see Chapter 13 under MENINGITIS.

192. Compare DPS III A obv. 5 ("calm temples," meaning calm temporal blood vessels; see Chapter 3.12); DPS IV B obv. 5b–6 = *TDP* 32:5b–6 ("collapsed temples," meaning collapsed temporal blood vessels; see Chapter 14.24), and the relatively common expression "pulating temples" meaning a sensation of pulsation in the temporal arteries (see Chapter 13.149).

193. Compare also DPS III C obv. 44 = *TDP* 22:44 (See Chapter 13.86).

194. Note also DPS XIX/XX:114′ (AOAT 43.233).

195. See also DPS V D i 5 = *TDP* 48 E i 5.

196. A possible example of the infant version is DPS XL A 57 = *TDP* 224:57, which describes a fever.

197. Heeßel, AOAT 43.241 suggests that DPS III C r. 9 = *TDP* 26:69 is also describing this fever. In addition to asking for water to bathe in, the patient of this text has a head that burns with fever; the fever is noticeably worse in the morning and evening than it is in the middle of the day.

198. See also DPS IV A obv. 59, 60//E ii 4, 5 = *TDP* 38:59, 60//*SpTU* 3.88 ii 4, 5; cf. DPS XIX/XX:9′, 29′ (AOAT 43.227).

199. Adamson, *JRAS* 1979.4 n. 25 cites this line as a possible reference to a malarial attack, but we do not concur. For possible ancient descriptions of malaria, see Chapter 3 under MALARIA.

200. Note also DPS XIX/XX:12′ (AOAT 43.227).

201. See DPS IV A obv. 56–57//E ii 2//G obv. 9–10 = *TDP* 38:56–57//*SpTU* 3.88 ii 2//*LKU* 94:9–10.

202. See DPS VI A r. 12//B_1 r. 9+B_2 r. 13 = *TDP* 60 r. 43′; cf. StBoT 36.40 obv. 7′.

203. See DPS XIX/XX:13′ (AOAT 43.227).

204. See DPS IV B obv. 24 = *TDP* 34:24.

205. The passage has been collated. The copy has ^{d}20.

206. Note also BM 77041:4′–5′ (AN.TA.ŠUB.BA and "hand" of Sîn).

207. See also DPS IV A obv. 59//E ii 4 = *TDP* 38:59//*SpTU* 3.88 ii 4; DPS XIX/XX:114′ (AOAT 43.233).

208. Note also DPS XV:19 (AOAT 43.151) and DPS XV:64b (AOAT 43.154) (cf. DPS XIV A_2 iv 11′//C_2 iii 36 = *TDP* 142 iv 11′) (with feet).

209. In all of the references in this sequence, the affliction "afflicts him in the evening" and the diagnosis is given as "affliction by a ghost."

210. Kinnier Wilson, *Diseases in Antiquity* 200 argues, and we agree, that the statement that the feet are "raised up" refers to flexion of the hips and knees, a position that commonly occurs in meningitis.

211. Kinnier Wilson, *Medical History* 34.187, 191, 195 believes this sequence of references to be describing nocturnal epilepsy. We do not believe that the findings are typical for seizures, and the presence of fever strongly suggests an infectious etiology.

212. DPS XVIII:3–4 (AOAT 43.218).

213. Kinnier Wilson, *Diseases in Antiquity* 200 suggests that this text is describing meningitis. We agree that this is a possible diagnosis, but the information is insufficient to be certain.

214. Compare also DPS III C obv. 28 = *TDP* 20:28.

215. Restoration follows a suggestion by Heeßel, AOAT 43.224, 255, 260.

216. The expression is used to describe applying plasters. Note Stol, *Epilepsy* 65 n. 31.

217. See also Heeßel, AOAT 43.269 for a discussion of ancient wordplays on the obvious similarity between the word for "ghost" (*eṭemmu*) and the human thought process (*ṭēmu*).

218. See also DPS XXII:53–54 (AOAT 43.256).

219. Note DPS X B r. 5 = *TDP* 88 r. 5 which mentions disorientation ("gazing at arms") and chills.

220. So Stol, *JEOL* 32.45, correcting *CAD* A/2.470a, which reads TAG-*te* and interprets this as a skin condition.

221. DPS XIII B ii 49–50//G_2 obv. 39+G_1 obv. 22 = *TDP* 120 ii 49–50 and DPS XVIII:38′ (AOAT 43.219) are two further texts with the diagnosis "hand" of Išḫara, which mention a rash on the abdomen and the

patient's being "overwhelmed." Since they also mention a month-long illness, however, they cannot be cases of meningococcal meningitis, but might possibly be mild or subacute meningococcemia, which can last for weeks and from which spontaneous recovery is possible.

222. Note also DPS IV A obv. 58//E ii 3 = *TDP* 38:58//*SpTU* 3.88 ii 3 (temples and ears lukewarm; patient dies); DPS IV A obv. 61//E ii 6 = *TDP* 38:61//*SpTU* 3.88 ii 6 (temples hurt; body hot; patient dies).

223. Lit. "his temple (feels) squeezed."

224. See also DPS IX A 54 = *TDP* 76:54 (with dizziness).

225. Kinnier Wilson, *Diseases in Antiquity* 200 argues, and we agree, that the statement that the feet are "raised up" refers to flexion of the hips and knees, a position that commonly occurs in meningitis.

226. Note also DPS XIX/XX:109′b (AOAT 43.232).

227. See also DPS III C r. 3–4//E_1 r. 4–5+E_2 r. 1 = *TDP* 24:63–64 (ghost of one who died of thirst); DPS III C r. 5–6//E_1 r. 6–7+E_2 r. 2–3 = *TDP* 26:65–66.

228. Lit. "his heart does not rise in him."

229. Note also DPS XXVII:27–28 (AOAT 43.299); DPS XIII B ii 13–14 = *TDP* 118 ii 13–14; DPS XIII G_2 r. 7–8 = *TDP* 122 iii 14, 15.

230. See also DPS XIII B i 7′ = *TDP* 110 i 11′.

231. Note also *BAM* 221 ii 5′//*AMT* 81/7:8 (with belching).

232. See also *BAM* 155 i 4′.

233. See also *BAM* 161 iii 19′.

234. See also DPS IV B obv. 10 = *TDP* 32:10.

235. See also *BAM* 482 iv 48′//*AMT* 19/1 iv! 31′.

236. See also DPS IX A 62//B r. 6–7 = *TDP* 76:62; cf. also DPS X A obv. 32b–33 = *TDP* 84:32b–33; *BAM* 216:59′–61′//*BAM* 470 obv. 12′–13′ (shortness of breath). Kinnier Wilson, *Diseases in Antiquity* 200 diagnoses *TDP* 76:62 and *TDP* 84:32 as meningitis, but we do not concur. The suggestion is based on a misinterpretation of the phrase "his breath is short" as "his neck is retracted." For possible ancient descriptions of meningitis, see Chapter 13 under MENINGITIS.

237. See also BM 42272 obv. 23, 25–26, 28–29; BM 67158 obv. 10′; BM 72246+72031+72008:15; *AMT* 31/4:14, 16; cf. *AMT* 29/13:9′; *BAM* 161 ii 11′, 15′.

238. W. Farber *BID* 227:1–14; see Chapter 4.

239. On the identification of *buʾšānu* with "scurvy," see Pangas, *Bull.Hist.Med.* 73.205–206.

240. Wiggerman in Stol, *Birth* 237–238.

241. For the Sumerian conjugation-prefix "a", see Thomsen, *Sumerian* 166–169.

242. DPS IX A 72–73//B r. 19–20 = *TDP* 78:72–73.

243. The wasting produced by ghosts (see below) seems to have been more rapid than that produced by curses.

244. Adamson, *RA* 87.153–154 interprets this phrase as referring to the rectus abdominus muscle.

245. Note also DPS XXII:28, 31–32 [AOAT 43.254].

246. The Aramaic cognate means "to sigh."

247. Another text that compares DÚR.GIG and "hand" of curse is *BAM* 49:32′–34′//*BAM* 579 iv 33–35//*BAM* 50 r. 7–10.

248. See *KAR* 73 obv. 1–5 (restored from 18–20).

249. Note also *BAM* 87:14–17.

250. Note also *BAM* 201:31′–32′ (conjunctival jaundice).

251. There is nothing in this reference to suggest botulism, rabies, or diabetes mellitus as offered in Fincke, *Augenleiden* 142. For possible ancient descriptions of rabies and diabetes, see Chapter 2 under ENVIRONMENTAL HAZARDS and Chapter 7 under DIABETES MELLITUS.

252. Labat, *TDP* 126 read this as "ghost." The text, however has NAM.ÉRIM: "curse."

253. The restoration is based on the surrounding entries in Tablet XIII.

254. *BAM* 174 r. 25 talks specifically about *ṣētu* "turning into" a curse. Note also *BAM* 579 i 40–41, 44//*BAM* 52:39–40, 44//*BAM* 67:1′–4′, 9′.

255. Note also DPS XXIII:2 (AOAT 43.272) (vomiting); *BAM* 201:23′–25′ (fever, bloating, and inability to eat); DPS XL A 119 = *TDP* 230:119 (choking, fever, and loss of appetite). Note also *BAM* 174 r. 15–16.

256. Mujais, *Am.J.Nephrology* 19.136–137 interprets this text to be a reference to generalized body swelling (anasarca). However, this interpretation is based on a faulty translation.

257. Lit. "he keeps changing his heads." Compare the expression "to change one's kidney" (meaning to roll over in bed). In this case, the patient is apparently lying on his back and rolling just the head rather than sleeping on his side as is implied by "changing" the kidney.

258. See also *BAM* 49:21′–24′.

259. That is, objects dedicated to the goddess to remind her of the supplicant's needs or to thank her for having healed him or her.

260. See the Introduction under Retrospective Diagnosis.

261. The N-stem of *saḫāru* in hendiadys with another verb implies that you "turn right around" and do something (often contrary to what you were doing before; for references, see *CAD* S 53–54). In this case, the infant seems to get better and then "turns right around" and gets sick again.

262. Since these references are sequenced, the restoration is fairly certain.

263. There may also be jaundice due to liver involvement; see below, DPS XL A 92, 93, 96 = *TDP* 228:92, 93, 96; DPS XL A 118 = *TDP* 230:118.

264. See also DPS XL A 75, 77 = *TDP* 226:75, 77.

265. Volk, *OrNS* 68.23 suggests that this is a reference to neonatal jaundice. However, the infant's yellow color is uneven (see Chapter 10), which makes jaundice an inappropriate diagnosis.

266. See also *STT* 89:202.

267. Cadelli, *Ktèma* 22.17 believes that the upper abdominal protrusion in this reference is due to a congenital malformation, rickets. Rickets is not a congenital malformation but an acquired deficiency disease (vitamin D). This condition occurs only rarely in sunny subtropical regions such as Mesopotamia. Moreover, the infant "hand" of Gula references appear to be sequenced (see Introduction under Retrospective Diagnosis) and other references in the sequence are not appropriate to this diagnosis.

268. See also DPS XL A 90 = *TDP* 228:90 (burning fever); DPS XL A 86 = *TDP* 226:86 (flushing and pallor). Compare also *BAM* 315 iii 39//*BAM* 314 obv. 4′–5′//*STT* 95 ii 63 (drawn face and chills but not an infant).

269. DPS XXXIII:106 [AOAT 43.358] (diarrhea). Other Gula references (DPS XL A 81, 83, 84 = *TDP* 226:81, 83, 84) are possibly complicating infections, but the descriptions are insufficient to suggest specific diseases.

270. See also DPS XL A 80 = *TDP* 226:80; DPS XL A 95, 96 = *TDP* 228:95, 96.

271. DPS XXXIII:103 (AOAT 43.357).

272. Kinnier Wilson, *Diseases in Antiquity* 205 and Cadelli, *Ktèma* 22.32 also suggest diphtheria for these infant "hand" of Gula references without, however, mentioning other possibilities. Volk, *OrNS* 68.27–28 mentions "leprosy" as a possibility for the infant *buʾšānu* references, while cautioning that the symptoms described are insufficient to confirm the diagnosis. In fact, many of the symptoms described (such as jaundice) are inappropriate and, since there is usually a long incubation period for leprosy, this disease is uncommon in the first four or five years of life.

273. According to the commentary, *SpTU* 1.41:5, BI.LU : *bu-šá-nu.*

274. Volk, *OrNS* 68.20 believes this text to be referring to tracheomalachia. Taken in isolation, this reference is compatible with this diagnosis, although the condition is infrequent. However, the infant "hand" of Gula references appear to be sequenced (see Introduction under Retrospective Diagnosis) and other references in the sequence are not appropriate.

275. See also DPS XL A 92, 94 = *TDP* 228:92, 94; DPS XL A 118 = *TDP* 230:118.

276. Volk, *OrNS* 68.22–23 interprets the "choking" as constipation secondary to meconium. Although we agree that "choking" can refer to tenesmus, laryngeal constriction is described in the immediately preceding reference. Kämmerer, RAI 44.168 considers this text to represent erythroblastosis fetalis (Rh factor incompatibility). Taken in isolation, this reference is compatible with this diagnosis. However, the infant "hand" of Gula references appear to be sequenced (see Introduction under Retrospective Diagnosis) and other references in the sequence are not appropriate to this diagnosis, as is tacitly admitted by Kämmerer, *RA* 94.71–75 when he states that it is "very difficult, if not impossible, to attribute any of the individual texts to erythroblastosis fetalis or neonatal jaundice." Nevertheless, he argues that if all of the "hand" of Gula texts could be made to refer to neonates in their first weeks of life, his diagnosis would be appropriate. This is then offered as "proof" that the term *infant* (LÚ.TUR) refers to neonates in their first weeks of life(!). LÚ.TUR can, in fact, refer to children as old as four years (see Chapter 17).

277. On this point, see also Römer, *Symb. Böhl* 311 n. 15; cf. Heeßel, AOAT 43.216.

278. Cadelli, *Ktèma* 22.17 believes that the upper abdominal protrusion in this reference is due to a congenital malformation, rickets. Rickets is not a congenital malformation but an acquired deficiency disease (vitamin D). This condition occurs only rarely in sunny subtropical regions such as Mesopotamia. Also rickets fails to explain the other findings in this sequence of references.

279. See also DPS XIII J 13 = *TDP* 126 iii 45. Volk, *OrNS* 68.22 n. 135 believes that the red and yellow color refers to a reddish-yellow jaundice caused by indirect bilirubin. The verb (*nadû*) used in this text, however, seems to refer to an uneven coloration of the skin (see p. 217). Cadelli, *Ktèma* 22.31 n. 143 interprets the red and yellow rash as jaundice with superimposed subcutaneous bleeding, and suggests congenital rubeola (measles) as the underlying cause. Since hepatitis and bleeding problems can occur in this condition, we agree that this would be a plausible cause if this were an isolated reference. However, these infant "hand" of Kūbu references appear to be sequenced (see Introduction under Retrospective Diagnosis) and other references in the sequence are not appropriate to this diagnosis.

280. See also DPS XIII B i 46′//F 7 = *TDP* 116 i 50′; DPS XIII G_2 2 = *TDP* 122 iii 10.

281. See also DPS XI A r. 29 = *TDP* 96 r. 29.

282. Lit. "his temple (feels) squeezed."

283. The commentary, *SpTU* 1.30 obv. 2 explains that AL.DU means *il-la-ku*: "they run."

284. Many ancient Mesopotamian names were miniature sentences that gave thanks to some divinity who patronized the name giver or his family. For example, Esarhaddon's name means "the god Aššur has given a brother" (to another male child already born).

285. Text E has: "his temples and his ears."

286. Note also [DIŠ UGU-*šú*] ⌜KÚM.KÚM⌝-*im* ŠU ^{d}*Nusku* "[If the top of his head] is continually feverish, 'hand' of Nusku" (DPS III A obv. 10). This is presumably what was meant. The text has ^{d}PA (long space) ^{d}×PA×KU. The latter sign appears as a KU with a tiny PA grafted onto the front of the bottom half of the sign and the two horizontal wedges of the DINGIR sharing a vertical with the spine of the KU.

287. The commentary *CT* 51.136:10–11 indicates that "hand" of his god could refer to the god of the patient's city.

288. The second reference below is attributed to Ištar in the parallel DPS XXII:14–15 [AOAT 43.252].

289. Possibly also describing a venereal disease is DPS XXXIII:84 [AOAT 43.357], which attributes the eruption of some sort of skin lesion in the inguinal region and on the base of the testicle to the personal goddess.

290. See above, Chapter 19.99n.

291. Note also DPS IV B obv. 27//E i 7 = *TDP* 34:27//*SpTU* 3.88 i 7.

292. Note also *BAM* 121:18.

293. DPS IX A 50//B obv. 49 = *TDP* 76:50.

294. DPS V G 11–12 = *TDP* 52 G 11–12 (see Chapter 9.73).

295. DPS X A obv. 28//B obv. 32 = *TDP* 84:28 (see Chapter 8.88).

296. DPS XIX/XX:109′a [AOAT 43.232].

297. DPS X A obv. 7//B obv. 7 = *TDP* 80:7; DPS XII D iii 37 = *TDP* 106 iii 37; DPS XIV C_2 iii 21//F 9; DPS XIV A_2 iv 8′//C_2 iii 33b = *TDP* 142 iv 8′; Böck, *Morphoskopie* 266:27–28.

298. DPS VII B obv. 2′ = *TDP* 64:41′ (coll.).

299. DPS XIV A ii 39//C ii 14 = *TDP* 134 ii 39.

300. DPS XXVIII:1–2 (AOAT 43.307); DPS XXVIII:7–8 (AOAT 43.308); DPS XXVIII:19 (AOAT 43.310).

301. Tsukimoto, *Priests and Officials* 199–200:61, 70.

302. Stol, *Epilepsy* 33–36 seems to suggest that "hand" of god in infants could be a single and specific modern disease (followed by Volk, *OrNS* 68.17 n. 104; cf. Cadelli, *Ktèma* 32.14 n. 27). He also seems to identify that disease with "spasms—so easily confused with epilepsy." Infantile spasms are not a single disease and were in any case usually attributed by the *āšipu* to Sîn and Ištar.

303. As, for example DPS IV A obv. 64//E ii 9 = *TDP* 38:64//*SpTU* 3.88 ii 9; DPS VI A obv. 22, 23 = *TDP* 56:22, 23.

304. For other references to fever, see DPS XVIII:2 (AOAT 43.218); DPS XXIII:11 (AOAT 43.272); DPS XXIII:16′ (AOAT 43.273).

305. See DPS IV B obv. 33//E i 13 = *TDP* 36:34//*SpTU* 3.88 i 13; DPS XIX/XX:100′ (AOAT 43.232).

306. See DPS XI A obv. 17//B 16 = *TDP* 90:17//*SpTU* 1.34:16.

307. See DPS XIII I 3–4 = *TDP* 122 iii 3–4; DPS XIX/XX:53′ (AOAT 43.229).

308. See DPS XIX/XX:108′b (AOAT 43.232).

309. See DPS XIX/XX:108′a (AOAT 43.232).

310. See DPS XIV C_2 iii 20//F 8.

311. Kinnier-Wilson, *Diseases in Antiquity* 726 suggests a diagnosis of "suicidal tendencies" for ZI.KU_5.RU.DA. However, there is nothing in any of the symptoms attributed to this form of sorcery that would suggest, let alone support, such an interpretation.

312. That this organ is the liver may be seen from Izbu comm. 203 (Leichty, *Izbu* 218): *ta-kal-tú* = *ga-bi-du*: "liver." See also Nougayrol, *RA* 44.3 and Goetze, *YOS* 10 p. 7. Note also *CAD* N 376a.

313. ⌜*i-ram-*⌝ coll. W. Lambert.

314. The passage has been collated.

315. These gods are by-forms of the plague and netherworld god Nergal, whose planet, Mars, was also associated with the kidneys in popular tradition according to a medical commentary (Civil, *JNES* 33.336–337:20–21).

316. See also DPS XII D iii 10, 11 = *TDP* 102 iii 10, 11. Note DPS XVII:19, 20 [AOAT 43.196].

317. Compare also DPS XVII:59 (AOAT 43.201); *STT* 93:106′–107′ (see Stol, *Epilepsy* 6) which mention another "deputy" of Anu, the "trembler," who caused people's lips to dribble while they slept.

318. Kinnier Wilson, *Iraq* 18.135, 144 interprets this to mean that he has an insatiable appetite, on the grounds that finding a condition in which the patient opens and closes his mouth for any other reason "would be too embarrassing a task." This does not seem sufficient grounds for such an inference.

319. As, for example, *STT* 95:16–18//*STT* 280 ii 1–3//*BAM* 205:19′–21′ (see Chapter 4.7) and DPS XIII B i 42′//F 4 = *TDP* 114 i 46′ (see Chapter 19.113).

320. DPS III A obv. 15–16//C obv. 6–7 = *TDP* 18:6–7 (see Chapter 7.17).

321. See DPS XXVI:85′ (AOAT 43.285).

322. See also DPS XIII B ii 22, 23, 24–25 = *TDP* 118 ii 22, 23, 24–25.

323. For this interpretation of ^{GIŠ}(NÍG).GIDRU/*ḫaṭṭu*: "scepter" as a pun for *ḫaṭṭu* from *ḫamāṭu*: "to burn," see *CAD* D 137 s.v. *dikšu* mng. 1a1′.

324. Text B has Ištar responsible for one side and Adad the other.

325. See above.

326. See also DPS IV B obv. 10 = *TDP* 32:10.

327. For this interpretation of ^{GIŠ}NÍG.GIDRU/*ḫaṭṭu*: "scepter" as a pun for *ḫaṭṭu* from *ḫamāṭu*: "to burn," see *CAD* D 137 s.v. *dikšu* mng. 1a1′.

328. See above, Chapter 19.99n.

329. For details, see Scurlock, *Ghost-Induced Illnesses*, Chapter 6.

330. This necessitated inclusion in the diagnostic/prognostic handbook of contrasting references (see Introduction) which explained the difference between the various syndromes attributed to the same causal agent, a sort of differential diagnosis for spirits. Examples of this include DPS III C obv. 34–35 = *TDP* 22:34–35 (Ištar's benign fever with headache versus Ištar's psychiatric headache), and DPS IV B obv. 7–11//D 7–11 = *TDP* 32:7–11 (ghost's alcoholic headache versus ghost's fatal headache) and (DPS IV B obv. 14–17 = *TDP* 34:14–17 (= ghost's alcoholic headache versus ghost's tension headache versus ghost's benign fever with headache).

331. For the suggestion that the association between goats and ghosts has to do with noises in the ears, see Heeßel, AOAT 43.223.

332. See also *BAM* 503 i 28′, 30′; cf. *STT* 281 i 21; Labat, *RSO* 32.112 v 13′; *BAM* 503 i 20′.

333. Kinnier Wilson, *Medical History* 34.187–188 interprets the "hand" of ghost in this text as referring to convulsions complicating a long-standing tapeworm infection. We see no basis for this conclusion.

334. See also DPS XIII B i 12′ = *TDP* 112 i 16′.

335. Another possible reference to Bornholm disease is DPS XIII B i 30′//D 3 = *TDP* 114 i 34′, which mentions a sore epigastrium that is interfering with the patient's breathing (he gets up and then has to sit down; see 8.29–8.30) in a context (affliction by a brother or sister's ghost) that suggests an epidemic.

336. See also *AMT* 76/1:15.

337. See also *AMT* 97/4:18; *BAM* 473 iv 16′; *AMT* 47/3 iii 20′.

338. Kinnier Wilson, *Diseases in Antiquity* 200 interprets painful neck as in this reference, pain in the back as in the preceding reference, and indeed all "hand" of ghost texts as descriptions of meningitis. However, neck stiffness is actually more prominent in meningitis than neck pain, so that nonfatal pain in the neck unaccompanied by other symptoms is unlikely to be meningitis. Also, although there are "hand" of ghost references which are suggestive of meningitis (see Chapter 13), many of the others have findings that are totally unrelated to this disease.

339. Labat, *TDP* 109 n. 194 (followed by *CAD* and *AHw*) understood [Z]U.GAM as a reading for *kurru*: "hip socket?" on the basis of the parallel between 108:23–24 and 236:49–50. However, ZU.GAM does not appear in 108:23–24. Where it does appear is in 108:19–20, which parallels 234:30–31. This parallel shows that the actual Akkadian reading for ZU.GAM is *šaḫātu*: "armpit."

340. Note also *BAM* 216:16′//*BAM* 217:1//*AMT* 97/5:9; *BAM* 216:29′–30′; *AMT* 96/1:14; *KAR* 56 r. 1. Note DPS XIV A_2 iv 6′//C_2 iv 32 = *TDP* 142 iv 6′ (one foot is shrunken).

341. These are *BAM* 482 ii 62′–63′, iii 1; cf. DPS IV B obv. 30–31//E i 10–11 = *TDP* 36:31–32//*SpTU* 3.88 i 10–11.

342. See also DPS IV A r. 5+A_4 4//B r. 17//E iv 1 = *TDP* 42 r. 38//*SpTU* 3.88 iv 1.

343. The commentary *STT* 403:21 explains this as *a-gap-pi* IGI^{II}-*šú*.

CHAPTER 20. PROGNOSTICS

1. It is important not to be confused by cases where the *āšipu* is being warned that the patient will die unless he speedily intervenes. In other words, we are here talking about cases where the "he will die" is *not* followed in short order by "in order for him not to die" you do x and y. Also not to be confused with hopeless cases is the not infrequent expression GÍD-*ma* GAM, which is often mistranslated as "he will linger and then die" or "after a long time he will die" (as, e.g., Labat, *TDP* 113:22′; Stol, *JEOL* 32.53). The correct translation is: "[if] it is prolonged, he will die"). The use of the enclitic *-ma* to indicate a subordinate "if" clause (Von Soden, *GAG* § 160 and Huehnergard, *A Grammar of Akkadian* § 7.4c) is very common in the diagnostic/prognostic handbook.

2. "If the ⌜sore⌝ [. . .], he will die; (the *āšipu*) shall not make a prognosis (as to his recovery). If [the sore . . .], (the *āšipu* may make a prognosis as to his recovery; to remove it. . ." (*BAM* 580 iii 4′–5′). Note also Labat, *MDP* 57.11 v 2′–20′, where two syndromes attributed to "hand" of Šulak appear side by side. The second syndrome has a treatment, whereas the first, whose prognosis is: "he will not get well; he will die" does not.

3. This rule applied also in Hippocratic, Vedic, and ancient Egyptian medicine. See Prioreschi, *Gesnerus* 49:341–350 who notes (pp. 345–346), "Far from being repugnant . . . witholding of treatment in hopeless cases should be considered rational and compassionate . . . By definition, to treat a disease that is untreatable . . . is ethically, medically, and logically unjustified."

4. See Herrero, *La thérapeutique* 35–37.

5. The number is restored from *Emar* VI/4.695:6.

6. DPS VIII (K 4080+) has *me-sír* IGI (coll.).

7. See also DPS XI A obv. 29, 31//B 28, 30 = *TDP* 92:29, 31//*SpTU* 1.34:28, 30; cf. DPS XV:17 (AOAT 43.151).

8. Note also DPS XXII:76 (AOAT 43.257) (the patient can answer questions).

9. See Adamson, *RA* 84.27–28.

10. The interpretation is based on restoration of the passage from DPS XI A obv. 45 = *TDP* 92:45 as suggested by Heeßel, AOAT 43.193.

11. See Adamson, *RA* 84.27–28.

12. See also DPS XIII B i 31′//D 5 = *TDP* 114 i 35′.

13. Compare DPS III A obv. 5 ("calm temples," meaning calm temporal blood vessels; see Chapter 3.12); DPS IV B obv. 5b–6 = *TDP* 32:5b–6 ("collapsed temples," meaning collapsed temporal blood vessels; see Chapter 14.24), and the relatively common expression "pulsating temples," meaning a sensation of pulsation in the temporal arteries (see Chapter 13.149).

14. Fincke, *Augenleiden* 152–153 believes this text to be describing cavernous sinus thrombosis. However, the reference does not provide enough information to reach this conclusion.

15. Note also DPS XI A r. 21 = *TDP* 96 r. 21 (coll.).

16. See *CAD* S 1a s.v. *sa*ʾ*ālu* mng. b.

17. Mujais, *Am.J.Nephrology* 19.137 suggests that this reference specifically describes the cardiac manifestations of fluid overload. However, this interpretation assumes that the *te-bi* refers to a literal elevation of the skin of the feet.

18. See also DPS X A obv. 34a = *TDP* 84:34a.

19. Also coming out of the mouth (DPS VI A obv. 32//C i 19 = TDP 56:32) or rising "up" (DPS VI C i 21 = *TDP* 56:34; cf. DPS X A obv. 32 = *TDP* 84:32a).

20. Also "violent" (DPS VI A obv. 33//C i 20 = *TDP* 56:33), "labored" (DPS VI A obv. 18//B_2 obv. 5//D 1 = *TDP* 56:18), "stifled" (DPS VI C i 22), or "massive and long" (DPS VI C i 23).

21. See also *SpTU* 3.86 obv. 9–10.
22. See also DPS X A obv. 30//B obv. 34 = *TDP* 84:30 (rapid breath and cramped insides).
23. Lit. "jumps."
24. The restoration is based on citation by the commentary *SpTU* 1.31:39.
25. For this interpretation of GIŠ(NÍG).GIDRU/*ḫaṭṭu*: "scepter" as a punning writing for *ḫaṭṭu*/*ḫanṭu* from *ḫamāṭu*, see *CAD* D 137 s.v. *dikšu* mng. 1a1′.
26. See Heeßel, AOAT 43.187.
27. For the reading, see ibid 190. The expression *ḫīṭu laššu* or *ḫīṭu yānu* appears not infrequently in Neo-Assyrian and Neo-Babylonian letters; it means something on the order of "no harm done" or "it is of no consequence." For references, see *CAD* Ḫ 210 s.v. *ḫīṭu* A mng. 1. For the interpretation, see also Ritter, *AS* 16.302 (quoting Landsberger).
28. Lit. "his temple (feels) squeezed."
29. See also DPS XVII:20 [AOAT 43.196).
30. The translation assumes that *ana* GÍR is equivalent to GÍR-*iš*, which means "quickly." For the latter expression, see Heeßel, AOAT 43.270.
31. See ibid. 224.
32. For the interpretation of GÍR-*iš* as *arḫiš*, see ibid. 270.
33. Ibid. 257, 261 interprets this as TAG-*ma* and translates "that patient was touched."
34. See also DPS XIV A ii 45//C ii 17 = *TDP* 136 ii 45.
35. Note also StBoT 36.23 r. 4′, 60:10.
36. For the reading, see Heeßel, AOAT 43.190. The expression *ḫīṭu laššu* or *ḫīṭu yānu* appears not infrequently in Neo-Assyrian and Neo-Babylonian letters; it means something on the order of "no harm done" or "it is of no consequence." For references, see *CAD* Ḫ 210 s.v. *ḫīṭu* A mng. 1. For the interpretation, see also Ritter, *AS* 16.302 (quoting Landsberger).
37. This was tentatively identified as malaria by Labat (see Heeßel, AOAT 43.212).
38. Text A has ŠUB (coll.); the TAK_4 found in text B would appear to fit the context much better.
39. Heeßel, AOAT 43.216 suggests that this refers to the patient and means something like "until the normal time (for the patient to go to bed)."
40. For the reading (but with *ba*), see ibid. 193.
41. 70 = U_4.MEŠ GÍD.DA.MEŠ (*STT* 400:46).
42. The N-stem of *saḫāru* in hendiadys with another verb implies that you "turn right around" and do something (often contrary to what you were doing before; for references, see *CAD* S 53–54). In this case, the infant seems to get better and then "turns right around" and gets sick again.
43. This reference appears in a sequence of texts all (or virtually all) of which end with "hand" of Gula, which makes the restoration fairly certain.
44. Compare DPS III A obv. 2//B 2 (see Chapter 13 with 13.286).
45. See Heeßel, AOAT 43.191.
46. See also DPS XVI:5 (AOAT 43.172).

CONCLUSION

1. This is described in *CT* 39.45:22 (Šumma Ālu); see 5.42.
2. DPS XXII:49–50 (AOAT 43.255) = *TDP* 182:49–50; see 13.252.

UNSOLVED PUZZLES APPENDIX

1. In both A and C, the word SAG.DU is omitted. However, the entries are aligned in such a way as to indicate that SAG.DU was meant to be read.
2. See also DPS III A obv. 27, 30//C obv. 18, 21 = *TDP* 20:18, 21.
3. Attia, *Histoire des Sciences Médicales* 34.8 believes that a diagnosis of venereal disease should only be made if the sexual organs are specifically mentioned. The sexual organs may, however, be free of findings in venereal diseases when the infection has spread to other parts of the body.
4. DPS XXII:12–13 (AOAT 43.252) (cf. DPS XIII B i 5′–6′ = *TDP* 110 i 9′–10′; see Chapter 4.35) and DPS XXII:14–15 (AOAT 43.252) (cf. DPS XIV A ii 34–36//C ii 9–10 = *TDP* 134 ii 34–36; see Chapter 4.34).

5. *Augenleiden* 88–89.

6. See Chapter 13 with 13.57–13.59.

7. See also DPS XII D iv 5–6 = *TDP* 106 iv 5–6.

8. The commentary *SpTU* 1.29:6′ suggests that "he has been sick for a month" was considered to mean that the illness was "going out" (resolving).

9. The passage has been collated. Also see the commentary *SpTU* 1.31:10.

10. See *CAD* K 175b; Labat, *Syria* 33.125 n. 11a.

11. Pangas, *Bull.Hist.Med.* 73.200 believes that this reference may be describing pituitary dwarfism.

12. The NÍG.GIG is visible on the tablet and on Ebeling's copy in *KMI.*

13. See also DPS IX A 37//B obv. 36 = *TDP* 74:37.

14. The reading follows CAD Ṣ 70b.

15. The opposite of "stand up"; the reference is presumably to the lack of response to light.

16. See also DPS XI A r. 18 = TDP 96 r. 18.

17. See also DPS IV A obv. 70–71+A_6 5–6//E ii 14–15 = *TDP* 38:70–71//*SpTU* 3.88 ii 14–15.

18. See also DPS III A r. 15′//C r. 38–39 = *TDP* 30:98–99; DPS IV A r. 2–3+A_4 1–2//B r. 15 = *TDP* 42 r. 35–36.

19. 70 = U_4.MEŠ GÍD.DA.MEŠ (*STT* 400:46).

20. Durand, *ARM* 26/1.573 restores "hand," but the traces favor "abdomen" and in any case pain in the hand is not a common complaint in heart attacks.

21. See also DPS XXII:18 (AOAT 43.253)

22. For this interpretation of ^{GIŠ}(NÍG).GIDRU/*ḫaṭṭu*: "scepter" as a pun for *ḫaṭṭu*/*ḫanṭu* from *ḫamāṭu*, see *CAD* D 137 s.v. *dikšu* mng. 1a1′.

23. See also DPS VII A obv. 8, 9 = *TDP* 62:9; DPS XI A obv. 36 = *TDP* 92:36.

24. This is the equivalent of Hebrew *peder*; see Milgrom, *Leviticus 1-16*.159.

25. Turning white and black is mentioned as a symptom in DPS IX A 17 = *TDP* 72:17 (see Chapter 19.321); DPS XL A 87 = *TDP* 226:87; and *STT* 89:202.

26. For the reading, see Heeßel, AOAT 43.164 (after a suggestion by Stol).

27. Kinnier Wilson, *Medical History* 34.187, 190, 195 argues that the patient must be an infant, but depression seems inappropriate in an infant.

28. Note also *BAM* 460:5′–10′ and Rm. 265:11′–12′, which are very fragmentary but which involve numbness. For the "bound" knees, see also *LKA* 102 obv. 18–22.

29. See also *BAM* 90:12′–13′.

30. In principle, this should have induced a seizure; see ND 5545:37 (Hulin, *Iraq* 21.46–53).

31. See also *BAM* 361:40–43.

32. Note *STT* 403 r. 44: *lu-ʾ-tum* = *kiš-pu*.

33. Wilhelm, StBoT 36.23 reads *a-na-at-m*[*e-e da-an* ŠÀ-*šu i-te-né*]-⸢*el*⸣-*la-a*. This would mean that the patient was having difficulty speaking and was nauseated.

34. Ibid. reads *lu-ʾa-*⸢*a*⸣-[*tu*] ŠU [^{d}*Išta*]*r*. For the restoration of the end of the line, see below.

35. For the reading, see Heeßel, AOAT 43.164.

36. For the reading, see ibid.163 (after a suggestion by Stol).

37. The passage has been collated. The copy has 150.

38. Restorations are based on DPS XVII:82 (AOAT 43.203); the passage has been collated.

39. See also DPS IX A 4 = *TDP* 72:4.

40. See Stol, *Epilepsy* 6.

41. See Heeßel, AOAT 43.188.

42. Ibid. 221 translates "sprinkled."

43. *MDP* 57.255.

CHART SHOWING THE ARRANGEMENT OF ENTRIES IN THE DIAGNOSTIC/PROGNOSTIC SERIES

1. Tablets I and II are omens taken by the *āšipu* on his way to the patient's house (see Chapter 1).

Bibliography

Abusch, Tzvi. "Dismissal by Authorities: *šuškunu* and Related Matters." *Journal of Cuneiform Studies* 37 (1985): 91–100.

———. "Magical and Medical Texts, Further Joins and Duplicates." *Revue d'Assyriologie* 78 (1984): 93–94.

———. *Mesopotamian Witchcraft*. Ancient Magic and Divination 5. Leiden: Styx, 2002.

———. *Toward a History and Understanding of Babylonian Witchcraft Beliefs and Literature*. Brown Judaic Studies 132. Atlanta: Scholars Press, 1987.

Adamson, P. B. "Anatomical and Pathological Terms in Akkadian: Part I." *Journal of the Royal Asiatic Society* 1974: 102–106.

———. "Anatomical and Pathological Terms in Akkadian: Part II." *Journal of the Royal Asiatic Society* 1979: 2–8.

———. "Anatomical and Pathological Terms in Akkadian: Part III." *Journal of the Royal Asiatic Society* 1981: 125–132.

———. "Anatomical and Pathological Terms in Akkadian: Part IV." *Journal of the Royal Asiatic Society* 1984: 3–18.

———. "An Assessment of Some Akkadian Medical Terms." *Revue d'Assyriologie* 87 (1993): 153–159.

———. "*Bubu'tu* and *birdu* Lesions in Akkadian Texts." *Journal of the Royal Asiatic Society* 1969: 10–12.

———. "The 'Bubu'tu' Lesion in Antiquity." *Medical History* 14 (1970): 313–318.

———. "Dracontiasis in Antiquity." *Medical History* 32 (1988): 204–209.

———. "Problems over Storing Food in the Ancient Near East." *Welt des Orients* 16 (1985): 5–15.

———. "Some Anatomical and Pathological Terms in Akkadian." *Revue d'Assyriologie* 84 (1990): 27–32.

———. "Some Infective and Allergic Conditions in Ancient Mesopotamia." *Revue d'Assyriologie* 82 (1988): 163–171.

———. "The Spread of Rabies into Europe and the Probable Origin of This Disease in Antiquity." *Journal of the Royal Asiatic Society* 1977: 140–144.

Admiralty War Staff Intelligence Division. *A Handbook of Mesopotamia*. Vol. 1. London: Admiralty War Staff, Intelligence Division, August 1916.

Alimurung, M., and C. Manahan. "Typhoid in Pregnancy." *Journal of the Philippine Medical Association* 28 (1952): 388.

Archi, Alfonso. "Lists of Tools." In *Vom alten Orient zum alten Testament: Festschrift für Wolfram Freiherrn von Soden zum 85. Geburtstag*. Ed. Manfried Dietrich and Oswald Loretz. Alter Orient und Altes Testament 240. Kevelaer/Neukirchen-Vluyn: Butzon & Bercker/Neukirchener Verlag, 1995.

Arnaud, Daniel. *Recherches au Pays d'Aštata Emar VI/3*. Recherche sur les Grandes Civilisations—Synthèse 18. Paris: Éditions Recherche sur les Civilizations, 1985–1986.

———. *Recherches au Pays d'Aštata Emar VI/4*. Recherche sur les Grandes Civilisations—Synthèse 28. Paris: Éditions Recherche sur les Civilizations, 1987.

The Assyrian Dictionary of the Oriental Institute of the University of Chicago. 26 vols. Chicago: The Oriental Institute, 1956– .

Attia, Annie. "A propos de la signification de šer'ânu dans les textes médicaux mésopotamiens: une question d'anatomie." *Histoire des Sciences Médicales* 34 (2000): 1–10.

———, and Gilles Buisson. "Du Bon Usage des Médecines en Assyriologie." *Le Journal des Médecines Cunéiformes* 4 (2004): 9–15.

Avalos, Hector. *Illness and Health Care in the Ancient Near East.* Harvard Semitic Museum Monographs 54. Atlanta: Scholars Press, 1995.

Becker, Kenneth L. *Principles and Practice of Endocrinology and Metabolism.* 2nd ed. Philadelphia: J. B. Lippincott, 1995.

Beckman, Gary. *Hittite Birth Rituals.* Studien zu den Boğazköy-Texten 29. Wiesbaden: Harrassowitz, 1983.

———, and Benjamin Foster. "Assyrian Scholarly Texts in the Yale Babylonian Collection." In *A Scientific Humanist: Studies in Memory of Abraham Sachs.* Ed. Erle Leichty, Maria deJ. Ellis, and Pamela Gerardi. Occasional Publications of the Samuel Noah Kramer Fund 9. Philadelphia: The University Museum, 1988. 1–26.

Beeson, Paul B., and Walsh McDermott. *Textbook of Medicine.* 14th ed. Philadelphia: W. B. Saunders, 1975.

Bellakhdar, Jamal. *Médicine traditionelle et toxicologie ouest-sahariennes. Contribution à l'étude de la pharmacopée marocaine.* Rabat: Éditions Techniques Nord-Africaines, 1978.

Bennett, J. Claude, and Fred Plum. *Cecil Textbook of Medicine.* 20th ed. Philadelphia: W. B. Saunders, 1996.

Biggs, Robert D. "Conception, Contraception, and Abortion in Ancient Mesopotamia." In *Wisdom, Gods and Literature: Studies in Assyriology in Honour of W. G. Lambert.* Ed. Andrew R. George and Irving L. Finkel. Winona Lake: Eisenbrauns, 2000. 1–13.

———. "Ergotism and Other Mycotoxicoses in Ancient Mesopotamia?" *Aula Orientalis* 9 (1991): 15–21.

———. "Kopfkrankheiten." In *Reallexikon der Assyriologie* 6. Berlin: Walter de Gruyter, 1981–1983. 210–211.

———. "Lepra." In *Reallexikon der Assyriologie* 6. Berlin: Walter de Gruyter, 1981–1983. 605.

———. "Medicine in Ancient Mesopotamia." *Journal of the History of Science* 8 (1969): 94–105.

———. "Medicine, Surgery, and Public Health in Ancient Mesopotamia." In *Civilizations of the Ancient Near East.* Ed. Jack M. Sasson. New York: Charles Scribner's Sons, 1995. 1911–1924.

———. "Medizin A, In Mesopotamien." In *Reallexikon der Assyriologie* 7. Berlin: Walter de Gruyter, 1987–1990. 623–629.

———. Review of *Studien zur altorientallischen und griechischen Heilkunde,* by Dietlinde Golz. *Journal of Near Eastern Studies* 36 (1977): 303–304.

———. Review of *The Healing Hand,* by Guido Majno. *Journal of Near Eastern Studies* 36 (1977): 302–303.

———. Review of *Medizinische Omina aus Ḫattuša in akkadischer Sprache,* Studien zu den Boğazköy-Texten 36, by Gernot Wilhelm. *Journal of Near Eastern Studies* 56 (1997): 230–231.

———. *ŠÀ.ZI.GA: Ancient Mesopotamian Potency Incantations.* Texts from Cuneiform Sources 1. Locust Valley: J. J. Augustin, 1967.

Black, Jeremy, and Donald J. Wiseman. *Literary Texts from the Temple of Nabû.* Cuneiform Texts from Nimrud 4. London: British School of Archaeology in Iraq, 1996.

Boardmen, John, et al. *The Cambridge Ancient History.* 2nd ed. Vol. III/2. Cambridge: Cambridge University Press, 1991.

Böck, Barbara. *Die babylonisch-assyrische Morphoskopie.* Archiv für Orientforschung, Beiheft 27. Horn: Ferdinand Berger & Söhne, 2000.

Boissier, Alfred. *Documents assyriens relatif aux présages.* Paris: E. Bouillon, 1894–1899.

Böllenrücher, Josef. *Gebete und Hymnen an Nergal.* Leipziger semitische Studien 1/6. Leipzig: J. C. Hinrichs, 1904.

Borger, Rykle. *Assyrisch-babylonische Zeichenliste.* Alter Orient und Altes Testament 33. Kevelaer/Neukirchen-Vluyn: Butzon & Bercker/Neukirchener Verlag, 1978.

———. "Die erste Teiltafel der ZI-PÀ-Beschwörungen (ASKT 11)." In *Lišān Mitḫurti: Festschrift Wolfram Freiherr von Soden.* Ed. Wolfgang Röllig. Alter Orient und Altes Testament 1. Kevelaer/Neukirchen-Vluyn: Butzon & Bercker/Neukirchener Verlag, 1969. 1–22.

———. "Gott Marduk und Gott-König Šulgi als Propheten: Zwei prophetische Texte." *Bibliotheca Orientalis* 28 (1971): 3–24.

———. "Vier Grenzsteinurkunden Merodachbaladans I." *Archiv für Orientforschung* 23 (1970): 1–26.

Bottéro, Jean. *Textes culinaires Mésopotamien.* Mesopotamian Civilizations 6. Winona Lake: Eisenbrauns, 1995.

Bradley, Walter G., et al. *Neurology in Clinical Practice.* Boston: Butterworth-Heinemann, 1991.

Brown, David. *Mesopotamian Planetary Astronomy-Astrology*. Cuneiform Monographs 18. Groningen: Styx, 2000.
Butler, Sally. *Mesopotamian Conceptions of Dreams and Dream Rituals*. Alter Orient und Altes Testament 258. Münster: Ugarit-Verlag, 1998.
Butz, Kilian. "Altbabylonishe Beschwörungen um den 'Blasensprung' bei Graviden herbeizuführen." *Oriens Antiquus* 21 (1982): 221–226.
Cadelli, Danielle. "Lorsque l'enfant paraît . . . malade." In Enfance et Éducation dans le Proche-orient Ancien. Ed. Brigitte Lion, Cécile Michel, and Pierre Villard. *Ktèma* 22 (1997): 11–33.
Campbell Thompson, Reginald. *Assyrian Medical Texts from the Originals in the British Museum*. Oxford: Humphrey Milford/Oxford University Press, 1923.
———. "Assyrian Medical Texts." *Proceedings of the Royal Society of Medicine: History of Medicine Section* 17 (1924): 2–34.
———. "Assyrian Prescriptions for Diseases of the Feet." *Journal of the Royal Asiatic Society* 1937: 265–286, 413–432.
———. "Assyrian Prescriptions for Diseases of the Urine." *Babyloniaca* 14 (1934): 57–151.
———. "A Babylonian Explanatory Text." *Journal of the Royal Asiatic Society* 1924: 452–457.
———. *Cuneiform Texts from Babylonian Tablets in the British Museum* 14. London: British Museum, 1902.
———. *Cuneiform Texts from Babylonian Tablets in the British Museum* 17. London: British Museum, 1903.
———. *Cuneiform Texts from Babylonian Tablets in the British Museum* 23. London: British Museum, 1906.
———. *A Dictionary of Assyrian Botany*. London: The British Academy, 1949.
Cavigneaux, Antoine. "A Scholar's Library in Meturan? With an Edition of the Tablet H 72 (Textes de Tell Haddad VII)." In *Mesopotamian Magic: Textual, Historical and Interpretative Perspectives*. Ed. Tzvi Abusch and Karel van der Toorn. Ancient Magic and Divination 1. Groningen: Styx, 1999. 251–273.
———. "Un texte médical bilingue." *Notes Assyriologiques Brèves et Utilitaires* 1988 no. 24.
———, and Farouk Al-Rawi. "Charmes de Sippar et de Nippur." In *Cinquante-deux réflexions sur le proche-orient ancien offertes en hommages à Léon De Meyer*. Mesopotamian History and Environment Occasional Publications 2. Leuven: Peeters, 1994. 73–89.
———, and ———. "New Sumerian Literary Texts from Tell Haddad (Ancient Meturan): A First Survey." *Iraq* 55 (1993): 91–105.
———, and ———. "Textes magiques de Tell Haddad (Textes de Tell Haddad II)." *Zeitschrift für Assyriologie* 83 (1993): 170–205.
Chadwick, John, and W. N. Mann. *The Medical Works of Hippocrates*. Oxford: Blackwell, 1950.
Charpin, Dominique. *Le Clergé d'Ur au siècle d'Hammurabi*. Genève: Droz, 1986.
Civil, Miguel. "Enlil and Ninlil: The Marriage of Sud." *Journal of the American Oriental Society* 103 (1983): 43–66.
———. "Medical Commentaries from Nippur." *Journal of Near Eastern Studies* 33 (1974): 329–338.
———. "Une nouvelle prescription médicale sumérienne." *Revue d'Assyriologie* 55 (1961): 91–94.
———. "Prescriptions médicales sumériennes." *Revue d'Assyriologie* 54 (1960): 57–72.
Clay, Albert T. *Babylonian Records in the Library of J. Pierpont Morgan* 4. New Haven: Yale University Press, 1923.
———. *Documents from the Temple Archives of Nippur Dated in the Reigns of Cassite Rulers*. Publications of the Babylonian Section 2/2. Philadelphia: University Museum, 1912.
Coleman, Mary. "Hyperthyroidism in Ancient Mesopotamia." *Thryoid* 12 (2002): 799.
Collins, Timothy J. *Natural Illness in Babylonian Medical Incantations*. Ph.D. diss., University of Chicago, 1999.
Cunningham, Graham. *Deliver me from Evil: Mesopotamian Incantations 2500-1500 B.C.* Studia Pohl: Series Maior 17. Rome: Pontifical Biblical Institute, 1997.
Dandamayev, Mohammed A. "About Life Expectancy in Babylonia in the First Millennium B.C." In *Death in Mesopotamia: Papers Read at the XXVI*[e] Rencontre assyriologique internationale. Ed. Bendt Alster. Mesopotamia 8. Copenhagen: Akademisk Forlag, 1980. 183–186.
Deller, Karlheinz. "*gurrudu* 'kahlköpfig' und *qerdu* 'abgeschabte' Wolle." *Notes Assyriologiques Brèves et Utilitaires* 1992 no. 79.
———. "*kurru* 'Mehlbrei.'" *Orientalia* N.S. 54 (1985): 327–330.
Denton, George B. "A New Interpretation of a Well Known Assyrian Letter." *Journal of Ancient Near Eastern Studies* 2 (1943): 314–315.
van Dijk, Jan. "Une incantation accompagnant la naissance de l'homme." *Orientalia* N.S. 44 (1975): 52–79.
———, Albrecht Goetze, and Mary I. Hussey. *Early Mesopotamian Incantations and Rituals*. Yale Oriental Series 11. New Haven: Yale University Press, 1985.

Dossin, Georges. *Archives Royales de Mari 10: Correspondance Féminine.* Paris: Librairie Orientaliste Paul Geuthner, 1978.

Dougherty, Raymond Philip. *Archives from Erech.* Goucher College Cuneiform Inscriptions. 2 vols. New Haven: Yale University Press, 1923, 1933.

Driver, Godfrey R., and John C. Miles. *The Assyrian Laws.* Oxford: Clarendon Press, 1935.

———, and ———. *The Babylonian Laws.* 2 vols. Oxford: Clarendon Press, 1952, 1955.

Drower, Ethel. "Woman and Taboo in Iraq." *Iraq* 5 (1938): 106–117.

Dunham, Sally. "The Monkey in the Middle." *Zeitschrift für Assyriologie* 75 (1985): 234–264.

Durand, Jean-Marie. *Documents cunéiformes de la quatrième section de l'École pratique des hautes études.* Geneva: Librairie Droz, 1982.

———. "Maladies et médecins." *Archives Royales de Mari* XXVI/1. Paris: Éditions Recherche sur les Civilisations, 1988. 543–584.

———. "Trois études sur Mari I.9: Maladies." *Mari, Annales de Recherches Interdisciplinaires* 3 (1984): 143–146.

Ebeling, Erich. "Anuskrankheiten." In *Reallexikon der Assyriologie* 1. Berlin: Walter de Gruyter, 1928–1932. 117–118.

———. "Augenkrankheiten." In *Reallexikon der Assyriologie* 1. Berlin: Walter de Gruyter, 1928–1932. 313–314.

———. "Aussatz." In *Reallexikon der Assyriologie* 1. Berlin: Walter de Gruyter, 1928–1932. 321.

———. "Epilepsie." In *Reallexikon der Assyriologie* 2. Berlin: Walter de Gruyter, 1933–1938. 409.

———. "Keilschrifttafeln medizinischen Inhalts." *Archiv für Geschichte der Medizin* 13 (1921): 1–42, 129–145.

———. "Keilschrifttafeln medizinischen Inhalts." *Archiv für Geschichte der Medizin* 14 (1922): 26–47, 65–78.

———. *Keilschrifttexte aus Assur religiösen Inhalts.* Wissenschaftliche Veröffentlichungen der Deutschen Orient-Gesellschaft 28, 34. Leipzig: J. C. Hinrichs, 1919–1923.

———. *Keilschrifttexte Medicinischen Inhalts.* Berlin: Erich Ebeling, 1922.

———. "Sammlungen von Beschwörungsformeln." *Archiv Orientální* 21 (1953): 357–423.

———, and Franz Köcher. *Literarische Keilschrifttexte aus Assur.* Berlin: Akademie-Verlag, 1953.

Edel, Elmar. *Die ägyptisch-hethitische Korrespondenz.* 2 vols. Abhandlungen der Rhenisch-Westfälischen Akademie der Wissenschaften 77. Opladen: Westdeutscher Verlag, 1994.

Edzard, Dietz Otto. "Keilschrift." In *Reallexikon der Assyriologie* 5. Berlin: Walter de Gruyter, 1976–1980. 544–568.

Ellison, Rosemary. "Diet in Mesopotamia: The Evidence of The Barley Ration Texts." *Iraq* 43 (1981): 35–45.

Englund, Robert K. "There's a Rat in my Soup," *Altorientalische Forschungen* 22 (1995): 37–55.

Fader, Robert C., and Michael R. McGinnis. "Infections Caused by Dermatiaceous Fungi: *Chromoblastomycosis* and *Phaeohyphomycosis.*" *Infectious Disease Clinics of North America* 2/4 (Dec. 1988): 925–937.

Fales, Frederick Mario, and J. Nicholas Postgate. *Imperial Administrative Records, Part 1.* State Archives of Assyria 7. Helsinki: Helsinki University Press, 1992.

Falkenstein, Adam. *Literarische Keilschrifttexte aus Uruk.* Berlin: Staatlichen Museen, 1931.

———. "Sumerische Beschwörungen aus Boğazköy." *Zeitschrift für Assyriologie* 45 (1939): 8–41.

Farber, Gertrud. "Another Old Babylonian Childbirth Incantation." *Journal of Near Eastern Studies* 43 (1984): 311–316.

Farber, Walter. "Akkadisch 'Blind.'" *Zeitschrift für Assyriologie* 75 (1985): 210–233.

———. *Beschwörungsrituale an Ištar und Dumuzi.* Wiesbaden: Franz Steiner, 1977.

———. "Early Akkadian Incantations: Addenda et Subtrahenda." *Journal of Near Eastern Studies* 43 (1984): 69–70.

———. "*Mannam lušpur ana Enkidu*: Some New Thoughts about an Old Motif." *Journal of Near Eastern Studies* 49 (1990): 299–321.

———. "*māra/ āt Anim* oder: Des Anu Töchterlein (In Singular und Plural, Text und Bild)." In *Festschrift für Rykle Borger zu seinem 65. Geburtstag am 24. Mai 1994.* Ed. Stefan Maul. Cuneiform Monographs 10. Groningen: Styx, 1998. 59–69.

——— Review of *Die babylonisch-assyrische Medizin in Texten und Untersuchungen* 5–6, by Franz Köcher. *Bibliotheca Orientalis* 39 (1982): 592–599.

———. *Schlaf, Kindchen, Schlaf!: Mesopotamische Baby-Beschwörungen und -Rituale.* Mesopotamian Civilizations 2. Winona Lake: Eisenbrauns, 1989.

———. "Vorzeichen aus der Waschschüssel." *Orientalia* N.S. 58 (1989): 86–101.

———. "(W)ardat-lilî(m)." *Zeitschrift für Assyriologie* 79 (1989): 14–25.

———. "Zur älteren akkadischen Beschwörungsliteratur." *Zeitschrift für Assyriologie* 71 (1981): 51–72.

———, and Helmut Freydank. "Zwei medizinische Texte aus Assur." *Altorientalische Forschungen* 5 (1977): 255–261.

Feigin, Ralph D., and James D. Cherry. *Textbook of Pediatric Infectious Diseases.* 4th ed. Philadelphia: W. B. Saunders, 1998.

Fincke, Jeanette. *Augenleiden nach keilschriftlichen Quellen.* Würzburger medizinhistorische Forschungen 70. Würzburg: Königshausen & Neumann, 2000.

Finet, André. "Les médecins au royaume de Mari." *Annuaire de l'Institut de Philologie et d'Histoire Orientales et Slaves* 14 (1954–1957): 123–144.

Finkel, Irving L. "The Crescent Fertile." *Archiv für Orientforschung* 27 (1980): 37–52.

———. "Magic and Medicine at Meskene." *Notes Assyriologiques Brèves et Utilitaires* 1999 no. 30.

———. "*Muššuʾu, Qutāru* and the Scribe Tanittu-Bēl." *Aula Orientalis* 9 (1991): 91–104.

——— "On Late Babylonian Medical Training." In *Wisdom, Gods and Literature: Studies in Assyriology in Honour of W. G. Lambert.* Ed. Andrew R. George and Irving L. Finkel. Winona Lake: Eisenbrauns, 2000. 137–223.

———. "On Some Dog, Snake and Scorpion Incantations." In *Mesopotamian Magic: Textual, Historical and Interpretative Perspectives.* Ed. Tzvi Abusch and Karel van der Toorn. Ancient Magic and Divination 1. Groningen: Styx, 1999. 213–250.

———. "On TDP Tablets XXIX and XXXI, and the Nature of SA.GIG." *Journal of Cuneiform Studies* 46 (1994): 87–88.

———. "A Study in Scarlet. Incantations against Samana." In *Festschrift für Rykle Borger zu seinem 65. Geburtstag am 24. Mai 1994.* Ed. Stefan Maul. Cuneiform Monographs 10. Groningen: Styx, 1998. 71–106.

Furlani, Giuseppe. "Sur la palmomantique chez les Babyloniens et les Assyriens." *Archiv Orientální* 17/1 (1949): 255–269.

Gadd, Cyril J. *Assyrian Sculptures in the British Museum: From Shalmaneser III to Sennacherib.* London: The British Museum, 1938.

Geller, Mark J. *Forerunners to Udug-Ḫul.* Freiburger Alt-orientalische Studien 12. Wiesbaden: Franz Steiner, 1985.

———. "Hippocrates, Galen and the Jews: Renal Medicine in the Talmud." *American Journal of Nephrology* 22 (2002): 101–106.

———. "An Incantation against Curses." In *Festschrift für Rykle Borger zu seinem 65. Geburtstag am 24. Mai 1994.* Ed. Stefan Maul. Cuneiform Monographs 10. Groningen: Styx, 1998. 127–140.

———. "Incipits and Rubrics." In *Wisdom, Gods and Literature: Studies in Assyriology in Honour of W. G. Lambert.* Ed. Andrew R. George and Irving L. Finkel. Winona Lake: Eisenbrauns, 2000. 225–257.

———. "The Last Wedge." *Zeitschrift für Assyriologie* 87 (1997): 43–95.

———. "A New Piece of Witchcraft." In *DUMU-É-DUB-BA-A Studies in Honor of Åke W. Sjöberg.* Ed. Hermann Behrens, Darlene Loding, and Martha T. Roth. Occasional Publications of the Samuel Noah Kramer Fund 11. Philadelphia: The University Museum, 1989. 193–205.

———. "A Recipe against ŠU.GIDIM." In *28. Rencontre assyriologique internationale in Wien.* Archiv für Orientforschung Beiheft 19. Horn: Ferdinand Berger & Söhne, 1982. 192–197.

———. Review of *La thérapeutique Mésopotamienne,* by Pablo Herrero. *Bibliotheca Orientalis* 43 (1986): 738–744.

———. Review of *Die babylonisch-assyrische Medizin in Texten und Untersuchungen* 6, by Franz Köcher. *Zeitschrift für Assyriologie* 74 (1984): 294–297.

———. "West Meets East: Early Greek and Babylonian Diagnosis." *Archiv für Orientforschung* 48–49 (2001–2002): 50–75.

———, and S. L. Cohen. "Kidney and Urinary Tract Disease in Ancient Babylonia, with Translations of the Cuneiform Sources." *Kidney International* 47 (1995): 1811–1815.

Goetze, Albrecht. "An Incantation against Diseases." *Journal of Cuneiform Studies* 9 (1955): 8–18.

———. *Old Babylonian Omen Texts.* Yale Oriental Series 10. New Haven: Yale University Press, 1947.

———. "Texts and Fragments 6." *Journal of Cuneiform Studies* 2 (1948): 305–306.

Goldsmith, Robert, and Donald Heyneman. *Tropical Medicine and Parasitology.* Norwalk: Appleton and Lange, 1989.

Golz, Dietlinde. *Studien zur altorientalischen und griechischen Heilkunde.* Sudhoffs Archiv Beiheft 16. Wiesbaden: Franz Steiner, 1974.

Gorbach, Sherwood L., John G. Bartlett, and Neil R. Backlow. *Infectious Diseases.* Philadelphia: W. B. Saunders, 1998.

Grmek, Mirko D. *Diseases in the Ancient Greek World.* Tr. Mireille and Leonard Muellner. Baltimore: Johns Hopkins University Press, 1989.

Guichard, Michael. "Présages fortuits à Mari (Copies et ajouts à ARMT XXVI/1)." *Mari Annales de Recherches Interdisciplinaires* 8 (1997): 305–328.

Gurney, Oliver R., and Jacob J. Finkelstein. *The Sultantepe Tablets* 1. Occasional Publications of the British Institute of Archaeology at Ankara 3. London: British Institute of Archaeology at Ankara, 1957.

———. and Peter Hulin, *The Sultantepe Tablets* 2. Occasional Publications of the British Institute of Archaeology at Ankara 7. London: British Institute of Archaeology at Ankara, 1964.

———. *Ur Excavations Texts 7: Middle Babylonian Legal Documents and Other Texts.* London: British Museum, 1974.

Gwaltney, W. C. *The Pennsylvania Old Assyrian Texts.* Hebrew Union College Annual: Supplement 3. Cincinnati: Hebrew Union College, 1983.

Hallo, William H. "More Incantations and Rituals from the Yale Babylonian Collection." In *Mesopotamian Magic: Textual, Historical and Interpretative Perspectives.* Ed. Tzvi Abusch and Karel van der Toorn. Ancient Magic and Divination 1. Groningen: Styx, 1999. 275–289.

Handcock, Percy. *Cuneiform Texts from Babylonian Tablets in the British Museum* 31. London: British Museum, 1911.

Harris, Rivkah. *Gender and Aging in Mesopotamia.* Norman: University of Oklahoma Press, 2000.

Harrison, Tinsley, Eugene Braunwald, et al. *Harrison's Principles of Internal Medicine.* 11th ed. New York: McGraw-Hill, 1987.

Harper, Robert Francis. *Assyrian and Babylonian Letters belonging to the K. Collection of the British Museum.* Chicago: University of Chicago Press, 1892–1914.

Haupt, Paul. *Akkadische und Sumerische Keilschrifttexte.* Leipzig: J. C. Hinrichs, 1881.

Haussperger, Martha. "Einige Anmerkungen zum 'Fachbuch der Abdominalerkrankungen.'" In *Variatio Delectat: Iran under der Westen: Gedenkschrift für Peter Calmeyer.* Ed. Reinhard Dittmann et al. Alter Orient und Altes Testament 272. Münster: Ugarit Verlag, 2000. 343–346.

———. "Einige medizinische Anmerkungen zum Text BAM 3." In *Studi sul vicino oriente antico dedicati alla memoria di Luigi Cagni.* Ed. Simonetta Graziani et al. Instituto Universitario Orientale Dipartimento di Studi Asiatici, Series Minor 61. Naples: Instituto Universitario Orientale, 2000. 439–450.

———. "Einige medizinische Anmerkungen zum Text *BAM* 393." *Collectanea Orientalia: Histoire arts de l'espace et industrie de la terre: Études offertes hommage à Agnès Spycket.* Ed. H. Gasche and Barthel Hrouda. Civilisations du Proche-Orient: Archeologie et Environnement 3. Neuchâtel: Recherches et publications, 1996. 129–132.

———. "Die mesopotamische Medizin und ihre Ärtze aus heutiger Sicht." *Zeitschrift für Assyriologie* 87 (1997): 196–218.

Hawkins, J. David. "Eunuchs among the Hittites." In *Sex and Gender in the Ancient Near East.* Ed. Simo Parpola and Robert M. Whiting. Proceedings of the XLVIIE Rencontre Assyriologique Internationale. Helsinki: The Neo-Assyrian Text Corpus Project, 2002. 217–233.

Heeßel, Nils P. *Babylonisch-assyrische Diagnostik.* Alter Orient und Altes Testament 43. Münster: Ugarit Verlag, 2000.

———. "Diagnostik in Babylonien und Assyrien." *Medizin Historisches Journal* 36 (2001): 247–266.

———. "Ein neubabylonisches Rezept zur Beraushung und Ausnüchterung." In *Mining the Archives: Festschrift for Christopher Walker.* Ed. Cornelia Wunsch. Babylonische Archive 1. Dresden: Islet, 2002. 99–106.

Heimpel, Wolfgang. "Maus." In *Reallexikon der Assyriologie* 7. Berlin: Walter de Gruyter, 1987–1990. 605–609.

Hélias, Pierre-Jakez. *The Horse of Pride: Life in a Breton Village.* Tr. June Guicharnaud. New Haven: Yale University Press, 1975.

Herrero, Pablo. "Une tablette médicale Assyrienne inédite." *Revue d'Assyriologie* 69 (1975): 41–53.

———. *La thérapeutique Mésopotamienne.* Éditions Recherche sur les civilizations, Mémoire 48. Paris: Éditions Recherche sur les civilizations, 1984.

Hojgaard, Karen. "Dilmun's Ancient Teeth." *Dilmun, Journal of the Bahrain Historical and Archaeological Society* 11 (1983): 11–13.

Holma, Harri. *Kleine Beiträge zum assyrischen Lexikon.* Annales Academiae Scientiarum Fennicae B 7/II. Helsinki: Finnischen Literaturgesellschaft, 1913.
Holmes, King K., et al. *Sexually Transmitted Diseases.* 3rd ed. New York: McGraw-Hill, 1999.
Hopkins, A., Simon D. Shorvon, and Gregory Cascino. *Epilepsy.* 2nd ed. New York: Chapman and Hall Medical, 1995.
Huehnergard, John. *A Grammar of Akkadian.* Harvard Semitic Museum Studies 45. Atlanta: Scholars Press, 1997.
Hulin, Peter. "A Hemerological Text from Nimrud." *Iraq* 21 (1959): 42–53.
Hunger, Hermann. "Noch einmal: Wachsstum eines Kindes vor der Geburt." *Notes Assyriologiques Brèves et Utilitaires* 1996 no. 39.
———. *Spätbabylonische Texte aus Uruk 1.* Ausgrabungen der Deutschen Forschungsgemeinschaft in Uruk-Warka 9. Berlin: Mann, 1976.
———. "Zur Ordnung der diagnostischen Omenserie." *Zeitschrift für Assyriologie* 65 (1975): 63–68.
———. "Wachsstum eines Kindes vor der Geburt." *Notes Assyriologiques Brèves et Utilitaires* 1994 no. 34.
Jacobsen, Thorkild. "Notes on Nintur." *Orientalia* N.S. 42 (1973): 274–298.
Jahier, Henri, and Noureddine Abdelkader, tr. ʿArib Ibn Saʿid al-Katib al Qurtʾubi. *Le Livre de la génération du foetus et le traitement des femmes enceintes et des nouveau-nés.* Algiers: Librairie Ferraris, 1956.
Jastrow, Morris. "An Assyrian Medical Tablet in the Possession of the College of Physicians." *Transactions of the College of Physicians of Philadelphia* (1913): 365–400.
Jensen, Peter. *Assyrisch-babylonische Mythen und Epen.* Keilschrift Bibliothek 6/1. Berlin: Reuther and Reichard, 1901.
Jones, Levy M. "Maps of Birth Defect Occurrences in the U.S." *Teratology* 48 (1993): 551–646.
Kämmerer, Thomas R. "Die erste Pockendiagnose stammt aus Babylonien." *Ugarit-Forschungen* 27 (1995): 129–168.
———. "Pathologisch Veränderungen an Leber und Galle. Das Krankheitsbild der Gelbsucht." *Revue d'Assyriologie* 94 (2000): 57–93.
———. "Zur Kenntnis der Erkrankungen von Leber und Galle im alten vorderen Orient." In *Landscapes: Territories Frontiers and Horizons in the Ancient Near East: Papers presented to the XLIV Rencontre Assyriologique Internationale.* Ed. Lucio Milano et al. History of the Ancient Near East Monographs 3. Padova: Sargon, 1999. 165–169.
King, Leonard W. *Babylonian Magic and Sorcery.* London: Luzac, 1896.
Kinnier Wilson, J. V. "Diseases of Babylon: An Examination of Selected Texts." *Journal of the Royal Society of Medicine* 89 (1996): 135–140.
———. "Gleanings from the Iraq Medical Journals." *Journal of Near Eastern Studies* 27 (1968): 243–247.
———. "An Introduction to Babylonian Psychiatry." In *Studies in Honor of Benno Landsberger on his Seventy-Fifth Birthday.* Assyriological Studies 16. Chicago: University of Chicago, 1965. 289–298.
———. "Leprosy in Ancient Mesopotamia." *Revue d'Assyriologie* 60 (1966): 47–58 with addendum *Revue d'Assyriologie* 61 (1967): 189–190.
———. "Medicine in the Land and Times of the Old Testament." In *Studies in the Period of David and Solomon and Other Essays.* Ed. Tomoo Ishida. Winona Lake: Eisenbrauns, 1982. 337–365.
———. "Mental Diseases of Ancient Mesopotamia." In *Diseases in Antiquity.* Ed. Don Brothwell and A. T. Sandison. Springfield, Ill.: Charles C. Thomas, 1967. 723–733.
———. "The Nimrud Catalogue of Medical and Physiognomical Omina." *Iraq* 24 (1962): 52–62.
———. "Organic Diseases of Ancient Mesopotamia." In *Diseases in Antiquity.* Ed. Don Brothwell and A. T. Sandison. Springfield, Ill.: Charles C. Thomas, 1967. 191–208.
———. "The *samānu* Disease in Babylonian Medicine." *Journal of Near Eastern Studies* 53 (1994): 111–115.
———. "Two Medical Texts from Nimrud." *Iraq* 18 (1956): 130–146.
———. "Two Medical Texts from Nimrud (Continued)." *Iraq* 19 (1957): 40–49.
———, and E. H. Reynolds. "Texts and Documents. Translation and Analysis of a Cuneiform Text Forming Part of a Babylonian Treatise on Epilepsy." *Medical History* 34 (1990): 185–198.
Köcher, Franz. "Ein akkadischer medizinischer Schülertext aus Boğazköy." *Archiv für Orientforschung* 16 (1952–1953): 47–56.
———. *Die babylonisch-assyrische Medizin in Texten und Untersuchungen.* 6 vols. Berlin: W. de Gruyter, 1963–1980.

———. *Keilschrifturkunden aus Boghazköi* 37. Berlin: Akademie-Verlag, 1953.
———. *Keilschrifttexte zur assyrisch-babylonischen Drogen- und Pflanzenkunde.* Deutsche Akademie der Wissenschaften zu Berlin, Institut für Orientforschung Veröffentlichung 28. Berlin: Akademie Verlag, 1955.
———. "Die Ritualtafel der magisch-medizinischen Tafelserie 'Einreibung.'" *Archiv für Orientforschung* 21 (1966): 13–20.
———. "*Saḫaršubbû*—zur Frage nach der Lepra im alten Zweistromland." In *Aussatz—Lepra—Hansen-Krankheit. Ein Menschheitsproblem im Wandel,* Part 2. Ed. Jörn Henning Wolf. Würzburg: Deutsches Aussätzigen-Hilfswerk, 1986. 27–34.
———. "Spätbabylonische medizinische Texte aus Uruk." In *Medizinsche Diagnostik in Geschichte und Gegenwart: Festschrift für Heinz Goerke.* Ed. Christa Habrich et al. Munich: Werver Fritsch, 1978. 17–39.
———. "Ein Text medizinischen Inhalts aus dem neubabylonischen Grab 405." In *Uruk: Die Gräber.* Ed. Rainer Michael Boehmer, F. Pedde, and Beate Salje. Ausgrabungen in Uruk-Warka Endberichte 10. Mainz: Philipp von Zabern, 1995. 203–216.
———. "Ein verkannter neubabylonischer Text aus Sippar." *Archiv für Orientforschung* 20 (1963): 156–158.
———, and A. Leo Oppenheim. "The Old-Babylonian Omen Text VAT 7525." *Archiv für Orientforschung* 18 (1957–1958): 62–80.
Krafeld-Daugherty, Maria. "Archäologie, Philologie und Anthropologie: eine Synthese." In *Ex Mesopotamia et Syria Lux: Festschrift für Manfred Dietrich.* Ed. Oswald Loretz, Kai Metzler and Hanspeter Schaudig. Alter Orient und Altes Testament 281. Münster: Ugarit Verlag, 2002. 245–287.
Kramer, Samuel Noah. "Lipit-Ištar Law Code." In *Ancient Near Eastern Texts Relating to the Old Testament.* Ed. James B. Pritchard. 3rd ed. Princeton: Princeton University Press, 1969. 159–161.
———. *The Sumerians: Their History, Culture, and Character.* Chicago: University of Chicago Press, 1963.
Kraus, Fritz R. "Verstreute Omentexte aus Nippur im Istanbuler Museum." *Zeitschrift für Assyriologie* 77 (1987): 194–206.
Labat, René. "À propos de la chirurgie babylonienne." *Journal Asiatique* 242 (1954): 207–218.
———. "AO 11447, AO 17617, AO 17624: note additionelle." *Revue d'Assyriologie* 55 (1961): 95.
———. "Frauenkrankheiten." In *Reallexikon der Assyriologie* 3. Berlin: Walter de Gruyter, 1957–1971. 109.
———. "Fußkrankheiten." In *Reallexikon der Assyriologie* 3. Berlin: Walter de Gruyter, 1957–1971. 126–127.
———. "Geburt." In *Reallexikon der Assyriologie* 3. Berlin: Walter de Gruyter, 1957–1971. 178–179.
———. "Geisteskrankheiten." In *Reallexikon der Assyriologie* 3. Berlin: Walter de Gruyter, 1957–1971. 196–197.
———. "Gelenkschmerz, Gliederkrankheiten." In *Reallexikon der Assyriologie* 3. Berlin: Walter de Gruyter, 1957–1971. 199–200.
———. "Geschlechtskrankheiten." In *Reallexikon der Assyriologie* 3. Berlin: Walter de Gruyter, 1957–1971. 221–223.
———. "Geschwulst, Geschwür, Hautkrankheiten." In *Reallexikon der Assyriologie* 3. Berlin: Walter de Gruyter, 1957–1971. 231–233.
———. *Hémérologies et ménologies d'Assur.* Paris: Librairie d'Amerique et d'Orient, Adrien Maisonneuve, 1939.
———. "Herz." In *Reallexikon der Assyriologie* 4. Berlin: Walter de Gruyter, 1972–1975. 367–368.
———. "Husten." In *Reallexikon der Assyriologie* 4. Berlin: Walter de Gruyter, 1972–1975. 523–524.
———. *Manuel d'Épigraphie Akkadienne.* Paris: Librairie Orientaliste Paul Geuthner, 1952. 6th ed. augmented by Florence Malbran-Labat. Paris: Librairie Orientaliste Paul Geuthner, 1995.
———. *Mémoires de la Délégation en Perse* 57. Paris: Geuthner, 1974.
———. "Une nouvelle tablette de pronostics médicaux." *Syria* 33 (1956): 119–130.
———. "Ordonnances médicales ou magiques." *Revue d'Assyriologie* 54 (1960): 169–176.
———. "Le premier chapitre d'un précis médical Assyrien." *Revue d'Assyriologie* 53 (1959): 1–18.
———. "Remèdes assyriens contre les affections de l'oreille d'après un inédit du Louvre (AO 6774)." *Revista degli Studi Orientali* 32 (1957): 109–122.
———. "Tabous de Tešrit et autres prescriptions." *Iraq* 23 (1961): 88–93.
———. *Traité akkadien de diagnostics et pronostics médicaux.* 2 vols. Paris: Academie Internationale d'Histoire des Sciences, 1951.
———, and J. Tournay. "Un texte médical inédit." *Revue d'Assyriologie* 40 (1945–1946): 113–122.
Lackenbacher, Sylvie. "Note sur l'*Ardat-lilî*." *Revue d'Assyriologie* 65 (1971): 119–154.
Lambert, Wilfred G. *Babylonian Wisdom Literature.* Oxford: Clarendon Press, 1975.

———. "The Gula Hymn of Bulluṭsa-rabi." *Orientalia* N.S. 36 (1967): 105–132.
———. "An Incantation of the Maqlû Type." *Archiv für Orientforschung* 18 (1957–1958): 288–299.
———. "A Middle Assyrian Medical Text." *Iraq* 31 (1969): 28–39.
———. "The Twenty-one 'Poultices.'" *Anatolian Studies* 30 (1980): 77–83.
Landsberger, Benno. "Corrections to the Article, 'An Old Babylonian Charm against *Merḫu.*'" *Journal of Ancient Near Eastern Studies* 17 (1958): 56–58.
———. "Einige unerkannt gebliebene oder verkannte Nomina des Akkadischen.5.*ḫa'attu* = Ohnmacht." *Welt des Orients* 3 (1964–1966): 48–79.
———. "Aus der 3.Tafel DIR = sijaku." *Zeitschrift für Assyriologie* 42 (1934): 155–163.
———. *Die Serie ana ittišu.* Materialien zum sumerischen Lexikon 1. Rome: Pontifical Biblical Institute, 1937.
———. *Die Serie ur-e-a = naqû.* Materialien zum sumerischen Lexikon 2. Rome: Pontifical Biblical Institute, 1951.
———, and Miguel Civil. *The Series ḪAR-ra = ḫubullu Tablet XV and Related Texts.* Materialien zum sumerischen Lexikon 2. Rome: Pontifical Biblical Institute, 1967.
———, and Thorkild Jacobsen. "An Old Babylonian Charm against *Merḫu.*" *Journal of Ancient Near Eastern Studies* 14 (1955): 14–21.
Lane, Edward W. *Arabic-English Lexicon.* London: Williams and Norgate, 1863–1893.
Langdon, Stephen. *Historical and Religious Texts from the Temple Library of Nippur.* The Babylonian Expedition of the University of Pennsylvania 31. Munich, 1914.
Larsen, Mogens Trolle, *The Aššur-nādā Archive.* Old Assyrian Archives 1. Publications de l'Institut historique et archéologique néerlandais de Stamboul 96. Leiden: Nederlands Instituut voor het Nabije Oosten, 2002.
Leichty, Erle. "Guaranteed to Cure." In *A Scientific Humanist: Studies in Memory of Abraham Sachs.* Ed. Erle Leichty, Maria deJ. Ellis, and Pamela Gerardi. Occasional Publications of the Samuel Noah Kramer Fund 9. Philadelphia: The University Museum, 1988. 261–264.
———. *The Omen Series Šumma Izbu.* Texts from Cuneiform Sources 4. Locust Valley: J. J. Augustin, 1970.
———. "Two Late Commentaries." *Archiv für Orientforschung* 24 (1973): 78–86.
Levine, Baruch. *The JPS Torah Commentary: Leviticus.* Philadelphia: The Jewish Publication Society, 1989.
Lewy, Hildegard. "Old Assyrian Texts in the University Museum." *Hebrew Union College Annual* 40 (1969): 45–85.
Littleton, J., and B. Fröhlich. "An Analysis of Dental Pathology and Diet in Historic Bahrain." *Paléorient* 15/2 (1989): 59–75.
Livingstone, Alasdair. *Court Poetry and Literary Miscellanea.* State Archives of Assyria 3. Helsinki: Helsinki University Press, 1989.
Lutz, Henry Frederick. *Selected Sumerian and Babylonian Texts.* Publications of the Babylonian Section 1/1. Philadelphia: University Museum, 1919.
Lyon, David Gordon. *Keilschrifttexte Sargon's.* Assyriologische Bibliothek 6. Leipzig: J. C. Hinrichs, 1883.
Majno, Guido. *The Healing Hand.* Cambridge, Mass.: Harvard University Press, 1975.
Mallowan, Max E. L. *Nimrud and its Remains.* 2 vols. London: Collins, 1966.
Maluszak, D., M. Sanders, J. Taylor, and M. Wasserman. "Toxic *Pfiesteria* and Human Health." *Maryland Medical Journal* 46 (1997): 515–520.
Mandell, Gerald L., John E. Bennett, and Raphael Dolin. *Principles and Practice of Infectious Diseases.* 4th ed. New York: Churchill Livingstone, 1995.
Massé, Henri. *Persian Beliefs and Customs.* New Haven: Human Relations Area Files, 1954.
Maul, Stefan. *Zukunftsbewältigung: Eine Untersuchung altorientalischen Denkens anhand der babylonisch-assyrischen Löserituale (Namburbi).* Baghdader Forschungen 18. Mainz am Rhein: Philipp von Zabern, 1994.
McEwan, Gilbert. "Lunge." In *Reallexikon der Assyriologie* 7. Berlin: Walter de Gruyter, 1987–1990. 170–172.
———. *Priest and Temple in Hellenistic Babylonia.* Freiburger Alt-orientalische Studien 4. Wiesbaden: Franz Steiner, 1981.
Meier, Gerhard. "Ein akkadisches Heilungsritual aus Boğazköy." *Zeitschrift für Assyriologie* 45 (1939): 195–215.
———. "Lexikalische Bemerkungen." *Orientalia* N.S. 8 (1939): 301–309.
Meissner, Bruno. *Supplement zu den assyrischen Wörterbuchern.* Leiden: E. J. Brill, 1898.

Michalowski, Piotr. "Carminative Magic: Towards an Understanding of Sumerian Poetics." *Zeitschrift für Assyriologie* 71 (1981): 1–18.

Milgrom, Jacob. *Leviticus 1-16.* The Anchor Bible 3. New York: Doubleday, 1991.

Miller, R. L. "Eye Surgery and *Ṣillu*, Pterygium, Conjunctival Degeneration.'" *Nouvelles Assyriologiques Brèves et Utilitaires* 1989 no. 10.

———. "*Šagbānu* 'Guinea Worm Disease, Dracunculiasis.'" *Nouvelles Assyriologiques Brèves et Utilitaires* 1988 no. 45.

Moran, William. "Some Akkadian Names of the Stomachs of Ruminants." *Journal of Cuneiform Studies* 21 (1967): 178–182.

Mujais, Salim. "The Future of the Realm: Medicine and Divination in Ancient Syro-Mesopotamia." *American Journal of Nephrology* 19 (1999): 133–139.

Müller, Reiner. "Die Sagalla- und die Kabartukrankheit der Keilschriften: Filaria medinensis und Mycetoma pedis." *Archiv für Geschichte der Medizin* 24 (1926): 189–192.

Myhrman, David W. "Die Labartu-Texte, babylonische Beschwörungsformeln nebst Zauberverfahren gegen die Dämonin Labartu." *Zeitschrift für Assyriologie* 16 (1902): 141–200.

Nelson, Waldo E., Richard E. Behrman, and Victor C. Vaughan III. *Nelson's Textbook of Pediatrics.* 13th ed. Philadelphia: W. B. Saunders, 1987.

Neufeld, Edward. "The Earliest Document of a Case of Contagious Disease in Mesopotamia (Mari Tablet ARM X, 129)." *Journal of Ancient Near Eastern Studies* 18 (1986): 52–66.

Newton, Charles R.J.C., and David A. Warrell. "Neurological Manifestations of Falciparum Malaria." *Annals of Neurology* 43 (1998): 695–702.

Nougayrol, Jean. "Conjuration ancienne contre Samana." *Archiv Orientální* 17/2 (1949): 213–226.

———. "La Lamaštu à Ugarit." *Ugaritica* 6 (1969): 393–408.

———. "Notes brèves no. 17." *Revue d'Assyriologie* 66 (1972): 191.

———. "Textes et documents figurés." *Revue d'Assyriologie* 41 (1947): 23–54.

———. "Textes hépatoscopiques d'époque ancienne conservés au Musée du Louvre (III)." *Revue d'Assyriologie* 44 (1950): 1–44.

———. "Textes religieux (II)." *Revue d'Assyriologie* 66 (1972): 141–145.

———. "Textes Suméro-Accadiens des archives et bibliothèques privées d'Ugarit." *Ugaritica* 5 (1968): 1–367.

Oates, Joan. "The Fall of Assyria." *The Cambridge Ancient History.* 2nd ed. Vol. III/2. Cambridge: Cambridge University Press, 1991. 162–193.

Oppenheim, A. Leo. "A Caesarian Section in the Second Millennium B.C." *Journal of the History of Medicine* (July 1960): 292–294.

———. *Letters from Mesopotamia.* Chicago: University of Chicago Press, 1967.

———. "On the Observation of the Pulse in Ancient Mesopotamian Medicine." *Orientalia* N.S. 31 (1962): 27–33.

al-Qurtʾubi, ʿArib Ibn Saʿid al-Katib. *Le livre de la génération du foetus et le traitement des femmes enceintes et des nouveau-nés.* Tr. Henri Jahier and Noureddine Abdelkader. Algiers: Librairie Ferraris, 1956.

Pangas, Julio César. "Birth Malformations in Babylon and Assyria." *American Journal of Medical Genetics* 91 (2000): 318–321.

———. "Dental Pathology in Ancient Mesopotamia." *Bulletin of the History of Medicine* 73 (1999): 197–207.

———. "La 'mano de un espectro.' Una enfermedad de la Antigua Mesopotamia." *Aula Orientalis* 7 (1989): 215–233.

Parpola, Simo. *Letters from Assyrian and Babylonian Scholars.* State Archives of Assyria 10. Helsinki: Helsinki University Press, 1993.

———. *Letters from Assyrian Scholars to the Kings Esarhaddon and Assurbanipal.* Alter Orient und Altes Testament 5/1–2. (Kevelaer/Neukirchen-Vluyn: Butzon & Bercker/Neukirchener Verlag, 1970, 1983.

Parrot, André. *Sumer: The Dawn of Art.* New York: Golden Press, 1961.

Pierce, Laurie. *Cuneiform Cryptography: Numerical Substitutions for Syllabic and Logographic Signs.* Ph.D. diss., Yale University, 1982.

Powell, Marvin. "Sumerian Area Measures and the Alleged Decimal Substratum." *Zeitschrift für Assyriologie* 62 (1972): 165–221.

Prechel, Doris, and Thomas Richter. "Abrakadabra oder Althurritisch. Betrachtungen zu einigen altbabylonischen Beschwörungstexten." In *Kulturgeschichten: altorientalische Studien für Volkert Haas*. Ed. Thomas Richter, Doris Prechel, and Jörg Klinger. Saarbrücken: Saarbrücker Druckerei und Verlag, 2001. 333–372.

Prioreschi, Plinio, "Did the Hippocratic Physician Treat Hopeless Cases?" *Gesnerus* 49 (1992): 341–350.

al-Rawi, Ali, and H. L. Chakravarty. *Medicinal Plants of Iraq*. 2nd ed. Baghdad: Ministry of Agriculture and Irrigation, 1988.

al-Rawi, Farouk N. H. "Cuneiform Inscriptions in the Collections of the John Rylands Library, University of Manchester." *Iraq* 62 (2000): 21–63.

Reiner, Erica. *Astral Magic in Babylonia*. Transactions of the American Philosophical Society 85/4. Philadelphia: American Philosophical Society, 1995.

———. "Babylonian Birth Prognoses." *Zeitschrift für Assyriologie* 72 (1982): 124–138.

———. "ME.UGU-*mēlu*." *Archiv für Orientforschung* 19 (1959–1960): 150–151.

Reisner, George A. *Sumerisch-babylonische Hymnen nach Thontafeln griechischer Zeit*. Berlin: W. Spemann, 1896.

Renfrew, Jane M. "Fruits from Ancient Iraq—The Palaeobotanical Evidence." *Bulletin of Sumerian Agriculture* 3 (1987): 157–161.

———. "Pulses Recorded from Ancient Iraq." *Bulletin of Sumerian Agriculture* 2 (1985): 67–71.

Ricci, James V., tr. *Aetios of Amida, The Gynaecology and Obstetrics of the 6th Century A.D.* Philadelphia: The Blakiston Co., 1950.

Ritter, Edith K. "Magical-expert (= *Āšipu*) and Physician (= *Asû*): Notes on Two Complementary Professions in Babylonian Medicine." In *Studies in Honor of Benno Landsberger on his Seventy-Fifth Birthday*. Assyriological Studies 16. Chicago: University of Chicago Press, 1965. 299–321.

———, and J. V. Kinnier Wilson. "Prescription for an Anxiety State: A Study of *BAM* 234." *Anatolian Studies* 30 (1980): 23–30.

Rochberg-Halton, Francesca. *Aspects of Babylonian Celestial Divination: The Lunar Eclipse Tablets of Enuma Anu Enlil*. Archiv für Orientforschung, Beiheft 22. Horn: Ferdinand Berger & Söhne, 1989.

Roderick, Lee Miles. "A Problem in the Coagulation of the Blood: Sweet Clover Disease of Cattle." *American Journal of Physiology* 96 (1931): 413–425.

Röllig, Wolfgang. "Der Mondgot und die Kuh: Ein Lehrstück zur Problematik der Textüberlieferung im Alten Orient." *Orientalia* N.S. 54 (1985): 260–273.

Römer, Willem H. Ph. "Einige Bemerkungen zum dämonischen Gotte ^{d}Kūbu(m)." In *Symbolae Biblicae et Mesopotamicae Francisco Mario Theodoro de Liagre Böhl Dedicatae*. Ed. M. Beek et al. Leiden: E. J. Brill, 1973. 310–319.

———. "Einige Beobachtungen zur Göttin Nini(n)sina auf Grund von Quellen der Ur III-Zeit und der altbabylonischen Periode." In *Lišān Mitḫurti: Festschrift Wolfram Freiherr von Soden*. Ed. Wolfgang Röllig. Alter Orient und Altes Testament 1. Kevelaer/Neukirchen-Vluyn: Butzon & Bercker/Neukirchener Verlag, 1969. 279–305.

Rose, F. Clifford. "The History of Migraine from Mesopotamian to Medieval Times." *Cephalalgia* 19 (1995): 1–3.

Ruffer, Marc Armand. "Studies in Paleopathology in Egypt." *Journal of Pathology and Bacteriology* 18 (1913–1914): 149–162. Republished as "On Pathological Lesions Found on Coptic Bodies." In *Studies in Paleopathology in Egypt*. Chicago: University of Chicago Press, 1921. 139–155.

Salo, Wilmar, Arthur C. Aufderheide, Jane E. Buikstra, and Todd Holcomb. "Identification of *Mycobacterium tuberculosis* DNA in a Pre-Columbian Peruvian Mummy." *Proceedings of the National Academy of Sciences (USA)* 91 (1994): 2091–2094.

Scheil, Vincent. "Notules." *Revue d'Assyriologie* 14 (1917): 87–96.

———. "Quelques remèdes pour les yeux." *Revue d'Assyriologie* 15 (1918): 75–80.

———. "Tablette de Pronostics Médicaux." *Revue d'Assyriologie* 14 (1917): 121–131.

Scott, Danny W. *Large Animal Dermatology*. Philadelphia: W. B. Saunders, 1986.

Scurlock, JoAnn. "Ancient Mesopotamian House Gods." *Journal of Ancient Near Eastern Religions* 3 (2003): 99–106.

———. "Baby-Snatching Demons, Restless Souls and the Dangers of Childbirth: Medico-Magical Means of Dealing with Some of the Perils of Motherhood in Ancient Mesopotamia." *Incognita* 2 (1991): 137–185.

———. "Fatally Sore Armpits: Marginalia on Labat, *TDP*." *Notes Assyriologiques Brèves et Utilitaires* 1993 no. 47.

———. "From Esagil-kin-apli to Hippocrates." *Le Journal des Médecines Cunéiformes.* 3 (2004): 10–30.

———. "The Interplay of 'Magic,' 'Religion' and 'Science' in Ancient Mesopotamian Medicine." In *Blackwell's Companion to the Ancient Near East.* Ed. Daniel Snell. Oxford: Blackwells (forthcoming).

———. *Magico-Medical Means of Treating Ghost-Induced Illnesses in Ancient Mesopotamia.* Groningen: Styx (forthcoming).

———. "Physician, Conjurer, Magician: A Tale of Two Healing Professionals." In *Mesopotamian Magic: Textual, Historical and Interpretative Perspectives.* Ed. Tzvi Abusch and Karel van der Toorn. Ancient Magic and Divination 1. Groningen: Styx, 1999. 69–79.

———. Review of *Die babylonisch-assyrische Morphoskopie,* by Barbara Böck. *Journal of the American Oriental Society* 123 (2003): 395–399.

———. Review of *Augenleiden nach keilschriftlichen Quellen: Untersuchungen zur altorientalischen Medizin,* by Jeanette C. Fincke. *Archiv für Orientforschung* 48–49 (2001–2002): 242–244.

———. Review of *Babylonisch-assyrische Diagnostik,* Alter Orient und Altes Testament 43, by Nils Heeßel. *Journal of the American Oriental Society* 123 (2003): 399–402.

———. Review of *Birth in Babylonia and the Bible: Its Mediterranean Setting,* by Marten Stol. *Nin* (forthcoming).

———. Review of *Epilepsy in Babylonia,* by Marten Stol. *Archiv für Orientforschung* 42–43 (1995–1996): 250–254.

———. Review of *Medizinische Omina aus Ḫattuša in akkadischer Sprache,* by Gernot Wilhelm. *Archiv für Orientforschung* 44–45 (1997–1998): 368.

———. "Some Thoughts on Ancient Mesopotamian Magic and Religion." (Review of *Mesopotamian Magic: Textual, Historical and Interpretative Perspectives,* ed. Tzvi Abusch and Karel van der Toorn). *Bibliotheca Orientalis* 59 (2002): 468–481.

———, and Mary Coleman. "Viral Haemorrhagic Fevers in Ancient Mesopotamia." *Tropical Medicine and International Health* (1997): 603–606.

Shaffer, Aaron. *Sumerian Sources of Tablet XII of the Epic of Gilgamesh.* Ph.D. diss., University of Pennsylvania, 1963.

Sigerist, Henry E. *A History of Medicine* I. Oxford: Oxford University Press, 1951.

Sjöberg, Åke W. "Der Vater und sein missratener Sohn." *Journal of Cuneiform Studies* 25 (1973): 105–169.

———. "Nungal in the Ekur." *Archiv für Orientforschung* 24 (1973): 19–46.

Smith, Sidney. *Cuneiform Texts from Babylonian Tablets in the British Museum* 37. London: The British Museum, 1923.

Soden, Wolfram Freiherr von. *Akkadisches Handwörterbuch.* Wiesbaden: Otto Harrassowitz, 1958–1981.

———. *Grundriss der akkadischen Grammatik.* Analecta Orientalia 33 and 47. Rome: Pontificium Institutum Biblicum, 1952, 1969.

———. "Krankheit und Unfall eines Kindes nach dem Karana-brief OBST Nr. 124." *Notes Assyriologiques Brèves et Utilitaires* 1991 no. 54.

Star, Ivan. *Queries to the Sungod.* State Archives of Assyria 4. Helsinki: Helsinki University Press, 1990.

Stol, Marten. *Birth in Babylonia and the Bible: Its Mediterranean Setting.* Cuneiform Monographs 14. Groningen: Styx, 2000.

———. "Blindness and Night-Blindness in Akkadian." *Journal of Near Eastern Studies* 45 (1986): 295–299.

———. "Diagnosis and Therapy in Babylonian Medicine." *Jaarbericht Ex Oriente Lux* 32 (1991–1992): 42–65.

———. "Einige kurze Wortstudien." In *Festschrift für Rykle Borger zu seinem 65. Geburtstag am 24. Mai 1994.* Ed. Stefan Maul. Cuneiform Monographs 10. Groningen: Styx, 1998. 343–352.

———. *Epilepsy in Babylonia.* Cuneiform Monographs 2. Groningen: Styx, 1993.

———. "Leprosy: New Light from Greek and Babylonian Sources." *Jaarbericht Ex Oriente Lux* 30 (1987–1988): 22–31.

———. "Milk, Butter and Cheese." *Bulletin of Sumerian Agriculture* 7 (1993): 99–113.

———. "Old Babylonian Ophthalmology." In *Reflets des deux fleuves: Volume de Mélanges offerts à André Finet.* Ed. Marc Lebeau and Philippe Talon. Akkadica Supplementum 6. Leuven: Peeters, 1989. 163–166.

———. "Private Life in Ancient Mesopotamia." In *Civilizations of the Ancient Near East.* Ed. Jack M. Sasson. New York: Charles Scribner's Sons, 1995. 485–515.

———. "Psychosomatic Suffering in Ancient Mesopotamia." In *Mesopotamian Magic: Textual, Historical and Interpretative Perspectives.* Ed. Tzvi Abusch and Karel van der Toorn. Ancient Magic and Divination 1. Groningen: Styx, 1999. 57–68.

———. Review of *Medicine and the Bible*, by B. Palmer et al. *Bibliotheca Orientalis* 46 (1989): 129–130.
Streck, Maximilian. *Assurbanipal*. 3 vols. Leipzig: J. C. Hinrichs, 1916.
Tasman, Allan, Jerald Kay, and Jeffrey A. Lieberman. *Psychiatry*. Philadelphia: W. B. Saunders, 1997.
Thomsen, Marie-Louise. "The Evil Eye in Mesopotamia." *Journal of Near Eastern Studies* 51 (1992): 19–32.
———. *The Sumerian Language*. Mesopotamia 10. Copenhagen: Akademisk Forlag, 1984.
Thureau-Dangin, François. *Rituels Accadiens*. Paris: Éditions Ernest Leroux, 1921.
———, and Maurice Dunand. *Til-Barsib*. Paris: Paul Geuthner, 1936.
van der Toorn, Karel. "Magic at the Cradle: A Reassessment." In *Mesopotamian Magic: Textual, Historical and Interpretative Perspectives*. Ed. Tzvi Abusch and Karel van der Toorn. Ancient Magic and Divination 1. Groningen: Styx, 1999. 139–147.
Townsend, C. C., and Evan Guest. *Flora of Iraq* 3. Baghdad: Ministry of Agriculture of the Republic of Iraq, 1974.
Tsukimoto, Akio. "'By the Hand of Madi-Dagan the Scribe and *Apkallu*-Priest'— A Medical Text from the Middle Euphrates Region." In *Priests and Officials in the Ancient Near East*. Ed. Kazuko Watanabe. Heidelberg: Universitätsverlag-C.Winter, 1999. 187–200.
Ungnad, Arthur. "Besprechungskunst und Astrologie in Babylonien." *Archiv für Orientforschung* 14 (1941–1944): 251–284.
———. "Zu den Labartu-Texten." *Zeitschrift für Assyriologie* 33 (1921): 69–71.
Veldhuis, Niek. "Comments on Igi-ḫul." *Notes Assyriologiques Brèves et Utilitaires* 1992 no. 43.
———. "Corrections to 'The Reading of GISSU in Ophthamological Context.'" *Notes Assyriologiques Brèves et Utilitaires* 1992 no. 32.
———. "The New Assyrian Compendium for a Woman in Childbirth." *Acta Sumerologica* 11 (1989): 239–260.
———. "The Poetry of Magic." In *Mesopotamian Magic: Textual, Historical and Interpretative Perspectives*. Ed. Tzvi Abusch and Karel van der Toorn. Ancient Magic and Divination 1. Groningen: Styx, 1999. 35–48.
———. "The Reading of GISSU in Ophthamological Context." *Notes Assyriologiques Brèves et Utilitaires* 1991 no. 106.
———. "An Ur III Incantation against the Bite of a Snake, a Scorpion, or a Dog." *Zeitschrift für Assyriologie* 83 (1993): 161–169.
Virolleaud, Charles. *L'astrologie chaldéenne, le livre intitulé "enuma Anu* ^{ILU}*Bêl"* and *L'astrologie chaldéenne* Supplement 2. Paris: Paul Geuthner, 1907–1912.
Volk, Konrad. "Kinderkrankheiten nach der Darstellung babylonisch-assyrischer Keilschrifttexte." *Orientalia* N.S. 68 (1999): 1–30.
Walker, Christopher B. F. *Cuneiform Texts from Babylonian Tablets in the British Museum* 51. London: British Museum, 1972.
———. "Some Mesopotamian Inscribed Vessels." *Iraq* 42 (1980): 84–86.
Wasserman, Nathan. "An Old Babylonian Medical Text Against the *kurārum* Disease." *Revue d'Assyriologie* 90 (1996): 1–5.
———. "An Old Babylonian Medical Text Against the *kurārum* Disease: Addition." *Revue d'Assyriologie* 91 (1997): 31–32.
Watanabe, Kazuko. "Die literarische Überlieferung eines babylonisch-assyrischen Fluchthemas mit Anrufung des Mondgottes Sîn." *Acta Sumerologica* 6 (1984): 99–119.
Weidner, Ernst F. "Neue Bruchstücke des Berichtes über Sargons achten Feldzug." *Archiv für Orientforschung* 12 (1937–1938): 144–148 w. pl. XI.
von Weiher, Egbert. *Der babylonische Gott Nergal*. Alter Orient und altes Testament 11. Kevelaer/Neukirchen-Vluyn: Butzon & Bercker/Neukirchener Verlag, 1971.
———. *Spätbabylonische Texte aus Uruk* 2. Ausgrabungen der Deutschen Forschungsgemeinschaft in Uruk-Warka 10. Berlin: Mann, 1983.
———. *Spätbabylonische Texte aus Uruk* 3. Ausgrabungen der Deutschen Forschungsgemeinschaft in Uruk-Warka 12. Berlin: Mann, 1988.
———. *Uruk: Spätbylonische Texte aus Planquadrat U18* 4. Ausgrabungen in Uruk-Warka Endberichte 12. Mainz: Philipp von Zabern, 1993.
———. *Uruk: Spätbylonische Texte aus Planquadrat U18* 5. Ausgrabungen in Uruk-Warka Endberichte 13. Mainz: Philipp von Zabern, 1998.
Whiting, Robert. "An Old Babylonian Incantation from Tell Asmar." *Zeitschrift für Assyriologie* 75 (1985): 179–187.

Wiggerman, Franz. "Lamaštu, Daughter of Anu. A Profile." In *Birth in Babylonia and the Bible.* Ed. Marten Stol. Groningen: Styx, 2000. 217–248.
Wilhelm, Gernot. *Medizinische Omina aus Ḫattuša in akkadischer Sprache.* Studien zu den Boğazköy-Texten 36. Wiesbaden: O. Harrassowitz, 1994.
Wolfert, Paula. *Couscous and Other Good Food from Morocco.* New York: Harper and Row, 1973.
Wulff, Hans E. *Traditional Crafts of Persia.* Cambridge, Mass.: MIT Press, 1966.
Yapp, Malcolm E. *The Making of the Modern Near East 1792–1923.* London: Longman, 1987.
Zakaria, Hanna. "Historical Study of *Schistosomiasis hematobium* and its Intermediate Host, *Bulinus truncatus,* in Central Iraq." *Journal of the Faculty of Medicine, Baghdad,* N.S. 1 (1959): 2–10.
al-Zeebari, Akram. *Altbabylonische Briefe des Iraq-Museums.* Ph.D. diss., University of Münster, 1964.

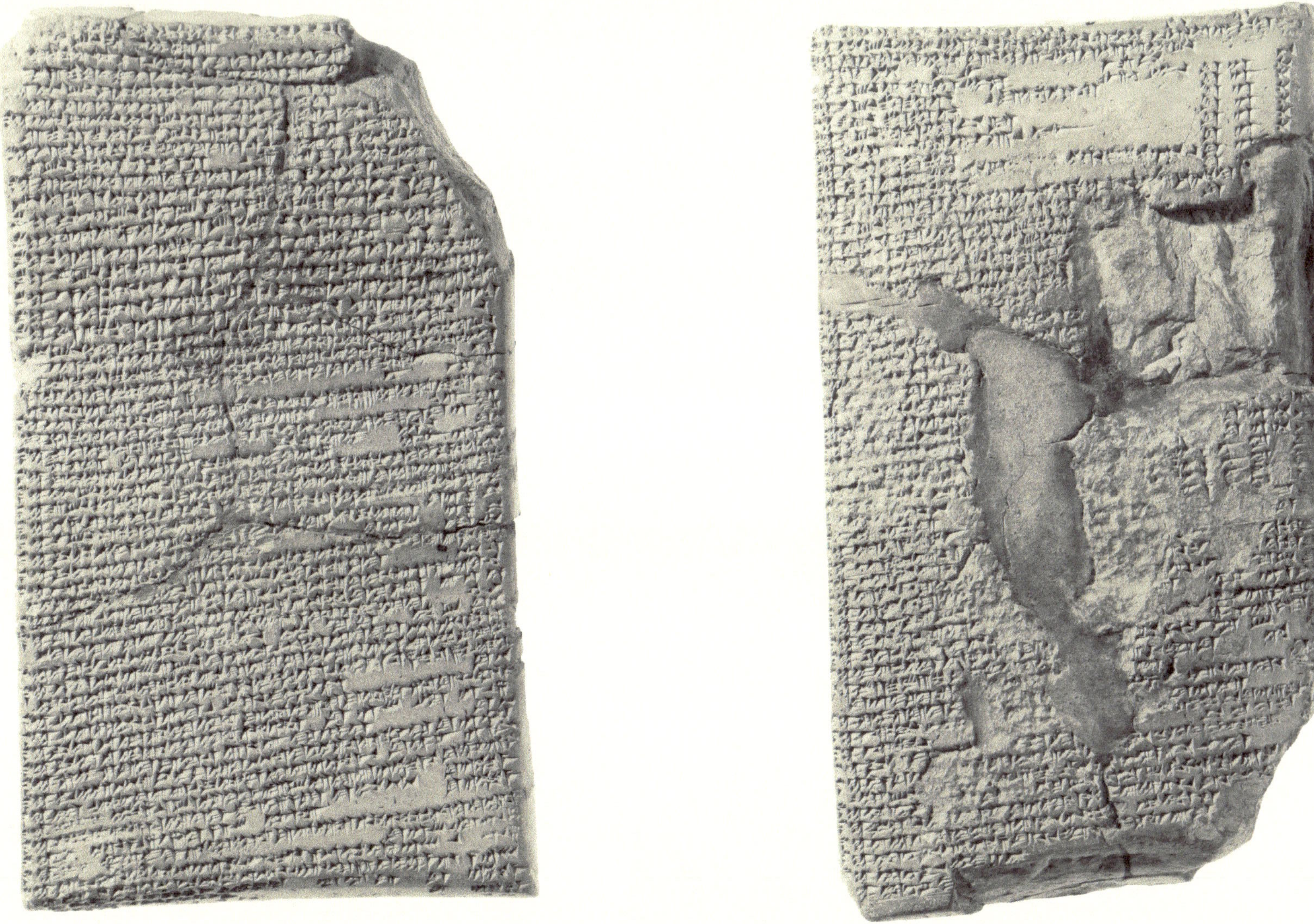

BM 46228 = DPS XL B (the pediatrics tablet)
Photo courtesy of the Trustees of the British Museum

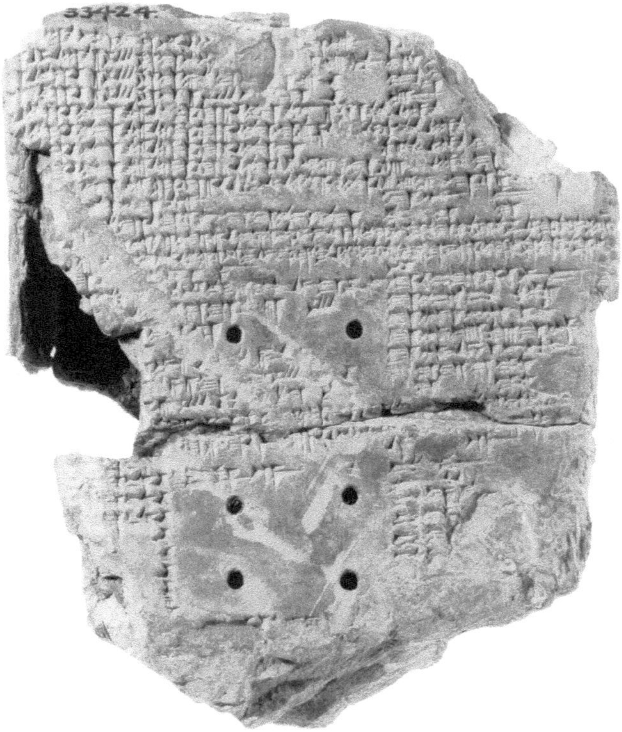

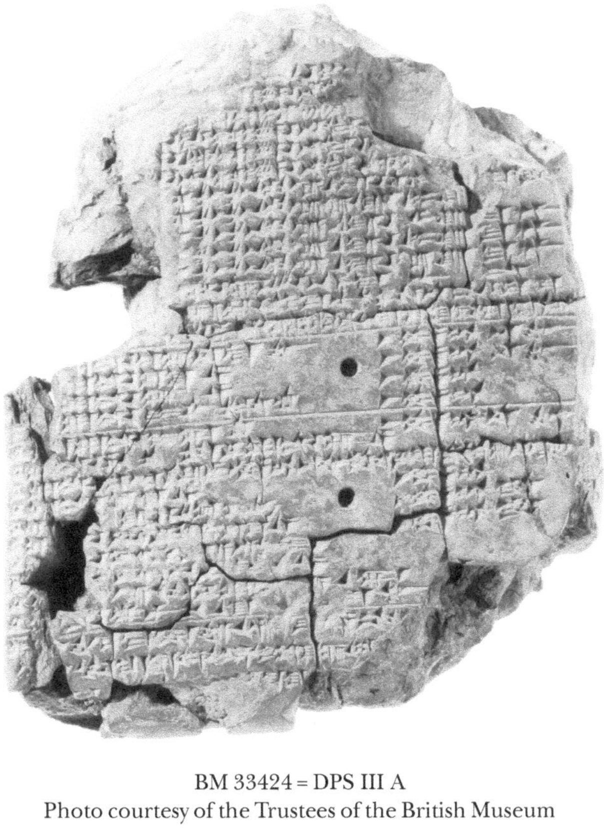

BM 33424 = DPS III A
Photo courtesy of the Trustees of the British Museum

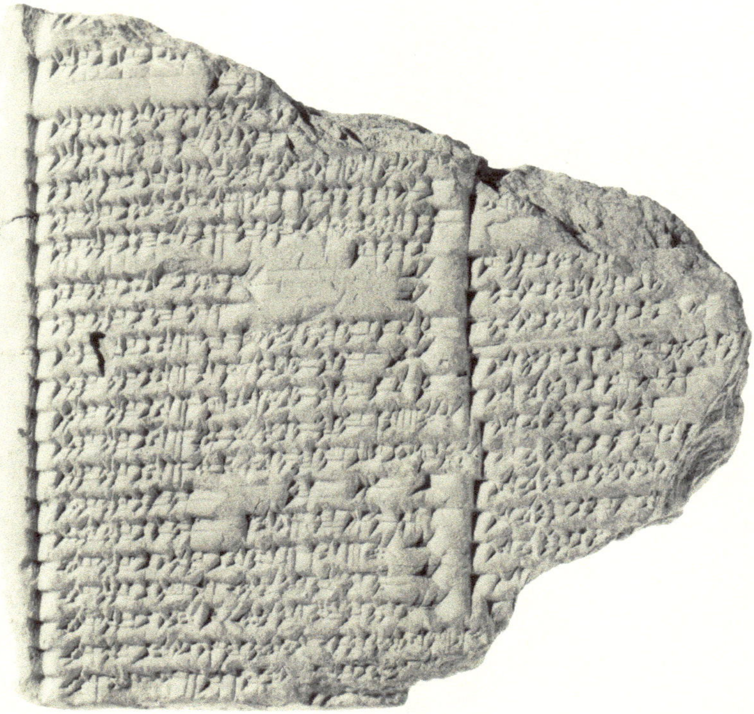

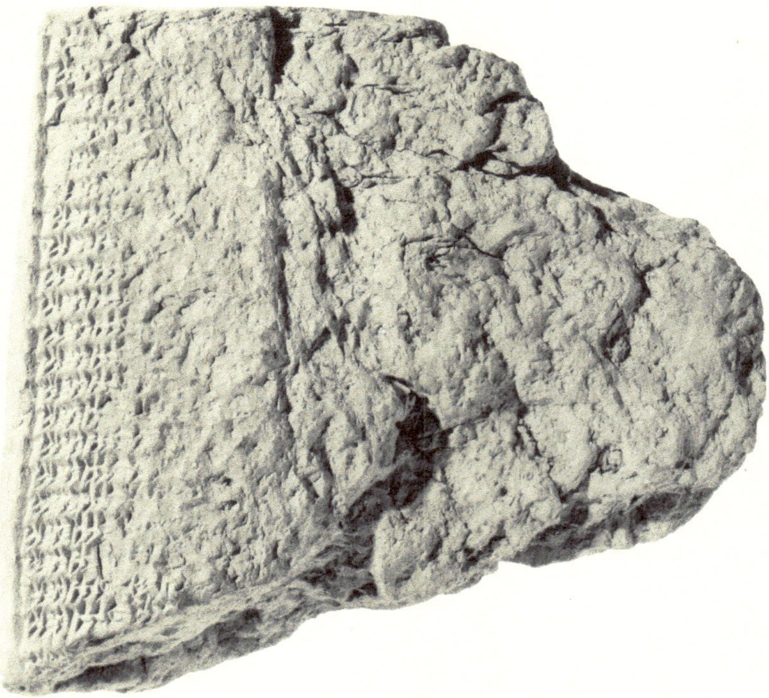

top: BM 34071 obv. = DPS VI C
bottom: BM 34071 rev. = DPS VII C
Photo courtesy of the Trustees of the British Museum

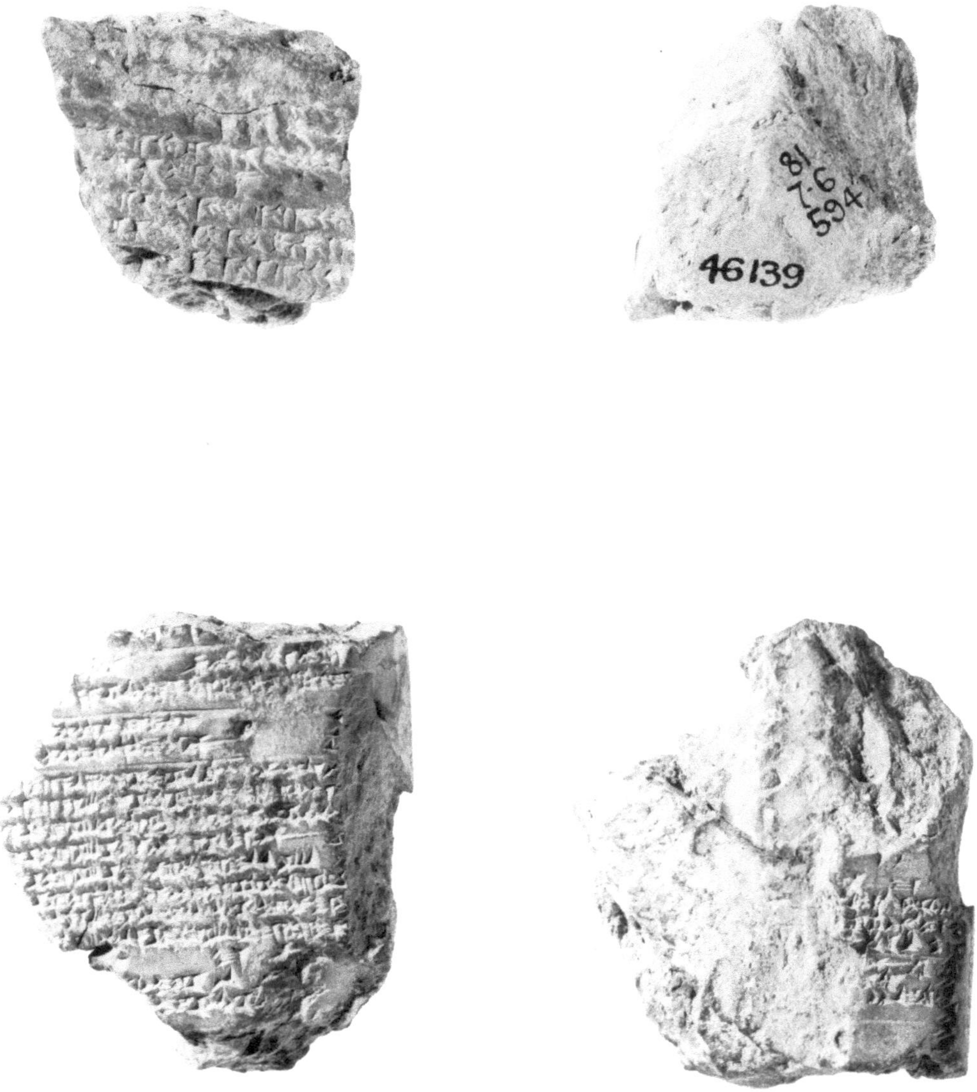

top: BM 46139 = DPS III B
bottom: BM 38655 = DPS XIV F
Photo courtesy of the Trustees of the British Museum

Indexes

Text Index

Note: The form of citations used in the right column of this index is explained in the introduction to the chart (p. 576).

Sumerian Words Treated

Akkadian Words Treated

English and Latin Words

JoAnn Scurlock is an internationally known scholar of the Ancient Near East. She holds a doctorate in Assyriology from the University of Chicago and is an adjunct professor of history at Elmhurst College.

Burton R. Andersen is a professor of medicine and microbiology and former chief of the Section of Infectious Diseases at the University of Illinois College of Medicine.

The University of Illinois Press
is a founding member of the
Association of American University Presses.

University of Illinois Press
1325 South Oak Street
Champaign, IL 61820-6903
www.press.uillinois.edu

Kolibri 360 GmbH
Ferdinand-Jühlke-Straße 7
99095 Erfurt, Deutschland
produktsicherheit@kolibri360.de